D0079873

Janice Thompson

Melinda Manore

NUTRITION

An Applied Approach

Fifth Edition

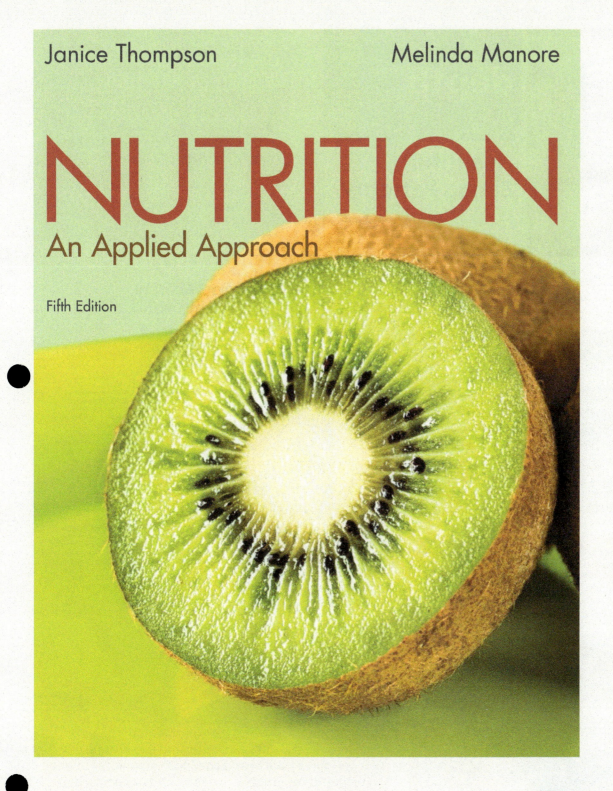

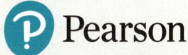
Pearson

Nutrition Concepts Applied to Students' Daily Lives

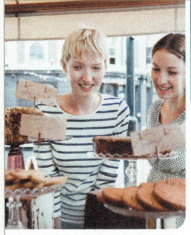

in depth 2.5

Healthful Eating Patterns

You and a friend have just finished dining at your favorite Thai restaurant. As you walk back toward your residence hall, you pass a bakery window displaying cakes and pies, each of wh looks more enticing than the last. You stop. Y not hungry, but . . . one little treat wouldn't h

learning outcomes
After studying this In Depth, you should be able to:

NEW! In Depth Chapters Obesity, Malnutrition, and Healthful Eating Patterns are three new mini-chapters that focus on topics such as the health and societal problems surrounding undernourishment; the effectiveness of lifestyle changes, medications, dietary supplements, and surgery in obesity treatment; and the components and principles of a healthful eating pattern.

NEW! Chapter 13: Food Equity, Sustainability, and Quality: The Challenge of "Good" Food
Focuses on current issues of food quality and availability that directly affect today's students. Topics include the disparities in availability of high-quality, nourishing food thought to contribute to the poverty-obesity paradox, unsafe working conditions in many U.S. farms and factories, and more.

13

Food Equity, Sustainability, and Quality
The challenge of "good food"

learning outcomes
After studying this chapter, you should be able to:

1. Compare and contrast levels of food insecurity globally and in the United States, pp. 4–5
2. Identify several ways in which human behavior contributes to food insecurity, pp. 5–9.
3. Discuss inequities in agricultural and food retail and service labor, and their effects on workers and the consumers they serve, pp. 9–10.
4. Discuss the effects of industrial agriculture on food security, food diversity, and the environment, pp. 10–13.
5. Discuss international, governmental, philanthropic, corporate, and local initiatives aimed at increasing the world's supply of and access to "good food," pp. 13–15.
6. Identify several steps you can take to promote production of and access to "good food," pp. 16–18.

In an affluent suburb in the United States, shoppers at a farmers market select organic meats, eggs, cheeses, produce, flour, and even freshly baked bread from nearby farms. When asked why they shop there, they say that they want to provide their families "good food." Across the globe in a village in Kenya, a group of neighbors are members of a farming cooperative that grows corn and beans, raises chickens for eggs and cows and goats for milk. Members boast of their ability to feed their families "good food" for breakfast, lunch, and dinner every day.

What is "good food"? Although farmers, chefs, and public health experts would likely propose very different definitions, in this chapter, we define "good food" as nutrient-dense food that is equitably and sustainably produced, distributed, and sold. That might sound like a tall order, but such foods do exist. The challenge is to make them in large enough quantities to feed the world, and make sure that consumers have the ability and the desire to obtain them.[1]

Equity means fairness, and we begin this chapter by looking at inequities in the production, distribution, and sale of the world's food supply. We then discuss the effects of industrial agriculture on our environment and on the quality and diversity of our food. Finally, we identify some ways that nations and organizations are meeting the challenge of "good food," and how you can help.

MasteringNutrition™
Go online for chapter quizzes, pre-tests, Interactive Activities, and more!

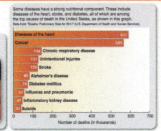
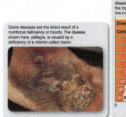

focus figure 1.2 The Relationship Between Nutrition and Human Disease

Some diseases have a strong nutritional component. These include diseases of the heart, stroke, and diabetes, all of which are among the top causes of death in the United States, as shown in this graph. Data from "Deaths: Preliminary Data for 2011" (U.S. Department of Health and Human Services).

Some diseases are the direct result of a nutritional deficiency or toxicity. The disease shown here, pellagra, is caused by a deficiency of a vitamin called niacin.

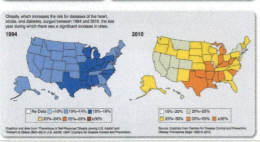

Obesity, which increases the risk for diseases of the heart, stroke, and diabetes, surged between 1994 and 2010, the last year during which there was a significant increase in rates.

NEW! Focus Figures
6 new Focus Figures on topics such as nutrition and human disease, the scientific method, the new nutrition facts panel, and more; and 8 new Meal Focus Figures have been added that graphically depict the differences in sets of meals, such as a comparison of nutrient density or a comparison of two high-carbohydrate meals, to engage students with relevant and practical information, and much more.

Help Students Master Tough
Concepts of the Course

NEW! Learning Outcomes Approach
New approach creates a clear learning path for students with numbered learning outcomes at the beginning of each chapter that are then tied to each major chapter section, helping students navigate each chapter and measure their progress against specific learning goals; this approach also helps instructors assess the key information and skills students are meant to take away from each chapter.

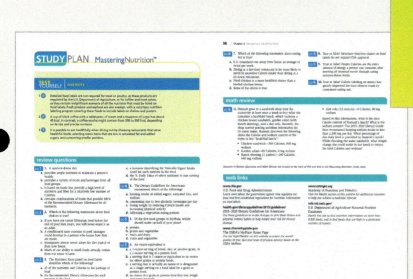

NEW! Study Plans
Study Plans conclude each chapter, tying the chapter learning outcomes to the review questions and math review questions, and also includes the test yourself t/f answers and web links.

NEW! Table of Contents Organization
To better streamline the coverage of the micronutrients, four former chapters (7-10 in the 4e) now become three (7-9 in the 5e) to help students better comprehend the role of vitamins and minerals in fluid and electrolyte balance (Ch. 7); key body functions (energy metabolism, antioxidant functions, and vision) (Ch. 8); and healthy body tissues (collagen, blood, and bone) (Ch. 9).

brief contents

Continuous Learning
Before, During, and After Class

BEFORE CLASS

Mobile Media and Reading Assignments Ensure Students Come to Class Prepared

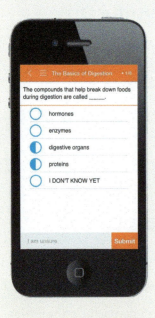

UPDATED! Dynamic Study Modules help students study effectively by continuously assessing student performance and providing practice in areas where students struggle the most. Each Dynamic Study Module, accessed by computer, smartphone or tablet, promotes fast learning and long-term retention.

NEW! Interactive eText 2.0 gives students access to the text whenever they can access the internet. eText features include:

- Now available on smartphones and tablets
- Seamlessly integrated videos and other rich media
- Accessible (screen-reader ready)
- Configurable reading settings, including resizable type and night reading mode
- Instructor and student note-taking, highlighting, bookmarking, and search
- Also available for offline use via Pearson's eText 2.0 app

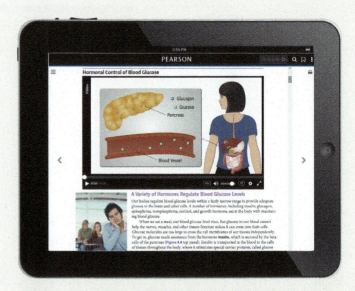

Pre-Lecture Reading Quizzes are easy to customize and assign

NEW! Reading Questions ensure that students complete the assigned reading before class and stay on track with reading assignments. Reading Questions are 100% mobile ready and can be completed by students on mobile devices.

with MasteringNutrition™

DURING CLASS

Engage students with Learning Catalytics

Learning Catalytics, a "bring your own device" student engagement, assessment, and classroom intelligence system, allows students to use their smartphone, tablet, or laptop to respond to questions in class.

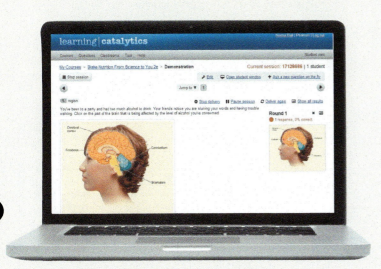

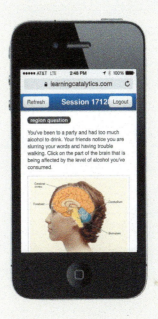

AFTER CLASS

MasteringNutrition Delivers Automatically Graded Nutrition Activities

UPDATED! Nutrition Animations explain big picture concepts that help students learn the hardest topics in nutrition. These animations, complete with a new design and compatible with Mastering and mobile devices, help students master tough topics and address students' common misconceptions, using assessment and wrong-answer feedback.

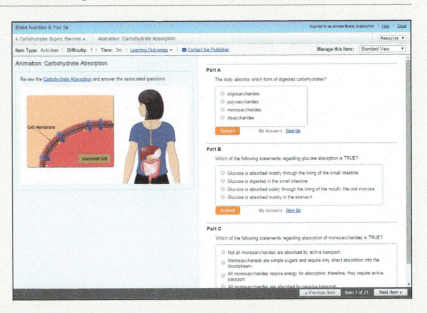

Continuous Learning
Before, During, and After Class

AFTER CLASS

Easy-to-Assign, Customize, Media-Rich, and Automatically Graded Assignments.

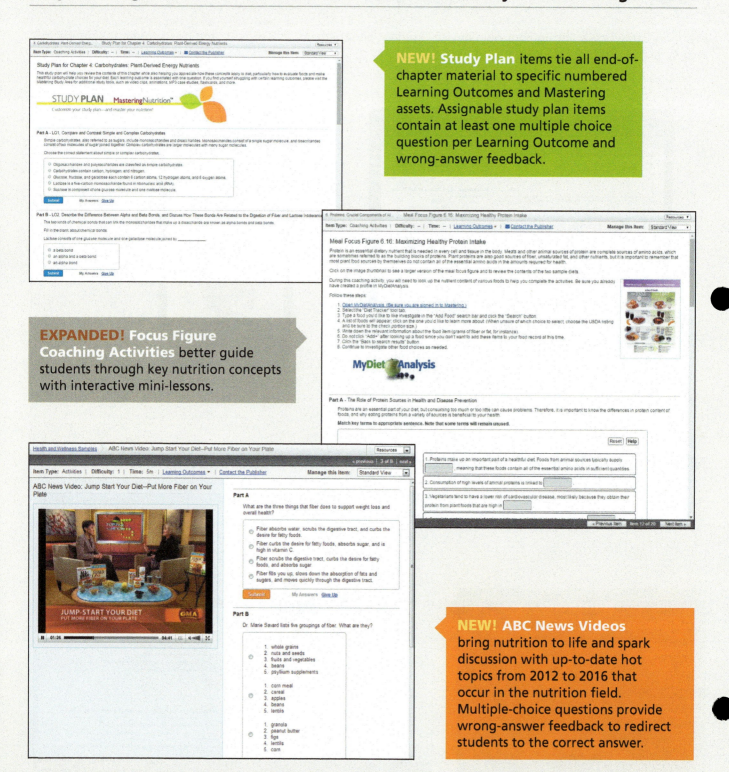

NEW! Study Plan items tie all end-of-chapter material to specific numbered Learning Outcomes and Mastering assets. Assignable study plan items contain at least one multiple choice question per Learning Outcome and wrong-answer feedback.

EXPANDED! Focus Figure Coaching Activities better guide students through key nutrition concepts with interactive mini-lessons.

NEW! ABC News Videos bring nutrition to life and spark discussion with up-to-date hot topics from 2012 to 2016 that occur in the nutrition field. Multiple-choice questions provide wrong-answer feedback to redirect students to the correct answer.

with MasteringNutrition™

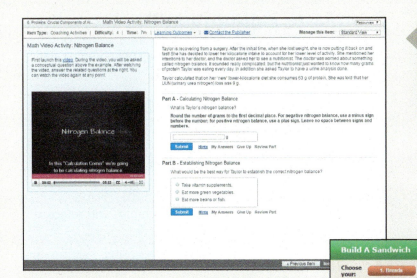

Math Coaching Activities provide hands-on practice of important nutrition-related calculations to help students understand and apply the material. Questions include wrong-answer feedback.

UPDATED! Nutritools Build-A-Meal Coaching Activities have been updated and allow students to combine and experiment with different food options and learn firsthand how to build healthier meals. The Build a Meal, Build a Pizza, Build A Salad, and Build A Sandwich tools have been carefully rethought to improve the user experience, making them easier to use and are now HTML5 compatible for mobile devices.

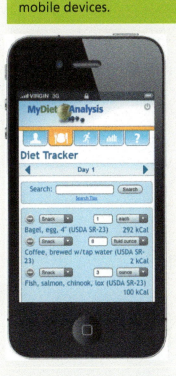

Single sign-on to MyDietAnalysis allows students to complete a diet assignment. Students keep track of their food intake and exercise and enter the information to create a variety of reports. A mobile version gives students 24/7 access via their smartphones to easily track food, drink, and activity on the go. MyDietAnalysis Case Study Activities with quizzing provide students with hands-on diet analysis practice that can also be automatically graded.

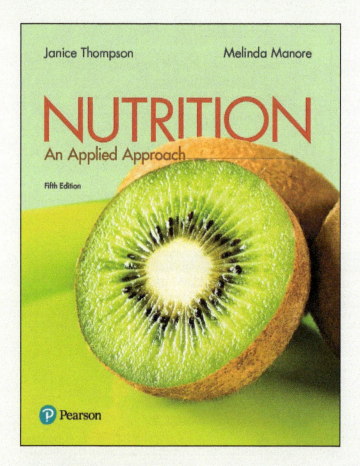

Janice Thompson   Melinda Manore

NUTRITION
An Applied Approach

Fifth Edition

P Pearson

MasteringNutrition™ provides you with everything you need to prep for your course and deliver a dynamic lecture, in one convenient place. Resources include:

Media Assets for Each Chapter

- *ABC News* Lecture Launcher videos
- Nutrition Animations
- PowerPoint Lecture Outlines
- PowerPoint clicker questions and Jeopardy-style quiz show questions
- Files for all illustrations and tables and selected photos from the text

Test Bank

- Test Bank in Microsoft, Word, PDF, and RTF formats
- Computerized Test Bank, which includes all the questions from the printed test bank in a format that allows you to easily and intuitively build exams and quizzes.

Teaching Resources

- Instructor Resource and Support Manual in Microsoft Word and PDF formats
- Teaching with Student Learning Outcomes
- Teaching with Web 2.0
- Learning Catalytics: Getting Started
- Getting Started with MasteringNutrition

Student Supplements

- Eat Right!
- Live Right!
- Food Composition Table

Measuring Student Learning Outcomes? All of the MasteringNutrition assignable content is tagged to book content and to Bloom's Taxonomy. You also have the ability to add your own learning outcomes, helping you track student performance against your learning outcomes. You can view class performance against the specified learning outcomes and share those results quickly and easily by exporting to a spreadsheet.

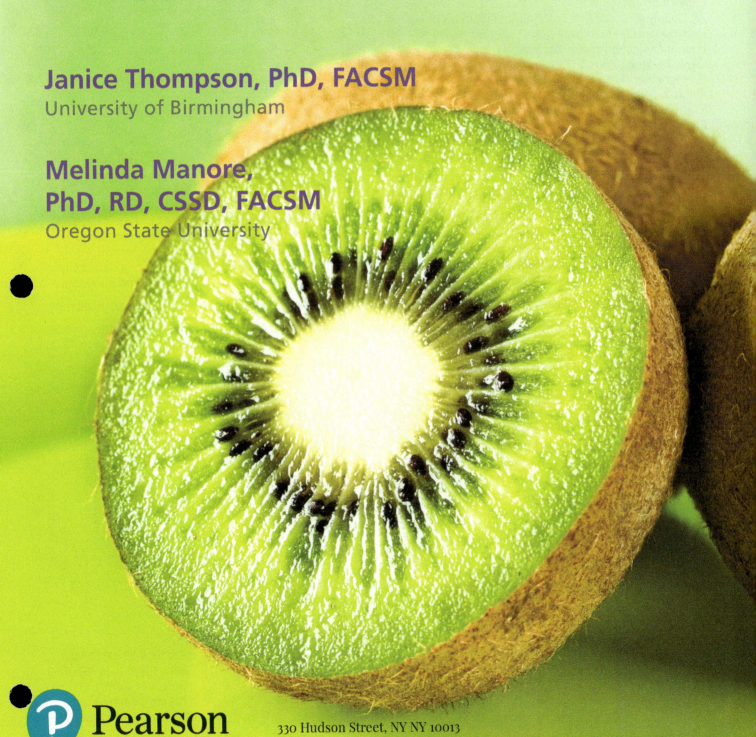

Nutrition

An Applied Approach

FIFTH EDITION

Janice Thompson, PhD, FACSM
University of Birmingham

**Melinda Manore,
PhD, RD, CSSD, FACSM**
Oregon State University

Pearson

330 Hudson Street, NY NY 10013

Courseware Portfolio Manager: Michelle Yglecias
Content Producer: Deepti Agarwal
Managing Producer: Nancy Tabor
Courseware Director, Content Development: Barbara Yien
Development Editor: Laura Bonazzoli
Art Development Editor: Jay McElroy
Courseware Editorial Assistant: Nicole Constantine
Rich Media Content Producer: Timothy Hainley, Lucinda Bingham
Mastering Content Developer, Science: Lorna Perkins
Full-Service Vendor: SPi Global
Copyeditor: Alyson Platt
Art Coordinator: Rebecca Marshall, Lachina Publishing Services
Design Manager: Mark Ong
Interior Designer: Preston Thomas
Cover Designer: Preston Thomas
Photographer: Renn Valo, CDV LLC
Rights & Permissions Project Manager: Matt Perry, Cenveo Publishing Services
Rights & Permissions Management: Ben Ferrini
Photo Researcher: Danny Meldung, Photo Affairs, Inc.
Manufacturing Buyer: Stacey Weinberger, LSC Communications
Executive Product Marketing Manager: Neena Bali
Senior Field Marketing Manager: Mary Salzman

Cover Photo Credit: portishead1/gettyimages

Library of Congress Cataloging-in-Publication Data
Names: Thompson, Janice, author. | Manore, Melinda, author.
Title: An applied approach / Janice Thompson, Ph.D., FACSM, University of
  Birmingham, Melinda Manore, Ph.D., RD, CSSD, FACSM, Oregon State
  University.
Description: Fifth edition. | New York, NY : Pearson, 2017.
Identifiers: LCCN 2016037778 | ISBN 0134516230
Subjects: LCSH: Nutrition.
Classification: LCC QP141 .T467 2017 | DDC 612.3–dc23
LC record available at https://lccn.loc.gov/2016037778

ISBN 10: 0-13-451623-0;
ISBN 13: 978-0-13-451623-3
(Student edition)
ISBN 10: 0-13-460828-3;
ISBN 13: 978-0-13-460828-0
(Instructor's Review Copy)

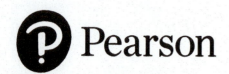

www.pearsonhighered.com

10 2021

This book is dedicated to my family, friends, and colleagues—you provide constant support, encouragement, and unconditional love. It is also dedicated to my students and the communities with which I work—you continue to inspire me, challenge me, and teach me. **—JLT**

This book is dedicated to my parents, for their consistent love, prayers, support, and encouragement. You helped me believe in myself. **—MMM**

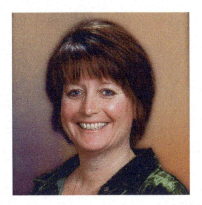

Janice Thompson, PhD, FACSM

University of Birmingham, UK

Janice Thompson earned a doctorate in exercise physiology and nutrition at Arizona State University. She is currently professor of public health nutrition and exercise at the University of Birmingham, UK, in the School of Sport and Exercise Sciences. Her research focuses on designing and assessing the impact of nutrition and physical activity interventions to reduce the risks for obesity, cardiovascular disease, and type 2 diabetes in high-risk populations. She also teaches nutrition and research methods courses and mentors graduate research students. Janice is a Fellow of the American College of Sports Medicine (ACSM), a member of the Scientific Committee of the European College of Sports Science, and a member of the American Society for Nutrition (ASN), the British Association of Sport and Exercise Science (BASES), and the Nutrition Society. Janice won an undergraduate teaching award while at the University of North Carolina, Charlotte, a Community Engagement Award while at the University of Bristol, and the ACSM Citation Award for her contributions to research, education, and service to the exercise sciences. In addition to *The Science of Nutrition*, Janice coauthored the Pearson textbooks *Nutrition: An Applied Approach* and *Nutrition for Life* with Melinda Manore. Janice loves hiking, yoga, traveling, and cooking and eating delicious food. She likes almost every vegetable except fennel and believes chocolate should be listed as a food group.

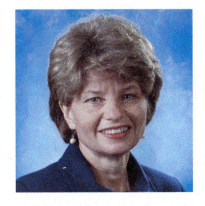

Melinda Manore, PhD, RD, CSSD, FACSM

Oregon State University

Melinda Manore earned a doctorate in human nutrition with minors in exercise physiology and health at Oregon State University (OSU). She is the past chair of the OSU Department of Nutrition and Food Management and is currently a professor of nutrition. Prior to OSU, she was a professor at Arizona State University. Melinda's area of expertise is nutrition and exercise, particularly the role of diet and exercise in health and prevention of chronic disease, exercise performance, and energy balance. She has a special focus on the energy and nutritional needs of active women and girls across the life cycle. Melinda is an active member of the Academy of Nutrition and Dietetics (AND) and the American College of Sports Medicine (ACSM). She is the past chair of the AND Research Dietetic Practice Group; served on the AND Obesity Steering Committee; and is an active member of the Sports, Cardiovascular, and Wellness Nutrition Practice Group. She is a fellow of ACSM, has served as vice president and on the Board of Trustees, and received the ACSM Citation Award for her contributions to research, education, and service to the exercise sciences. Melinda is also a member of the American Society of Nutrition (ASN) and the Obesity Society. She is the past chair of the U.S. Department of Agriculture (USDA) Nutrition and Health Committee for Program Guidance and Planning and currently is chair of the USDA, ACSM, AND Expert Panel Meeting, Energy Balance at the Crossroads: Translating Science into Action. She serves on the editorial board of numerous research journals and has won awards for excellence in research and teaching. Melinda also coauthored the Pearson textbooks *Nutrition: An Applied Approach* and *Nutrition for Life* with Janice Thompson. Melinda is an avid walker, hiker, and former runner who loves to garden, cook, and eat great food. She is also an amateur birder.

Welcome to *Nutrition: An Applied Approach,* Fifth Edition!

Why We Wrote This Book

Nutrition gets a lot of press. Go online or pick up a magazine and you'll read the latest debate over which weight-loss diet is best; turn on the TV or stream a video and you'll hear a celebrity describe how she lost 50 pounds without exercising; scan the headlines or read some blogs and you'll come upon the latest "super foods" and the politics surrounding the creation of new, enhanced "designer" foods. How can you evaluate these sources of nutrition information and find out whether the advice they provide is reliable? How do you navigate through seemingly endless recommendations and arrive at a way of eating that's right for *you*—one that supports your physical activity, allows you to maintain a healthful weight, and helps you avoid chronic diseases?

Nutrition: An Applied Approach began with our conviction that students and instructors would both benefit from an accurate and clear textbook that links nutrients to their functional benefits. As authors and instructors, we know that students have a natural interest in their bodies, their health, their weight, and their success in sports and other activities. By demonstrating how nutrition relates to these interests, this text empowers students to reach their personal health and fitness goals. Throughout the text, material is presented in a lively narrative that continually links the facts to students' circumstances, lifestyles, and goals. Information on current events and research keeps the inquisitive spark alive, illustrating that nutrition is truly a "living" science, and a source of considerable debate. The content of *Nutrition: An Applied Approach* is appropriate for non-nutrition majors, but also includes information that will challenge students who have a more advanced understanding of chemistry and math. We present the "science side" in a contemporary narrative style that's easy to read and understand, with engaging features that reduce students' apprehensions and encourage them to apply the material to their lives. Also, because this book is not a derivative of a major text, the writing and the figures are cohesive and always level appropriate.

As teachers, we are familiar with the myriad challenges of presenting nutrition information in the classroom, and we have included the most comprehensive ancillary package available to assist instructors in successfully meeting these challenges. We hope to contribute to the excitement of teaching and learning about nutrition—a subject that affects all of us, and a subject so important and relevant that correct and timely information can make the difference between health and disease.

New to the Fifth Edition

Retaining its hallmark applied approach, the new fifth edition takes personal nutrition concepts a step further with dynamic new features that help students realize that they think about their nutrition daily. The most noteworthy changes include:

- **NEW! Focus Figures** (two new) in Chapter 1, one focusing on nutrition and human disease, the other on the six groups of nutrients found in food.
- **NEW! Meal Focus Figures** (four new) graphically depict the differences in sets of meals, such as a comparison of nutrient density or a comparison of two high-carbohydrate meals, to engage students with useful information.
- **UPDATED! Nutrition Facts Panel and Dietary Guidelines for Americans** offer the latest nutritional guidelines (Chapter 2).
- **NEW! Chapter 13: Food Equity, Sustainability, and Quality: The Challenge of "Good" Food** focuses on current issues of food quality and availability that directly affect today's students. Topics include the disparities in availability of high-quality,

nourishing food thought to contribute to the poverty-obesity paradox, unsafe working conditions in many U.S. farms and factories, and more.

- **NEW! In Depth Chapters: Obesity, Malnutrition, and Healthful Eating Patterns,** these three new mini-chapters focus on topics such as the health and societal problems surrounding undernourishment; the effectiveness of lifestyle changes, medications, dietary supplements, and surgery in obesity treatment; and the components and principles of a healthful eating pattern.
- **NEW!** *ABC News* **Videos** bring nutrition to life and spark discussion with up-to-date hot topics from 2012 to 2016. MasteringNutrition activities tied to the videos include multiple-choice questions that provide wrong-answer feedback to redirect students to the correct answer.

To help students master tough concepts of the course, updates include:

- **NEW! Table of Contents organization to better streamline the coverage of the micronutrients** where four former chapters [7 to 10 in the 4th edition] now become three [7 to 9 in the 5th edition] to reduce duplicate coverage and help students better comprehend the role of vitamins and minerals in fluid and electrolyte balance (Chapter 7); key body functions (energy metabolism, antioxidant functions, and vision) (Chapter 8); and healthy body tissues (collagen, blood, and bone) (Chapter 9).
- **NEW! Learning Outcomes approach** creates a clear learning path for students with numbered learning outcomes at the beginning of each chapter that are then tied to each major chapter section, helping students navigate each chapter and measure their progress against specific learning goals, and helping instructors assess the key information and skills students are meant to take away from each chapter.
- **NEW! Study Plans** conclude each chapter, tying the chapter learning outcomes to the review questions and math review questions, and also includes the Test Yourself true/false answers and Web Links.
- **NEW! Offline access to the eText anytime with eText 2.0.** Complete with embedded *ABC News* videos and animation, eText 2.0 is mobile friendly and ADA accessible.
  - ☐ Now available on smartphones and tablets.
  - ☐ Seamlessly integrated videos.
  - ☐ Accessible (screen-reader ready).
  - ☐ Configurable reading settings, including sizable type and night reading mode.
  - ☐ Instructor and student note taking, highlighting, bookmarking, and search.

This fifth edition of *Nutrition: An Applied Approach* also features the **Mastering-Nutrition**™ online homework, tutorial, and assessment system, which delivers self-paced tutorials and activities that provide individualized coaching, a focus on course objectives, and tools enabling instructors to respond individually to each student's progress. The proven Mastering system provides instructors with customizable, easy-to-assign, automatically graded assessments that motivate students to learn outside of class and arrive prepared for lecture.

The Visual Walkthrough located at the front of this text provides an overview of these and other important features in the fifth edition. For specific changes to each chapter, see the following.

Chapter 1 Nutrition: Linking Food and Health

- Restructured headings throughout the chapter to improve organization and flow of the chapter.
- Expanded narrative text on wellness and the role that a healthy diet plays in promoting wellness.
- Revised Figure 1.1 (previously titled "Components of Wellness") to figure illustrating how a nutritious diet contributes to wellness in numerous ways.
- Deleted the Nutrition Myth or Fact and incorporated discussion of pellagra into the narrative text.
- Deleted the Hot Topic on spam and incorporated it into the narrative text.

- New Focus Figure 1.2 on the relationship between nutrition and human disease, which consolidated the previous Figures 1.2 to 1.4.
- New Focus Figure 1.3 on the six groups of nutrients found in foods, which consolidated the previous Figures 1.6 to 1.8, and added in new information and graphics on vitamins and minerals.
- Deleted previous Table 1.4 on AMDRs, as this information is provided in Focus Figure 1.4.
- New Focus Figure 1.5 on the scientific method—improves upon previous figure.
- Added new narrative text for epidemiological studies, prevalence, and incidence.
- New Figure 1.6 on types of research studies—combines narrative and decorative photos.
- New end-of-chapter Nutrition Debate on "Conflict of Interest"; included a new Critical Thinking Question that requires students to conduct research into the topic.

In Depth 1.5 New Frontiers in Nutrition and Health

- Slightly expanded the discussion of epigenetics and added a new figure illustrating the effect of epigenetic factors on gene expression.
- Deleted the Hot Topic on PB&J.

Chapter 2 Designing a Healthful Diet

- Restructured chapter headings and subheadings to improve organization, flow, and readability.
- Revised the chapter opener Test Yourself questions.
- Included new Meals Focus Figure (now Figure 2.1) illustrating the concept of nutrient density, which is now discussed as one of the characteristics of a healthful diet.
- Expanded narrative on nutrient density to include an example of the NuVal system in supermarkets.
- Complete rewrite of section on "What's Behind Our Food Choices?" which moved here from the former In Depth 2.5.
- Updated section on food labels, and included updated and enhanced figures on food labels (now Figure 2.3) and the Nutrition Facts panel (now Focus Figure 2.4).
- Deleted the previous Figure 2.3 (Health Claims Report Card) as it was repetitive and not particularly helpful.
- Updated section on Dietary Guidelines for Americans to include the latest 2015–2020 DGAs. Deleted previous Table 2.3 (Ways to Incorporate the Dietary Guidelines for Americans into your Daily Life) as it was outdated and inconsistent with the new DGAs.
- Moved the discussion and figure of the Mediterranean-style eating pattern and the Exchange System to the new In Depth on Healthful Eating Patterns, and tightened up the section on "Ethnic Variations and Other Eating Plans."
- Added in a new section on "Get Some High-Tech Help" in designing a healthful diet.
- Expanded the section "Can Eating Out Be Part of a Healthful Diet?" to include recent evidence related to nutrition labeling on menus, and whether this has changed the menu choices of Americans when eating out.
- Deleted the Nutrition Label Activity on "How Realistic Are the Serving Sizes Listed on Food Labels?" as it was repetitive and did not add any additional information to what is already included in the narrative and figures.
- Revised the Nutrition Debate on "Nutrition Advice from the U.S. Government: Is Anyone Listening?"

In Depth 2.5 Healthful Eating Patterns

- This is an entirely new In Depth, teaching students the components and principles of a healthful eating pattern as recommended by the *2015–2020 Dietary Guidelines for Americans*, and providing some examples, such as the Mediterranean diet.

Chapter 3 The Human Body: Are We Really What We Eat?

- Reorganized opening section to improve text-art integration.
- Split discussion of gastrointestinal anatomy and physiology so that the journey of food through the GI tract is discussed in its own A-section, followed by an A-section covering the accessory organs and special features.
- Deleted the Hot Topic on GI simulators.
- Added discussion and a figure of the four mechanisms by which nutrients are absorbed across enterocytes.
- Expanded discussion and added figure of peristalsis and segmentation.

In Depth 3.5 Disorders Related to Specific Foods

- Tightened narrative on food allergies.
- Added discussion of non-celiac gluten sensitivity.

Chapter 4 Carbohydrates: Plant-Derived Energy Nutrients

- Incorporated the information on health properties of various forms of sugars into the chapter narrative (previously in Nutrition Myth or Fact box).
- Expanded information on types of soluble fibers.
- Added more detail on how fructose is metabolized differently from glucose, and the impact of these differences on insulin release, satiety, and associations with obesity.
- Incorporated information on hypoglycemia into the narrative (previously included in a Hot Topic).
- Updated the recommendations on added sugars based on the new 2015–2020 Dietary Guidelines for Americans in the narrative and Table 4.1.
- Added information on Advantame, a new artificial sweetener.
- Fully revised the section on the role artificial sweeteners play in weight management.
- Updated the end-of-chapter Nutrition Debate on whether added sugars are the cause of the obesity epidemic.
- Revised Figure 4.1 to more clearly show the results that occur from the chemical reactions that take place in photosynthesis.
- Enhanced Figure 4.11 on the glycemic index to include a graph showing the surge in blood glucose with high versus low glycemic index foods, along with the glycemic index values for specific foods.
- Added new Meals Focus Figure 4.16 comparing the food and fiber content of two diets, one high in fiber-rich carbohydrates and one high in refined carbohydrates.

In Depth 4.5 Diabetes

- Added historical information on the discovery of the role of insulin in diabetes.
- Added a figure identifying and allowing comparison of lab values for normal blood glucose, prediabetes, and diabetes for the FPG, OGT, and A1C tests.
- Expanded the information on lifestyle changes (including dietary strategies and smoking cessation) to reduce the risk for type 2 diabetes.

Chapter 5 Fats: Essential Energy-Supplying Nutrients

- Reorganized opening pages of the chapter: The first main section now provides an overview of the three main types of lipids. The second main section discusses triglycerides in detail.
- Updated the discussion of *trans* fatty acids to cover the recent FDA ruling to eliminate partially hydrogenated oils (PHOs) from the food supply by 2018.
- Updated all content to reflect the 2015–2020 Dietary Guidelines.
- Updated Figure 5.11 on micelle transport.

- Added a new Meals Focus Figure comparing a day's meals high and low in saturated fat.
- Deleted Table 5.2.
- Expanded recommendations for consuming beneficial fats.
- Emphasized the role of a diet high in added sugars in cardiovascular disease.
- Replaced the Nutrition Debate on fat blockers with a new debate on the controversy about the role of saturated fats in cardiovascular disease.

In Depth 5.5 Cardiovascular Disease

- Updated throughout, including and especially on role of different types of dietary fats and blood lipids in CVD.
- Replaced calculation matrix (former Figure 4) with a link to a web-based risk assessment, replacing the lab data on blood lipids with a table from the NHLBI.
- Modestly expanded the information on medications for CVD.

Chapter 6 Proteins: Crucial Components of All Body Tissues

- Revised chapter introduction to make it more pertinent to the target audience.
- Revised Figure 6.6 to include exclusively red blood cells.
- Expanded section on nitrogen balance to include a discussion of the limitations of the method.
- Deleted previous Table 6.2 (protein needs) to reflect most up-to-date evidence that is now discussed in the text.
- Updated section on protein needs, including new evidence that protein needs of many groups may be higher than the RDA.
- Streamlined and updated the section on potential harmful effects of high protein intakes.
- Added a Nutrition Label Activity on assessing your protein intake.
- Expanded the information on vegan diets, including more information on health benefits as compared to vegetarian diets.
- Included a new Meal Focus Figure comparing a day's meals that are comprised of nutrient-dense protein sources to meals that are less nutrient dense (Figure 6.13).
- Included a new figure comparing the protein content of a vegan meal with a meat-based meal (Figure 6.15).
- Deleted section on "Disorders Related to Genetic Abnormalities."
- Replaced the Nutrition Debate with a more current topic, "Are Current Protein Recommendations High Enough?"

In Depth 6.5 Vitamins and Minerals: Micronutrients with Macro Powers

- Added information on ultra-trace minerals.
- Added QuickTips on retaining vitamins in foods.

Chapter 7 Nutrients Essential to Fluid and Electrolyte Balance

- Added a new figure on fluid balance.
- Expanded the description of the regulation of fluid balance.
- Updated information on the dangers of energy drinks.
- Changed feature box on bottled water to a Nutrition Label Activity.
- Added a Nutrition Debate on controversy related to current sodium intake guidelines.

In Depth 7.5 Alcohol

- Added a new figure showing caloric content of popular alcoholic drinks.
- Added a new figure describing levels of impairment related to blood alcohol concentration.

Chapter 8 Nutrients Essential to Key Body Functions

- This chapter combines the content from Chapters 8 and 10 of the fourth edition that focuses on the role of micronutrients in supporting three key body functions, namely, energy metabolism, antioxidant function, and vision. The micronutrients covered here are: for energy metabolism, the B-vitamins, choline, iodine, chromium, manganese, and sulphur; for antioxidant function, vitamin E, vitamin C's antioxidant role, selenium, and the antioxidant functions of the carotenoids; and for vision, vitamin A. To maintain a chapter of reasonable length, content has been condensed modestly throughout.
- The chapter includes a Focus Figure on vision, two QuickTips features, a Nutri-Case, several Nutrition Online links, and a Nutrition Debate on the importance of deriving antioxidants from foods and not supplements.

In Depth 8.5 Cancer

- Expanded the description of cancer progression (Initiation, Promotion, and Progression).
- Updated the discussion and debate around the potential contribution of "bad luck" to causing cancer.
- Added in information on how exercise can reduce risks for various forms of cancer.
- Updated information on the role of tanning beds in increasing the risk for skin cancer.
- Updated information on the role of phytochemicals in cancer prevention.

Chapter 9 Nutrients Essential to Healthy Tissues

- This chapter combines the content from Chapters 8, 9, and 10 of the fourth edition that focuses on the role of micronutrients in supporting connective tissues; namely, blood, the collagen component of connective tissues, and bone. The micronutrients covered here are: for blood, the trace minerals iron, zinc, and copper, and vitamins B6, folate, B12, and K; for collagen synthesis, vitamin C; and for bone, calcium, phosphorus, magnesium, fluoride, and vitamins D and K. To maintain a chapter of reasonable length, content has been condensed modestly throughout.
- The chapter includes a new figure on the role of vitamin C in collagen synthesis; a new Focus Figure on regulation of blood calcium; a You Do the Math on calculating iron intake; three QuickTips features, a Nutri-Case, several Nutrition Online links, and a Nutrition Debate on the surge in vitamin D deficiency.

In Depth 9.5 Osteoporosis

- Updated opening story on bone health to discuss mother-daughter with osteoporosis and osteopenia.
- Expanded information on the role of calcium and vitamin D supplements in promoting bone health.
- Included a more age-appropriate figure for kyphosis (now Figure 3).
- Added a new figure on the reduction in bone density with age (now Figure 4).
- Updated research on the impact of caffeine on risk for fractures.
- Tightened up section on nutritional influences on osteoporosis risk, and updated information on the role of protein in promoting bone health.
- Updated the research into whether calcium and vitamin D supplementation can prevent osteoporosis.
- Included new information addressing the latest controversy on whether exercise can strengthen bone and reduce risk for fractures.
- Added new information on pharmaceutical treatments for osteoporosis.
- Discussed the controversy on whether taking calcium supplements increases the risk for myocardial infarction.

Chapter 10 Achieving and Maintaining a Healthful Body Weight

- Reorganized chapter headings and content to improve flow and clarity.
- Deleted three figures to update and reduce clutter: (a) variations in lean body mass (previously Figure 11.7); (b) the goal-setting card (previously 11.9); and (c) graph of childhood obesity rates (previously 11.11).
- Replaced the previous Figure 11.8 with a new Meal Focus Figure (now Figure 10.7).
- Incorporated updated information on whether being overweight is associated with decreased risks for premature mortality and various chronic diseases.
- Added two new sections on the factors that influence body weight: (a) the protein leverage hypothesis; and (b) the drifty gene hypothesis.
- Integrated the information on sociocultural factors affecting food choice and body weight to reduce repetition.
- Expanded information on non-exercise activity thermogenesis (NEAT), and added as a boldface term and margin definition.
- Moved all information on obesity (why it is harmful, why it occurs, and how it is treated) into In Depth 11.5.
- Condensed the narrative on the effect of macronutrient composition of the diet on weight loss to reduce repetition.
- Included a discussion of mindful eating in the section on behavioral modification.
- Updated the Nutrition Debate on high-carbohydrate, moderate-fat diets, and included a discussion of the effects of the Paleo diet on weight loss.

In Depth 10.5 Obesity

- Extracted, updated, and expanded information that had been in the weight chapter in the fourth edition.
- Included new information on the pro-inflammatory role of adipokines and the relationship between abdominal obesity, metabolic syndrome, and cardiometabolic risk. To support this discussion, we altered Figure 1, which depicts abdominal obesity and its inflammatory effects.
- Added a new Focus Figure 2 and accompanying discussion on the more than 100 variables that directly or indirectly influence energy balance and body weight.
- Expanded the discussion of how people in the National Weight Control Registry succeed in losing weight and keeping it off.
- Added more information on prescription weight-loss medications, on weight-loss dietary supplements, and on the risks and benefits of bariatric surgery.

Chapter 11 Nutrition and Physical Fitness: Keys to Good Health

- Incorporated the discussion of the inactivity levels of Americans into the section on "How Can You Improve Your Fitness?"
- Added in a link to the President's Challenge Adult Fitness Test to the end-of-chapter Web Links.
- Incorporated the latest information on the roles of lactic acid as a key fuel source into the section, "The Breakdown of Carbohydrates Provides Energy for Both Brief and Long-Term Exercise."
- Revised Figure 11.9 (illustration of use of carbohydrate and fat across levels of exercise intensity) to include an additional bar graph illustrating the absolute amount of kcal from fat and carbohydrate that are expended during exercise of low and moderate intensity.
- Added in new information and references related to intrinsic and extrinsic motivation to be active and high intensity interval training (HIIT).
- Incorporated the latest sports nutrition guidance for macronutrient, micronutrient, and fluid replacement that was recently published in the 2016 ACSM Position Stand on Nutrition and Exercise Performance.
- Included a new Meal Focus Figure (Figure 11.10) illustrating examples of one day of high-carbohydrate meals differing in total energy content.

- Incorporated updated section on ergogenic aids into the chapter narrative.
- Updated the Nutrition Debate on "How Much Physical Activity Is Enough?"

In Depth 11.5 Disorders Related to Body Image, Eating, and Exercise

- Expanded the information on body image, explaining how it can affect eating and exercise patterns, as well as physical and mental health.
- Included a discrete discussion of excessive exercise (also called exercise addiction or exercise dependence).
- Included a discrete narrative discussion of body dysmorphic disorder and the subtype called muscle dysmorphia.
- Included information about relative energy deficiency in sports (RED-S), which encompasses numerous health problems associated with inadequate energy consumption to meet the energy needs of active men and women. The female athlete triad is one form of RED-S.
- Removed discussion of talking to a friend about disordered eating.

Chapter 12 Food Safety and Technology: Protecting Our Food

- Replaced Fight Bac! Logo with the food safety logo from the USDA's Foodsafety.gov.
- Added information on the Hazard Analysis Critical Control Point (HACCP) system.
- Identified percentages of foodborne illness outbreaks by setting (restaurants, homes, etc.).
- Added a QuickTips for food safety for packed lunches.
- Expanded narrative on benefits and concerns of GM foods, placing the entire discussion in the narrative section instead of covering part in narrative and part in the Nutrition Debate.
- Expanded the discussion of persistent organic pollutants, including types and health concerns.
- Briefly explained how food animals become reservoirs for antibiotic-resistant pathogens.
- Changed the Nutrition Debate topic to question organic foods: are they worth the cost?

In Depth 12.5 The Safety and Effectiveness of Dietary Supplements

- Throughout, emphasized safety concerns with dietary supplements.
- Tightened the structure of the chapter to eliminate repetition.
- Completely rewrote the table on herbal supplements.

Chapter 13 Food Equity, Sustainability, and Quality: The Challenge of "Good Food"

This is an entirely new chapter for the fifth edition. It covers global and domestic food insecurity, inequities in farm, food service, and food retail labor, the role of the food industry in limiting food diversity and influencing our food choices, sustainability (use of natural resources and emission of greenhouse gases and other forms of pollution) and aspects of the food movement such as local food, fair trade, and others.

In Depth 13.5 Malnutrition

This is a new In Depth. It covers severe acute malnutrition (SAM), micronutrient deficiencies, the nutrition paradox in countries transitioning out of poverty, and the poverty–obesity paradox, emphasizing hypotheses attempting to explain why it occurs.

Chapter 14 Nutrition Through the Life Cycle: Pregnancy and the First Year of Life

- Expanded the discussion of the roles of mothers' and fathers' preconception health and pregnancy outcomes.
- Updated guidelines to reflect *2015–2020 Dietary Guidelines for Americans*.
- New figure on foods at risk for bacterial contamination.
- Added discussion on "older" mothers.
- Added Meal Focus Figure comparing nonpregnant and lactating diets.
- Added discussion of *Cronobacter* contamination of infant formula.
- New Nutrition Debate on new approaches to preventing pediatric food allergies.

In Depth 14.5 The Fetal Environment

Updated research throughout, especially on the effects of maternal obesity on offspring.

Chapter 15 Nutrition Through the Life Cycle: Childhood to Late Adulthood

- Expanded information on the federal School Breakfast and School Lunch Programs, as well as in-class breakfasts, replacing the former Nutrition Myth or Fact box on breakfast.
- Added discussion of Class 2 and Class 3 obesity in pediatric populations, and of the health effects of pediatric obesity.
- Expanded the discussion on the family's role in the prevention and management of pediatric obesity.
- Replaced the Tufts University plate for older adults with a plate based on the USDA MyPlate.
- Expanded the discussion on nutrition/medication interactions for older adults.
- Updated information on federal food programs for older adults.

In Depth 15.5 Searching for the Fountain of Youth

Updated all research throughout, especially in the discussion on Calorie restriction and other dietary approaches, "anti-aging" supplements, and the CDC's guidelines for healthy lifestyle and chronic disease prevention.

Teaching and Learning Package

Available with *Nutrition: An Applied Approach*, Fifth Edition, is a comprehensive set of ancillary materials designed to enhance learning and to facilitate teaching.

Instructor Supplements

- **MasteringNutrition with Pearson eText 2.0 and MyDietAnalysis**
  MasteringNutrition is an online homework, tutorial, and assessment product designed to improve results by helping students quickly master concepts. Students will benefit from self-paced tutorials that feature immediate wrong answer feedback and hints that emulate the office-hour experience to help keep them on track. With a wide range of interactive, engaging, and assignable activities, students will be encouraged to actively learn and retain tough course concepts:

  ☐ **Before class,** assign adaptive Dynamic Study Modules and reading assignments from the eText with Reading Quizzes to ensure that students come prepared to class, having done the reading.

□ **During class,** Learning Catalytics, a "bring your own device" student engagement, assessment and classroom intelligence system, allows students to use their smartphone, tablet, or laptop to respond to questions in class. With Learning Catalytics, you can assess students in real time using open-ended question formats to uncover student misconceptions and adjust lectures accordingly.

□ **After class** assign, an array of assignments such as Focus Figure Coaching Activities, *ABC News* Videos, Nutrition Animations, Nutri-Tool Activities, and much more. Students receive wrong-answer feedback personalized to their answers, which will help them get back on track.

□ **MyDietAnalysis** is available as a single sign-on to MasteringNutrition. Developed by the nutrition database experts at ESHA Research, Inc., and tailored for use in college nutrition courses, MyDietAnalysis provides an accurate, reliable, and easy-to-use program for students' diet analysis needs. Featured is a database of nearly 20,000 foods and multiple reports.

For more information on MasteringNutrition, please visit www.masteringhealthand nutrition.com

- *ABC News* **Nutrition and Wellness Lecture Launcher Videos.** Twenty-seven brand-new brief videos help instructors stimulate critical discussion in the classroom. Videos are provided already linked within PowerPoint lectures and are available separately in large-screen format with optional closed captioning through MasteringNutrition.

- *Instructor Resource and Support Manual.* Easier to use than a typical instructor's manual, this key guide provides a step-by-step visual walk-through of all the resources available to you for preparing your lectures. Also included are tips and strategies for new instructors, sample syllabi, and suggestions for integrating MasteringNutrition into your classroom activities and homework assignments.

- **Test Bank.** The Test Bank incorporates Bloom's Taxonomy, or the Higher Order of Learning, to help instructors create exams that encourage students to think analytically and critically, rather than simply to regurgitate information.

- *Great Ideas! Active Ways to Teach Nutrition.* This manual provides ideas for classroom activities related to specific nutrition topics, as well as suggestions for activities that can be adapted to various topics and class sizes.

Student Supplements

- **MasteringNutrition Student Study Area** also provides students with self-study material like access to the eText 2.0, practice quizzes, flashcards, videos, MP3s, and much more to help them get the best grade in your course at their own pace.

- **Dynamic Study Modules in MasteringNutrition** assess students' performance and activity in real time. They use data and analytics that personalize content to target students' particular strengths and weaknesses. And, because we know students are always on the go, Dynamic Study Modules can be accessed from any computer, tablet, or smartphone.

- **MyDietAnalysis** (www.mydietanalysis.com). Powered by ESHA Research, Inc., MyDietAnalysis features a database of nearly 20,000 foods and multiple reports. It allows students to track their diet and activity using up to three profiles and to generate and submit reports electronically.

- *Eat Right! Healthy Eating in College and Beyond.* This handy, full-color booklet provides students with practical guidelines, tips, shopper's guides, and recipes that turn healthy eating principles into blueprints for action. Topics include healthy eating in the cafeteria, dorm room, and fast-food restaurants; planning meals on a budget; weight management; vegetarian alternatives; and how alcohol affects health.

- **Food Composition Table** available via PDF and posted in the MasteringNutrition Study Area for students to access easily.

nutri-case | YOU PLAY THE EXPERT!

Our Nutri-Case scenarios enable students to evaluate the nutrition-related beliefs and behaviors of five people representing a range of backgrounds and nutritional challenges. Take a moment to get acquainted with our Nutri-Case characters here.

HANNAH

Hi, I'm Hannah. I'm 18 years old and in my first year at Valley Community College. I'm 5'6" and right now I weigh 171 lbs. I haven't made up my mind yet about my major. All I know for sure is that I don't want to work in a hospital like my mom! I got good grades in high school, but I'm a little freaked out by college so far. There's so much homework, plus one of my courses has a lab, plus I have to work part time because my mom doesn't have the money to put me through school. . . . Sometimes I feel like I just can't handle it all. And when I get stressed out, I eat. I've already gained 10 pounds and I haven't even finished my first semester!

THEO

Hi, I'm Theo. Let's see, I'm 21, and my parents moved to the Midwest from Nigeria 11 years ago. I'm 6'8" tall and weigh in at 200 lbs. The first time I ever played basketball, in middle school, I was hooked. I won lots of awards in high school and then got a full scholarship to the state university, where I'm a junior studying political science. I decided to take a nutrition course because, last year, I had a hard time making it through the playing season, plus keeping up with my classes and homework. I want to have more energy, so I thought maybe I'm not eating right. Anyway, I want to figure out this food thing before basketball season starts again.

LIZ

I'm Liz, I'm 20, and I'm a dance major at the School for Performing Arts. I'm 5'4" and currently weigh about 103 lbs. Last year, two other dancers from my class and I won a state championship and got to dance in the New Year's Eve celebration at the governor's mansion. This spring, I'm going to audition for the City Ballet, so I have to be in top condition. I wish I had time to take a nutrition course, but I'm too busy with dance classes, rehearsals, and teaching a dance class for kids. But it's okay, because I get lots of tips from other dancers and from the Internet. Like last week, I found a website especially for dancers that explained how to get rid of bloating before an audition. I'm going to try it for my audition with the City Ballet!

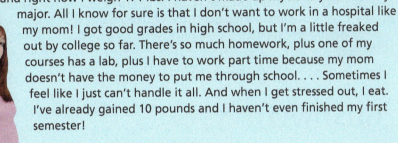

JUDY

I'm Judy, Hannah's mother. I'm 38 years old and a nurse's aide at Valley Hospital. I'm 5'5" and weigh 200 lbs. Back when Hannah was a baby, I dreamed of going to college so I could be a registered nurse. But then my ex and I split up, and Hannah and me, we've been in survival mode ever since. I'm proud to have raised my daughter without any handouts, and I do good work, but the pay never goes far enough and it's exhausting. I guess that's partly because I'm out of shape, and my blood sugar is high. Most nights I'm so tired at the end of my shift that I just pick up some fast food for supper. I know I should be making home-cooked meals, but like I said, I'm in survival mode.

GUSTAVO

Hello. My name is Gustavo. I'm 69 years young at the moment, but when I was 13 years old I came to the United States from Mexico with my parents and three sisters to pick crops in California. Now I manage a large vineyard. They ask me when I'm going to retire, but I can still work as hard as a man half my age. Health problems? None. Well, maybe my doctor tells me my blood pressure is high, but that's normal for my age! I guess what keeps me going is thinking about how my father died 6 months after he retired. He had colon cancer, but he never knew it until it was too late. Anyway, I watch the nightly news and read the papers, so I keep up on what's good for me, "Eat less salt" and all that stuff. I'm doing great! I'm 5'5" tall and weigh 166 lbs.

Throughout this text, students will follow these five characters as they grapple with various nutrition-related challenges. As they do, the characters might remind students of themselves, or of people they may know. Our hope is that by applying the information learned in this course to their own circumstances, students will deepen their understanding of the importance of nutrition in achieving a healthful life.

acknowledgments

It is always eye-opening to author a textbook and to realize that the work of so many people contributes to the final product. There are numerous people to thank, and we'd like to begin by extending our gratitude to our contributors. Our deepest gratitude and appreciation goes to Dr. Linda Vaughan of Arizona State University. Linda revised and updated the fluid and electrolyte balance chapter and the life cycle chapters. She also revised the In Depth features on alcohol, the fetal environment, and strategies to promote healthy aging. Our enduring thanks as well goes to the many contributors and colleagues who made important and lasting contributions to earlier editions of this text. We also extend our sincere thanks to the able reviewers who provided much important feedback and guidance for this revision. These reviewers help to ensure our content is up-to-date and that the presentation of this information meets the needs of instructors and students.

We would like to thank the fabulous staff at Pearson for their incredible support and dedication to this book. Our Acquisitions Editor, Michelle Yglecias, has provided unwavering support and guidance throughout the entire process of writing and publishing this book. We could never have written this text without the exceptional skills of our Developmental Editor, Laura Bonazzoli, whom we have been fortunate enough to have had on board for multiple editions. In addition to providing content guidance, Laura revised and updated the chapters on the human body, food safety, and food security, as well as the In Depth features on new frontiers in nutrition, disorders related to specific foods, dietary supplements, and malnutrition. Laura's energy, enthusiasm, and creativity significantly enhanced the quality of this textbook. Deepti Agarwal, our Project Editor, kept us on course and sane with her humor, organizational skills, and excellent editorial instincts, and made revising this book a pleasure rather than a chore. We are also deeply indebted to Art Development Editor Jay McElroy for his work on the Focus Figures in this edition. Nicole Constantine, Editorial Assistant, provided invaluable editorial and administrative support that we would have been lost without. Multiple talented players helped build this book in the production and design processes as well. Rebecca Marshall supervised the photo program, assisted by Matt Perry, who researched the important photo permissions. Preston Thomas created both the beautiful interior design and our glorious cover, under the expert guidance of Mark Ong. We would also like to thank the professionals at SPi Global, especially our Project Manager Karen Berry, for their important contributions to this text. Our thanks as well to Laura Bonazzoli for her excellent work on developing and updating the comprehensive Test Bank.

We also can't go without thanking the marketing and sales teams, especially Neena Bali, Executive Marketing Manager, and Mary Salzman, Field Marketing Manager, who ensured that we directed our writing efforts to meet the needs of students and instructors. The team at Pearson is second to none, and their hard work and targeted efforts ensure that this book will get out to those who will benefit most from it.

We would also like to thank the many colleagues, friends, and family members who helped us along the way. Janice would like to thank her coauthor Melinda Manore, who has provided unwavering support and guidance throughout her career and is a wonderful life-long friend and colleague. She would also like to thank her family and friends, who have been so incredibly supportive throughout her career. They are always there to offer a sympathetic ear and endless encouragement, and lovingly tolerate the demands of juggling a full-time job and authoring multiple textbooks. She would also like to thank her students because they are the reason she loves her job so much. They provide critical feedback on her teaching approaches, and help her to understand the issues and challenges they face related to learning and application of knowledge.

Melinda would specifically like to thank her husband, Steve Carroll, for the patience and understanding he has shown through this process—once again. He has learned that there is always another chapter due! Melinda would also like to thank her family, friends, graduate students, and professional colleagues for their support and listening ear throughout this whole process. They all helped make life a little easier during this incredibly busy time. Finally, she would like to thank Janice, a great friend and colleague, who makes working on the book fun and rewarding.

Janice Thompson
Melinda Manore

reviewers

Ann Marie Afflerbach
University of North Texas

April Graveman
Marshalltown Community College

Christina Minges
Miami University of Ohio

George Delahunty
Goucher College

Irving Smith
Coppin State University

Lisa Murray
Pierce College

Mallory Brown
Eastern Kentucky University

Monica Esquivel
University of Hawaii—Manoa

Theresa Martin
College of San Mateo

Zhenhua Liu
University of Massachusetts—Amherst

focus group participants

Priscilla Connors
University of North Texas

Emily Shupe
Western Illinois University

Donna Louie
University of Colorado, Boulder

Elizabeth Sussman
California State University, Northridge

Lisa Kenyon
Wright State University

Joanne Tippin
Shasta College

Pei-Yang Liu
University of Akron

Elisabeth De Jonge
George Mason University

Sherry Stewart
Navarro College

Linda Friend
Wake Technical Community College

Joann Burnett
Indiana University, Purdue

Julia Rieck
Indiana University, Purdue

Heidi Wengreen
Utah State University

Serah Theuri
University of Southern Indiana

Sherry Fletcher
Palm Beach Community College

Lisa Herzig
California State University, Fresno

Nancy Hunt
Lipscomb University

Betty Joynes
Camden County Community College

Erika Ireland
California State University, Fresno

brief contents

contents

1

Nutrition: Linking food and health 2

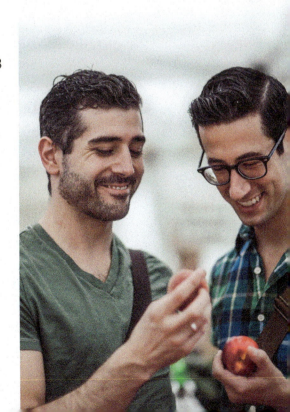

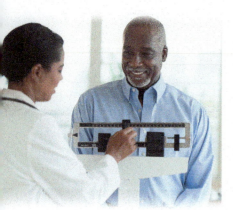

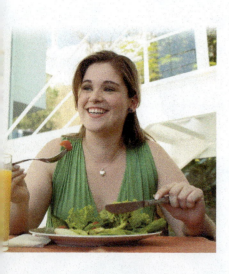

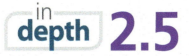

in depth 2.5

Healthful Eating Patterns   59

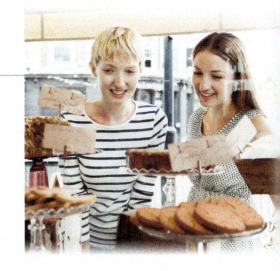

3

The Human Body: Are we really what we eat?   64

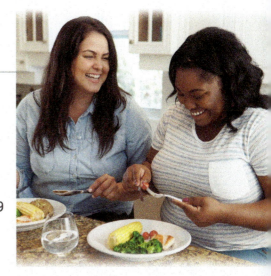

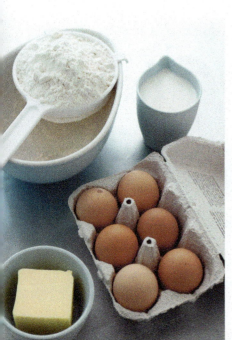

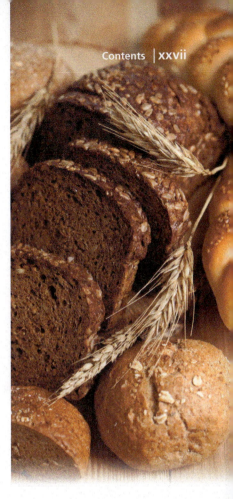

4

Carbohydrates: Plant-derived energy nutrients 98

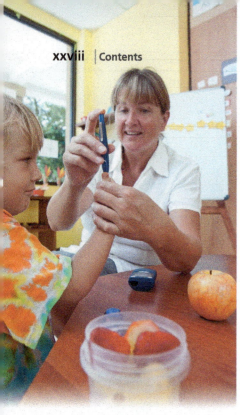

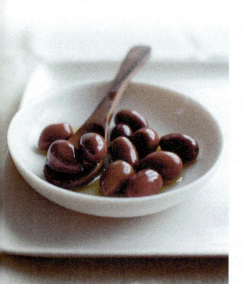

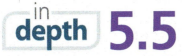

in depth 5.5

Cardiovascular Disease   167

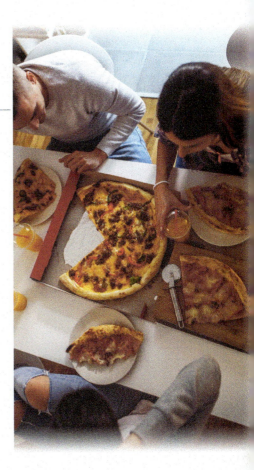

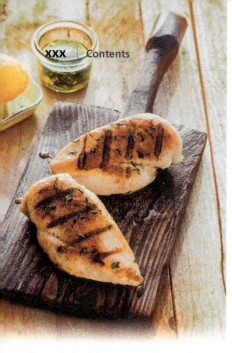

6

Proteins: Crucial Components of All Body Tissues   178

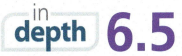

depth 6.5
Vitamins and Minerals: Micronutrients with Macro Powers   211

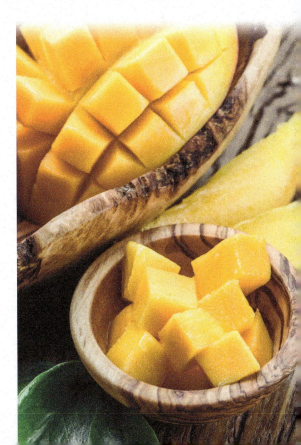

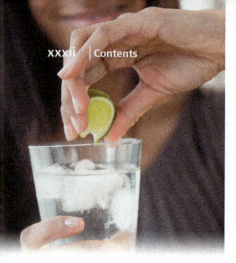

7

Nutrients Essential to Fluid and Electrolyte Balance   222

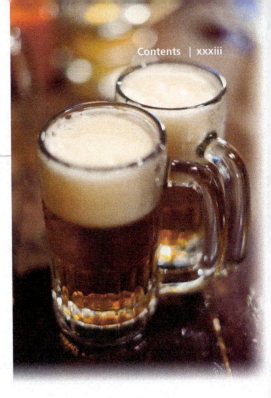

8

Nutrients Essential to Key Body Functions   260

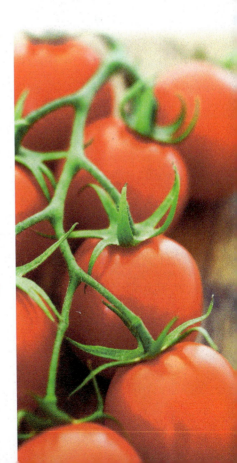

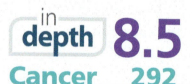

in depth 8.5

Cancer 292

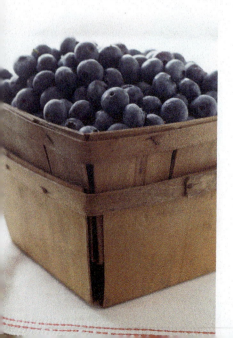

9

Nutrients Essential to Healthy Tissues 300

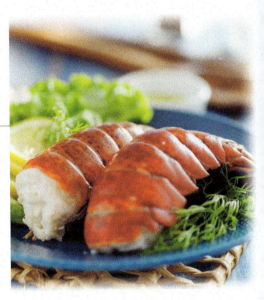

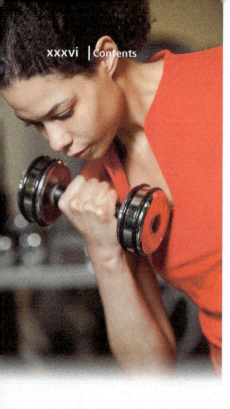

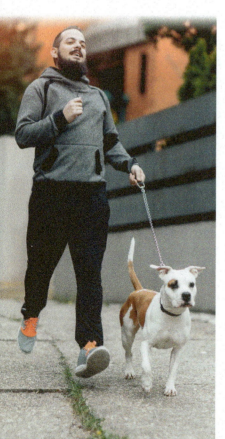

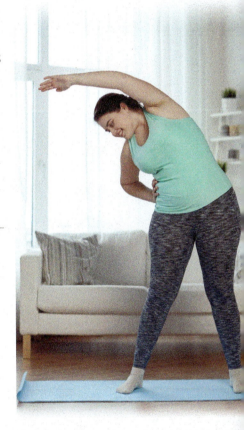

11

Nutrition and Physical Fitness: Keys to good health   380

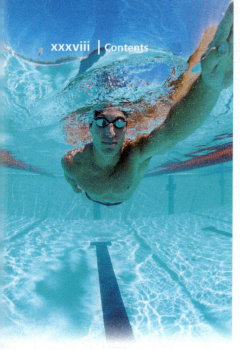

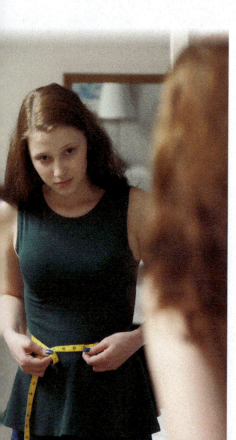

in
depth 11.5

Disorders Related to Body Image, Eating, and Exercise   413

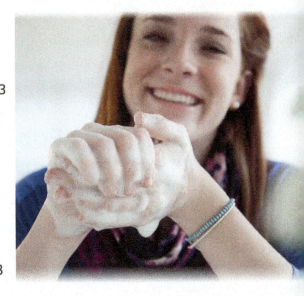

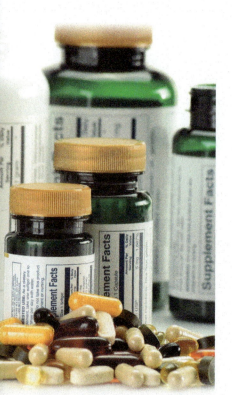

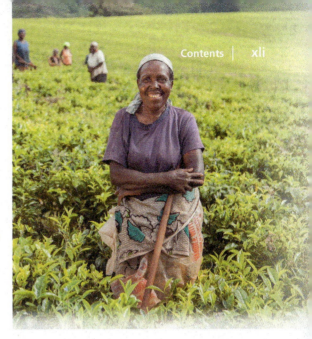

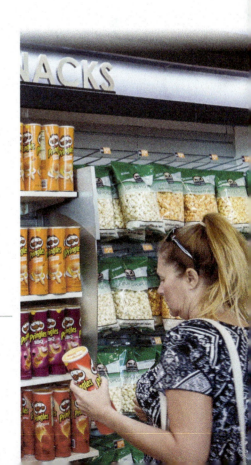

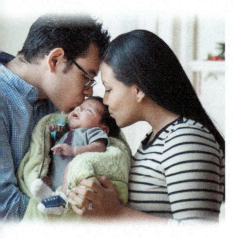

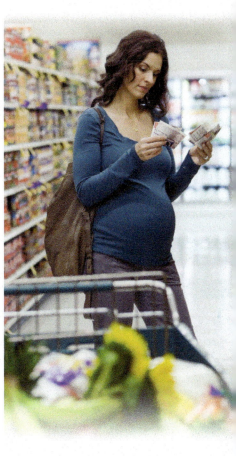

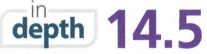

depth 14.5
The Fetal Environment 524

15
Nutrition Through the Life Cycle: Childhood to late adulthood 528

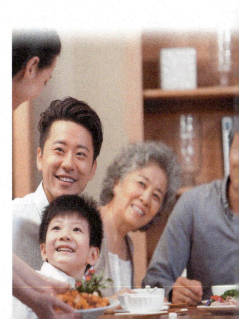

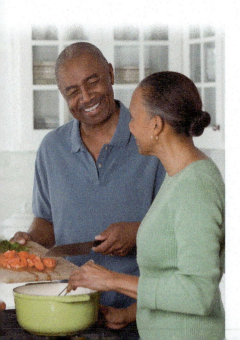

in depth 15.5
Searching for the Fountain of Youth 562

Appendices

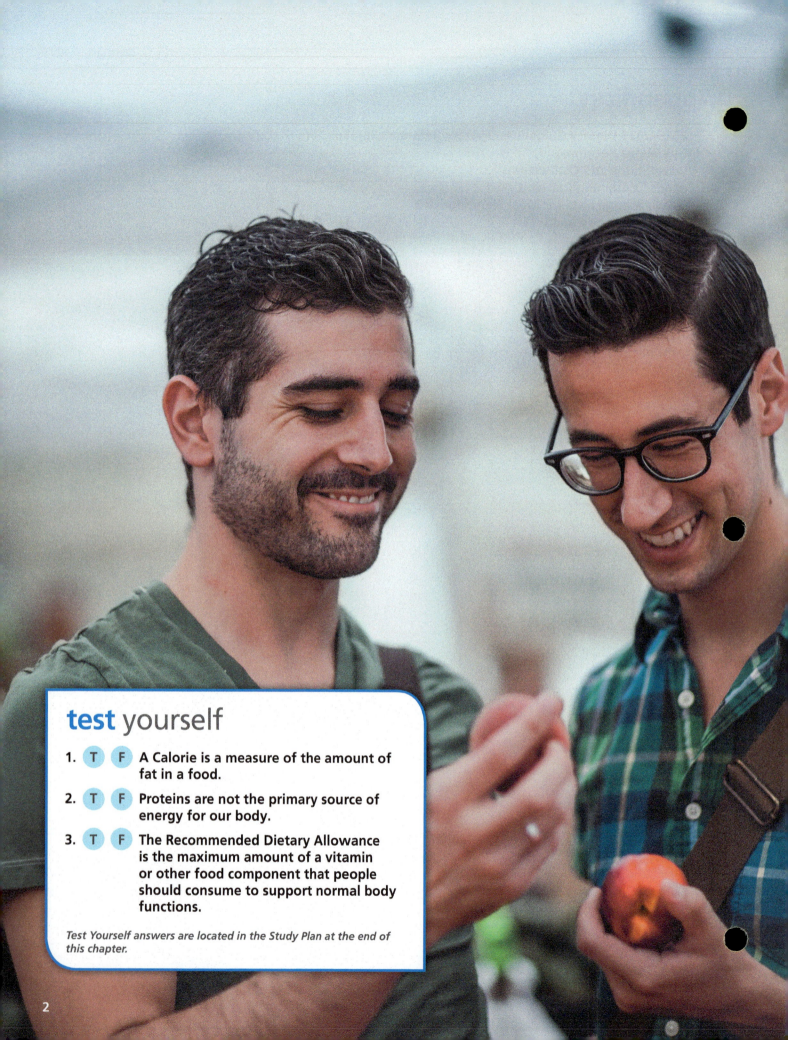

test yourself

1. T F A Calorie is a measure of the amount of fat in a food.

2. T F Proteins are not the primary source of energy for our body.

3. T F The Recommended Dietary Allowance is the maximum amount of a vitamin or other food component that people should consume to support normal body functions.

Test Yourself answers are located in the Study Plan at the end of this chapter.

1

Nutrition
Linking food and health

Miguel hadn't expected college life to make him feel so tired. After classes, he just wanted to go back to his dorm and sleep. Scott, his roommate, had little sympathy. "It's all that junk food you eat!" he insisted. "Let's go down to the organic market for some real food." Miguel dragged himself to the market with Scott. They bought fresh vegetables and fish, and were heading to the checkout when they noticed a woman in a white lab coat promoting a variety of "energy-boosting" supplements. Miguel was intrigued and told her that he had been feeling tired lately. She nodded sympathetically. "You look pale. I'd recommend taking an iron supplement." She handed him a bottle of tablets. "This one is easy to absorb, and it's on special this week." Miguel bought the supplement and began taking it that night. A week later, he didn't feel any better, so he visited the campus health clinic. The physician there ran some tests and told him that his thyroid gland wasn't functioning properly. She prescribed a medication and congratulated Miguel for catching the problem early. "If you had waited," she said, "you could have become seriously ill." Miguel asked if he should continue taking his iron supplement. The doctor looked puzzled. "Where did you get the idea that you needed an iron supplement?"

Like Miguel, you've probably been offered nutrition-related advice from well-meaning friends and self-professed "experts." Perhaps you found the advice helpful, or maybe, as in Miguel's case, it turned out to be all wrong. Where can you go for reliable advice about nutrition? What exactly is nutrition, and how does what we eat influence our health? In this chapter, we'll begin to answer these questions.

MasteringNutrition™
Go online for chapter quizzes, pre-tests, interactive activities, and more!

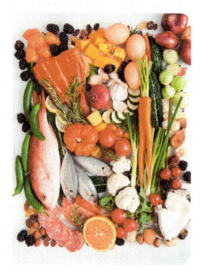

↖ Nutrition is the science that studies all aspects of food and its influence on our body and health.

What is nutrition?

Although many people think that food and nutrition mean the same thing, they don't. **Food** refers to the plants and animals we consume. It provides the chemicals our body need to maintain life and support growth and health. **Nutrition**, in contrast, is the science that studies food and how food nourishes our body and influences our health. It encompasses how we consume, digest, absorb, and store the chemicals in food, and how these chemicals affect our body. Nutrition also involves studying the factors that influence our eating patterns, making recommendations about the amount we should eat of each type of food, attempting to maintain food safety, and addressing issues related to the global food supply. You can think of nutrition, then, as the science that encompasses everything about food.

When compared with other scientific disciplines such as chemistry, biology, and physics, nutrition is a relative newcomer. Although food production has played a defining role in the evolution of the human species, an appreciation of the importance of nutrition to our health has developed only within the past 400 years. Early research in nutrition focused on making the link between dietary deficiencies and illness. For instance, in the mid-1700s, it was discovered that regular consumption of citrus fruits could prevent a potentially fatal disease called scurvy. But two centuries would pass before a deficiency of vitamin C was identified as the precise culprit. Another early discovery in nutrition is related to pellagra, a disease characterized by a skin rash, diarrhea, and mental impairment. In the early 20th century it afflicted more than 50,000 people each year, and in about 10% of the cases it resulted in death. Originally thought to be an infectious disease, experiments conducted by Dr. Joseph Goldberger and colleagues found that pellagra could be effectively treated by changing the diet of those affected from one that was predominantly corn-based to one that included a variety of nutritious foods. Although Goldberger could not identify the precise component in the new diet that cured pellagra, he eventually found an inexpensive and widely available substance, brewer's yeast, that when added to the diet prevented or reversed the disease. Shortly after Goldberger's death in 1937, scientists identified the component that is deficient in the diet of pellagra patients: a vitamin called niacin, which is plentiful in brewer's yeast.

Nutrition research continued to focus on identifying and preventing deficiency diseases through the first half of the 20th century. Then, as the higher standard of living after World War II led to an improvement in the American diet, nutrition research began pursuing a new objective: supporting health and preventing and treating **chronic diseases**—that is, diseases that come on slowly and can persist for years, often despite treatment. Chronic diseases of particular interest to nutrition researchers include obesity, cardiovascular disease, type 2 diabetes, and various cancers. This new research has raised as many questions as it has answered, and we still have a great deal to learn about the relationship between nutrition and chronic disease.

In recent decades, advances in technology have contributed to the emergence of several exciting new areas of nutrition research. For example, reflecting our growing understanding of genetics, nutrigenomics seeks to uncover links between our genes, our environment, and our diet. The **In Depth** following this chapter describes this and other new frontiers in nutrition research and health.

food The plants and animals we consume.

nutrition The science that studies food and how food nourishes our body and influences our health.

chronic diseases Diseases that come on slowly and can persist for years, often despite treatment.

recap Food refers to the plants and animals we consume, whereas nutrition is the scientific study of food and how food affects our body and our health. An appreciation of the importance of nutrition to our health has developed only within the past 400 years. Early research in nutrition focused on making the link between dietary deficiencies and illness. Contemporary nutrition research typically studies the influence of nutrition on chronic disease.

How does nutrition support health?

LO 2 Explain how nutrition supports health.

Think about it: If you eat three meals a day, by this time next year, you'll have had more than a thousand chances to influence your body's makeup! As you'll learn in this text, you really are what you eat: the substances you take into your body are broken down and reassembled into your brain cells, bones, muscles—all of your tissues and organs. The foods you eat also provide your body with the energy it needs to function properly. These are just two of the ways that proper nutrition supports your health. Let's look at two more.

A Nutritious Diet Contributes to Wellness

Wellness can be defined in many ways. Traditionally defined as simply the absence of disease, wellness is now considered an active process we work on every day. Consuming a nutritious diet contributes to wellness in a variety of ways, including by providing the energy and functional chemicals that help us to perform activities of daily living, support our ability to concentrate and perform mental tasks, and boost our ability to ward off infections **(FIGURE 1.1)**.

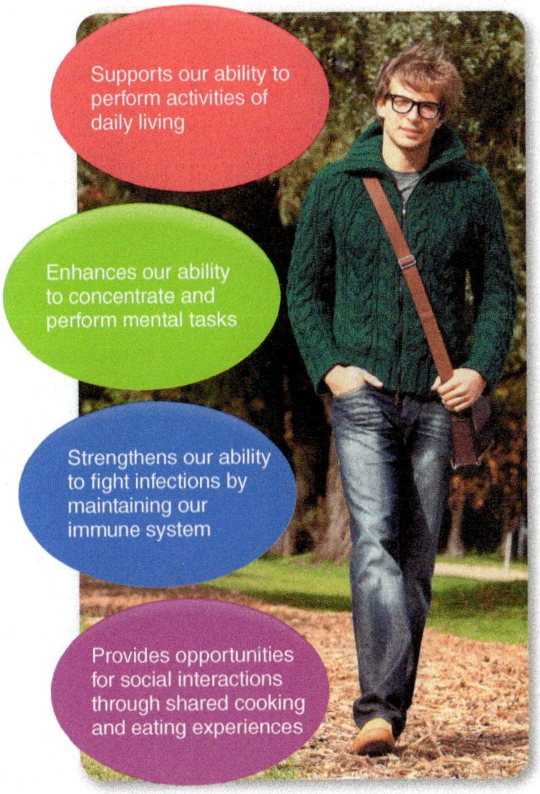

In this book, we focus on two critical aspects of physical health: nutrition and physical activity. The two are so closely related that you can think of them as two sides of the same coin: our overall state of nutrition is influenced by how much energy we expend doing daily activities, and our level of physical activity has a major impact on how we use the food we eat. We can perform more strenuous activities for longer periods when we eat a nutritious diet, whereas an inadequate or excessive food intake can make us lethargic. A poor diet, inadequate or excessive physical activity, or a combination of these also can lead to serious health problems. Finally, several studies have suggested that healthful nutrition and regular physical activity can increase feelings of well-being and reduce feelings of anxiety and depression. In other words, wholesome food and physical activity just plain feel good!

Because of its importance to the wellness of all Americans, nutrition has been included in the national health promotion and disease prevention plan of the United States. Called *Healthy People*, the plan is revised every decade. *Healthy People 2020*, launched in January 2010, identifies a set of goals and objectives (as an agenda) that we hope to reach as a nation by the year 2020.[1] This agenda was developed by a team of experts from a variety of federal agencies under the direction of the Department of Health and Human Services.

The four overarching goals of *Healthy People* are to "1) attain high-quality, longer lives free of preventable disease, disability, injury, and premature death; 2) achieve health equity, eliminate disparities, and improve the health of all groups; 3) create social and physical environments that promote good health for all; and 4) promote quality of life, healthy development, and healthy behaviors across all life stages." These overarching goals are supported by hundreds of specific goals, including many related to nutrition. Others address physical activity and the problems of overweight and obesity, which are, of course, influenced by nutrition. **TABLE 1.1** identifies some objectives related to weight, nutrition, and physical activity from *Healthy People 2020*.

A Nutritious Diet Reduces the Risk for Disease

Nutrition appears to play a role—from a direct cause to a mild influence—in the development of many diseases **(FOCUS FIGURE 1.2)**. As we noted, poor nutrition is a direct cause of deficiency diseases, such as scurvy and pellagra. Early nutrition

Supports our ability to perform activities of daily living

Enhances our ability to concentrate and perform mental tasks

Strengthens our ability to fight infections by maintaining our immune system

Provides opportunities for social interactions through shared cooking and eating experiences

FIGURE 1.1 Consuming a nutritious diet contributes to our wellness in numerous ways.

wellness A multidimensional, active process by which people make choices that enhance their lives.

TABLE 1.1 Weight, Nutrition, and Physical Activity Objectives from *Healthy People 2020*

Topic	Objective Number and Description
Weight status	NWS-8. Increase the proportion of adults who are at a healthy weight from 30.8% to 33.9%.
	NWS-9. Reduce the proportion of adults who are obese from 34.0% to 30.6%.
	NWS-10.2. Reduce the proportion of children aged 6 to 11 years who are considered obese from 17.4% to 15.7%.
Food and nutrient composition	NWS-14. Increase the contribution of fruits to the diets of the population aged 2 years and older.
	NWS-15. Increase the variety and contribution of vegetables to the diets of the population aged 2 years and older.
Physical activity	PA–1. Reduce the proportion of adults who engage in no leisure-time physical activity from 36.2% to 32.6%.
	PA–2.1. Increase the proportion of adults who engage in aerobic physical activity of at least moderate intensity for at least 150 minutes per week, or 75 minutes per week of vigorous intensity, or an equivalent combination from 43.5% to 47.9%.
	PA–2.3. Increase the proportion of adults who perform muscle-strengthening activities on 2 or more days of the week from 21.9% to 24.1%.

Data adapted from: Healthy People 2020 (U.S. Department of Health and Human Services).

research focused on identifying the missing vitamin or other food substance behind such diseases and on developing guidelines for intake levels that are high enough to prevent them. Over the years, nutrition scientists successfully lobbied for the fortification of foods with the substances of greatest concern. These measures, along with a more abundant and reliable food supply, have almost completely wiped out the majority of nutritional deficiency diseases in developed countries. However, they are still major problems in many developing nations.

In addition to causing disease directly, poor nutrition can have a subtle influence on our health. For instance, it can contribute to the development of brittle bones (a disease called osteoporosis) as well as to the progression of some forms of cancer. These associations are considered mild; however, poor nutrition is also strongly associated with three chronic diseases—heart disease, stroke, and diabetes—which are among the top 10 causes of death in the United States (see Focus Figure 1.2).

It probably won't surprise you to learn that the primary link between poor nutrition and early death is obesity. Fundamentally, obesity is a consequence of eating more Calories than are expended. At the same time, obesity is a well-established risk factor for heart disease, stroke, and the most common form of diabetes. Unfortunately, the prevalence of obesity has dramatically increased throughout the United States during the past 30 years (see Focus Figure 1.2). Throughout this text, we will discuss in detail how nutrition and physical activity affect the development of obesity.

Want to see how the prevalence of obesity differs across various ethnic groups in the United States? Go to www.cdc.gov and enter "obesity data trend maps" into the search bar.

recap Nutrition is an important component of wellness and is strongly associated with physical activity and body weight. *Healthy People 2020* is a health promotion and disease prevention plan for the United States. One goal of a healthful diet is to prevent deficiency diseases, such as scurvy and pellagra; a second goal is to lower the risk for chronic diseases, including heart disease, stroke, and the most common form of diabetes, all of which are linked to obesity.

focus figure 1.2 The Relationship Between Nutrition and Human Disease

Some diseases are the direct result of a nutritional deficiency or toxicity. The disease shown here, pellagra, is caused by a deficiency of a vitamin called niacin.

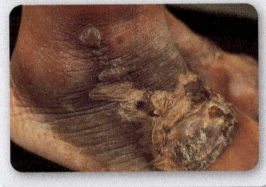

Some diseases have a strong nutritional component. These include diseases of the heart, stroke, and diabetes, all of which are among the top causes of death in the United States, as shown in this graph.
Data from: "Deaths: Preliminary Data for 2011" (U.S. Department of Health and Human Services).

Disease	Number of deaths (in thousands)
Diseases of the heart	611
Cancer	585
Chronic respiratory disease	149
Unintentional injuries	131
Stroke	129
Alzheimer's disease	85
Diabetes mellitus	76
Influenza and pneumonia	57
Inflammatory kidney disease	47
Suicide	41

Obesity, which increases the risk for diseases of the heart, stroke, and diabetes, surged between 1994 and 2010, the last year during which there was a significant increase in rates.

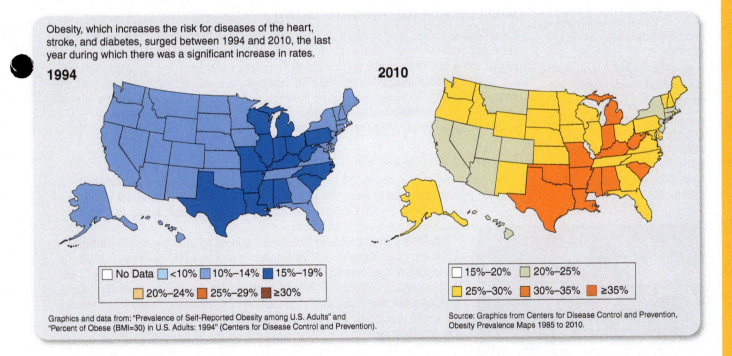

1994

2010

No Data <10% 10%–14% 15%–19% 20%–24% 25%–29% ≥30%

15%–20% 20%–25% 25%–30% 30%–35% ≥35%

Graphics and data from: "Prevalence of Self-Reported Obesity among U.S. Adults" and "Percent of Obese (BMI=30) in U.S. Adults: 1994" (Centers for Disease Control and Prevention).

Source: Graphics from Centers for Disease Control and Prevention, Obesity Prevalence Maps 1985 to 2010.

Nutrition also plays a minor role in some diseases, such as certain types of cancer, some joint diseases such as osteoarthritis, and a disease called osteoporosis, which can cause loss of bone mass, as shown here.

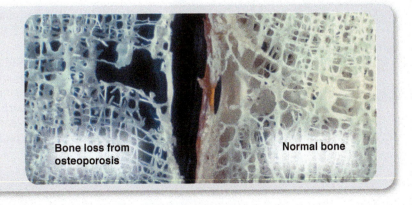

Bone loss from osteoporosis   Normal bone

LO 3 Identify the six classes of nutrients essential for health.

What are nutrients?

We enjoy eating food because of its taste, its smell, and the pleasure and comfort it gives us. However, we rarely stop to think about what our food actually contains. Foods are composed of many chemical substances, some of which are not useful to the body and others of which are critical to our growth and function. These latter chemicals are referred to as *nutrients*. The six groups of **nutrients** found in foods are (FOCUS FIGURE 1.3):

- carbohydrates
- fats and oils (two types of lipids)
- proteins
- vitamins
- minerals
- water

The term *organic* is commonly used to describe foods that are grown with little or no use of synthetic chemicals. But when scientists describe individual nutrients as **organic**, they mean that these nutrients contain both carbon and hydrogen, fundamental units of matter that are common to all living organisms. Carbohydrates, lipids, proteins, and vitamins are organic. Minerals and water are **inorganic**. Organic and inorganic nutrients are equally important for sustaining life but differ in their structures, functions, and basic chemistry. You will learn more about these nutrients in subsequent chapters; a brief review is provided here.

Macronutrients Provide Energy

Carbohydrates, fats, and proteins are the only nutrients that provide energy. By this we mean that our body breaks down these nutrients and reassembles their components into a fuel that supports physical activity and basic functioning. Although taking a multivitamin might be beneficial in other ways, it will not provide you with the energy for a 20-minute session on the stair-climber! The energy-yielding nutrients are also referred to as **macronutrients**. Macro means "large," and our body need relatively large amounts of these nutrients to support normal function and health.

Energy Is Measured in Kilocalories

The energy in foods is measured in units called *kilocalories* (*kcal*). A kilocalorie is the amount of heat required to raise the temperature of 1 kilogram (about 2.2 pounds) of water by 1 degree Celsius. We can say that the energy found in 1 gram of carbohydrate is equal to 4 kcal.

Kilo- is a prefix used in the metric system to indicate 1,000 (think of *kilometer*). Technically, 1 kilocalorie is equal to 1,000 calories. A kilocalorie is also sometimes referred to as a *large calorie* or as a *Calorie*, written with a capital C. Because they're designed for the public, nutrition labels typically use the term *calories* to indicate kilocalories. Thus, if the wrapper on an ice cream bar states that it contains 150 calories, it actually contains 150 kilocalories.

In this textbook, we use the term *energy* when referring to the general concept of energy intake or energy expenditure. We use the term *kilocalories* (*kcal*) when discussing units of energy. We use the term *Calories* with a capital "C" when presenting information about foods and food labels.

Both carbohydrates and proteins provide 4 kcal per gram, alcohol provides 7 kcal per gram, and fats provide 9 kcal per gram. Thus, for every gram of fat we consume, we obtain more than twice the energy derived from a gram of carbohydrate or protein. Refer to the **You Do the Math** box on page 10 to learn how to calculate the energy contribution of carbohydrates, fats, and proteins in a given food.

nutrients Chemicals found in foods that are critical to human growth and function.

organic A substance or nutrient that contains the elements carbon and hydrogen.

inorganic A substance or nutrient that does not contain carbon and hydrogen.

macronutrients Nutrients that our body need in relatively large amounts to support normal function and health. Carbohydrates, fats, and proteins are energy-yielding macronutrients.

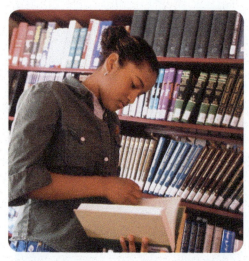

Carbohydrates are the primary source of fuel for our body, particularly for our brain.

Carbohydrates

Functions: Primary energy source for the body
Composed of: Chains of carbon, hydrogen, and oxygen
Best Food Sources: Whole grains, vegetables, fruits

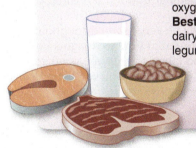

Fats and oils

Functions: Important source of energy at rest and during low-intensity exercise
Composed of: Carbon, hydrogen, and oxygen
Best Food Sources: Vegetable oils, butter, and dairy products

Proteins

Functions: Support tissue growth, repair, and maintenance
Composed of: Amino acids made up of carbon, hydrogen, oxygen, and nitrogen
Best Food Sources: Meats, dairy products, seeds, nuts, legumes

Vitamins

Functions: Assist with release of macronutrients; critical to building and maintaining bone, muscle, and blood; support immune function and vision
Composed of: Fat-soluble and water-soluble compounds
Best Food Sources: Fruits, vegetables, dairy products, meats

Minerals

Functions: Assist with fluid regulation and energy production; maintain health of blood and bones; rid body of harmful by-products of metabolism
Composed of: Single elements such as sodium, potassium, calcium, or iron
Best Food Sources: Fruits, vegetables, dairy products, meats

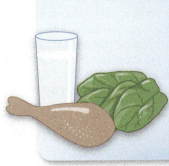

Water

Functions: Ensures proper fluid balance; assists in regulation of nerve impulses, body temperature, and muscle contractions
Composed of: Hydrogen and oxygen
Best Food Sources: Water, juices, soups, fruits, vegetables

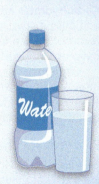

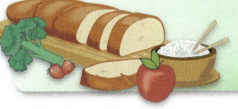
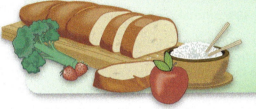

Calculating the Energy Contribution of Carbohydrates, Fats, and Proteins

The energy in food is used for everything from maintaining normal body functions—such as breathing, digesting food, and repairing damaged tissues and organs—to enabling you to perform physical activity and even to read this text. So how much energy is produced from the foods you eat?

To answer this question, you need to know the following information:

- Carbohydrates should make up the largest percentage of your nutrient intake, about 45–65%; they provide 4 kcal of energy per gram of carbohydrate consumed.

- Proteins also provide 4 kcal of energy per gram; they should be limited to 10–35% of your daily energy intake.

- Fats provide the most energy, 9 kcal per gram; they should make up 20–35% of your total energy intake.

In order to figure out whether you're taking in the appropriate percentages of carbohydrates, fats, and proteins, you will need to use a little math.

1. Let's say you have completed a personal diet analysis, and you consume 2,500 kcal per day. You consume 300 g of carbohydrates, 90 g of fat, and 123 g of protein.

2. To calculate your percentage of total energy that comes from carbohydrate, you must do two things:

   a. Multiply your total grams of carbohydrate by the energy value for carbohydrate.

   300 g of carbohydrate × 4 kcal/g
   = 1,200 kcal of carbohydrate consumed

   b. Take the kcal of carbohydrate consumed, divide this by the total kcal consumed, and multiply by 100. This will give you the percentage of the total energy you consume that comes from carbohydrate.

   (1,200 kcal/2,500 kcal) × 100
   = 48% of total energy comes from carbohydrate

3. To calculate your percentage of total energy that comes from fat, you follow the same steps but incorporate the energy value for fat:

   a. 90 g of fat × 9 kcal/g = 810 kcal of fat
   b. (810 kcal/2,500 kcal) × 100 = 32.4% of total energy comes from fat

Now try these steps to calculate the percentage of the total energy you consume that comes from protein.

Also, have you ever heard that alcohol provides "empty Calories"? Alcohol contributes 7 kcal per gram. You can calculate the percentage of kcal from alcohol in your daily diet, but remember that it is not considered an energy nutrient.

These calculations will be very useful throughout this course as you learn more about how to design a healthful diet and how to read labels to help you meet your nutritional goals. Later in this book you will learn how to estimate your unique energy needs.

Carbohydrates Are a Primary Fuel Source

Carbohydrates are the primary source of fuel for our body, particularly for our brain and during physical exercise (see Focus Figure 1.3). *Carbo-* refers to carbon, and *hydrate* refers to water. You may remember that water is made up of hydrogen and oxygen. Thus, carbohydrates are composed of chains of carbon, hydrogen, and oxygen.

Carbohydrates are found in a wide variety of foods, including rice, wheat, and other grains, as well as vegetables and fruits. Carbohydrates are also found in legumes (foods that include lentils, beans, and peas), seeds, nuts, and milk and other dairy products. (Carbohydrates and their role in health are the subject of Chapter 4.)

Fats Provide Energy and Other Essential Nutrients

Fats are another important source of energy for our body (see Focus Figure 1.3). They are a type of lipids, a diverse group of organic substances that are insoluble in water. Like carbohydrates, fats are composed of carbon, hydrogen, and oxygen; however, they contain proportionally much less oxygen and water than carbohydrates do. This quality allows them to pack together tightly, which explains why they yield more energy per gram than either carbohydrates or proteins.

carbohydrates The primary fuel source for our body, particularly for our brain and for physical exercise.

fats An important energy source for our body at rest and during low-intensity exercise.

proteins The only macronutrient that contains nitrogen; the basic building blocks of proteins are amino acids.

Fats are an important energy source for our body at rest and during low-intensity exercise. Our body is capable of storing large amounts of fat as adipose tissue. These fat stores can then be broken down for energy during periods when we are not eating—for example, while we are asleep. Foods that contain fats are also essential for the transportation of certain vitamins that are soluble only in fat into our body.

Dietary fats come in a variety of forms. Solid fats include such things as butter, lard, and margarine. Liquid fats, referred to as *oils,* include vegetable oils, such as canola and olive oils. Cholesterol is a form of lipid that our body can produce independently, and it can also be consumed in the diet. (Chapter 5 provides a thorough discussion of lipids.)

Proteins Support Tissue Growth, Repair, and Maintenance

Proteins also contain carbon, hydrogen, and oxygen, but they differ from carbohydrates and fats in that they contain the element *nitrogen* (see Focus Figure 1.3). Within proteins, these four elements assemble into small building blocks known as amino acids. We break down dietary proteins into amino acids and reassemble them to build our own body proteins—for instance, the proteins in our muscles and blood.

Although proteins can provide energy, they are not usually a primary energy source. Proteins play a major role in building new cells and tissues, maintaining the structure and strength of bone, repairing damaged structures, and assisting in regulating the breakdown of foods and fluid balance.

Proteins are found in many foods. Meats and dairy products are primary sources, as are seeds, nuts, and legumes. We also obtain small amounts from vegetables and whole grains. (Proteins are the subject of Chapter 6.)

Micronutrients Assist in the Regulation of Body Functions

Vitamins and minerals are referred to as **micronutrients**. That's because we need relatively small amounts of these nutrients to support normal health and body functions.

Vitamins are organic compounds that help regulate our body' functions. Contrary to popular belief, vitamins do not contain energy (kilocalories); however, they are essential to energy **metabolism**, the process by which the macronutrients are broken down into the smaller chemicals that our body can absorb and use. So vitamins assist with releasing and using the energy in carbohydrates, fats, and proteins. They are also critical in building and maintaining healthy bone, muscle, and blood; supporting our immune system so that we can fight infection and disease; and ensuring healthy vision (see Focus Figure 1.3).

Vitamins are classified as two types: **fat-soluble vitamins** and **water-soluble vitamins** (TABLE 1.2). This classification reflects how vitamins are absorbed, transported, and stored in our body. Both types of vitamins are essential for health and are found in a variety of foods. (Learn more about vitamins in the **In Depth** essay following Chapter 6. Chapters 7 through 9 discuss individual vitamins in detail.)

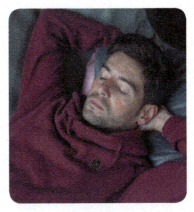

⬥ Fats are an important source of energy for our body, especially when we are at rest.

micronutrients Nutrients needed in relatively small amounts to support normal health and body functions. Vitamins and minerals are micronutrients.

vitamins Organic compounds that assist in the regulation of many body processes and the maintenance of many body tissues.

metabolism The chemical reactions by which large compounds, such as carbohydrates, fats, and proteins, are broken down into smaller units the body can use. Also refers to the assembly of smaller units into larger compounds.

fat-soluble vitamins Vitamins that are not soluble in water but are soluble in fat. These are vitamins A, D, E, and K.

water-soluble vitamins Vitamins that are soluble in water. These include vitamin C and the B vitamins.

TABLE 1.2 Overview of Vitamins

Type	Names	Distinguishing Features
Fat soluble	A, D, E, K	Soluble in fat
		Stored in the human body
		Toxicity can occur from consuming excess amounts, which accumulate in the body
Water soluble	C, B-vitamins (thiamin, riboflavin, niacin, vitamin B_6, vitamin B_{12}, pantothenic acid, biotin, folate)	Soluble in water
		Not stored to any extent in the human body
		Excess excreted in urine
		Toxicity generally only occurs as a result of vitamin supplementation

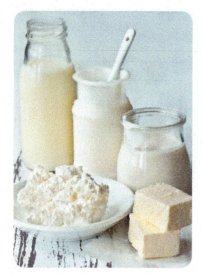

▲ Fat-soluble vitamins are found in a variety of fat-containing foods, including dairy products.

TABLE 1.3 Overview of Minerals

Type	Names	Distinguishing Features
Major minerals	Calcium, phosphorus, sodium, potassium, chloride, magnesium, sulfur	Needed in amounts greater than 100 mg/day in our diet
		Amount present in the human body is greater than 5 g (5,000 mg)
Trace minerals	Iron, zinc, copper, manganese, fluoride, chromium, molybdenum, selenium, iodine	Needed in amounts less than 100 mg/day in our diet
		Amount present in the human body is less than 5 g (5,000 mg)

Minerals include sodium, calcium, iron, and over a dozen more. They are classified as inorganic because they do not contain carbon and hydrogen. In fact, they do not "contain" other substances at all. Minerals are single elements, so they already exist in the simplest possible chemical form. Thus, they cannot be broken down during digestion or when our body use them to promote normal function; unlike certain vitamins, they can't be destroyed by heat or light. All minerals maintain their structure no matter what environment they are in. This means that the calcium in our bones is the same as the calcium in the milk we drink, and the sodium in our cells is the same as the sodium in our table salt.

Minerals have many important functions in our body. They assist in fluid regulation and energy production, are essential to the health of our bones and blood, and help rid our body of the harmful by-products of metabolism (see Focus Figure 1.3).

Minerals are classified according to the amounts we need in our diet and according to how much of the mineral is found in our body. The two broad categories are the **major minerals** and the **trace minerals** (TABLE 1.3). (Learn more about minerals in the **In Depth** following Chapter 6. Chapters 7 through 9 discuss individual minerals in detail.)

Water Supports All Body Functions

Water is an inorganic nutrient (it contains oxygen and hydrogen, but not carbon) that is vital for our survival. We consume water from many sources: in its pure form; in juices, soups, and other liquids; and in solid foods, such as fruits and vegetables. Adequate water intake ensures the proper balance of fluid both inside and outside our cells, and assists in the regulation of nerve impulses and body temperature, muscle contractions, nutrient transport, and the excretion of waste products (see Focus Figure 1.3). (Chapter 7 focuses on water and its functions in our body.)

minerals Inorganic elements that assist in the regulation of many body processes and the maintenance of many body tissues.

major minerals Minerals we need to consume in amounts of at least 100 mg per day and of which the total amount in our body is at least 5 g.

trace minerals Minerals we need to consume in amounts less than 100 mg per day and of which the total amount in our body is less than 5 g.

recap The six essential nutrient groups are carbohydrates, fats, proteins, vitamins, minerals, and water. Carbohydrates, fats, and proteins are macronutrients that provide energy. Carbohydrates and fats are our main energy sources; proteins primarily support tissue growth, repair, and maintenance. Vitamins and minerals are micronutrients. Vitamins are organic compounds that assist in breaking down the macronutrients for energy and in many other functions. Minerals are elements—fundamental units of matter essential to virtually all aspects of human health. Water is critical for regulating nerve impulses, body temperature, muscle contractions, nutrient transport, and the excretion of wastes.

LO 4 Distinguish among six groups of Dietary Reference Intakes for nutrients.

Dietary Reference Intakes (DRIs) A set of nutritional reference values for the United States and Canada that applies to healthy people.

How much of each nutrient do most people need?

Now that you know what the six classes of nutrients are, you're probably wondering how much of each you need each day. The United States and Canada share a set of standards defining the recommended intake values for various nutrients. These are called the **Dietary Reference Intakes (DRIs)** (FOCUS FIGURE 1.4). The DRIs are dietary

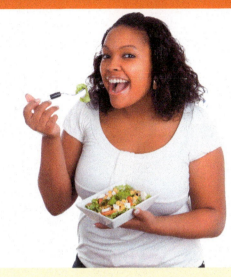

Dietary Reference Intakes (DRIs) are specific reference values for each nutrient issued by the United States National Academy of Sciences, Health and Medicine Division. They identify the amounts of each nutrient that one needs to consume to maintain good health.

DRIs FOR MOST NUTRIENTS

EAR The Estimated Average Requirement (EAR) is the average daily intake level estimated to meet the needs of half the people in a certain group. Scientists use it to calculate the RDA.

RDA The Recommended Dietary Allowance (RDA) is the average daily intake level estimated to meet the needs of nearly people in a certain group. Aim for this amount!

AI The Adequate Intake (AI) is the average daily intake level assumed to be adequate. It is used when an EAR cannot be determined. Aim for this amount if there is no RDA!

UL The Tolerable Upper Intake Level (UL) is the highest average daily intake level likely to pose no health risks. Do not exceed this amount on a daily basis!

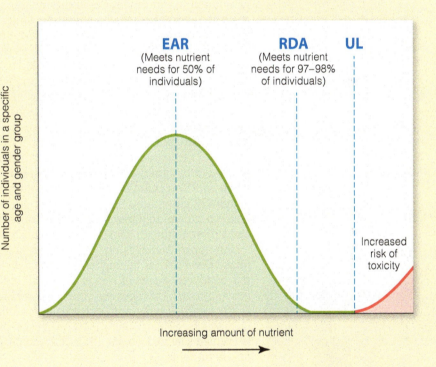

DRIs RELATED TO ENERGY

AMDR The Acceptable Macronutrient Distribution Range (AMDR) is the recommended range of carbohydrate, fat, and protein intake expressed as a percentage of total energy.

EER The Estimated Energy Requirement (EER) is the average daily energy intake predicted to meet the needs of healthy adults.

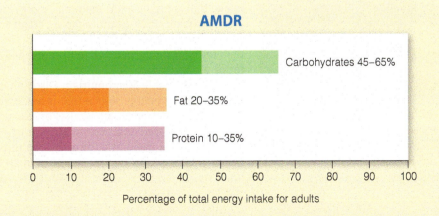

standards for healthy people only; they do not apply to people with diseases or to those who are suffering from nutrient deficiencies.

The DRIs for most nutrients consist of four values:

- Estimated Average Requirement (EAR)
- Recommended Dietary Allowance (RDA)
- Adequate Intake (AI)
- Tolerable Upper Intake Level (UL)

When nutrition scientists determine nutrient requirements, they first calculate the EAR (see Focus Figure 1.4). The Estimated Average Requirement (EAR) represents the average daily intake level estimated to prevent deficiency diseases in half the healthy individuals in a particular life stage and gender group.[2] As an example, the EAR for iron for women between the ages of 19 and 30 years represents the average daily intake of iron that meets the requirement of half the women in this age group. Scientists use the EAR to define the Recommended Dietary Allowance (RDA) for a given nutrient. Obviously, if the EAR meets the needs of only half the people in a group, then the recommended intake will be higher.

Recommended Dietary Allowance (RDA) was the term previously used to refer to all nutrient recommendations in the United States. The RDA is now considered one of many reference standards within the larger umbrella of the DRIs. The RDA represents the average daily nutrient intake level that meets the requirements of 97–98% of healthy individuals in a particular life stage and gender group.[2] The graph in Focus Figure 1.4 compares the RDA to the EAR. For example, the RDA for iron is 18 mg per day for women between the ages of 19 and 50 years. This amount of iron will meet the nutrient requirements of almost all women in this age group.

Again, scientists use the EAR to establish the RDA. In fact, if an EAR cannot be determined for a nutrient, then this nutrient cannot have an RDA. When this occurs, an Adequate Intake value is determined for the nutrient. The Adequate Intake (AI) value is a recommended average daily nutrient intake level assumed to be adequate. It is based on observations or experiments involving healthy people, and it is used when an RDA cannot be determined.[2] Many nutrients have an AI value, including vitamin K, chromium, fluoride, and certain types of fats. More research needs to be done on human requirements for the nutrients assigned an AI value so that an EAR, and subsequently an RDA, can be established.

An upper level of safety for nutrients has also been defined. The Tolerable Upper Intake Level (UL) is the highest average daily nutrient intake level likely to pose no risk of adverse health effects to almost all individuals in a particular life stage and gender group.[2] This does not mean that we should consume this intake level! In fact, as our intake of a nutrient increases beyond the UL, the potential for toxic effects increases (see Focus Figure 1.4). Again, the UL is the highest average intake level that is deemed safe to consume. Note that there is not enough research to define the UL for all nutrients.

Two DRIs apply to energy specifically:

- Estimated Energy Requirement (EER)
- Acceptable Macronutrient Distribution Range (AMDR)

The Estimated Energy Requirement (EER) is defined as the average dietary energy intake that is predicted to maintain energy balance in a healthy individual. This dietary intake varies according to a person's age, gender, weight, height, and level of physical activity (see Focus Figure 1.4).[3] Thus, the EER for an active person is higher than the EER for an inactive person, even if all the other factors (age, gender, and so forth) are the same.

The Acceptable Macronutrient Distribution Range (AMDR) is a range of intakes for a particular energy source that is associated with a reduced risk for chronic disease but provides adequate intakes of essential nutrients (see Focus Figure 1.4).[3] The AMDR is expressed as a percentage of total energy or as a percentage of total kilocalories. The AMDR also has a lower and an upper boundary; if we consume nutrients below or above this range, there is potential for increasing our risk for poor health.

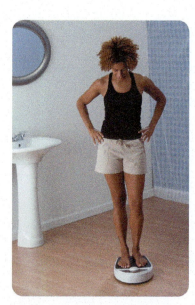

▲ Knowing your daily Estimated Energy Requirement (EER) is a helpful way to maintain an optimal body weight.

By eating foods that give you nutrient intakes that meet the DRIs, you help your body maintain a healthful weight, support your daily physical activity, prevent nutrient deficiencies and toxicities, and reduce your risk for chronic disease.

Throughout this text, the DRI values are reviewed with each nutrient as it is introduced. (They are presented in full in Appendix A at the back of this text.) Find your life stage group and gender in the left-hand column; then simply look across to see each nutrient's value for you. Using the DRIs in conjunction with the diet-planning tools discussed in Chapter 2 will help you develop a healthful diet.

recap The Dietary Reference Intakes (DRIs) are nutrient standards established for healthy people in a particular life stage and gender group. Whereas the Estimated Average Requirement (EAR) meets the requirements of half the healthy individuals in a group, the Recommended Dietary Allowance (RDA) meets the requirements of 97–98% of healthy individuals in a group. The Adequate Intake (AI) is an intake level assumed to be adequate. It is used when there is not enough information to set an RDA. The Tolerable Upper Intake Level (UL) is the highest daily nutrient intake level that likely poses no health risk. The Estimated Energy Requirement (EER) is the average daily energy intake that is predicted to maintain energy balance in a healthy adult. The Acceptable Macronutrient Distribution Range (AMDR) is a range of macronutrient intakes expressed as a percentage of total energy.

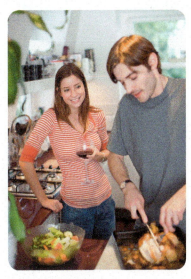

▲ Eating foods that provide the recommended nutrients helps promote optimal wellness.

How do nutrition scientists evaluate claims?

When confronted with a claim about any aspect of our world, from "The Earth is flat" to "Carbohydrates cause obesity," scientists must first consider whether the claim can be tested. In other words, can evidence be presented to substantiate the claim and, if so, what data would qualify as evidence? Scientists worldwide use a standardized method of looking at evidence called the **scientific method**. This method ensures that certain standards and processes are used in evaluating claims. The scientific method usually includes the following steps, which are described in more detail next and summarized in **FOCUS FIGURE 1.5**, on page 16:

LO 5 Describe the steps of the scientific method.

1. The researcher first makes an observation and a description of a phenomenon.
2. The researcher proposes a hypothesis, or an educated guess, to explain why the phenomenon occurs.
3. The researcher then develops an experimental design that will test the hypothesis.
4. The researcher collects and analyzes data that will either support or reject the hypothesis.
5. If the data do not support the original hypothesis, then an alternative hypothesis is proposed and tested.
6. If the data support the original hypothesis, then a conclusion is drawn.
7. The experiment must be repeatable so that other researchers can obtain similar results.
8. Finally, a theory is proposed offering a conclusion drawn from repeated experiments that have supported the hypothesis time and time again.

The Scientific Method Enables Researchers to Test a Hypothesis

The first step in the scientific method is to observe and describe a phenomenon. As an example, let's say you are working in a healthcare office that caters to mostly older clients. You have observed that many of these clients have high blood

scientific method The standardized, multistep process scientists use to examine evidence and test hypotheses.

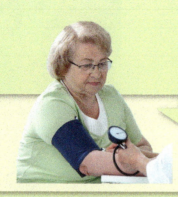

OBSERVATIONS

A pattern is observed in which older adults who are more active appear to have lower blood pressure than those who are less active.

HYPOTHESIS

Adults over age 65 with high blood pressure who participate in a program of 45 minutes per day of aerobic exercise will experience a decrease in blood pressure.

EXPERIMENT
Randomized Clinical Trial

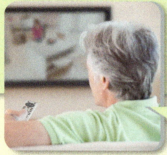

Control group:
No exercise

Modified hypothesis

Experimental group:
45 minutes of daily aerobic exercise

OBSERVATIONS

Data support hypothesis
Average blood pressure was reduced by 8 mmHg for systolic blood pressure and 5 mmHg for diastolic blood pressure in the experimental group.
The control group experienced a slight increase in blood pressure.

Data do not support hypothesis

Reject hypothesis

Modify hypothesis

REPEAT EXPERIMENT

ACCEPT HYPOTHESIS

A hypothesis supported by repeated experiments over many years may be accepted as a theory.

THEORY

pressure, but some have normal blood pressure. After talking with a large number of clients, you notice a pattern developing in that those who report being more physically active are also those with lower blood pressure readings. This observation leads you to question the relationship that might exist between physical activity and blood pressure.

Your next step is to develop a **hypothesis**, a possible explanation for your observation. A hypothesis is also sometimes referred to as a *research question*. In this example, your hypothesis might be "Adults over age 65 with high blood pressure who begin and maintain a program of 45 minutes of aerobic exercise daily will experience a decrease in blood pressure." A hypothesis must be stated so that it can be either supported or rejected. In other words, it must be testable.

After developing a hypothesis, scientists conduct an *experiment,* or scientific study, to test it. A well-designed experiment should have several key elements:

- The *sample size*—the number of people being studied—should be adequate to ensure that the results obtained are not due to chance alone. Would you be more likely to believe a study that tested 5 people or 500?
- Having a *control group* is essential for comparing treated to untreated individuals. A control group consists of people who are as much like the treated group as possible, except with respect to the *condition* being tested. For instance, in your study, 45 minutes of daily aerobic exercise would be the condition; the experimental group would consist of people over age 65 with high blood pressure who exercise, and the control group would consist of similar people who do not exercise. Using a control group helps a researcher judge whether a particular treatment has worked or not.
- A good experimental design also attempts to control for other factors that may coincidentally influence the results. For example, what if someone in your study is on a diet, smokes, or takes blood pressure–lowering medication? Because any of these factors can affect the results, researchers try to design experiments that have as many constants as possible. In doing so, they increase the chance that their results will be *valid*. To use an old saying, you can think of validity as "comparing apples to apples."

As part of the design of the experiment, the researcher must determine the type of data to collect—such as blood pressure readings—and how to collect them most accurately. For example, an automatic blood pressure gauge would provide more reliable and consistent data than blood pressure measurements taken by research assistants.

Once the data have been collected, they must be analyzed and interpreted. Often, the data will begin to make sense only after they have been organized into different forms, such as tables or graphs, that reveal patterns. In your study, you can create a graph comparing blood pressure readings from both your experimental group and your control group to see if there was a significant difference between the blood pressure readings of those who exercised and those who did not.

Repetition of Research Is Required to Develop Theories

Remember that a hypothesis is basically a guess as to what causes a particular phenomenon. Rarely do scientists get it right the first time. The original hypothesis is often refined after the initial results are obtained, usually because the answer to the question is not clear and leads to more questions. When this happens, an alternative hypothesis is proposed, a new experiment is designed, and the new hypothesis is tested.

One research study does not prove or disprove a hypothesis. Ideally, multiple experiments are conducted over many years to thoroughly test a hypothesis. Indeed, repeatability is a cornerstone of scientific investigation. Supporters and skeptics alike must be able to replicate an experiment and arrive at similar conclusions, or the hypothesis becomes invalid. Have you ever wondered why the measurements used in scientific textbooks are always in the metric system? The answer is repeatability. Scientists use the metric system because it is a universal system and thus allows repeatability in any research facility worldwide.

hypothesis An educated guess as to why a phenomenon occurs.

Unfortunately, media reports on the findings of a research study that has just been published rarely include a thorough review of the other studies conducted on that topic. Thus, you should never accept one report in a newspaper, magazine, or online source as absolute fact on any topic.

If the results of multiple experiments consistently support a hypothesis, then scientists may advance a **theory**. A theory represents a scientific consensus (agreement) as to why a particular phenomenon occurs. Although theories are based on data drawn from repeated experiments, they can still be challenged and changed as the knowledge within a scientific discipline evolves. For example, at the beginning of this chapter, we said that the prevailing theory held that pellagra was an infectious disease. Experiments were conducted over several decades before their consistent results finally confirmed that the disease is due to niacin deficiency. We continue to apply the scientific method to test hypotheses and challenge theories today.

recap The steps in the scientific method include observing a phenomenon; creating a hypothesis; designing and conducting an experiment; and collecting and analyzing data that support or refute the hypothesis. If the data are rejected, then an alternative hypothesis is proposed and tested. If the data support the original hypothesis, then a conclusion is drawn. A hypothesis that is supported after repeated experiments may be called a theory.

LO 6 Discuss the design and primary goals of three basic types of nutrition research.

Why do nutrition scientists use different types of research?

Understanding the role of nutrition in health requires constant experimentation. Different research study designs yield different types of information that tells different stories. Let's take a look at the various types of research.

Animal Studies Can Inform Human Studies

Studies involving animals frequently provide preliminary information that assists scientists in designing human studies **(FIGURE 1.6)**. Animal studies also are used to conduct research that cannot be done with humans. For instance, researchers can cause a nutrient deficiency in an animal and study its adverse health effects over the animal's life span, but this type of experiment with humans is not acceptable. Drawbacks of animal studies include ethical concerns and the fact that the results may not apply directly to humans.

Over the past century, animal studies have advanced our understanding of many aspects of nutrition, from micronutrients to obesity. Still, some hypotheses can only be investigated using human subjects. The primary types of studies conducted with humans are epidemiological studies, which include observational and case control studies, and clinical trials.

Epidemiological Studies Explore Patterns Within Populations

Epidemiological studies examine patterns of health and disease in defined populations (see Figure 1.6). They commonly report the prevalence and incidence of disease. **Prevalence** refers to the actual percentage of the population that has a particular disease at a given period of time. **Incidence** refers to the rate of new (or newly diagnosed) cases of a disease within a period of time.

Observational studies are a type of epidemiological study used to assess dietary habits, disease trends, and other health phenomena of large populations and to determine the factors that may influence these phenomena. However, these studies can only indicate *relationships* between factors; they do not prove or suggest that the data are linked by cause and effect. For example, smoking and low vegetable intake appear to be related in some studies, but this does not mean that smoking cigarettes

theory A conclusion, or scientific consensus, drawn from repeated experiments.

epidemiological studies Studies that examine patterns of health and disease in defined populations.

prevalence The percentage of the population that is affected with a particular disease at a given time.

incidence The rate of new (or newly diagnosed) cases of a disease within a period of time.

observational studies Studies that indicate relationships between nutrition habits, disease trends, and other health phenomena of large populations of humans.

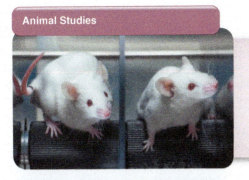

Animal Studies

- Provide information to assist with designing human studies
- Used when research cannot be done with humans
- Limitations include ethical concerns and results that may not apply directly to humans

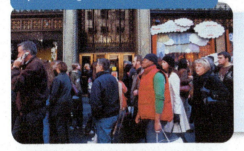

Epidemiological Studies

- Examine patterns of, and factors associated with, health and disease in defined populations
- Includes observational and case control studies
- Can only indicate relationships between factors influencing dietary and other lifestyle habits, health, and disease

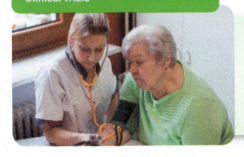

Clinical Trials

- Controlled experiments that test the effect of an intervention on a certain disease or health condition
- Includes an intervention group and a control group into which participants are randomly assigned
- May involve single-or-double blinding
- Results indicate whether or not intervention may be effective

FIGURE 1.6 Types of research studies.

causes people to eat fewer vegetables or that eating fewer vegetables causes people to smoke.

Case control studies are more complex epidemiological studies with additional design features that allow scientists to gain a better understanding of things that may influence disease. They involve comparing a group of individuals with a particular condition (for instance, 1,000 elderly people with high blood pressure) to a similar group without this condition (for instance, 1,000 elderly people with normal blood pressure). This comparison allows the researcher to identify factors other than the defined condition that differ between the two groups. For example, researchers may find that 75% of the people in their normal blood pressure group are physically active but that only 20% of the people in their high blood pressure group are physically active. Again, this would not prove that physical activity prevents high blood pressure. It would merely suggest a significant relationship between these two factors.

Clinical Trials Examine Cause and Effect

Clinical trials are tightly controlled experiments in which an intervention is given to determine its effect on a certain disease or health condition (see Figure 1.6). Interventions include medications, nutritional supplements, controlled diets, and exercise programs. In clinical trials, people in the experimental group are given the intervention, but people in the control group are not. The responses of the two groups are

case control studies Observational studies that compare groups with and without a condition, allowing researchers to gain a better understanding of factors that may influence disease.

clinical trials Tightly controlled experiments in which an intervention is given to determine its effect on a certain disease or health condition.

compared. In the case of the blood pressure experiment, researchers could assign one group of elderly people with high blood pressure to an exercise program and assign a second group of elderly people with high blood pressure to a program in which no exercise is done. Over the next few weeks, months, or even years, researchers could measure the blood pressure of the people in each group. If the blood pressure of those who exercised decreased and the blood pressure of those who did not exercise rose or remained the same, the influence of exercise on lowering blood pressure would not be proven, but it would be supported.

Two important questions to consider when evaluating the quality of a clinical trial are whether the subjects were randomly chosen and whether the researchers and subjects were blinded:

- **Randomized trials.** Ideally, researchers should *randomly* assign research participants to intervention groups (who get the treatment) and control groups (who do not get the treatment). Randomizing participants is like flipping a coin or drawing names from a hat; it reduces the possibility of showing favoritism toward any participants and ensures that the groups are similar on the factors or characteristics being measured in the study. These types of studies are called *randomized clinical (controlled) trials*.
- **Single- and double-blind experiments.** If possible, it is also important to blind both researchers and participants to the treatment being given. A *single-blind experiment* is one in which the participants are unaware of or blinded to the treatment they are receiving, but the researchers know which group is getting the treatment and which group is not. A *double-blind experiment* is one in which neither researchers nor participants know which group is really getting the treatment. Double blinding helps prevent the researcher from seeing only the results he or she wants to see. In the case of testing medications or nutrition supplements, the blinding process can be assisted by giving the control group a placebo. A **placebo** is an imitation treatment that has no effect on participants; for instance, a sugar pill may be given in place of a vitamin supplement. Studies like this are referred to as *placebo-controlled double-blind randomized clinical trials*.

There has been substantial interest in the "placebo effect." This refers to an improvement in health—for instance, pain reduction—in people given a placebo treatment. Although the placebo effect does not occur for all people or across the range of health conditions and diseases affecting the population, it is an intriguing phenomenon that researchers continue to explore to better understand how personal beliefs and expectations can influence one's response to research and medical treatments.

> **Want to learn more about the placebo effect and how it may lead to improvements in health?** Go to www.cbsnews.com and type "Placebo Phenomenon" to be directed to the video.

recap Different types of research studies can be used to gather a different types of data. Studies involving animals provide preliminary information that assists scientists in designing human studies. Human studies include epidemiological studies, which examine patterns of health and disease in large populations. They include observational studies and case control studies. Another type of human study is the clinical trial, a tightly controlled experiment in which an intervention is given to determine its effect. The most rigorous type of study is a placebo-controlled double-blind randomized clinical trial.

LO 7 Explain how to discern the truth or fallacy of nutrition-related claims.

placebo An imitation treatment having no active ingredient that is sometimes used in a clinical trial.

How can you use your knowledge of research to evaluate nutrition claims?

Now that you've increased your understanding of scientific research, you're better equipped to discern the truth or fallacy of nutrition-related claims. Keep the nearby **Quick Tips** in mind when evaluating the findings of research studies and the claims made on commercial websites.

QuickTips

Detecting Media Hype

✅ **Consider the source of the information.** If a report is written or broadcast by a person or group who may financially benefit from selling the products being studied, you should be skeptical. Also, many people who write for popular magazines and newspapers are not trained in science and are capable of misinterpreting research results.

✅ **Find out who conducted the research and who paid for it.** Was the study funded by a company or entity that stands to profit from certain results? Do the researchers have investments in such a company, or are they receiving money or perks from the research sponsor? If the answer to any of these questions is yes, there exists a conflict of interest between the researchers and the funding agency.

✅ **Evaluate the content.** Is the report based on reputable research studies? Did the research follow the scientific method, and were the results reported in a reputable scientific journal? Ideally, the journal is peer-reviewed; that is, the articles are critiqued by other specialists working in the same scientific field. A reputable report should include the reference, or source of the information, and should identify researchers by name.

✅ **Watch for red flags.** Is the report based on testimonials about personal experiences? Testimonials are fraught with bias. Are sweeping conclusions made from only one study? Remember that one study cannot prove any hypothesis. Are the claims made in the report too good to be true? If something sounds too good to be true, it probably is.

Watch for Conflict of Interest and Bias

You probably wouldn't think it strange to see an ad from your favorite brand of ice cream encouraging you to "Go ahead. Indulge." It's just an ad, right? But what if you were to read about a research study in which people who ate your favorite brand of ice cream improved the density of their bones? Could you trust the study results more than you would the ad?

To answer that question, you'd have to ask several more, such as who conducted the research and who paid for it. Specifically:

- Was the study funded by a company that stands to profit from certain results?
- Are the researchers receiving a stipend (payment), goods, personal travel funds, or other perks from the research sponsor, or do they have investments in companies or products related to their study?

If the answer to either of these questions was yes, a **conflict of interest** would exist between the researchers and the funding agency. A *conflict of interest* refers to a situation in which a person is in a position to derive personal benefit and unfair advantage from actions or decisions made in their official capacity. A conflict of interest can seriously compromise the researchers' ability to conduct impartial research and report the results in an accurate and responsible manner. That's why, when researchers submit their results for publication in scientific journals, they are required to reveal any conflicts of interest they may have that could be seen as affecting the integrity of their research. In this way, people who review and eventually read and interpret the study are better able to consider if there are any potential researcher *biases* influencing the results. A bias is any factor—such as investment in the product being studied or gifts from the product manufacturer—that might influence the

conflict of interest A situation in which a person is in a position to derive personal benefit and unfair advantage from actions or decisions made in their official capacity.

researcher to favor certain results. The **Nutrition Debate** at the end of this chapter focuses on issues surrounding conflicts of interests, and examines whether researchers and industry can, and should, work together to conduct research.

Recent media investigations have reported widespread bias in studies funded by pharmaceutical companies testing the effectiveness of their drugs for medical treatment. In addition, journals in both the United States and Europe have been found less likely to publish negative results (that is, study results suggesting that a therapy is not effective). Also, clinical trials funded by pharmaceutical companies are more likely to report positive results than are trials that were independently financed.[4] This lack of *transparency*, or failure to openly present all research findings, has serious implications: if ineffectiveness and side effects are not fully reported, healthcare providers may be prescribing medications that are not helpful or may even be harmful.

Evaluate a Website's Credibility

The Internet is increasingly becoming the repository of almost all credible scientific information, including health and nutrition information. But it's simultaneously the source of some of the most unreliable and even dangerous pseudoscience. How can you determine if the information published on a website is credible? Here are some tips to assist you in separating Internet fact from fiction:

- Look at the credentials of the people providing information for the website. Are the names and credentials of those contributing to the website available? If so, examine their credentials. Are the individuals qualified professionals in this topic? Are experts reviewing the content of the website for accuracy and currency?
- Look at the date of the website. Is it fairly recent? Because nutrition and medical information are constantly changing, websites should be updated frequently, and the date of the most recent update should be clearly identified on the site.
- Look at the web address. The three letters following the "dot" in a World Wide Web address can provide some clues as to the credibility of the information. Government addresses (ending in ".gov"), academic institutions (ending in ".edu"), and professional organizations (ending in ".org") are typically considered to be relatively credible sources of information. However, lecture notes, PowerPoint slides, student assignments, and similar types of documents that can be found on university websites may not be current, accurate, or credible sources of information. Addresses ending in ".com" designate commercial and business sites. Many of these are credible sources, but many are not. It is important to consider if the site sponsor's primary motivation is to encourage you to buy a product or service.
- Look at the bottom line. What is the message being highlighted on the site? Is it consistent with what is reported by other credible sources? If the message contradicts what would be considered as common knowledge, then you should question its validity and intent. An additional clue that a website may lack credibility includes strong and repeated claims of conspiracy theories designed to breed distrust of existing reputable sites.

quackery The promotion of an unproven remedy, such as a supplement or other product or service, usually by someone unlicensed and untrained.

These suggestions can also be applied to spam. If you have an e-mail account, you're probably familiar with spam ads that make promises such as "Weight-loss miracles for only $19.99!" Do you delete them unread? Or are you tempted to open them to see if you might find something worth exploring? A recent study found that, in the course of 1 year, 42% of college students with weight problems had opened spam e-mails touting weight-loss products, and almost 19% had placed an order! Lead researchers were shocked by the findings and advised physicians to discuss with patients the potential risks of using weight-loss products marketed via spam e-mails.[5]

As you may know, **quackery** is the promotion of an unproven remedy, usually by someone unlicensed and untrained, for financial gain. Miguel, the young man from our opening story, was a victim of quackery. He probably would not have purchased that iron supplement if he had understood that it was not the correct treatment for his medical condition.

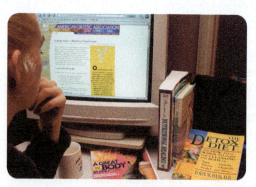

To become a more educated consumer and informed critic of nutrition reports in the media, you need to understand the research process and how to interpret study results.

nutri-case | LIZ

"Am I ever sorry I caught the news last night right before going to bed! They reported on this study that just came out, saying that ballet dancers are at some super-high risk for fractures! I couldn't sleep, thinking about it, and then today in dance class every move I made was freaking me out about breaking my ankle. I can't go on being afraid like this!"

What information should Liz find out about the fracture study to evaluate its merits? Identify *at least two factors* she should evaluate. Let's say that her investigation of these factors leads her to conclude that the study is trustworthy: what else should she keep in mind about the research process that might help her take a more balanced perspective when thinking about this single study?

Throughout this text we provide you with information to assist you in becoming a more educated consumer regarding nutrition. You will learn about labeling guidelines, the proper use of supplements, and whether various nutrition topics are myths or facts. Armed with the information in this book, plus plenty of opportunities to test your knowledge, you will become more confident when evaluating nutrition claims.

> To learn more about how to spot quackery, go to www .quackwatch.com, enter "spot quack" in the search box, and then click on "Critiquing Quack Ads."

recap When evaluating research studies, consider whether a conflict of interest exists, and check the credentials, date, and URL of websites. Quackery is the promotion of an unproven remedy, usually by someone unlicensed and untrained, for financial gain.

Which sources of nutrition advice are trustworthy?

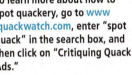 **LO 8** List several professionals, government agencies, and organizations that are trustworthy sources of nutrition information.

Many people claim to be nutrition experts, but are they? If you're wondering how to determine whether an "expert" is trustworthy, the following discussion should help.

Trustworthy Experts Are Educated and Credentialed

It is not possible to list here all of the types of health professionals who provide reliable and accurate nutrition information. The following are the most common types:

- *Registered dietitian (RD):* To become a **registered dietitian (RD)** requires, minimally, a bachelor's degree, completion of a supervised clinical experience, a passing grade on a national examination, and maintenance of registration with the Academy of Nutrition and Dietetics (formerly the American Dietetic Association). There is now an optional change to the RD designation—*RD/Nutritionist*. This designation indicates that anyone who has earned an RD is also a qualified nutritionist; however, not all nutritionists are qualified RDs (see below). Individuals who complete the education, experience, exam, and registration are qualified to provide nutrition counseling in a variety of settings. For a reliable list of RDs in your community, contact the Academy of Nutrition and Dietetics (see **Web Links**).
- *Licensed dietitian:* A licensed dietitian is a dietitian meeting the credentialing requirement of a given state in the United States to engage in the practice of dietetics.[6] Each state has its own laws regulating dietitians. These laws specify which types of licensure or registration a nutrition professional must obtain in order to provide nutrition services or advice. Individuals who practice nutrition and dietetics without the required license or registration can be prosecuted for breaking the law.
- *Professional with an advanced degree (a master's degree [MA or MS] or doctoral degree [PhD]) in nutrition:* Many individuals hold an advanced degree in nutrition and have years of experience in a nutrition-related career. For instance, they may

registered dietitian (RD) A professional designation that requires a minimum of a bachelor's degree in nutrition, completion of a supervised clinical experience, a passing grade on a national examination, and maintenance of registration with the Academy of Nutrition and Dietetics (in Canada, the Dietitians of Canada). RDs are qualified to work in a variety of settings.

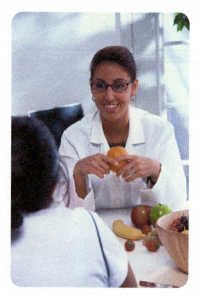

⬆ Your medical doctor may have limited experience and training in the area of nutrition but can refer you to a registered dietitian (RD) or licensed nutritionist to assist you in meeting your dietary needs.

For a list of registered dietitians in your community, visit the Academy of Nutrition and Dietetics at www.eatright.org.

teach at colleges or universities or work in fitness or healthcare settings. Unless these individuals are licensed or registered dietitians, they are not certified to provide clinical dietary counseling or treatment for individuals with disease. However, they are reliable sources of information about nutrition and health.

- *Physician:* The term *physician* encompasses a variety of healthcare professionals. A medical doctor (MD) is educated, trained, and licensed to practice medicine in the United States. However, MDs typically have very limited experience and training in the area of nutrition. Medical students in the United States are not required to take any nutrition courses throughout their academic training, although some may take courses out of personal interest. On the other hand, a number of individuals who started their careers in nutrition go on to become medical doctors and thus have a solid background in nutrition. Nevertheless, if you require a dietary plan to treat an illness or a disease, most medical doctors will refer you to an RD. In contrast, an osteopathic physician, referred to as a doctor of osteopathy (DO), may have studied nutrition extensively, as may a naturopathic physician. Thus, it is prudent to determine a physician's level of expertise rather than assuming that he or she has extensive knowledge of nutrition.

In contrast to the above discussion, the term *nutritionist* generally has no definition or laws regulating it. In some cases, it refers to a professional with academic credentials in nutrition who may also be an RD.[6] In other cases, the term may refer to anyone who thinks he or she is knowledgeable about nutrition. There is no guarantee that a person calling himself or herself a nutritionist is necessarily educated, trained, and experienced in the field of nutrition. It is important to research the credentials and experience of any individual calling himself or herself a nutritionist.

Government Agencies Are Usually Trustworthy

Many government health agencies have come together to address the growing problem of nutrition-related disease in the United States. These agencies are funded with taxpayer dollars, and many provide financial support for research in the areas of nutrition and health. Thus, these agencies have the resources to organize and disseminate the most recent and reliable information related to nutrition and other areas of health and wellness. A few of the most recognized and respected of these government agencies are discussed here.

The National Institutes of Health

The **National Institutes of Health (NIH)** is the world's leading medical research center, and it is the focal point for medical research in the United States. The NIH is one of the agencies of the Public Health Service, which is part of the U.S. Department of Health and Human Services. The mission of the NIH is to uncover new knowledge that leads to better health for everyone. Many institutes within the NIH conduct research into nutrition-related health issues. Some of these institutes are:

- National Cancer Institute (NCI)
- National Heart, Lung, and Blood Institute (NHLBI)
- National Institute of Diabetes and Digestive and Kidney Diseases (NIDDK)
- National Center for Complementary and Alternative Medicine (NCCAM)

To find out more about the NIH, see **Web Links** at the end of this chapter.

The Centers for Disease Control and Prevention

National Institutes of Health (NIH) The world's leading medical research center and the focal point for medical research in the United States.

Centers for Disease Control and Prevention (CDC) The leading federal agency in the United States that protects the health and safety of people.

The **Centers for Disease Control and Prevention (CDC)** is considered the leading federal agency in the United States that protects human health and safety. Located in Atlanta, Georgia, the CDC works in the areas of health promotion, disease prevention and control, and environmental health. The CDC's mission is to promote health and quality of life by preventing and controlling disease, injury, and disability. Among its many activities, the CDC supports two large national surveys that provide important nutrition and health information.

The National Health and Nutrition Examination Survey (NHANES) is conducted by the National Center for Health Statistics and the CDC. The NHANES tracks the food and nutrient consumption of Americans. Nutrition and other health information is gathered from interviews and physical examinations. The database for the NHANES survey is extremely large, and an abundance of research papers have been generated from it. To learn more about the NHANES, see **Web Links** at the end of this chapter.

The Behavioral Risk Factor Surveillance System (BRFSS) was established by the CDC to track lifestyle behaviors that increase our risk for chronic disease. The world's largest telephone survey, the BRFSS gathers data related to injuries and infectious diseases, especially the health behaviors that increase the risk for heart disease, stroke, cancer, and diabetes. These health behaviors include:

- Not consuming enough fruits and vegetables
- Being overweight
- Leading a sedentary lifestyle
- Using tobacco and abusing alcohol
- Not getting medical care that is known to save lives, such as regular flu shots and screening exams

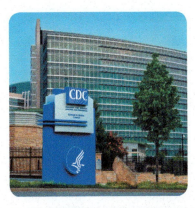

▲ The Centers for Disease Control and Prevention (CDC) is the leading federal agency in the United States that protects human health and safety.

Professional Organizations Provide Reliable Nutrition Information

A number of professional organizations represent nutrition professionals, scientists, and educators. These organizations publish cutting-edge nutrition research studies and educational information in journals that are accessible in most university and medical libraries. Some of these organizations are:

- *The Academy of Nutrition and Dietetics*: This is the largest organization of food and nutrition professionals in the world. Their mission is to promote nutrition, health, and well-being. (The Canadian equivalent is Dietitians of Canada.) The Academy of Nutrition and Dietetics publishes a professional journal called the *Journal of the Academy of Nutrition and Dietetics* (formerly the *Journal of the American Dietetic Association*).
- *The American Society for Nutrition (ASN)*: The ASN is the premier research society dedicated to improving quality of life through the science of nutrition. It supports nutrition-related research, publishing a professional journal called the *American Journal of Clinical Nutrition*.
- *The American College of Sports Medicine (ACSM)*: The ACSM is the leading sports medicine and exercise science organization in the world. Many members are nutrition professionals who combine their nutrition and exercise expertise to promote health and athletic performance. *Medicine and Science in Sports and Exercise* is the professional journal of the ACSM.
- *The Obesity Society (TOS)*: TOS is the leading scientific society dedicated to the study of obesity. It is committed to improving the lives of people with obesity, nurturing careers of obesity scientists and healthcare providers, and promoting interdisciplinary obesity research, management, and education. The official TOS journal is *Obesity Journal*.

For more information on these organizations, see the **Web Links** at the end of this chapter.

recap A registered dietitian (RD) is qualified to provide nutrition counseling. The optional designation RD/Nutritionist indicates that anyone who has earned an RD is also a qualified nutritionist; however, a nutritionist is not necessarily an RD. Licensed dietitians, individuals who hold an advanced degree in nutrition, and some physicians may be able to provide trustworthy nutrition information. The CDC is the leading federal agency in the United States that protects human health and safety. The CDC supports two large national surveys that provide important nutrition and health information: the NHANES and the BRFSS. The NIH is the leading medical research agency in the world. The Academy of Nutrition and Dietetics, the American Society for Nutrition, the American College of Sports Medicine, and The Obesity Society are examples of professional organizations that provide reliable nutrition information.

Conflict of Interest: Should Scientists and Industry Collaborate in Research?

In August 2015, an article published in the *New York Times* exposed the myriad links between the Coca-Cola Company and influential scientists and public health organizations.[7] The article observed that Coca-Cola's sales had begun to fall in recent years as consumers became increasingly aware of the role that sugar-sweetened beverages play in obesity. It then claimed that, as a result, the company began funding health researchers to spread the message that obesity is not caused by overconsumption of foods or beverages, but by inadequate exercise. The article was particularly critical of the Global Energy Balance Network (GEBN), a nonprofit organization whose stated mission was "to connect and engage multi-disciplinary scientists and other experts around the globe dedicated to applying and advancing the science of energy balance to achieve healthier living."[8] Coca-Cola donated $1.5 million to help start the organization and pay for its website; a major issue was not only the amount donated, but the fact that Coca-Cola's role and funding were not acknowledged on the GEBN website. Once questioned about its sources of funding, the GEBN acknowledged this oversight and published all funding sources on their website.

The funding of health research by the food and beverage industries is not a new phenomenon. In addition to Coca-Cola, companies such as PepsiCo, Kraft Foods, McDonald's, and Mars have a long history of funding nutrition- and exercise-related research. As discussed in this chapter, a conflict of interest can seriously compromise a researcher's ability to design, conduct, analyze, and report data from a study without bias. In fact, a recent systematic review of research into the role of sugar-sweetened beverages in obesity found that studies funded by the beverage or sugar industries were five times more likely to find no link between sugar-sweetened beverages and weight gain than studies in which the authors reported no financial ties to a food or beverage industry.[9]

The release of the article in the *New York Times* prompted a major backlash. In response, Coca-Cola pledged full transparency and published a list of all of the organizations it had funded over the previous 5 years. During this period, $118.6 million was awarded to various organizations, of which $21.8 million funded scientific research and $96.8 million went toward supporting health and well-being partnerships. Among the top 50

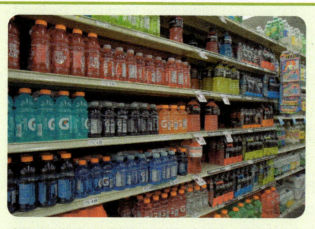

There is a long history of industry funding nutrition- and exercise-related research, particularly in relation to the formulation of sport performance products.

organizations that were awarded funding from Coca-Cola were universities and public health organizations, including the American Academy of Family Physicians, the American College of Cardiology, the American Academy of Pediatrics, the American Cancer Society, the Academy of Nutrition and Dietetics, and the American College of Sports Medicine.[10] The negative press following this release resulted in many of these organizations cutting all ties with Coca-Cola. The GEBN discontinued its operations "due to resource limitations," as indicated via a brief message on its now defunct website.[8]

Does this recent controversy suggest that scientists and industry should never collaborate? Not necessarily. Some experts advise the scientific community to avoid accepting funding where there is a major conflict of interest, but they suggest that industry sponsorship does not have to be completely avoided.[9] Recommended actions include establishing enforceable guidelines that prevent industry sponsors from participating in the research design, data analysis, or interpretation; and creating conditions that allow the public health sector to work independently of the industry sponsor. Such controlled collaborations could lead to important research that is far less vulnerable to the threat of bias. This approach would also provide food and beverage companies with a mechanism to fulfill their social and corporate responsibilities toward their customers and the environment.

CRITICAL THINKING QUESTIONS

1. Do you believe that scientists can partner with industry and conduct research in a relatively unbiased way? Why or why not?
2. What are some reasons researchers might feel pressured to design research studies and interpret the results differently if the study is funded by the food or beverage industry?
3. Coca-Cola's support of prominent health researchers has been compared to tactics used in the past by the tobacco industry. Conduct your own research into this claim to: identify the commonalities between the approach taken by Coca-Cola and that of the tobacco industry related to the health hazards of their products.

TEST YOURSELF | ANSWERS

1 F A Calorie is a measure of the energy in a food. More precisely, a kilocalorie is the amount of heat required to raise the temperature of 1 kilogram of water by 1 degree Celsius.

2 T Carbohydrates and fats are the primary energy sources for our body.

3 F The Recommended Dietary Allowance is the average daily intake of a vitamin or other food component that meets the requirements of 97–98% of healthy individuals in a particular group.

review questions

LO 1 **1.** Early nutrition research focused on
  a. improving crop yields.
  b. classifying plants as edible or inedible.
  c. identifying and preventing diseases caused by dietary deficiencies.
  d. uncovering links between genes, environment, and diet.

LO 2 **2.** Which of the following statements is true?
  a. Pellagra is caused by a nutrient deficiency.
  b. Cancer is caused by a nutrient deficiency.
  c. A nourishing diet can prevent cardiovascular disease.
  d. There is a mild association between inadequate intake of vitamin C and scurvy.

LO 3 **3.** Vitamins A and C, thiamin, calcium, and magnesium are considered
  a. water-soluble vitamins.
  b. fat-soluble vitamins.
  c. energy-yielding nutrients.
  d. micronutrients.

LO 4 **4.** For good health, you should aim to consume
  a. the EAR for vitamin C.
  b. the RDA for vitamin C.
  c. the UL for vitamin C.
  d. within the AMDR for vitamin C.

LO 5 **5.** Which of the following statements about hypotheses is true?
  a. Hypotheses can be proven by clinical trials.
  b. "Many inactive people have high blood pressure" is an example of a hypothesis.

  c. If the results of multiple experiments consistently support a hypothesis, it is confirmed as fact.
  d. "A high-protein diet increases the risk for porous bones" is an example of a hypothesis.

LO 6 **6.** Researchers wish to determine the percentage of U.S. college undergraduates who regularly eat at least five servings of fruits and vegetables a day. To do so, they conduct
  a. an animal experiment.
  b. an observational study.
  c. a case control study.
  d. a clinical trial.

LO 7 **7.** The researchers in a study of the health benefits of coffee consumption received money as well as stock in the coffee company funding the study. This is an example of
  a. lack of transparency.
  b. quackery.
  c. conflict of interest.
  d. a testimonial.

LO 8 **8.** The world's leading medical research agency is the
  a. Centers for Disease Control and Prevention.
  b. National Institutes of Health.
  c. American Medical Association.
  d. National Health and Nutrition Examination Survey.

LO 2 9. **True or false?** Nutrition can significantly influence a person's wellness.

LO 4 10. **True or false?** The Adequate Intake represents the average daily intake level known to meet the requirements of almost all healthy individuals in a group.

math review

LO 4 11. Kayla meets with a registered dietitian recommended by her doctor to design a weight-loss diet plan. She is shocked when a dietary analysis reveals that she consumes an average of 2,200 kcal and 60 grams of fat each day. What percentage of Kayla's diet comes from fat, and is this percentage within the AMDR for fat?

Answers to Review Questions and Math Review are located at the back of this text and in the MasteringNutrition Study Area.

web links

www.eatright.org
The Academy of Nutrition and Dietetics (formerly the American Dietetic Association)
Obtain a list of registered dietitians in your community from the largest organization of food and nutrition professionals in the United States.

www.cdc.gov
Centers for Disease Control and Prevention
Visit this site for additional information about the leading federal agency in the United States that protects the health and safety of people.

www.cdc.gov/nchs/
National Center for Health Statistics
Visit this site to learn more about the National Health and Nutrition Examination Survey (NHANES) and other national health surveys.

www.nih.gov
National Institutes of Health
Find out more about the National Institutes of Health, an agency under the U.S. Department of Health and Human Services.

www.ncbi.nlm.nih.gov/pmc/
PubMed Central
Search for PubMed at the National Library of Medicine for summaries of research studies on health topics of your choice.

www.nutrition.org
American Society for Nutrition
Learn more about the American Society for Nutrition and its goal to improve quality of life through the science of nutrition.

www.acsm.org
American College of Sports Medicine
Obtain information about the leading sports medicine and exercise science organization in the world.

www.obesity.org/home
The Obesity Society
Learn about this interdisciplinary society and its work to understand, prevent, and treat obesity to improve the lives of those affected through research, education, and advocacy.

www.nationalacademies.org/hmd/
The National Academies of Sciences, Engineering and Medicine—Health and Medicine Division
Learn about the Health and Medicine Division (formerly the Institute of Medicine) and its history of examining the nation's nutritional well-being and providing sound information about food and nutrition. Select "Food and Nutrition" from the drop-down menu in the Explore by Topic bar to learn more.

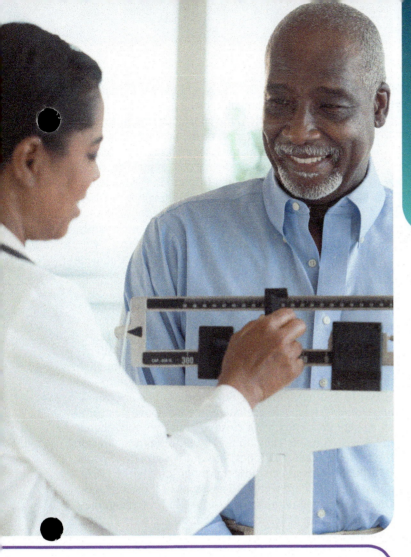

New Frontiers in Nutrition and Health

learning outcomes

After studying this In Depth, you should be able to:

1 Discuss the potential benefits and challenges of nutrigenomics, pp. 30–31.

2 Explain how research into the human microbiome is influencing our understanding of nutrition and health, pp. 32–33.

3 Identify several health benefits of phytochemicals, pp. 33–35.

Imagine a patient visiting his physician for his annual exam. He is 20 pounds overweight and his blood pressure is elevated. The physician takes a blood sample for genetic testing, then sends the patient to a technician to extract a sample of the microbes living in his colon. At the close of the visit, she hands her patient a prescription: *2 servings of fresh fruits, 2 servings of fresh vegetables, a bowl of oatmeal, a cup of soy milk, and 2 cups of yogurt daily.* The patient accepts the prescription gratefully, assuring his physician as he says goodbye, "I'll stop at the market on my way home!"

Sound unreal? As researchers uncover more evidence of a link between our genes, microbes, phytochemicals, and health, it's possible that scenarios like this could become familiar. Here, we explore these new frontiers **In Depth**. Who knows? When you finish reading, you might find yourself writing up your own health-promoting grocery list!

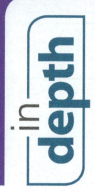
How does our diet affect our genes?

LO 1 Discuss the potential benefits and challenges of nutrigenomics.

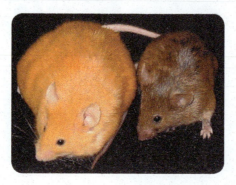

▲ **FIGURE 1** Prompted only by a change in her diet before she conceived, an inbred agouti mouse (*left*) gave birth to a young mouse (*right*) that differed not only in appearance but also in its susceptibility to disease.

Agouti mice are specifically bred for scientific studies. These mice are normally yellow in color, obese, and prone to cancer and diabetes, and they typically have a short life span. When agouti mice breed, these traits are passed on to their offspring. Look at the picture of the agouti mice in **FIGURE 1**; do you see a difference? The mouse on the right is obviously brown and of normal weight; but what you can't see is that it did not inherit its parents' susceptibility to disease and therefore will live a longer, healthier life. What caused this dramatic difference between parent and offspring? The answer is diet!

The Foods We Eat Can Influence Gene Expression

In 2003, researchers at Duke University reported that, when they changed the mother's diet just before conception, they could "turn off" the agouti gene, and any offspring born to

that mother would appear normal.[1] As you might know, a *gene* is a segment of DNA, the substance responsible for inheritance, or the passing on of traits from parents to offspring. An organism's *genome* is its complete set of DNA, which is found in the nucleus of its cells. Genes are regions of DNA that encode instructions for assembling specific proteins. In other words, genes are *expressed* in proteins; for instance, one way that the agouti gene is expressed is in the pigment proteins that produce yellow fur.

The Duke University researchers interfered with normal gene expression in their agouti mice by manipulating the mice's diet. Specifically, they fed the mother mice a diet that was high in methyl donors, compounds that can donate a methyl group (CH3) to another molecule. Such compounds are called *epigenetic factors*. The prefix *epi-* means above or near, so epigenetic factors work close to genes without changing the DNA itself. They do this by binding to regions on the proteins (called histones) around which DNA spools **(FIGURE 2)**. This affects how tightly or loosely the DNA and its histones are wound: The genes in loosely wound DNA are accessible to the cell for use in protein synthesis, whereas the genes in tightly bound regions cannot be read.

In the agouti mice, the methyl donors in the mothers' diet made the agouti gene unreadable. In essence, they

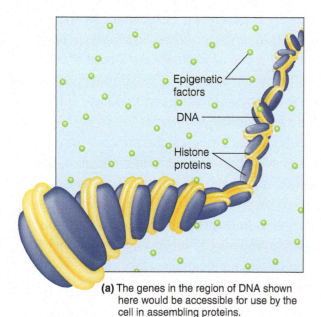

(a) The genes in the region of DNA shown here would be accessible for use by the cell in assembling proteins.

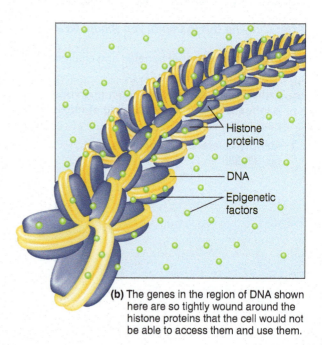

(b) The genes in the region of DNA shown here are so tightly wound around the histone proteins that the cell would not be able to access them and use them.

▲ **FIGURE 2** The binding of epigenetic factors to histone proteins causes physical and functional changes. **(a)** When DNA is loosely wrapped around its histones, its genes are more accessible for use in protein synthesis. **(b)** When DNA is tightly wound around its histones, its genes are inaccessible; thus, these genes are not expressed as proteins.

turned it off. When the mothers conceived, their offspring still carried the agouti gene on their DNA, but their cells no longer used the gene to make proteins. Thus, the traits, such as obesity, that were linked to the agouti gene did not appear in the offspring. These Duke University studies were some of the first to directly link a dietary intervention to a genetic modification and contributed significantly to the emerging science of *nutrigenomics* (*nutritional genomics*).

Nutrigenomics Studies Food-Gene Interactions

Nutrigenomics is a scientific discipline studying the interactions among genes, the environment, and nutrition. Until the late 20th century, scientists believed that the genes a person is born with determined his or her traits rigidly, but we now know that genetic expression is influenced by diet, body weight, substance use, and many other factors. This helps explain why the appearance and health of identical twins—who have the same DNA—commonly change as the twins age.

In addition, as we saw with the agouti mice, epigenetic factors can affect gene expression not only in our own body but also in our offspring. In the Duke University study, switching off the agouti gene caused beneficial changes in the offspring mice. But sometimes flipping the switch can be harmful, as when paternal obesity causes epigenetic changes in sperm cells that increase the risk for certain types of cancer in the offspring.[2]

Several commonly observed phenomena are now thought to be due at least in part to epigenetics. For example, it has long been noted that some people will lose weight on a specific diet and exercise program, whereas others following the same program will not. Some people who smoke develop cardiovascular disease or cancer, whereas others do not. And in some people, moderate alcohol consumption appears to reduce the risk of cardiovascular disease, whereas in other people, it does not. These varying results are now thought to depend to a certain extent on how these factors affect genetic expression.[3,4]

Nutrigenomics Could Lead to Personalized Nutrition

Recently, a working group of the American Society for Nutrition published a list of urgent research needs, one of which was for research into nutrigenomics.[5] One goal of this research would be to increase our understanding of how specific foods or nutrients interact with specific genes. This could help reduce the prevalence of diet-related diseases and possibly even treat existing conditions through diet alone.[6]

Nutrigenomics research could also lead to personalized nutrition. Today, dietary advice is based primarily on observations of large populations. But advice that is generally appropriate for a population might not be appropriate for every individual within that population. Advances in nutrigenomics could eliminate this concern by making it possible to provide each individual with a personalized diet. In this future world, analysis of your DNA would guide an RD in creating a diet tailored to your genetic makeup. By identifying both foods to eat and foods to avoid, this personalized diet would help you turn on beneficial genes and turn off genes that could be harmful.

If the promises of nutrigenomics strike you as pie in the sky, you're not alone. Many researchers caution, for example, that dietary "prescriptions" to prevent or treat chronic diseases would be extremely challenging, because multiple genes may be involved, as well as countless nutritional and environmental factors. In addition, genetics researchers currently believe that there are about 21,000 to 25,000 genes in human DNA, but that these genes represent only a fraction of the DNA in body cells.[7] The remaining regions of DNA are considered noncoding but are thought to have other functions, many of which may influence nutrition and health. Moreover, the pathways for genetic expression are extremely complex, and turning on a gene may have a beneficial effect on one body function but a harmful effect on another. To complicate the matter further, other factors such as age, gender, and lifestyle will also affect how different foods interact with these different genetic pathways. In short, the number of variables that would have to be considered in order to develop a "personalized diet" is staggering.

We might first encounter nutrigenomics in diagnostic testing. In this process, a blood or tissue sample of DNA would be genetically analyzed to predict how foods and dietary supplements might interact with that individual's genes and how a change in diet might affect those interactions. Genetic counseling would be required to help consumers understand the meaning and recommendations suggested by their genetic profile.

We might also begin to see more specialized foods promoted for specific conditions. For example, consumers currently have an array of foods to choose from if they want to lower their cholesterol or enhance their bone health. More such foods will likely be developed, and food packages of the future might even be coded for certain genetic profiles.

We may be decades away from a "personalized diet," but one thing is clear right now. Research into nutrigenomics is changing not only the way we look at food but also the science of nutrition itself.

---

nutrigenomics A scientific discipline studying the interactions between genes, the environment, and nutrition.

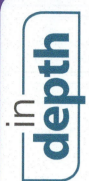

How does our diet affect our microbiome?

LO 2 Explain how research into the human microbiome is influencing our understanding of nutrition and health.

We like to think of ourselves as discrete, individual organisms, but it's not true. The human body is a lush microbial ecosystem containing about 40 trillion *microorganisms* (microscopic organisms such as bacteria)—that's more than the number of our human body cells![8] These microorganisms and their genes, both of which are referred to as the **human microbiome**, interact with our human cells and genes in a dizzying number of ways that affect our health.

A Healthy Microbiome Promotes a Healthy Body

Research suggests that a healthy microbiome fulfills many functions in the body that promote human health. For example, our microbiome enables us to digest foods and absorb nutrients that otherwise would be unavailable to us. This may be in part because genes in our microbiome may complement the functions of human genes required for digestion—genes that may be missing or incompletely encoded in the human genome.[9] Moreover, the microbiome is thought to:[9-14]

- Supply compounds used to replace worn-out tissues of the intestine
- Produce certain essential vitamins
- Protect against intestinal infections
- Provide some protection against the development of obesity and type 2 diabetes

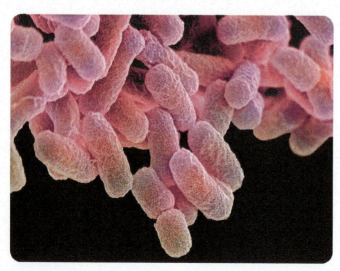

The human body is a microbial ecosystem containing about 40 trillion microorganisms, such as this gut bacteria.

- Degrade potential carcinogens (cancer-causing agents) in foods
- Produce anti-inflammatory chemicals, thereby providing some protection against eczema, asthma, and allergies, as well as certain inflammatory disorders of the esophagus, stomach, and small and large intestine.

Taking a broad-spectrum antibiotic prescribed to fight an infection not only kills the invading bacteria but also depletes the healthful bacteria in our microbiome. In fact, overuse of antibiotics is increasingly linked to intestinal disorders, asthma, and many other health problems. Given this research, you're probably wondering how you can build and maintain a robust microbiome. That's where probiotics and prebiotics come in.

Probiotics and Prebiotics Nourish the Microbiome

Probiotics and prebiotics are two groups of **functional foods**; that is, foods with biologically active ingredients that provide health benefits beyond basic nutrition. They qualify as functional foods because, in addition to the nutrients they provide, they help grow your microbiome.

Probiotics are foods or supplements that contain live microorganisms that benefit human health. Interest in probiotic foods was sparked in the early 1900s with the work of Elie Metchnikoff, a Nobel Prize–winning scientist. Dr. Metchnikoff linked the long, healthy lives of Bulgarian peasants with their consumption of fermented

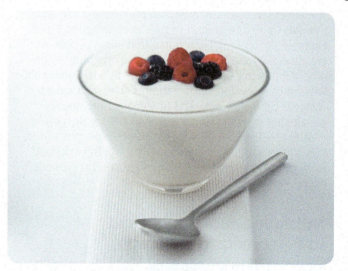

Beneficial bacteria, such as those found in yogurt or kefir, are a part of probiotic foods.

human microbiome The complete population of microorganisms, including their genes, that inhabit the human body.

functional foods Foods that may have biologically active ingredients that provide health benefits beyond basic nutrition.

probiotics Foods, beverages, or supplements containing living microorganisms that beneficially affect consumers by improving the intestinal microbial balance.

milk products, such as yogurt and a creamy beverage called kefir. Subsequent research identified the bacteria in fermented milk products—typically *Lactobacillus* and *Bifidobacterium*—as the factor that promoted health.

When a person consumes probiotics, the bacteria survive in the large intestine for a few days. There, they're thought to exert many beneficial actions. For example, studies support a reduction in "transit time" of wastes through the large intestine in people who regularly consume yogurt, reducing their risk for constipation.[15] The probiotics in yogurt may also reduce the risk for diabetes.[16] And some laboratory studies have shown that probiotics can help reduce infection and inflammation, an effect that may reduce college students' susceptibility to colds! In a recent randomized, double-blind, placebo-controlled study, nearly 600 college students were given either a probiotic supplement or a placebo. Those who consumed the probiotic supplement experienced significantly fewer cold/flu symptoms and significantly more healthy days than students who received the placebo.[17]

Again, probiotic bacteria live only for a short time. This means that probiotic foods and supplements should be consumed on a daily basis to be most effective. They must also be properly stored and consumed within a relatively brief period of time to confer maximal benefit. In general, refrigerated foods containing probiotics have a shelf life of 3 to 6 weeks, whereas refrigerated supplements keep about 12 months. However, because the probiotic content of foods is much more stable than that of supplements, yogurt and other probiotic foods may be a better health bet.

Now that you know a little more about probiotics, you may be wondering how they're related to prebiotics. We've said that probiotic foods and supplements contain living and helpful bacteria. In contrast, **prebiotics** are nondigestible food ingredients (typically carbohydrates) that support the growth and/or activity of probiotic bacteria. In other words, prebiotics don't feed you, but they do feed your microbiome. An example is inulin, a carbohydrate found in a few fruits, onions, certain green vegetables, and some grains. Many **processed foods**—that is, foods manipulated in some way before being sold—also claim to be prebiotic. For example, inulin is added to certain brands of yogurt, milk, and cottage cheese, some fruit juices, cookies, and energy bars and supplements. Watch out, though, that your desire to feed your microbiome doesn't cause you to overindulge. Products touted as prebiotic may have just as many Calories as regular versions of the same foods.

How do phytochemicals enhance our health?

LO 3 Identify several health benefits of phytochemicals.

As you'll discover throughout this text, plant foods are loaded with nutrients, including carbohydrates, vitamins, minerals, and water. Many also contain healthful fats

and protein. They're also a great source of dietary fiber, a nondigestible carbohydrate that promotes body functioning. But another advantage of plants is their phytochemicals. *Phyto* means "plant," so **phytochemicals** are literally plant chemicals. While plants are growing, these naturally occurring compounds are believed to protect them from pests, the UV radiation they capture, and the oxygen they produce. What makes them important to nutrition scientists is that phytochemicals are believed to have health-promoting properties for humans who consume them.

Thousands of different phytochemicals have been identified.[18] They're present in **whole foods**—foods such as fruits and vegetables sold in their natural state—as well as in many processed foods such as soy products, chocolate, coffee, tea, wine, and beer. Any one food can contain hundreds. **FIGURE 3** on page 34 identifies a few of the most common phytochemical groups.

nutri-case | HANNAH

"On my way home from school today, I was really hungry, and when I passed a convenience store about halfway home, I just had to go in. I looked around for something healthy, like a banana or an apple, but they didn't have anything fresh. So I bought some pretzels. I know pretzels aren't exactly a health food, but at least they're low fat, right?"

Hannah and her mother live in an urban neighborhood that has 11 different fast-food outlets and four convenience stores but lacks a grocery store. There is no local farmer's market or community garden. In order to buy fresh produce, they have to travel to a more affluent neighborhood several miles away. Given the importance of phytochemicals to a healthful diet, can you think of at least two strategies Hannah and her mother could use to increase their access to affordable produce?

prebiotics Nondigestible food compounds that support the growth and/or activity of one or a limited number of bacteria in the large intestine.

processed foods Foods that have been manipulated in some way to transform raw ingredients into products for consumption.

phytochemicals Naturally occurring plant compounds believed to have health-promoting effects in humans.

whole foods Foods that have been modified as little as possible, remaining in or near their natural state.

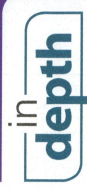

Phytochemical	Health Claims	Food Source	
Carotenoids: alpha-carotene, beta-carotene, lutein, lycopene, zeaxanthin, etc.	Diets with foods rich in these phytochemicals may reduce the risk for cardiovascular disease, certain cancers (e.g., prostate), and age-related eye diseases (cataracts, macular degeneration).	Red, orange, and deep-green vegetables and fruits, such as carrots, cantaloupe, sweet potatoes, apricots, kale, spinach, pumpkin, and tomatoes	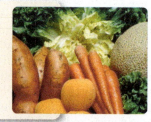
Flavonoids:[1] flavones, flavonols (e.g., quercetin), catechins (e.g., epigallocatechin gallate or EGCG), anthocyanidins, isoflavonoids, etc.	Diets with foods rich in these phytochemicals are associated with lower risk for cardiovascular disease and cancer, possibly because of reduced inflammation, blood clotting, and blood pressure and increased detoxification of carcinogens or reduction in replication of cancerous cells.	Berries, black and green tea, chocolate, purple grapes and juice, citrus fruits, olives, soybeans and soy products (soy milk, tofu, soy flour, textured vegetable protein), flaxseed, whole wheat	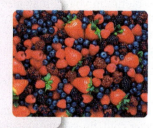
Phenolic acids:[1] ellagic acid, ferulic acid, caffeic acid, curcumin, etc.	Similar benefits as flavonoids.	Coffee beans, fruits (apples, pears, berries, grapes, oranges, prunes, strawberries), potatoes, mustard, oats, soy	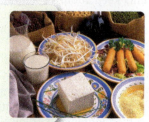
Phytoestrogens:[2] genistein, diadzein, lignans	Foods rich in these phytochemicals may provide benefits to bones and reduce the risk for cardiovascular disease and cancers of reproductive tissues (e.g., breast, prostate).	Soybeans and soy products (soy milk, tofu, soy flour, textured vegetable protein), flaxseed, whole grains	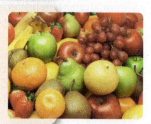
Organosulfur compounds: allylic sulfur compounds, indoles, isothiocyanates, etc.	Foods rich in these phytochemicals may protect against a wide variety of cancers.	Garlic, leeks, onions, chives, cruciferous vegetables (broccoli, cabbage, cauliflower), horseradish, mustard greens	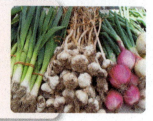

[1] Flavonoids, phenolic acids, and stilbenes are three groups of phytochemicals called phenolics. The phytochemical Resveratrol is a stilbene. Flavonoids and phenolic acids are the most abundant phenolics in our diet.
[2] Phytoestrogens include phytochemicals that have mild or anti-estrogenic action in our body. They are grouped together based on this similarity in biological function, but they also can be classified into other phytochemical groups, such as isoflavonoids.

FIGURE 3 Health claims and food sources of phytochemicals.

Like probiotics and prebiotics, phytochemicals are not classified as nutrients—that is, substances necessary for sustaining life. Yet eating an abundance of phytochemical-rich foods has been shown to protect against a number of diseases. Here are just a few examples of the proposed benefits of phytochemicals:[19-24]

- Reduce inflammation linked to the development of cardiovascular disease, cancer, and Alzheimer's disease, allergies, and arthritis.
- Protect against unhealthful blood cholesterol levels associated with cardiovascular disease.
- Impede the initiation and progression of cancer by helping to detoxify carcinogens, slow tumor growth, inhibit communication among cancer cells, and provoke cancer cells to self-destruct.
- Combat infections by enhancing our immune function and acting as antibacterial and antiviral agents.

Although you might assume that the more phytochemicals you consume the better, that's somewhat simplistic. They appear to be beneficial in the low doses commonly provided by foods, but they may be ineffective or even harmful when consumed as supplements. This may be due to their mode of action: instead of *protecting* our cells, phytochemicals might benefit our health by *stressing* our cells, causing them to rev up their internal defense systems. Cells are very well equipped to deal with minor stresses, but not with excessive stress, which may explain why clinical trials with phytochemical supplements may not show the same benefits as high intakes of plant foods, and can even be harmful. For example, a classic study found that supplementing with 20 to 30 mg/day of a phytochemical called beta-carotene for 4 to 6 years *increased* lung cancer risk by 16% to 28% in smokers.[25,26] In short, whereas there is ample evidence to support the health

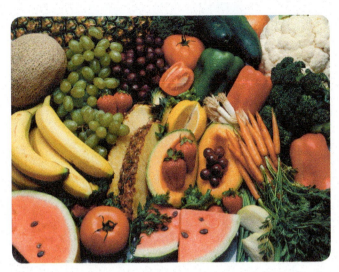

Avoid phytochemical supplements in favor of whole foods.

benefits of a plant-based diet, phytochemical supplements should be avoided.

So what's the take-home message from all this new research? Eat sensibly—for your genes, your microbiome, and your health. To increase your prebiotic and phytochemical intake, build a rainbow of colors on your plate; for instance, black beans, onions, peppers, and tomatoes over brown rice, a green salad sprinkled with nuts or seeds—and why not fruit salad for dessert! Oats and wheat are also rich in prebiotics and phytochemicals, as are tofu and soy milk, and many dark green vegetables. Probiotics, too, should be part of your daily diet. Try Greek yogurt drizzled with honey, or pour yourself a glass of kefir, which tastes like a yogurt smoothie. In short, a probiotic-rich plant-based diet may be just the prescription you need for better health.

web links

www.commonfund.nih.gov
The Human Microbiome Project

Click on "HMP" in the search box to find out more about the microbes that live within you—and help you live!

www.isapp.net
International Scientific Association for Probiotics and Prebiotics

Click on links from the home page to find consumer guides to probiotic and prebiotic foods.

www.aicr.org
American Institute for Cancer Research

Search for "phytochemicals" to learn about the AICR's stance and recommendations on the role of these substances in cancer prevention.

http://lpi.oregonstate.edu
Linus Pauling Institute

This extensive website covers phytochemicals as well as nutrients and other cutting-edge health and nutrition topics.

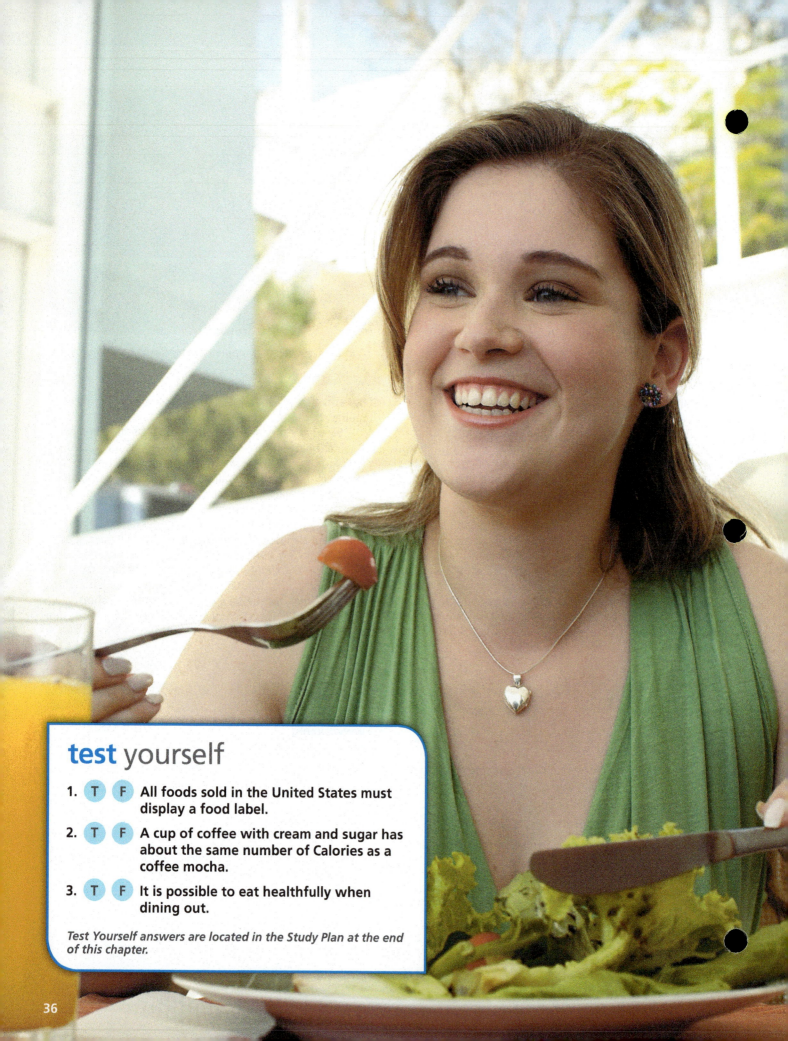

test yourself

1. (T) (F) **All foods sold in the United States must display a food label.**

2. (T) (F) **A cup of coffee with cream and sugar has about the same number of Calories as a coffee mocha.**

3. (T) (F) **It is possible to eat healthfully when dining out.**

Test Yourself answers are located in the Study Plan at the end of this chapter.

2

Designing a Healthful Diet

learning outcomes

After studying this chapter you should be able to:

1 Identify five characteristics of a healthful diet, pp. 38–40.

2 Discuss the influence of sensory data, sociocultural cues, emotions, and learning on food choices, pp. 40–42.

3 Explain how to read a food label, including the Nutrition Facts panel and label claims, to determine the nutritional profile of a given food, pp. 42–46.

4 Summarize the key messages of the *2015–2020 Dietary Guidelines for Americans*, pp. 47–48.

5 Explain how to use the USDA Food Patterns to design a healthful diet, pp. 48–53.

6 Describe several ways to make healthful meal choices when eating out, pp. 53–55.

Sigrid and her parents moved to the United States from Scandinavia when she was 6 years old. At first, she continued to eat her accustomed healthful diet and enjoyed riding her bike in her new neighborhood. But by the time she entered college, she was overweight. Sigrid explains, "My parents' diet is largely fish and vegetables, and desserts are only for special occasions. When we moved to America, I wanted to eat like all the other kids: hamburgers, french fries, sodas, and sweets. I gained a lot of weight on that diet, so I've started eating more like my parents again, choosing soups and salads, for instance, instead of pizza, in the campus dining hall."

There is no one right way to eat that is healthful and acceptable for everyone. Each of us is an individual with unique needs, food preferences, and cultural influences. Still, a variety of nutritional tools can guide you in designing a healthful diet that's right for you. In this chapter, we introduce these tools, including food labels, the Dietary Guidelines for Americans, the U.S. Department of Agriculture Food Patterns (and its accompanying graphic, MyPlate), and others. Before exploring the question of how to design a healthful diet, however, it is important to understand what a healthful diet *is*.

LO 1 Identify five characteristics of a healthful diet.

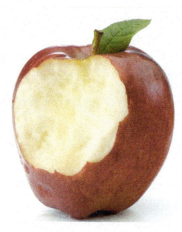

▲ A healthful diet can help prevent disease.

What is a healthful diet?

A **healthful diet** provides the proper combination of energy and nutrients. It is adequate, moderate, nutrient-dense, balanced, and varied. If you keep these characteristics in mind, you will be able to select foods that provide you with the optimal combination of nutrients and energy each day.

A Healthful Diet Is Adequate

An *adequate diet* provides enough of the energy, nutrients, and fiber (a nondigestible carbohydrate that promotes body functioning) to maintain a person's health. A diet may be adequate in one area, and inadequate in another. For example, many Americans have an adequate intake of protein, fat, and carbohydrate, but because they don't eat enough vegetables, their intake of fiber and certain micronutrients is inadequate. In fact, some people who eat too few vegetables are overweight or obese, which means that their diet, although inadequate in one area, exceeds their energy needs.

A diet that is adequate for one person may not be adequate for another. For example, a small woman who is lightly active needs approximately 1,700 to 2,000 kilocalories (kcal) each day, whereas a highly active male athlete may require more than 4,000 kcal each day to support his body's demands. These two individuals require very different levels of fat, carbohydrate, protein, and other nutrients to support their daily needs.

A Healthful Diet Is Moderate

The amount of any particular food you eat should be *moderate*—not too much and not too little. Eating too much or too little of certain foods can derail your health goals. For example, some people drink as many as three 20-oz bottles (a total of 765 kcal) of soft drinks on an average day. In order to allow for these extra kcal and avoid weight gain, most people would need to reduce their food intake significantly. This could mean eliminating many healthful foods. In contrast, people who drink mostly water and low-Calorie beverages can consume more nourishing foods.

A Healthful Diet Is Nutrient-Dense

A *nutrient-dense* diet is made up of foods and beverages that supply the highest level of nutrients for the lowest number of Calories. **MEAL FOCUS FIGURE 2.1** compares 1 day of meals that are high and low in **nutrient density**. As you can see in this figure, a turkey sandwich on whole-grain bread provides a high level of fiber-rich carbohydrates, healthful fats, and micronutrients, for a low "cost" in Calories. In contrast, a cheeseburger is lower in nutrients and fiber and higher in Calories. Thus, the turkey sandwich is more nutrient dense. Compare the other meals shown in the figure for help selecting nutrient-dense foods throughout the day.

Another tool for selecting nutrient-dense foods is in your supermarket! Have you ever wondered why there are numbers or stars on the shelf labels under everything from produce to canned goods? They are there to help shoppers make more healthful choices. Higher numbers or more stars indicate foods with a higher nutrient density. For example, in one system, kale gets the highest possible numerical score, whereas a can of spaghetti and meatballs scores near the bottom. Although a few nutritional guidance systems are in use in U.S. supermarkets, by far the most common is the NuVal system.

A Healthful Diet Is Balanced

A *balanced diet* contains the combinations of foods that provide the proper proportions of nutrients. As you will learn in this course, the body needs many types of foods in varying amounts to maintain health. For example, fruits and vegetables are excellent sources of fiber, vitamin C, potassium, and magnesium. Meats don't provide much of these, but they are excellent sources of protein, iron, zinc, and copper.

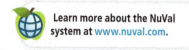

Learn more about the NuVal system at www.nuval.com.

healthful diet A diet that provides the proper combination of energy and nutrients and is adequate, moderate, nutrient-dense, balanced, and varied.

nutrient density The relative amount of nutrients and fiber per amount of energy (or number of Calories).

a day of meals

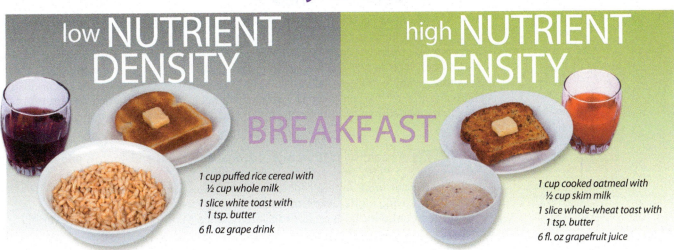

low NUTRIENT DENSITY

high NUTRIENT DENSITY

BREAKFAST

1 cup puffed rice cereal with
 ½ cup whole milk
1 slice white toast with
 1 tsp. butter
6 fl. oz grape drink

1 cup cooked oatmeal with
 ½ cup skim milk
1 slice whole-wheat toast with
 1 tsp. butter
6 fl. oz grapefruit juice

LUNCH

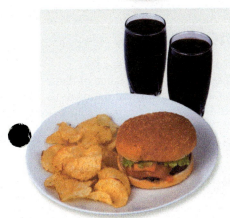

Cheeseburger
3 oz regular ground beef
1.5 oz cheddar cheese
1 white hamburger bun
2 tsp. Dijon mustard
2 leaves iceberg lettuce
1 snack-sized bag potato chips
32 fl. oz cola soft drink

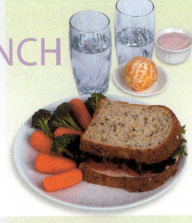

Turkey sandwich
3 oz turkey breast
2 slices whole-grain bread
2 tsp. Dijon mustard
3 slices fresh tomato
2 leaves red leaf lettuce
1 cup baby carrots with
 broccoli crowns
20 fl. oz (2.5 cups) water
1 peeled orange
1 cup nonfat yogurt

DINNER

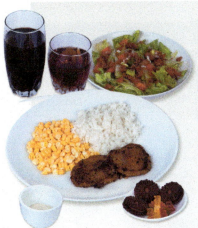

Green salad
1 cup iceberg lettuce
¼ cup diced tomatoes
1 tsp. green onions
¼ cup bacon bits
1 tbsp. regular Ranch salad dressing
3 oz beef round steak, breaded and fried
½ cup cooked white rice
½ cup sweet corn
8 fl. oz (1 cup) iced tea
3 chocolate sandwich cookies
1 12-oz can diet soft drink
10 Gummi Bears candy

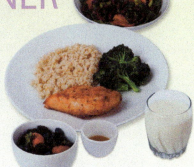

Spinach salad
1 cup fresh spinach leaves
¼ cup sliced tomatoes
¼ cup diced green pepper
½ cup kidney beans
1 tbsp. fat-free Italian salad
 dressing
3 oz broiled chicken breast
½ cup cooked brown rice
½ cup steamed broccoli
8 fl. oz (1 cup) skim milk
1-1/2 cup mixed berries

nutrient analysis

3,319 kcal
11.4% of energy from saturated fat
11.6 grams of dietary fiber
3,031 milligrams of sodium
83 milligrams of vitamin C
18.2 milligrams of iron
825 milligrams of calcium

Provides
more
nutrients
and fewer
calories!

nutrient analysis

1,753 kcal
3% of energy from saturated fat
53.1 grams of dietary fiber
2,231 milligrams of sodium
372 milligrams of vitamin C
15.2 milligrams of iron
1,469 milligrams of calcium

Eating the proper balance of nutrient-dense foods from each food group is important to maintain your health.

A Healthful Diet Is Varied

Variety refers to eating many different foods from the different food groups on a regular basis. With thousands of healthful foods to choose from, trying new foods is a fun and easy way to vary your diet. Eat a new vegetable each week or substitute one food for another, such as raw spinach on your turkey sandwich in place of iceberg lettuce. Selecting a variety of foods increases the likelihood that you will consume the multitude of nutrients your body needs. As an added benefit, eating a varied diet prevents boredom and helps you avoid getting into a "food rut."

recap A healthful diet provides adequate nutrients and energy, and it includes moderate amounts—neither too much nor too little—of any particular food. A healthful diet is nutrient-dense, composed mostly of foods that provide higher levels of nutrients and fiber for fewer Calories. A healthful diet also includes an appropriate balance of nutrients and a wide variety of foods.

LO 2 Discuss the influence of sensory data, sociocultural cues, emotions, and learning on food choices.

What's behind our food choices?

Do the food choices you make each day contribute to a healthful diet? Let's take a look at the factors that commonly influence our choices of what to eat. Some of them might surprise you! After that, we'll discuss tools such as food labels and national guidelines that can help you make better choices.

Sensory Data Influence Food Choices

appetite A psychological desire to consume specific foods.

Whereas hunger is a basic biological urge to eat, **appetite** is a psychological desire to consume specific foods. Appetite is commonly triggered by sensory data; that is, cues that stimulate our five senses **(FIGURE 2.2)**. Artfully decorated foods, for

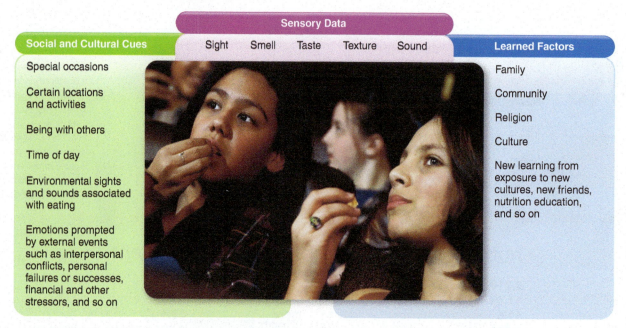

Sensory Data

| Social and Cultural Cues | Sight Smell Taste Texture Sound | Learned Factors |

Social and Cultural Cues:
Special occasions

Certain locations and activities

Being with others

Time of day

Environmental sights and sounds associated with eating

Emotions prompted by external events such as interpersonal conflicts, personal failures or successes, financial and other stressors, and so on

Learned Factors:
Family

Community

Religion

Culture

New learning from exposure to new cultures, new friends, nutrition education, and so on

▲ **FIGURE 2.2** The factors that drive food choices include social and cultural cues and sensory data, in addition to learning.

example, stimulate your sense of sight and can prompt you to choose a slice of chocolate cake instead of a bran muffin. The aroma of foods such as freshly brewed coffee and baked goods can also be powerful stimulants. **Olfaction**—our sense of smell—plays a key role in the stimulation of appetite. Much of our ability to taste foods actually comes from our sense of smell. This is why foods are not as appealing when we have a stuffy nose. Certain tastes, such as sweetness, are almost universally appealing, while others, such as the astringent taste of some foods (for instance, spinach and kale), are quite individual. **Mouthfeel**, the tactile sensation of food in the mouth, is also important in food choices because it stimulates nerve endings sensitive to touch in our mouth and on our tongue. Even our sense of hearing can be stimulated by foods, from the fizz of cola to the crunch of pretzels.

Sociocultural Cues and Emotions Influence Food Choices

In addition to sensory data, our brain's association with certain social events can influence food choices. At holiday gatherings, for example, our culture gives us permission to eat "forbidden" foods, whereas food choices may be more cautious when we're out on a date. Being in a certain location, such as at a baseball game or a movie theater, or engaging in certain activities, such as watching television, can also influence choices.

The cultural group with which we identify strongly influences our food choices. A Japanese American, for example, might regularly cook with white rice, fish, and seaweed because these foods are readily available in, and part of the cuisine of, Japan. But even for recent immigrants, the dominant American food culture strongly influences food choices, mainly through food advertisements and availability, that is, the types of foods available in restaurants, supermarkets, convenience stores, vending machines, farm stands, and other vendors in the community. The "culture" on a school campus can also encourage or discourage certain choices, inducing us to favor a popular brand of energy drink, for instance, or to snub the meals offered in the campus dining hall.

In some people, food choices are influenced by emotions. For example, a person might crave "comfort food" after arguing with a friend, or when feeling worried or bored. Others subconsciously seek food as a "reward," such as heading out for a burger and fries after turning in a term paper.

Learning Influences Food Choices

Would you eat pigs' feet? What about blood sausage, stewed octopus, or grasshoppers? If you had grown up in certain cultures, you might. That's because your preference for particular foods is largely a learned response. The culture in which you are raised teaches you what plant and animal products are appropriate or desirable to eat. If your parents fed you cubes of plain tofu throughout your toddlerhood, then you are probably still eating tofu.

That said, early introduction to foods is not essential; we can learn to enjoy new foods at any point in our lives. For instance, you may never have tasted Ethiopian food before a restaurant opened in your neighborhood, but now it's your favorite cuisine.

Many immigrants adopt the diet typical of their new home, or develop a blended diet of some of their traditional foods and foods found in their adopted country.

We can also "learn" to dislike foods we once enjoyed. For example, a **conditioned taste aversion** to foods can occur as a result of illness, even if there is no relationship between the food and the illness. If we experience an episode of food poisoning after eating scrambled eggs, we might develop a strong distaste for all types of eggs. Additionally, many adults who become vegetarians do so after learning about the treatment of animals in slaughterhouses: they might have eaten meat daily when young but no longer have any appetite for it.

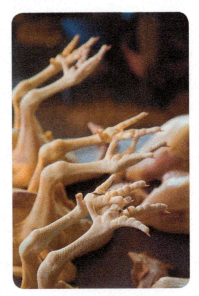

▲ Food preferences are influenced by the family and culture in which you're raised.

olfaction Our sense of smell, which plays a key role in the stimulation of appetite.

mouthfeel The tactile sensation of food in the mouth; derived from the interaction of physical and chemical characteristics of the food.

conditioned taste aversion Avoidance of a food as a result of a negative experience, such as illness, even if the illness has no relationship with the food consumed.

recap Appetite is a psychological desire to consume specific foods. Sensory data, including the sight, smell, and taste of foods, commonly influence our food choices. The people we're with, the setting and activities we're engaged in, and the culture with which we identify also influence food choices, as do our emotions, especially when we seek "comfort foods." Moreover, preference for particular foods is a learned response. The family and society in which we were raised teaches us what foods are appropriate, but we can learn to enjoy—or dislike—foods at any point in our lives.

LO 3 Explain how to read a food label, including the Nutrition Facts panel and label claims, to determine the nutritional profile of a given food.

How can reading food labels help you improve your diet?

To design and maintain a healthful diet, it's important to read and understand food labels. It may surprise you to learn that a few decades ago there were no federal regulations for including nutrition information on food labels! The U.S. Food and Drug Administration (FDA) first established label regulations in 1973. These provided general information and were not required for many available foods. More detailed regulations were established in 1990 under the Nutrition Labeling and Education Act. This act specifies which foods require a food label, what information must be included on the label, and the companies and food products that are exempt. For example, detailed food labels are not required for meat, poultry, fish, coffee, fresh produce, and most spices.

Five Components Must Be Included on Food Labels

Five primary components of information must be included on food labels (FIGURE 2.3):

1. **A statement of identity.** The common name of the product or an appropriate identification of the food product must be prominently displayed on the label. This information tells us very clearly what the product is.
2. **The net contents of the package.** The quantity of the food product in the entire package must be accurately described. Information may be listed as weight (such as grams), volume (fluid ounces), or numerical count (4 each).
3. **Ingredient list.** The ingredients must be listed by their common names, in descending order by weight. This means that the first product listed is the

The **Nutrition Facts panel** lists standardized serving sizes and specific nutrients, and shows how a serving of the food fits into a healthy diet by stating its contribution to the percentage of the Daily Value for each nutrient.

The **name** of the product must be displayed on the front label.

The **ingredients** must be listed in descending order by weight. Whole-grain wheat is the predominant ingredient in this cereal.

The **information** of food manufacturer, packer, or distributor is also located at the bottom of the package.

The **net weight** of the food in the box is located at the bottom of the package.

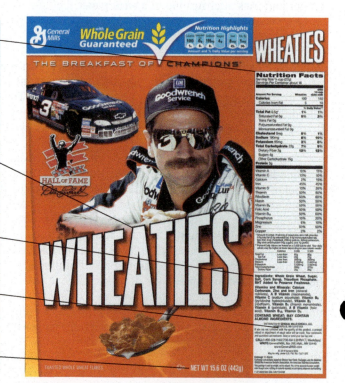

FIGURE 2.3 The five primary components that are required for food labels.

(Source: © ConAgra Brands, Inc. Reprinted by permission)

predominant ingredient in that food. This information can be very useful in many situations, such as when you are looking for foods that are lower in sugar or contain whole-grain flour instead of processed wheat flour.

4. **The name and address of the food manufacturer, packer, or distributor.** You can use this information to find out more details about a food product and to contact the company if there is something wrong with the product or you suspect that it has caused an illness.

5. **Nutrition information.** The **Nutrition Facts panel** contains the nutrition information required by the FDA. This panel is the primary tool to assist you in choosing more healthful foods. An explanation of the components of the Nutrition Facts panel follows.

Use the Nutrition Facts Panel to Evaluate and Compare Foods

In May 2016, the FDA finalized the new Nutrition Facts panel for packaged foods. Manufacturers are required to use the new panel by July 26, 2018. **FOCUS FIGURE 2.4** on page 44 compares the old Nutrition Facts panel with the new design. You can use the information on this panel to learn more about an individual food, and you can use the panel to compare one food to another. Let's start at the top of the new panel and work our way down to better understand how to use this information.

1. **Serving size and servings per container:** describes the serving size in a common household measure (such as cup) and a metric measure (grams), as well as how many servings are contained in the package. For packages of foods that are commonly consumed in one sitting, this information reflects the amount in the entire package. Serving size information has been updated to be more realistic to amounts typically consumed. It is important to factor in how much of the food you eat when determining the amount of nutrients that this food contributes to your diet.

2. **Calories per serving:** describes the total number of Calories in larger, bolder print. In the new panel, the total number of Calories that come from fat per one serving of that food has been removed. However, the grams of fat, carbohydrate, and protein per serving are all indicated, allowing you to calculate Calorie information for these nutrients.

3. **Percent Daily Values (%DVs):** tells you how much a serving of food contributes to an average individual's overall intake of the nutrient indicated. For example, 1 gram of saturated fat constitutes 5% of an average individual's total daily recommended saturated fat intake. When defining the %DV, the FDA based its calculations on a 2,000-Calorie diet. Even if you don't consume 2,000 Calories each day, you can use the %DV to figure out whether a food is high or low in a given nutrient. Foods that contain less than 5% DV of a nutrient are considered low in that nutrient, while foods that contain more than 20% DV are considered high in that nutrient. If you are trying to increase your intake of calcium, for example, select foods that contain more than 20% DV for calcium. In contrast, if you are trying to reduce your sodium intake, select foods that contain less than 5% sodium. You can also compare the %DV of key nutrients in different brands of foods to see which is higher or lower in those nutrients. The new panel includes the %DVs and amounts for added sugars, vitamin D, calcium, iron, and potassium; identifying the %DV for vitamins A and C is now voluntary.

4. **Footnote (lower part of the panel):** provides a simple definition of %DV and tells you that the %DV are based on a 2,000-Calorie diet.

Food Labels Can Display a Variety of Claims

Have you ever noticed a food label displaying a claim such as "This food is low in sodium" or "This food is part of a heart-healthy diet"? The claim may have influenced you to buy the food, even if you weren't sure what it meant. Let's take a look.

Want to find out more about how to use food labels to maintain a healthful weight? Go to www.fda.gov and type in the search bar "Make Your Calories Count."

Nutrition Facts panel The label on a food package that contains the nutrition information required by the FDA.

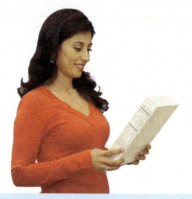

The U.S. Food and Drug Administration (FDA) has made changes to the 20-year-old nutrition labels on packaged foods. The changes to the nutrition label provide information to help compare products and make healthy food choices.

OLD LABEL

GRANOLA

Nutrition Facts
Serving Size 2/3 cup (55 g)
Servings Per Container About 8

Amount Per Serving

Calories 230	Calories from Fat 72	
		% Daily Value*
Total Fat 8 g		**12%**
Saturated Fat 1 g		**5%**
Trans Fat 0 g		
Cholesterol 0 mg		**0%**
Sodium 160 mg		**7%**
Total Carbohydrates 37 g		**12%**
Dietary Fiber 4 g		**16%**
Sugars 12 g		
Protein 3 g		
Vitamin A		10%
Vitamin C		8%
Calcium		20%
Iron		45%

* Percent Daily Values are based on a 2,000 calorie diet. Your daily value may be higher or lower depending on your calorie needs.

		Calories:	2,000	2,500
Total Fat	Less than		65 g	80 g
Sat Fat	Less than		20 g	25 g
Cholesterol	Less than		300 mg	300 mg
Sodium	Less than		2,400 mg	2,400 mg
Total Carbohydrate			300 g	375 g
Dietary Fiber			25 g	30 g

SERVINGS

- Serving sizes are standardized, making comparison shopping easier.

NEW
- Serving sizes are larger and bolder.
- Serving sizes updated and more realistic.

CALORIES

- Calories per serving and the number of servings in the package are listed.

NEW
- Calories are larger to stand out more.
- "Calories from fat" is removed.

DAILY VALUES

- Daily Values are general reference values based on a 2,000 Calorie diet.
- The %DV can tell you if a food is high or low in a nutrient or dietary substance.

NEW
- Daily Values are updated.
- A shorter footnote that more clearly explains %DV is included.
- The %DV for added sugar is included.

ADDED SUGARS

NEW
- Added sugars are listed.

VITAMINS & MINERALS

- Vitamin A, vitamin C, calcium, and iron are required.
- Other vitamins and minerals are voluntary.

NEW
- Vitamin D and potassium are required, in addition to calcium and iron.
- Vitamins A and C are voluntary.
- Actual amounts of each nutrient are listed as well as the %DV.

NEW LABEL

GRANOLA

Nutrition Facts
8 servings per container
Serving size   2/3 cup (55g)

Amount per serving

Calories		**230**
		% Daily Value*
Total Fat 8g		**12%**
Saturated Fat 1g		**5%**
Trans Fat 0g		
Cholesterol 0mg		**0%**
Sodium 160mg		**7%**
Total Carbohydrate 37g		**12%**
Dietary Fiber 4g		**16%**
Total Sugars 12g		
Includes 10g Added Sugars		**20%**
Protein 3g		
Vitamin D 2mcg		10%
Calcium 260mg		20%
Iron 8mg		45%
Potassium 235mg		6%

* The % Daily Value (DV) tells you how much a nutrient in a serving of food contributes to a daily diet. 2,000 calories a day is used for general nutrition advice.

The FDA regulates two types of claims that food companies put on food labels: nutrient claims and health claims. Food companies are prohibited from using a nutrient or health claim that is not approved by the FDA.

The %Daily Values on the food labels serve as a basis for nutrient claims. For instance, if the label states that a food is "low in sodium," the food contains 140 mg or less of sodium per serving. **TABLE 2.1** defines the terms approved for use in nutrient claims.

TABLE 2.1 U.S. Food and Drug Administration (FDA)–Approved Nutrient-Related Terms and Definitions

Nutrient	Claim	Meaning
Energy	Calorie free	Less than 5 kcal per serving
	Low Calorie	40 kcal or less per serving
	Reduced Calorie	At least 25% fewer kcal than reference (or regular) food
Fat and Cholesterol	Fat free	Less than 0.5 g of fat per serving
	Low fat	3 g or less fat per serving
	Reduced fat	At least 25% less fat per serving than reference food
	Saturated fat free	Less than 0.5 g of saturated fat *and* less than 0.5 g of *trans* fat per serving
	Low saturated fat	1 g or less saturated fat and less than 0.5 g *trans* fat per serving *and* 15% or less of total kcal from saturated fat
	Reduced saturated fat	At least 25% less saturated fat *and* reduced by more than 1 g saturated fat per serving as compared to reference food
	Cholesterol free	Less than 2 mg of cholesterol per serving *and* 2 g or less saturated fat and *trans* fat combined per serving
	Low cholesterol	20 mg or less cholesterol *and* 2 g or less saturated fat per serving
	Reduced cholesterol	At least 25% less cholesterol than reference food *and* 2 g or less saturated fat per serving
Fiber and Sugar	High fiber	5 g or more fiber per serving*
	Good source of fiber	2.5 g to 4.9 g fiber per serving
	More or added fiber	At least 2.5 g more fiber per serving than reference food
	Sugar free	Less than 0.5 g sugars per serving
	Low sugar	Not defined; no basis for recommended intake
	Reduced/less sugar	At least 25% less sugars per serving than reference food
	No added sugars or without added sugars	No sugar or sugar-containing ingredient added during processing
Sodium	Sodium free	Less than 5 mg sodium per serving
	Very low sodium	35 mg or less sodium per serving
	Low sodium	140 mg or less sodium per serving
	Reduced sodium	At least 25% less sodium per serving than reference food
Relative Claims	Free, without, no, zero	No or a trivial amount of given nutrient
	Light (lite)	This term can have three different meanings: (1) a serving provides one-third fewer kcal than or half the fat of the reference food; (2) a serving of a low-fat, low-Calorie food provides half the sodium normally present; or (3) lighter in color and texture, with the label making this clear (for example, light molasses)
	Reduced, less, fewer	Contains at least 25% less of a nutrient or kcal than reference food
	More, added, extra, or plus	At least 10% of the Daily Value of nutrient as compared to reference food (may occur naturally or be added); may be used only for vitamins, minerals, protein, dietary fiber, and potassium
	Good source of, contains, or provides	10% to 19% of Daily Value per serving (may not be used for carbohydrate)
	High in, rich in, or excellent source of	20% or more of Daily Value per serving for protein, vitamins, minerals, dietary fiber, or potassium (may not be used for carbohydrate)

*High-fiber claims must also meet the definition of low fat; if not, then the level of total fat must appear next to the high-fiber claim.

Data adapted from: "Food Labeling Guide" (U.S. Food and Drug Administration).

TABLE 2.2 U.S. Food and Drug Administration–Approved Health Claims on Labels

Disease/Health Concern	Nutrient	Example of Approved Claim Statement
Osteoporosis	Calcium	Regular exercise and a healthful diet with enough calcium help teens and young white and Asian women maintain good bone health and may reduce their high risk for osteoporosis later in life.
Coronary heart disease	Saturated fat and cholesterol Fruits, vegetables, and grain products that contain fiber, particularly soluble fiber Soluble fiber from whole oats, psyllium seed husk, and beta glucan soluble fiber from oat bran, rolled oats (or oatmeal), and whole-oat flour Soy protein Plant sterol/stanol esters Whole-grain foods	Diets low in saturated fat and cholesterol and rich in fruits, vegetables, and grain products that contain some types of dietary fiber, particularly soluble fiber, may reduce the risk for heart disease, a disease associated with many factors.
Cancer	Dietary fats Fiber-containing grain products, fruits, and vegetables Fruits and vegetables Whole-grain foods	Low-fat diets rich in fiber-containing grain products, fruits, and vegetables may reduce the risk for some types of cancer, a disease associated with many factors.
Hypertension and stroke	Sodium Potassium	Diets containing foods that are a good source of potassium and that are low in sodium may reduce the risk of high blood pressure and stroke.*
Neural tube defects	Folate	Healthful diets with adequate folate may reduce a woman's risk of having a child with a brain or spinal cord defect.
Dental caries	Sugar alcohols	Frequent between-meal consumption of foods high in sugars and starches promotes tooth decay. The sugar alcohols in [name of food] do not promote tooth decay.

*Required wording for this claim. Wordings for other claims are recommended model statements but not required verbatim.

Data adapted from: "Food Labeling Guide" (U.S. Food and Drug Administration).

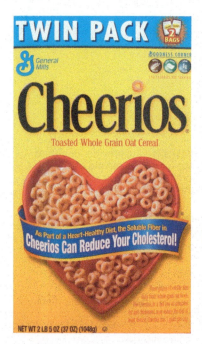

▲ The health claim on this box of cereal is approved by the FDA.

The FDA also allows food labels to display certain claims related to health and disease **(TABLE 2.2)**. If current scientific evidence about a particular health claim is not convincing, the label may have to include a disclaimer so that consumers are not misled.

In addition to nutrient and health claims, labels may also contain structure–function claims. These are claims that can be made without approval from the FDA. Although these claims can be generic statements about a food's impact on the body's structure and function, they cannot refer to a specific disease or symptom. Examples of structure–function claims include "Builds stronger bones," "Improves memory," "Slows signs of aging," and "Boosts your immune system." It is important to remember that these claims can be made with no proof, and thus there are no guarantees that any benefits identified in structure–function claims are true about that food. So, just because something is stated on the label doesn't guarantee it is always true!

recap The ability to read and interpret food labels is important for planning and maintaining a healthful diet. Food labels must identify the food, the net contents of the package, the contact information for the food manufacturer or distributor, and the ingredients in the food. They must also include a Nutrition Facts panel providing information about Calories, macronutrients, and selected vitamins and minerals. The FDA is currently revising the Nutrition Facts panel. The FDA also allows food labels to display approved nutrient and health claims. Generic claims regarding body structure and function are allowed but not regulated.

nutri-case | GUSTAVO

"Until last night, I hadn't been inside a grocery store in about 10 years. But then my wife broke her hip and had to go to the hospital. On my way home from visiting her, I realized I needed to do some food shopping. Was I ever in for a shock! I don't know how my wife does it, choosing between all the different brands, and reading those long labels. She never went to school past the sixth grade, and she doesn't speak English very well, either! I bought a frozen chicken pie for dinner, but it didn't taste right, so I got the package out of the trash and read all the labels, and that's when I saw there wasn't any chicken in it at all . . . it was made out of tofu! This afternoon, my daughter is picking me up, and we're going to do our grocery shopping together."

Given what you've learned about FDA food labels, what parts of a food package would you advise Gustavo to be sure to read before he makes a choice? What other advice might you give him to make his grocery shopping easier? Imagine that you have only limited skills in reading and mathematics. In that case, what other strategies might you use when shopping for nutritious foods?

How do the Dietary Guidelines for Americans promote a healthful diet?

LO 4 Summarize the key messages of the *2015–2020 Dietary Guidelines for Americans*.

The **Dietary Guidelines for Americans** are a set of principles developed by the U.S. Department of Agriculture and the U.S. Department of Health and Human Services and updated approximately every 5 years. Their goal is to make recommendations about the components of a healthful and nutritionally adequate diet to help promote health and prevent chronic disease.[1] The *2015–2020 Dietary Guidelines for Americans* reflect current evidence indicating that healthful eating patterns and regular physical activity together help people to achieve and maintain good health and reduce their risks for chronic diseases and obesity across the lifespan. Whereas the previous Dietary Guidelines focused primarily on individual food groups and nutrients, the 2015–2020 Guidelines encourage a healthful eating pattern that you can tailor to your personal preferences.

The five Guidelines are as follows:

1. **Follow a healthful eating pattern across the lifespan.** All food and beverage choices influence health. Choose a healthful eating pattern at an appropriate energy level to enable you to achieve and maintain a healthful body weight, consume an adequate level of nutrients, and reduce your risks for chronic diseases. For information on how to follow a healthful eating pattern, see the **In Depth** essay following this chapter.
2. **Focus on variety, nutrient density, and amount.** To meet nutrient needs within an energy-intake level that allows you to maintain a healthful body weight, choose a variety of nutrient-dense foods across and within all food groups in recommended amounts. (See Meal Focus Figure 2.1 on page 39.)
3. **Limit Calories from added sugars and saturated fats, and reduce your sodium intake.**
   - Added sugars are any sweeteners that do not occur naturally in foods. They are commonly added to soft drinks and other sugary drinks, desserts, and some yogurts, breakfast cereals, and other processed foods. A diet high in added sugars is associated with an increased risk for obesity and its related chronic diseases. Follow an eating pattern that limits your intake of foods and beverages containing added sugars, ensuring no more than 10% of total Calories comes from added sugars.
   - Saturated fats are a type of fat abundant in meats and other animal-based foods. A diet high in saturated fats is associated with an increased risk for

Dietary Guidelines for Americans A set of principles developed by the U.S. Department of Agriculture and the U.S. Department of Health and Human Services to assist Americans in designing a healthful diet and lifestyle.

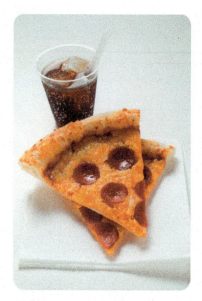

The Dietary Guidelines recommend limiting added sugars, saturated fats, and sodium. A soft drink and a slice of pepperoni pizza are, unfortunately, loaded with all three.

cardiovascular disease. Cut back on your consumption of fatty meats, butter and lard, packaged meals, and other foods high in saturated fats. It is recommended we consume no more than 10% of total Calories from saturated fats.

- Sodium is an essential mineral, but high intake is linked to an increased risk for high blood pressure in some people. Although table salt contains sodium, most of our intake is from processed foods, especially processed meats, canned vegetables and vegetable juices, salty condiments such as soy sauce and salad dressings, and packaged meals. Your sodium intake should remain below 2,300 mg per day.

4. **Shift to more healthful food and beverage choices.** Choose nutrient-dense foods and beverages across and within all food groups.
5. **Support healthful eating patterns for everyone.** Recognize your role in creating and supporting healthful eating patterns at home, on campus, in your workplace, and within your community.

The Guidelines also recommend consuming alcohol in moderation, if at all; that is, no more than one drink per day for women and two per day for men. In tandem with these recommendations, all Americans should engage in recommended levels of physical activity (identified in Chapter 11). A healthful diet and regular physical activity together contribute to Calorie management and maintenance of a healthful body weight.[1]

recap The goal of the Dietary Guidelines for Americans is to make recommendations about the components of a healthful and nutritionally adequate diet to help promote health and prevent chronic disease. The five Guidelines encourage Americans to follow a healthful eating pattern; focus on a variety of nutrient-dense foods in recommended amounts; limit added sugars, saturated fats, and sodium; shift to more healthful choices; and support healthful eating patterns for everyone. The Guidelines also recommend consuming alcohol in moderation, if at all, and engaging in regular physical activity.

LO 5 Explain how to use the USDA Food Patterns to design a healthful diet.

How can the USDA Food Patterns help you design a healthful diet?

The **USDA Food Patterns** were developed to help Americans incorporate the *Dietary Guidelines* into their everyday lives. They identify daily amounts of foods, and nutrient-dense choices, to eat from the five major food groups and their subgroups. The food groups emphasized in the USDA Food Patterns are grains, vegetables, fruits, dairy, and protein foods. **FIGURE 2.5** illustrates each of these food groups and provides detailed information on the nutrients they provide and recommended servings each day. Notice that legumes (beans, peas, and lentils) are included in both the vegetables and the protein foods groups, and that processed soy products, nuts and seeds, and eggs are also considered protein foods.

Log Onto MyPlate

MyPlate is the visual representation of the USDA Food Patterns. Notice that the plate is divided into colored segments that represent the five food groups (**FIGURE 2.6**) (see page 50). Moreover, MyPlate is a web-based, interactive, personalized guide to diet and physical activity. When you log onto MyPlate, you can assess your current diet and physical activity level and plan healthful changes. The MyPlate website helps Americans:

- Eat in moderation to balance calories.
- Eat a variety of foods.
- Consume the right proportion of each recommended food group.
- Personalize their eating plan.

USDA Food Patterns A set of recommendations for types and amounts of foods to consume from the five major food groups and subgroups to help people meet the Dietary Guidelines for Americans.

MyPlate The visual representation of the USDA Food Patterns and the website supporting their implementation.

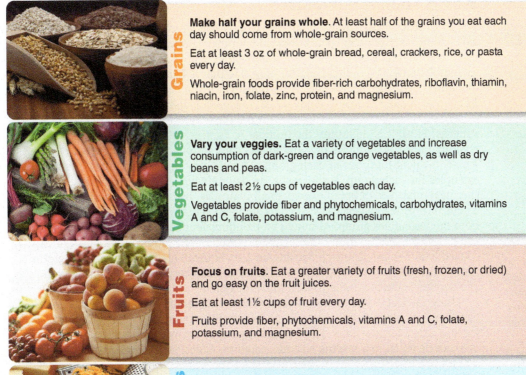

Grains

Make half your grains whole. At least half of the grains you eat each day should come from whole-grain sources.

Eat at least 3 oz of whole-grain bread, cereal, crackers, rice, or pasta every day.

Whole-grain foods provide fiber-rich carbohydrates, riboflavin, thiamin, niacin, iron, folate, zinc, protein, and magnesium.

Vegetables

Vary your veggies. Eat a variety of vegetables and increase consumption of dark-green and orange vegetables, as well as dry beans and peas.

Eat at least 2½ cups of vegetables each day.

Vegetables provide fiber and phytochemicals, carbohydrates, vitamins A and C, folate, potassium, and magnesium.

Fruits

Focus on fruits. Eat a greater variety of fruits (fresh, frozen, or dried) and go easy on the fruit juices.

Eat at least 1½ cups of fruit every day.

Fruits provide fiber, phytochemicals, vitamins A and C, folate, potassium, and magnesium.

Dairy Foods

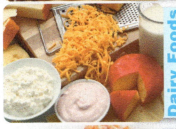

Get your calcium-rich foods. Choose low-fat or fat-free dairy products, such as milk, yogurt, and cheese. People who can't consume dairy foods can choose lactose-free dairy products or other sources, such as calcium-fortified juices and soy and rice beverages.

Get 3 cups of low-fat dairy foods, or the equivalent, every day.

Dairy foods provide calcium, phosphorus, riboflavin, protein, and vitamin B_{12} and are often fortified with vitamins D and A.

Protein Foods

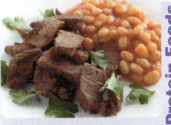

Go lean with protein. Choose low-fat or lean meats and poultry. Switch to baking, broiling, or grilling more often, and vary your choices to include more fish, eggs, processed soy products, beans, nuts, and seeds. Legumes, including beans, peas, and lentils, are included in both the protein and the vegetable groups.

Eat about 5½ oz of lean protein foods each day.

These foods provide protein, phosphorus, vitamin B_6, vitamin B_{12}, magnesium, iron, zinc, niacin, riboflavin, and thiamin.

◄ **FIGURE 2.5** Food groups of the USDA Food Patterns.

- Increase their physical activity.
- Set goals for gradually improving their food choices and lifestyle.

Limit Empty Calories

One concept emphasized in the USDA Food Patterns is that of **empty Calories**. These are Calories from solid fats or added sugars that provide few or no nutrients. The USDA recommends that you limit the empty Calories you eat. Foods that contain the greatest amount of empty Calories include cakes, cookies, pastries, ice cream, sugary drinks, cheese, pizza, sausages, hot dogs, bacon, and ribs. A few foods that contain empty Calories also provide important nutrients. Examples are sweetened applesauce, sweetened breakfast cereals, and regular ground beef. To reduce your intake of empty Calories but ensure you get adequate nutrients, choose the unsweetened, lean, or nonfat versions of these foods.

empty Calories Calories from solid fats or added sugars that provide few or no nutrients.

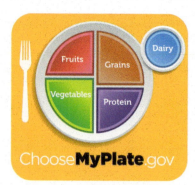

FIGURE 2.6 The USDA MyPlate graphic. MyPlate is an interactive food guidance system based on the Dietary Guidelines for Americans and the Dietary Reference Intakes from the National Academy of Sciences. Eating more fruits, vegetables, and whole grains and choosing foods low in added sugars, saturated fat, and sodium from the five food groups in MyPlate will help you balance your Calories and consume a healthier overall food pattern.
(Data from: MyPlate graphic, U.S. Department of Agriculture.)

Watch Your Serving Sizes

The USDA Food Patterns also helps you decide *how much* of each food you should eat. The number of servings is based on your age, gender, and activity level. A term used when defining serving sizes that may be new to you is **ounce-equivalent (oz-equivalent)**. It is defined as a serving size that is 1 ounce, or that is equivalent to an ounce, for the grains and protein groups. For instance, both a slice of bread and 1/2 cup of cooked brown rice qualify as ounce-equivalents.

What is considered a serving size for the foods recommended in the USDA Food Patterns? **FIGURE 2.7** identifies the number of cups or oz-equivalent servings recommended for a 2,000-Calorie diet and gives examples of amounts equal to 1 cup or 1 oz-equivalent for foods in each group. As you study this figure, notice the variety of examples for each group. For instance, an oz-equivalent serving from the grains group can mean one slice of bread or two small pancakes. Because of their low density, 2 cups of raw, leafy vegetables, such as spinach, actually constitute a 1-cup serving from the vegetables group. Although an oz-equivalent serving of meat is actually 1 oz, 1/2 oz of nuts also qualifies. One egg, 1 tablespoon of peanut butter, and 1/4 cup cooked legumes are also each considered 1 oz-equivalents from the protein group. Although it may seem inconvenient to measure food servings, understanding the size of a serving is crucial to planning a nutritious diet.

Using the USDA Food Patterns (and their visual representation, MyPlate) does have some challenges. For example, no nationally standardized definition for a serving size exists for any food. Thus, a serving size as defined in the USDA Food Patterns may not be equal to a serving size identified on a food label. For instance, the serving size for crackers suggested in the USDA Food Patterns is three to four small crackers, whereas a serving size for crackers on a food label can range from five to 18 crackers, depending on the size and weight of the cracker.

Also, for food items consumed individually—such as muffins, frozen burgers, and bottled juices—the serving sizes in the USDA Food Patterns are typically much smaller than the items we actually buy and eat. In addition, serving sizes in restaurants, cafés, and movie theaters have grown substantially over the past 30 years. This "supersizing" phenomenon, now widespread, is an important contributor to the rise in obesity rates around the world. Thus, when using diet-planning tools, such as the USDA Food Patterns, learn the definition of a serving size for the tool you're using and measure your portions. If you don't want to gain weight, it's important to become informed about portion size.

How much physical activity do you think you'd need to perform in order to burn off the extra Calories in a larger portion size? Try the **You Do the Math** on page 52 and find out.

Despite their efforts to improve their nutrition and physical activity recommendations for Americans, the USDA and HHS have met with some criticism for the *2015–2020 Dietary Guidelines for Americans* and the MyPlate graphic. Refer to the **Nutrition Debate** at the end of this chapter to learn more about this controversy.

Consider Ethnic Variations and Other Eating Plans

As you know, the population of the United States is culturally and ethnically diverse, and this diversity influences our food choices. **FIGURE 2.9** (page 53) is a Spanish-language version of MyPlate. Like the English-language version, it recommends food groups, not specific food choices. MyPlate easily accommodates foods that we may consider part of an ethnic diet. You can also easily incorporate into MyPlate foods that match a vegetarian diet or other lifestyle preferences.

The Mediterranean diet is a healthful eating plan associated in many research studies with a reduced risk for cardiovascular disease. In fact, MyPlate incorporates many features of the Mediterranean diet. It is discussed in detail in the **In Depth** essay following this chapter. Another healthful eating plan is the DASH diet, which stands for "Dietary Approaches to Stop Hypertension." (Hypertension is high blood pressure.) This low-sodium diet emphasizes fruits, vegetables, and whole grains. For details about the DASH diet, see the **In Depth** essay following Chapter 5.

ounce-equivalent (oz-equivalent) A serving size that is 1 ounce, or equivalent to an ounce, for the grains and the protein foods sections of MyPlate.

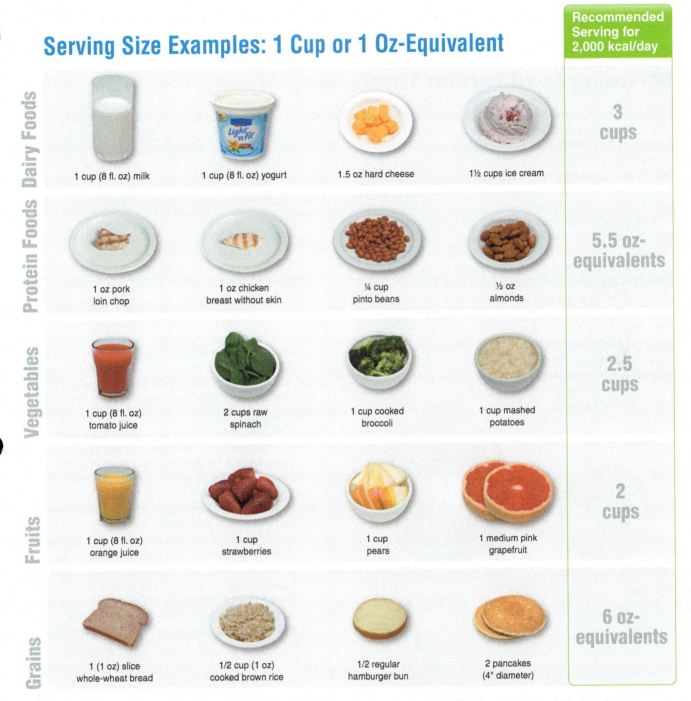

Serving Size Examples: 1 Cup or 1 Oz-Equivalent

				Recommended Serving for 2,000 kcal/day
Dairy Foods	1 cup (8 fl. oz) milk	1 cup (8 fl. oz) yogurt	1.5 oz hard cheese	1½ cups ice cream	**3 cups**
Protein Foods	1 oz pork loin chop	1 oz chicken breast without skin	¼ cup pinto beans	½ oz almonds	**5.5 oz-equivalents**
Vegetables	1 cup (8 fl. oz) tomato juice	2 cups raw spinach	1 cup cooked broccoli	1 cup mashed potatoes	**2.5 cups**
Fruits	1 cup (8 fl. oz) orange juice	1 cup strawberries	1 cup pears	1 medium pink grapefruit	**2 cups**
Grains	1 (1 oz) slice whole-wheat bread	1/2 cup (1 oz) cooked brown rice	1/2 regular hamburger bun	2 pancakes (4" diameter)	**6 oz-equivalents**

FIGURE 2.7 Examples of equivalent amounts for foods in each food group of MyPlate for a 2,000-kcal food intake pattern. Here are some examples of household items that can help you estimate amounts: 1.5 oz of hard cheese is equal to 4 stacked dice, 3 oz of meat is equal in size to a deck of cards, and half of a regular hamburger bun is the size of a yo-yo.

Get Some High-Tech Help

Many diet analysis programs are available to help you evaluate the quality of your diet. One example of a web-based tool available to the public is MyPlate Supertracker (see the **Web Links** at the end of this chapter). This tool allows you to analyze your current dietary intake and physical activity and to create personalized eating and physical activity plans. It also provides access to information on the nutrient content

you do the math

How Much Exercise Is Needed to Combat Increasing Food Portion Sizes?

Although the causes of obesity are complex, expanding food portion sizes and reduced physical activity certainly contribute. This math activity should help you better understand how portion sizes have increased over the past 20 years and how much physical activity you would need to do to expend the excess energy resulting from these larger portion sizes.

The two sets of photos in **FIGURE 2.8** give examples of foods whose portion sizes have increased substantially. A bagel 20 years ago had a diameter of approximately 3 inches and contained 140 kcal. A bagel today is about 6 inches in diameter and contains 350 kcal. Similarly, a cup of coffee 20 years ago was 8 fl. oz and was typically served with a small amount of whole milk and sugar. It contained about 45 kcal. A standard coffee mocha commonly consumed today is 16 fl. oz and contains 350 kcal; this excess energy comes from the addition of a sweet flavored syrup and a larger amount of whole milk.

20 Years Ago   **Today**

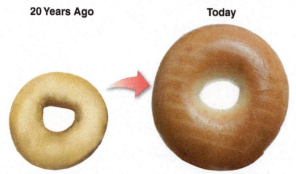

3-inch diameter, 140 Calories   6-inch diameter, 350 Calories
(a) Bagel

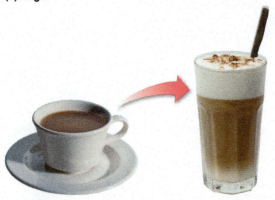

8 fluid ounces, 45 Calories   16 fluid ounces, 350 Calories
(b) Coffee

⬆ **FIGURE 2.8** Examples of increases in food portion sizes over the past 20 years. **(a)** A bagel has increased in diameter from 3 inches to 6 inches; **(b)** a cup of coffee has increased from 8 fl. oz to 16 fl. oz and now commonly contains Calorie-dense flavored syrup as well as steamed whole milk.

On her morning break at work, Judy routinely consumes a bagel and a coffee mocha. Judy has type 2 diabetes, and her doctor has advised her to lose weight. How much physical activity would Judy need to do to "burn" this excess energy? Let's do the math.

1. Calculate the excess energy Judy consumes from both of these foods:

   a. Bagel: 350 kcal in larger bagel − 140 kcal in smaller bagel = 210 kcal extra

   b. Coffee: 350 kcal in large coffee mocha − 45 kcal in small regular coffee = 305 kcal extra

   Total excess energy for these two larger portions = 515 kcal

2. Judy has started walking each day in an effort to lose weight. Judy currently weighs 200 lb. She walks at a slow pace (approximately 2 miles per hour), expending about 1.2 kcal per pound of body weight per hour. How long does Judy need to walk each day to expend 515 kcal?

   a. First, calculate how much energy Judy expends if she walks for a full hour by multiplying her body weight by the energy cost of walking per hour = 1.2 kcal/lb body weight × 200 lb = 240 kcal.

   b. Next, calculate how much energy she expends each minute she walks by dividing the energy cost of walking per hour by 60 = 240 kcal/hour ÷ 60 minutes/hour = 4 kcal/minute.

   c. To determine how many minutes she would need to walk to expend 515 kcal, divide the total amount of energy she needs to expend by the energy cost of walking per minute = 515 kcal ÷ 4 kcal/minute = 128.75 minutes.

   Thus, Judy would need to walk for about 129 minutes (2 hours and 9 minutes) to expend the excess energy in the larger bagel and coffee. If she wanted to burn off all of the energy in her morning snack, she would have to walk even longer, especially if she enjoyed her bagel with cream cheese!

   Now use your own weight in these calculations to determine how much walking you would have to do if you consumed the same foods:

   a. 1.2 kcal/lb × (your weight in pounds) = _____ kcal/hour
   (If you walk at a brisk pace, use 2.4 kcal/lb.)

   b. _____ kcal/hour ÷ 60 minutes/hour = _____ kcal/minute

   c. 515 extra kcal in bagel and coffee ÷ _____ kcal/minute = _____ minutes

of more than 8,000 foods as well as tips to support you in making more healthful choices. Using MyPlate Supertracker, you can track your current food intake and physical activity and compare it to targets you've set.

Students using this textbook also have access to MyDietAnalysis, a diet analysis software package developed by the nutrition database experts at ESHA Research. MyDietAnalysis is tailored for use in college nutrition courses, and it features a database of nearly 20,000 foods and multiple report options. This program is accurate, reliable, and easy to use in calculating the quality of your dietary intake.

In addition, anyone can access the USDA's Nutrient Database for Standard Reference to find nutrient information on more than 8,000 foods (see **Web Links** at the end of this chapter). You can also search on a specific nutrient (for instance, iron) to find out how much of that nutrient is present in a vast number of foods. The database even provides information on components of foods that are not classified as essential nutrients and are thus not typically included in diet analysis programs. These include, for example, caffeine, certain phytochemicals, and binders such as oxalic acid that can inhibit nutrient absorption. The USDA's Nutrient Database is updated annually, and any errors are identified, corrected, and highlighted for users.

Now even your cell phone can help you to eat more healthfully! Numerous apps can help you plan and keep track of healthful dietary changes. Some have you scan a barcode to get a broad nutritional profile of the food. Others help you track Calories or food additives, or to create a healthful shopping list or meal plans. Some send you a daily nutrition tip. What's more, many of these apps are free—as long as you don't mind putting up with the on-screen ads.

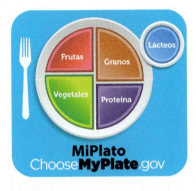

FIGURE 2.9 MiPlato is the Spanish language version of MyPlate.
(Data from: MiPlato graphic, U.S. Department of Agriculture.)

To find reviews of more than two dozen nutrition-related apps, visit the Academy of Nutrition and Dietetics at www .eatrightpro.org. In the search bar, type "App reviews."

recap The USDA Food Patterns identify daily amounts of foods and nutrient-dense choices to eat from the five major food groups: grains, vegetables, fruits, dairy, and protein foods. MyPlate is both the visual representation of the USDA Food Patterns and its accompanying website, which assists consumers in designing a personalized healthful diet. The USDA recommends that you limit the empty Calories you eat—that is, Calories from solid fats and added sugars—and that you watch your serving sizes. MyPlate easily accommodates ethnic and other diet variations. Many diet analysis programs are available online to help you evaluate the quality of your diet. One example is MyPlate Supertracker. In addition, numerous apps are available to help you design a healthful diet.

Can eating out be part of a healthful diet?

LO 6 Describe several ways to make healthful meal choices when eating out.

How many times each week do you eat out? Data from the USDA indicate that buying foods away from home now accounts for about half of all food expenditures,[2] and U.S. consumers eat away from home an average of almost five times per week.[3] Full-service restaurants and fast-food outlets are the most common sources of foods eaten away from home. Given that almost 35% of all adults in the United States are classified as obese,[4] it is imperative that we learn how to eat more healthfully when eating out.

Avoid Large Portions

TABLE 2.3 on page 54 shows an example of foods served at McDonald's and Burger King restaurants. As you can see, a regular McDonald's hamburger has only 240 kcal, whereas the Big Mac has 530 kcal. A meal of a Big Mac, large french fries, and a small McCafé Chocolate Shake provides 1,600 kcal. This meal has enough energy to support an entire day's needs for a small, lightly active woman! Similar meals at Burger King and other fast-food chains are similarly high in Calories.

Fast-food restaurants are not alone in serving large portions. Most sit-down restaurants also serve large meals, which may include bread with butter, a salad with dressing, sides of vegetables and potatoes, and free refills of sugary drinks. Combined with a popular appetizer like potato skins, fried onions, fried mozzarella sticks, or buffalo wings, it is easy to eat more than 2,000 kcal at one meal!

TABLE 2.3 Nutritional Value of Selected Fast Food

Menu Item	kcal	Fat (g)	Fat (% kcal)	Sodium (mg)
McDonald's				
Hamburger	240	8	30	480
Cheeseburger	290	11	34	680
Quarter Pounder with Cheese	520	26	45	1100
Big Mac	530	27	46	960
French fries, small	230	11	43	130
French fries, medium	340	16	42	190
French fries, large	510	24	42	290
Coke, large	280	0	0	5
McCafé Chocolate Shake (small)	560	16	26	240
McCafé Chocolate Shake (large)	850	23	24	380
Burger King				
Hamburger	230	9	35	460
Cheeseburger	270	12	40	630
Whopper	650	37	51	910
Double Whopper	900	56	56	980
Bacon Double Cheeseburger	390	21	48	790
French fries, small	340	15	40	480
French fries, medium	410	18	40	570
French fries, large	500	22	40	710

Sources: McDonald's Nutrition Choices. http://www.mcdonalds.com/us/en/food/food_quality/nutrition_choices. html; and Burger King Nutrition Information. http://www.bk.com/.

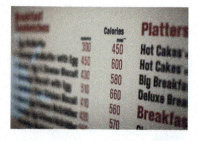

From 2016, nutritional labeling is required in chain restaurants and other food retail outlets, including Calorie information for standard menu items.

With a little education, you can avoid large portions and still enjoy eating out. Most restaurants, even fast-food restaurants, offer smaller menu items that you can choose. For instance, eating a regular McDonald's hamburger, a side salad with oil and vinegar dressing, and a diet beverage or water provides 310 kcal. Most restaurants offer smaller portions, including child's portions, or you can split your meal with a friend, or eat half and take the rest home for another meal.

Use Nutrition Information

After years of lobbying by health and nutrition professionals, the FDA has agreed to require nutrition labeling in chain restaurants and many other retail food outlets beginning in 2016. Calorie information must be posted for standard menu items on menus and menu boards, along with a brief statement about suggested daily energy intake. Other nutrient information, such as Calories from saturated fat, sodium content, and so forth must be provided in writing upon request.

A number of restaurant chains across the country have been printing nutrition information on their menus for several years, and some cities have taken the additional step of mandating menu labeling in restaurants within city limits. Have these actions influenced Americans to make more healthful food choices when eating out? Recent reviews of the research conducted in this area indicate that Calorie-labeling has not resulted in any consistent or substantive changes in food choices made by adults or children.[5,6] It also has not appeared to significantly increase the number of healthful menu options or reduce the Caloric-content of foods offered. Although some restaurants have reduced the Calories, added sugars, saturated fat, and sodium content of menu items, in most cases these foods still exceed the levels recommended for promoting health.

There is some evidence, however, that providing contextual or interpretive information may affect Calorie consumption. For example, a study conducted in adolescents examined consumption of sugar-sweetened beverages. Researchers provided easy-to-understand information about Calories, number of teaspoons of sugar, and number of minutes that one would need to run or walk to expend the Calories in the beverage. Posting this information reduced the size and number of sugar-sweetened beverages that the adolescents purchased, and these changes persisted for 6 weeks after the signs were removed.[7]

Next time you eat out, examine the menu before ordering. Look for "lite" menu items, such as grilled or broiled chicken or fish with vegetables. Avoid fried meats. If you're ordering a sandwich, ask for whole-grain bread, and for a salad instead of french fries or chips as a side. The nearby **Quick Tips** provide more suggestions on how to eat right when you're eating out.

recap Healthful ways to eat out include choosing smaller menu portions, splitting a meal with a friend, or taking part of the meal home. Order meats that are grilled or broiled, avoiding meats that are fried. Choose meals accompanied with vegetables or a salad, and avoid energy-rich appetizers, beverages such as sugary drinks, desserts. Although posting Calorie and other nutrition information on menus does not appear to reduce energy intake, providing interpretive information, such as by identifying how much exercise would be needed to burn the Calories in a sugary drink, may help consumers choose more wisely.

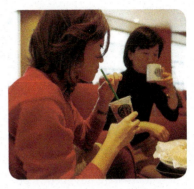

◆ When ordering your favorite coffee drink, avoid flavored syrups, cream, and whipping cream and request reduced-fat or skim milk instead.

Quick Tips

Eating Right When You're Eating Out

✔ Avoid all-you-can-eat buffet-style restaurants.

✔ Avoid appetizers that are breaded, fried, or filled with cheese or meat, or skip the appetizer altogether.

✔ Order a healthful appetizer instead of a larger meal as an entrée.

✔ Order your meal from the children's menu or share it with a friend.

✔ Order broth-based soups instead of cream-based soups.

✔ If you order meat, select a lean cut and ask that it be grilled or broiled rather than fried or breaded.

✔ Instead of a beef burger, order a chicken burger, fish burger, or veggie burger.

✔ Order a meatless dish filled with vegetables and whole grains. Avoid dishes with cream sauces and a lot of cheese.

✔ Order a salad with low-fat or nonfat dressing served on the side.

✔ Order steamed vegetables on the side instead of potatoes or rice. If you order potatoes, make sure to get a baked potato (with very little butter or sour cream on the side).

✔ Order beverages with few or no Calories, such as water, tea, or diet drinks. Avoid coffee drinks made with syrups as well as those made with cream or topped with whipped cream.

✔ Don't feel you have to eat everything you're served. If you feel full, take the rest home for another meal.

✔ Skip dessert or share one dessert with a lot of friends, or order fresh fruit for dessert.

✔ Watch out for those "yogurt parfaits" offered at some fast-food restaurants. Many are loaded with added sugar and Calories.

Nutrition Advice from the U.S. Government: Is Anyone Listening?

The *2015–2020 Dietary Guidelines for Americans* (DGAs) were released in January 2016. They continue to be accompanied by the MyPlate graphic and website (www.chooseMyPlate.gov) that were released in 2011 to support the 2010 DGAs. These tools were designed to be practical and user-friendly, so that they would help people to eat more healthfully and reduce their risk for obesity and other chronic diseases. But are they based on scientific consensus? And do people actually consult them for meal planning, shopping, or eating out? Moreover, is there any evidence that the DGAs and MyPlate improve the health of Americans?

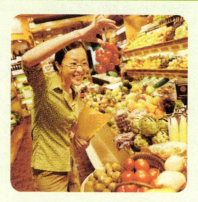

The Dietary Guidelines for Americans can help consumers make healthful food choices—if consumers actually use them.

To begin to answer these questions, let's review the changes made in revising the 2010 DGAs into the 2015–2020 DGAs:[8]

- Instead of focusing on food groups and nutrients, the updated DGAs recommend following a healthful eating pattern. They remind consumers that every food and beverage choice influences their health.

- Specifically, the updated DGAs advise limiting intake of added sugars to less than 10% of total daily energy intake.

- They also suggest consuming less than 10% of total energy from saturated fat; however, in recognition of the health benefits of unsaturated fats, the 2010 upper limit for total energy intake from fat is gone.

- The 2010 recommendation to limit dietary cholesterol intake to 300 mg per day is also gone; the recommendation now states that individuals should consume as little dietary cholesterol as possible.

Despite these updates, concerns are being expressed about the failure of the 2015–2020 DGAs to include all of the recommendations put forth in the report of the Dietary Guidelines Advisory Committee, which is the committee that reviewed the current scientific evidence on the impact of diet and health. Two omissions of concern are the following:[8]

- A recommendation to reduce consumption of red and processed meat. This recommendation was made because of the association of red and processed meat intake with increased risk for cardiovascular disease and some cancers, as well as to support a more sustainable and secure food supply. (For more information on the environmental costs of beef production, see Chapter 13.)

- A recommendation to reduce consumption of sugar-sweetened beverages. This recommendation reflects the association of high intake of sugar-sweetened beverages with increased risks for obesity and type 2 diabetes.

A further concern is the potential for conflicts of interest to arise within the UDSA when developing the guidelines. In other words, do industry groups such as the National Cattlemen's Beef Association and the American Beverage Association "purchase" recommendations—or limitations on recommendations—that favor their profits over public health? Experts have argued that, to protect their profit margin, lobbyists from the food and agricultural industries exert undue influence over the Guidelines, and that this influence has prompted officials from the USDA to disregard or minimize scientific evidence of the benefits or health risks of various foods.[8]

No matter what the strengths and limitations of the DGAs and MyPlate might be, a bigger question arises—is anyone listening? Early research examining this question in the context of the 2005 DGAs found that less than half of Americans 17 years of age and older had even heard of them.[9] A more recent study exploring this question after the publication of the 2010 DGAs and 2011 MyPlate found that, despite media coverage, awareness of these tools was less than 25% in those sampled, including only about 6% in college students![10]

The goal of the DGAs and MyPlate is to help reduce obesity and chronic disease in the United States. The primary assumption made is that people will actually use these tools to design their diets; however, the limited evidence currently available suggests that only a minority of people are even aware of them, let alone use them in their daily lives. Clearly, more research is needed to determine whether Americans follow the DGA and MyPlate recommendations, and if so, whether these changes have a positive impact on public health. Until such evidence is assessed, the debate about their value will continue.

CRITICAL THINKING QUESTIONS

1. How would you redesign and market MyPlate to make it more useful and accessible to the general public?
2. Do you think any federal guidelines can make a difference in how Americans eat? If so, why? If not, how might the money used to develop these guidelines be better spent?
3. Conduct your own research into how well the 2015–2020 DGAs[11] follow the recommendations put forth in the *Scientific Report* of the 2015 Dietary Guidelines Advisory Committee.[12] Identify at least two areas of discrepancy not discussed in this debate.

STUDY PLAN MasteringNutrition™

1 F Detailed food labels are not required for meat or poultry, as these products are regulated by the U.S. Department of Agriculture, or for coffee and most spices, as they contain insignificant amounts of all the nutrients that must be listed on food labels. Fresh produce and seafood are also exempt, with a voluntary nutrition labeling program covering these foods to include labels on shelves and posters.

2 F A cup of black coffee with a tablespoon of cream and a teaspoon of sugar has about 45 kcal. In contrast, a coffee mocha might contain from 350 to 500 kcal, depending on its size and precise contents.

3 T It is possible to eat healthfully when dining out by choosing restaurants that serve healthful foods, selecting menu items that are low in saturated fat and added sugars, and consuming smaller portions.

review questions

LO 1 **1.** A nutrient-dense diet
- **a.** provides ample nutrients to maintain a person's health.
- **b.** provides a variety of foods and beverages from all food groups.
- **c.** is based on foods that provide a high level of nutrients and fiber for a relatively low number of Calories.
- **d.** contains combinations of foods that provide 100% of the Recommended Dietary Allowance for all nutrients.

LO 2 **2.** Which of the following statements about food choices is true?
- **a.** If you have not tasted Ethiopian food before the end of your teen years, you will never enjoy it as an adult.
- **b.** A conditioned taste aversion to pork sausages could develop in a person who learns how they are made.
- **c.** Immigrants almost never adopt the diet typical of their new home.
- **d.** Much of our ability to smell foods actually comes from our sense of taste.

LO 3 **3.** The Nutrition Facts panel on food labels identifies which of the following?
- **a.** all of the nutrients and Calories in the package of food
- **b.** the Recommended Dietary Allowance for each nutrient in the food

- **c.** a footnote identifying the Tolerable Upper Intake Level for each nutrient in the food
- **d.** the % Daily Value of select nutrients in one serving of the food

LO 4 **4.** The Dietary Guidelines for Americans recommend which of the following?
- **a.** limiting intake of added sugars, saturated fats, and sodium
- **b.** consuming one to two alcoholic beverages per day
- **c.** losing weight by reducing Calorie intake and increasing physical activity
- **d.** following a vegetarian eating pattern

LO 5 **5.** Of the five food groups in MyPlate, which should make up half of your plate?
- **a.** protein
- **b.** grains and vegetables
- **c.** fruits and dairy
- **d.** fruits and vegetables

LO 5 **6.** An ounce-equivalent is
- **a.** a 1-ounce serving of bread, rice, or another grain, or a 1-ounce serving of a protein food.
- **b.** a serving that is 1 ounce or equivalent to an ounce for either grains or protein foods.
- **c.** a serving that is actually an ounce or is designated as a single serving on a food label for a grain or protein food.
- **d.** an ounce of a grain or protein food that you weigh and serve yourself.

LO 6   **7.** Which of the following statements about eating out is true?

    a. U.S. consumers eat away from home an average of twice per week.

    b. Dining at a fast-food restaurant is far more likely to result in excessive Calorie intake than dining at a sit-down restaurant.

    c. Fried chicken is a more healthful choice than a broiled chicken breast.

    d. None of the above is true.

LO 3   **8.** True or false? Structure–function claims on food labels do not require FDA approval.

LO 5   **9.** True or false? Empty Calories are the extra amount of energy a person can consume after meeting all essential needs through eating nutrient-dense foods.

LO 6   **10.** True or false? Calorie labeling on menus has greatly improved the food choices made by consumers eating out.

math review

LO 6   **11.** Hannah goes to a sandwich shop near the university at least once a week to buy what she considers a healthful lunch, which includes a chicken breast sandwich, garden salad (with Ranch dressing), and a diet cola. Recently, the shop started posting nutrition information for its menu items. Hannah discovers the following about the Calorie and sodium content of the items in her "healthful lunch":

- Chicken sandwich—360 Calories, 960 mg sodium
- Garden salad—49 Calories, 0 mg sodium
- Ranch dressing (1 packet)—290 Calories, 656 mg sodium

- Diet cola (12 ounces)—0 Calories, 40 mg sodium

Based on this information, what is the total Calorie content of Hannah's lunch? What is the sodium content? The 2015–2020 Dietary Guidelines recommend keeping sodium intake to less than 2,300 mg per day. What percentage of this daily limit is provided by Hannah's lunch? While choosing the same sandwich, what simple change she could make in her lunch to reduce the total Calories and sodium?

Answers to Review Questions and Math Review are located at the back of this text and in the Mastering Nutrition Study Area.

web links

www.fda.gov
U.S. Food and Drug Administration
Learn more about the government agency that regulates our food and first established regulations for nutrition information on food labels.

health.gov/dietaryguidelines/2015/guidelines/
2015–2020 Dietary Guidelines for Americans
Use these guidelines to make changes in your food choices and physical activity habits to help reduce your risk for chronic disease.

www.choosemyplate.gov
The USDA's MyPlate Home Page
Use the SuperTracker on this website to assess the overall quality of your diet and level of physical activity based on the USDA MyPlate.

www.eatright.org
Academy of Nutrition and Dietetics
Visit the Health section of this website for additional resources to help you achieve a healthful lifestyle.

ndb.nal.usda.gov/
U.S. Department of Agriculture National Nutrient Databases
Search this site to find nutrition information on more than 8,000 foods, and to find foods that are high in a particular nutrient of interest.

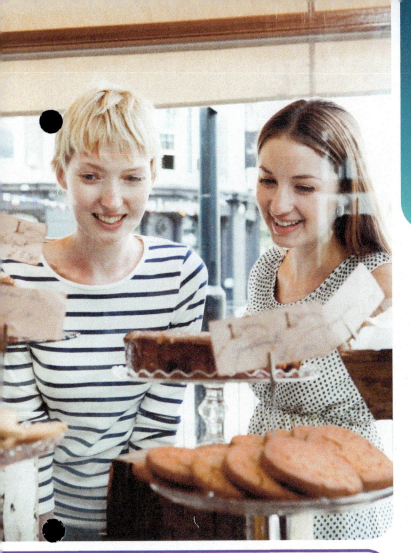

Healthful Eating Patterns

learning outcomes

After studying this In Depth, you should be able to:

1 Identify the components and principles of a healthful eating pattern, pp. 60–61.

2 Describe at least two healthful eating patterns recommended by public health experts, pp. 61–63.

You and a friend have just finished dining at your favorite Thai restaurant. As you walk back toward your residence hall, you pass a bakery window displaying cakes and pies, each of which looks more enticing than the last. You stop. You're not hungry, but . . . one little treat wouldn't hurt, would it?

Although an occasional treat doesn't harm us, every food choice we make influences our health—by boosting our body's supply of important nutrients, fiber, and phytochemicals, or contributing added sugars, saturated fats, and Calories. When empty-Calorie foods frequently replace nutrient-dense choices, we've fallen into an eating pattern that's associated with obesity and chronic disease. How do we get out of this pattern? Here we take an **In Depth** look at the components and principles of a healthful eating pattern and explore several healthful patterns supported by extensive research and widely recommended by public health experts.

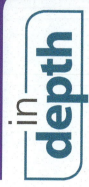
What is a healthful eating pattern?

LO 1 Identify the components and principles of a healthful eating pattern

The *2015–2020 Dietary Guidelines for Americans* (DGAs)[1] reflect current evidence that healthful eating patterns are critical to achieving and maintaining good health and reducing the risks for obesity and chronic disease across the lifespan. But what exactly is a healthful eating pattern? Let's explore its food components and underlying principles.

The DGAs identify the following components of a healthful eating pattern:

- A variety of vegetables, including dark green, orange, red, legumes (beans and peas), and starchy vegetables such as yams, sweet potatoes, and corn
- Fruits, particularly whole fruits
- Whole grains and cereals
- Low-fat and fat-free dairy products or alternatives, including milk, yogurt, cheese, and fortified soy beverages
- A variety of protein foods such as fish, lean meats, eggs, poultry, legumes, nuts and seeds, and soy products
- Oils

As discussed in more detail in Chapter 2 (page 38), a healthful eating pattern is also limited in added sugars, saturated and *trans* fats, sodium, and alcohol.

Additionally, a healthful eating pattern is founded on three dietary principles **(FIGURE 1)**:[1]

- An eating pattern includes all foods and beverages consumed. As a result, everything you consume "counts" and needs to be considered when you follow a healthful eating pattern.
- Nutrient needs should be met primarily from nutrient-dense foods. Although there are situations when it is acceptable, appropriate, or even necessary to include empty-Calorie foods, processed foods, or dietary supplements into a healthful eating pattern, you should meet as many of your nutritional needs as possible from nutrient-dense foods.
- Healthful eating patterns are adaptable, which means that there are many ways to achieve a healthful pattern within your sociocultural environment, budget, and personal preferences.

Unfortunately, most Americans do not follow a healthful eating pattern. Consider the following examples:[2]

- Overall, nearly 90% of Americans

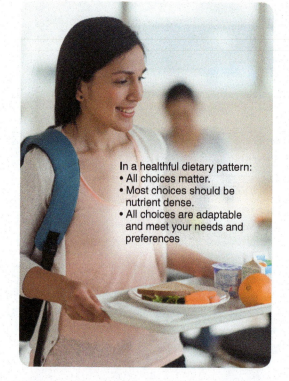

In a healthful dietary pattern:
- All choices matter.
- Most choices should be nutrient dense.
- All choices are adaptable and meet your needs and preferences

⬆ **FIGURE 1** Principles of a healthful eating pattern.

fail to meet their daily intake recommendations for vegetables, and 80% fail to meet their intake recommendations for fruits.
- Nearly 100% of Americans fail to meet their daily intake recommendations for whole grains.
- Nearly 90% of Americans consume more than the recommended levels of added sugars and saturated fats.

nutri-case | JUDY

"Ever since I was diagnosed with type 2 diabetes, I've felt like there's a 'food cop' always spying on me. Sometimes I feel like I have to look over my shoulder when I pull into the Dunkin' Donuts parking lot. My doctor says I'm supposed to eat fresh fruits and vegetables, fish, brown bread, brown rice . . . but I didn't tell him I don't like that stuff, and I don't have the money to buy it or the time to cook it even if I did. Besides, that kind of diet is for movie stars. All the real people I know eat the same way I do."

What do you think? Is the diet Judy's doctor described really just for movie stars and celebrities? If you could suggest a few strategies to help Judy begin to follow a more healthful eating pattern, what would they be?

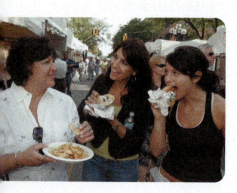

Thus, it's not surprising that more than two-thirds of American adults are overweight or obese, and about half have one or more preventable chronic diseases related to an unhealthful dietary pattern and low levels of physical activity.[2]

What are some healthful eating patterns?

LO 2 Describe at least two healthful eating patterns recommended by public health experts.

In Chapter 2, you learned how to design a healthful diet by reading food labels and following the Dietary Guidelines for Americans and the USDA Food Patterns. Here, we provide an overview of the Mediterranean diet and other tools that can guide you in following a healthful eating pattern. In the **In Depth** essay following Chapter 5, you'll learn more about another healthful eating pattern introduced in Chapter 2, the DASH diet.

A Mediterranean-Style Eating Pattern Is Healthful

The Mediterranean diet has received significant attention for many years, largely because the rates of cardiovascular disease in many Mediterranean countries are substantially lower than rates in the United States.[3] There is actually not a single Mediterranean diet because this region of the world includes Portugal, Spain, Italy, France, Greece, Turkey, and Israel. Each of these countries has different dietary patterns; however, there are many similarities. Aspects of the Mediterranean-style pattern seen as more healthful than the typical U.S. diet include the following (FIGURE 2):

- Red meat is eaten only monthly, and eggs, poultry, fish, and sweets are eaten weekly, making the diet low in saturated fats and refined sugars.
- The primary fat used for cooking and flavor is olive oil, making the diet high in monounsaturated fats.
- Foods eaten daily include grains, such as bread, pasta, couscous, and bulgur; fruits; beans and other legumes; nuts; vegetables; and cheese and yogurt. These choices make this diet high in vitamins and minerals, fiber, phytochemicals, probiotics, and prebiotics.
- Wine is included, in moderation.

If you were following a Mediterranean-style eating pattern, you'd consume beans, other legumes, and nuts as daily sources of protein; fish, poultry, and eggs weekly; and red meat only about once each month. For dairy choices, you would eat cheese and yogurt in moderation, and you'd drink water or wine (in moderation) rather than milk.

What does research say about the health benefits of a Mediterranean-style eating pattern? Studies over many years indicate that this type of eating plan reduces the risks for cardiovascular disease, even when Calories are not restricted,[3,4] with some evidence suggesting it may also reduce the risks for cognitive decline and Alzheimer's disease.[5]

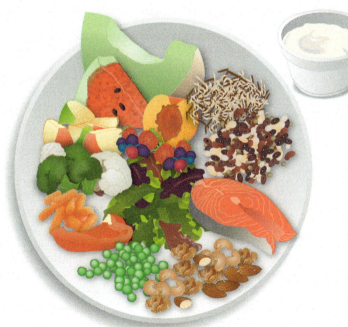

- Vegetables, fruits, nuts, beans and other legumes, whole grains, cheese and yogurt consumed daily.

- Eggs, poultry, and fish consumed weekly.

- Red meat consumed once per month.

- Olive oil is the predominant fat used for cooking and flavor.

- Wine is consumed in moderation.

◆ **FIGURE 2** Foods associated with a Mediterranean-style eating pattern.

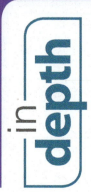

The Exchange System Can Help You Follow a Healthful Eating Pattern

The **exchange system** is another tool you can use to follow a healthful eating pattern. This system was originally designed for people with diabetes by the American Dietetic Association (now known as the Academy of Nutrition and Dietetics) and the American Diabetes Association. It has also been used successfully in weight-loss programs. Exchanges, or portions, of food are organized into six lists according to the amount of carbohydrate, protein, fat, and Calories in each. The six exchange lists are starch/bread, meat and meat substitutes, vegetables, fruits, milk, and fat. In addition to these lists, others include free foods (any food or drink less than 20 Calories per serving), combination foods (foods such as soups, casseroles, and pizza), and special-occasion foods (desserts such as cakes, cookies, and ice cream). Refer to the **Web Links** at the end of this essay to locate an interactive tool that can help you use the exchange system.

The Healthy Eating Plate and Power Plate Are Also Healthful Eating Patterns

Two alternatives to MyPlate have been developed to assist people with designing and following a healthful eating pattern. These include the Healthy Eating Plate developed by the Harvard School of Public Health and the Power Plate from the Physicians Committee for Responsible Medicine.

The Healthy Eating Plate recommends using plant oils and avoiding *trans* fat; consuming virtually all grains as whole grains; consuming more vegetables (potatoes and

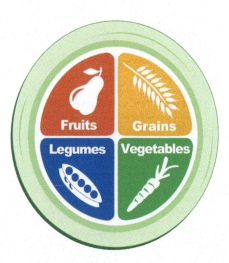

▲ **FIGURE 3** The Power Plate has been proposed by the Physicians Committee for Responsible Medicine.

QuickTips

Following a Healthful Eating Pattern

✓ Focus on all the foods and beverages you consume, as all choices "count"!

✓ Instead of eating mostly tomatoes and potatoes, try vegetables across the range of colors and textures.

✓ Choose to eat a whole peeled orange instead of opting for orange juice.

✓ Select unsweetened whole-grain foods, such as regular oatmeal or whole-grain pasta, instead of flavored oatmeal and white pasta.

✓ Try unsweetened yogurt instead of a flavored yogurt that contains added sugars, and top with a few fresh blueberries or peach slices for a naturally sweet treat.

✓ Incorporate legumes, nuts, and seeds into two meals per week in place of meat, poultry, or eggs to increase your intake of these nutrient-dense protein foods.

✓ Instead of salting your food during cooking, try adding different herbs and spices.

✓ If you eat meat, avoid processed and cured meats to reduce your sodium intake and your risk for certain types of cancer.

✓ Try following a Mediterranean-style eating pattern for a week.

French fries don't count!); selecting lean protein sources from fish, poultry, beans and nuts; and drinking water, tea, or coffee with little or no added sugar. It also emphasizes daily physical activity. Check the **Web Links** at the end of this **In Depth** essay to find out more.

The Power Plate emphasizes the "four food groups": fruits, legumes, other vegetables, and whole grains **(FIGURE 3)**. Nuts and seeds are also allowed. This eating pattern is low in added sugars, saturated fats, and sodium, and high in fiber. The Physicians Committee for Responsible Medicine claims that the Power Plate is "powerful" in helping reduce your risk for obesity, cardiovascular disease, diabetes, and cancer.[6] The website listed in the **Web Links** provides more information, including recipes for increasing your intake of the "four food groups."

exchange system A diet planning tool in which exchanges, or portions, are organized according to the amount of carbohydrate, protein, fat, and Calories in each food.

Include Regular Physical Activity

The DGAs include a key recommendation that people should meet the current Physical Activity Guidelines for Americans. They state that adults should engage in at least 150 minutes per week of moderate intensity physical activity, and should perform muscle-strengthening exercises on 2 or more days per week.

The benefits of physical activity are numerous. In addition to assisting with maintaining a healthful body weight and reducing our risks for cardiovascular disease, type 2 diabetes, some cancers, and osteoporosis, regular physical activity supports digestion, improves sleep, enhances mood, and even promotes a longer life. The Physical Activity Guidelines for Americans, and the benefits of physical activity, are discussed in more detail in Chapter 11.

web links

www.eatright.org
Academy of Nutrition and Dietetics

Explore a range of tips to help you eat more healthfully throughout the year.

health.gov/dietaryguidelines/2015/guidelines/
2015–2020 Dietary Guidelines for Americans

Use these guidelines to help you design and follow a healthful eating pattern.

www.diabetes.org
American Diabetes Association

Access an interactive tool that can help you use the exchange system to design a healthful eating pattern. Click on the "Food and Fitness" tab at the top of the home page, select "Food," and then select "Planning Meals." Click on "Create Your Plate."

www.hsph.harvard.edu
Harvard School of Public Health

Scroll down to "The Nutrition Source" on this site to learn more about the Healthy Eating Plate, an alternative to the USDA MyPlate.

www.pcrm.org
Physicians Committee for Responsible Medicine

Visit this site to learn more about the Power Plate, a vegetarian alternative to the USDA MyPlate. Choose "Health and Nutrition" from the left-hand menu, then select "Vegetarian and Vegan Diets" for details.

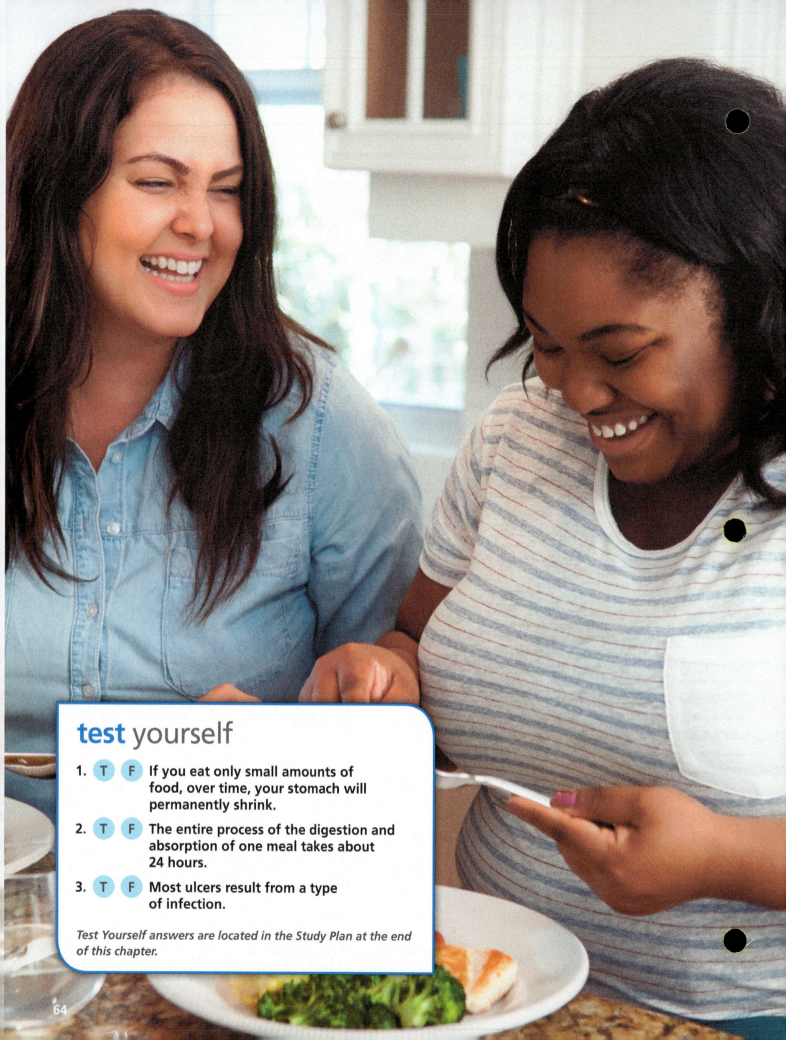

test yourself

1. **T F** If you eat only small amounts of food, over time, your stomach will permanently shrink.

2. **T F** The entire process of the digestion and absorption of one meal takes about 24 hours.

3. **T F** Most ulcers result from a type of infection.

Test Yourself answers are located in the Study Plan at the end of this chapter.

3

The Human Body
Are we really what we eat?

learning outcomes

After studying this chapter you should be able to:

1 Describe the structures of the human body from smallest to largest, pp. 66–68.

2 Identify the mechanisms that contribute to our sense of hunger, pp. 68–70.

3 Identify each organ food encounters on its way through the gastrointestinal tract, and its primary function, pp. 70–79.

4 Describe the specialized organs and features that contribute to gastrointestinal function, pp. 79–85.

5 Discuss the causes, symptoms, and treatments of several common disorders affecting digestion, absorption, and elimination, pp. 85–89.

Two months ago, Andrea's dream of becoming a lawyer came one step closer to reality: she moved out of her parents' home in Michigan to study political science at a university in Washington, DC. Unfortunately, adjusting to a new city and a full load of college classes was more stressful than she'd imagined, and her always "sensitive stomach" began to act up: after eating, she'd get painful abdominal cramps and sometimes diarrhea. Suspecting that the problem was related to stress, she enrolled in a stress-management seminar that helped her prioritize her workload. There, she made friends with another stressed-out student from Michigan, and they've begun studying, exercising, and just hanging out together. Now that she's more relaxed, her symptoms rarely bother her anymore.

Almost everyone experiences brief episodes of abdominal pain and diarrhea from time to time. They're often caused by an infection, but stress is a common culprit, too. To understand why, it helps to know the structures and steps involved in the digestion of food, absorption of nutrients, and elimination of wastes, including the points at which the process can break down.

MasteringNutrition™
Go online for chapter quizzes, pre-tests, interactive activities, and more!

LO 1 Describe the structures of the human body from smallest to largest.

How do food molecules build body structure?

You've no doubt heard the saying "You are what you eat." Is this scientifically true? To answer that question, and to better understand how we digest and process foods, we'll need to look at how the body is organized (FIGURE 3.1).

Atoms Bond to Form Molecules

The human body is made up of atoms, tiny units of matter that cannot be broken down by natural means. Atoms almost constantly bind to each other in nature. When they do, they form groups called molecules. For example, a molecule of water is composed of two atoms of hydrogen and an atom of oxygen, which is abbreviated H_2O.

Not only the liquids we drink, but every bite of food we eat is composed of molecules. Rice, for instance, is composed of atoms of carbon, hydrogen, and oxygen grouped into large carbohydrate molecules. The actions of digestion break food down into molecules small enough to be absorbed easily through the wall of the intestine and transported in the bloodstream to every part of the body. We convert these molecules into the energy we need to live and the chemicals our body needs to function. We also use them to build, maintain, and repair body structures, the smallest of which are the components of individual body cells.

Molecules Join to Form Cells

Cells are the smallest units of life. That is, cells can grow, reproduce, and perform certain basic functions, such as taking in nutrients, producing chemicals, and excreting wastes. The human body is composed of trillions of cells, many of which have short

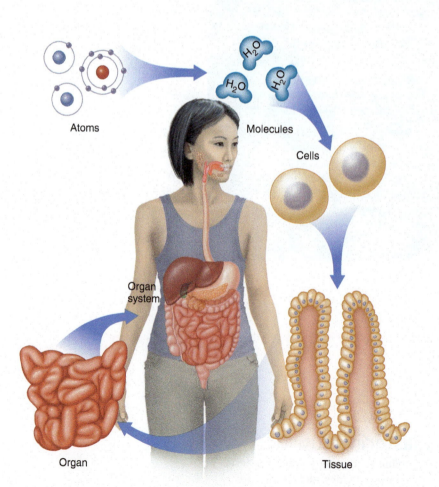

▶ **FIGURE 3.1** The organization of the human body. Atoms bond to form molecules. Body cells are composed of molecules of the foods we eat. Cells join to form tissues, which combine to form organs, such as the small intestine. Body systems, such as the gastrointestinal system, are made up of several organs, each of which performs a discrete function within that system.

Atoms

Molecules

Cells

Organ system

Organ

Tissue

life spans and must be replaced continually. For example, **enterocytes**, the cells lining the intestine, live only a few days (*entero-* is a prefix referring to the intestine, and *-cyte* means cell). To support this demand for new cells, we need a ready supply of nutrient molecules to serve as building blocks. All cells, whether of the intestine, bones, or brain, are made of the same basic nutrient molecules, which are derived from the foods we eat.

From Cells to Systems

Cells of a single type, such as enterocytes, join to form functional sheets or cords of cells called **tissues**. In general, several types of tissues join together to form **organs**, which are sophisticated structures that perform unique body functions. The stomach and the small intestine are examples of organs.

Organs are further grouped into **systems** that perform integrated functions. The stomach, for example, is part of the gastrointestinal system (*gastro-* refers to the stomach). It holds and partially digests a meal, but achieving all of the system's functions—digestion, absorption, and elimination—requires the cooperation of several organs.

The Cell Membrane

Cells are encased by a thin covering called a **cell membrane** (FIGURE 3.2). This membrane defines the cell's boundaries: it encloses the cell's contents and acts as a gatekeeper, either allowing or denying the entry and exit of molecules, such as nutrients and wastes.

cell The smallest unit of matter that exhibits the properties of living things, such as growth and metabolism.

enterocytes The cells lining the wall of the intestine.

tissue A grouping of like cells that performs a function; for example, muscle tissue.

organ A body structure composed of two or more tissues and performing a specific function; for example, the esophagus.

system A group of organs that work together to perform a unique function; for example, the gastrointestinal system.

cell membrane The boundary of an animal cell that separates its internal cytoplasm and organelles from the external environment.

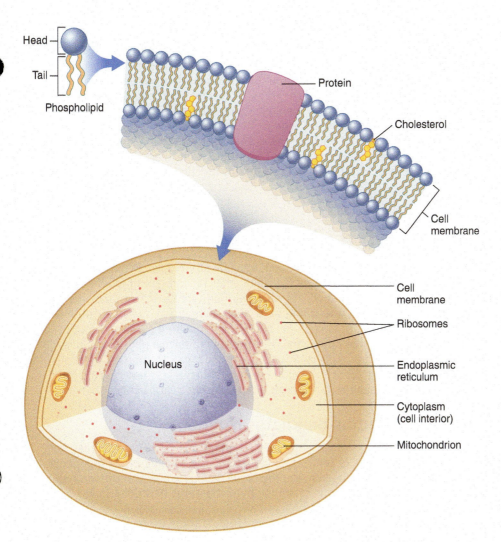

FIGURE 3.2 Representative enterocyte, showing the cell membrane, cytoplasm, and a variety of organelles. The cell membrane is a double layer of phospholipid molecules, aligned such that the lipid tails form a water-repellant interior, whereas the phosphate heads interact with the fluids inside and outside the cell. The fluid inside the cell is the cytoplasm. Within it are many different organelles.

Cell membranes are composed of two layers of molecules called phospholipids, which consist of a long lipid "tail" that repels water, bound to a round phosphate "head" that interacts with water. Located throughout the membrane are molecules of another lipid, cholesterol, which helps keep the membrane flexible. The membrane is also studded with various proteins, which assist in the gatekeeper function, allowing the transport of nutrients and other substances across the cell membrane.

Cytoplasm and Key Organelles

The cell membrane encloses the semiliquid **cytoplasm** (see Figure 3.2), which includes a variety of **organelles**. These tiny structures accomplish some surprisingly sophisticated functions. In terms of nutrition, the most important organelles are the following:

- **Nucleus.** The nucleus is where our genetic information, in the form of deoxyribonucleic acid (DNA), is located. The cell nucleus is darkly colored because DNA is a huge molecule that is tightly packed within it. A cell's DNA contains the instructions that the cell uses to make certain proteins.
- **Ribosomes.** Ribosomes use the instructions from DNA to assemble proteins.
- **Endoplasmic reticulum (ER).** Proteins assembled on the ribosomes enter this network of channels and are further processed and packaged for transport. The ER is also responsible for the synthesis of lipids and many other cell functions.
- **Mitochondria.** Often called the cell's powerhouses, mitochondria produce the energy molecule adenosine triphosphate (ATP) from basic food components. ATP can be thought of as a stored form of energy that can be drawn upon as cells need it. Cells that have high energy needs—such as muscle cells—contain more mitochondria than do cells with low energy needs.

recap The smallest units of matter are atoms—such as carbon, hydrogen, and oxygen—which join to form molecules. The body uses food molecules for energy, for the production of functional chemicals, and for building, maintaining, and repairing body structures. Molecules are the building blocks of cells, the smallest units of life. Different cell types give rise to different tissue types and ultimately to all of the different organs of the body. A system is a group of organs that together accomplish a body function. Cells are encased in a membrane, which helps the cell regulate the entry and exit of various molecules. The cell membrane encloses a fluid called cytoplasm, which contains functional units called organelles.

LO 2 Identify the mechanisms that contribute to our sense of hunger.

Why do we feel the urge to eat?

Two mechanisms prompt us to seek food: appetite and hunger. Whereas appetite is a desire to eat that is stimulated by the sight, smell, or thought of food, **hunger** is a physiologic drive to eat that occurs when our body senses that we need food. If you've recently finished a nourishing meal, then hunger won't compel you toward dessert. Instead, the culprit is appetite, which we commonly experience in the absence of hunger. On the other hand, it is possible to have a physiologic need for food yet have no appetite. This state, called **anorexia**, can accompany a variety of illnesses, from infectious diseases to mood disorders. It can also occur as a side effect of certain medications, such as the chemotherapy used in treating cancer patients.

The Hypothalamus Regulates Hunger

Because hunger is a physiologic stimulus that drives us to find food and eat, we often feel it as a negative or unpleasant sensation. The primary organ producing that sensation is not the stomach, but the brain. The region of brain tissue responsible for prompting us to seek food is called the **hypothalamus (FIGURE 3.3)**. It's located above the pituitary gland in the forebrain, a region that regulates many types of involuntary activity.

cytoplasm The interior of an animal cell, not including its nucleus.

organelle A tiny "organ" within a cell that performs a discrete function necessary to the cell.

hunger A physiologic drive for food.

anorexia An absence of appetite.

hypothalamus A region of the forebrain above the pituitary gland, where visceral sensations, such as hunger and thirst, are regulated.

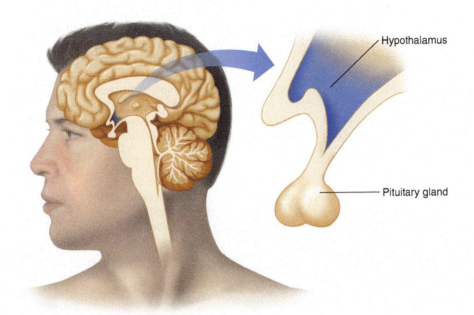

◀ **FIGURE 3.3** The hypothalamus triggers hunger by integrating signals from nerve cells throughout the body as well as from messages carried by hormones.

The hypothalamus contains a cluster of nerve cells known collectively as the *feeding center*. Stimulation of the feeding center triggers feelings of hunger that drive us to eat. In contrast, signals from a cluster of cells called the *satiety center* (**satiety** means fullness) inhibit the feeding center cells. This prompts us to stop eating.

The feeding and satiety centers work together to regulate food intake by integrating signals from three sources: nerve cells in the gastrointestinal system, chemicals called *hormones*, and the amount and type of food we eat.

Nerve Cells in the Gastrointestinal System Signal the Hypothalamus

One important signal for both hunger and satiety comes from nerve cells lining the stomach and small intestine. These cells detect changes in pressure according to whether the organ is empty or distended with food. The cells then relay these data to the hypothalamus. For instance, if you have not eaten for many hours and your stomach and small intestine do not contain food, signals transmitted to the hypothalamus will suppress the satiety center, allowing the feeding center to dominate. This in turn will cause you to experience the sensation of hunger.

Nerve cells in the mouth, pharynx (throat), and esophagus (the tube leading to the stomach) also contribute to our feelings of hunger and satiety. Chewing and swallowing food, for example, stimulates these nerve cells, which then relay data to the satiety center in the hypothalamus. As a result, we begin to feel full.

Hormones Send Chemical Messages to the Hypothalamus

Hormones are molecules, usually proteins or lipids, that are secreted into the bloodstream by one of the many *glands* of the body. In the bloodstream, they act as chemical messengers, binding to and triggering a response in target cells far away from the gland in which they were produced. The relative levels of different hormones in the blood help regulate many body functions. Of the many hormones involved in food intake, the following are the most significant.

Insulin and Glucagon

Insulin and glucagon are two hormones responsible for maintaining blood glucose levels. Glucose (a carbohydrate) is our body's most readily available fuel supply.

satiety A physiologic sensation of fullness (from the Latin *satis* meaning enough, as in *satisfied*).

hormone A chemical messenger secreted into the bloodstream by a gland. Hormones regulate physiologic processes at sites distant from the glands that secrete them.

It's not surprising, then, that its level in the blood is an important signal affecting hunger. When we have not eaten for a while, our blood glucose levels fall, prompting a decrease in the level of insulin and an increase in glucagon. This chemical message is relayed to the hypothalamus, which then prompts us to eat in order to supply our body with more glucose.

After we eat, the hypothalamus picks up the sensation of distention in the stomach and intestine. In addition, as our body begins to absorb the nutrients from a meal, blood glucose levels rise. This triggers an increase in insulin secretion and a decrease in glucagon. When the hypothalamus integrates these signals, we experience satiety.

Ghrelin, CCK, and Leptin

The hormone ghrelin, which is produced by the stomach, is considered a physiologic "hunger hormone." Immediately after a meal, ghrelin levels plummet. As time since our last meal elapses, ghrelin levels begin to rise, eventually triggering the hypothalamus to induce us to eat. As you might suppose, dramatically restricting our food intake, as when dieting for weight loss, causes ghrelin levels to surge.

Opposite in action to ghrelin is the hormone cholecystokinin (CCK), which is produced in the small intestine in response to food entry. CCK causes the transmission of signals to the hypothalamus that trigger satiety, reducing both how long we eat and how much.

The hormones we've discussed so far act in short-term regulation of food intake. But our body produces other hormones that regulate food intake over time. One of the most important of these is leptin, a protein hormone. When we consume more energy than we burn, whether as carbohydrate, fat, or protein, the excess is converted to fat and stored in adipose cells (fat cells). These cells produce leptin, which acts on the hypothalamus to induce satiety. Unfortunately, obese people appear to have higher-than-average levels of leptin in their bloodstream, suggesting that they are resistant to leptin's effects.[1]

The Amount and Type of Food Play a Role

Protein-rich foods have the highest satiety value.[2] This means that a ham and egg breakfast will trigger satiety sooner and maintain it longer than will pancakes with maple syrup, even if both meals have exactly the same number of Calories. Bulky meals high in fiber and water tend to stretch the stomach and small intestine, which send signals back to the hypothalamus telling us that we are full, so we stop eating. Beverages tend to be less satisfying than semisolid foods, and semisolid foods have a lower satiety value than solid foods. For example, if you were to eat a bunch of grapes, you would feel a greater sense of fullness than if you drank a glass of grape juice providing the same number of Calories.

recap Hunger is a drive to eat triggered by the physiologic need for food. The feeding and satiety centers in the hypothalamus regulate food intake in response to nerve signals from the mouth, stomach, and other organs, and the levels of certain hormones, including insulin and glucagon. Foods rich in protein have the highest satiety value, and bulky meals fill us up quickly, causing the distention that signals us to stop eating.

digestion The process by which foods are broken down into their component molecules, either mechanically or chemically.

absorption The physiologic process by which molecules of food cross from the gastrointestinal tract into the circulation.

elimination The process by which undigested portions of food and waste products are removed from the body.

LO 3 Identify each organ food encounters on its way through the gastrointestinal tract, and its primary function.

How does food travel through the gastrointestinal tract?

When we eat, the food is digested, then the useful nutrients are absorbed, and the waste products are eliminated (**FOCUS FIGURE 3.4**). **Digestion** is the process by which foods are broken down into their component molecules, either mechanically or chemically. **Absorption** is the process of taking these products of digestion through the wall of the small intestine into the circulation. **Elimination** is the process by which the remaining waste is removed from the body.

The digestive system consists of the organs of the gastrointestinal (GI) tract and associated accessory organs. The processing of food in the GI tract involves ingestion, mechanical digestion, chemical digestion, propulsion, absorption, and elimination.

ORGANS OF THE GI TRACT

MOUTH

Ingestion Food enters the GI tract via the mouth.

Mechanical digestion Mastication tears, shreds, and mixes food with saliva.

Chemical digestion Salivary amylase and lingual lipase begin the breakdown of carbohydrates and lipids.

PHARYNX AND ESOPHAGUS

Propulsion Swallowing and peristalsis move food from mouth to stomach.

STOMACH

Mechanical digestion Mixes and churns food with gastric juice into a liquid called chyme.

Chemical digestion Pepsin begins digestion of proteins, and gastric lipase begins to break lipids apart.

Absorption A few fat-soluble substances are absorbed through the stomach wall.

SMALL INTESTINE

Mechanical Digestion and **Propulsion** Segmentation mixes chyme with digestive juices; peristaltic waves move it along tract.

Chemical digestion Digestive enzymes from pancreas and brush border digest most classes of nutrients.

Absorption Nutrients are absorbed into blood and lymph through enterocytes.

LARGE INTESTINE

Chemical digestion Some remaining food residues are digested by bacteria.

Absorption Reabsorbs salts, water, and vitamins.

Propulsion Compacts waste into feces and propels it toward the rectum.

RECTUM

Elimination Temporarily stores feces before voluntary release through the anus.

ACCESSORY ORGANS

SALIVARY GLANDS

Produce saliva, a mixture of water, mucus, enzymes, and other chemicals.

LIVER

Produces bile to emulsify fats.

GALLBLADDER

Stores bile before release into the small intestine through the bile duct.

PANCREAS

Produces digestive enzymes and bicarbonate, which are released into the small intestine via the pancreatic duct.

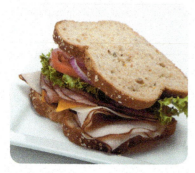

⬆ Digestion of a sandwich starts before you even take a bite.

gastrointestinal (GI) tract A long, muscular tube consisting of several organs: the mouth, pharynx, esophagus, stomach, small intestine, and large intestine and rectum.

sphincter A tight ring of muscle separating some of the organs of the GI tract and opening in response to nerve signals indicating that food is ready to pass into the next section.

accessory organs of digestion The salivary glands, liver, gallbladder, and pancreas, which contribute to GI function but are not anatomically part of the GI tract.

cephalic phase The earliest phase of digestion, in which the brain thinks about and prepares the digestive organs for the consumption of food.

Digestion, absorption, and elimination occur in the **gastrointestinal (GI) tract**, the organs of which work together to process foods. The GI tract is a long tube that begins at the mouth and ends at the anus: if held out straight, an adult GI tract would be close to 30 feet long. It is composed of several distinct organs, including the mouth, pharynx, esophagus, stomach, small intestine, and large intestine and rectum (see Focus Figure 3.4). The flow of food between these organs is controlled by muscular **sphincters**, which are tight rings of muscle that open when a nerve signal indicates that food is ready to pass into the next section.

Assisting the GI tract are four **accessory organs of digestion**. These play essential roles in GI function, but are not anatomically part of the GI tract. They include the salivary glands, liver, gallbladder, and pancreas (see Focus Figure 3.4). We'll discuss these accessory organs in more detail later in this chapter. For now, imagine that you ate a turkey sandwich for lunch today. It contained two slices of bread spread with mayonnaise, some turkey, two lettuce leaves, and a slice of tomato. Let's accompany the sandwich as it travels through your GI tract.

Digestion Begins in the Mouth

Believe it or not, the first step in the digestive process is not your first bite of that sandwich. It is your first thought about what you want for lunch and your first whiff of freshly baked bread as you stand in line at the deli. In this **cephalic phase** of digestion, hunger and appetite work together to prepare the GI tract to digest food. The nervous system stimulates the release of digestive juices in preparation for food entering the GI tract, and sometimes we experience some involuntary movement commonly called "hunger pangs."

Now let's stop smelling that sandwich and take a bite and chew! Chewing moistens the food and breaks it down into pieces small enough to swallow **(FIGURE 3.5)**. Thus, chewing initiates the mechanical digestion of food. The tough coating surrounding the lettuce fibers and tomato seeds is also broken open, facilitating digestion. This is especially important when we're eating foods that are high in fiber, such as grains, fruits, and vegetables. Chewing also mixes everything in your sandwich together: the protein in the turkey; the carbohydrates in the bread, lettuce, and tomato; the fat in the mayonnaise; and the vitamins, minerals, and water in all of the foods.

The presence of food in your mouth also initiates chemical digestion. As your teeth cut and grind the different foods in your sandwich, more surface area is

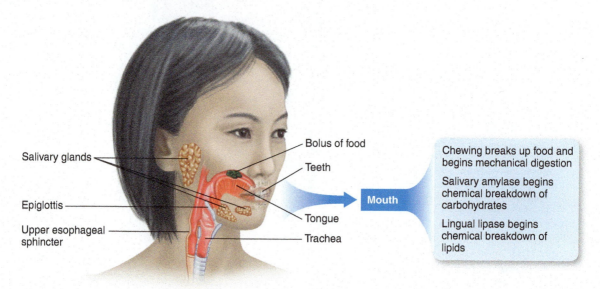

Salivary glands
Epiglottis
Upper esophageal sphincter

Bolus of food
Teeth
Tongue
Trachea

Mouth

Chewing breaks up food and begins mechanical digestion

Salivary amylase begins chemical breakdown of carbohydrates

Lingual lipase begins chemical breakdown of lipids

⬆ **FIGURE 3.5** Where your food is now: the mouth. Chewing moistens food and mechanically breaks it down into pieces small enough to swallow, while salivary amylase and lingual lipase initiate chemical digestion.

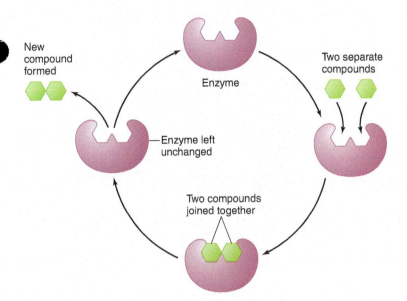

New compound formed

Enzyme

Enzyme left unchanged

Two separate compounds

Two compounds joined together

FIGURE 3.6 Enzymes speed up the body's chemical reactions, including many reactions essential to the digestion and absorption of food. Here, an enzyme joins two small compounds to create a larger compound. Notice that the enzyme itself is not changed in this process.

exposed to the digestive juices in your mouth. Foremost among these is **saliva**, which you secrete from your **salivary glands**, an accessory organ of digestion. Saliva not only moistens your food but also begins the process of chemical breakdown. One component of saliva, salivary *amylase*, starts the process of carbohydrate digestion. Saliva also contains other components, such as antibodies that protect the body from foreign bacteria entering the mouth and keep the oral cavity free from infection.

Salivary amylase is the first of many **enzymes** that assist the body in digesting and absorbing food. Because we will encounter enzymes throughout our journey through the GI tract, let's discuss them briefly here. Enzymes are small chemicals, usually proteins, that act on other chemicals to speed up body processes **(FIGURE 3.6)**. Imagine them as facilitators: a chemical reaction that might take an hour to occur independently might happen in a single second with the help of one or more enzymes. Because they remain essentially unchanged by the chemical reactions they facilitate, enzymes can be reused repeatedly. The action of enzymes can result in the production of new substances or can assist in breaking substances apart. The process of digestion—as well as many other biochemical processes that go on in our body—could not happen without enzymes. Another enzyme active in the mouth is lingual lipase, which is secreted by tongue cells during chewing and begins the breakdown of fats. By the way, enzyme names typically end in *-ase* (as in *amylase*), so they are easy to recognize as we look at the digestive process.

In reality, very little digestion occurs in the mouth. This is because we do not hold food in the mouth for very long and because the most powerful digestive enzymes are secreted further along in the GI tract.

The Esophagus Transports Food from the Pharynx into the Stomach

The mass of food that has been chewed and moistened in the mouth is referred to as a **bolus**. This bolus moves from the mouth to the **pharynx**, the region of the GI tract extending from the back of the mouth, where it is swallowed **(FIGURE 3.7)** (see page 74) and propelled into the esophagus.

Most of us take swallowing for granted. However, it is a complex process involving voluntary and involuntary motion. A tiny flap of tissue called the *epiglottis* acts as a trapdoor covering the entrance to the trachea (windpipe). The epiglottis is normally open, allowing us to breathe freely even while chewing (Figure 3.7a). As a food bolus moves toward the pharynx, the brain is sent a signal to temporarily

saliva A mixture of water, mucus, enzymes, and other chemicals that moistens the mouth and food, binds food particles together, and begins the digestion of carbohydrates.

salivary glands A group of glands found under and behind the tongue and beneath the jaw that release saliva continually as well as in response to the thought, sight, smell, or presence of food.

enzymes Small chemicals, usually proteins, that act on other chemicals to speed up body processes but are not apparently changed during those processes.

bolus A mass of food that has been chewed and moistened in the mouth.

pharynx Segment of the GI tract connecting the back of the nose and mouth to the top of the esophagus.

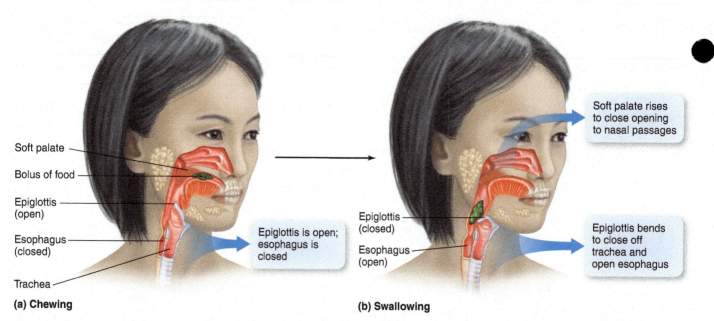

Soft palate

Bolus of food

Epiglottis
(open)

Esophagus
(closed)

Trachea

(a) Chewing

Epiglottis is open;
esophagus is
closed

Soft palate rises
to close opening
to nasal passages

Epiglottis
(closed)

Esophagus
(open)

Epiglottis bends
to close off
trachea and
open esophagus

(b) Swallowing

FIGURE 3.7 Chewing and swallowing are complex processes. **(a)** During the process of chewing, the epiglottis is open and the esophagus is closed, so that we can continue to breathe as we chew. **(b)** During swallowing, the epiglottis closes, so that food does not enter the trachea and obstruct our breathing. Also, the soft palate rises to seal off our nasal passages, preventing the aspiration of food or liquid into them.

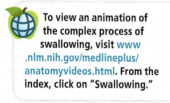

To view an animation of the complex process of swallowing, visit www .nlm.nih.gov/medlineplus/ anatomyvideos.html. From the index, click on "Swallowing."

esophagus A muscular tube of the GI tract connecting the pharynx to the stomach.

peristalsis Waves of squeezing and pushing contractions that move food in one direction through the length of the GI tract.

stomach A J-shaped organ where food is partially digested, churned, and stored until it is released into the small intestine.

raise the soft palate and close the openings to the nasal passages, preventing the aspiration of food or liquid into the nasal passages (Figure 3.7b). The brain also signals the epiglottis to close during swallowing, so that food and liquid cannot enter the trachea.

Sometimes this protective mechanism goes awry—for instance, when we try to eat and talk at the same time. When this happens, food or liquid enters the trachea. Typically, this forces us to cough until the food or liquid is expelled.

As the trachea closes, the sphincter muscle at the top of the esophagus, called the *upper esophageal sphincter*, opens to allow the passage of food. The **esophagus** is a muscular tube that connects and transports food from the pharynx to the stomach **(FIGURE 3.8)**. It does this by contracting two sets of muscles: inner sheets of circular muscle squeeze the food while outer sheets of longitudinal muscle push food along the length of the tube. Together, these rhythmic waves of squeezing and pushing are called **peristalsis**. We will see later in this chapter that peristalsis occurs throughout the GI tract.

Gravity also helps transport food down the esophagus, which explains why it is wise to sit or stand upright while eating. Together, peristalsis and gravity can transport a bite of food from the mouth to the opening of the stomach in 5 to 8 seconds. At the end of the esophagus is a sphincter muscle, the *gastroesophageal sphincter*, which is normally tightly closed. When food reaches the end of the esophagus, this sphincter relaxes to allow the food to pass into the stomach. In some people, this sphincter is continually somewhat relaxed. Later in the chapter, we'll discuss this disorder and the unpleasant symptoms it causes.

The Stomach Mixes, Digests, and Stores Food

The **stomach** is a J-shaped organ. Its size varies with different individuals; in general, its volume is about 6 fluid ounces (or 3/4 cup) when it is empty. The stomach wall contains four layers, the innermost of which is crinkled into large folds called *rugae* that flatten progressively to accommodate food. This allows the stomach to expand to hold as much as 1 gallon of food and liquid. As food is

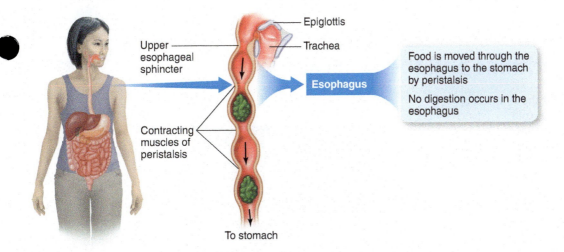

Epiglottis

Trachea

Upper esophageal sphincter

Contracting muscles of peristalsis

To stomach

Esophagus

Food is moved through the esophagus to the stomach by peristalsis

No digestion occurs in the esophagus

◄ **FIGURE 3.8** Where your food is now: the esophagus. Peristalsis, the rhythmic contraction and relaxation of both circular and longitudinal muscles in the esophagus, propels food toward the stomach. Peristalsis occurs throughout the GI tract.

released into the small intestine, the rugae reform, and the stomach gradually returns to its baseline size.

Before any food reaches the stomach, the brain sends signals to the stomach to stimulate and prepare it to receive food. For example, the hormone *gastrin*, secreted by stomach-lining cells called *G cells*, stimulates gastric glands to secrete a digestive fluid referred to as **gastric juice**. Gastric glands are lined with two important types of cells—parietal cells and chief cells—that secrete the various components of gastric juice.

The parietal cells secrete:

- *Hydrochloric acid (HCl)*, which keeps the stomach interior very acidic. To be precise, the pH of HCl is 1.0, which means that it is 10 times more acidic than pure lemon juice and a hundred times more acidic than vinegar! For a review of the calculations behind the pH scale, see the **You Do the Math** box (on page 76). The acidic environment of the stomach interior kills any bacteria that may have entered with the sandwich. HCl is also extremely important for digestion because it starts to **denature** proteins, which means it breaks the bonds that maintain their structure. This is an essential preliminary step in protein digestion.
- *Intrinsic factor*, a protein critical to the absorption of vitamin B_{12}, which is present in the turkey.

The chief cells secrete:

- *Pepsinogen*, an inactive enzyme, which HCl converts into the active enzyme *pepsin*. Pepsin begins the digestion of protein and is considered one of the principal protein-digesting enzymes in the GI tract.
- *Gastric lipase*, which minimally digests the lipids in the turkey and mayonnaise in your sandwich.

Because gastric juice is already present in the stomach, chemical digestion of proteins and lipids begins as soon as food enters **(FIGURE 3.10)** (see page 77). The stomach also plays a role in mechanical digestion by mixing and churning the food with the gastric juice until it becomes a liquid called **chyme**. This mechanical digestion facilitates chemical digestion because enzymes can access the liquid chyme more easily than solid forms of food.

Despite the acidity of gastric juice, the stomach itself is not eroded because cells in gastric glands and in the stomach lining secrete a protective layer of mucus. Any disruption of this mucus barrier can cause gastritis (inflammation of the stomach lining)

For a fun animation explaining the concept of pH, visit www.johnkyrk.com. Choose "pH" on the first-page menu and click through the animation.

gastric juice Acidic liquid secreted within the stomach; it contains hydrochloric acid and other compounds.

denature The action of the unfolding of proteins in the stomach. Proteins must be denatured before they can be digested.

chyme A semifluid mass consisting of partially digested food, water, and gastric juices.

Negative Logarithms and the pH Scale

Have you ever been warned that the black coffee, orange juice, or cola you enjoy is corroding your stomach? If so, relax. It's an urban myth. How can you know for sure? Take a look at the pH scale (FIGURE 3.9). As you can see, the scale shows that hydrochloric acid (HCl) has a pH of 1.0 and gastric juice is 2.0, whereas soft drinks (including cola) are 3.0, orange juice is 4.0, and black coffee is 5.0. Not sure what all of these numbers mean?

An abbreviation for the *potential of hydrogen,* pH is a measure of the hydrogen ion concentration of a solution, or more precisely, the potential of a substance to release or to take up hydrogen ions in solution. Given that an acid by definition is a compound that releases hydrogen ions, and a base (an alkali) is a compound that binds them, we can also say that pH is a measure of a compound's acidity or alkalinity. The precise measurements of pH range from 0 to 14, with 7.0 designated as pH neutral. Pure water is exactly neutral, and human blood is close to neutral, normally ranging from about 7.35 to 7.45.

The pH scale is a negative base-10 logarithmic scale. As you may recall from high school math classes, a base-10 logarithm ($\log_{10}$) tells you how many times you multiply by 10 to get the desired number. So for example, $\log_{10} (1,000) = 3$ because to get 1,000 you have to multiply 10 three times ($10 \times 10 \times 10$). The pH scale is a negative scale because an *increased* number on the scale identifies a corresponding *decrease* in concentration. These facts taken together mean that:

- for every increase of a single digit, the concentration of hydrogen ions decreases by tenfold.

- for every decrease of a single digit, the concentration of hydrogen ions increases by tenfold.

So, for example, milk has a pH of 6, which is one digit lower than 7. Milk is therefore 10 times more acidic than pure water. Baking soda, at pH 9, is two digits higher than 7, and thus baking soda is 100 times less acidic (more alkaline) than pure water: $2 = \log_{10} (100)$.

Now you do the math:

1. Is the pH of blood normally slightly acidic or slightly alkaline?

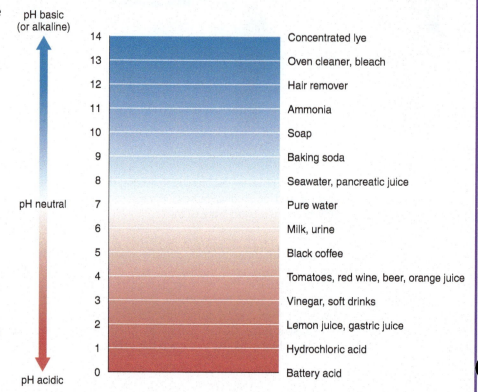

pH basic (or alkaline)

pH neutral

pH acidic

pH	Substance
14	Concentrated lye
13	Oven cleaner, bleach
12	Hair remover
11	Ammonia
10	Soap
9	Baking soda
8	Seawater, pancreatic juice
7	Pure water
6	Milk, urine
5	Black coffee
4	Tomatoes, red wine, beer, orange juice
3	Vinegar, soft drinks
2	Lemon juice, gastric juice
1	Hydrochloric acid
0	Battery acid

▲ FIGURE 3.9 The pH scale identifies the levels of acidity or alkalinity of various substances. More specifically, pH is defined as the negative logarithm of the hydrogen–ion concentration of any solution. Each one-unit change in pH from high to low represents a tenfold increase in the concentration of hydrogen ions. This means that gastric juice, which has a pH of 2, is 100,000 times more acidic than pure water, which has a pH of 7.

2. Identify the relative acidity of black coffee as compared to pure water; as compared to HCl.

3. Identify the relative acidity of soft drinks as compared to pure water; as compared to HCl.

If you answered correctly, you can appreciate the fact that, because the tissues lining your stomach wall are adequately protected (by mucus and bicarbonate) from the acidity of HCl, they are not likely to be damaged by coffee, cola, or any other standard beverage. On the other hand, if you were to down an entire bottle of pure lemon juice (pH 2.0, the same as gastric juice), the release of all those additional hydrogen ions into the already acidic environment of your stomach would likely make you very sick. Your blood pH would drop, your breathing rate would increase, and you would almost certainly vomit. However, the juice would not corrode your stomach.

Answers to these questions can be found in the MasteringNutrition Study Area.

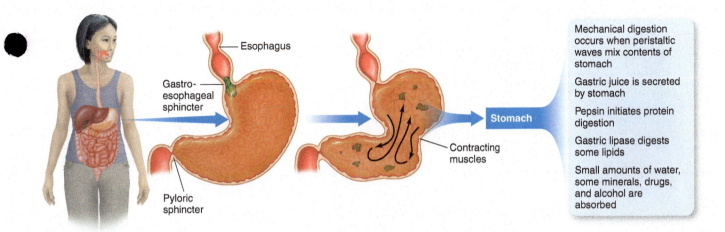

- **FIGURE 3.10** Where your food is now: the stomach. Protein digestion begins in the stomach, and some lipid digestion occurs there. Your meal is churned into chyme and stored until released into the small intestine.

or an ulcer (a condition that is discussed later in this chapter). Other lining cells secrete bicarbonate, an alkaline compound, which neutralizes acid near the surface of the stomach's lining.

Although most absorption occurs in the small intestine, some substances are absorbed through the stomach lining and into the blood. These include water, fluoride, some lipids, and some lipid-soluble drugs, including aspirin and alcohol.

Another of the stomach's jobs is to store chyme while the next part of the digestive tract, the small intestine, gets ready for the food. Remember that the capacity of the stomach is as much as 1 gallon. If this amount of chyme were to move into the small intestine all at once, it would overwhelm it. Chyme stays in the stomach for about 2 hours before it is released periodically in spurts into the duodenum, which is the first part of the small intestine. Regulating this release is the *pyloric sphincter* (see Figure 3.10).

Most Digestion and Absorption Occur in the Small Intestine

The **small intestine** is the longest portion of the GI tract, accounting for about two-thirds of its length. However, it is called "small" because it is only an inch in diameter.

The small intestine is composed of three sections **(FIGURE 3.11)** (see page 78). The *duodenum* is the section that is connected via the pyloric sphincter to the stomach. The *jejunum* is the middle portion, and the last portion is the *ileum*. It connects to the large intestine at another sphincter, called the *ileocecal valve*.

Most digestion and absorption takes place in the small intestine. Here, food is broken down into its smallest components, molecules that the body can then absorb into the circulation. In the next section, we'll discuss the unique anatomical features of the small intestine that facilitate gastrointestinal function. But first, let's continue our journey through the GI tract.

The Large Intestine Stores Food Waste Until It Is Excreted

The **large intestine** (also called the *colon*) is a thick, tubelike structure that frames the small intestine on three-and-a-half sides **(FIGURE 3.12)** (see page 79). It begins with a tissue sac called the *cecum*, which explains the name of the sphincter—the *ileocecal valve*—that connects it to the ileum of the small intestine. From the cecum, the large intestine continues up along the right side of the small intestine as the

small intestine The longest portion of the GI tract, where most digestion and absorption take place.

large intestine The terminal region of the GI tract, in which most water is absorbed and feces are formed.

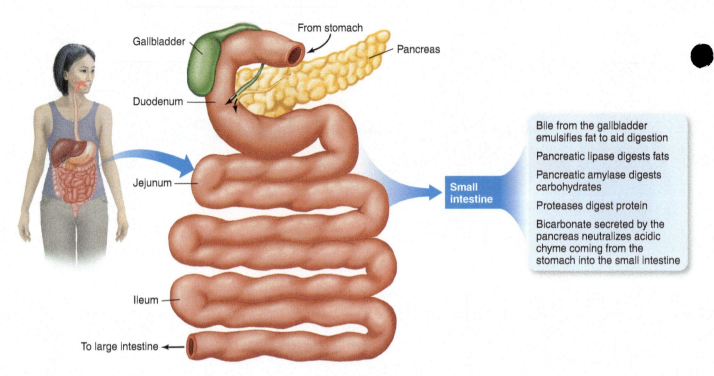

Gallbladder

From stomach

Pancreas

Duodenum

Jejunum

Ileum

To large intestine

Small intestine

Bile from the gallbladder emulsifies fat to aid digestion

Pancreatic lipase digests fats

Pancreatic amylase digests carbohydrates

Proteases digest protein

Bicarbonate secreted by the pancreas neutralizes acidic chyme coming from the stomach into the small intestine

◀ **FIGURE 3.11** Where your food is now: the small intestine. Here, most digestion and absorption takes place.

ascending colon. Beneath the liver, it flexes nearly 90° to continue as the *transverse colon* along the top of the small intestine. It then flexes downward, and continues as the *descending colon* along the left side of the small intestine. The *sigmoid colon* is the last segment of the colon; it extends from the bottom left corner to the *rectum.* The last segment of the large intestine is the *anal canal,* which is about an inch and a half long.

When the digestive mass finally reaches the large intestine, it does not resemble the chyme that left the stomach several hours before. This is because most of the nutrients have been absorbed, leaving mainly nondigestible food material and water. As in the stomach, cells lining the large intestine secrete mucus, which helps protect it from the abrasive materials passing through it.

The main functions of the large intestine are to store the digestive mass for 12 to 24 hours and, during that time, to absorb water and any other nutrients from it, leaving a semisolid mass called *feces.* Peristalsis occurs weakly to move the feces through the colon, except for one or more stronger waves of peristalsis each day, which force the feces more powerfully toward the rectum for elimination through the anus.

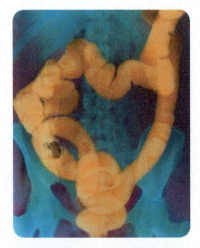

◀ The large intestine is a thick, tubelike structure that stores the undigested mass exiting the small intestine and also absorbs any remaining nutrients, including water.

recap Digestion, absorption, and elimination take place in the gastrointestinal (GI) tract. In the cephalic phase of digestion, hunger and appetite work together to prepare the GI tract. Chewing initiates mechanical digestion by breaking the food mass apart and mixing it together. The release of salivary amylase and lingual lipase begins chemical digestion of carbohydrates and lipids. Swallowing occurs in the pharynx, and the esophagus transports food to the stomach via waves of peristalsis. The stomach secretes a highly acidic gastric juice, components of which begin to digest proteins and lipids. It also secretes mucus and bicarbonate to protect its lining. The stomach also churns food into a liquid called chyme, which it releases gradually into the small intestine through the pyloric sphincter. Most digestion and absorption occurs in the small intestine. Its three sections are the duodenum, the jejunum, and the ileum. The large intestine is composed of seven sections: the cecum, ascending, transverse, descending, and

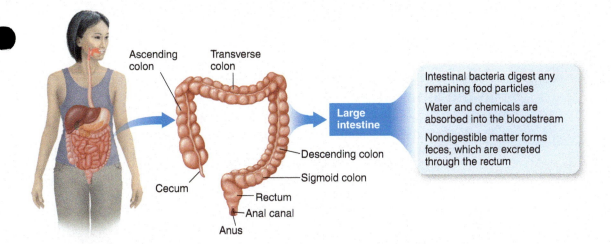

Intestinal bacteria digest any remaining food particles

Water and chemicals are absorbed into the bloodstream

Nondigestible matter forms feces, which are excreted through the rectum

◆ **FIGURE 3.12** Where your food is now: the large intestine. Most water absorption occurs here, as does the formation of food wastes into semisolid feces. Peristalsis propels the feces to the body exterior.

sigmoid colon, rectum, and anal canal. The main functions of the large intestine are to store the digestive mass and to absorb any remaining nutrients, including water. A semisolid mass, called feces, is then eliminated from the body.

What else contributes to gastrointestinal function?

LO 4 Describe the specialized organs and features that contribute to gastrointestinal function.

To digest a meal and absorb its nutrients, your GI tract relies on a variety of specialized organs, features, and processes, including the contributions of trillions of helpful bacteria. Let's take a look.

The Gallbladder and Pancreas Aid in Digestion

Recall that the stomach releases chyme into the small intestine. In response to the presence of protein and fat in the chyme, glandular cells in the duodenum secrete the hormone CCK, mentioned earlier for its role in promoting satiety. The release of CCK signals the **gallbladder**, an accessory organ located beneath the liver (see Figures 3.4 and 3.11), to contract. The gallbladder stores a greenish fluid called **bile**, which the liver produces, and its contraction propels bile through the *common bile duct* into the duodenum. Bile then *emulsifies* the fat; that is, it reduces the fat into smaller globules and disperses them, so that they are more accessible to digestive enzymes. If you've ever noticed how a drop of liquid detergent breaks up a film of fat floating at the top of a basin of greasy dishes, you understand the function of bile.

The **pancreas**, another accessory organ, manufactures, holds, and secretes different digestive enzymes. It is located behind the stomach (see Figures 3.4 and 3.11). Enzymes secreted by the pancreas include *pancreatic amylase,* which continues the digestion of carbohydrates, and *pancreatic lipase,* which continues the digestion of fats. *Proteases* secreted in pancreatic juice digest proteins. The pancreas is also responsible for manufacturing hormones that are important in metabolism. Earlier we mentioned insulin and glucagon, two pancreatic hormones that help regulate the amount of glucose in the blood.

Recall that the stomach lining cells secrete bicarbonate, a base, which helps protect it from the acidic chyme. Similarly, the pancreas secretes bicarbonate into the duodenum, ensuring that its lining is not eroded. This action also helps the pancreatic enzymes work more effectively.

gallbladder A saclike accessory organ of digestion, which lies beneath the liver; it stores bile and secretes it into the small intestine.

bile Fluid produced by the liver and stored in the gallbladder; it emulsifies fats in the small intestine.

pancreas An accessory organ of digestion located behind the stomach; it secretes digestive enzymes and bicarbonate as well as hormones that help regulate blood glucose.

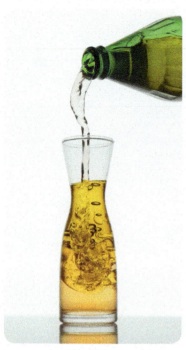

A small amount of vinegar emulsifies the oil in this container.

The small intestine also releases its own digestive enzymes, which help to break down carbohydrates, fats, and proteins. For example, lactase is an intestinal enzyme that helps break down a sugar in milk called lactose.

A Specialized Lining Boosts Absorption in the Small Intestine

Aided by the action of bile and enzymes from the pancreas and small intestine, the chyme in the duodenum is processed into nutrient molecules small enough for absorption. As this molecular "soup" moves along the small intestine, it encounters the absorptive enterocytes of the intestinal lining.

Also referred to as the *mucosal membrane,* the lining of the small intestine has several features that facilitate absorption **(FOCUS FIGURE 3.13)**. First, it is heavily folded. This feature increases the surface area of the small intestine and allows it to absorb more nutrients than if it were smooth. Within these larger folds are even smaller, fingerlike projections called *villi,* whose constant movement helps them encounter and trap nutrient molecules. Inside each villus are *capillaries,* or tiny blood vessels, and a **lacteal**, which is a small lymph vessel. The capillaries absorb water-soluble nutrients directly into the bloodstream, whereas lacteals absorb fat-soluble nutrients into a watery fluid called *lymph.*

Covering the villi are enterocytes whose cell membrane is carpeted with hairlike projections called *microvilli.* Because this makes the cells look like tiny scrub brushes, the microvilli are sometimes referred to collectively as the **brush border**. The carpet of microvilli multiplies the surface area of the small intestine more than 500 times, tremendously increasing its absorptive capacity.

Vitamins, minerals, and water are so small that they're not "digested" in the same way that macronutrients are. The fat-soluble vitamins A, D, E, and K are readily absorbed into the enterocytes along with the fats in our foods. The water-soluble vitamins—the B vitamins and vitamin C—typically use some type of transport process (discussed next) to cross the intestinal lining. Minerals are already the smallest possible units of matter; thus, they're absorbed all along the small intestine, and in some cases in the large intestine as well, by a wide variety of mechanisms. Water is readily absorbed along the entire length of the GI tract because it is a small molecule that can easily pass through the cell membrane.

Four Types of Absorption Occur in the Small Intestine

Nutrients are absorbed across the mucosal membrane and into the bloodstream or lymph via four mechanisms: passive diffusion, facilitated diffusion, active transport, and endocytosis. These are illustrated in **FIGURE 3.14** on page 82.

Passive diffusion is a simple process in which lipids, some minerals, and water cross into the enterocytes along their "concentration gradient." That is, these nutrients diffuse from the GI tract where they are highly concentrated to an area of lower concentration in the enterocytes.

Facilitated diffusion occurs when nutrients in high concentration in the GI tract are carried across the enterocyte membrane with the help of a protein. Fructose (a carbohydrate composed of a single sugar unit) is transported via facilitated diffusion.

Active transport requires both a carrier protein and energy (in the form of ATP) to transport nutrients against their concentration gradient, meaning the nutrients move from areas of low to high concentration. Glucose, amino acids, and certain minerals are among the nutrients absorbed via active transport. Vitamin C may be absorbed via passive diffusion but is more commonly absorbed via active transport.

Endocytosis is a form of active transport by which a small amount of the intestinal contents is engulfed by the enterocyte's cell membrane and incorporated into the cell. Some proteins are absorbed in this way.

Blood and Lymph Transport Nutrients

We noted earlier that, within the intestinal villi, capillaries and lacteals absorb water-soluble and fat-soluble nutrients, respectively, into blood and lymph.

lacteal A small lymph vessel located inside the villi of the small intestine.

brush border The microvilli projecting from the membrane of enterocytes of the small intestine's villi. These microvilli tremendously increase the small intestine's absorptive capacity.

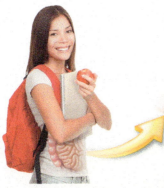

The small intestine is highly adapted for absorbing nutrients. Its length—about 20 feet—provides a huge surface area, and its wall has three structural features—circular folds, villi, and microvilli—that increase its surface area by a factor of more than 600.

CIRCULAR FOLDS

The lining of the small intestine is heavily folded, resulting in increased surface area for the absorption of nutrients.

VILLI

The folds are covered with villi, thousands of finger-like projections that increase the surface area even further. Each villus contains capillaries and a lacteal for picking up nutrients absorbed through the enterocytes and transporting them throughout the body.

MICROVILLI

The cells on the surface of the villi, enterocytes, end in hairlike projections called microvilli that together form the brush border through which nutrients are absorbed.

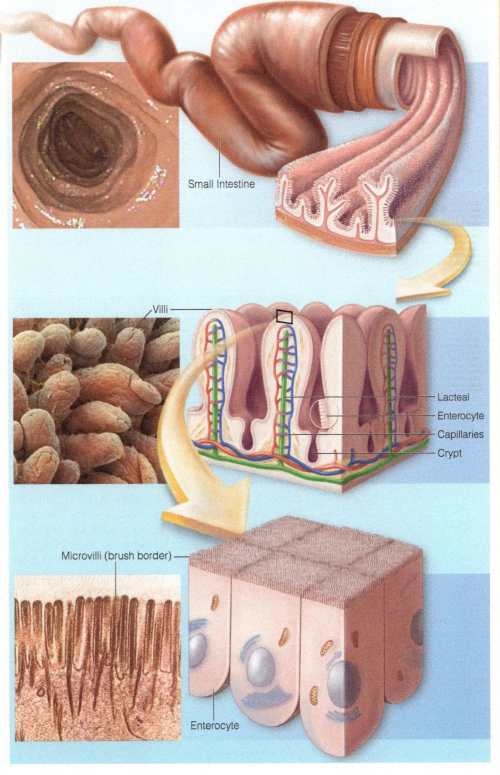

Small Intestine

Villi

Lacteal
Enterocyte
Capillaries
Crypt

Microvilli (brush border)

Enterocyte

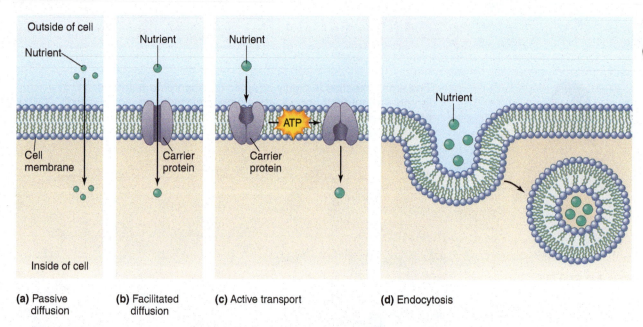

(a) Passive diffusion

(b) Facilitated diffusion

(c) Active transport

(d) Endocytosis

◆ **FIGURE 3.14** The four types of absorption that occur in the small intestine. **(a)** In passive diffusion, nutrients at a higher concentration outside the enterocytes diffuse readily along their concentration gradient into the enterocytes. **(b)** In facilitated diffusion, nutrients are shuttled into the enterocytes with the help of a carrier protein. **(c)** In active transport, both a carrier protein and energy (in the form of ATP) are needed to transport nutrients against their concentration gradient. **(d)** In endocytosis, nutrients are engulfed by the cell membrane of the enterocyte and released into its interior.

These two fluids then transport the nutrients throughout the body. Blood travels through the cardiovascular system, and lymph travels through the lymphatic system (**FIGURE 3.15**).

The cardiovascular system includes the heart, which pumps blood, and the blood vessels, which carry blood to all of our tissues to deliver nutrients, oxygen, and other substances and to pick up wastes. As blood travels through the GI tract, it picks up most of the nutrients, including water, that are absorbed through the brush border into the capillaries. This nutrient-rich blood is then transported to the liver for further processing.

The lymphatic system consists of a network of lymphatic vessels, including the lacteals that pick up fats and fat-soluble vitamins in the intestinal villi, as well as lymphatic capillaries that absorb fluids that have escaped from the cardiovascular system. Lymph traveling through the lymphatic vessels encounters *lymph nodes,* clusters of immune and other cells that filter out particles and destroy harmful microbes. Eventually, lymph returns to the bloodstream in an area near the heart where the lymphatic and blood vessels join together.

Bear in mind that circulation also allows for the elimination of metabolic wastes. Many waste products picked up by the blood as it circulates around the body are filtered and excreted by the kidneys in urine. Carbon dioxide, which is a waste product of energy metabolism, is transported in the blood to the lungs, where it is exhaled into the outside air, making room for oxygen to attach to the red blood cells and repeat this cycle of circulation.

The Liver Regulates Blood Nutrients

liver The largest accessory organ of digestion and one of the most important organs of the body. Its functions include the production of bile and the processing of nutrient-rich blood from the small intestine.

Once nutrients are absorbed from the small intestine, most enter the *portal vein,* which carries them to the **liver**. The liver is a triangular, wedge-shaped organ weighing about 3 pounds and resting almost entirely within the protection of the rib cage on the right side of the body (see Figure 3.4). It is not only the largest digestive organ but also one of the most important organs in the body, performing more than 500 discrete functions.

One function of the liver is to receive the products of digestion and then release into the bloodstream those nutrients needed throughout the body. The liver also processes and stores carbohydrates, fats, and amino acids and plays a major role in regulating their levels in the bloodstream. For instance, after we eat a meal, the liver picks up excess glucose from the blood and stores it as glycogen, releasing it into the bloodstream when we need energy later in the day. It also stores certain vitamins. But the liver is more than a nutrient warehouse: it also manufactures blood proteins and can even make glucose when necessary to keep our blood glucose levels constant.

Have you ever wondered why people who abuse alcohol are at risk for liver damage? It's because another of the liver's functions is to filter the blood, removing wastes and toxins such as alcohol, medications, and other drugs. When you drink, your liver works hard to break down the alcohol; but with heavy drinking over time, liver cells become damaged and scar tissue forms. The scar tissue blocks the free flow of blood through the liver, so that any further toxins accumulate in the blood, causing confusion, coma, and ultimately death.

Another important job of the liver is to synthesize many of the chemicals the body uses to carry out metabolic processes. For example, the liver synthesizes bile, which, as we just discussed, is then stored in the gallbladder until the body needs it to emulsify fats.

The GI Flora Perform Several Beneficial Functions

The GI tract is host to trillions of bacterial cells. Collectively called the *GI flora,* they are the largest constituents of the human microbiome, discussed **In Depth** on pages 32–33. Most of the GI flora live in the large intestine, where they perform several beneficial functions. First, they finish digesting some of the nutrients remaining in food residues. The by-products of this bacterial digestion are then absorbed into the bloodstream, which transports them to the liver where they are either stored or used as needed. In addition, the GI flora synthesize certain vitamins, including vitamin K and some of the B vitamins.[3] The GI flora also compete with—and thereby inhibit the growth of—harmful bacteria and yeasts (a type of fungus).[4] They are also thought to stimulate the immune system, oppose inflammation, and reduce the risk of diarrhea.[4]

These bacteria are so helpful that many people consume them deliberately in *probiotic* foods such as yogurt. On the other hand, they can be wiped out by the use of broad-spectrum antibiotics. A recent study found that, in the colon of people who had taken any of several common antibiotics for as little as one week, the population of GI flora was depleted for up to a full year.[5]

The Neuromuscular System Regulates the Activities of the GI Tract

Now that you can identify the organs involved in digestion, absorption, and elimination, and the job each performs, you might be wondering—who's the boss? In other words, what organ or system directs and coordinates all of these interrelated processes? The answer is the neuromuscular system. Its two components, the nervous and muscular systems, partner to regulate the activities of the GI tract.

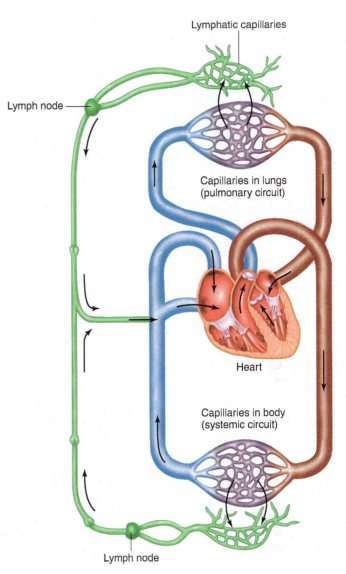

FIGURE 3.15 Blood travels through the cardiovascular system to transport water-soluble nutrients and pick up waste products. Lymph travels through the lymphatic system and transports most fats and fat-soluble vitamins.

▶ **FIGURE 3.16** Peristalsis and segmentation. **(a)** Peristalsis occurs through the actions of circular and longitudinal muscles that run along the entire GI tract. These muscles continuously contract and relax, pushing the tract contents along. **(b)** Segmentation is unique to the small intestine, and occurs through the rhythmic contraction of its circular muscles. This action squeezes the chyme, mixes it, and enhances its contact with digestive enzymes and enterocytes.

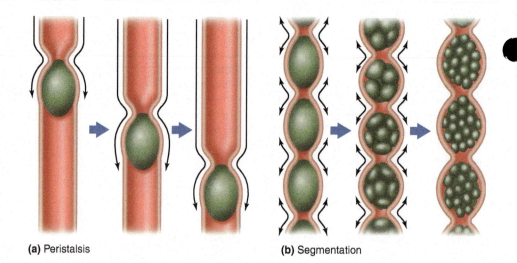

(a) Peristalsis   (b) Segmentation

Muscles of the GI Tract

To process the food we eat, we use voluntary and involuntary muscles. Chewing and swallowing are, of course, voluntary actions; that is, they are under conscious control. However, once we swallow, nerves respond to the stretching of the GI tract walls and send signals to its circular and longitudinal muscles, stimulating peristalsis, which is involuntary **(FIGURE 3.16a)**. As you've learned, peristalsis pushes food along the entire GI tract. In addition, in the small intestine, a unique type of involuntary movement called *segmentation* occurs (see Figure 3.16b). Segmentation enhances the contact of the chyme with digestive enzymes and enterocytes, thereby boosting both digestion and absorption. Both peristalsis and segmentation continue while we're working, exercising, even sleeping.

Nerves Controlling the GI Tract

The contractions and secretions of the gastrointestinal tract are controlled by three types of nerves:

- The **enteric nervous system (ENS)**, which is localized in the wall of the GI tract and is part of the *autonomic nervous system*, a group of nerves that regulates many unconscious, internal functions;
- Other branches of the autonomic nervous system outside the GI tract;
- The central nervous system (CNS), which includes the brain and spinal cord.

Some digestive functions are carried out entirely within the ENS. For instance, control of peristalsis is enteric, occurring without assistance from beyond the GI tract. In addition, enteric nerves regulate the secretions of the various digestive glands whose roles we have discussed in this chapter.

Enteric nerves also work in collaboration with other autonomic nerves and with the CNS. For example, we noted earlier in this chapter that in response to fasting, nerves in the stomach and intestinal walls (ENS nerves) trigger signals that travel along nerves beyond the GI tract all the way to the hypothalamus, which is part of the CNS. We then experience the sensation of hunger.

Finally, some functions, such as the secretion of saliva, are achieved without any enteric involvement. A variety of stimuli from the smell, sight, taste, and tactile sensations from food trigger special salivary cells in the CNS; these cells then stimulate increased activity of the salivary glands.

recap Many specialized organs, features, and processes contribute to the functioning of the GI system. The gallbladder stores bile, which emulsifies fats, and the pancreas and small intestine secrete digestive enzymes that break down carbohydrates, fats, and proteins. The lining of the small intestine is heavily folded and the surface area expanded by villi and microvilli. Nutrients are absorbed across the mucosal membrane by passive and facilitated diffusion,

enteric nervous system (ENS) The autonomic nerves in the walls of the GI tract.

active transport, and endocytosis. The liver processes all the nutrients absorbed from the small intestine and stores and regulates energy nutrients. The cardio-vascular and lymphatic system transport nutrients. The GI flora contribute to digestion, synthesize certain vitamins, and perform many other beneficial functions. The coordination and regulation of GI functions are directed by the neuro-muscular system. Voluntary muscles assist us with chewing and swallowing. The involuntary processes of peristalsis and segmentation transport food and facilitate gastrointestinal functions. The enteric nerves of the GI tract work independently and in partnership with other nerves of the body to achieve the digestion of food, absorption of nutrients, and elimination of wastes.

What disorders are related to digestion, absorption, and elimination?

LO 5 Discuss the causes, symptoms, and treatments of several common disorders affecting digestion, absorption, and elimination.

Considering the complexity of digestion, absorption, and elimination, it's no wonder that sometimes things go wrong. Certain GI problems can affect food intake, digestion, or the absorption of nutrients and, over time, malnutrition can result. Let's look at some GI tract disorders and what you might be able to do if they affect you.

Heartburn and Gastroesophageal Reflux Disease (GERD) Are Caused by Reflux of Gastric Juice

We noted earlier that, even as you're chewing your first bite of food, your stomach is starting to secrete gastric juice to prepare for digestion. When you swallow, the food is propelled along the esophagus. The gastroesophageal sphincter relaxes, and the food enters the stomach. As this occurs, a small amount of gastric juice may flow "backwards" into the lower esophagus for a moment. This phenomenon is technically known as gastroesophageal reflux (GER), and is common.

However, in some people, peristalsis in the esophagus is weak and the food exits too slowly, or the gastroesophageal sphincter is overly relaxed and stays partially open. In either case, gastric juice isn't cleared from the lower esophagus quickly and completely. Although the stomach is protected from the highly acidic gastric juice by a thick coat of mucus, the esophagus does not have this coating; thus, the gastric juice burns it **(FIGURE 3.17)** (see page 86). When this happens, the person experiences a painful sensation in the region of the chest behind the sternum (breastbone). This symptom is commonly called **heartburn**.

Many people take over-the-counter antacids to raise the pH of the gastric juice, thereby relieving the heartburn. A nondrug approach is to repeatedly swallow: this action causes any acid pooled in the esophagus to be swept down into the stomach, eventually relieving the symptoms.

Occasional heartburn is common and not a cause for concern; however, heartburn is also the most common symptom of **gastroesophageal reflux disease (GERD)**, a chronic disease in which episodes of GER cause heartburn or other symptoms more than twice per week. These other symptoms of GERD include chest pain, trouble swallowing, burning in the mouth, the feeling that food is stuck in the throat, and hoarseness in the morning.

The exact causes of GERD are unknown. However, a number of factors may contribute, including the following:[6]

- A hiatal hernia. The *hiatus* is the opening in the diaphragm—a sheet of muscle that separates the stomach from the chest cavity—through which the lower esophagus passes. Normally, the hiatus is tight, helping to keep gastric juice from flowing into the esophagus. In a hiatal hernia, the upper part of the stomach slides through and above the hiatus. Gastric juice can more easily enter the esophagus in people with a hiatal hernia.
- Overweight, obesity, and pregnancy.
- Cigarette smoking.
- A variety of medications, from pain relievers to antidepressants.

heartburn A painful sensation that occurs over the sternum when gastric juice pools in the lower esophagus.

gastroesophageal reflux disease (GERD) A chronic disease in which episodes of gastroesophageal reflux cause heartburn or other symptoms more than twice per week.

▶ **FIGURE 3.17** The mechanism of heartburn and gastroesophageal reflux disease is the same: acidic gastric juices seep backward through the gastroesophageal sphincter into the lower portion of the esophagus and pool there, burning its lining. The pain is felt behind the sternum (breastbone), over the heart.

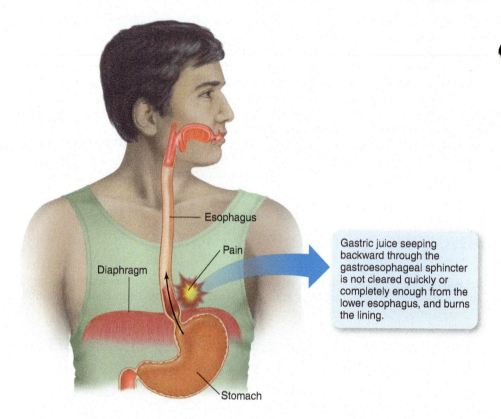

Esophagus

Pain

Diaphragm

Gastric juice seeping backward through the gastroesophageal sphincter is not cleared quickly or completely enough from the lower esophagus, and burns the lining.

Stomach

One way to reduce the symptoms of GERD is to identify the types of foods or situations that trigger episodes, and then avoid them. Eating smaller meals also helps. After a meal, wait at least 3 hours before lying down. Staying upright helps keep gastric juice from backing up. Some people relieve their nighttime symptoms by elevating the head of their bed 4 to 6 inches—for instance, by placing a wedge between the mattress and the box spring, to keep the chest area elevated. People with GERD who smoke should stop, and, if they are overweight, they should lose weight. Taking an antacid before a meal can help prevent symptoms, and many other over-the-counter and prescription medications are now available to treat GERD.

It is important to treat GERD because it can lead to bleeding and erosion of the esophagus. Scar tissue can develop in the esophagus, making swallowing very difficult. Some people can also develop a condition called Barrett's esophagus, which can lead to cancer. Asthma can also be aggravated or even caused by GERD.

An Ulcer Is an Area of Erosion in the GI Tract

A **peptic ulcer** is an area of the GI tract that has been eroded away by a combination of hydrochloric acid and the enzyme pepsin **(FIGURE 3.18)**. In almost all cases, it is located in the stomach area (*gastric ulcer*) or the part of the duodenum closest to the stomach (*duodenal ulcer*). It causes a burning pain in the abdominal area, typically 1 to 3 hours after eating a meal. In serious cases, eroded blood vessels bleed into the GI tract, causing vomiting of blood and/or blood in the stools as well as anemia. If the ulcer entirely perforates the tract wall, stomach contents can leak into the abdominal cavity, causing a life-threatening infection.

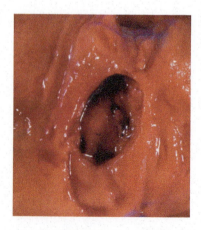

◆ **FIGURE 3.18** A peptic ulcer.

peptic ulcer An area of the GI tract that has been eroded away by the acidic gastric juice of the stomach.

For decades, physicians believed that experiencing high levels of stress, drinking alcohol, and eating spicy foods were the primary factors responsible for ulcers. But in 1982, Australian gastroenterologists J. Robin Warren and Barry Marshall detected the same species of bacteria, *Helicobacter pylori* (*H. pylori*), in the majority of the stomachs of their patients with ulcers. Treatment with an antibiotic cured the ulcers. It is now known that *H. pylori* plays a key role in the development of most peptic ulcers. The hydrochloric acid in gastric juice kills most bacteria, but *H. pylori* thrives in acidic environments.

Although most peptic ulcers are caused by *H. pylori* infection, some are caused by prolonged use of nonsteroidal anti-inflammatory drugs (NSAIDs); these drugs include the common pain relievers aspirin, ibuprofen, and naproxen sodium. They promote ulcers by suppressing the activity of enzymes active in the stomach's production of mucus and bicarbonate, which normally protect the stomach from its acidic gastric juice.[7]

H. pylori is implicated not only in peptic ulcers, but also in stomach cancer and other disorders. So eradicating it with antibiotics would be a good idea, right? Find out in the **Nutrition Debate** at the end of this chapter.

Some Disorders Affect Intestinal Function

GERD and ulcers involve the upper GI tract. In this section, we'll discuss disorders affecting intestinal function.

Vomiting

Vomiting is the involuntary expulsion of the contents of the stomach and duodenum from the mouth. The reflex is triggered when substances or sensations stimulate a cluster of cells in the brain stem to signal a strong wave of "backwards" peristalsis that begins in the small intestine and surges upward. The sphincter muscles of the GI tract relax, allowing the chyme to pass.

One or two episodes of vomiting often accompany a gastrointestinal infection, typically with the norovirus, which is often spread via contaminated water or food. Vomiting triggered by infection is classified as one of the body's innate defenses because it removes harmful agents before they are absorbed. Certain medical procedures, medications, illicit drugs, motion sickness, the hormonal changes of pregnancy, and severe pain can also trigger vomiting.

In contrast, *cyclic vomiting syndrome* (CVS) is a chronic condition characterized by recurring cycles of nausea and vomiting severe enough to cause dehydration. Anxiety, allergies, infections, and a variety of other disturbances may trigger CVS. The person may need to be hospitalized.

Diarrhea

Diarrhea is the frequent passage (more than three times in 1 day) of loose, watery stools. Other symptoms may include cramping, abdominal pain, bloating, nausea, fever, and blood in the stools. Diarrhea is usually caused by an infection of the gastrointestinal tract, a chronic disease, stress, or reactions to medications.[8] It can also occur as a reaction to a particular food or food ingredient. Disorders related to specific foods include food intolerances, allergies, and celiac disease. For a discussion of these disorders, see the **In Depth** essay following this chapter.

Whatever the cause, diarrhea can be harmful if it persists for a long period because the person can lose large quantities of water and minerals and become severely dehydrated. **TABLE 3.1** reviews the signs and symptoms of dehydration, which is particularly dangerous in infants, young children, and older adults. A doctor should be seen immediately if diarrhea persists for more than 24 hours in children or more than 3 days in adults, or if diarrhea is bloody, fever is present, or there are signs of dehydration.

Traveler's diarrhea is experienced by people traveling to countries outside of their own and is usually caused by viral or bacterial infections, often a species of bacteria

vomiting The involuntary expulsion of the contents of the stomach and duodenum from the mouth.

diarrhea A condition characterized by the frequent passage of loose, watery stools.

TABLE 3.1   Signs and Symptoms of Dehydration in Adults and Children

Symptoms in Adults	Symptoms in Children
Thirst	Dry mouth and tongue
Light-headedness	No tears when crying
Less frequent urination	No wet diapers for 3 hours or more
Dark-colored urine	High fever
Fatigue	Sunken abdomen, eyes, or cheeks
Dry skin	Irritable or listless
	Skin does not rebound when pinched and released

Data adapted from: Diarrhea, National Digestive Diseases Information Clearinghouse, www.niddk.nih.gov.

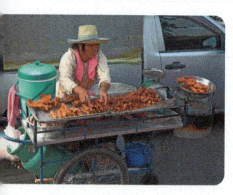

⬆ When traveling, it is wise to avoid food from street vendors.

called *E. coli*. The large intestine and even some of the small intestine become irritated by the microbes and the body's defense against them. This irritation leads to increased secretion of fluid and increased motility of the large intestine, causing watery and frequent bowel movements.

People generally get traveler's diarrhea from consuming water or food that is contaminated with fecal matter. Very risky foods include any raw or undercooked fish, meats, and raw fruits and vegetables. Tap water, ice made from tap water, and unpasteurized milk and dairy products are also common sources of infection.

What can you do to prevent traveler's diarrhea? The accompanying **Quick Tips** from the National Institutes of Health should help.[8]

Constipation

Constipation is typically defined as a condition in which no stools are passed for 2 or more days; however, some people normally experience bowel movements only every

nutri-case | THEO

"My parents and I went to visit our family in Nigeria two years ago, during my winter break. We're planning to go again this year, but I'm not sure I'm looking forward to it. Don't get me wrong, I had a great time—after I got over being sick. We'd been there a couple of days when I came down with gut pain, nausea, and diarrhea so bad I had to stay within a few feet of a toilet. And it lasted for days! I'm thinking maybe I'll ask my doctor if I should start taking some antibiotics now so I can clean out my gut before we leave. I'd hate to go through all that again."

What do you think of Theo's idea about taking antibiotics to "clean out his gut" before he goes on his trip? Identify any potential benefits or drawbacks of such treatment. Is there a better approach Theo could take to reducing his risk for traveler's diarrhea? If so, what?

constipation A condition characterized by the absence of bowel movements for a period of time that is significantly longer than normal for the individual, and stools that are small, hard, and difficult to pass.

second or third day. Thus, the definition varies from one person to another. In addition to being infrequent, the stools are usually hard, small, and difficult to pass.

Many people experience temporary constipation at some point, such as when they travel, if they change their diet, or if they are on certain medications. Many healthcare providers suggest increasing fiber and fluid in the diet. Five to nine servings of fruits and vegetables each day and six or more servings of whole grains are recommended, as is ample fluid. (The dietary recommendation for fiber and the role it plays in maintaining healthy elimination are discussed in detail in Chapter 4.) Regular exercise may also help reduce your risk for constipation.

Irritable Bowel Syndrome

Irritable bowel syndrome (IBS) is a group of symptoms caused by changes in the normal functions of the GI tract. It is one of the most common medical diagnoses, and it affects about twice as many women as men.[9] Symptoms include abdominal cramps, bloating, and either diarrhea or constipation: in some people with IBS, food moves too quickly through the GI tract, and in others, the movement is too slow.

IBS shows no sign of underlying disease that can be observed or measured. However, it appears that the GI tract is more sensitive to stress in people with IBS than in healthy people. Some researchers believe that the problem stems from conflicting messages between the central nervous system and the enteric nervous system. Infection may also trigger the syndrome, and an imbalance in the GI flora may also be a factor. Many people with IBS report that certain foods and beverages trigger episodes. These include coffee, alcohol, fatty foods, and foods high in carbohydrates. Genetics may also play a role.[9]

If you think you have IBS, it is important to have a complete physical examination to rule out celiac disease. (See the **In Depth** essay following this chapter.) Treatment options include medications, stress management, regular physical activity, eating a diet high in fiber and low in sugars, and consuming probiotics.[9]

Cancer Can Develop in Any Gastrointestinal Organ

Cancer can develop in any organ of the gastrointestinal system. Commonly affected are the oral cavity and pharynx, the esophagus, stomach, liver, pancreas, and the colon and rectum. Of these, the most common is colorectal cancer—cancer affecting the colon or rectum. It is diagnosed in about 135,000 Americans annually, making it the third most common cancer in men as well as in women. It is also the third most deadly, killing about 50,000 Americans annually.[10]

Risk factors include obesity, low levels of physical activity, smoking, and moderate to heavy alcohol consumption. Research also implicates high consumption of red and processed meats.[10] A diet high in whole grains, fruits, and vegetables appears to reduce the risk.

Symptoms of colorectal cancer include a persistent change in bowel habits, blood in the stool, unexplained weight loss, and abdominal pain. Either of two screening tests are recommended for Americans beginning at age 50. They include an annual stool test that looks for occult blood (hidden blood) in a stool sample, and an internal imaging test called a *colonoscopy* that looks for polyps—small masses of malignant but noninvasive cells—as well as cancerous tumors. Polyps are typically removed during a colonoscopy. Larger tumors require surgery.

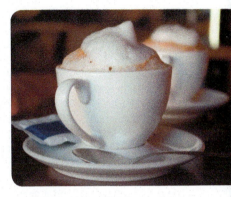

Consuming coffee is one of several factors that have been linked with irritable bowel syndrome.

To learn more about IBS, watch a short video at www.mayoclinic.org. In the search bar, enter "Video: Irritable bowel syndrome." Then click on the link, "How Irritable Bowel Syndrome Affects You."

recap Gastroesophageal reflux is the seepage of gastric juices into the esophagus. Peptic ulcers are erosions of the GI tract by hydrochloric acid and pepsin. Most ulcers are caused by bacterial infection or use of nonsteroidal anti-inflammatory drugs. Cyclic vomiting syndrome is a pattern of recurring episodes of severe vomiting. Diarrhea is the frequent passage of loose stools. Constipation is failure to have a bowel movement within a time period that is normal for the individual. Irritable bowel syndrome causes abdominal cramps, bloating, and constipation or diarrhea. The causes are unknown. Cancer can develop in any GI organ; however, colorectal cancer is the most common type.

irritable bowel syndrome (IBS) A group of symptoms caused by changes in the normal functions of the GI tract.

H. pylori: Could the Same Germ Make Us Sick and Keep Us Well?

The bacterium *Helicobacter pylori* has resided in the GI tract of humans for at least tens of thousands of years.[11] In developed nations, about 20% of the population has colonies of *H. pylori* inhabiting the stomach, whereas in the developing world, infection rates are about 90%.[11] The difference in prevalence can be explained largely by the "miracle of antibiotics," which are prescribed routinely in the United States and other industrialized nations to relieve childhood pain and suffering from strep throat, ear infections, and a variety of other common bacterial diseases. These *broad-spectrum antibiotics*—medications effective against a wide variety of bacterial species—kill not only the targeted microbes in the throat or other organs, but also the *H. pylori* residing in the child's stomach. Although healthcare providers in the United States have been reducing their antibiotic prescribing rate for the past two decades, American children still receive an average of at least one course of antibiotics per year through age 6.[12]

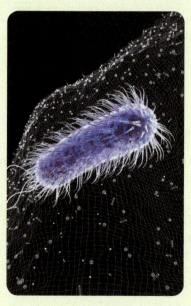

The *Helicobacter pylori* (*H. pylori*) bacterium plays a key role in the development of most peptic ulcers.

Not long ago, the decline in prevalence of *H. pylori* infection was considered a triumph of modern medicine. After all, the bacterium increases the risk not only for ulcers, but also for stomach cancer, iron deficiency anemia, and possibly a host of other disorders from skin rashes to cardiovascular disease.[11] But over the past 20 years, researchers have become increasingly convinced that—at least throughout childhood—*H. pylori* can be a helpful, healthful member of our GI flora. Studies suggest that colonization of the GI tract with *H. pylori* might protect children against at least the following diseases:

- *Asthma and allergies.* Several epidemiological studies have found an inverse correlation between childhood *H. pylori* infection and childhood-onset asthma and allergies.[11] That is, children whose GI tract is populated with *H. pylori* are less likely to suffer from these immune hypersensitivities. Animal studies have provided experimental evidence that *H. pylori* colonization protects against the airway inflammation and other immune responses that are the hallmark of asthma. In one study, among mice exposed to dust mites and other allergens, all mice without *H. pylori* became ill, whereas mice with *H. pylori* did not.[13] These animal studies lend support to a popular theory that the rise in asthma and allergies in industrialized nations is due to the disappearance of our ancestral GI flora, including *H. pylori*. However, not all researchers agree, and the link between *H. pylori* and asthma and allergies is still the subject of considerable debate.[13]

- *Gastroesophageal reflux disease and esophageal cancer.* Studies in the United States, Europe, and Asia have also found an inverse correlation between *H. pylori* colonization and both gastroesophageal reflux disease and esophageal cancer.[11] Although the precise mechanism for this relationship is not clear, some experimental studies suggest that the effect may occur because *H. pylori* reduces both the amount and acidity of gastric juice. Other researchers propose that, because obesity increases the risk for GERD, another contributing factor may be the role of *H. pylori* infection in protecting against obesity.[11]

- *Overweight and obesity.* Studies have shown that, in stomachs colonized by *H. pylori*, levels of the hormone ghrelin are lower than in stomachs lacking *H. pylori*.[11] Recall that ghrelin stimulates the hypothalamus to strongly induce us to eat. Population studies have shown that children given antibiotics during early infancy (age 0 to 6 months) are 22% more likely to be overweight at age 3 than children not given antibiotics in early infancy.[14]

Despite these findings, no one denies that, in adults, *H. pylori* infection increases the risk of serious disease, from peptic ulcers to stomach cancer. Indeed, especially as we age, *H. pylori* infection can pose a serious threat. But some researchers contend that, during childhood, its presence confers no risk and might be beneficial. In fact, whereas some researchers are proposing developing a vaccine against *H. pylori*, others are suggesting that children as well as obese people be injected with a therapeutic dose of the microbe, fostering its colonization in their GI tract. For now, the relative benefits and harms of *H. pylori* is a subject for which there appear to be more questions than answers.[11]

CRITICAL THINKING QUESTIONS

1. Until recently, many ranchers fed antibiotics to livestock to quickly increase the animals' weight. Explain a possible mechanism for this weight gain.
2. At the beginning of this debate, we referred to the "miracle of antibiotics." Are antibiotics a miracle cure? Why or why not?
3. Visit www.cdc.gov and type "antibiotics quiz" in the search bar. From the menu, click on the quiz and answer the questions. After reading the answers, list at least three ways you can prevent antibiotic resistant infections, and three negative consequences of developing an infection with a resistant strain of bacteria.

TEST YOURSELF | ANSWERS

1 F Even extreme food restriction, such as near-starvation, does not cause the stomach to shrink permanently. Likewise, the stomach doesn't stretch permanently. The folds in the wall of the stomach flatten as it expands to accommodate a large meal, but they re-form over the next few hours as the food empties into the small intestine. Only after gastric surgery, when a very small stomach "pouch" remains, can stomach tissue stretch permanently.

2 T Although there are individual variations in how we respond to food, the entire process of digestion and absorption of one meal usually takes about 24 hours.

3 T Most ulcers result from an infection of the bacterium *Helicobacter pylori* (*H. pylori*). Contrary to popular belief, ulcers are not caused by stress or spicy food.

review questions

LO 1 1. Which of the following represents the levels of organization in the human body from smallest to largest?
a. cells, molecules, atoms, tissues, organs, systems
b. atoms, molecules, cells, organs, tissues, systems
c. atoms, molecules, cells, tissues, organs, systems
d. molecules, atoms, cells, tissues, organs, systems

LO 1 2. The cell membrane is composed of
a. a somewhat rigid layer of cholesterol molecules and proteins.
b. two flexible layers of phospholipid molecules.
c. a flexible layer of cholesterol molecules studded with multiple organelles.
d. repeating atoms of various lipids.

LO 2 3. The region of brain tissue that is responsible for prompting us to seek food is the
a. pituitary gland.
b. cephalic phase.
c. hypothalamus.
d. autonomic nervous system.

LO 3 4. The jejunum is
a. the first segment of the esophagus.
b. the main portion of the stomach.
c. the middle segment of the small intestine.
d. the first segment of the large intestine.

LO 4 5. Most digestion of carbohydrates, fats, and proteins takes place in the
a. mouth.
b. stomach.
c. small intestine.
d. large intestine.

LO 4 6. The nerves of the GI tract are
a. collectively known as the enteric nervous system.
b. part of the central nervous system.
c. incapable of acting independently of the brain.
d. all of the above.

LO 5 7. Heartburn is caused by pooling of
a. gastric juice in the esophagus.
b. pepsin in the cardiac muscle.
c. bile in the stomach.
d. salivary amylase in the stomach.

LO 3 8. **True or false?** Food encounters the pharynx before it encounters the esophagus.

LO 4 9. **True or false?** Bile is produced by the gallbladder.

LO 5 10. **True or false?** Diarrhea can be a normal, protective response to infection.

math review

LO 3 **11.** Some people use baking soda as an antacid. The pH of baking soda is 9.0. The pH of gastric juice is 2.0. Baking soda is how many times more alkaline than gastric juice?

Answers to Review Questions and Math Review are located at the back of this text and in the MasteringNutrition Study Area.

web links

www.niddk.nih.gov
National Institute of Diabetes and Digestive and Kidney Diseases (NIDDK)
Explore this site to learn more about disorders involving the gastrointestinal system.

www.cancer.gov
National Cancer Institute
Search this site to learn more about cancers affecting the gastrointestinal tract and its accessory organs.

www.ibsgroup.org
Irritable Bowel Syndrome Self-Help and Support Group
Visit this site for information on self-help measures and support for people diagnosed with IBS.

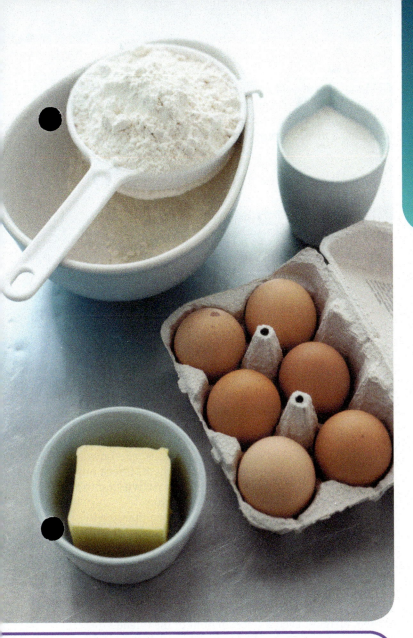

Disorders Related to Specific Foods

learning outcomes

After studying this In Depth, you should be able to:

1 Identify the most common physiologic problem underlying food intolerances, including lactose intolerance, p. 94.

2 Describe how an immune hypersensitivity to food proteins can produce the symptoms characteristic of an allergic reaction, pp. 94–95.

3 Compare and contrast the risk factors and health problems associated with celiac disease and non-celiac gluten sensitivity, pp. 96–97.

You're at a snack bar on campus, trying to decide between two brands of energy bars. You compare their lists of ingredients. One of the bars, although it contains no nuts, says, "Produced in a facility that processes peanuts." The other warns, "Contains wheat, milk, and soy." Why all the warnings? The reason is that, for some people, consuming these normally healthful food ingredients can provoke gastrointestinal distress, itching, nasal congestion, or other uncomfortable symptoms. For others, these ingredients can impair body functions and tissues so dramatically that consuming them—even in minute amounts—can be life-threatening.

Disorders related to specific foods can be clustered into three main groupings: food intolerances, food allergies, and two disorders specifically related to consumption of a protein called gluten. Many people confuse these disorders, and even physicians sometimes misdiagnose them. In this **In Depth** essay, we'll identify their significant differences and the potential impact of those differences on your health.

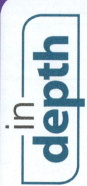

in depth

What are food intolerances?

LO 1 Identify the most common physiologic problem underlying food intolerances, including lactose intolerance.

A **food intolerance** is a cluster of GI symptoms (often gas, pain, and diarrhea) that occur following the consumption of a particular food. Commonly, intolerance results when the body does not produce enough of the enzymes it needs to break down certain food components before they reach the colon. A common example is **lactose intolerance**, in which the small intestine does not produce sufficient amounts of the enzyme lactase to digest the milk sugar *lactose,* which is present in milk and many other dairy products. Lactose intolerance should not be confused with a milk allergy. People who are allergic to milk experience an immune reaction to the proteins found in cow's milk, whereas the immune system plays no role in food intolerances. Symptoms of lactose intolerance include intestinal gas, bloating, cramping, nausea, diarrhea, and discomfort. These symptoms resolve spontaneously within a few hours—typically once the offending food has been eliminated from the GI tract.

Many people who are lactose intolerant are able to tolerate multiple small servings of dairy products without symptoms.[1] They may also be able to digest aged cheese and yogurt with live and active cultures, because the molds or bacteria used in these products break down the lactose during processing. Other people will experience symptoms after consuming even minute amounts of lactose. These individuals should avoid not only all dairy products but also hidden sources of lactose in processed foods. If any of the following ingredients appears on a food label, the product contains lactose: milk, lactose, whey, curds, milk by-products, dry milk solids, nonfat dry milk powder.

People with lactose intolerance need to find foods that can supply enough calcium for normal growth, development, and maintenance of bones. Many can tolerate specially formulated milk products that are low in lactose, whereas others take pills or use drops that contain the lactase enzyme when they eat dairy products. Calcium-fortified soy milk is an excellent substitute for cow's milk.

How can you tell if you are lactose intolerant? Many people discover that they have problems digesting dairy products by trial and error. But because intestinal gas, bloating, and diarrhea may indicate other health

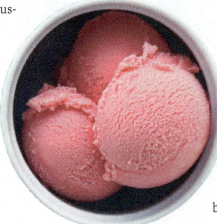

For those who are lactose intolerant, milk products, such as ice cream, are difficult to digest.

problems, you should consult a physician to determine the cause. If you're diagnosed with lactose intolerance, a consultation with a registered dietitian may help in designing a diet that provides adequate nutrients.

What are food allergies?

LO 2 Describe how an immune hypersensitivity to food proteins can produce the symptoms characteristic of an allergic reaction.

A **food allergy** is a hypersensitivity reaction of the immune system to a particular component (usually a protein) in a food. This reaction causes the immune cells to release chemicals that cause inflammation. Wheat, soy, egg, and other proteins are technically referred to as *allergens* because they are capable of prompting an allergic reaction in susceptible people. What are the eight most common food allergens, and how can you recognize them? Check out the **Nutrition Label Activity** on the next page to learn more.

Although food allergies are less common than food intolerances, they can be far more serious. Approximately 30,000 consumers require emergency department treatment and 150 Americans die each year because of allergic reactions to foods.[2] How can peanuts, milk, or other foods that most people consume regularly cause another person's immune system to react so violently? In food allergies, even a trace amount of the offending protein can stimulate immune cells to release their inflammatory chemicals. In some people, the inflammation is localized, so the damage is limited. For instance, some people's mouths and throats itch when they eat cantaloupe, whereas others develop a rash whenever they eat eggs. But in some people, the inflammation is widespread, affecting essentially all body systems. This response, called *anaphylaxis,* can cause a sudden drop in blood pressure, difficulty breathing, and even loss of consciousness. Anaphylaxis is life-threatening, so many people with known food allergies carry with them a kit (called an EpiPen®) containing an injection of a powerful

food intolerance Gastrointestinal discomfort caused by certain foods that is not a result of an immune system reaction.

lactose intolerance A disorder in which the small intestine does not produce enough lactase enzyme to break down the sugar lactose, which is found in milk and milk products.

food allergy An inflammatory reaction to food caused by an immune system hypersensitivity.

Recognizing Common Allergens in Foods

Beginning on January 1, 2006, the U.S. Food and Drug Administration (FDA) required food labels to clearly identify any ingredients containing protein derived from the eight major allergenic foods.[2] Manufacturers were required to identify "in plain English" the presence of ingredients that contain protein derived from milk, eggs, fish, crustacean shellfish (crab, lobster, shrimp, and so on), tree nuts (almonds, pecans, walnuts, and so on), peanuts, wheat, or soybeans.

Although more than 160 foods have been identified as causing food allergies in sensitive individuals, the FDA requires labeling for only these eight foods because together they account for over 90% of all documented food allergies in the United States and represent the foods most likely to result in severe or life-threatening reactions.[2]

These eight allergenic foods must be indicated in the list of ingredients; alternatively, adjacent to the ingredients list, the label must say "Contains" followed by the name of the food. For example, the label of a product containing the milk-derived protein casein must use the term *milk* in addition to the term *casein,* so that those who have milk allergies can clearly understand the presence of an allergen they need to avoid.[2] Any food product found to contain an undeclared allergen is subject to recall by the FDA.

Look at the ingredients list from an energy bar, listed below. How many of the FDA's eight allergenic foods does this bar contain? If you were allergic to peanuts, would you eat this bar? Would you eat it if you were lactose intolerant? Explain your answers.

Ingredients: Soy protein isolate, rice flour, oats, milled flaxseed, brown rice syrup, evaporated cane juice, sunflower oil, soy lecithin, cocoa, nonfat milk solids, salt.
Contains soy and dairy. May contain traces of peanuts and other nuts.

---

stimulant called epinephrine. This drug can reduce symptoms long enough for the victim to get to emergency medical care.

Physicians use a variety of tests to diagnose food allergies. Usually, the physician orders a skin test, commonly known as a "scratch test," in which a small amount of fluid containing the suspected allergen is swabbed onto the patient's skin, which is then lightly scratched. Redness and/or swelling indicates that the patient is allergic to the substance. Some physicians perform a blood test, in which a sample of the patient's blood is tested for the presence of unique proteins, called *antibodies,* that the immune system produces in a person with an allergy.

The simplest way to avoid an allergic reaction to a food component is to avoid consuming foods that contain it. This may sound easier than it is in practice, as allergenic proteins can be listed on food labels by several different names. This is why FDA labeling is so important. Dozens of foods are recalled annually not because they contain bacteria or other harmful microbes, but because they contain allergens such as milk or wheat proteins that have not been identified on the label.

If mild signs and symptoms of a food allergy do occur, taking an over-the-counter antihistamine may help. For severe reactions, an injection of epinephrine and emergency treatment are essential. Researchers are studying the potential benefits and risks of introducing infants and children to minute amounts of allergenic foods (such as peanut butter) to prevent them from developing food allergies. However, this research is experimental at this time.

Beware of e-mail spam, Internet websites, and ads in popular magazines attempting to link a vast assortment of health problems to food allergies. Typically, these ads offer allergy-testing services for exorbitant fees, then make even more money by selling "nutritional counseling" and sometimes supplements and other products they say will help you cope with your allergies. If you suspect you might have a food allergy, consult an MD.

For some people, eating a meal of grilled shrimp with peanut sauce would cause a severe allergic reaction.

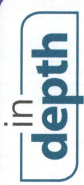

Is celiac disease the same as gluten sensitivity?

LO 3 Compare and contrast the risk factors and health problems associated with celiac disease and nonceliac gluten sensitivity.

Gluten is a protein found in wheat, rye, and barley. Until recently, it was challenging for consumers to locate breads, breakfast cereals, pasta, and other grain foods that didn't contain gluten. But in the last decade, "gluten-free" has become a craze. Why?

Celiac Disease Is an Inherited Immune Disease

Celiac disease, also known as *celiac sprue,* is a disease that severely damages the lining of the small intestine and interferes with the absorption of nutrients.[3] As in food allergy, the body's immune system causes the disorder. There is a strong genetic predisposition to celiac disease, with the risk now linked to specific gene markers.

nutri-case | LIZ

"I'm allergic to peanuts. I used to think of my allergy as no big deal, but about a year ago, I was having lunch in a restaurant when I started to itch and wheeze. I didn't realize that the dressing on the salad I was eating was made with peanut oil. Fortunately, I had my EpiPen® with me and was able to get to my doctor before things got out of control. For a long time after that, I didn't eat anything I hadn't prepared myself. I eat out again now, but always insist on talking with the chef first. Food shopping is hard, too, because I have to check every label. The worst, though, is eating at my friends' houses. I have to ask them if they have peanuts or peanut butter or oil in their house. Some of them are sympathetic, but others look at me like I'm a hypochondriac! I wish I could think of something to say to make them understand this isn't something I have any control over!"

What could Liz say in response to friends who don't understand the cause and seriousness of her food allergy? Do you think it would help Liz to share her fears with her doctor and to discuss possible strategies? If so, why? In addition to shopping, dining out, and eating at friends' houses, what other situations might require Liz to be cautious about her food choices, and sources?

Approximately 1 in every 141 Americans is thought to have celiac disease, but among those with a close family member with the disease, the rate is much higher.[3]

Whereas many foods prompt food allergies, in celiac disease the offending food component is always *gliadin,* a fraction of the protein gluten. When people with celiac disease eat a food containing gluten, their immune system triggers an inflammatory response that erodes the villi of the small intestine. If the person is unaware of the disorder and continues to eat gluten, repeated immune reactions cause the villi to become greatly decreased, so that there is less absorptive surface area. In addition, the enzymes secreted at the brush border of the small intestine become reduced. As a result, the person becomes unable to absorb certain nutrients properly—a condition known as *malabsorption*. Over time, malabsorption can lead to malnutrition (poor nutrient status). Deficiencies of fat-soluble vitamins A, D, E, and K, as well as iron, folic acid, and calcium, are common in those suffering from celiac disease, as are inadequate intakes of protein and total energy.[3]

Symptoms of celiac disease often mimic those of other intestinal disturbances, such as irritable bowel syndrome, so the condition is often misdiagnosed. Some of the symptoms of celiac disease include fatty stools (due to poor fat absorption) with an odd odor; abdominal bloating and cramping; diarrhea, constipation, or vomiting; and weight loss. However, other puzzling symptoms do not appear to involve the GI tract. These include an intensely itchy rash called *dermatitis herpetiformis,* unexplained anemia, fatigue, osteoporosis (poor bone density), arthritis, infertility, seizures, anxiety, irritability, and depression, among others.[3]

Diagnostic tests for celiac disease include a variety of blood tests that screen for the presence of antigliadin antibodies or for the genetic markers of the disease.

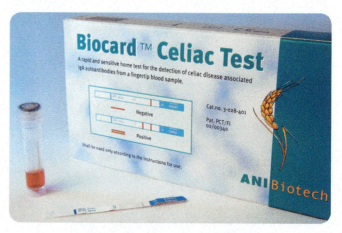

A simple blood test can identify celiac disease.

celiac disease An inherited disorder characterized by inflammation of the lining of the small intestine upon consumption of gluten.

Definitive diagnosis requires a biopsy of the small intestine showing atrophy of the villi. Because long-term complications of undiagnosed celiac disease include an increased risk for intestinal cancer, early diagnosis can be life-saving.

Currently, there is no cure for celiac disease. Treatment is with a special diet that excludes all forms of wheat, rye, and barley. Oats are allowed, as long as they are not contaminated with wheat flour from processing, as even a microscopic amount of wheat can cause an immune response. Although many gluten-free foods are now available, and the FDA now regulates the labeling of such foods, a gluten-free diet is challenging and nutritional counseling is essential.

Someday, gluten-free foods may be unnecessary. Earlier, we discussed the beneficial functions of certain types of bacteria in the GI tract. Now, researchers have discovered that beneficial mouth bacteria are able to degrade gluten.[3,4] Thus, researchers are looking into the potential of developing probiotic breads and other gluten-containing foods that would be safe for people with celiac disease to consume.

Nonceliac Gluten Sensitivity Is the Subject of Research

Recent surveys suggest that as many as 100 million Americans consume at least some foods specifically formulated to be gluten-free.[5] Many of these Americans consume gluten-free products believing that they're more healthful, or will help them lose weight. These claims are largely unfounded. However, there is "undisputable and increasing evidence" for a disorder that is related to gluten consumption but is not celiac disease.[5] This is called *nonceliac gluten sensitivity* (*NCGS*). Signs and symptoms of the disorder can vary greatly, from abdominal bloating and diarrhea to bone and joint pain to depression and confusion; however, the common factor is that patients improve on a gluten-free diet.[6,7] Research into the factors contributing to NCGS is ongoing. In the meantime, if you believe that you might be "gluten sensitive," don't stop eating gluten-containing foods without consulting your doctor to determine whether or not you have celiac disease. That's because antibody tests for celiac disease are not sensitive in people who aren't currently consuming gluten.

web links

www.medlineplus.gov
MEDLINE Plus Health Information

Search for "food allergies" to obtain additional resources as well as the latest news about food allergies.

www.foodallergy.org
The Food Allergy and Anaphylaxis Network

Visit this site to learn more about common food allergens.

www.csaceliacs.org
Celiac Sprue Association—National Celiac Disease Support Group

Get information on the Celiac Sprue Association, a national educational organization that provides information and referral services for persons with celiac disease.

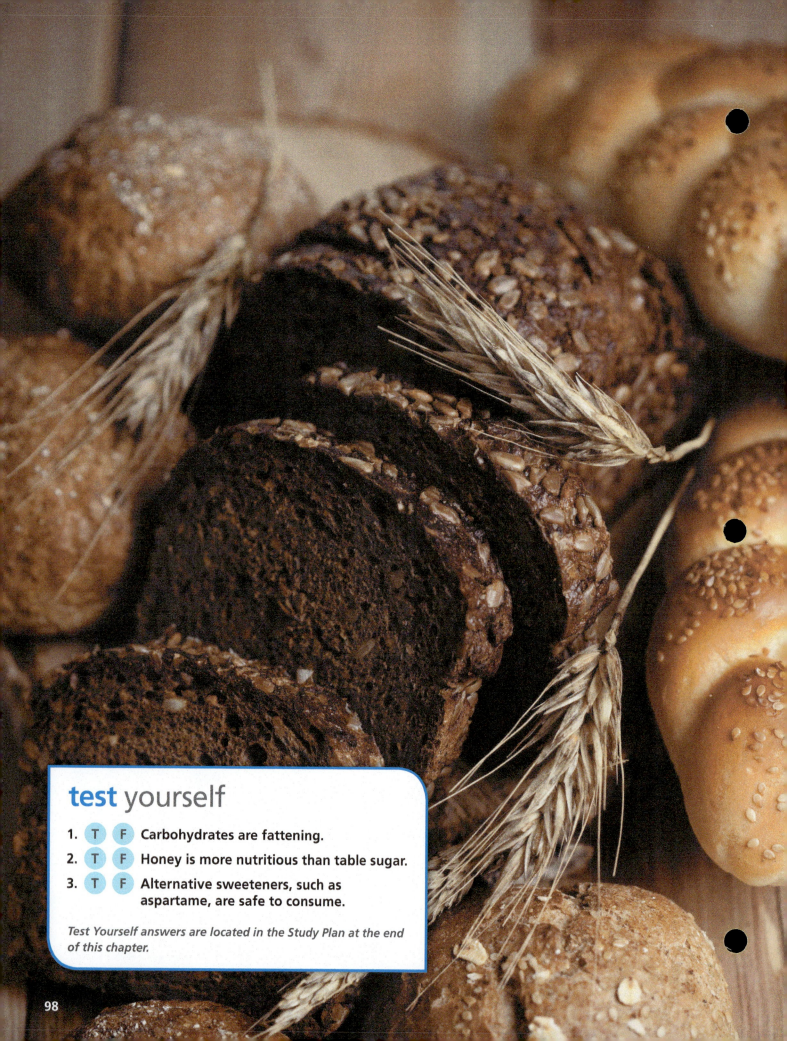

test yourself

1. **T** **F** Carbohydrates are fattening.
2. **T** **F** Honey is more nutritious than table sugar.
3. **T** **F** Alternative sweeteners, such as aspartame, are safe to consume.

Test Yourself answers are located in the Study Plan at the end of this chapter.

4 Carbohydrates
Plant-derived energy nutrients

When Khalil lived at home, he snacked on whatever was around. That typically meant fresh fruit or his mom's homemade flatbread and either plain water or skim milk. His parents never drank soda, and the only time he ate sweets was on special occasions. Now Khalil is living on campus. When he gets hungry between classes, he visits the snack shack in the Student Union for one of their awesome chocolate-chunk cookies and washes it down with a large cola. Studying at night, he munches on cheese curls or corn chips and drinks more cola to help him stay awake. Not surprisingly, Khalil has noticed lately that his clothes feel tight. When he steps on the scale, he's shocked to discover that, since starting college 3 months ago, he has gained 7 pounds!

Several popular diets—including the Paleo Diet, Zone Diet, and Dr. Atkins' New Diet Revolution—claim that carbohydrates are bad for your health. They recommend eating a higher ratio of protein and fat. Is this good advice? Are carbohydrates a health menace, and is one type of carbohydrate "better" or "worse" than another?

In this chapter, we'll explore different types of carbohydrates and learn why some really are better than others. We'll also learn how the human body breaks down carbohydrates and uses them to maintain our health and to fuel activity and exercise. In the **In Depth** essay following this chapter, we'll discuss the relationship between carbohydrate intake and diabetes.

What are carbohydrates?

The term **carbohydrate** literally means "hydrated carbon." When something is said to be *hydrated*, it contains water, which is made of hydrogen and oxygen (H_2O). Thus, the chemical abbreviation for carbohydrate (CHO) indicates the atoms it contains: **c**arbon, **h**ydrogen, and **o**xygen.

We obtain carbohydrates predominantly from plant foods, such as fruits, vegetables, and grains. Plants make the most abundant form of carbohydrate, called **glucose**, through a process called **photosynthesis**. During photosynthesis, the green pigment of plants, called *chlorophyll*, absorbs sunlight, which provides the energy needed to fuel the manufacture of glucose. As shown in **FIGURE 4.1**, water absorbed from the earth by the roots of plants combines with the carbon dioxide present in the leaves to produce glucose. Oxygen is released into the atmosphere as a by-product of these reactions. As discussed shortly, plants continually store glucose as starch and use it to support their own growth. Then, when we eat plant foods, our body digests the starch and absorbs and uses the stored glucose.

Carbohydrates can be classified as *simple* or *complex*. These terms are used to describe carbohydrates based on the number of molecules of sugar present. Simple carbohydrates contain either one or two molecules, whereas complex carbohydrates contain hundreds to thousands of molecules.

Simple Carbohydrates Include Monosaccharides and Disaccharides

Simple carbohydrates are commonly referred to as *sugars*. Three of these sugars are called **monosaccharides** because they consist of a single sugar molecule (*mono* means "one," and *saccharide* means "sugar"). The other three sugars are **disaccharides**, which consist of two molecules of sugar joined together (*di* means "two").

Monosaccharides

Glucose, fructose, and *galactose* are the three most common monosaccharides in our diet. Each of these monosaccharides contains six carbon atoms, twelve hydrogen atoms, and six oxygen atoms **(FIGURE 4.2)**. Very slight differences in the arrangement

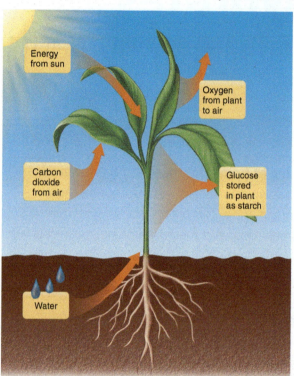

▲ **FIGURE 4.1** Plants make carbohydrates through the process of photosynthesis. Water, carbon dioxide, and energy from the sun are combined to produce glucose. The plant stores glucose in long chains known as starch. As a by-product of photosynthesis, oxygen is released into the atmosphere.

carbohydrate One of the three macronutrients, a compound made up of carbon, hydrogen, and oxygen, that is derived from plants and provides energy.

glucose The most abundant sugar molecule, a monosaccharide generally found in combination with other sugars; it is the preferred source of energy for the brain and an important source of energy for all cells.

photosynthesis The process by which plants use sunlight to fuel a chemical reaction that combines carbon and water into glucose, which is then stored in their cells.

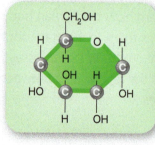

Glucose
Most abundant sugar molecule in our diet; good energy source

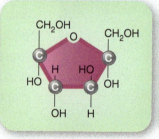

Fructose
Sweetest natural sugar; found in fruit, high-fructose corn syrup

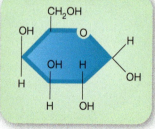

Galactose
Does not occur alone in foods; binds with glucose to form lactose

▲ **FIGURE 4.2** The three most common monosaccharides. Notice that all three monosaccharides contain identical atoms: 6 carbon, 12 hydrogen, and 6 oxygen. It is only the arrangement of these atoms that differs.

of the atoms in these three monosaccharides cause major differences in their levels of sweetness.

Given what you've just learned about how plants manufacture and store carbohydrate in the form of glucose, it probably won't surprise you to discover that glucose is the most abundant sugar molecule in our diets and in our body. Glucose does not generally occur by itself in foods, but attaches to other sugars to form disaccharides and complex carbohydrates. In our body, glucose is the preferred source of energy for the brain, and it is a very important source of energy for all cells.

Fructose, the sweetest natural sugar, is found in fruits and vegetables. Fructose is also called *levulose*, or *fruit sugar*. In many processed foods, it comes in the form of **high-fructose corn syrup**. This syrup is manufactured from corn and is used to sweeten soft drinks, desserts, candies, and jellies.

Galactose does not occur alone in foods. It joins with glucose to create lactose, one of the three most common disaccharides.

Disaccharides

The three most common disaccharides found in foods are *lactose, maltose*, and *sucrose* (**FIGURE 4.3**). **Lactose** (also called *milk sugar*) consists of one glucose molecule and one galactose molecule. Interestingly, human breast milk has more lactose than cow's milk, making human breast milk taste sweeter. Like all carbohydrates, the lactose in dairy products is derived from plants. Dairy cows, sheep, and goats produce lactose from the plants they eat.

Maltose (also called *malt sugar*) consists of two molecules of glucose. It does not generally occur by itself in foods but, rather, is bound together with other molecules. As our body breaks down these larger molecules, maltose results as a by-product. Maltose is also the sugar that is formed during the fermentation of the carbohydrates in grains and other foods into alcohol. **Fermentation** is a process in which an agent, such as yeast, causes an organic substance to break down into simpler substances, resulting in the production of the energy molecule adenosine triphosphate (ATP). Very little maltose remains in alcoholic beverages after the fermentation process is complete; thus, they are not good sources of carbohydrate.

Sucrose is composed of one glucose molecule and one fructose molecule. Because sucrose contains fructose, it is sweeter than lactose or maltose. Sucrose provides much of the sweet taste found in honey, maple syrup, fruits, and vegetables. Table sugar, brown sugar, powdered sugar, and many other products are made by refining the sucrose found in sugarcane and sugar beets.

simple carbohydrate Commonly called *sugar*; can be either a monosaccharide (such as glucose) or a disaccharide.

monosaccharide The simplest of carbohydrates, consisting of one sugar molecule, the most common form of which is glucose.

disaccharide A carbohydrate compound consisting of two sugar molecules joined together.

fructose The sweetest natural sugar; a monosaccharide that occurs in fruits and vegetables; also called levulose, or fruit sugar.

high-fructose corn syrup A highly sweet syrup that is manufactured from corn and is used to sweeten soft drinks, desserts, candies, and jellies.

galactose A monosaccharide that joins with glucose to create lactose, one of the three most common disaccharides.

lactose A disaccharide consisting of one glucose molecule and one galactose molecule. It is found in milk, including human breast milk; also called *milk sugar*.

maltose A disaccharide consisting of two molecules of glucose. It does not generally occur independently in foods but results as a by-product of digestion; also called *malt sugar*.

fermentation A process in which an agent causes an organic substance to break down into simpler substances resulting in the production of ATP.

sucrose A disaccharide composed of one glucose molecule and one fructose molecule; sucrose is sweeter than lactose or maltose.

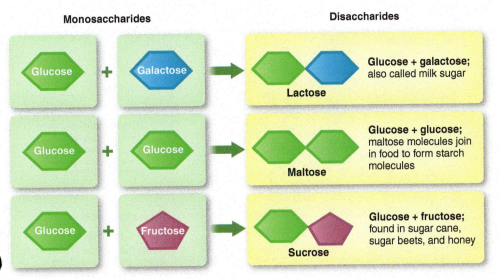

FIGURE 4.3 Galactose, glucose, and fructose join together in different combinations to make the disaccharides lactose, maltose, and sucrose.

Polysaccharides Are Complex Carbohydrates

Complex carbohydrates, the second major type of carbohydrate, generally consist of long chains of glucose molecules called **polysaccharides** (*poly* means "many"). They include starch, glycogen, and most fibers **(FIGURE 4.4)**.

Starch

Plants store glucose not as single molecules but as polysaccharides in the form of **starch**. Excellent food sources of starch include grains (wheat, rice, corn, oats, and barley), legumes (peas, beans, and lentils), and tubers (potatoes and yams). Our cells cannot use the complex starch molecules exactly as they occur in plants. Instead, our body must break them down into the monosaccharide glucose from which we can then fuel our energy needs.

Our body easily digests most starches; however, some starches in plants are not digestible and are called *resistant*. Technically, resistant starch is classified as a type of fiber. When our intestinal bacteria ferment resistant starch, a fatty acid called *butyrate* is produced. Consuming resistant starch may be beneficial: some research suggests that butyrate consumption reduces the risk for cancer.[1] Legumes contain more resistant starch than do other vegetables, fruits, or grains. This quality, plus their high protein and fiber content, makes legumes an especially healthful food.

Glycogen

Glycogen is the storage form of glucose for animals, including humans. After an animal is slaughtered, most of the glycogen is broken down by enzymes found in animal tissues. Thus, very little glycogen exists in meat. As plants contain no glycogen, it is not a dietary source of carbohydrate. We store glycogen in our muscles and liver; our body can metabolize this stored glycogen to glucose when we need energy. The storage and use of glycogen are discussed in more detail shortly.

Fiber

Like starch, fiber is composed of long polysaccharide chains; however, our body does not easily break down the bonds that connect fiber molecules. This means that most fibers pass through the gastrointestinal tract without being digested and absorbed, so they contribute no energy to our diet. However, fiber offers many other health benefits, as we will see shortly.

There are currently a number of definitions of fiber. The Food and Nutrition Board of the Health and Medicine Division of the National Academies of Science propose three distinctions: *dietary fiber, functional fiber,* and *total fiber*.[2]

- **Dietary fiber** is the nondigestible parts of plants that form the support structures of leaves, stems, and seeds (see Figure 4.4). In a sense, you can think of dietary fiber as a plant's "skeleton."

▲ Tubers, such as these sweet potatoes, are excellent food sources of starch.

complex carbohydrate A nutrient compound consisting of long chains of glucose molecules, such as starch, glycogen, and fiber.

polysaccharide A complex carbohydrate consisting of long chains of glucose.

starch A polysaccharide stored in plants; the storage form of glucose in plants.

glycogen A polysaccharide; the storage form of glucose in animals.

dietary fiber The nondigestible carbohydrate parts of plants that form the support structures of leaves, stems, and seeds.

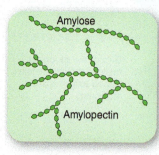

Starch
Storage form of glucose in plants; found in grains, legumes, and tubers

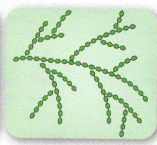

Glycogen
Storage form of glucose in animals; stored in liver and muscles

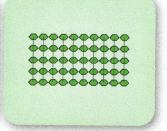

Fiber
Forms the support structures of leaves, stems, and plants

▲ **FIGURE 4.4** Polysaccharides, also referred to as complex carbohydrates, include starch, glycogen, and fiber.

- **Functional fiber** consists of the nondigestible forms of carbohydrates that are extracted from plants or manufactured in a laboratory and have known health benefits. Functional fiber is added to foods and is the form used in fiber supplements. Examples of functional fiber sources you might see on nutrition labels include cellulose, guar gum, pectin, and psyllium.
- **Total fiber** is the sum of dietary fiber and functional fiber.

Fiber can also be classified according to its chemical and physical properties as soluble or insoluble.

Soluble Fibers **Soluble fibers** dissolve in water. They are also **viscous**, forming a gel when wet, and fermentable; that is, they are easily digested by bacteria in the colon. Soluble fibers are typically found in citrus fruits, berries, oat products, and beans. Research suggests that the regular consumption of soluble fibers reduces the risks for cardiovascular disease and type 2 diabetes by lowering blood cholesterol and blood glucose levels. Soluble fibers include the following:

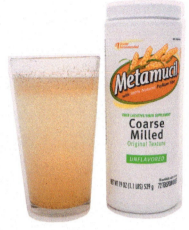

- *Pectins,* which are found in many fruits and berries. They can be isolated and used to thicken foods, such as jams and yogurts.
- *Fructans,* which are found in the stems of many vegetables and grasses, including artichokes, asparagus, leeks, onions, garlic, and wheat. One commonly isolated fructan is inulin, which is used to alter the texture and stability of foods and can be used to replace sugar, fat, and flour. Inulin is also added to foods as a prebiotic.
- *Gums,* which are viscous polysaccharides typically isolated from seeds and used as thickening, gelling, and stabilizing agents. Guar gum and gum arabic are common gums used as food additives.
- *Mucilages,* which are similar to gums. Two examples are psyllium and carrageenan. Psyllium is the husk of psyllium seeds, which are also known as plantago or flea seeds. Carrageenan comes from seaweed. Mucilages are used as food stabilizers.

▲ Dissolvable laxatives are examples of soluble fiber.

Insoluble Fibers **Insoluble fibers** are those that do not typically dissolve in water. These fibers are usually nonviscous and typically cannot be fermented by bacteria in the colon. Insoluble fibers are generally found in whole grains, such as wheat, rye, and brown rice as well as in many vegetables. These fibers are not associated with reducing cholesterol levels but are known for promoting regular bowel movements, alleviating constipation, and reducing the risk for a bowel disorder called diverticulosis (discussed later in this chapter).

Examples of insoluble fibers include the following:

- *Lignins,* which are found in the woody parts of plant cell walls and in carrots and the seeds of fruits and berries. Lignins are also found in brans (the outer husk of grains such as wheat, oats, and rye) and other whole grains.
- *Cellulose,* which is the main structural component of plant cell walls. Cellulose is a chain of glucose units similar to those in starch, but the bonds between the units in cellulose cannot be digested by humans. Cellulose is found in whole grains, fruits, vegetables, and legumes. It can also be extracted from wood pulp or cotton, and it is added to foods as an agent for anticaking, thickening, and texturizing.
- *Hemicelluloses,* which are found in plant cell walls, where they surround cellulose. They are the primary component of cereal fibers and are found in whole grains and vegetables. Although many hemicelluloses are insoluble, some are also classified as soluble.

Fiber-Rich Carbohydrates Materials written for the general public usually don't refer to the carbohydrates found in foods as complex or simple; instead, resources such as the *2015–2020 Dietary Guidelines for Americans* emphasize eating *fiber-rich carbohydrates,* such as fruits, vegetables, and whole grains.[3] This term is important because fiber-rich carbohydrates are known to contribute to good health, but not all complex carbohydrate foods are fiber rich. For example, potatoes that have been processed into frozen hash browns retain very little of their original fiber. On the other

functional fiber The nondigestible forms of carbohydrates that are extracted from plants or manufactured in a laboratory and have known health benefits.

total fiber The sum of dietary fiber and functional fiber.

soluble fibers Fibers that dissolve in water.

viscous Having a gel-like consistency; viscous fibers form a gel when dissolved in water.

insoluble fibers Fibers that do not dissolve in water.

hand, some foods rich in simple carbohydrates (such as fruits) are also rich in fiber. So when you're reading labels, it pays to check the grams of dietary fiber per serving. And if the food you're considering is fresh produce and there's no label to read, that almost guarantees it's fiber rich.

recap Carbohydrates contain carbon, hydrogen, and oxygen. Plants make one type of carbohydrate, glucose, through the process of photosynthesis. Simple carbohydrates include monosaccharides and disaccharides. Glucose, fructose, and galactose are monosaccharides; lactose, maltose, and sucrose are disaccharides. The three types of polysaccharides are starch, glycogen, and fiber. Starch is the storage form of glucose in plants, whereas glycogen is the storage form of glucose in humans and other animals. Fiber forms the support structures of plants. Soluble fibers dissolve in water, are viscous, and can be digested by bacteria in the colon, whereas insoluble fibers do not dissolve in water, are not viscous, and cannot be digested. Fiber-rich carbohydrates are known to contribute to good health.

LO 2 Identify three functions of carbohydrates.

Why do we need carbohydrates?

We have seen that carbohydrates are an important energy source for our body. Let's learn more about this and other functions of carbohydrates.

Carbohydrates Provide Energy for Daily Activities and Exercise

Carbohydrates, an excellent source of energy for all our cells, provide 4 kilocalories (kcal) of energy per gram. Some of our cells can also use fat and even protein for energy if necessary. However, our red blood cells can use only glucose, and our brain and other nervous tissues rely primarily on glucose. This is why you get tired, irritable, and shaky when you haven't eaten any carbohydrate for a prolonged period.

Carbohydrates Fuel Daily Activity

Many popular diets—such as the Paleo Diet and Dr. Atkins' New Revolution Diet—are based on the idea that our body actually "prefers" to use fat and/or protein for energy. They claim that current carbohydrate recommendations are much higher than we really need.

In reality, we rely mostly on both carbohydrates and fat for energy. In fact, as shown in **FIGURE 4.5**, our body always uses some combination of carbohydrates and fat to fuel daily activities. Fat is the predominant energy source used at rest and during low-intensity activities, such as sitting, standing, and walking. Even during rest, however, our brain cells and red blood cells rely on glucose.

Carbohydrates Fuel Exercise

When we exercise, whether running, briskly walking, bicycling, or performing any other activity that causes us to breathe harder and sweat, we begin to use more glucose than fat. Whereas fat breakdown is a slow process and requires oxygen, we can break down glucose very quickly either with or without oxygen. Even during very intense exercise, when less oxygen is available, we can still break down glucose very quickly for energy. That's why when you are exercising at maximal effort carbohydrates are providing almost 100% of the energy your body requires.

If you are physically active, it is important to eat enough carbohydrates to provide energy for your brain, red blood cells, and muscles. In general, if you do not eat enough carbohydrate to support regular exercise, your body will have to rely on fat and protein as alternative energy sources. One advantage of training for endurance-type events, such as marathons and triathlons, is that it boosts the

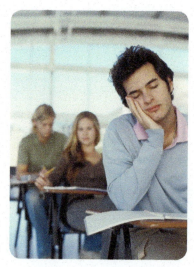

Our red blood cells, brain, and nerve cells primarily rely on glucose. This is why we get tired, irritable, and shaky when we have not eaten for a prolonged period.

muscles' capacity to store glycogen, which provides more glucose for use during exercise. (See Chapter 11 for more information on how exercise affects our need, use, and storage of carbohydrates.)

Carbohydrates Spare Protein and Prevent Ketoacidosis

If the diet does not provide enough carbohydrate, the body will make its own glucose from protein. This involves breaking down the proteins in blood and tissues into amino acids, then converting them to glucose. This process is called **gluconeogenesis** ("generating new glucose").

When our body uses proteins for energy, the amino acids from these proteins cannot be used to make new cells, repair tissue damage, support our immune system, or perform any other function. During periods of starvation or when eating a diet that is very low in carbohydrate, our body will take amino acids from the blood first, and then from other tissues, such as muscles and the heart, liver, and kidneys. Using amino acids in this manner over a prolonged period can cause serious, possibly irreversible, damage to these organs. (See Chapter 6 for more details on using protein for energy.)

Whenever carbohydrate intake is inadequate to supply glucose to the brain, our body seeks an alternative source of fuel and begins to break down stored fat. This process, called **ketosis**, produces an alternative fuel called **ketones**. Ketosis is an important mechanism for providing energy to the brain during sleep, vigorous exercise, and other situations that deplete glycogen stores. However, if inadequate carbohydrate intake continues for an extended period, the body will produce excessive amounts of ketones. Because many ketones are acids, high ketone levels cause the blood to become very acidic, leading to a condition called **ketoacidosis**. The high acidity of the blood interferes with basic body functions, causes the loss of lean body mass, and damages many body tissues. People with untreated diabetes are at high risk for ketoacidosis, which can lead to coma and even death(see the **In Depth** essay on diabetes following this chapter).

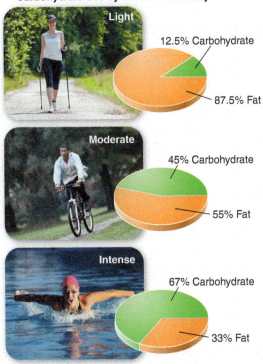

Carbohydrate Use by Exercise Intensity

Light — 12.5% Carbohydrate — 87.5% Fat

Moderate — 45% Carbohydrate — 55% Fat

Intense — 67% Carbohydrate — 33% Fat

🔺 **FIGURE 4.5** Amounts of carbohydrate and fat used during light, moderate, and intense exercise.

Data adapted from: "Regulation of endogenous fat and carbohydrate metabolism in relation to exercise intensity and duration" by Romijn et al., from *American Journal of Physiology*, September 1, 1993. Copyright © 1993 by The American Physiological Society. Reprinted with permission.

Fiber Helps Us Stay Healthy

Although we cannot digest fiber, research indicates that it helps us stay healthy and may prevent many digestive and chronic diseases. The following are potential benefits of fiber consumption:

- Promotes bowel health by helping to prevent hemorrhoids, constipation, and other intestinal problems by keeping our stools moist and soft. Fiber gives gut muscles "something to push on" and makes it easier to eliminate stools.
- Reduces the risk for *diverticulosis*, a condition that is caused in part by trying to eliminate small, hard stools. A great deal of pressure must be generated in the large intestine to pass hard stools. This increased pressure weakens intestinal walls, causing them to bulge outward and form pockets **(FIGURE 4.6)** (see page 106). Feces and fibrous materials can get trapped in these pockets, which become infected and inflamed. This is a painful condition that must be treated with antibiotics or surgery.
- May reduce the risk of colon cancer. The mechanism by which fiber is proposed to reduce our risk of colon cancer is that fiber binds cancer-causing substances and speeds their elimination from the colon.[4] However, recent studies of colon cancer and fiber have shown that their relationship is not as strong as previously thought.[5]

gluconeogenesis The generation of glucose from the breakdown of proteins into amino acids.

ketosis The process by which the breakdown of fat during fasting states results in the production of ketones.

ketones Substances produced during the breakdown of fat when carbohydrate intake is insufficient to meet energy needs. Ketones provide an alternative energy source for the brain when glucose levels are low.

ketoacidosis A condition in which excessive ketones, which are acidic, lower the pH of blood, altering basic body functions and damaging tissues.

▶ **FIGURE 4.6** Diverticulosis occurs when bulging pockets form in the wall of the colon. These pockets become infected and inflamed, demanding proper treatment.

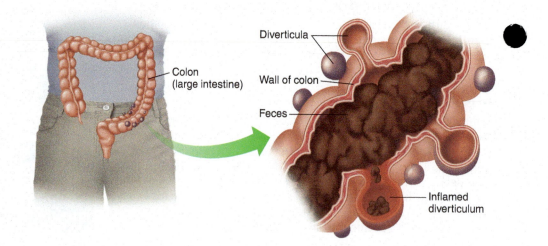

■ May enhance weight loss, as eating a high-fiber diet causes a person to feel more full. Fiber absorbs water, expands in our large intestine, and slows the movement of food through the upper part of the gastrointestinal tract. Also, people who eat a fiber-rich diet tend to eat fewer fatty and sugary foods.

■ May reduce the risk of cardiovascular disease by delaying or blocking the absorption of dietary cholesterol into the bloodstream, a process depicted in **FIGURE 4.7**. In addition, when bacteria in the colon ferment soluble fiber, they produce short-chain fatty acids, types of fat that are thought to reduce the production

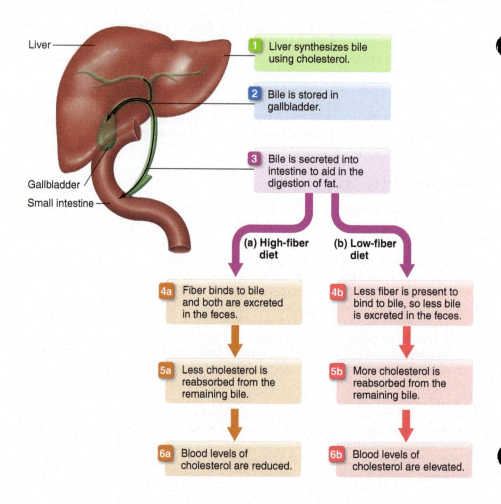

▶ **FIGURE 4.7** How fiber may help decrease blood cholesterol levels. **(a)** When eating a high-fiber diet, fiber binds to the bile that is produced from cholesterol, resulting in relatively more cholesterol being excreted in the feces. **(b)** When a lower-fiber diet is consumed, less fiber (and thus less cholesterol) is bound to bile and excreted in the feces.

of low-density lipoproteins (LDLs), which are compounds associated with cardiovascular disease.

- May lower the risk for type 2 diabetes. In slowing digestion and absorption, fiber also slows the release of glucose into the blood. It thereby improves the body's regulation of insulin production, a factor in diabetes. As discussed shortly, insulin is a hormone that enables cells to clear glucose from the blood.

recap Carbohydrates are an important energy source at rest and during exercise, providing 4 kcal of energy per gram. Adequate intake is important to spare body protein and prevent ketoacidosis. Complex carbohydrates contain fiber and other nutrients that may reduce the risk for obesity, cardiovascular disease, and diabetes. Fiber also helps prevent hemorrhoids, constipation, and diverticulosis, and may reduce the risk for colon cancer.

How does the body process carbohydrates?

LO 3 Describe the steps involved in carbohydrate digestion, absorption, and transport.

Glucose is the form of sugar that our body uses for energy, and the primary goal of carbohydrate digestion is to break down polysaccharides and disaccharides into monosaccharides, which can then be converted to glucose. FOCUS FIGURE 4.8 (page 108) provides a visual tour of carbohydrate digestion.

Digestion Breaks Down Most Carbohydrates into Monosaccharides

Carbohydrate digestion begins in the mouth as the starch in the foods you eat mixes with your saliva during chewing (see Focus Figure 4.8). Saliva contains an enzyme called **salivary amylase**, which breaks starch into smaller particles and eventually into the disaccharide maltose. The next time you eat a piece of bread, notice that you can actually taste it becoming sweeter; this indicates the breakdown of starch into maltose. Disaccharides are not digested in the mouth.

As the bolus of food leaves the mouth and enters the stomach, all digestion of carbohydrates ceases. This is because the acid in the stomach inactivates salivary amylase.

The majority of carbohydrate digestion occurs in the small intestine. As the contents of the stomach enter the small intestine, the pancreas secretes an enzyme called **pancreatic amylase** into the small intestine. Pancreatic amylase continues to digest any remaining starch into maltose. Additional enzymes found in the microvilli of the enterocytes that line the intestinal tract work to break down disaccharides into monosaccharides:

- Maltose is broken down into glucose by the enzyme **maltase**.
- Sucrose is broken down into glucose and fructose by the enzyme **sucrase**.
- Lactose is broken down into glucose and galactose by the enzyme **lactase**.

Once digestion of carbohydrates is complete, all monosaccharides are then absorbed into the enterocytes, where they pass through and enter into the bloodstream.

The Liver Converts Most Nonglucose Monosaccharides into Glucose

Once the monosaccharides enter the bloodstream, they travel to the liver, where fructose and galactose are converted to glucose. If needed immediately for energy, the glucose is released into the bloodstream, where it can travel to the cells to provide

salivary amylase An enzyme in saliva that breaks starch into smaller particles and eventually into the disaccharide maltose.

pancreatic amylase An enzyme secreted by the pancreas into the small intestine that digests any remaining starch into maltose.

maltase A digestive enzyme that breaks maltose into glucose.

sucrase A digestive enzyme that breaks sucrose into glucose and fructose.

lactase A digestive enzyme that breaks lactose into glucose and galactose.

The primary goal of carbohydrate digestion is to break down polysaccharides and disaccharides into monosaccharides that can then be converted to glucose.

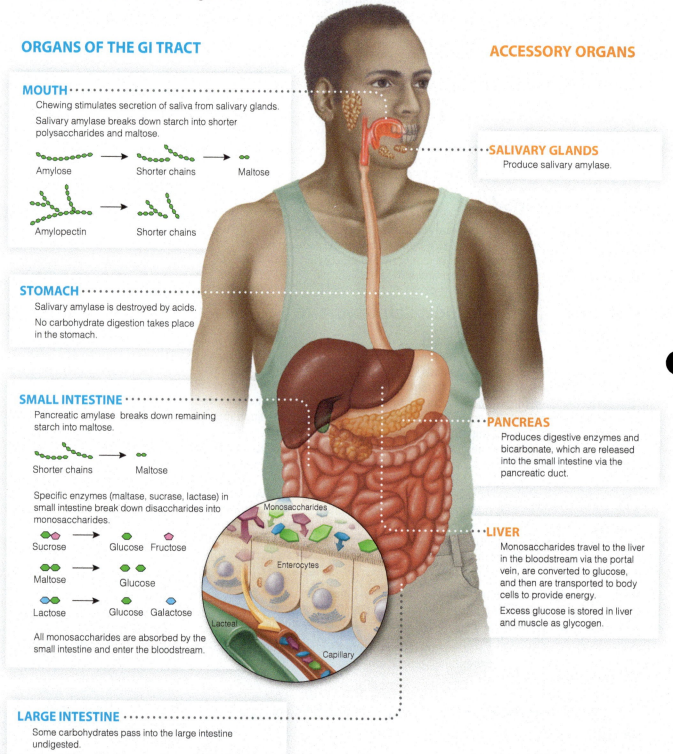

ORGANS OF THE GI TRACT

MOUTH

Chewing stimulates secretion of saliva from salivary glands.

Salivary amylase breaks down starch into shorter polysaccharides and maltose.

Amylose → Shorter chains → Maltose

Amylopectin → Shorter chains

STOMACH

Salivary amylase is destroyed by acids.

No carbohydrate digestion takes place in the stomach.

SMALL INTESTINE

Pancreatic amylase breaks down remaining starch into maltose.

Shorter chains → Maltose

Specific enzymes (maltase, sucrase, lactase) in small intestine break down disaccharides into monosaccharides.

Sucrose → Glucose Fructose

Maltose → Glucose

Lactose → Glucose Galactose

All monosaccharides are absorbed by the small intestine and enter the bloodstream.

LARGE INTESTINE

Some carbohydrates pass into the large intestine undigested.

Bacteria ferment some undigested carbohydrate.

Remaining fiber is excreted in feces.

ACCESSORY ORGANS

SALIVARY GLANDS

Produce salivary amylase.

PANCREAS

Produces digestive enzymes and bicarbonate, which are released into the small intestine via the pancreatic duct.

LIVER

Monosaccharides travel to the liver in the bloodstream via the portal vein, are converted to glucose, and then are transported to body cells to provide energy.

Excess glucose is stored in liver and muscle as glycogen.

Monosaccharides

Enterocytes

Lacteal

Capillary

energy. If glucose is not needed immediately for energy, it is stored as glycogen in the liver and muscles. Enzymes in liver and muscle cells combine glucose molecules to form glycogen in an anabolic, or building, process called *glycogenesis*. On average, the liver can store 70 g (280 kcal) and the muscles can store about 120 g (480 kcal) of glycogen. Stored glycogen can then be converted back into glucose in a catabolic, or destructive, process called *glycogenolysis* to supply the body's energy needs. Between meals, for example, our body draws on liver glycogen reserves to maintain blood glucose levels and support the needs of our cells, including those of our brain, spinal cord, and red blood cells (**FIGURE 4.9**).

The glycogen stored in our muscles continually provides energy to our muscle cells, particularly during intense exercise. Endurance athletes can increase their storage of muscle glycogen from two to four times the normal amount through a process called *carbohydrate loading* (see Chapter 11). Any excess glucose is stored as glycogen in the liver and muscles and saved for such future energy needs as exercise. Once the storage capacity of the liver and muscles is reached, any excess glucose can be stored as fat in adipose tissue (fat tissue).

Fiber Is Excreted from the Large Intestine

As previously mentioned, humans do not possess enzymes in the small intestine that can break down fiber. Thus, fiber passes through the small intestine undigested and enters the large intestine, or colon. There, bacteria ferment soluble fibers, causing the production of gases and a few short-chain fatty acids. The cells of the large intestine use these short-chain fatty acids for energy and, as noted earlier, their production may reduce the level of low-density lipoproteins linked to cardiovascular disease. Insoluble fiber in the colon adds bulk to our stools and is excreted in feces (see Focus Figure 4.8). In this way, fiber assists in maintaining bowel regularity.

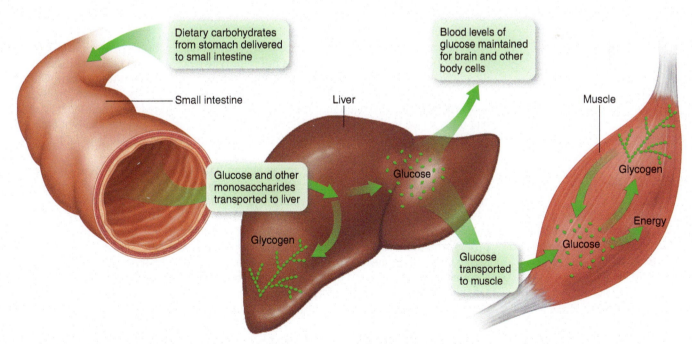

◄ **FIGURE 4.9** In the process of glycogenesis, glucose is stored as glycogen in both the liver and muscle. In the process of glycogenolysis, the glycogen stored in the liver is metabolized to maintain blood glucose between meals; muscle glycogen provides immediate energy to the muscle during exercise.

recap Carbohydrate digestion starts in the mouth with salivary amylase and continues in the small intestine with the help of pancreatic amylase and the intestinal enzymes maltase, sucrase, and lactase. Glucose and other monosaccharides are absorbed into the bloodstream and travel to the liver, where nonglucose sugars are converted to glucose. Glucose either is used by the cells for energy or is converted to glycogen and stored in the liver and muscle for later use. Fiber passes through the small intestine undigested. Bacteria in the colon can ferment soluble fiber, whereas insoluble fiber is excreted in feces.

LO 4 Explain how the body regulates blood glucose levels.

How does the body regulate blood glucose levels?

The body regulates blood glucose levels within a fairly narrow range to provide adequate glucose to the brain and other cells. Let's look at the hormones involved.

Insulin and Glucagon Regulate Blood Glucose Levels

Among the hormones contributing to blood glucose regulation, insulin and glucagon are the key players. When we eat a meal, our blood glucose level rises. But glucose in our bloodstream cannot help our nerves, muscles, and other organs to function unless it can cross into their cells. Glucose molecules are too large to cross cell membranes independently. To get in, glucose needs assistance from the hormone **insulin**, which is secreted into the bloodstream by pancreatic cells called *beta cells* (**FOCUS FIGURE 4.10**, top panel). Insulin is transported in the blood throughout the body, where it stimulates special molecules called *glucose transporters*, which are located in cells, to travel to the cell membrane and transport glucose into the cell. Insulin can therefore be thought of as a key that opens the gates of the cell membrane, enabling the transport of glucose into the cell interior, where it can be used for energy. Insulin also stimulates the liver and muscles to take up glucose and store it as glycogen.

When you have not eaten for some time, your blood glucose level declines. This decrease in blood glucose stimulates a different type of cells of the pancreas, called *alpha cells*, to secrete the hormone **glucagon** (Focus Figure 4.10, bottom panel). Glucagon acts in an opposite way to insulin. It triggers glycogenolysis, in which the liver converts its stored glycogen into glucose, which is then secreted into the bloodstream and transported to the cells for energy. Glucagon also assists in the breakdown of body proteins to amino acids, so that the liver can stimulate gluconeogenesis, the production of new glucose from amino acids.

Normally, the effects of insulin and glucagon balance each other to maintain blood glucose within a healthy range. An alteration in this balance can lead to diabetes (discussed **In Depth** following this chapter) or to a condition known as **hypoglycemia**, in which blood glucose falls to lower-than-normal levels. This commonly occurs in people with diabetes who aren't getting proper treatment, but it can also happen in people who don't have diabetes if their pancreas secretes too much insulin after a high-carbohydrate meal. The characteristic symptoms usually appear about 1 to 4 hours after the meal and occur because the body clears glucose from the blood too quickly. People with this form of hypoglycemia must eat smaller meals more frequently to level out their blood insulin and glucose levels.

Fructose Does Not Stimulate Insulin Release

Fructose is metabolized differently from glucose, and this difference has important implications for hunger, satiety, and body weight. Because it is absorbed farther down in the small intestine, it does not stimulate insulin release from the pancreas. Insulin release inhibits food intake; thus, people consuming fructose might consume more

insulin The hormone secreted by the beta cells of the pancreas in response to increased blood levels of glucose; it facilitates the uptake of glucose by body cells.

glucagon The hormone secreted by the alpha cells of the pancreas in response to decreased blood levels of glucose; it causes the breakdown of liver stores of glycogen into glucose.

hypoglycemia A condition marked by blood glucose levels that are below normal fasting levels.

Our body regulates blood glucose levels within a fairly narrow range to provide adequate glucose to the brain and other cells. Insulin and glucagon are two hormones that play a key role in regulating blood glucose.

HIGH BLOOD GLUCOSE

1 **Insulin secretion:** When blood glucose levels increase after a meal, the pancreas secretes the hormone insulin from the beta cells into the bloodstream.

2 **Cellular uptake:** Insulin travels to the tissues. There, it stimulates glucose transporters within cells to travel to the cell membrane, where they facilitate glucose transport into the cell to be used for energy.

3 **Glucose storage:** Insulin also stimulates the storage of glucose in body tissues. Glucose is stored as glycogen in the liver and muscles (glycogenesis), and is stored as triglycerides in adipose tissue (lipogenesis).

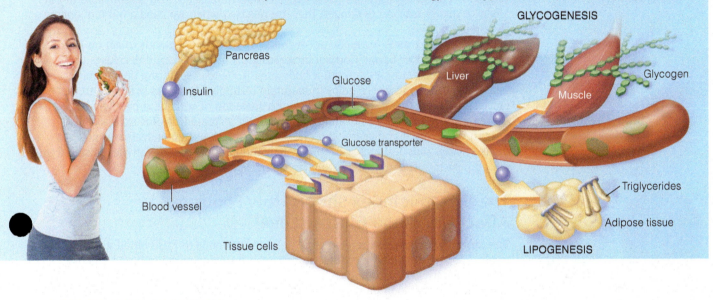

LOW BLOOD GLUCOSE

1 **Glucagon secretion:** When blood glucose levels are low, the pancreas secretes the hormone glucagon from the alpha cells into the bloodstream.

2 **Glycogenolysis:** Glucagon stimulates the liver to convert stored glycogen into glucose, which is released into the blood and transported to the cells for energy.

3 **Gluconeogenesis:** Glucagon also assists in the breakdown of proteins and the uptake of amino acids by the liver, which creates glucose from amino acids.

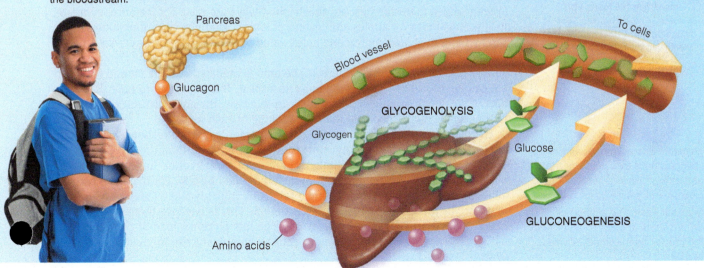

total Calories in a meal than they would if they had consumed the same amount of carbohydrate as glucose. In addition, fructose enters body cells via a transport protein not present in brain cells; thus, unlike glucose, fructose cannot enter brain cells and stimulate satiety signals. If we don't feel full, we are likely to continue eating or drinking. The links between added sugars, particularly those that contain fructose, and the obesity epidemic are discussed in more detail in the **Nutrition Debate** at the end of this chapter.

Other Hormones Increase Blood Glucose Levels

Epinephrine, norepinephrine, cortisol, and growth hormone work to increase blood glucose. Epinephrine and norepinephrine are secreted by the adrenal glands and nerve endings when blood glucose levels are low. They trigger glycogen breakdown in the liver, resulting in a subsequent increase in the release of glucose into the bloodstream. They also increase gluconeogenesis. These two hormones are also responsible for our "fight-or-flight" reaction to danger; they are released when we need a burst of energy to respond quickly.

Cortisol and growth hormone are secreted by the adrenal glands to act on liver, muscle, and adipose tissue. Cortisol increases gluconeogenesis and decreases the use of glucose by muscles and other body organs. Its release during the second phase of the stress response helps to maintain a supply of glucose sufficient to fuel our response to a threat; however, long-term secretion of cortisol in people who are chronically stressed has been implicated in an increased risk for excessive body weight, cardiovascular disease, and diabetes.[6,7] Growth hormone decreases glucose uptake by our muscles, increases our mobilization and use of the fatty acids stored in our adipose tissue, and increases our liver's output of glucose.

The Glycemic Index Shows How Foods Affect Our Blood Glucose Level

The term **glycemic index** refers to the potential of foods to raise blood glucose levels. Foods with a high glycemic index cause a sudden surge in blood glucose. This in turn triggers a large increase in insulin, which may be followed by a dramatic drop in blood glucose. The line graph in **FIGURE 4.11a** compares the effect on blood sugar of a high versus a low glycemic-index food. Foods with a low glycemic index cause low to moderate fluctuations in blood glucose. When foods are assigned a glycemic index value, they are often compared to the glycemic effect of pure glucose.

The glycemic index of a food is not always easy to predict. Figure 4.11b ranks certain foods according to their glycemic index. Do any of these rankings surprise you? Most people assume that foods containing simple sugars have a higher glycemic index than starches, but this is not always the case. For instance, compare the glycemic index for apples and instant potatoes. Although instant potatoes are a starchy food, they have a glycemic index value of 85, whereas the value for an apple is only 38!

The type of carbohydrate, the way the food is prepared, and its fat and fiber content can all affect how quickly the body absorbs it. It is important to note that we eat most of our foods combined into a meal. In this case, the glycemic index of the total meal becomes more important than the ranking of each food.

For determining the effect of a food on a person's glucose response, some nutrition experts believe that the **glycemic load** is more useful than the glycemic index. A food's glycemic load is the number of grams of carbohydrate the serving contains multiplied by the food's glycemic index, and divided by 100. For instance, carrots are recognized as a vegetable having a relatively high glycemic index of about 68; however, the glycemic load of carrots is only 3. This is because there is very little total carbohydrate in a serving of carrots. The low glycemic load of carrots means that carrot consumption is unlikely to cause a significant rise in glucose and insulin levels.

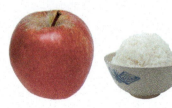

An apple has a much lower glycemic index value (38) than a serving of white rice (56).

To find out the glycemic index and glycemic load of more than 100 foods, visit www.health.harvard.edu/. Type "glycemic index 100 foods" in the search bar, then click on the link.

glycemic index The system that assigns ratings (or values) for the potential of foods to raise blood glucose and insulin levels.

glycemic load The amount of carbohydrate in a food multiplied by the food's glycemic index, divided by 100.

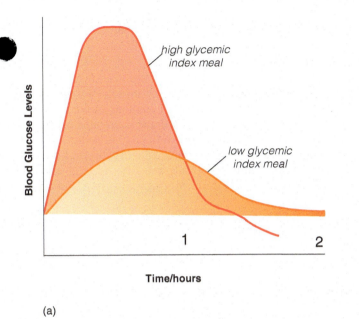

(a)

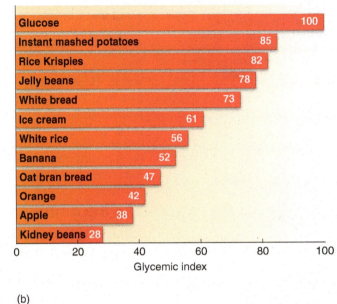

(b)

FIGURE 4.11 The glycemic index is a rating of the potential for a food to raise blood glucose. **(a)** Surge in blood glucose after consuming a food with a high versus a low glycemic index. **(b)** Glycemic index values for various foods as compared to pure glucose.

Data adapted from: "International Table of Glycemic Index and Glycemic Load Values," by Foster-Powell, K., S. H. A. Holt, and J. C. Brand-Miller from *American Journal of Clinical Nutrition*, 2002.

Why do we care about the glycemic index and glycemic load? Foods and meals with a lower glycemic load are better choices for someone with diabetes because they will not trigger dramatic fluctuations in blood glucose. They may also reduce the risk for cardiovascular disease because they generally contain more fiber, and fiber helps decrease cholesterol levels in the blood. A recent systematic review has shown that eating a lower glycemic index diet decreases total blood cholesterol and low-density lipoproteins, which we noted earlier are associated with increased risk for cardiovascular disease.[8]

Despite some encouraging research findings, the glycemic index and glycemic load remain controversial. Many nutrition researchers feel that the evidence supporting their health benefits is weak. In addition, many believe the concepts of the glycemic index/load are too complex for people to apply to their daily lives. Other researchers insist that helping people choose foods with a lower glycemic index/load is critical in the prevention and treatment of many chronic diseases. Until this controversy is resolved, people are encouraged to eat a variety of fiber-rich and less-processed carbohydrates, such as beans and lentils, fresh vegetables, and whole-wheat bread, because these forms of carbohydrates have a lower glycemic load and they contain a multitude of important nutrients.

recap Various hormones are involved in regulating blood glucose. Insulin lowers blood glucose levels by facilitating the entry of glucose into cells. Glucagon raises blood glucose levels by triggering glycogenolysis and gluconeogenesis. Altered blood glucose regulation can lead to hypoglycemia. Epinephrine, norepinephrine, cortisol, and growth hormone raise blood glucose levels by a variety of mechanisms. The glycemic index is a value that indicates the potential of foods to raise blood glucose and insulin levels. The glycemic load is the amount of carbohydrate in a food multiplied by the glycemic index of the carbohydrate in that food. Foods with a high glycemic index/load cause surges in blood glucose and insulin, whereas foods with a low glycemic index/load cause more moderate fluctuations in blood glucose. Diets with a low glycemic index/load are associated with a reduced risk for chronic diseases.

How much total carbohydrate and added sugar should you eat?

Proponents of low-carbohydrate diets claim that eating carbohydrates makes you gain weight. However, anyone who consumes more Calories than he or she expends will gain weight, whether those Calories are in the form of simple or complex carbohydrates, protein, or fat. Moreover, fat is twice as "fattening" as carbohydrate: it contains 9 kcal per gram, whereas carbohydrate contains only 4 kcal per gram. In fact, as we noted earlier, eating fiber-rich carbohydrates has been shown to reduce the overall risk for obesity, cardiovascular disease, and diabetes. Thus, all carbohydrates are not bad, and even foods with added sugars—in limited amounts—can be included in a healthful diet.

The Recommended Dietary Allowance for Total Carbohydrate Reflects Glucose Use by the Brain

The Recommended Dietary Allowance (RDA) for carbohydrate is based on the amount of glucose the brain uses.[2] The current RDA for adults 19 years of age and older is 130 g of carbohydrate per day. It is important to emphasize that this RDA does not cover the amount of carbohydrate needed to support daily activities; it covers only the amount of carbohydrate needed to supply adequate glucose to the brain.

Recall from Chapter 1 that carbohydrates have been assigned an Acceptable Macronutrient Distribution Range (AMDR) of 45% to 65% of total energy intake. This is the range of intake associated with a decreased risk for chronic diseases. TABLE 4.1 compares the RDA and AMDR recommendations from the Health and Medicine Division of the National Academies of Science with the *2015–2020 Dietary Guidelines for Americans* related to carbohydrate-containing foods.[2,3] As you can see, the Health and Medicine Division of the National Academies of Science provides specific numeric recommendations, whereas the Dietary Guidelines focus on consumption of a healthful eating pattern. Most health agencies agree that most of the carbohydrates you eat each day should be high in fiber, whole-grain, and unprocessed. As recommended in the USDA Food Guide, eating at least half your grains as whole grains and eating the suggested amounts of fruits and vegetables each day will ensure that you get enough fiber-rich carbohydrates in your diet. Although fruits are predominantly composed of simple sugars, they are good sources of vitamins, some minerals, and fiber.

▲ The RDA for carbohydrate is based on the amount the brain uses. Exercise, or even routine activity, increases our need for carbohydrate beyond the RDA.

Most Americans Eat Too Much Added Sugar

The average carbohydrate intake per person in the United States is approximately 50% of total energy intake. For some people, almost half of this amount consists of sugars. Where does all this sugar come from? Some sugar comes from healthful food sources, such as fruit and milk. Some comes from foods made with refined grains, such as soft white breads, saltine crackers, and pastries. Much of the rest comes from **added sugars**—that is, sugars and syrups that are added to foods during processing or preparation. For example, many processed foods include high-fructose corn syrup

added sugars Sugars and syrups that are added to food during processing or preparation.

TABLE 4.1 Dietary Recommendations for Carbohydrates

Health and Medicine Division of the National Academies of Science Recommendations*	2015–2020 Dietary Guidelines for Americans†
Recommended Dietary Allowance (RDA) for adults 19 years of age and older is 130 g of carbohydrate per day.	Consume a healthful eating pattern that accounts for all foods and beverage within an appropriate Calorie level. A healthful eating pattern includes: a variety of vegetables from all subgroups (dark green, red and orange, legumes, starch and other); fruits (especially whole fruits); grains (at least half of which are whole grains); fat-free or low-fat dairy; a variety of protein foods; and oils.
The Acceptable Macronutrient Distribution Range (AMDR) for carbohydrate is 45–65% of total daily energy intake.	
Added sugar intake should be 25% or less of total energy intake each day.	Consume less than 10% of Calories per day from added sugars.

*Data from: Health and Medicine Division of the National Academies of Science, Food and Nutrition Board, 2005. *Dietary Reference Intakes for Energy, Carbohydrates, Fiber, Fat, Fatty Acids, Cholesterol, Protein, and Amino Acids (Macronutrients)*. Washington, DC: The National Academy of Sciences. Reprinted with permission.

†Data from: U.S. Department of Health and Human Services and U.S. Department of Agriculture. *2015–2020 Dietary Guidelines for Americans,* 8th edn.

(HFCS), an added sugar. Note in Table 4.1 that the *2015–2020 Dietary Guidelines for Americans* recommend consuming less than 10% of our total energy from added sugars. As discussed in Chapter 2, the Nutrition Facts panel being revised by the FDA will include the % Daily Values for added sugars, which will be an additional tool to help consumers identify foods that are high in added sugars.

The most common source of added sugars in the U.S. diet is sweetened soft drinks; we drink an average of 40 gallons per person each year. Consider that one 12-oz cola contains 38.5 g of sugar, or almost 10 teaspoons. The average American consumes more than 16,420 g of sugar (about 267 cups) in sweetened soft drinks each year. Other common sources of added sugars include cookies, cakes, pies, fruit drinks, fruit punches, and candy. Even many nondessert items, such as peanut butter, yogurt, flavored rice mixes, and even salad dressing, contain added sugars.

If you want a quick way to figure out the amount of sugar in a processed food, check the Nutrition Facts panel for the line that identifies "Sugars." You'll notice that the amount of total and added sugars in a serving is identified in grams. Divide the total grams by 4 to get teaspoons. For instance, one national brand of yogurt contains 21 grams of sugar in a half-cup serving. That's more than 5 teaspoons of sugar! Doing this simple math before you buy may help you choose among different, more healthful versions of the same food.

There is also confusion about whether some types of sweeteners are more healthful than others, with claims that sweeteners such as honey, molasses, or raw sugar are more natural and nutritious than table sugar. Is there any evidence to back these claims?

Remember that sucrose consists of one glucose molecule and one fructose molecule joined together. From a chemical perspective, honey is almost identical to sucrose because honey also contains glucose and fructose molecules in almost equal amounts. However, enzymes in bees' "honey stomachs" separate some of the glucose and fructose molecules, and bees fan honey with their wings to reduce its moisture content; as a result, honey looks and tastes slightly different.

Honey does not contain any more nutrients than sucrose, so it is not a more healthful choice. In fact, per tablespoon, honey has more Calories (energy) than table sugar. This is because the crystals in table sugar take up more space on a spoon than the liquid form of honey, so a tablespoon contains less sugar. However, some people argue that honey is sweeter, so you use less.

Is raw sugar more healthful than table sugar? Actually, the "raw sugar" available in the United States has gone through more than half of the same steps in the refining process used to make table sugar. Raw sugar has a coarser texture than white sugar and is unbleached; in most markets, it is also significantly more expensive. Nevertheless, it's still sugar. What about molasses? The syrup that remains when sucrose is made from sugarcane, molasses has a distinctive taste that is less sweet than table sugar. It does contain some iron, but this iron does not occur naturally. It is a contaminant from the machines that process the sugarcane!

As you can see, all added sugars are chemically similar, and foods and beverages with added sugars have lower levels of vitamins, minerals, and fiber than foods that naturally contain simple sugars. Moreover, increasing concerns about the contribution of added sugars to obesity and chronic disease have led many public health agencies to recommend that we limit our consumption of added sugars. In addition to checking the Nutrition Facts panel for information on added sugars, you should also read the ingredients list to help you distinguish between added sugars and naturally occurring sugars. Refer to **TABLE 4.2** on page 116 for a list of terms indicating added sugars. To maintain a diet low in added sugars, limit foods in which a form of added sugar is listed as one of the first few ingredients on the label.

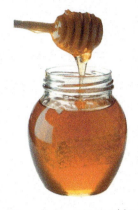

◄ Honey is no more nutritious than table sugar.

Sugars Are Blamed for Many Health Problems

Why do added sugars have such a bad reputation? First, they are known to contribute to tooth decay. Second, eating a lot of sugar could increase the levels of unhealthful lipids in our blood, increasing our risk for cardiovascular disease. High intakes of added sugars have also been blamed for diabetes and obesity. Let's learn the truth about these accusations.

TABLE 4.2 Forms of Sugar Commonly Added to Foods

Name of Sugar	Definition
Brown sugar	A highly refined sweetener made up of approximately 99% sucrose and produced by adding to white table sugar either molasses or burnt table sugar for coloring and flavor.
Cane sugar	Sucrose that has been extracted from sugarcane, a tropical plant naturally rich in sugar.
Concentrated fruit juice sweetener	A form of sweetener made with concentrated fruit juice, commonly pear juice.
Confectioner's sugar	A highly refined, finely ground white sugar; also referred to as powdered sugar.
Corn sweeteners	A general term for any sweetener made with corn starch.
Corn syrup	A syrup produced by the partial hydrolysis of corn starch.
Dextrose	An alternative term for glucose.
Fructose	A monosaccharide that occurs in fruits and vegetables; also called levulose, or fruit sugar.
Galactose	A monosaccharide that joins with glucose to create lactose.
Granulated sugar	Another term for white sugar, or table sugar.
High-fructose corn syrup	A type of corn syrup in which part of the sucrose is converted to fructose, making it sweeter than sucrose or regular corn syrup; most high-fructose corn syrup contains 42% to 55% fructose.
Honey	A sweet, sticky liquid sweetener made by bees from the nectar of flowers; contains glucose and fructose.
Invert sugar	A sugar created by heating a sucrose syrup with a small amount of acid; inverting sucrose results in its breakdown into glucose and fructose, which reduces the size of the sugar crystals; because of its smooth texture, it is used in making candies and some syrups.
Levulose	Another term for fructose, or fruit sugar.
Mannitol	A type of sugar alcohol.
Maple sugar	A sugar made by boiling maple syrup.
Molasses	A thick, brown syrup that is separated from raw sugar during manufacturing; it is considered the least refined form of sucrose.
Natural sweeteners	A general term used for any naturally occurring sweeteners, such as fructose, honey, and raw sugar.
Raw sugar	The sugar that results from the processing of sugar beets or sugarcane; it is approximately 96% to 98% sucrose; true raw sugar contains impurities and is not stable in storage; the raw sugar available to consumers has been purified to yield an edible sugar.
Sorbitol	A type of sugar alcohol.
Turbinado sugar	The form of raw sugar that is purified and safe for human consumption; sold as "Sugar in the Raw" in the United States.
White sugar	Another name for sucrose, or table sugar.
Xylitol	A type of sugar alcohol.

Sugar and Tooth Decay

Sugars do play a role in dental problems, because the bacteria that cause tooth decay thrive on sugar. These bacteria produce acids, which eat away at tooth enamel and can eventually cause cavities and gum disease (FIGURE 4.12). Eating sticky foods that adhere to teeth—such as caramels, crackers, sugary cereals, and licorice—and slowly sipping sweetened beverages over time are two behaviors that should be avoided because they increase the risk for tooth decay. People also shouldn't put babies to bed with a bottle unless it contains water. As we have seen, even breast milk contains sugar, which can slowly drip onto the baby's gums. As a result, infants should not routinely be allowed to fall asleep at the breast.

To reduce your risk for tooth decay, brush your teeth after each meal, after drinking sugary drinks, and after snacking on sweets. Drinking fluoridated water and using a fluoride toothpaste will also help protect your teeth.

Sugar and Blood Lipids

Research evidence does suggest that consuming a diet high in added sugars is associated with unhealthful changes in blood lipids. For example, higher intakes of added sugars are associated with changes in lipoproteins that are risk factors for cardiovascular disease. Two recent studies have shown that people who consume sugar-sweetened beverages have an increased risk of and premature mortality from cardiovascular disease.[9,10] Although the Health and Medicine Division of the National Academies of Science has yet to set a UL for added sugars, the growing body of evidence suggests that eating high amounts may be harmful. Again, the *2015–2020 Dietary Guidelines for Americans* recommends we should consume less than 10% of our total Calories as added sugars. Because added sugars are a component of many processed foods and beverages, careful label reading is advised.

Sugar and Diabetes

Recent studies suggest that eating a diet high in added sugars is associated with a higher risk for diabetes; the relationship is particularly strong between higher intakes of sugar-sweetened beverages and diabetes. An observational study examined the relationship between diabetes and sugar intake across 175 countries and found that for every 150 kcal per person per day increase in availability of sugar (equivalent to about one can of soft drink per day), the prevalence of diabetes increased by 1.1%.[11] Although the exact mechanisms explaining this relationship are not clear, experts have speculated that the surges in glucose and insulin levels that occur when we consume high amounts of rapidly absorbable carbohydrates (which includes any forms of sugar, including fructose as discussed earlier) may stimulate appetite, increase food intake, and promote weight gain, which increases our risk for diabetes. High-fructose corn syrup in particular has negative effects on how we metabolize and store body fat; this can lead to us being more resistant to the normal actions of insulin and increase our risk for diabetes.

Sugar and Obesity

There is also evidence linking added sugar intake with obesity. For example, a recent systematic review of randomized controlled trials and observational studies found that reducing intake of added sugars in adults results in weight loss and increasing intake of added sugars results in weight gain.[12] This increase in weight is due to the excess Calorie intake and not due to the sugars per se. This same review found that children who consume one or more servings of sugar-sweetened beverages per day had a 1.55 times higher risk of being overweight than those children consuming none or very little.

It is important to emphasize that if you consume more energy than you expend, you will gain weight. It makes intuitive sense that people who consume extra energy from high-sugar foods are at risk for obesity, just like people who consume extra energy from fat or protein. However, more evidence is accumulating to indicate that the type of carbohydrates consumed may play a role in increasing one's risk for obesity. The precise relationship between added sugars and obesity is discussed in more detail in the **Nutrition Debate** (page 127).

If you're concerned about the amount of added sugars you consume, what can you do to cut down? See the **Quick Tips** feature on page 118 for answers.

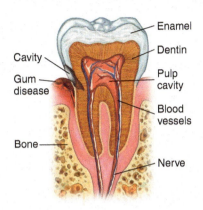

▲ **FIGURE 4.12** Eating sugars can cause an increase in cavities and gum disease. This is because bacteria in the mouth consume sugars present on the teeth and gums and produce acids, which eat away at these tissues.

recap The RDA for carbohydrate is 130 g per day; this amount is only sufficient to supply adequate glucose to the brain. The AMDR for carbohydrate is 45% to 65% of total energy intake. The *2015–2020 Dietary Guidelines for Americans* recommend consuming less than 10% of Calories per day as added sugars; that is, sugars and syrups added to foods during processing or preparation. The most common source of added sugars in the U.S. diet is sweetened soft drinks. Sugar causes tooth decay. High intakes of added sugars are associated with increases in unhealthful blood lipids and increased risks for cardiovascular disease, diabetes, and obesity.

QuickTips

Slashing Your Sugar Intake

✓ Switch from sugary drinks to diet drinks, milk or soymilk, unsweetened tea or coffee, fruit juice highly diluted with sparkling water, or plain water.

✓ Limit the number of specialty coffees flavored with syrup that you drink—have these as an occasional treat.

✓ Reduce the amount of sugar you put into your coffee, tea, and cereal—try cutting the amount to half, then a quarter. Or consider using an alternative sweetener instead of sugar.

✓ When buying fruit, go for fresh, frozen, dried, or canned options packed in water or their own juice. Avoid fruits packed in syrup.

✓ Switch from fruit-flavored yogurts, ice cream, or sherbet to plain yogurt topped with fresh fruit.

✓ Choose desserts such as cookies, candies, and cakes less often, replacing them with fresh or dried fruit, nuts and seeds, or a small piece of dark chocolate.

✓ Read food labels to increase your awareness of the sugar content of the foods you normally buy.

LO 6 Identify the Adequate Intake for fiber and list several foods that are good sources of fiber-rich carbohydrates.

How much fiber do you need, and what are the best sources?

Do you get enough dietary fiber each day? Most Americans don't.[13] The Adequate Intake (AI) for fiber is 25 g per day for women and 38 g per day for men, or 14 g of fiber for every 1,000 kcal per day that a person eats.[2] Most people in the United States eat only 15 g (females) and 18 g (males) of fiber each day, which is only about half of the fiber they need.[13] Although fiber supplements are available, it is best to get fiber from your diet because foods rich in fiber also provide vitamins, minerals, and phytochemicals. So what foods qualify?

Whole Grains Are Excellent Sources of Fiber

Whole-grain foods have many benefits. In addition to being excellent sources of fiber, they're rich in micronutrients and phytochemicals. They also have a lower glycemic index than refined carbohydrates; thus, they prompt a more gradual release of insulin and result in less severe fluctuations in both insulin and glucose.

TABLE 4.3 lists the terms commonly used on nutrition labels to identify the type of grains in breads and cereals. Read the label for the bread you eat—does it list *whole-wheat flour* or just *wheat flour*? The term *wheat flour* actually refers to refined white flour. So make sure to choose products with the word *whole* in the first ingredient listed. To appreciate exactly what you'll be buying, let's look at what makes a whole grain whole.

Grains are grasses that produce edible kernels. A kernel of grain is the seed of the grass. If you were to plant a kernel of barley, a blade of grass would soon shoot up. Kernels of different grains all share a similar design. As shown in FIGURE 4.13, they consist of three parts:

- The outermost covering, called the *bran*, is very high in fiber and contains most of the grain's vitamins and minerals.
- The *endosperm* is the grain's midsection and contains most of the grain's carbohydrates and protein.
- The *germ* sits deep in the base of the kernel, surrounded by the endosperm, and is rich in healthful fats and some vitamins.

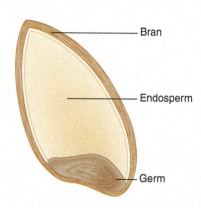

Bran

Endosperm

Germ

▲ **FIGURE 4.13** A whole grain includes the bran, endosperm, and germ.

TABLE 4.3 Terms Used to Describe Grains and Cereals on Nutrition Labels

Term	Definition
Brown bread	Bread that may or may not be made using whole-grain flour. Many brown breads are made with white flour with brown (caramel) coloring added.
Enriched (or fortified)	Enriching or fortifying involves adding nutrients back to refined foods. In order to use this term in grain products in the United States, a minimum amount of iron, folate, niacin, thiamin, and riboflavin must be added. Other nutrients can also be added.
Refined	Refining involves removing the coarse parts of food products; refined wheat flour is flour in which all but the internal part of the kernel has been removed.
Stone ground	This term refers to a milling process in which limestone is used to grind any grain. Stone ground does not mean that bread is made with whole grain because refined flour can be stone ground.
Unbleached flour	Unbleached flour has been refined but not bleached; it is very similar to refined white flour in texture and nutritional value.
Wheat flour	This term refers to any flour made from wheat; it includes white flour, unbleached flour, and whole-wheat flour.
White flour	White flour has been bleached and refined. All-purpose flour, cake flour, and enriched baking flour are all types of white flour.
Whole-grain flour	This flour is made from grain that is not refined; whole grains are milled in their complete form with only the husk removed.
Whole-wheat flour	Whole-wheat flour is an unrefined, whole-grain flour made from whole-wheat kernels.

Whole grains are kernels that retain all three of these parts. The kernels of some grains also have a *husk* (hull): a thin, dry coat that is inedible. Removing the husk is always the first step in milling (grinding) these grains for human consumption.

People worldwide have milled grains for centuries, usually using heavy stones. A little milling removes only a small amount of the bran, leaving a crunchy grain suitable for cooked cereals. For example, cracked wheat and hulled barley retain much of the kernel's bran. Whole-grain flours are produced when whole grains are ground and then recombined. Because these hearty flours retain a portion of the bran, endosperm, and germ, foods such as breads made with them are rich in fiber and a wide array of vitamins and minerals.

With the advent of modern technology, processes for milling grains became more sophisticated, with seeds being repeatedly ground and sifted into increasingly finer flours, retaining little or no bran and therefore little fiber and few vitamins and minerals. For instance, white wheat flour, which consists almost entirely of endosperm, is high in carbohydrate but retains only about 25% of the wheat's fiber, vitamins, and minerals.

In the United States, manufacturers of breads and other baked goods made with white flour are required by law to enrich their products with vitamins and minerals to replace some of those lost in processing. **Enriched foods** are foods in which nutrients that were lost during processing have been added back, so the food meets a specified standard. However, enrichment replaces only a handful of nutrients and leaves the product low in fiber. Notice that the terms *enriched* and *fortified* are not synonymous: **fortified foods** have nutrients added that did not originally exist in the food (or existed in insignificant amounts). For example, some breakfast cereals have been fortified with iron, a mineral that is not naturally present in cereals.

Again, when choosing cereals, breads, and crackers and other baked goods, look for whole wheat, whole oats, or similar whole grains on the ingredient list. This ensures that the product contains the fiber and micronutrients that nature packed into the plant's seed. Try the **Nutrition Label Activity** on page 120 to learn how to recognize various carbohydrates on food labels.

Other Good Sources of Fiber Are Vegetables, Fruits, Nuts, and Seeds

Most people in the United States eat less than three servings of fruits or vegetables each day.[14] This is true of college students as well: fewer than 6% eat the recommended five or more servings of fruits and vegetables each day.[15]

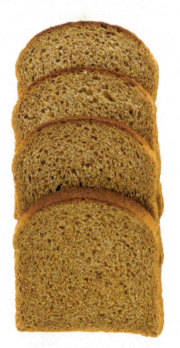

◀ Whole-grain breads provide more nutrients and fiber than breads made with enriched flour.

enriched foods Foods in which nutrients that were lost during processing have been added back, so that the food meets a specified standard.

fortified foods Foods in which nutrients are added that did not originally exist in the food, or which existed in insignificant amounts.

nutrition label activity

Recognizing Carbohydrates on the Label

FIGURE 4.14 shows labels for two breakfast cereals. The cereal on the left (a) is processed and sweetened, whereas the one on the right (b) is a whole-grain product with no added sugar. Which is the better breakfast choice? Fill in the label data below to find out!

■ Check the center of each label to locate the amount of total carbohydrate.
  1. For the sweetened cereal, the total carbohydrate is _____ g.
  2. For the whole-grain cereal, the total carbohydrate is _____ g for a smaller serving size.

■ Look at the information listed as subgroups under Total Carbohydrate. The label for the sweetened cereal lists all types of carbohydrates in the cereal: dietary fiber, sugars, and other carbohydrate (which refers to starches). Notice that this cereal contains 13 g of sugar—half of its total carbohydrates.
  3. How many grams of dietary fiber does the sweetened cereal contain? _____

■ The label for the whole-grain cereal lists only 1 g of sugar, which is 4% of its total carbohydrates.
  4. How many grams of dietary fiber does the whole-grain cereal contain?

■ To calculate the percentage of Calories that comes from carbohydrate, do the following:
  a. Calculate the *Calories* in the cereal that come from carbohydrate. Multiply the total grams of carbohydrate per serving by the energy value of carbohydrate:

    26 g of carbohydrate × 4 kcal/g = 104 kcal from carbohydrate

  b. Calculate the *percentage of Calories* in the cereal that comes from carbohydrate. Divide the Calories from carbohydrate by the total Calories for each serving:

    (104 kcal ÷ 120 kcal) × 100 = 87% Calories from carbohydrate

Which cereal should you choose to increase your fiber intake? Check the ingredients for the sweetened cereal. Remember that they are listed in order from highest to lowest amount. The second and third ingredients listed are sugar and brown sugar, and the corn and oat flours are not whole grain. Now look at the ingredients for the other cereal—it contains whole-grain oats. Although the sweetened product is enriched with more B-vitamins, iron, and zinc, the whole-grain cereal packs 4 g of fiber per serving, not to mention 5 g of protein, and it contains no added sugars. Overall, it is a more healthful choice.

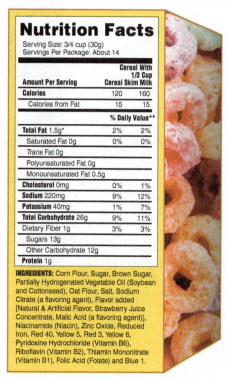

Nutrition Facts

Serving Size: 3/4 cup (30g)
Servings Per Package: About 14

Amount Per Serving	Cereal	Cereal With 1/2 Cup Skim Milk
Calories	120	160
Calories from Fat	15	15

	% Daily Value**	
Total Fat 1.5g*	2%	2%
Saturated Fat 0g	0%	0%
Trans Fat 0g		
Polyunsaturated Fat 0g		
Monounsaturated Fat 0.5g		
Cholesterol 0mg	0%	1%
Sodium 220mg	9%	12%
Potassium 40mg	1%	7%
Total Carbohydrate 26g	9%	11%
Dietary Fiber 1g	3%	3%
Sugars 13g		
Other Carbohydrate 12g		
Protein 1g		

INGREDIENTS: Corn Flour, Sugar, Brown Sugar, Partially Hydrogenated Vegetable Oil (Soybean and Cottonseed), Oat Flour, Salt, Sodium Citrate (a flavoring agent), Flavor added [Natural & Artificial Flavor, Strawberry Juice Concentrate, Malic Acid (a flavoring agent)], Niacinamide (Niacin), Zinc Oxide, Reduced Iron, Red 40, Yellow 5, Red 3, Yellow 6, Pyridoxine Hydrochloride (Vitamin B6), Riboflavin (Vitamin B2), Thiamin Mononitrate (Vitamin B1), Folic Acid (Folate) and Blue 1.

(a)

Nutrition Facts

Serving Size: 1/2 cup dry (40g)
Servings Per Container: 13

Amount Per Serving		
Calories		150
Calories from Fat		25

		% Daily Value*
Total Fat 3g		5%
Saturated Fat 0.5g		2%
Trans Fat 0g		
Polyunsaturated Fat 1g		
Monounsaturated Fat 1g		
Cholesterol 0mg		0%
Sodium 0mg		0%
Total Carbohydrate 27g		9%
Dietary Fiber 4g		15%
Soluble Fiber 2g		
Insoluble Fiber 2g		
Sugars 1g		
Protein 5g		

INGREDIENTS: 100% Natural Whole Grain Rolled Oats.

(b)

◄ **FIGURE 4.14** Labels for two breakfast cereals: **(a)** processed and sweetened cereal; **(b)** whole-grain cereal with no sugar added.

That's unfortunate, because fruits and vegetables are excellent sources of dietary fiber. **FIGURE 4.15** shows the fiber content of some common legumes, other vegetables, fruits, and whole grains. Eating a variety of these foods will help ensure that you eat enough fiber.

Notice that, among vegetables, legumes are particularly high in fiber. Add them to soups and salads, chili, tacos and burritos, or eat them on their own as a side dish. Leafy or crunchy greens like spinach, kale, and cabbage are also rich in fiber, as are baked potatoes with the skin on. For fruits, all berries are particularly high in fiber, as are apples and pears—as with potatoes, eat the skin.

Although not shown in Figure 4.15, nuts and seeds can be excellent sources of fiber. An ounce of almonds provides 4 g, and pistachio nuts, pumpkin seeds, and sunflower seeds all provide 3 g per ounce. Quinoa (pronounced keen-wah), a seed that is cooked and served as a grain, is very high in fiber—about 5 grams per serving. For more suggestions on selecting healthful carbohydrate sources rich in fiber, see the **Quick Tips** feature (page 123).

MEAL FOCUS FIGURE 4.16 on page 122 compares the food and fiber content of two diets, one high in fiber-rich carbohydrates and one high in refined carbohydrates. Notice that the meals on the right provide more than double the fiber.

It's important to drink plenty of fluid as you increase your fiber intake because fiber binds with water to soften stools. Inadequate fluid intake with a high-fiber diet can actually result in hard, dry stools that are difficult to pass through the colon. At least eight 8-oz glasses of fluid each day are commonly recommended.

Also, be aware that it's possible to eat too much fiber. Excessive fiber consumption can lead to intestinal gas, bloating, and constipation, and because fiber causes

To see a vast menu of high-fiber choices and find out how much fiber various foods provide, visit the Fiber-o-Meter at www.webmd.com. Type "fiber-o-meter" in the search bar, then click on the link.

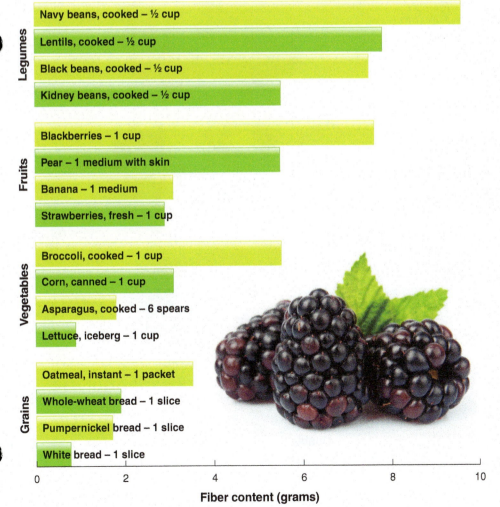

◀ **FIGURE 4.15** Fiber content of common foods. *Note:* The Adequate Intake for fiber is 25 g per day for women and 38 g per day for men.

Data from: U.S. Department of Agriculture, Agricultural Research Service, Nutrient Data Laboratory. 2015. USDA National Nutrient Database for Standard Reference, Release 28. http://www.ars.usda.gov/nea/bhnrc/ndl.

a day of meals

about **15.6** grams of dietary fiber

about **32** grams of dietary fiber

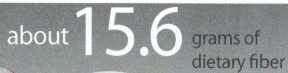

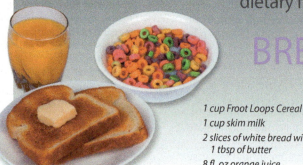

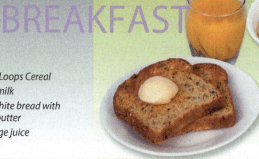

BREAKFAST

1 cup Froot Loops Cereal
1 cup skim milk
2 slices of white bread with
   1 tbsp of butter
8 fl. oz orange juice

1 cup Cheerios
1 cup skim milk
1 medium banana
2 slices whole-wheat toast with
   1 tbsp light margarine
8 fl. oz orange juice

LUNCH

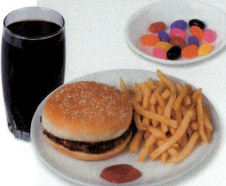

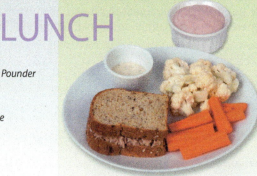

McDonald's Quarter Pounder
1 small French Fries
1 packet ketchup
16 fl oz cola beverage
15 jelly beans

Tuna Sandwich with:
2 slices of whole wheat bread
3 oz tuna packed in water,
   drained
1 tsp Dijon mustard
1 tbsp reduced-calorie
   mayonnaise
1 large carrot, sliced
1 cup raw cauliflower
2 tbsp fat-free ranch dressing
8 fl oz non-fat fruit yogurt

DINNER

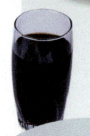

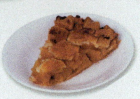

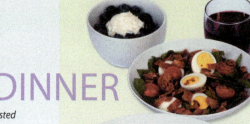

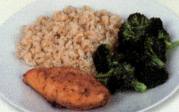

½ chicken breast, roasted
1 cup mashed potatoes
½ cup sliced cooked carrots
12 fl oz cola beverage
Apple pie (1/8 of 9-inch pie)

1/2 chicken breast, roasted
1 cup brown rice
1 cup steamed broccoli
Spinach salad:
  1 cup chopped spinach
  1 boiled egg
  2 slices turkey bacon
  3 cherry tomatoes
  2 tbsp cream poppyseed
    dressing
1 cup fresh blueberries with
  ½ cup whipped cream
8 fl oz cranberry juice

nutrient analysis

nutrient analysis

2,410 kcal
58.3% of energy from carbohydrates
29.2% of energy from fat
12.5% of energy from protein
15.6 grams of dietary fiber

Double the fiber intake!

2,181 kcal
58.5% of energy from carbohydrates
22.3% of energy from fat
19.2% of energy from protein
32 grams of dietary fiber

QuickTips

Hunting for Fiber

✓ Select breads made with *whole* grains, such as wheat, oats, barley, and rye. Two slices of whole-grain bread provide 4–6 grams of fiber.

✓ Switch from a low-fiber breakfast cereal to one that has at least 4 grams of fiber per serving.

✓ For a mid-morning snack, stir ground flaxseed meal, chia seeds, or chopped almonds (about 4 grams of fiber) into a cup of plain yogurt. Or choose an apple or a pear, with the skin left on (about 5 grams of fiber).

✓ Instead of potato chips with your lunchtime sandwich, have a side of carrot or celery sticks (about 2 grams of fiber).

✓ Eat legumes every day, if possible (about 5 to 6 grams of fiber per serving). Have them as your main dish, as a side, or in soups and other dishes.

✓ Choose brown rice instead of white rice, and whole-wheat or quinoa pasta instead of regular pasta.

✓ Don't forget the greens! A cup of cooked leafy greens provides about 4 grams of fiber, and a salad is rich in fiber.

✓ Snack on a mixture of nuts and dried fruit.

✓ For dessert, try a baked apple or pear or a high-fiber granola with soymilk.

✓ When shopping, choose fresh, frozen, and canned fruits and vegetables. Check the labels of frozen and canned selections to make sure there is no sugar or salt added, or rinse before serving.

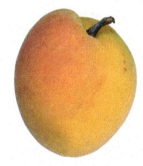

▲ Eating five or more servings of vegetables and fruits, such as apricots, will help you get enough fiber in your diet.

the body to eliminate more water in the feces, a very-high-fiber diet could result in dehydration. Fiber also binds many vitamins and minerals; thus, a diet with too much fiber could reduce absorption of iron, zinc, calcium, and vitamin D. In children, some elderly, the chronically ill, and other at-risk populations, extreme fiber intake can even lead to malnutrition—they feel full before they have eaten enough to provide adequate energy and nutrients. Although there is no UL for fiber, most Americans find it difficult to tolerate more than about 50 g of fiber per day.

recap The Adequate Intake for fiber is 25 g per day for women and 38 g per day for men. Most Americans eat only about half of the fiber they need each day. A whole grain retains the bran, which is rich in fiber and micronutrients, the endosperm, and the germ. Foods high in fiber and nutrient density include whole grains and products made with whole grains; legumes and other vegetables; fruits; and nuts and seeds. The more processed the food, the fewer fiber-rich carbohydrates it contains. It's important to drink plenty of fluid as you increase your fiber intake, and to avoid consuming more than about 50 g of fiber a day.

What's the story on alternative sweeteners?

LO 7 Compare and contrast a variety of alternative sweeteners.

Most of us love sweets but want to avoid the extra Calories and tooth decay that go along with them. Remember that all carbohydrates, whether simple or complex, contain 4 kcal of energy per gram. Because sweeteners such as sucrose, fructose, honey, and brown sugar contribute energy, they are called **nutritive sweeteners**.

nutritive sweeteners Sweeteners, such as sucrose, fructose, honey, and brown sugar, that contribute Calories (energy).

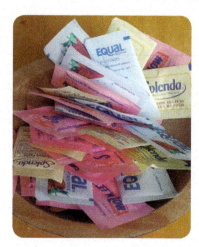

▲ Contrary to media reports claiming severe health consequences related to the consumption of alternative sweeteners, major health agencies have determined that these products are safe for us to consume.

Other nutritive sweeteners include the *sugar alcohols* such as mannitol, sorbitol, isomalt, and xylitol. Popular in sugar-free gums, mints, and diabetic candies, sugar alcohols are less sweet than sucrose. Foods with sugar alcohols have health benefits that foods made with sugars do not have, such as a reduced glycemic response and decreased risk of dental caries. Also, because sugar alcohols are absorbed slowly and incompletely from the intestine, they provide less energy than sugar, usually 2 to 3 kcal of energy per gram. However, because they are not completely absorbed from the intestine, they can attract water into the large intestine and cause diarrhea.

A number of other products have been developed to sweeten foods without promoting tooth decay and weight gain. Because these products provide little or no energy, they are called **nonnutritive,** or *alternative*, **sweeteners.**

Limited Use of Alternative Sweeteners Is Not Harmful

Research has shown alternative sweeteners to be safe for adults, children, and individuals with diabetes. Women who are pregnant should discuss the use of alternative sweeteners with their healthcare provider. In general, it appears safe for pregnant women to consume alternative sweeteners in amounts within the Food and Drug Administration (FDA) guidelines.[16] These amounts, known as the **Acceptable Daily Intake (ADI)**, are estimates of the amount of a sweetener that someone can consume each day over a lifetime without adverse effects. The estimates are based on studies conducted on laboratory animals, and they include a 100-fold safety factor. It is important to emphasize that actual intake by humans is typically well below the ADI.

Saccharin

Discovered in the late 1800s, *saccharin* is about 300 times sweeter than sucrose. Concerns arose in the 1970s that saccharin could cause cancer; however, more than 20 years of subsequent research failed to link saccharin to cancer in humans, and in 2000, the National Toxicology Program of the U.S. government removed saccharin from its list of products that may cause cancer. No ADI has been set for saccharin, and it is used in foods and beverages and as a tabletop sweetener. It is sold as Sweet n' Low (also known as "the pink packet") in the United States.

Acesulfame-K

Acesulfame-K (acesulfame potassium) is marketed under the names Sunette and Sweet One. It is a Calorie-free sweetener that is 200 times sweeter than sugar. It is used to sweeten gums, candies, beverages, instant tea, coffee, gelatins, and puddings. The taste of acesulfame-K does not change when it is heated, so it can be used in cooking. The body does not metabolize acesulfame-K, so it is excreted unchanged by the kidneys. The ADI for acesulfame-K is 15 mg per kg body weight per day. For example, the ADI in an adult weighing 150 pounds (or 68 kg) would be 1,020 mg.

Aspartame

Aspartame, also called Equal ("the blue packet") and NutraSweet, is one of the most popular alternative sweeteners currently in use. Aspartame is composed of two amino acids: phenylalanine and aspartic acid. When these amino acids are separate, one is bitter and the other has no flavor—but joined together, they make a substance that is 180 times sweeter than sucrose. Although aspartame contains 4 kcal of energy per gram, it is so sweet that only small amounts are used, thus it ends up contributing little or no energy. Heat destroys the bonds that bind the two amino acids in aspartame. Therefore, it cannot be used in cooking because it loses its sweetness.

Although there are numerous claims that aspartame causes headaches and dizziness, and can increase a person's risk for cancer and nerve disorders, studies do not support these claims.[17] A significant amount of research has been done to test the safety of aspartame.

The ADI for aspartame is 50 mg per kg body weight per day. For an adult weighing 150 pounds (or 68 kg), the ADI would be 3,400 mg. **TABLE 4.4** shows how many servings of aspartame-sweetened foods would have to be consumed to exceed the ADI. Because the ADI is a very conservative estimate, it would be difficult for adults

nonnutritive sweeteners Manufactured sweeteners that provide little or no energy; also called *alternative sweeteners*.

Acceptable Daily Intake (ADI) An FDA estimate of the amount of a nonnutritive sweetener that someone can consume each day over a lifetime without adverse effects.

TABLE 4.4   Foods and Beverages That a Child and an Adult Would Have to Consume Daily to Exceed the ADI for Aspartame

Foods and Beverages	50-lb Child	150-lb Adult
12 fl. oz carbonated diet soft drink *or*	5.6	17
8 fl. oz powdered soft drink *or*	11	34
4 fl. oz gelatin dessert *or*	14	42
Packets of tabletop sweetener	32	97

Data from: Academy of Nutrition and Dietetics. 2015. "Sugar Substitutes: How Much Is Too Much?" http://www.eatright.org/resource/food/nutrition/dietary-guidelines-and-myplate/sugar-substitutes-how-much-is-too-much.

or children to exceed this amount of aspartame intake. However, drinks sweetened with aspartame, which are extremely popular among children and teenagers, are very low in nutritional value. They should not replace more healthful beverages such as milk, water, and 100% fruit juice.

There are some people who should not consume aspartame at all: those with the disease *phenylketonuria* (*PKU*). This is a genetic disorder that prevents the breakdown of the amino acid phenylalanine. Because the person with PKU cannot metabolize phenylalanine, it builds up to toxic levels in the tissues of the body and causes irreversible brain damage. In the United States, all newborn babies are tested for PKU; those who have it are placed on a phenylalanine-limited diet. Some foods that are common sources of protein and other nutrients for many growing children, such as meats and milk, contain phenylalanine. Thus, it is critical that children with PKU not waste what little phenylalanine they can consume on nutrient-poor products sweetened with aspartame.

Sucralose

Sucralose is marketed under the brand name Splenda and is known as "the yellow packet." It is made from sucrose, but chlorine atoms are substituted for the hydrogen and oxygen normally found in sucrose, and it passes through the gastrointestinal tract unchanged, without contributing any energy. It is 600 times sweeter than sucrose and is stable when heated, so it can be used in cooking. It has been approved for use in many foods, including chewing gum, salad dressings, beverages, gelatin and pudding products, canned fruits, frozen dairy desserts, and baked goods. Studies have shown sucralose to be safe. The ADI for sucralose is 5 mg per kg body weight per day. For example, the ADI of sucralose in an adult weighing 150 pounds (or 68 kg) would be 340 mg.

Neotame, Stevia, and Advantame

Neotame is an alternative sweetener that is 7,000 times sweeter than sugar. Manufacturers use it to sweeten a variety of products, such as beverages, dairy products, frozen desserts, and chewing gums.

Stevia was approved as an alternative sweetener by the FDA in 2008. It is produced from a purified extract of the stevia plant, native to South America. Stevia is 200 times sweeter than sugar. It is currently used commercially to sweeten beverages and is available in powder and liquid for tabletop use. Stevia is also called Rebiana, Reb-A, Truvia, and Purevia.

Advantame was approved as an alternative sweetener in 2014. It is Calorie-free and 20,000 times sweeter than sugar. Although derived from aspartame, it is so much sweeter that very little is used; therefore, it is considered safe for people with phenylketonuria to consume. Advantame is used to sweeten foods such as frozen desserts, beverages, and chewing gum.

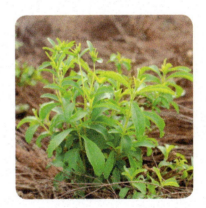

◄ A purified extract of the stevia plant, native to South America, is the source of the alternative sweetener stevia.

The Effect of Alternative Sweeteners on Body Weight Is Unclear

Although alternative sweeteners are used to reduce the energy content of various foods, their role in weight loss and weight maintenance is unclear. Although the popular media have recently linked drinking diet soft drinks with weight gain, a recent review concluded that there is no evidence that alternative sweeteners cause weight gain, and they may help people to lose weight.[18] In addition, a recent randomized controlled trial found that participants in a behavioral weight loss program who consumed at least 24 fluid ounces per day of an artificially sweetened beverage lost more weight after 12 weeks than participants who drank only water, suggesting that alternative sweeteners can be an effective part of a weight loss program.[19]

However, this doesn't mean that consuming alternative sweeteners will necessarily help you maintain a healthful body weight. To prevent weight gain, you need to balance the total number of kcal you consume against the number you expend. If you're expending an average of 2,000 kcal a day and you consume about 2,000 kcal per day, then you'll neither gain nor lose weight. But if, in addition to your normal diet, you regularly indulge in "treats," you're bound to gain weight, whether they are sugar free or not. Consider the Calorie count of these artificially sweetened foods:

- One cup of nonfat chocolate frozen yogurt with artificial sweetener = 199 Calories
- One sugar-free chocolate cookie = 100 Calories
- One serving of no-sugar-added hot cocoa = 55 Calories

Does the number of Calories in these foods surprise you? *Remember, sugar free doesn't mean Calorie free.* Make it a habit to check the Nutrition Facts panel to find out how much energy is really in your food!

recap Alternative sweeteners can be used in place of sugar to sweeten foods. Most of these products do not promote tooth decay and contribute little or no energy. The alternative sweeteners approved for use in the United States are considered safe when consumed in amounts less than the Acceptable Daily Intake, an estimate of the amount of a sweetener that someone can consume each day over a lifetime without adverse effects. People with phenylketonuria should avoid foods and beverages sweetened with aspartame. Other approved sweeteners commonly used are saccharin, acesulfame-K, sucralose, neotame, stevia, and advantame. Products that are sugar free are not necessarily low in Calories; thus, consuming foods and beverages made with alternative sweeteners will not necessarily help you maintain a healthful body weight.

nutri-case | HANNAH

"Last night, my mom called and said she'd be late getting home from work, so I made dinner. I made vegetarian quesadillas with flour tortillas, canned green chilies, cheese, and sour cream, plus a few baby carrots on the side. Later on while I was studying, I got really hungry, so I had some sugar-free cookies. They're sweetened with sorbitol and taste just like regular cookies! I ate maybe three or four, but I didn't think it was a big deal because they're sugar free. When I checked the package label this morning, I found out that each cookie has 90 Calories! I'm so mad at myself for blowing my diet!"

Without knowing the exact ingredients in Hannah's dinner and snack, would you agree that, prior to the cookies, she'd been making healthy choices? Why or why not? How might she have changed the ingredients in her quesadillas to increase their fiber content? And, if the cookies were sugar free, how can you explain the fact that each cookie still contained 90 Calories?

Are Added Sugars the Cause of the Obesity Epidemic?

Over the past 40 years, obesity rates in the United States have increased dramatically for both adults and children. At the same time, the risk for many chronic diseases, such as type 2 diabetes, cardiovascular disease, and arthritis, has also increased. We cannot blame genetics for America's rapid rise in obesity rates. Our genes have evolved over thousands of years; humans who lived even 100 years ago had a similar genetic makeup to humans today. Instead, we need to look at the effect of our lifestyle changes over the last four decades.

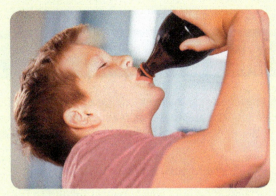

It is estimated that the rate of overweight in children has doubled since the mid-1970s.

One lifestyle factor that has come to the forefront of obesity research is our increased consumption of added sugars.[20] The *2015–2020 Dietary Guidelines for Americans* recommend limiting added sugars to less than 10% of total Calories; however, Americans currently consume about 16% of their total energy from added sugars.[21] The primary source of the added sugars in our diet is sugary drinks—soft drinks, fruit drinks, energy drinks, bottled coffees and teas, and vitamin waters. It is estimated that children's intake of sugary drinks has increased threefold since the late 1970s, with approximately 10% of children's energy intake coming from these beverages.[22]

High-fructose corn syrup (HFCS), in particular, has garnered a great deal of attention because until recently it was the sole caloric sweetener used in sugary drinks, and was also added to many other foods and beverages in the United States. More than a decade ago, researchers linked the increased use and consumption of HFCS with the rising rates of obesity since the 1970s, when HFCS first appeared.[23] HFCS is made by converting the starch in corn to glucose and then converting some of the glucose to fructose, which is sweeter. As described earlier in this chapter, fructose is metabolized differently from glucose, and these differences could affect appetite control, decrease feelings of satiety, and increase storage of body fat. The "fructose hypothesis" now dominating both the scientific and popular media proposes that fructose is associated with, and may even cause, obesity, cardiovascular disease, type 2 diabetes, and nonalcoholic fatty liver disease.[24–26]

The growing evidence linking the consumption of added sugars with overweight and obesity in children has led to a decline in consumption in schools and at school-sponsored events. In 2006, the beverage industry agreed to a voluntary ban on sales of all sweetened soft drinks in U.S. schools. Then, the Healthy, Hunger-Free Kids Act of 2010 required the U.S. Department of Agriculture to issue new nutrition standards for competitive foods and beverages—those sold outside of the school meals program. The new standards limited the amount of energy, salt, fat, and sugar in these products. Unfortunately, state policies regulating the availability and content of competitive foods vary. Thus, despite these positive changes, foods and beverages containing added sugars are still widely available in America's schools.

Although the evidence pinpointing added sugars and HFCS as major contributors to the obesity epidemic may appear strong, some nutrition professionals disagree. It has been proposed that soft drinks and other foods high in added sugars would have contributed to the obesity epidemic whether the sweetener was sucrose or fructose, and that their contribution to obesity is due to increased consumption as a result of advertising, increases in serving sizes, and virtually unlimited access. It is also possible that the obesity epidemic has resulted from increased consumption of energy from all sources, along with a reduction in physical activity levels, and that added sugars themselves are not to blame.

This issue is extremely complex, and more research needs to be done before we can fully understand how added sugars contribute to our diet, our weight, and our health.

CRITICAL THINKING QUESTIONS

1. After reading this debate, do you think added sugars in foods and beverages should be tightly regulated, or even banned? Why or why not?
2. Should reducing consumption of sugary drinks be up to individuals, or should it be encouraged via sales taxes and/or bans on promotions such as coupons, two-for-one pricing, and free refills in restaurants that would make these drinks more expensive overall? Defend your answer.
3. Make a list of your five favorite "sweet" snack foods. Using the USDA National Nutrient Database for Standard Reference (https://ndb.nal.usda.gov/), search for each of these foods and determine how much total sugar is in the amount of each snack food you would normally consume. After considering this information, do you feel you should identify alternative snack foods that are more healthful? Why or why not?

review questions

LO 1 1. Glucose, fructose, and galactose are
a. monosaccharides.
b. disaccharides.
c. polysaccharides.
d. complex carbohydrates.

LO 2 2. Which of the following statements about carbohydrates is true?
a. Carbohydrates are our main energy source during light activity and while we are at rest.
b. Simple carbohydrates are higher in energy (kcals per gram) than complex carbohydrates.
c. Excessive intake of carbohydrates can lead to ketoacidosis.
d. Consuming a diet high in fiber-rich carbohydrates may reduce the level of cholesterol in the blood.

LO 3 3. Glucose not immediately needed by the body
a. is converted to cholesterol and stored in abdominal fat.
b. is converted to glycogen and stored in the liver and muscles.
c. passes into the large intestine and is fermented by bacteria.
d. All of the above are possible fates of excess glucose.

LO 4 4. The glycemic index rates
a. the acceptable amount of alternative sweeteners to consume in 1 day.
b. the potential of foods to raise blood glucose and insulin levels.
c. the risk of a given food for causing diabetes.
d. the ratio of soluble to insoluble fiber in a complex carbohydrate.

LO 5 5. The Health and Medicine Division of the National Academies of Science recommends that adults consume
a. up to 14 grams of carbohydrate a day.
b. at least 25% of our daily energy intake as added sugars.
c. up to 65% of our daily energy intake as carbohydrate.
d. all grains as whole grains.

LO 5 6. The most common source of added sugars in the American diet is
a. table sugar.
b. white flour.
c. alcohol.
d. sweetened soft drinks.

LO 6 7. Which of the following is a reliable source of fiber-rich carbohydrate?
a. gluten-free pasta
b. unbleached flour
c. whole-oat cereal
d. enriched 9-grain bread

LO 7 8. Aspartame should not be consumed by people who have
a. phenylketonuria.
b. hypoglycemia.
c. lactose intolerance.
d. diverticulosis.

LO 1 9. **True or false?** In the process of photosynthesis, plants produce glucose and store it as fiber.

LO 4 10. **True or false?** Both glucagon and cortisol cause an increase in blood glucose.

math review

LO 5 **11.** Simon is trying to determine the minimum amount of carbohydrate he should consume in his diet to meet the AMDR for health. The total energy intake needed to maintain his current weight is 3,500 kcal per day. How many (a) kcal and (b) grams of carbohydrate should Simon consume each day?

Answers to Review Questions and Math Review are located at the back of this text and in the MasteringNutrition Study Area.

web links

www.foodinsight.org
Food Insight—International Food Information Council Foundation
Search this site to find out more about sugars and low-Calorie sweeteners.

www.ada.org/en/
American Dental Association
Go to this site to learn more about tooth decay as well as other oral health topics.

www.choosemyplate.gov
The USDA's MyPlate Home Page
Click on the various food groups in MyPlate on this website to learn more about foods that are high in fiber.

caloriecontrol.org
Calorie Control Council
This site provides information about reducing energy and fat in the diet, achieving and maintaining a healthy weight, and eating various low-Calorie, reduced-fat foods and beverages.

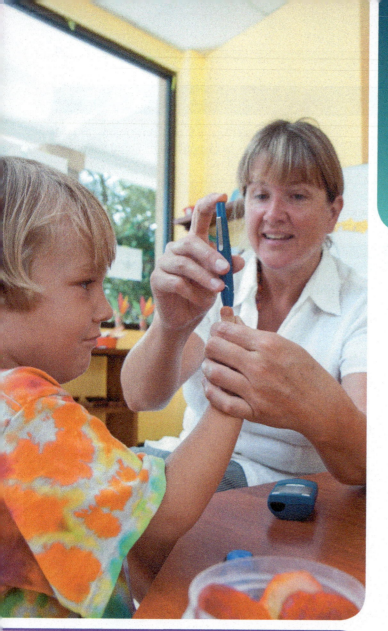

Diabetes

In 2012, the most recent year for which statistics are available, about 1.7 million Americans were newly diagnosed with diabetes.[1] Despite the image of diabetes as a disease of aging, these diagnoses weren't limited to the elderly: an estimated 24,000 were in children and adolescents, and another 371,000 were in adults younger than age 45.

Patients with diabetes have two to four times the risk for heart disease and stroke seen in people without the disease. Moreover, nearly half the cases of kidney failure as well as the majority of amputations and new cases of blindness occur among people with diabetes.[1] These complications typically develop about 10 to 15 years after the onset of the disease, and until recently, were almost exclusively seen in people over age 60. Now, as more and more children and adolescents are being diagnosed with diabetes, these complications are increasingly affecting young adults.[1]

What is diabetes, and how does it lead to kidney failure, blindness, and death? Why are diagnoses soaring, especially among young people? Can you reduce your risk? In this **In Depth** essay, we explore these questions.

learning outcomes

After studying this In Depth, you should be able to:

1 Define diabetes and explain how it damages cells and tissues, p. 131.

2 Distinguish between type 1 diabetes, type 2 diabetes, and prediabetes, pp. 132–134.

3 Identify the risk factors for type 2 diabetes and the lifestyle choices that can help you reduce that risk, pp. 134–137.

What is diabetes?

LO 1 Define diabetes and explain how it damages cells and tissues.

Diabetes is a chronic disease in which the body can no longer regulate glucose within normal limits. As a result, **hyperglycemia**—a condition in which the level of glucose in the blood is abnormally high—becomes chronic. It is imperative to detect and treat the disease as soon as possible because, as we explain shortly, hyperglycemia injures tissues throughout the body.

Approximately 29.1 million people in the United States—9.3% of the total population, including adults and children—live with diabetes. Of these, 21 million have been diagnosed, and it is speculated that another 8.1 million have diabetes but do not know it.[1] **FIGURE 1** shows the percentage of adults with diabetes from various ethnic groups in the United States. As you can see, diabetes is much more common in American Indians/Alaska Natives than in members of other ethnic and racial groups.[2]

Diabetes causes disease when chronic exposure to elevated blood glucose levels damages the body's blood vessels, and this in turn damages other body tissues. As the concentration of glucose in the blood increases, a shift in the body's chemical balance allows glucose to attach to certain body proteins, including ones that make up blood vessels. Glucose coats these proteins like a sticky glaze, causing damage and dysfunction.

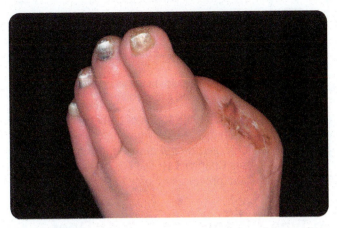

◆ **FIGURE 2** Amputations are a common complication of uncontrolled diabetes.

Damage to large blood vessels results in problems referred to as *macrovascular complications*. These include cardiovascular disease, which occurs because damage to artery walls allows fatty plaque to accumulate and narrow or block the vessels.

Damage to small blood vessels results in *microvascular complications*. For example, the kidneys' microscopic blood vessels, which filter blood and produce urine, become thickened. This impairs their function and can lead to kidney failure. Blood vessels that serve the eyes can swell and leak, leading to blindness.

When blood vessels that supply nutrients and oxygen to nerves are affected, *neuropathy*, damage to the nerves, can also occur. This condition leads to a loss of sensation, most commonly in the hands and feet. At the same time, circulation to the limbs is reduced overall. Together, these changes increase the risk of injury, infection, and tissue death (necrosis), leading to a greatly increased number of toe, foot, and lower leg amputations in people with diabetes **(FIGURE 2)**.

> Watch any of several videos on diabetic eye diseases at https://nei.nih.gov/youtube/ded/.

Because uncontrolled diabetes impairs carbohydrate metabolism, the body begins to break down stored fat, producing ketones for fuel. A buildup of excessive ketones can lead to ketoacidosis, a condition in which the brain cells do not get enough glucose to function properly. The person will become confused and lethargic and have trouble breathing. If left unchecked, ketoacidosis may result in coma and death. Indeed, as a result of cardiovascular disease, kidney failure, ketoacidosis, and other complications, diabetes is the seventh leading cause of death in the United States.[3]

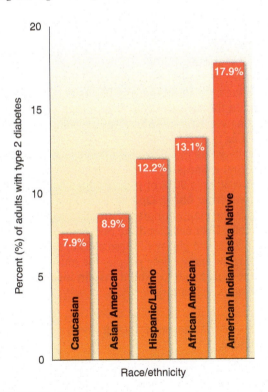

◆ **FIGURE 1** The percentage of adults from various ethnic and racial groups with type 2 diabetes.

Data from: Blackwell, D. L., J. W. Lucas, and T. C. Clarke. 2014. Summary Health Statistics for U.S. Adults: National Health Interview Survey, 2012. National Center for Health Statistics. *Vital and Health Stat.* 10(260).

diabetes A chronic disease in which the body can no longer regulate glucose normally.

hyperglycemia A condition in which blood glucose levels are higher than normal.

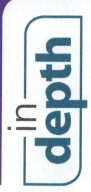

How is diabetes classified?

LO 2 Distinguish between type 1 diabetes, type 2 diabetes, and prediabetes.

The two main forms of diabetes are type 1 and type 2. Some women develop a third form, *gestational diabetes*, during pregnancy (see Chapter 14). See **FOCUS FIGURE 3** for an overview of the processes involved in type 1 and type 2 diabetes.

In Type 1 Diabetes, the Body Does Not Produce Enough Insulin

Approximately 5% of people with diabetes have **type 1 diabetes**, in which the body cannot produce enough insulin.[1] Most cases are diagnosed in adolescents around 10 to 14 years of age, although the disease can appear in infants, young children, and adults. It has a genetic link, so siblings and children of those with type 1 diabetes are at greater risk.[4]

When people with type 1 diabetes eat a meal and their blood glucose rises, the pancreas is unable to secrete insulin in response. Glucose therefore cannot move into body cells and remains in the bloodstream. The kidneys try to expel the excess blood glucose by excreting it in the urine. In fact, the medical term for the disease is *diabetes mellitus* (from the Greek *diabainein*, "to pass through," and Latin *mellitus*, "sweetened with honey"), and frequent urination is one of its warning signs (see **TABLE 1** for other symptoms). If blood glucose levels are not controlled, a person with type 1 diabetes can develop potentially fatal ketoacidosis.

Type 1 diabetes is classified as an *autoimmune disease*. This means that the body's immune system attacks and destroys its own tissues—in this case, the insulin-producing beta cells of the pancreas.[4]

TABLE 1 Symptoms of Type 1 and Type 2 Diabetes

Type 1 Diabetes	Type 2 Diabetes*
Increased or frequent urination	Any of the type 1 signs and symptoms
Excessive thirst	Greater frequency of infections
Constant hunger	Sudden vision changes
Unexplained weight loss	Slow healing of wounds or sores
Extreme fatigue	Tingling or numbness in the hands or feet
Blurred vision	Very dry skin

*Some people with type 2 diabetes experience no symptoms.

Data adapted from: U.S. Dept. of Health and Human Services, National Diabetes Information Clearinghouse (NDIC). Available at http://www.niddk.nih.gov/health-information/health-topics/Diabetes/your-guide-diabetes/Pages/index.aspx#signs and from the Centers for Disease Control and Prevention, Basics about Diabetes, available at http://www.cdc.gov/diabetes/basics/diabetes.html.

By the late 19th century, scientists had discovered that some type of abnormality of the pancreas triggered diabetes. Experiments had shown that, without a pancreas, an otherwise healthy animal would develop the disease quickly. Still, no one knew how to treat diabetes: nutritional therapies ranged from low-carbohydrate diets to starvation. For children, a diagnosis of diabetes was essentially a death sentence.

Then, in 1921, Canadian surgeon Frederick Banting had an idea. He and his medical assistant removed the pancreas from a dog, thereby inducing diabetes. They then injected the diabetic dog with secretions extracted from the pancreatic islets (or *islets of Langerhans*), which are clusters of hormone-secreting cells, including beta cells, in the pancreas. They called their extraction *isletin*. A few injections of isletin a day cured the dog of diabetes. They then purified the substance—which we now call insulin—and repeated their experiment several times before trying it on a 14-year-old boy dying of diabetes. The injections reversed all signs of the disease in the boy. Banting published a paper on his research in 1922 and received a Nobel Prize the following year.

To this day, the only treatment for type 1 diabetes is the administration of insulin by injection or pump several times daily. Insulin is a hormone composed of protein, so it would be digested in the intestine if taken as a pill. Individuals with type 1 diabetes must also monitor their blood glucose levels closely to ensure that they remain within a healthful range (**FIGURE 4** on page 134).

In Type 2 Diabetes, Cells Become Less Responsive to Insulin

In **type 2 diabetes**, body cells become resistant (less responsive) to insulin. This type of diabetes develops progressively, meaning that the biological changes resulting in the disease occur over a long period. Approximately 90% to 95% of all cases of diabetes are classified as type 2.[1]

Obesity is the most common trigger for a cascade of changes that eventually results in this disorder. It is estimated that 80% to 90% of people with type 2 diabetes are overweight or obese. One factor linking obesity to diabetes is the inappropriate accumulation of lipids in muscle cells, liver cells, and the beta cells of the pancreas, which reduces the ability of these cells to respond to insulin. That is, in many obese people, the muscle, liver, and pancreatic cells begin to exhibit **insulin insensitivity** (also called *insulin resistance*).

type 1 diabetes A disorder in which the body cannot produce enough insulin.

type 2 diabetes A progressive disorder in which body cells become less responsive to insulin.

insulin insensitivity (*insulin resistance*) A condition in which the body becomes less sensitive (or more resistant) to a given amount of insulin, resulting in insulin having a biological effect that is less than expected.

Diabetes is a chronic disease in which the body can no longer regulate glucose within normal limits, and blood glucose becomes dangerously high.

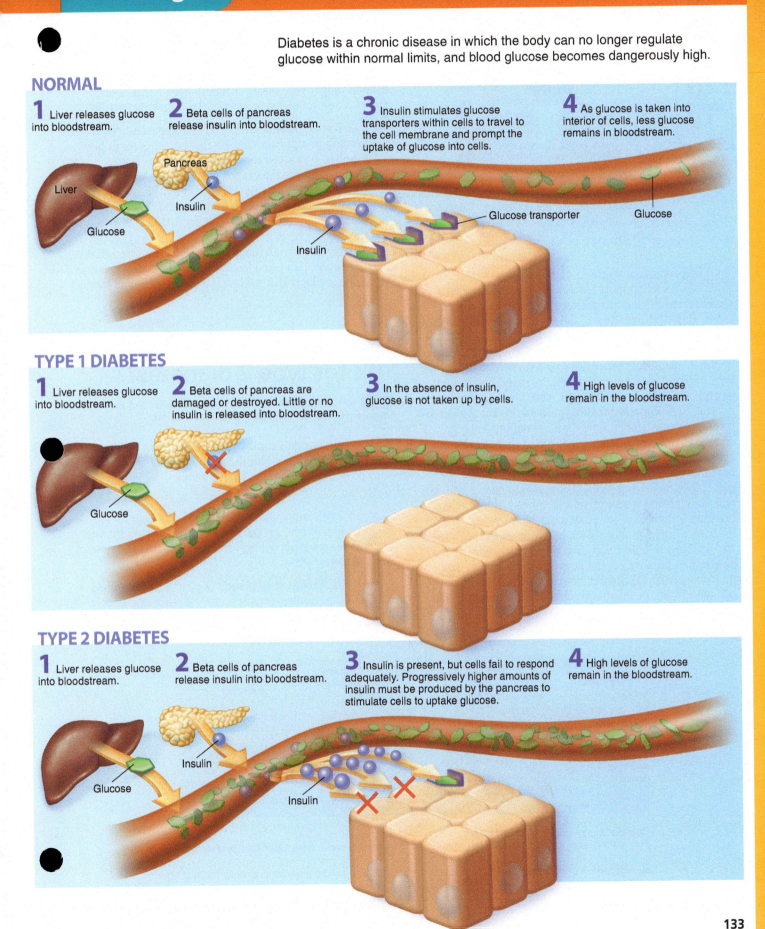

NORMAL

1 Liver releases glucose into bloodstream.

2 Beta cells of pancreas release insulin into bloodstream.

3 Insulin stimulates glucose transporters within cells to travel to the cell membrane and prompt the uptake of glucose into cells.

4 As glucose is taken into interior of cells, less glucose remains in bloodstream.

Pancreas

Liver

Insulin

Glucose

Insulin

Glucose transporter

Glucose

TYPE 1 DIABETES

1 Liver releases glucose into bloodstream.

2 Beta cells of pancreas are damaged or destroyed. Little or no insulin is released into bloodstream.

3 In the absence of insulin, glucose is not taken up by cells.

4 High levels of glucose remain in the bloodstream.

Glucose

TYPE 2 DIABETES

1 Liver releases glucose into bloodstream.

2 Beta cells of pancreas release insulin into bloodstream.

3 Insulin is present, but cells fail to respond adequately. Progressively higher amounts of insulin must be produced by the pancreas to stimulate cells to uptake glucose.

4 High levels of glucose remain in the bloodstream.

Insulin

Glucose

Insulin

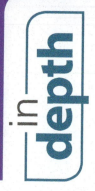

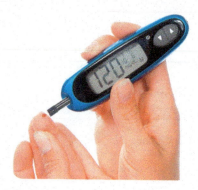

FIGURE 4 Monitoring blood glucose usually requires pricking the fingers and measuring the blood using a glucometer multiple times each day.

The pancreas attempts to compensate for this insensitivity by secreting more insulin. At first, the increased secretion is sufficient to maintain normal blood glucose levels. However, over time, a person who is insulin insensitive will have to circulate very high levels of insulin to use glucose for energy. Eventually, this excessive production becomes insufficient for preventing a persistently high level of blood glucose, even when the individual has not recently consumed carbohydrate. The resulting condition is referred to as **impaired fasting glucose**, meaning glucose levels are persistently higher than normal but not high enough to indicate a diagnosis of type 2 diabetes. Health care providers typically refer to this condition as **prediabetes**, because people with impaired fasting glucose are more likely to develop type 2 diabetes than people with normal fasting blood glucose levels. Ultimately, the pancreas becomes incapable of secreting these excessive amounts of insulin and stops producing the hormone altogether.

In short, in type 2 diabetes, blood glucose levels may be elevated because (1) the person has developed insulin insensitivity, (2) the pancreas can no longer secrete enough insulin, or (3) the pancreas has entirely stopped insulin production.

Three Blood Tests Are Used to Diagnose Diabetes

Diabetes is diagnosed when two or more tests of a person's blood glucose indicate values in the clinically defined range. Three tests currently used to diagnose diabetes and prediabetes include the following **(FIGURE 5)**:

- The fasting plasma glucose (FPG) test measures blood glucose in a person who has been fasting for at least 8 hours. It is a common and inexpensive test.
- The oral glucose tolerance (OGT) test is more reliable than the FPG test, but less convenient. It requires the person to fast for at least 8 hours, and then to drink a glucose solution. After two hours, blood is drawn and the glucose level measured.
- The glycosylated hemoglobin test (abbreviated HbA1c, or simply A1c) provides information about a person's average blood glucose levels over the previous three months.

How can you reduce your risk for type 2 diabetes?

LO 3 Identify the risk factors for type 2 diabetes and the lifestyle choices that can help you reduce that risk.

Certain factors significantly increase your risk for diabetes. Some of these are not modifiable, but others are within your power to change. Let's have a look.

---

impaired fasting glucose Fasting blood glucose levels that are higher than normal but not high enough to lead to a diagnosis of type 2 diabetes.

prediabetes A term used synonymously with *impaired fasting glucose*; it is a condition considered to be a major risk factor for both type 2 diabetes and heart disease.

Diagnosis	Fasting Plasma Glucose (mg/dL)	Oral Glucose Tolerance Test (mg/dL)	A1C (percent)
Diabetes	126 or above	200 or above	6.5 or above
Prediabetes	100 to 125	140 to 199	5.7 to 6.4
Normal	99 or below	139 or below	About 5

Definitions: mg = milligram, dL = deciliter
For all three tests, within the prediabetes range, the higher the test result, the greater the risk of diabetes.

FIGURE 5 Blood test levels for diagnosing diabetes and prediabetes according to the fasting plasma glucose, oral glucose tolerance, and HbA1c tests.

Some Diabetes Risk Factors Are Modifiable

Increased age is a significant risk factor for type 2 diabetes: most cases develop after age 45, and 26% of Americans 65 years and older have diabetes.[1] In fact, type 2 diabetes used to be referred to as *adult-onset diabetes* because it was virtually unheard of in children and adolescents until about 20 years ago. Unfortunately, the prevalence of the disease in young people has been increasing dramatically. In the United States, about 208,000 people younger than 20 years of age are estimated to have diagnosed diabetes, which is about 0.25% of that population group.[1]

A family history of type 2 diabetes increases your own risk. Your race/ethnicity is another significant influence: Among Native Americans age 20 or older, the prevalence of diabetes is more than double that of Caucasian Americans (see Figure 1). African Americans, Hispanic Americans, and Asian Americans also have an increased prevalence of diabetes as compared to Caucasian Americans.

In addition, a cluster of potentially modifiable risk factors referred to as the *metabolic syndrome* is known to increase the risk for type 2 diabetes. The criteria for metabolic syndrome include:

- Abdominal obesity; that is, a waist circumference greater than 88 cm (35 in.) for women and 102 cm (40 in.) for men
- Elevated blood pressure
- Elevated blood glucose (FPG 110 mg/dL or higher)
- Unhealthful levels of certain blood lipids (identified in the In Depth essay following Chapter 5).

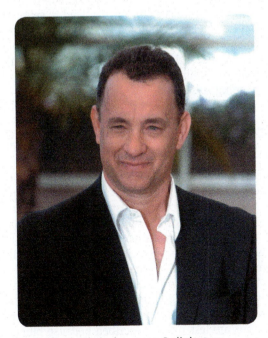

Actor Tom Hanks has type 2 diabetes.

Because these criteria for metabolic syndrome can be reduced significantly by following a healthful eating pattern and engaging in regular physical activity, they are modifiable.

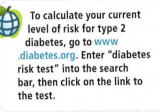

To calculate your current level of risk for type 2 diabetes, go to www.diabetes.org. Enter "diabetes risk test" into the search bar, then click on the link to the test.

Lifestyle Changes Can Reduce Your Risk

Type 2 diabetes is thought to have become an epidemic in the United States because of a combination of an aging population and our increased rates of obesity. We can't control our age, but we can and do control how much and what types of foods we eat and how much physical activity we engage in—and that, in turn, influences our risk for obesity. Currently, about 35% of American college students are either overweight or obese.[5]

Dietary changes specifically recommended to reduce your risk for type 2 diabetes include the following:

- Limit your intake of added sugars. A recent study examining the influence of availability of sugar on type 2 diabetes risk in 175 countries found that for every 150 kcal per person per day of sugar availability (which is equivalent to approximately one 12-ounce soft drink), the prevalence of type 2 diabetes increased by 1.1%.[6] This increase was independent of levels of overweight and obesity.
- Choose fiber-rich whole grains and whole-grain products in place of refined and processed carbohydrate foods. The evidence is strong that consuming a dietary pattern rich in fiber and whole grains is protective against type 2 diabetes, while a dietary pattern high in refined grains and processed carbohydrates increases type 2 diabetes risk.[7,8]
- Limit your consumption of red meats and processed meats. Overall, an increased intake of red and processed meats is associated with an elevated risk for type 2 diabetes.[9] Moreover, a study examining changes in intake of red meat over a 4-year period found that increasing red meat consumption by more than half a serving size was associated with a 48% elevated risk for type 2 diabetes.[10] Correspondingly, the study found that a reduction of at least half a serving size of red meat was associated with a 14% decreased risk for type 2 diabetes.

Although adopting a healthful diet is important, moderate daily exercise may prevent the onset of type 2 diabetes more effectively than dietary changes alone. In a recent study, researchers

To download a family history tree that you can fill out to determine your family history of diabetes, visit www.heart.org. Enter "my family health tree" into the search box, and then click on the link that appears.

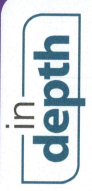

followed more than 1.5 million young men over 26 years and found that those who were defined as unfit (according to their muscle strength and aerobic capacity) at 18 years of age were three times more likely to develop type 2 diabetes by 44 years of age as compared to men who were defined as fit at 18 years of age.[11] This higher risk was observed regardless of the person's body weight and family history of type 2 diabetes. Exercise will also assist in weight loss, and studies show that losing only 10 to 30 pounds can reduce or eliminate the symptoms of type 2 diabetes.[12] (See Chapter 11 for examples of moderate exercise programs.)

Avoiding or stopping smoking can also reduce a person's risk for type 2 diabetes. Evidence indicates that smokers are 30% to 40% more likely to develop type 2 diabetes than nonsmokers, and people with type 2 diabetes who smoke have greater difficulty controlling their disease than nonsmokers with type 2 diabetes.[13]

In summary, by eating a healthy diet, staying active, maintaining a healthful body weight, and avoiding smoking, you should be able to keep your risk for type 2 diabetes low.

Dietary Counseling Can Help People Living with Diabetes

What if you've already been diagnosed with type 2 diabetes? The Academy of Nutrition and Dietetics emphasizes that there is no *single* diet or eating plan for people with diabetes. You should follow a healthful eating pattern just as you would to reduce your risk for heart disease, cancer, and obesity. One difference is that you may need to eat fewer carbohydrates and slightly more fat or protein to help regulate your blood glucose levels. Carbohydrates are still an important part of the diet, so, if you're eating less, make sure your choices are rich in micronutrients and fiber. Because precise nutritional recommendations vary according to each individual's responses to foods, consulting with a registered dietitian/ nutritionist is essential.

The Academy of Nutrition and Dietetics identifies the following basic strategies for eating more healthfully while living with diabetes:[14]

- Eat meals and snacks regularly and at planned times throughout the day.
- Try to eat about the same amount and types of food at each meal or snack.
- Follow the Dietary Guidelines for Americans or the USDA Food Patterns to guide your food choices (see Chapter 2).
- Seek the expert advice of a registered dietitian/nutritionist to assist you with carbohydrate counting and using the exchange system.

nutri-case | JUDY

"My daughter, Hannah, has been pestering me about changing how we eat and getting more exercise. She says she's just trying to lose weight, but ever since we found out I have type 2 diabetes I know she's been worried about me. What I didn't get until last night is that she's worried about herself, too. All through dinner she was real quiet; then all of a sudden she says, 'Mom, I had my blood sugar tested at the health center, and guess what? They said I have prediabetes.' She said that's kind of like the first step toward diabetes and that, if she doesn't make some serious changes, she'll end up just like me. So I guess we both need to change some things. Trouble is, I don't really know where to start."

Are you surprised to learn that Hannah has prediabetes? What are her risk factors? Given what you know about Judy's and Hannah's lifestyle, what kind of small changes could both mother and daughter make immediately to start addressing their high blood glucose levels?

In addition, people with diabetes should avoid alcoholic beverages, which can cause hypoglycemia, a drop in blood glucose that can cause confusion, clumsiness, and fainting. If left untreated, this can lead to seizures, coma, and death. The symptoms of alcohol intoxication and hypoglycemia are very similar. People with diabetes, their companions, and even healthcare providers may confuse these conditions; this can result in a potentially life-threatening situation.

Prescription Medications or Surgery May Be Advised

When blood glucose levels can't be adequately controlled with lifestyle changes, oral medications may be required. The prescription medication most commonly prescribed is metformin. It works both by increasing body cells' sensitivity to insulin and by reducing the amount of glucose the liver produces. Possible side effects include nausea and diarrhea, but these typically resolve as the body adapts to the drug. Two other classes of medications (sulfonylureas and meglitinides) work by stimulating the pancreas to increase its secretion of insulin. These medications are less often prescribed because blood glucose can drop too low, and weight gain is a possible side effect. Another group of medications (GLP-1 receptor agonists) work by slowing digestion, and can actually contribute to weight loss. Finally, a new class of medications (SGLT2 inhibitors) works by increasing the body's excretion of glucose in the urine. If both lifestyle changes and prescription medications cannot adequately control blood glucose, then people with type 2 diabetes must have daily insulin injections, just like people with type 1 diabetes.

web links

www.eatright.org
Academy of Nutrition and Dietetics

Visit this website to learn more about diabetes, low- and high-carbohydrate diets, and healthy eating guidance for people with diabetes.

www.diabetes.org
American Diabetes Association

Find out more about the nutritional needs of people living with diabetes.

www.niddk.nih.gov
National Institute of Diabetes and Digestive and Kidney Diseases (NIDDK)

Learn more about diabetes, including treatment, complications, U.S. statistics, clinical trials, recent research, and the National Diabetes Education Program.

www.cdc.gov/diabetes/home/
Centers for Disease Control and Prevention (CDC)

Explore the latest research and statistics about diabetes, find out if you are at risk, and learn about the National Diabetes Prevention Program.

www.joslin.org/
Joslin Diabetes Center

Learn more about type 1 diabetes and the latest research regarding treatments and a potential cure.

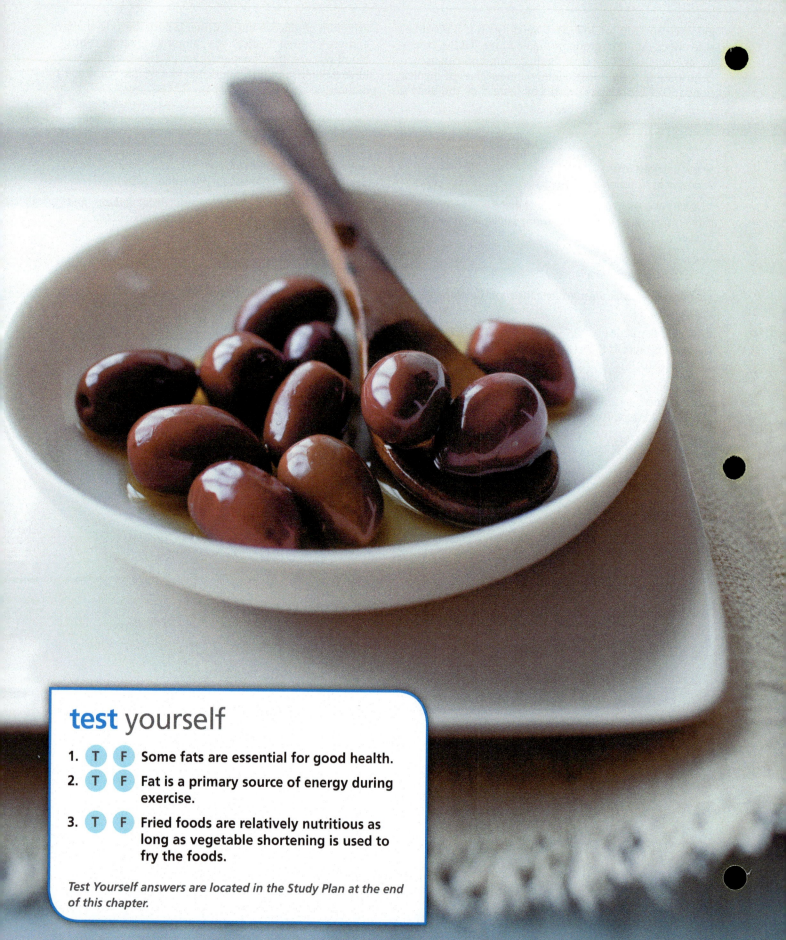

test yourself

1. **T** **F** Some fats are essential for good health.

2. **T** **F** Fat is a primary source of energy during exercise.

3. **T** **F** Fried foods are relatively nutritious as long as vegetable shortening is used to fry the foods.

Test Yourself answers are located in the Study Plan at the end of this chapter.

5

Fats
Essential energy-supplying nutrients

Wyatt and John are sharing an apartment off-campus this year and often shop for groceries together. They don't always agree on what to buy, however: Wyatt describes himself as a "health freak," whereas John is a "meat and potatoes" guy. At the market this evening, John said he was too tired to fix a meal from scratch, and suggested picking up some prepared ribs and potato salad from the deli. Wyatt said no way—ribs were loaded with saturated fat! He'd compromise on the potato salad if John would agree to have it with chicken or fish—and a green vegetable on the side. "Fine with me," John laughed, "but you're cooking it!"

Is saturated fat really such a menace? If so, why? What is saturated fat, anyway? And are other types of fat—*trans* fats, for instance—just as bad?

Although some people think that all dietary fat should be avoided, a certain amount of fat is essential for life and health. In fact, consuming adequate amounts of certain healthful fats can reduce your risk for cardiovascular disease. In this chapter, we'll explore several types of dietary fat and discuss their critical functions in the human body. We'll also identify changes you can make to shift your diet toward more healthful fats. The role of dietary fats in cardiovascular disease is discussed in the **In Depth** essay following this chapter.

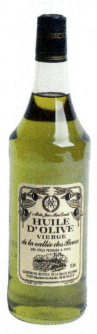

Some fats, such as olive oil, are liquid at room temperature.

What are fats?

Fats are just one form of a much larger and more diverse group of organic substances called **lipids**, which are distinguished by the fact that they are insoluble in water. Think of a salad dressing made with vinegar, which is mostly water, and olive oil, which is a lipid. Shaking the bottle *disperses* the oil but doesn't *dissolve* it: that's why it separates back out again so quickly. Lipids are found in all sorts of living things, from bacteria to plants to human beings. In fact, their presence on your skin explains why you can't clean your face with water alone: you need some type of soap to break down the insoluble lipids before you can wash them away. In this chapter, we focus on the small group of lipids that are found in foods.

We can distinguish two different types of food lipids according to their state at room temperature: Fats, such as butter, are solid at room temperature, whereas oils, such as olive oil, are liquid. Because most people are familiar with the term *fats*, we will use that term generically throughout this book, including when referring to oils. We can also distinguish three types of food lipids according to their chemical structure. These are triglycerides, phospholipids, and sterols. Let's take a look at each.

Triglycerides Are the Most Common Food-Based Fat

About 95% of the fat we eat is in the form of triglycerides (also called *triacylglycerols*). As reflected in the prefix *tri-*, a **triglyceride** is a molecule consisting of *three* fatty acids attached to a *three*-carbon glycerol backbone. **Fatty acids** are long chains of carbon atoms bound to each other as well as to hydrogen atoms. They are acids because they contain an acid group (carboxyl group) at one end of their chain. **Glycerol**, the backbone of a triglyceride molecule, is an alcohol composed of three carbon atoms. One fatty acid attaches to each of these three carbons to make the triglyceride (FIGURE 5.1).

Triglycerides are not only the most common form of fat in our diet, but also the form in which most of our body fat is stored. Body fat, clinically referred to as *adipose tissue* from the Latin root *adip-* meaning fat, is not inert. Rather, it is a metabolically active tissue that can contribute to or reduce our health. (We discuss the influence of body fat on health later in this chapter.)

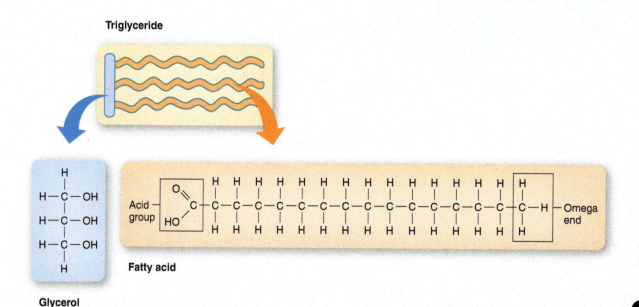

FIGURE 5.1 A triglyceride consists of three fatty acids attached to a three-carbon glycerol backbone.

Phospholipids Combine Lipids with Phosphate

Phospholipids are found in a limited number of foods, including egg yolks, liver, peanuts, soybeans, and some processed foods. They consist of two fatty acids and a glycerol backbone bound to another compound that contains phosphate **(FIGURE 5.2)**. This addition of a phosphate compound makes phospholipids soluble in water, a property that enables phospholipids to assist in transporting fats in our bloodstream. Also, phospholipids in our cell membranes regulate the transport of substances into and out of the cell. Phospholipids also help with the digestion of dietary fats: the liver uses phospholipids called *lecithins* to make bile. The body manufactures phospholipids, so they are not essential nutrients. What *is* essential is phosphorus, a mineral that combines with oxygen to make phosphate.

Sterols Have a Ring Structure

Sterols are lipids with a multiple-ring structure **(FIGURE 5.3a)**. They are found in both animal and plant foods and are produced in the body.

Cholesterol is the most commonly occurring sterol in the diet (see Figure 5.3b). It is found only in the fatty part of animal products such as butter, egg yolks, whole milk, meats, and poultry. Low- or reduced-fat animal products, such as lean meats and skim milk, have little cholesterol.

We don't need to consume cholesterol in our diet because our body continually synthesizes it, mostly in the liver and intestines. This continuous production is essential because cholesterol is part of every cell membrane, where it works in conjunction with fatty acids to help maintain cell membrane integrity. It is particularly plentiful in the neural cells that make up our brain, spinal cord, and nerves. The body also uses cholesterol to synthesize several important compounds, including sex hormones (estrogen, androgen, and progesterone), bile, adrenal hormones, and vitamin D. Given these important functions of cholesterol, you might be wondering why it has such a bad reputation. The answer is that a high level of cholesterol circulating in the blood is associated with cardiovascular disease, the subject of the **In Depth** essay following this chapter.

As just noted, plants also contain some sterols. Plant sterols are not very well absorbed; nevertheless, they may confer a health benefit because they appear to block the absorption of dietary cholesterol. Nuts are especially rich in plant sterols.

recap Fats and oils are two forms of lipids, compounds that are insoluble in water. Three types of lipids are found in foods and in the body. These are triglycerides, phospholipids, and sterols. Triglycerides are the most common. A triglyceride is made up of a glycerol backbone and three fatty acids. Phospholipids combine two fatty acids and a glycerol backbone with a phosphate-containing

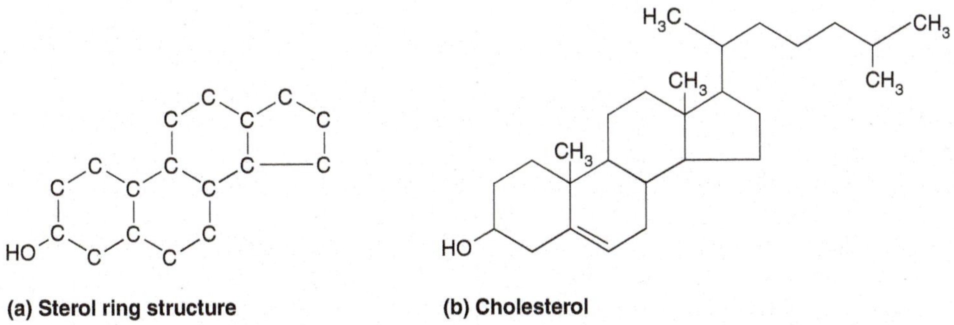

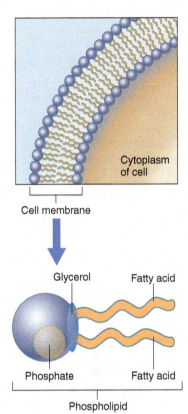

FIGURE 5.2 Structure of a phospholipid. Phospholipids consist of a glycerol backbone with two fatty acids and a compound that contains phosphate.

lipids A diverse group of organic substances that are insoluble in water; lipids include triglycerides, phospholipids, and sterols.

triglyceride A molecule consisting of three fatty acids attached to a three-carbon glycerol backbone.

fatty acids Long chains of carbon atoms bound to each other as well as to hydrogen atoms.

glycerol An alcohol composed of three carbon atoms; it is the backbone of a triglyceride molecule.

phospholipid A type of lipid in which a fatty acid is combined with another compound that contains phosphate; unlike other lipids, phospholipids are soluble in water.

sterol A type of lipid found in foods and the body that has a ring structure; cholesterol is the most common sterol in our diets.

(a) Sterol ring structure

(b) Cholesterol

FIGURE 5.3 Sterol structure. **(a)** Sterols are lipids that contain multiple-ring structures. **(b)** Cholesterol is the most commonly occurring sterol in our diets.

Learn more about plant sterols and how to incorporate them into your diet at www.webmd.com. Type "plant sterols" in the search bar to get underway.

LO 2 Compare and contrast types of triglycerides, explaining why some are more healthful than others.

compound, making them soluble in water. Sterols have a multiple-ring structure. Cholesterol is the most commonly occurring sterol in our diet, and is used by the body to build many essential compounds. Cholesterol is found only in animal-based foods. Plant foods provide plant sterols.

Why are some triglycerides better than others?

Now that you know how triglycerides differ from phospholipids and sterols, let's compare the various types of triglycerides to find out why some are better than others. In general, triglycerides can be classified by:

- their chain length, which is the number of carbons in each fatty acid.
- their level of saturation; that is, how much hydrogen, H, is attached to each carbon atom in the fatty acid chain.
- their shape, which is determined in some cases by how they are commercially processed.

All of these factors influence how the body uses triglycerides.

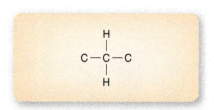

(a) Saturated fatty acid

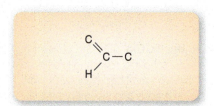

(b) Unsaturated fatty acid

▲ **FIGURE 5.4** An atom of carbon has four attachment sites. In fatty acid chains, two of these sites are filled by adjacent carbon atoms. **(a)** In saturated fatty acids, the other two sites are always filled by two hydrogen atoms. **(b)** In unsaturated fatty acids, at one or more points along the chain, a double bond to an adjacent carbon atom takes up one of the attachment sites that would otherwise be filled by hydrogen.

Fatty Acid Chain Length Affects Digestion and Absorption

The fatty acids attached to the glycerol backbone can vary in the number of carbons they contain, referred to as their *chain length.*

- Short-chain fatty acids are usually fewer than 6 carbon atoms in length.
- Medium-chain fatty acids are 6 to 12 carbons in length.
- Long-chain fatty acids are 14 or more carbons in length.

Fatty acid chain length determines how the fat is digested, absorbed, and transported in the body. For example, short- and medium-chain fatty acids are digested and absorbed more quickly than long-chain fatty acids. We discuss the digestion, absorption, and transport of fats in more detail later in this chapter.

Level of Hydrogen Saturation Influences Health Effects

Triglycerides can also vary by their level of saturation, which is determined by the types of bonds found in the fatty acid chains. **FIGURE 5.4** shows two types of carbon bonds found in fatty acid chains. Notice that the central carbon can bond with single bonds to two hydrogens and two other carbons (Figure 5.4a). Alternatively, the central carbon can bond with single bonds to one hydrogen and a second carbon, and with a double bond to a third carbon (Figure 5.4b).

If a fatty acid chain has no carbons bonded together with a double bond, it is referred to as a **saturated fatty acid (SFA).** This is because every carbon atom in the chain is *saturated* with hydrogen: each has the maximum amount of hydrogen bound to it. The fatty acid chain in Figure 5.1 is saturated, as is the one in the top row of **FIGURE 5.5a**, which looks a bit different because it's represented with a more succinct chemical formula. Some foods that are high in saturated fatty acids are coconut oil, palm oil, palm kernel oil, butter, cream, whole milk, lard, and beef.

If, within the chain of carbon atoms, two carbons are bound to each other with a double bond, then this double carbon bond excludes hydrogen. This lack of hydrogen at *one* part of the molecule results in a fat that is referred to as *monounsaturated* (recall from Chapter 4 that the prefix *mono-* means "one"). A **monounsaturated fatty acid (MUFA)** is usually liquid at room temperature (see

saturated fatty acid (SFA) A fatty acid that has no carbons joined together with a double bond; SFAs are generally solid at room temperature.

monounsaturated fatty acid (MUFA) A fatty acid that has two carbons in the chain bound to each other with one double bond; MUFAs are generally liquid at room temperature.

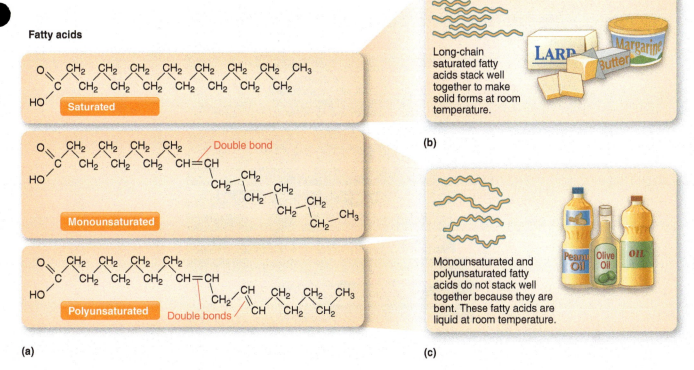

Fatty acids

(a)

(b) Long-chain saturated fatty acids stack well together to make solid forms at room temperature.

(c) Monounsaturated and polyunsaturated fatty acids do not stack well together because they are bent. These fatty acids are liquid at room temperature.

◆ **FIGURE 5.5** Examples of levels of saturation among fatty acids and how these levels of saturation affect the shape of fatty acids. **(a)** Saturated fatty acids are saturated with hydrogen, meaning they have no carbons bonded together with a double bond. Monounsaturated fatty acids contain two carbons bound by one double bond. Polyunsaturated fatty acids have more than one double bond linking carbon atoms. **(b)** Saturated fats have straight fatty acids packed tightly together and are solid at room temperature. **(c)** Unsaturated fats have "kinked" fatty acids at the area of the double bond, preventing them from packing tightly together; they are liquid at room temperature.

the middle row of Figure 5.5a). Foods that are high in MUFAs are olive oil, canola oil, and cashew nuts.

If the fat molecule has *more than one* double bond, it contains even less hydrogen and is referred to as a **polyunsaturated fatty acid (PUFA)** (see the bottom row of Figure 5.5a). Polyunsaturated fatty acids are also liquid at room temperature. Canola, corn, and safflower oils are rich in PUFAs.

Although foods vary in the types of fatty acids they contain, in general we can say that animal-based foods tend to be high in saturated fats and plant foods tend to be high in unsaturated fats. Specifically, animal fats provide approximately 40–60% of their energy from saturated fats, whereas plant fats provide 80–90% of their energy from monounsaturated and polyunsaturated fats. Most oils are a good source of both MUFAs and PUFAs. **FIGURE 5.6** on page 144 compares the percentages of the different types of fats in a variety of foods.

In general, saturated fats have a detrimental effect on our health, whereas unsaturated fats are protective. It makes sense, therefore, that diets high in plant foods—because they're low in saturated fats—are more healthful than diets high in animal products. We discuss the influence of various types of fatty acids on your risk for cardiovascular disease in the **In Depth** essay immediately following this chapter.

Carbon Bonding Influences Shape

Have you ever noticed how many toothpicks are packed into a small box? A hundred or more! But if you were to break a bunch of toothpicks into V shapes anywhere along their length, how many could you then fit into the same box? It would be very few because the bent toothpicks would jumble together, taking up much more space.

polyunsaturated fatty acid (PUFA) A fatty acid that has more than one double bond in the chain; PUFAs are generally liquid at room temperature.

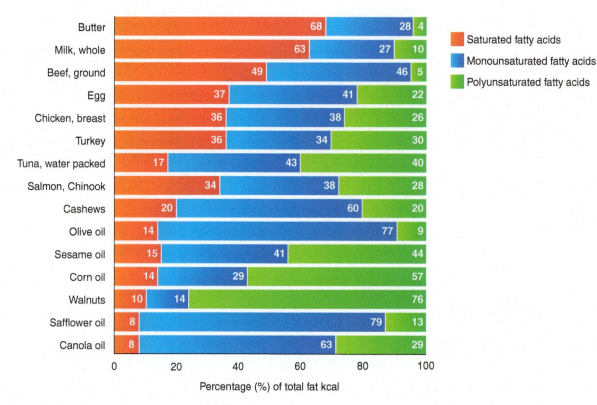

FIGURE 5.6 Major sources of dietary fat.

Molecules of saturated fat are like straight toothpicks: they have no double carbon bonds and always form straight, rigid chains. Because they have no kinks, these chains can pack together tightly (see Figure 5.5b). That is why saturated fats, such as the fat in meats, are solid at room temperature.

In contrast, each double carbon bond of unsaturated fats gives them a kink along their length (see Figure 5.5c). This means that they're unable to pack together tightly—for example, to form a stick of butter—and instead are liquid at room temperature.

Unsaturated fatty acids are kinked when they occur naturally, but they can be manipulated by food manufacturers to create a straight fatty acid called a *trans* fat. Let's take a look at this process.

Trans Fatty Acids Are Especially Harmful

Unsaturated fatty acids can occur in either a *cis* or a *trans* shape. The prefix *cis-* means things are located on the same side or near each other, whereas *trans-* is a prefix that denotes across or opposite. These terms describe the positioning of the hydrogen atoms around the double carbon bond as follows:

- A *cis fatty acid* has both hydrogen atoms located on the same side of the double bond **(FIGURE 5.7a)**. This positioning gives the *cis* molecule a pronounced kink at the double carbon bond. We typically find the *cis* fatty acids in nature and, thus, in whole foods.
- In a *trans fatty acid,* the hydrogen atoms are attached on diagonally opposite sides of the double carbon bond (see Figure 5.7b). This positioning makes the fatty acid straighter and more rigid, just like saturated fats. Thus, "*trans* fats" is a collective term used to define fats with *trans* double bonds. Although *trans* fatty acids occur in limited amounts in cow's milk and meat, the majority of *trans* fatty acids in foods are produced by manipulating the fatty acids during food processing.

This process, called **hydrogenation**, was developed in the early 1900s to produce a type of cheap fat that could be stored in a solid form and would resist rancidity.

hydrogenation The process of adding hydrogen to unsaturated fatty acids, making them more saturated and thereby more solid at room temperature.

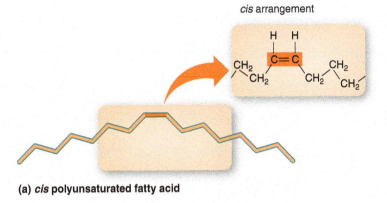

(a) *cis* polyunsaturated fatty acid

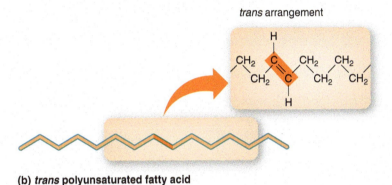

(b) *trans* polyunsaturated fatty acid

◀ **FIGURE 5.7** Structure of **(a)** a *cis* and **(b)** a *trans* polyunsaturated fatty acid. Notice that *cis* fatty acids have both hydrogen atoms located on the same side of the double bond. This positioning makes the molecule kinked. In the *trans* fatty acids, the hydrogen atoms are attached on diagonally opposite sides of the double carbon bond. This positioning makes them straighter and more rigid.

During hydrogenation, pressurized hydrogen is added directly to unsaturated fatty acids, such as those found in corn and safflower oils. This alters the arrangement of their double bonds and thereby straightens the fatty acid chains. The degree of hydrogenation can make an oil more or less saturated, resulting in a *partially hydrogenated oil* (PHO).

The *Dietary Guidelines for Americans* suggest that you keep your *trans* fat intake as low as possible. This recommendation is grounded in an overwhelming body of evidence associating *trans* fats with an increased risk for cardiovascular disease. In fact, *trans* fats are considered the most harmful fat for your health.

Be aware that products labeled as having "zero" *trans* fats can still contain *trans* fatty acids! That's because the U.S. Food and Drug Administration (FDA) allows products that have less than 1 g of *trans* fat per serving to claim that they are *trans* fat free. So, even if the Nutrition Facts panel states 0 g *trans* fats, the product can still have 1/2 g of *trans* fat per serving.

How can you tell if a food contains *trans* fats? Check the ingredients list. If it states that the product contains PHOs, it contains *trans* fats. However, new regulations from the FDA mean that you'll rarely need to take this precaution in coming years. Because of the negative effect *trans* fatty acids have on health, especially cardiovascular health, in 2015 the FDA removed PHOs from a list of food components "generally recognized as safe."[1] Thus, all food manufacturers must remove PHOs from their products by the middle of 2018. Even after this date, you might still consume some *trans* fatty acids since they occur naturally in meat and dairy.

Essential Fatty Acids Have Unique Health Benefits

There has been a lot of press lately about "omega" fatty acids, so you might be wondering what they are and why they're so important. First, let's explain the Greek name. As illustrated in **FIGURE 5.8** on page 146, one end of a fatty acid chain (where it attaches to glycerol in a triglyceride) is designated the α (alpha) end (α is the first letter in the Greek alphabet). The other end of a fatty acid chain is called the ω (omega) end (ω is the last letter in the Greek alphabet). When synthesizing fatty acids, the

FIGURE 5.8 Two essential fatty acids: linoleic acid (an omega-6 fatty acid) and alpha-linolenic acid (an omega-3 fatty acid).

Essential fatty acids

Linoleic acid

Alpha-linolenic acid

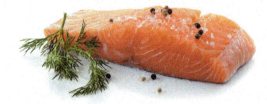

Salmon is high in omega-3 fatty acid content.

essential fatty acids (EFAs) Fatty acids that must be consumed in the diet because they cannot be made by our body.

linoleic acid An essential fatty acid found in vegetable and nut oils; one of the omega-6 fatty acids.

alpha-linolenic acid (ALA) An essential fatty acid found in leafy green vegetables, flaxseed oil, soy oil, and other plant foods; an omega-3 fatty acid.

eicosapentaenoic acid (EPA) An omega-3 fatty acid available from marine foods and as a metabolic derivative of alpha-linolenic acid.

body has no mechanism for inserting double bonds before the ninth carbon from the omega end. This means that, when our body needs types of fatty acids having a double bond close to the omega end, it has to obtain them from the foods we eat. These are considered **essential fatty acids (EFAs)** because the body cannot make them, yet it requires them for healthy functioning. The EFAs are classified into two groups: omega-6 fatty acids and omega-3 fatty acids.

Omega-6 Fatty Acids

Fatty acids that have a double bond six carbons from the omega end (at ω-6) are known as *omega-6 fatty acids*. One omega-6 fatty acid, **linoleic acid**, is essential to human health. It is found in vegetable and nut oils, such as sunflower, safflower, corn, soy, and peanut oil. If you eat lots of vegetables or use vegetable-oil-based margarines or vegetable oils, you are probably getting adequate amounts of this EFA in your diet.

Omega-3 Fatty Acids

Fatty acids with a double bond three carbons from the omega end (at ω-3) are known as *omega-3 fatty acids*. The most common omega-3 fatty acid in our diet is **alpha-linolenic acid (ALA)**. It is derived primarily from plants, especially dark green, leafy vegetables, flaxseeds and flaxseed oil, soybeans and soybean oil, walnuts and walnut oil, and canola oil.

You may also have read news reports of the health benefits of the two omega-3 fatty acids found in many fish. These are **eicosapentaenoic acid (EPA)** and **docosahexaenoic acid (DHA)**. Although our body can use ALA to assemble the chains of EPA and DHA, the amount that can be converted is limited;[2] therefore, it is important to consume them directly from marine sources. They are found in fish, shellfish, and fish oils. Fish that naturally contain more oil, such as salmon and tuna, are higher in EPA and DHA than lean fish, such as cod or flounder.

Functions of Essential Fatty Acids

As a group, EFAs are essential to growth and health because they are precursors to important biological compounds called *eicosanoids*, which are produced in nearly every cell in the body. Eicosanoids get their name from the Greek word *eicosa*, which means "twenty," because they are synthesized from fatty acids with 20 carbon atoms. In the body, eicosanoids are potent regulators of cellular function. For example, they help regulate gastrointestinal tract motility, blood clotting, blood pressure, the permeability of our blood vessels to fluid and large molecules, and the regulation of inflammation and gene expression.[3]

Each EFA also has one or more unique roles. For example, linoleic acid is metabolized in the body to arachidonic acid, which is a precursor to a number of eicosanoids. Linoleic acid is also needed for cell membrane structure and is required for the lipoproteins—lipid-protein compounds—that transport fats in our blood. In contrast, research indicates that diets high in the omega-3 fatty acids stimulate the production of eicosanoids that reduce inflammation, improve blood lipid profiles, and otherwise reduce an individual's risk for cardiovascular disease and cardiac death.[3,4]

> **Want to boost your omega-3 intake but not sure what foods to buy? Download an omega-3 shopping list at www.webmd.com. To find it, type "omega-3 shopping list" in the search bar.**

recap Triglycerides are made up of a molecule of glycerol bonded to three fatty acid chains, which can be classified based on chain length, level of saturation, and shape. Saturated fatty acids have no double carbon bonds and are straight. Monounsaturated fatty acids have one double carbon bond, and poly-unsaturated fatty acids have two or more double bonds. Both are kinked. Most *trans* fatty acids are produced by food manufacturers in a process called hydroge-nation, in which the unsaturated fatty acids in a plant oil are straightened by the addition of hydrogen. In 2015, the FDA ruled that partially hydrogenated oils are no longer "generally recognized as safe." The essential fatty acids, linoleic acid (an omega-6 fatty acid) and alpha-linolenic acid (an omega-3 fatty acid), cannot be synthesized by the body and yet are necessary for health; thus, they must be consumed in the diet. Both saturated and *trans* fatty acids increase our risk for cardiovascular disease, whereas unsaturated fatty acids, including the essential fatty acids, are protective.

Why do we need fats?

LO 3 Identify five functions of fat.

Although dietary fat has been demonized for decades, fat is critical to body function and survival.

Fats Provide Energy

Dietary fat is a primary source of energy because fat has more than twice the energy (9 kcal per gram) of carbohydrate or protein (4 kcal per gram). This means that fat is much more energy dense. For example, 1 tbsp. of butter or oil contains approxi-mately 100 kcal, whereas it takes 2.5 cups of steamed broccoli or 1 slice of whole-wheat bread to provide 100 kcal.

Fats Sustain Us at Rest

Just as a candle needs oxygen for the flame to burn the tallow, our cells need oxygen to burn fat for energy. At rest, we are able to deliver plenty of oxygen to our cells, and approximately 30–70% of the energy we use comes from fat. The exact percentage varies, according to how much fat you are eating in your diet, how physically active you are, and whether you are gaining or losing weight. If you are dieting, more fat will be used for energy than if you are gaining weight. During times of weight gain, more of the fat consumed in the diet is stored in the adipose tissue, and the body uses more dietary protein and carbohydrate as fuel sources at rest.

docosahexaenoic acid (DHA) An omega-3 fatty acid available from marine foods and as a metabolic derivative of alpha-linolenic acid.

Fats Fuel Physical Activity

Fat is a major energy source during physical activity, and one of the best ways to lose body fat and increase energy expenditure is to exercise. During exercise such as running and cycling, fat can be mobilized from any of the following sources: muscle tissue, adipose tissue, blood lipids, and/or any dietary fat consumed shortly before or during exercise.

A number of hormonal changes signal the body to break down stored energy to fuel the working muscles. The hormonal responses, and the amount and source of the fat used, depend on your level of fitness; the type, intensity, and duration of the exercise; and how well fed you are before you exercise. For example, the hormone adrenaline strongly stimulates the breakdown of stored fat. Blood levels of adrenaline rise dramatically within seconds of beginning exercise. This in turn activates additional hormones within the fat cell to begin breaking down fat.

Adrenaline also signals the pancreas to *decrease* insulin production. This is important because insulin inhibits fat breakdown. Thus, when the need for fat as an energy source is high, blood insulin levels are typically low. As you might guess, blood insulin levels are high after eating, when our need for getting energy from stored fat is low and the need for fat storage is high.

Once fatty acids are released from the adipose cell, they travel in the blood attached to a protein, *albumin*, to the muscles, where they enter the mitochondria and use oxygen to produce ATP, which is the cell's energy source. Becoming more physically fit means you can deliver more oxygen to the muscle to use the fat that is delivered there. In addition, you can exercise longer when you are fit. Since the body has only a limited supply of stored carbohydrate as glycogen in muscle tissue, the longer you exercise, the more fat you use for energy. This point is illustrated in **FIGURE 5.9**. In this example, an individual is running for 4 hours at a moderate intensity. The longer the individual runs, the more depleted the muscle glycogen levels become and the more fat from adipose tissue is used as a fuel source for exercise.

Body Fat Stores Energy for Later Use

Our adipose tissue gives us ready access to energy even when we choose not to eat (or are unable to eat), when we are exercising, and while we are sleeping. The body has little stored carbohydrate—only enough to last about 1 to 2 days—and there is no place where our body can store extra protein. We cannot consider our muscles and organs as a place where "extra" protein is stored! For these reasons, although we don't want excessive adipose tissue, a moderate amount is absolutely essential to

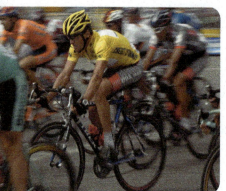

The longer you exercise, the more fat you use for energy. Cyclists in long-distance races use fat stores for energy.

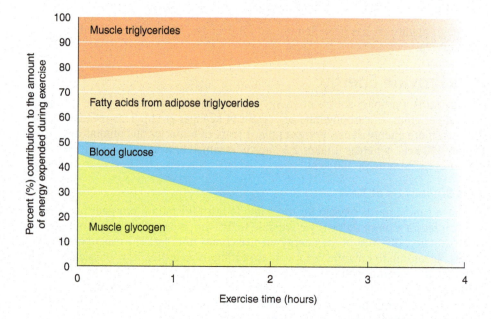

▶ **FIGURE 5.9** Various sources of energy used during exercise. As a person exercises for a prolonged period, fatty acids from adipose cells contribute relatively more energy than do carbohydrates stored in the muscle or circulating in our blood.

Data adapted from: Substrate utilization during exercise in active people. *Am. J. Clin. Nutr.* 6(suppl):958S–979S.

good health. Incidentally, muscle tissue also stores some triglycerides; however, the amount is much less than in body fat. This fat is readily used during exercise to fuel the working muscle.

Fats Enable the Transport of Fat-Soluble Vitamins

Dietary fat enables the transport of the fat-soluble vitamins (A, D, E, and K) our body needs for many essential metabolic functions. Vitamin A is essential for vision; vitamin D helps maintain bone health; vitamin E protects cell membranes from potentially harmful by-products of metabolism; and vitamin K is important for proteins involved in blood clotting and bone health. (These vitamins are discussed in detail in Chapters 8 and 9.)

Fats Help Maintain Cell Function

Phospholipids, cholesterol, and fatty acids—especially PUFAs—are critical components of every cell membrane. These various lipids help maintain membrane integrity, determine what substances are transported into and out of the cell, and regulate what substances can bind to the cell; thus, they strongly influence the function of the cell.

In addition, fats help maintain cell membrane fluidity and flexibility. For example, wild salmon live in very cold water and have high levels of omega-3 fatty acids in their cell membranes. These fats stay fluid and flexible even in very cold environments, allowing the fish to swim in extremely cold water. In the same way, fats help our membranes stay fluid and flexible. For example, they enable our red blood cells to bend and move through the smallest capillaries in our body, delivering oxygen to all our cells.

Fatty acids, especially PUFAs, are also primary components of the tissues of the brain and spinal cord, where they facilitate the transmission of information from one cell to another. We also need fats for the development, growth, and maintenance of these tissues.

Body Fat Provides Protection

Many people think of body fat as "bad," but it helps keep us healthy. Besides being the primary site of stored energy, adipose tissue pads our body and protects our organs, such as the kidneys and liver, when we fall or are bruised. The fat under our skin also acts as insulation to help us retain body heat.

Although some stored fat is essential to life, too much, especially in the abdominal region, is a risk factor for metabolic syndrome, which increases the risk for type 2 diabetes and cardiovascular disease. That's because adipose cells overloaded with triglycerides can malfunction, secreting proteins and other compounds that promote insulin resistance and blood vessel inflammation. (Obesity and metabolic syndrome are discussed in the **In Depth** essay following Chapter 10.)

Dietary Fats Contribute to the Flavor, Texture, and Satiety of Foods

Dietary fat helps food taste good because it contributes to texture and flavor. Fat makes salad dressings smooth and ice cream "creamy," and it gives cakes and cookies their moist, tender texture. Frying foods in melted butter, lard, or oils gives them a crisp, flavorful coating; however, eating fried foods regularly is unhealthful because these foods are high in saturated and *trans* fatty acids.

Although protein is the most satiating nutrient, fats are more satiating than carbohydrates, so we stop eating sooner and can go a longer time before we feel hungry again. This is in part due to fat's higher energy density. In addition, fat takes longer to digest because more steps are involved in the digestion process. This may help you feel fuller for a longer period of time as energy is slowly released into your bloodstream.

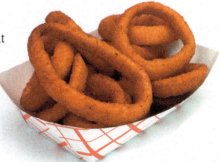

▲ Fat adds texture and flavor to foods.

Unfortunately, you can eat a lot of fat without feeling overfull because fat is so compact. For example, one medium apple weighs 117 g (approximately 4 oz) and has 70 kcal, but the same number of Calories of butter—two pats—would hardly make you feel full! Looked at another way, an amount of butter weighing the same number of grams as a medium apple would contain 840 kcal.

recap Dietary fats provide more than twice the energy of protein and carbohydrate, at 9 kcal per gram. They provide the majority of the energy required at rest, and are a major fuel source during exercise, especially endurance exercise. Dietary fats help transport the fat-soluble vitamins into the body and help regulate cell function and maintain membrane integrity. Stored body fat in the adipose tissue helps protect vital organs and pad the body. Fats contribute to the flavor and texture of foods and the satiety we feel after a meal.

LO 4 Describe the steps involved in fat digestion, absorption, and transport.

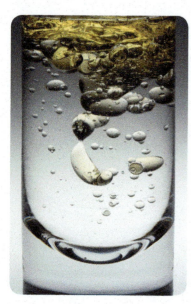

⬆ Fats and oils do not dissolve readily in water.

How does the body process fats?

Because fats are not soluble in water, they cannot enter our bloodstream easily from the digestive tract. Thus, fats must be digested, absorbed, and transported within the body differently than carbohydrates and proteins, which are water-soluble substances. The digestion and absorption of fat were discussed in Chapter 3, but we review the process here, and the steps are illustrated in **FOCUS FIGURE 5.10**.

Salivary enzymes released during chewing have a limited role in the breakdown of fats, so most fat reaches the stomach intact. The primary role of the stomach in fat digestion is to mix and break up the fat into small droplets. Because they are not soluble in water, these fat droplets typically float on top of the watery digestive juices in the stomach until they are passed into the small intestine.

The Gallbladder, Liver, and Pancreas Assist in Fat Digestion

Because fat is not soluble in water, its digestion requires the help of bile from the gallbladder and digestive enzymes from the pancreas. The gallbladder is a sac attached to the underside of the liver, and the pancreas is an oblong-shaped organ sitting below the stomach. Both have a duct connecting them to the small intestine.

As fat enters the small intestine from the stomach, the gallbladder contracts and releases bile, a compound synthesized in the liver and stored in the gallbladder until needed. Bile contains cholesterol, certain amino acids, and the mineral sodium in compounds referred to as *bile salts*. As shown in **FIGURE 5.11a** (page 152), bile salts act somewhat like soap, emulsifying large fat droplets into smaller and smaller droplets. At the same time, pancreatic lipases—lipid-digesting enzymes produced in the pancreas—travel through the pancreatic duct into the small intestine. By emulsifying the fat into small droplets, bile has exposed more surface area to the action of pancreatic lipases, which now begin digesting the triglycerides. Each triglyceride molecule is broken down into two free fatty acids and one *monoacylglyceride*, a glycerol backbone with one fatty acid still attached.

Absorption of Fat Occurs Primarily in the Small Intestine

The majority of fat absorption occurs in the enterocytes with the help of micelles (see Figures 5.10 and 5.11b). A *micelle* is a spherical compound made up of bile and phospholipids that can trap the free fatty acids and monoacylglycerides, as well as cholesterol and phospholipids, and transport these products to the enterocytes for absorption.

focus figure 5.10 Lipid Digestion Overview

The majority of lipid digestion takes place in the small intestine, with the help of bile from the liver and digestive enzymes from the pancreas. Micelles transport the end products of lipid digestion to the enterocytes for absorption and eventual transport via the blood or lymph.

ORGANS OF THE GI TRACT

MOUTH
Lingual lipase secreted by tongue cells and mixed with saliva digests some triglycerides.

Little lipid digestion occurs here.

STOMACH
Most fat arrives intact at the stomach, where it is mixed and broken into droplets.

Gastric lipase digests some triglycerides.

SMALL INTESTINE
Bile from the gallbladder breaks fat into smaller droplets.

Lipid-digesting enzymes from the pancreas break triglycerides into monoacylglycerides and fatty acids.

Lipid-digesting enzymes from the pancreas break dietary cholesterol esters and phospholipids into their components.

Products of fat digestion combine with bile salts to form micelles.

Micelles transport lipid digestion products to the enterocytes.

Within enterocytes, components from micelles reform triglycerides and are repackaged as chylomicrons for transport into the lymphatic system.

Shorter fatty acids can be absorbed directly into the bloodstream.

ACCESSORY ORGANS

SALIVARY GLANDS
Produce saliva.

LIVER
Produces bile, which is stored in the gallbladder.

GALLBLADDER
Contracts and releases bile into the small intestine.

PANCREAS
Produces lipid-digesting enzymes, which are released into the small intestine.

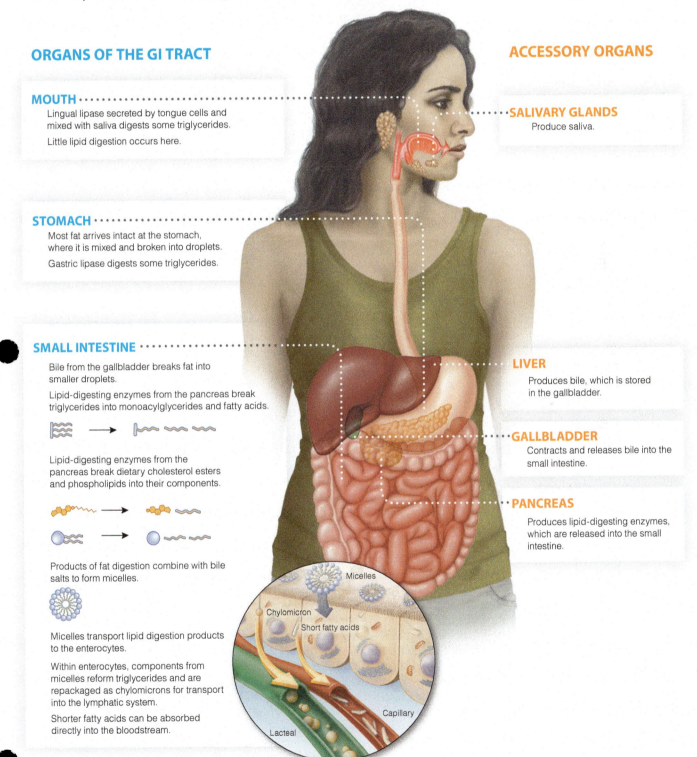

Micelles

Chylomicron

Short fatty acids

Capillary

Lacteal

151

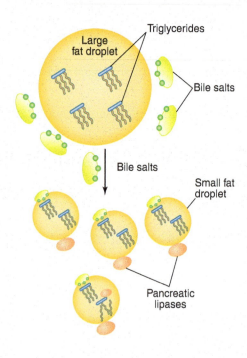

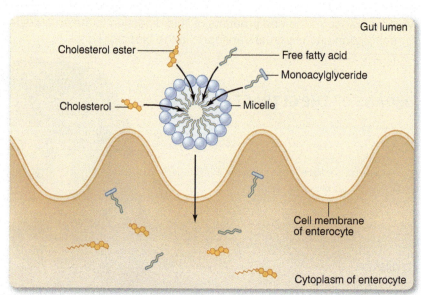

(a) Fat is emulsified by bile salts, then triglycerides are broken apart by pancreatic lipase.

(b) Micelle transports lipid digestion products to the enterocyte for absorption.

🔺 **FIGURE 5.11** Action of bile salts, pancreatic lipase, and micelles in fat emulsification, digestion, and absorption. **(a)** Large fat droplets filled with triglycerides are emulsified by bile into smaller and smaller droplets. Pancreatic lipase can then access the triglycerides and break them apart into free fatty acids and monoacylglycerides. **(b)** These products, along with cholesterol, are trapped in micelles, spherical compounds made up of bile salts and phospholipids. Micelles transport lipid digestion products to the enterocytes. Bile salts are taken up in the lower intestine and recycled by the liver.

lipoprotein A spherical compound in which fat clusters in the center and phospholipids and proteins form the outside of the sphere.

chylomicron A lipoprotein produced in the enterocyte; transports dietary fat out of the intestinal tract.

lipoprotein lipase (LPL) An enzyme that sits on the outside of cells and breaks apart triglycerides in chylomicrons, so that their fatty acids can be removed and taken up by the cell.

Given that fats do not mix with water, how does the absorbed fat get into the bloodstream? As the micelle nears the surface of the enterocytes, the fatty acids, monoacylglycerides, phospholipids, and cholesterol are released and absorbed. At this point the micelle itself is not absorbed; instead, it is absorbed later in the ileum of the small intestine, at which point it can be recycled back to the liver.

Once inside the enterocytes, the free fatty acids and monoacylglycerides are reformulated into triglycerides, and then packaged into lipoproteins. A **lipoprotein** is a spherical compound in which the fat clusters in the center and phospholipids and proteins form the outside of the sphere **(FIGURE 5.12)**. The specific lipoprotein produced in the enterocyte to transport fat from a meal is called a **chylomicron**. Again, this unique compound is soluble in water because phospholipids and proteins are soluble in water. Once chylomicrons are formed, they are transported from the intestinal lining to the lymphatic system through the lacteals. Lymphatic vessels eventually drain into the left subclavian vein, a large vein beneath the left collarbone (clavicle). In this way, dietary fat finally arrives in your blood.

How does the fat get out of the chylomicrons in the bloodstream and into body cells? This process occurs with the help of an enzyme called **lipoprotein lipase (LPL)**, which sits outside of cells, including adipose and muscle cells. LPL comes into contact with the chylomicrons when they touch the surface of a cell. As a result of this contact, LPL breaks apart the triglycerides in the core of the chylomicrons. The free fatty acids then move out of the chylomicrons and cross into the cell, whereas the glycerol is transported back to the liver or kidney.

As the cells take up the free fatty acids, the chylomicrons shrink in size and become more dense. These smaller chylomicrons, called *chylomicron remnants*, are now filled

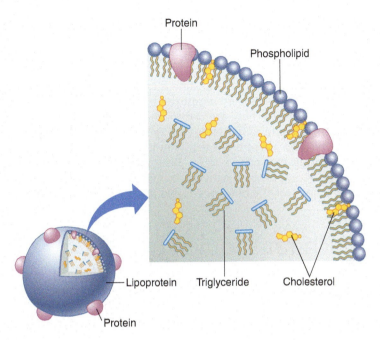

◄ FIGURE 5.12 Structure of a lipoprotein. Notice that the fat clusters in the center of the molecule and the phospholipids and proteins, which are water soluble, form the outside of the sphere. This enables lipoproteins to transport fats in the bloodstream.

with cholesterol, phospholipids, and protein. As they pass through the liver, these remnants are removed from the bloodstream and their contents are recycled. The liver also synthesizes two other types of lipoproteins that play important roles in cardiovascular disease. They are discussed in the **In Depth** essay following this chapter.

For most individuals, the chylomicrons that appear in the blood after the consumption of a moderate fat meal can easily be cleared by the body within 6 to 8 hours. This is why you are asked to fast for at least 8 hours before having blood drawn for a laboratory analysis for blood lipid levels.

As mentioned earlier, short- and medium-chain fatty acids (those fewer than 14 carbons in length) can be transported in the body more readily than the long-chain fatty acids. When short- and medium-chain fatty acids are digested and transported to the enterocytes, they do not have to be incorporated into chylomicrons. Instead, they can travel bound to either a transport protein, such as albumin, or a phospholipid. For this reason, shorter-chain fatty acids can get into the bloodstream more quickly than long-chain fatty acids.

Fat Is Stored in Adipose Tissues for Later Use

As described earlier, with the help of LPL, the chylomicrons deliver their load of fatty acids to body cells. There are three primary fates of these fatty acids:

1. Body cells, especially muscle cells, can take them up and use them as a source of energy.
2. Cells can use them to make lipid-containing compounds needed by the body.
3. If the body doesn't need the fatty acids for immediate energy, muscle and adipose cells can re-create the triglycerides (using glucose for the glycerol backbone) and store them for later use.

The primary storage site for triglycerides is the adipose cell **(FIGURE 5.13)**, which is the only body cell with significant fat-storage capacity. However, if you are physically active, your body will preferentially store this extra fat in muscle cells, so the next time you work out, the fat is readily available for energy. Thus, people who engage in regular physical activity are more likely to have fat stored in the muscle tissue and

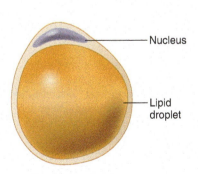

◄ FIGURE 5.13 Diagram of an adipose cell.

to have less body fat—something many of us would prefer. Of course, fat stored in the adipose tissue can also be used for energy during exercise, but it must be broken down first and then transported to the muscle cells.

recap Fat entering the small intestine is emulsified into droplets by bile. Pancreatic lipases then digest the triglycerides into two free fatty acids and one monoacylglyceride. These are transported into the enterocytes with the help of micelles. Once inside, triglycerides are re-formed and packaged into lipoproteins called *chylomicrons*. These enter the lymph, then the bloodstream, in which they travel to body cells that need energy. Fat stored in the muscle tissue is used as a source of energy during physical activity. Excess fat is stored in the adipose tissue and can be used whenever the body needs energy.

LO 5 Identify the DRIs for fats and common food sources of unhealthful and beneficial fats.

How much fat should you eat?

Now that you know which fats are healthful and which are harmful, you may be wondering how much—or how little—of each type to consume, and how that translates into specific foods. To make the switch to more healthful fats, it helps to be aware of exactly where the fat in your diet is coming from.

Recognize the Fat in Foods

We add fats—such as butter, cream, mayonnaise, and salad oils—to foods because they make them taste good. This type of fat is called **visible fat** because we can easily see what we're adding and approximately how much. Still, we may not be aware of the type of fat we're using and the number of Calories it adds to the food. For instance, it's easy to make a slice of whole-grain toast even more healthful by spreading it with peanut butter, which is rich in unsaturated fats, but spreading it with 1/2 tablespoon of butter adds about 4 grams of saturated fat. When adding visible fats, use moderation and, when possible, select oils, such as canola oil, soybean oil, or olive oil, over solid fats such as butter or margarine. When selecting butter or margarine, use those made with or mixed with healthful oils.[5]

Also be on the lookout for **hidden fats**—that is, fats added to processed and prepared foods to improve taste and texture. Their invisibility often tricks us into choosing them over more healthful foods. For example, a blueberry scone is much higher in saturated fat (about 12 grams) than two blueberry waffles (about 1.5 grams), yet consumers assume that the saturated fat content of these foods is the same because they are both bread products. The majority of the fat in the average American diet is invisible. Foods that can be high in invisible saturated fats are baked goods, regular-fat dairy products, processed meats or meats that are highly marbled or not trimmed, and most convenience and fast foods, such as hamburgers, hot dogs, chips, ice cream, and french fries and other fried foods. When purchasing packaged foods, read the Nutrition Facts panel! The nearby **Nutrition Label Activity** shows you how to calculate the amount of fat hidden in packaged foods.

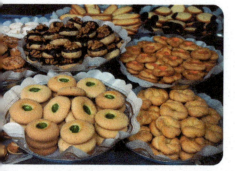

▲ Baked goods are often high in hidden fats and may contain *trans* fats.

visible fats Fats that are clearly present and visible in our food, or visibly added to food, such as butter, margarine, cream, shortening, salad dressings, chicken skin, and untrimmed fat on meat.

hidden fats Fats that are not apparent, or "hidden" in foods, such as the fats found in baked goods, regular-fat dairy products, marbling in meat, and fried foods.

Decipher Label Claims

The FDA and the U.S. Department of Agriculture (USDA) have set specific regulations on allowable label claims for reduced-fat products. The following claims are defined for one serving:

- Fat free = less than 0.5 g of fat
- Low fat = 3 g or less of fat
- Reduced or less fat = at least 25% less fat as compared to a standard serving
- Light = one-third fewer Calories or 50% less fat as compared with a standard serving amount

There are now thousands of fat-modified foods in the market. However, if you're choosing such foods because of a concern about your weight, let the buyer beware!

How Much Fat Is in This Food?

How can you figure out how much fat is in a food you might buy? One way is to read the Nutrition Facts panel on the label. Two cracker labels are shown in **FIGURE 5.14**; one cracker is higher in fat than the other. Let's use the label to find out what percentage of energy is coming from fat in each product. The calculations are relatively simple.

1. Divide the total Calories from fat by the total Calories per serving, and multiply the answer by 100.
   - For the regular wheat crackers:
     50 kcal/150 kcal = 0.33 × 100 = 33%.
   Thus, for the regular crackers, the total energy coming from fat is 33%.
   - For the reduced-fat wheat crackers:
     35 kcal/130 kcal = 0.269 × 100 = 27%.
   Thus, for the reduced-fat crackers, the total energy coming from fat is 27%.

   Although the energy per serving is not very different between these two crackers, the percentage from fat is quite different.

2. If the total Calories per serving from fat are not given on the label, you can quickly calculate this value by multiplying the grams of total fat per serving by 9 (because there are 9 kcal per gram of fat).
   - For the regular wheat crackers:
     6 g fat × 9 kcal/gram = 54 kcal of fat.
   - To calculate the percentage of Calories from fat:
     54 kcal/150 kcal = 0.36 × 100 = 36%.

   This value is not exactly the same as the 50 kcal reported on the label or the 33% of Calories from fat calculated in example 1. That's because the values on food labels are rounded off.

   In summary, you can quickly calculate the percentage of fat per serving for any packaged food in three steps: (1) multiply the grams of fat per serving by 9 kcal per gram; (2) divide this number by the total kcal per serving; (3) multiply by 100.

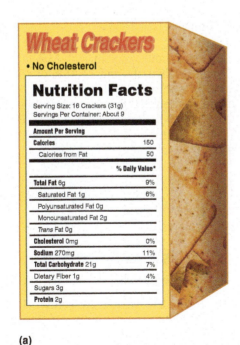

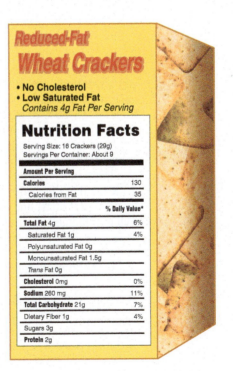

▲ **FIGURE 5.14** Labels for two types of wheat crackers. **(a)** Regular wheat crackers. **(b)** Reduced-fat wheat crackers.

nutri-case | LIZ

"Lately I'm hungry all the time. I read online that if I limit my total fat intake to no more than 10% of my total Calories, I can eat all the carbs and protein that I want, and I won't gain weight. So, when I felt hungry after my last class, I stopped at the yogurt shop in the Student Union and ordered a sundae with nonfat vanilla yogurt and fat-free chocolate syrup. I have to admit, though, that about an hour after I ate it I was hungry again. Maybe it's stress."

What do you think of Liz's approach to her persistent hunger? What have you learned in this chapter about the role of fats—and sugars—that would be important information to share with her?

Concerned about the saturated fat and cholesterol in the beef you eat? Use the guide to choosing the leanest cuts at www.mayoclinic.org. From the home page, type "lean cuts of beef" in the search bar to find it.

Lower-fat versions of foods may not always be lower in Calories. The reduced fat is often replaced with added simple carbohydrate, resulting in a very similar total energy intake. For example, one national brand of chocolate ice cream contains 10 grams of saturated fat per serving, whereas a low-fat brand contains 3 grams of saturated fat for the same size serving. Choosing the lower-fat ice cream will save you only 30 Calories, however, because the low-fat brand is higher in sugars. Bear in mind that when saturated fat is replaced by added sugars, risk factors for chronic disease can actually increase.[6,7] There are strong data linking added sugars to a number of chronic diseases including obesity, cardiovascular disease, and cancer.[7,8]

Keep Your Fat Intake Within the AMDR

The Acceptable Macronutrient Distribution Range (AMDR) for fat is 20–35% of total energy intake.[9] This recommendation is based on evidence indicating that higher intakes of fat increase the risk for obesity and its complications, especially cardiovascular disease, but that diets too low in fat and too high in carbohydrate can also increase the risk for cardiovascular disease if they cause blood triglycerides to increase.

If you're an athlete, you've probably been advised to consume less fat and more carbohydrate to replenish your glycogen stores, especially if you participate in endurance activities. Specifically, you should consume 20–25% of your total energy from fat, 55–60% of energy from carbohydrate, and 12–15% of energy from protein.[10] This percentage of fat intake is still within the AMDR.

Although many people trying to lose weight consume less than 20% of their energy from fat, this practice may do more harm than good, especially if they are also limiting energy intake (eating fewer than 1,500 kcal per day). There is no clear evidence that diets with less than 15% of energy from fat have advantages over moderate-fat diets, and they are usually very difficult to follow. In fact, most people trying to manage their weight find they are more successful if they keep their fat within the AMDR recommendations for fat. For example, the DASH diet provides 28–30% of energy from fat on a 2,000-Calorie diet.[11] (The DASH diet is discussed in the **In Depth** essay following this chapter.)

Aim for a Balance of the Essential Fatty Acids

The Dietary Reference Intakes (DRIs) for the two essential fatty acids are as follows:[9]

- **Linoleic acid.** The Adequate Intake (AI) for linoleic acid (an omega-6 fatty acid) is 14 to 17 g per day for adult men and 11 to 12 g per day for women 19 years and older.
- **Alpha-linolenic acid.** The AI for ALA (an omega-3 fatty acid) is just 1.6 g per day for adult men and 1.1 g per day for adult women.

It is unrealistic for most Americans to keep track of the number of grams of linoleic acid and ALA they consume each day. Overall, we appear to get adequate amounts of linoleic acid in our diets because of the salad dressings, vegetable oils, margarines, and mayonnaise we eat. In contrast, our consumption of ALA, including

EPA, and DHA, is more variable and can be low in the diet of people who do not eat dark green, leafy vegetables; walnuts; soy products; canola oil; flax seeds or their oils; or fish or fish oils. So rather than attempting to monitor your linoleic acid to ALA intake, focus on consuming healthful amounts of the foods listed in TABLE 5.1.

Reduce Your Intake of Saturated Fats

Research over the last two decades has shown that diets high in saturated and *trans* fatty acids can increase the risk for cardiovascular disease. Thus, the recommended intake of saturated fats is less than 10% of total energy.[12] Let's look at the primary sources of saturated fats in the American diet.

- **Mixed dishes.** The majority of our saturated fat (36%) comes from the consumption of pizza, tacos, burgers, sandwiches, and other mixed dishes with animal protein, especially red meat and cheese.[13]
- **Animal products.** Meats and dairy products that are not part of mixed dishes are also a primary source of saturated fat in our diet (28%).[13] Meats contain a mixture of fatty acids, and the precise amount of saturated fat will depend on the cut of the meat and how it is prepared. For example, red meats, such as beef, pork, and lamb, typically have more fat than skinless chicken or fish. Lean red meats are lower in saturated fat than regular cuts. In addition, broiled, grilled, or baked meats have less saturated fat than fried meats. Dairy products may also be high in saturated fat. Whole-fat milk and yogurt has three times the saturated fat as low-fat milk products, and nearly twice the energy. As a group, eggs contribute to only 3% of our saturated fat intake.

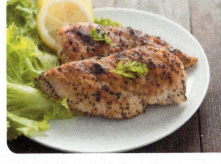

This skinless roasted chicken breast provides less than 1 g saturated fat and 131 kcal; with the skin, it would provide 3 g saturated fat and 235 kcal.

TABLE 5.1   Omega-3 Fatty Acid Content of Selected Food

Food Item	Total Omega-3	DHA grams	EPA
		per serving	
Flaxseed oil, 1 tbsp.	7.25	0.00	0.00
Salmon oil (fish oil), 1 tbsp.	4.39	2.48	1.77
Sardine oil, 1 tbsp.	3.01	1.45	1.38
Flaxseed, whole, 1 tbsp.	2.50	0.00	0.00
Herring, Atlantic, broiled, 3 oz	1.83	0.94	0.77
Salmon, Coho, steamed, 3 oz	1.34	0.71	0.46
Canola oil, 1 tbsp.	1.28	0.00	0.00
Sardines, Atlantic, w/ bones & oil, 3 oz	1.26	0.43	0.40
Trout, rainbow fillet, baked, 3 oz	1.05	0.70	0.28
Walnuts, English, 1 tbsp.	0.66	0.00	0.00
Halibut, fillet, baked, 3 oz	0.53	0.31	0.21
Shrimp, Canned, 3 oz	0.47	0.21	0.25
Tuna, white, in oil, 3 oz	0.38	0.19	0.04
Crab, Alaska King, steamed, 3 oz	0.36	0.10	0.25
Scallops, broiled, 3 oz	0.31	0.14	0.17
Smart Balance Omega-3 Buttery Spread (1 tbsp.)	0.32	0.01	0.01
Tuna, light, in water, 3 oz	0.23	0.19	0.04
Avocado, Calif., fresh, whole	0.22	0.00	0.00
Spinach, cooked, 1 cup	0.17	0.00	0.00
Eggland's Best, 1 large egg, with omega-3	0.12	0.06	0.03

Note: EPA = Eicosapentaenoic acid; DHA = docosahexaenoic acid.

Data adapted from: Food Processor SQL, Version 10.3, ESHA Research, Salem, OR, and manufacturer labels.

QuickTips

Reducing Saturated Fats When Cooking

✅ Trim visible fat from meats before cooking.

✅ Remove the skin from poultry before cooking.

✅ Instead of frying meats, poultry, fish, or potatoes or other vegetables, grill, bake, or broil them.

✅ Cook with olive oil or canola oil instead of butter.

✅ Use oil instead of butter when stir-frying.

✅ Substitute hard cheeses (such as parmesan), which are naturally lower in fat, for softer cheeses that are higher in fat (such as cheddar).

✅ Substitute low-fat or nonfat yogurt for cream, cream cheese, mayonnaise, or sour cream in recipes; also on baked potatoes, tacos, salads, and in dips.

- **Baked goods, sweets, and snack foods.** Muffins, pastries, cookies, and brownies may be filled with saturated fats. Tortilla chips, microwave and movie-theater popcorn, snack crackers, and packaged rice and pasta mixes may also be high in saturated fat. Overall this category contributes to 22% of our saturated fat intake.[13]
- **Prepared vegetables, salad dressings, and condiments.** We often don't think of plant foods as having high amounts of saturated fats, but if these foods are fried, breaded, or drenched in sauces they can become a source of saturated fat. For example, a small baked potato (138 g) has no fat and 134 kcal, whereas a medium serving (134 g) of french fries cooked in vegetable oil has 427 kcal, 23 g of fat, and 5.3 g of saturated fat. This is one-fourth of the saturated fat recommended for an entire day for a person on a 2,000-kcal/day diet.

You can significantly reduce your intake of saturated fats by making smart choices when you prepare and cook foods. The **Quick Tips** feature on this page will help.

Avoid *Trans* Fatty Acids

The Institute of Medicine (IOM; which is now the Health and Medicine Division of the National Academies of Sciences, Engineering, and Medicine) and the *2015–2020 Dietary Guidelines for Americans* recommend that we keep our intake of *trans* fatty acids to an absolute minimum.[9,12] This is because diets high in *trans* fatty acids are thought to increase the risk for cardiovascular disease even more than diets high in saturated fats.[14,15] A research review that involved more than 140,000 individuals showed that for every 2% increase in energy intake from *trans* fatty acids, there was a 23% increase in incidence of cardiovascular disease.[14]

Currently, the majority of *trans* fats in the American diet comes from deep-fried fast or frozen foods, snacks, and bakery products.[16] A 2012 review of top-selling packaged foods in the United States showed that 9% of these foods contained PHOs, yet 84% of these products reported they had no *trans* fatty acids.[16] As discussed earlier, the only way to find out if a food contains *trans* fats is to read the ingredients list on the label. If the food contains PHOs, it contains *trans* fats even if the label says it does not. Also, remember that manufacturers have until the middle of 2018 to remove all PHOs from processed foods. Next time you shop, let the **Quick Tips** feature on page 159 help guide your choices.

What About Dietary Cholesterol?

Consumers are confused about whether they should avoid dietary cholesterol. This confusion is understandable given that health experts have changed their message over the years as they have learned more about saturated fat and cholesterol metabolism and their relationship to cardiovascular disease.[5,17] Here are some points to keep in mind:

- Recall that the body can make cholesterol; moreover, the body recycles cholesterol. Thus, you don't have to worry about getting enough in your diet. When you consume cholesterol, your body typically reduces its internal production, which keeps its total cholesterol pool constant.
- The body absorbs only about 40–60% of the cholesterol consumed.[18] It excretes the rest in feces. The precise percentage of cholesterol absorbed can vary according to genetics, body size, health status, and the other components of the diet.[17,19]
- One of the dietary components that influences cholesterol metabolism is saturated fat. By keeping your intake of saturated fat low, you can avoid excessive levels of harmful cholesterol in your blood. Because saturated fat and cholesterol are typically found in the same foods, namely, fatty animal products, keeping saturated fat low also keeps dietary cholesterol low.
- Although the Health and Medicine Division of the National Academies of Sciences, Engineering, and Medicine (formerly the Institute of Medicine, or IOM)[9] recommends consuming less than 300 mg/d of dietary cholesterol, there appears to be no direct link between dietary cholesterol and cardiovascular disease.[20] The *2015–2020 Dietary Guidelines for Americans* recommends consuming as little dietary cholesterol as possible.[12] However, if you follow a healthful eating pattern, as recommended in the Guidelines, your cholesterol intake should range from 100–300 mg/day.

QuickTips

Shopping for Foods Low in Saturated and *Trans* Fats

✔ Read food labels. Look for foods low in saturated fats and avoid foods with PHOs in the ingredients list.

✔ Select liquid or tub margarine/butters over stick forms. Fats that are solid at room temperature are usually high in *trans* or saturated fats. Also, select margarines made from healthful fats, such as canola oil.

✔ Buy naturally occurring oils, such as olive and canola oil. These provide healthful unsaturated fatty acids.

✔ Select 100% whole-grain baked products made with unsaturated oils instead of butter.

✔ Cut back on packaged pastries, such as Danish, croissants, donuts, cakes, and pies. These baked goods are typically high in saturated and *trans* fatty acids. Read the ingredients list to see if PHOs have been used.

✔ Select salad dressings made with healthful fats, such as olive oil and vinegar. Also select lower fat mayonnaise and dressings when available.

✔ Add fish, especially those high in omega-3 fatty acids, to your shopping list. For example, select salmon, line-caught tuna, herring, and sardines.

✔ For other healthful sources of protein, select lean cuts of meat and skinless poultry, meat substitutes made with soy, or beans or lentils.

✔ Select lower-fat versions of dairy products such as milk, cheese, yogurt, sour cream, and cream cheese. Soy milk is naturally low in saturated fat.

Select Beneficial Fats

As mentioned earlier, it's best to switch to healthful fats without increasing your total fat intake. The following suggestions will help you find foods rich in the beneficial fats you need.

Pick Plants

Plant oils are excellent sources of unsaturated fats, as are avocados, olives, nuts and nut butters, and seeds. An easy way to shift your diet toward these healthful fats—without increasing your total fat intake—is to replace animal-based foods with versions derived from plants. For example, drink calcium-fortified soy milk instead of cow's milk. Order your Chinese takeout with tofu instead of beef. Use thin slices of avocado in a sandwich in place of cheese, or serve tortilla chips with guacamole instead of nachos. Use beans, peas, and lentils more frequently as the main source of protein in your meal, or add them to your meat-based dish, so that you use less meat overall.

Many nuts and seeds are high in mono- and polyunsaturated fatty acids, and walnuts, almonds, flax seeds, and chia seeds are a rich source of ALA specifically. Nuts and seeds also provide protein, minerals, vitamins, antioxidant phytochemicals, and fiber. However, a 1-oz serving of nuts (about 4 tablespoons) typically contains 160–180 kcal and could contribute to a high energy intake. So do their benefits outweigh their cost in Calories? Research shows that people who consume nuts have a reduced risk for chronic disease[3] and maintain a lower body weight.[21,22] The mechanisms contributing to these associations are not fully understood. However, two factors might be contributing to this effect.

- Nuts contain healthful fats that may contribute to lowering our risk of chronic disease. They may also substitute for less healthful snacks, such as chips, that are higher in saturated fat and sodium.
- The energy available from nuts is lower than the number of Calories typically identified. For example, the energy from consumption of 1 oz (28 g) of walnuts is only 146 kcal, which is 39 kcal less than attributed.[23]

However, even if nuts contain healthful oils and their energy content is lower than expected, we still need to eat them in moderation. One approach is to by sprinkling a few on your salad, yogurt, or breakfast cereal. Spread a nut butter on your morning toast instead of butter, or pack a peanut butter and jelly sandwich instead of a meat sandwich for lunch. Finally, add nuts or seeds to raisins and pretzel sticks for a quick trail mix.

Switch to Fish

To increase your intake of EPA and DHA, replace a meat-based meal with fish at least twice a week, or look for foods fortified with an adequate amount of EPA and DHA per serving. It's important to recognize, however, that there are risks associated with eating large amounts of certain fish on a regular basis. Depending on the species and the level of pollution in the water in which it is caught, the fish may contain mercury, polychlorinated biphenyls (PCBs), and other environmental contaminants. Types of fish that are currently considered safe to consume include salmon (except from the Great Lakes region), farmed trout, flounder, sole, *mahi mahi,* and cooked shellfish. Line-caught tuna, either fresh or canned, is low in mercury. These tuna are smaller, usually less than 20 pounds, and have had less exposure to mercury in their lifetime. Line-caught cod and rock fish and Pacific sardines are also good choices. Fish more likely to be contaminated are shark, swordfish, golden bass, golden snapper, marlin, bluefish, and largemouth and smallmouth bass. Women who are pregnant or breastfeeding, women who may become pregnant, and small children should avoid these fish species entirely. (For more information on seafood safety, see Chapter 12.)

As you can see, substituting beneficial fats for saturated or *trans* fats isn't difficult. See the **MEAL FOCUS FIGURE 5.15** to compare a day of meals high and low in saturated fats.

a day of meals

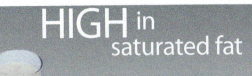

HIGH in saturated fat

LOW in saturated fat

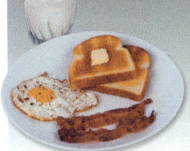

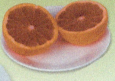

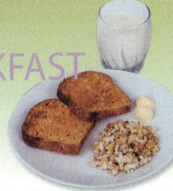

BREAKFAST

1 egg, fried
2 slices bacon
2 slices white toast with
   2 tsp. butter
8 fl. oz whole milk

2 egg whites, scrambled
2 slices whole-wheat toast
   with 2 tsp. olive oil spread
1 grapefruit
8 fl. oz skim milk

McDonald's Quarter Pounder
   with cheese
McDonald's French fries, small
12 fl. oz cola beverage

Tuna Sandwich

3 oz tuna (packed in water)
2 tsp. reduced fat mayonnaise
2 leaves red leaf lettuce
2 slices rye bread
1 large carrot, sliced with
   1 cup raw cauliflower with
   2 tbsp. low-fat Italian salad
   dressing
1 1-oz bag of salted potato chips
24 fl. oz water

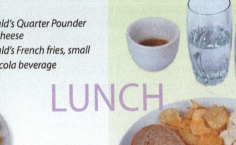

LUNCH

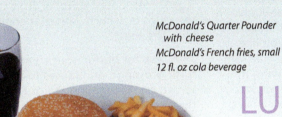

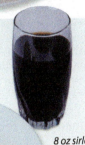

DINNER

1 cup minestrone soup
4 oz grilled salmon
1 cup brown rice with 2 tsp.
   slivered almonds
1 cup steamed broccoli
1 dinner roll with 1 tsp. butter
12 fl. oz iced tea

8 oz sirloin steak, grilled
1 large baked potato with
   1 tbsp. butter
   and 1 tbsp. sour cream
½ cup sweet corn
12 fl. oz diet cola beverage

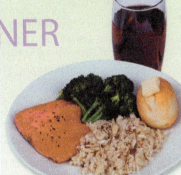

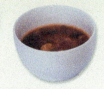

nutrient analysis

2,316 kcal
36.6% of energy from carbohydrates
39.1% of energy from fat
16% of energy from saturated fat
15.3% of energy from unsaturated fat
23% of energy from protein
15.3 grams of dietary fiber
3,337 milligrams of sodium

**11%
LESS**
saturated
fat

nutrient analysis

2,392 kcal
46.6% of energy from carbohydrates
28.1% of energy from fat
5% of energy from saturated fat
18.8% of energy from unsaturated fat
17.5% of energy from protein
28 grams of dietary fiber
2,713 milligrams of sodium

Watch Out When You're Eating Out

Many college students eat most of their meals in dining halls and fast-food restaurants or buy to-go foods from the grocery delicatessen. If that describes you, watch out! The menu items you choose each day may be increasing your intake of saturated and *trans* fats. The 2015 Dietary Guidelines Advisory Committee found that intakes of total energy, total fat, and saturated fat are higher among Americans who frequently eat fast food.[13] And although many fast-food restaurants have eliminated commercially produced *trans* fatty acids from certain menu items, some burgers, breakfast sandwiches, desserts, and shakes may still contain them until the middle of 2018. The **Quick Tips** on this page provide specific strategies for choosing healthful fats when eating out.

QuickTips

Selecting Healthful Fats When Eating Out

When deciding where to eat out, choose a restaurant that allows you to order alternatives to the usual menu items. For instance, if you like burgers, look for a restaurant that will grill your burger instead of frying it, offers whole-grain rolls, and will let you substitute a salad for french fries.

Before you order, compare the saturated fat and Calorie content of the menu items you're considering.

Select healthful appetizers, such as salads, broth-based soups, vegetables, or fruit, over white bread with butter, nachos, or fried foods such as chicken wings.

Select broth-based soups, which are lower in fat and Calories than cream-based soups, which are typically made with cream, cheese, and/or butter.

Ask that all visible fat be trimmed from meats and that poultry be served without the skin.

Select menu items that use cooking methods that add little or no additional fat, such as broiling, grilling, steaming, and sautéing. Be alert to menu descriptions such as *fried, crispy, creamed, buttered, au gratin, escalloped,* and *parmesan*. Also avoid foods served in sauces such as butter sauce, alfredo, and hollandaise. All of these types of food preparation typically add saturated fat to a meal.

Avoid meat and vegetable pot pies, quiches, and other items with a pastry crust because these may be high in *trans* fats.

Substitute a salad, veggies, broth-based soup, or fruit for the chips or french fries that come with the meal.

Ask for butter, sour cream, salad dressings, and sauces to be served on the side instead of added in the kitchen. Select salsa as a condiment over higher-fat options.

Request low-fat spreads on your sandwiches, such as mustards, chutneys, or low-fat mayonnaise.

Select fruit for dessert, or share a traditional dessert with friends or family members.

Keep counting at your favorite café! Many specialty coffee drinks contain 5–10 grams of saturated fat, as compared to about 1 gram in a regular cup of coffee made with low-fat milk.

Select lower-fat options to accompany your coffee drink. For example, choose a biscotti or a small piece of dark chocolate instead of a croissant, a scone, a muffin, coffee cake, or a cookie.

Be Aware of Fat Replacers

One way to lower the fat content of processed foods is by using a *fat replacer*. Snack foods have been the primary target for fat replacers because it is difficult to simply reduce or eliminate the fat in these foods without dramatically changing their texture and taste. In the mid-1990s, the food industry promoted fat replacers as the answer to the growing obesity problem. They claimed that substituting fat replacers for traditional fats in snack and fast foods might reduce both energy and fat intake and help Americans manage their weight better.

Products such as olestra (brand name *Olean*) hit the market in 1996 with a lot of fanfare, but the hype was short-lived. Only a limited number of foods in the marketplace contain olestra. It is also evident from our growing obesity problem that fat replacers, such as olestra, do not help Americans lose weight or even maintain their current weight.

More recently, a new group of fat replacers has been developed using proteins, such as the whey protein found in milk. Like their predecessors, these new fat replacers lower the fat content of food, but in addition they improve the food's total nutrient profile and decrease its Calorie content. This means we can have a low-fat ice cream with the mouth-feel, finish, and texture of a full-fat ice cream that is also higher in protein and lower in Calories than traditional ice cream. So don't be surprised if you see more products containing protein-based fat replacers on your supermarket shelves in the next few years.

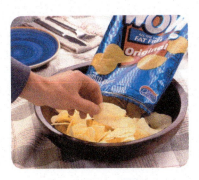

Snack foods have been the primary target for fat replacers, such as Olean, because it is more difficult to eliminate the fat from these types of foods without dramatically changing the taste.

Fat Blockers Contribute Minimally to Weight Loss

To help them lose weight, many people turn to so-called fat blockers, dietary supplements and medications said to block the absorption of dietary fat and eliminate it in the stool. Two popular fat blockers are chitosan and orlistat. Chitosan is a dietary supplement containing a purified shellfish extract, which is supposed to trap fat in the GI tract and prevent its absorption. Orlistat, an over-the-counter medication sold under the brand name Alli, is a lipase inhibitor that prevents intestinal digestion and absorption of about 25% of the fat consumed.

Reviews of extensive research using double-blind randomized clinical trials has shown that, when chitosan is used alone without changing diet or physical activity, the weight loss produced is minimal (<2 pounds over 8–12 weeks).[24–26] In 2014, an extensive systematic review of research studies combining the use of orlistat with changes in diet and physical activity found an average weight loss of 4 pounds in 12 months.[27] Thus, these products contribute only minimally to weight loss for their cost and side effects, the most significant of which is gastrointestinal distress.

recap Visible fats are those we add to foods ourselves. Hidden fats are added to processed and prepared foods to improve taste and texture. The AMDR for total fat is 20–35% of total energy. An AI has also been set for linoleic acid, found in vegetable oils, and ALA, found in fish, flax seeds, walnuts, and leafy vegetables. No DRIs have been set for DHA or EPA. The recommended intake of saturated fats is less than 10% of total energy. Following a healthful eating pattern will limit consumption of both saturated fats and cholesterol. You should keep your intake of *trans* fats to an absolute minimum. By making simple substitutions when shopping, cooking, and eating out, such as by replacing meats with plants or fish, you can reduce the quantity of saturated and *trans* fatty acids in your diet and increase your intake of healthful fats. Fat replacers are substances used to replace the typical fats found in foods.

Are Saturated Fats Bad or Benign?

Decades of research have suggested that diets high in saturated fatty acids (SFAs) are associated with increased risk of coronary heart disease (CHD), the most common form of cardiovascular disease (CVD). However, some recent studies have suggested that saturated fats don't deserve their bad rap. Let's look at the studies involved in this controversy.

In 2014, a meta-analysis of 32 studies specifically examining the relationship between SFA intake and the risk of CHD concluded that no clear evidence supports high consumption of polyunsaturated fatty acids (PUFAs) and low consumption of total SFA.[28] Immediately upon the publication of this article, researchers from the American Heart Association (AHA) and other public health organizations around the world began reviewing the methodology, data, and conclusions of this analysis. The following key criticisms emerged from these reviews:

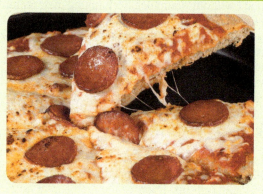

A body of research links high intake of saturated fat with an increased risk for CVD—but not all experts agree.

- Two-thirds of the studies included in the analysis were observational and relied on self-reported diets. This means the researchers had asked people what they typically ate, and then looked at CHD outcomes 5–23 years later. These types of studies do not provide information about cause and effect. To determine whether or not a high-SFA diet increases the risk for CHD, researchers need to conduct randomized clinical trials (RCTs) in which they feed participants diets higher and lower in SFAs and monitor the occurrence of CHD or cardiac death in subsequent years. In fact, an earlier meta-analysis of eight such RCTs had found that replacing SFAs with PUFAs reduced CHD risk by 10%.[29]

- The researchers included studies that other scientists thought were inappropriate, such as some in which margarines containing *trans* fatty acids were consumed as part of the intervention.[30,31] Given the established link between *trans* fatty acid consumption and CHD, such studies should have been excluded.

- The researchers made some minor calculation errors, which required them to rerun their data after the original article was published.[32] They also tried to generalize their results to the whole population, which is inappropriate.[30] Your risk of developing CHD is based on genetics, diet, physical activity, and many other factors.

Despite these limitations of the 2014 study, significant debate about the relationship between SFA consumption and CHD remains. The current recommendation to limit SFAs is based on two key assumptions:[33,34]

1. Higher intakes of SFAs increase blood lipids associated with increased risk for CHD.
2. Lowering these blood lipids will reduce the risk of CHD.

As our understanding of the relationship between diet and CVD grows, these simple assumptions are being challenged. Researchers now recognize that only certain blood lipids are able to easily penetrate the wall of blood vessels and become oxidized, which is an early step in the development of CHD. Factors clearly associated with increased levels of these harmful blood lipids are obesity, inactivity, and a high intake of refined sugars.[35–37] Specifically, the evidence linking diets high in refined sugars with CVD is derived from a global assessment of sugar-sweetened beverage (SSB) consumption and its contribution to body weight and chronic disease mortality.[8] These researchers estimated that the SSB consumption contributed to approximately 45,000 CVD deaths globally per year.[7]

So what's the bottom line? National dietary recommendations are not based on one study, but on a body of research evidence. This doesn't mean the current SFA recommendations won't change, but until more conclusive research is available, eating a variety of whole foods while limiting SFAs and added sugars is currently the best recommendation for lowering your risk of CHD.

CRITICAL THINKING QUESTIONS

1. You want dessert. You avoid the ice cream in your freezer—too much saturated fat!—and go for the fat-free mango sorbet, which has no saturated fat, *trans* fat, or cholesterol, but does have 36 grams of added sugar in a half-cup serving. Why do researchers suggest that such trade-offs aren't as smart as you might think?

2. Look at your own diet. What whole-food dietary changes are you willing to make to help lower your lifetime risk of CHD? How much effort and cost would it take to make these changes?

3. Visit the AHA at www.heart.org/HEARTORG and type "saturated fats" in the search bar. Read the page and watch the video. What percentage of your total energy intake does the AHA recommend you consume as SFAs? Does the AHA discussion convince you consumption of SFAs increases your risk for CHD? Why or why not?

TEST YOURSELF | ANSWERS

1 T Although eating too much fat, or too much of unhealthful fats (such as saturated and *trans* fatty acids), can increase our risk for diseases such as cardiovascular disease and obesity, some fats are essential to good health. We need to consume a certain minimum amount to provide adequate levels of essential fatty acids and fat-soluble vitamins.

2 T Fat is our primary source of energy when we are at rest and engaging in low- and moderate-intensity exercise. Fat is also an important fuel source during prolonged exercise. During periods of high-intensity exercise, carbohydrate becomes the dominant fuel source.

3 F Even foods fried in vegetable shortening can be unhealthful because they are high in *trans* fatty acids, in total fat, and in energy and can contribute to overweight and obesity.

review questions

LO 1 1. Cholesterol is
 a. a triglyceride.
 b. a phospholipid.
 c. available from a wide variety of plant- and animal-based foods.
 d. produced by the body.

LO 2 2. Fatty acids with one double bond in part of the chain are
 a. saturated.
 b. monounsaturated.
 c. polyunsaturated.
 d. essential fatty acids.

LO 2 3. Most plant oils contain
 a. only saturated fats.
 b. only unsaturated fats.
 c. both saturated and unsaturated fats.
 d. both EPA and DHA.

LO 2 4. Alpha-linolenic acid (ALA) is
 a. converted by the body to linoleic acid.
 b. metabolized in the body to arachidonic acid.
 c. synthesized in the liver and small intestine.
 d. found in leafy green vegetables, flaxseeds, soy milk, walnuts, and almonds.

LO 3 5. Fats
 a. do not provide as much energy, gram for gram, as carbohydrates.
 b. are a major source of fuel for the body at rest.
 c. enable the emulsification and digestion of fat-soluble vitamins.
 d. keep foods from turning rancid.

LO 4 6. What compound in the blood breaks apart the triglycerides in chylomicrons, freeing their fatty acids for uptake by body cells?
 a. lipoprotein lipase
 b. micelles
 c. bile salts
 d. pancreatic lipase

LO 5 7. Saturated fat intake should be
 a. 0.5 g/kg of body weight.
 b. less than 300 mg/day.
 c. less than 10% of total energy.
 d. 20–35% of total energy.

LO 5 8. Three healthful foods rich in beneficial fats are
 a. skim milk, lean meats, and fruits.
 b. fruits, vegetables, and low-fat yogurt.
 c. vegetables, fish, and nuts.
 d. whole milk, egg whites, and stick margarine.

LO 2   **9. True or false?** The essential fatty acids linoleic acid and alpha-linolenic acid are polyunsaturated fatty acids.

LO 4   **10. True or false?** When fatty chyme enters the small intestine, bile causes the fat droplets to dissolve in water.

math review

LO 5   11. Getting adequate amounts of the omega-3 fatty acids can be tricky. Study Table 5.1. What food or combination of foods would you need to eat today to reach 250 mg of EPA and DHA?

LO 5   12. Your friend Maria has determined that she needs to consume about 2,000 kcal per day to maintain her healthful weight. Create a list for Maria showing the recommended maximum number of Calories she should consume in each of the following forms: total fat; saturated fat; unsaturated fat; and *trans* fatty acids.

Answers to Review Questions and Math Review are located at the back of this text, and in the MasteringNutrition Study Area.

web links

www.heart.org/HEARTORG/
American Heart Association
Learn the best way to help lower your blood cholesterol level. Access the AHA's online cookbook for healthy-heart recipes and cooking methods.

www.nhlbi.nih.gov
National Heart, Lung, and Blood Institute
Visit this site for resources on diet, physical activity, and other lifestyle choices that can lower your risk for cardiovascular disease.

www.nih.gov
The National Institutes of Health, U.S. Department of Health and Human Services
Go to this clearinghouse for a wide range of information and useful tools on the subjects we cover in this chapter.

www.nlm.nih.gov/medlineplus/
MEDLINE Plus Health Information
Search for "fats" or "lipids" to locate resources and learn the latest news on dietary fats.

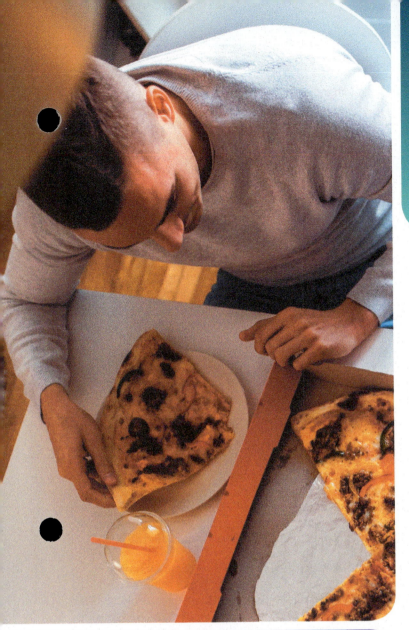

Cardiovascular Disease

learning outcomes

After studying this In Depth, you should be able to:

1 Describe cardiovascular disease, including the major types and contributing mechanisms, pp. 168–170.

2 Explain the role of modifiable factors and blood lipids in the development of cardiovascular disease, pp. 170–174.

3 Identify several lifestyle choices that can reduce your risk for cardiovascular disease, pp. 174–177.

Pizza can be a nutritious food—if it's made with a whole-grain crust, loaded with vegetables, and only lightly sprinkled with low-fat cheese. But the pizza that most Americans enjoy, a refined-flour crust, topped with pepperoni or sausage and high-fat cheese, provides 25–35% of an average adult's recommended daily intake of saturated fat—in a single slice. Why does this matter?

As you learned (in Chapter 5), many researchers have linked diets high in saturated fat with an increased risk for diseases of the heart and blood vessels. These diseases together account for more than 29% of all deaths of Americans.[1] The deaths can result from a sudden cardiac arrest, heart attack, or stroke, or occur after many years of chronic, progressive heart failure.

What role does a diet high in saturated fats play in these diseases? Are genetics also to blame? What about obesity, smoking, or failure to engage in recommended levels of physical activity? We'll explore the factors behind cardiovascular disease **In Depth** here, and identify steps you can take to reduce your risk.

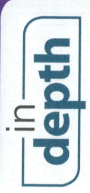

What is cardiovascular disease?

LO 1 Describe cardiovascular disease, including the major types and contributing mechanisms.

Cardiovascular disease (CVD) is a general term used to refer to any abnormal condition involving dysfunction of the heart (*cardio-* means "heart") and blood vessels (*vasculature*). Among the many forms of this disease, the two with the highest mortality rates are the following:

- Coronary heart disease (CHD), also known as coronary artery disease (CAD), occurs when blood vessels supplying the heart (the coronary arteries) become blocked or constricted. Such blockage reduces the flow of blood—and the oxygen and nutrients it carries—to the heart muscle. This can result in chest pain, called *angina pectoris*. It can lead to a heart attack (also called a myocardial infarction, or MI), which is a loss of blood to, and death of, a region of heart muscle. It can also lead to sudden cardiac arrest, in which the heart suddenly stops beating. CHD causes about 600,000 deaths annually.[1]

> Knowing the warning signs of a heart attack could save your life. Download the wallet card from the National Institutes of Health at www.nhlbi.nih.gov. From the home page, type "heart attack wallet card" in the search bar to find it.

- Stroke, also known as *cerebrovascular disease*, is caused by a blockage of one of the blood vessels supplying the brain (the cerebral arteries). When this occurs, the region of the brain that depends on that artery for oxygen and nutrients cannot function. As a result, the movement, speech, or other body functions controlled by that part of the brain suddenly stop. Stroke causes about 129,000 deaths annually.[1]

> To view a brief animation of a stroke, visit MedlinePlus at www.nlm.nih.gov/medlineplus. From the home page, select "Videos and Tools," then "Health Videos," then click on "Stroke" in the index.

To understand CVD, we need to look at two conditions, atherosclerosis and hypertension, which underlie CHD and stroke.

Atherosclerosis Is Narrowing of Arteries

Atherosclerosis is a disease in which arterial walls accumulate deposits of lipids and scar tissue that build up to such

a degree that they impair blood flow. It's a complex process that begins with injury to the cells that line the insides of all arteries **(FOCUS FIGURE 1)**. Factors that commonly promote such injury are the forceful pounding of blood under high pressure and blood-vessel damage from irritants, such as the nicotine in tobacco, the excessive blood glucose in people with poorly controlled diabetes, or even the immune response associated with chronic infection.

Whatever the cause, the injury leads to vessel inflammation, which is increasingly being recognized as an important marker of CVD.[2] Inflamed lining cells release chemicals that cause certain blood lipids to accumulate at the site. These lipids are mainly low-density lipoproteins, or LDLs, described shortly. LDLs invade beneath the lining of the artery wall and become oxidized. As they do, they attract the attention of immune cells that move to the site, squeeze between the lining cells, and ingest the lipids beneath, becoming foam cells. Accumulated foam cells form *fatty streaks* that are the first visible sign of atherosclerosis.

Over time, foam cells, along with proteins, calcium, platelets (cell fragments found in blood), and other substances, form thick, grainy deposits called *plaque*. The term *atherosclerosis* reflects the presence of these deposits: *athere* is a Greek word meaning "a thick porridge." As plaques form, they narrow the interior of the blood vessel (see Figure 1). This slowly diminishes the blood supply to any tissues "downstream." As a result, these tissues wither, and gradually lose their ability to function. The person may experience angina, shortness of breath, and fatigue.

Alternatively, the blockage may occur suddenly; this happens when an enlarging plaque ruptures and the blood vessel tears. *Platelets,* substances in blood that promote clotting, stick to the damaged area. This quickly obstructs the artery, causing the death of the tissue it supplies. As a result, the person experiences a heart attack or stroke.

Arteries damaged by atherosclerosis become not only narrow, but also stiff; that is, they lose their ability to stretch and spring back with each heartbeat. This characteristic is often referred to as "hardening of the arteries." As you can imagine, atherosclerosis strains the heart, forcing it to exert increased pressure to eject each burst of blood into narrowed, stiffened vessels. Physicians refer to this increased pressure as *systolic hypertension*, as we explain next.

---

cardiovascular disease (CVD) A general term for abnormal conditions involving dysfunction of the heart and blood vessels, which can result in heart attack or stroke.

atherosclerosis A condition characterized by accumulation of cholesterol-rich plaque on artery walls; these deposits build up to such a degree that they impair blood flow.

focus figure 1 Atherosclerosis

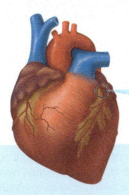

Plaque accumulation within coronary arteries narrows their interior and impedes the flow of oxygen-rich blood to the heart.

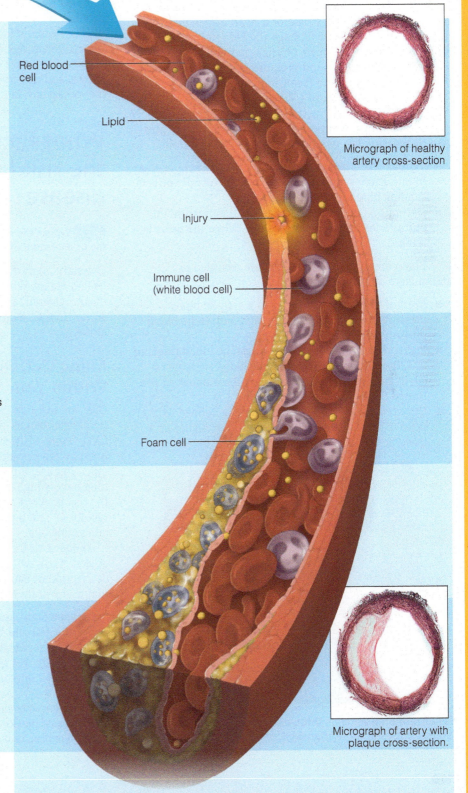

HEALTHY ARTERY

Blood flows unobstructed through normal, healthy artery.

ARTERIAL INJURY

The artery's lining is injured, attracting immune cells, and prompting inflammation.

LIPIDS ACCUMULATE IN WALL

Lipids, particulary cholesterol-containing LDLs, seep beneath the wall lining. The LDLs become oxidized. Immune cells, attracted to the site, engulf the oxidized LDLs and are transformed into foam cells.

FATTY STREAK

The foam cells accumulate to a form a fatty streak, which releases more toxic and inflammatory chemicals.

PLAQUE FORMATION

The foam cells, along with platelets, calcium, protein fibers, and other substances, form thick deposits of plaque, stiffening and narrowing the artery. Blood flow through the artery is reduced or obstructed.

Red blood cell

Lipid

Injury

Immune cell (white blood cell)

Foam cell

Micrograph of healthy artery cross-section

Micrograph of artery with plaque cross-section.

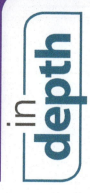

Hypertension Increases the Risk for Heart Attack and Stroke

Hypertension (HTN) is one of the major chronic diseases in the United States. It affects over 29% of all adults in the United States and more than 64% of people over the age of 65.[3] Although HTN itself is often without symptoms, it is a warning sign that a person's risk for a heart attack or stroke is increased. It can also damage the kidneys, reduce brain function, and impair physical mobility. In addition, chronically elevated blood pressure is one of the criteria for metabolic syndrome (see Chapter 4), which dramatically increases the risk of CVD and diabetes.

When we define hypertension as blood pressure above the normal range, what exactly do we mean? Blood pressure is measured in two phases, systolic and diastolic.

- *Systolic blood pressure* represents the pressure exerted in our arteries at the moment that the heart contracts, sending blood into our blood vessels.
- *Diastolic blood pressure* represents the pressure in our arteries between contractions, when the heart is relaxed.

Blood pressure measurements are recorded in millimeters of mercury (mmHg).

- *Normal blood pressure* includes a systolic blood pressure *less than* 120 mmHg, and a diastolic blood pressure *less than* 80 mmHg.
- *Prehypertension* is defined as a systolic blood pressure of 120–139 mmHg, or a diastolic blood pressure of 80–89 mmHg. About one of every three adults in the United States has prehypertension.[3]
- *Hypertension or high blood pressure* is defined as a systolic blood pressure of 140 mmHg or higher or a diastolic blood pressure of 90 mmHg or higher.

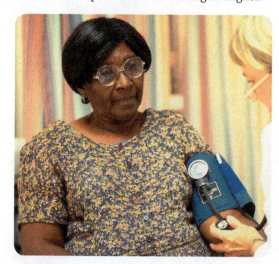

Hypertension is a major chronic disease in the United States, affecting more than 64% of adults over 65 years old.

What causes HTN? For about 45–55% of people, the condition is hereditary. This type is referred to as *primary* or *essential hypertension*. For the other 45% of people with HTN, a variety of factors may contribute. In addition to underlying atherosclerosis, as just explained, anything that increases the volume or viscosity (thickness) of blood forces the heart to beat harder, increasing the pressure of the ejected blood against the vessel walls. Because salt draws water, high blood sodium can increase the volume of blood and, thus, blood pressure. Other factors implicated in HTN include age, race or ethnicity, family history of HTN, genetic factors, sleep apnea (a sleep disorder that affects breathing), psychosocial stressors, tobacco use, obesity, low levels of physical activity, excessive alcohol intake, and dietary factors, including sensitivity to salt and low potassium intake.[3,4]

What factors influence the risk for cardiovascular disease?

LO 2 Explain the role of modifiable factors and blood lipids in the development of cardiovascular disease.

Coronary heart disease is the leading cause of death in the United States, while stroke is the fourth leading cause of death.[1] Overall, about 92.2 million Americans of all ages suffer from CVD or the after effects of stroke.[4] So, who's at risk?

Many CVD Risk Factors Are Within Your Control

Over the last two decades, researchers have identified a number of factors that contribute to an increased risk for CVD. Some of these risk factors are nonmodifiable, meaning they are beyond your control. These include age—the older you are, the higher your risk. Until about age 60, men have a higher risk for CVD than women. After that, the risk is about equal. At any age, you have an increased risk for CVD if a parent suffered a heart attack, especially at a young age.

Other risk factors are modifiable—meaning they are at least partly within your control. Following is a brief description of each of these modifiable risk factors. Notice that many of them have a dietary component.[4–6]

- **Overweight and Obesity** Being obese is associated with CVD and higher rates of death from CVD than being overweight or normal weight. The risk is due primarily to a greater occurrence of high blood pressure, inflammation, abnormal blood lipids (discussed

hypertension A chronic condition characterized by above-average blood pressure levels—specifically, systolic blood pressure over 140 mmHg, or diastolic blood pressure over 90 mmHg.

in more detail shortly), and type 2 diabetes in people who are overweight or obese, with the prevalence highest in the obese. (See Chapter 10 for information on body weight.)

- **Inactivity**   A sedentary lifestyle increases the risk of CVD. Conversely, numerous research studies have shown that regular physical activity can protect against several risk factors associated with the disease. Physical activity can also significantly reduce the risk for type 2 diabetes, a major CVD risk factor in itself.[5] According to the 2008 U.S. Physical Activity Guidelines,[6] physical activity can reduce your risk for heart disease by 20–30%, stroke by 25–30%, and type 2 diabetes by 25–35%.
- **Smoking**   There is strong evidence that smoking increases your risk for blood-vessel injury and atherosclerosis. Research indicates that smokers die 13–14 years earlier than nonsmokers, with one-third of deaths from CHD attributable to smoking or second-hand smoke.[4] Smokers also have two to four times increased risk of stroke than nonsmokers, depending on age and gender.[4] People who stop smoking at 25–34 years of age gain 10 years of life compared to those who continue to smoke.[4]
- **Type 2 Diabetes Mellitus**   For many people with type 2 diabetes, the condition is directly related to being overweight or obese, which is also associated with abnormal blood lipids and high blood pressure. The risk for CVD is three times higher in women with diabetes and two times higher in men with diabetes compared to individuals without diabetes.
- **Inflammation**   We noted earlier that inflammation plays a role in atherosclerosis. C-reactive protein (CRP) is a nonspecific marker of inflammation somewhere in the body. Its level can be measured with a simple blood test. Risk for CVD appears to be higher in individuals who have an elevated CRP level in addition to other risk factors, such as abnormal blood lipids.[7,8] Obesity, a diet low in omega-3 fatty acids, and a high intake of saturated fats promote inflammation. Thus, reducing these factors can lower your risk for CVD.
- **Abnormal Blood Lipids**   As we explain next, abnormal levels of cholesterol and triglycerides in the blood are associated with an increased risk for CVD. A diet high in added sugars and saturated and *trans* fat, and low in soluble fiber, overweight and obesity, and low levels of physical activity are all associated with abnormal blood lipids. Conversely, omega-3 fatty acids reduce blood triglycerides, and increase levels of lipids that protect the health of blood vessels.[9,10]

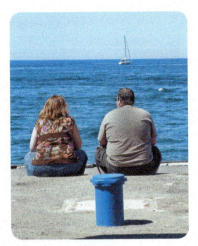

Obesity is associated with higher rates of death from cardiovascular disease.

Blood Lipids Play a Significant Role in Cardiovascular Disease

Recall that lipids are transported in the blood by lipoproteins made up of a lipid center and a protein outer coat. The names of lipoproteins reflect their proportion of lipid, which is less dense, to protein, which is very dense. For example, very-low-density lipoproteins (VLDLs) are only 10% protein, whereas high-density lipoproteins (HDLs) are 50% protein (**FIGURE 2**).

Because lipoproteins are soluble in blood, they are commonly called *blood lipids.* The mechanisms by which blood lipids are produced and transported in the body are illustrated in **FOCUS FIGURE 3** (page 173).

Chylomicrons

Recall (from Chapter 5) that chylomicrons are produced in the small intestine to transport dietary fat into the lymphatic vessels and from there into the bloodstream. At 85% triglyceride, chylomicrons have the lowest density. However, your blood contains chylomicrons only for a short time after you have consumed a meal.

Very-Low-Density Lipoproteins

More than half of the substance of very-low-density lipoproteins (VLDLs) is triglyceride. The liver is the primary source of VLDLs, but they are also produced in the intestines. VLDLs are primarily transport vehicles ferrying triglycerides from their source to the body's cells, including to adipose tissues for storage. The enzyme lipoprotein lipase (LPL) frees most of the triglyceride from the VLDL molecules, resulting in its uptake by the body's cells.

Diets high in fat, simple sugars, and extra Calories can increase the body's production of VLDLs, whereas diets high in omega-3 fatty acids can help reduce their production. In addition, exercise can reduce VLDLs because they're readily used for energy instead of remaining to circulate in the blood.

Low-Density Lipoproteins

The molecules resulting when VLDLs release their triglyceride load are higher in cholesterol, phospholipids, and protein and therefore somewhat more dense. These low-density lipoproteins (LDLs) circulate in the blood, delivering their cholesterol to cells.

LDLs not removed from the bloodstream are left to circulate in the blood. The more LDL-cholesterol circulating in the blood, the greater the risk that some of it will adhere to the walls of the blood vessels, contributing to the development of atherosclerosis. Because high blood levels of LDL-cholesterol increase the risk for CVD, it is

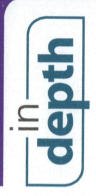

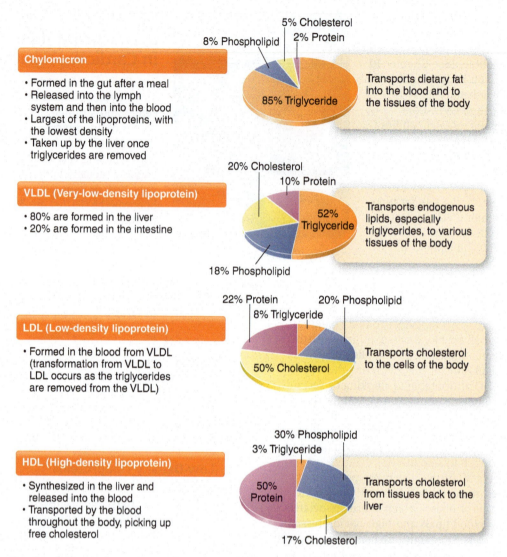

Chylomicron

- Formed in the gut after a meal
- Released into the lymph system and then into the blood
- Largest of the lipoproteins, with the lowest density
- Taken up by the liver once triglycerides are removed

8% Phospholipid
5% Cholesterol
2% Protein
85% Triglyceride

Transports dietary fat into the blood and to the tissues of the body

VLDL (Very-low-density lipoprotein)

- 80% are formed in the liver
- 20% are formed in the intestine

20% Cholesterol
10% Protein
52% Triglyceride
18% Phospholipid

Transports endogenous lipids, especially triglycerides, to various tissues of the body

LDL (Low-density lipoprotein)

- Formed in the blood from VLDL (transformation from VLDL to LDL occurs as the triglycerides are removed from the VLDL)

22% Protein
20% Phospholipid
8% Triglyceride
50% Cholesterol

Transports cholesterol to the cells of the body

HDL (High-density lipoprotein)

- Synthesized in the liver and released into the blood
- Transported by the blood throughout the body, picking up free cholesterol

30% Phospholipid
3% Triglyceride
50% Protein
17% Cholesterol

Transports cholesterol from tissues back to the liver

FIGURE 2 The chemical components of various lipoproteins. Notice that chylomicrons contain the highest proportion of triglycerides, making them the least dense, whereas high-density lipoproteins (HDLs) have the highest proportion of protein, making them the most dense.

often labeled the "bad cholesterol." Diets lower in simple carbohydrate and saturated fats, along with regular physical activity, can reduce LDL-cholesterol.[11,12]

High-Density Lipoproteins

As their name indicates, high-density lipoproteins (HDLs) are small, dense lipoproteins with a very low cholesterol content and a high protein content. They are released from the liver and intestines to circulate in the blood. As they do, they pick up cholesterol from dying cells and arterial plaques and transfer it to other lipoproteins, which return it to the liver. The liver takes up the cholesterol and uses it to synthesize bile, thereby removing it from the circulatory system. High blood levels of HDL-cholesterol are therefore associated with a low risk for CVD. That's why HDL-cholesterol is often referred to as the "good cholesterol." There is some evidence that diets high in omega-3 fatty acids and participation in regular

physical exercise can modestly increase HDL-cholesterol levels.[13,14]

Total Serum Cholesterol

Normally, as the dietary level of cholesterol increases, the body decreases the amount of cholesterol it makes and the amount of cholesterol it absorbs, which keeps the body's level of cholesterol constant. Unfortunately, this feedback mechanism does not work well in everyone. For some individuals, eating dietary cholesterol doesn't decrease the amount of cholesterol produced in the body, and their total body cholesterol level—including the level in their blood—rises. These individuals benefit from reducing their intake of saturated and *trans* fats, because doing so also decreases the intake of dietary cholesterol.

For most Americans, the Dietary Guidelines suggest focusing on limiting saturated fat intake.[15] By limiting

Lipids are transported in the body via several different lipoprotein compounds, such as chylomicrons, VLDLs, LDLs, and HDLs.

CHYLOMICRONS

Chylomicrons are produced in the enterocytes to transport dietary lipids. The enzyme lipoprotein lipase (LPL), found on the endothelial cells in the capillaries, hydrolyzes the triglycerides in the chylomicrons into fatty acids and glycerol, which enter body cells (such as muscle and adipose cells), leaving a chylomicron remnant. Chylomicron remnants are dismantled in the liver.

VLDLS

VLDLs (very-low-density lipoproteins) are produced primarily in the liver to transport endogenous fat in the form of triglycerides into the bloodstream. The enzyme lipoprotein lipase (LPL), found on the endothelial cells in the capillaries, breaks apart the triglycerides in the chylomicrons. The fatty acids can then enter the body cells, especially the muscle and adipose cells, leaving a chylomicron remnant. Glycerol is also released and is transported back to the liver.

LDLS

LDLs (low-density lipoproteins) are created with the removal of most of the VLDLs' triglyceride load. LDLs are rich in cholesterol, which they deliver to body cells with LDL receptors. LDLs not taken up by the cells are primarily taken up by the liver for degradation.

HDLS

HDLs (high-density lipoproteins) are produced in the liver and circulate in the blood, picking up cholesterol from dying cells, other lipoproteins, and arterial plaques. They return this cholesterol to the liver, where it can be recycled or eliminated from the body through bile.

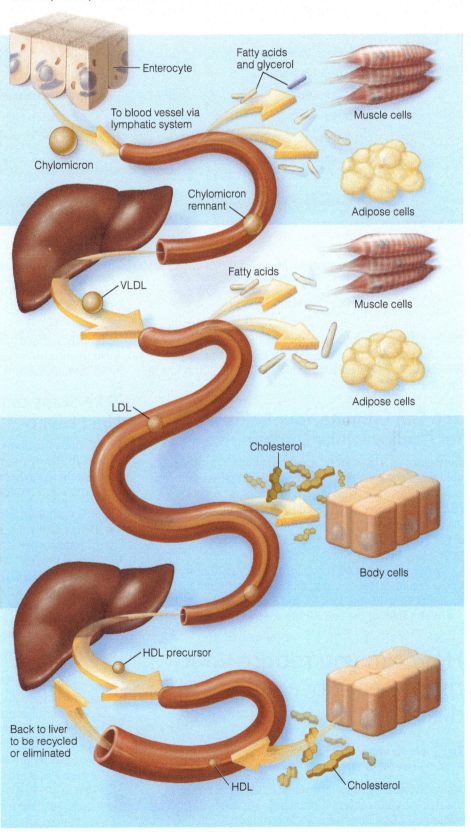

173

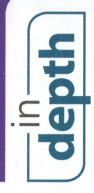

TABLE 1 Interpreting Blood Cholesterol Levels

Total Cholesterol Level	Category
Less than 200 mg/dL	Desirable
200–239 mg/dL	Borderline high
240 mg/dL and above	High

LDL (Bad) Cholesterol Level	LDL Cholesterol Category
Less than 100 mg/dL	Optimal
100–129 mg/dL	Near optimal/above optimal
130–159 mg/dL	Borderline high
160–189 mg/dL	High
190 mg/dL and above	Very High

HDL (Good) Cholesterol level	HDL Cholesterol Category
Less than 40 mg/dL	A major risk factor for heart disease
40–59 mg/dL	The higher, the better
60 mg/dL and higher	Considered protective against heart disease

Source: National Institutes of Health. 2012, Summer. Cholesterol levels: What you need to know. *NIH Medline Plus Magazine* 7(2):6–7. www.nlm.nih.gov/medlineplus

intake of animal products or selecting low-fat versions, you can reduce your intake of both saturated fat and cholesterol. (See the suggestions for choosing healthful fats in Chapter 5.)

You Can Estimate Your Risk for Cardiovascular Disease

Now that you know more about blood lipids, you're probably wondering what your levels look like. If so, you can have them measured by your physician. See **TABLE 1** (above) to compare your blood lipid levels to optimal levels. You also need to know your blood pressure. Especially if you have a family history of CVD, it's important to have your blood pressure checked regularly.

After you've found this information, visit the website of the National Heart, Lung, and Blood Institute (NHLBI) to assess your 10-year risk for having a heart attack. See the **Web Links** at the end of this chapter.

How can you reduce your risk for cardiovascular disease?

LO 3 Identify several lifestyle choices that can reduce your risk for cardiovascular disease.

Many diet and exercise interventions aimed at reducing the risk for CVD center on reducing high levels of triglycerides and LDL-cholesterol while raising HDL-cholesterol.

Approaches aimed specifically at reducing blood pressure include most of the same recommendations, along with strict monitoring of sodium intake.

Take Steps to Improve Your Blood Lipid Levels

The Centers for Disease Control and Prevention and the American Heart Association have made the following dietary and lifestyle recommendations to improve blood lipid levels and reduce the risk for CVD.[4,16]

- Keep fat intake to within 20–35% of total energy intake.[17]
- Decrease dietary saturated fat to less than 7–10% of total energy intake and keep *trans* fatty acids as low as possible.[11,15] (For dietary strategies, see the Quick Tips in Chapter 5.)
- Increase your intake of the omega-3 fatty acid ALA from dark green, leafy vegetables, soybeans or soybean oil, walnuts or walnut oil, flaxseed meal or oil, or canola oil. Also, consume fish, especially oily fish, at least twice a week to increase your intake of the omega-3 fatty acids EPA and DHA.
- Consume the RDA for vitamin B_6, B_{12}, and folate, because these B vitamins help maintain low blood levels of the amino acid homocysteine. High homocysteine levels in the blood are associated with increased risk for CVD.
- Increase dietary intakes of whole grains, fruits, and legumes and other vegetables, so that total dietary fiber is 20–30 g per day. Include oat bran, beans, and fruits, as these foods contain a type of fiber that helps to reduce LDL-cholesterol specifically.[18]

- High blood glucose levels are associated with high blood triglycerides. To help maintain normal blood glucose, consume whole foods high in fiber (see the above bullet); select lean meats and low-fat dairy products; and limit your intake of foods high in added sugars and/or saturated fat.
- Eat meals throughout the day instead of eating most of your Calories in the evening before bed. This approach decreases the load of fat entering the body at any one time. Exercising after a meal also helps keep blood lipids and glucose within normal ranges.
- Consume no more than two alcoholic drinks per day for men and one drink per day for women. Because heavy alcohol consumption can worsen high blood pressure, it is suggested that people with HTN abstain from drinking alcohol entirely. (Alcohol consumption is discussed **In Depth** following Chapter 7.)
- If you smoke, stop. As noted earlier, smoking significantly increases the risk for CVD.
- Exercise most days of the week for 30 to 60 minutes if possible. Exercise will increase HDL-cholesterol while lowering blood triglyceride levels. Exercise also helps you maintain a healthful body weight and a lower blood pressure and reduces your risk for type 2 diabetes.
- Maintain a healthful body weight. Obesity promotes inflammation; thus, keeping body weight within a healthful range helps keep inflammation low.[19] In addition, blood pressure values have been shown to decrease 7–8% in people who have lost several pounds of body weight (~13 pounds).[20]

Take Steps to Manage Your Blood Pressure

We noted earlier that HTN is a risk factor in the development of atherosclerosis, CHD, and stroke. Therefore, the lifestyle changes just identified are appropriate for anyone diagnosed with hypertension or prehypertension. In addition, recommendations for reducing blood pressure include limiting dietary sodium intake and following the DASH diet.

Limit Dietary Sodium

Many people with HTN are sensitive to sodium; that is, when they consume a high-sodium diet, their blood pressure increases. We know, however, that not everyone with HTN is sensitive to sodium, and it is impossible to know who is sensitive and who is not because there is

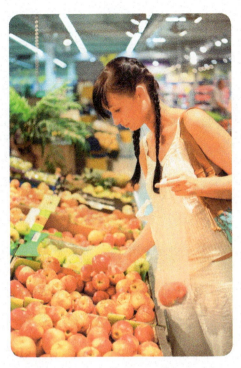

Consuming whole fruits and vegetables can reduce your risk for cardiovascular disease.

no ready test for sodium sensitivity. Moreover, lowering sodium intake does not reduce blood pressure in all people with hypertension. Thus, there is significant debate over whether everyone—or even everyone with HTN—can benefit from eating a lower-sodium diet.

Despite this debate, the leading health organizations, including the American Heart Association and the NHLBI, continue to support a reduction in dietary sodium to less than 2,300 mg/day, as recommended in the *2015–2020 Dietary Guidelines for Americans*.[15] Currently, the average sodium intake in the United States is about 3,300 mg/day.

Follow the DASH Diet

The impact of diet on reducing the risk for cardiovascular disease—including hypertension—was clearly demonstrated in a study from the National Institutes of Health (NIH) called Dietary Approaches to Stop Hypertension (DASH). The **DASH diet** is an eating plan that is high in several minerals that have been shown to help reduce hypertension, including calcium, magnesium, and potassium. At the same time, it is moderately low in sodium (2,300 mg/day on a 2000 kcal/d diet), low in saturated fat, and high in fiber, and it includes 10 servings of fruits and vegetables each day. **FIGURE 4** shows the DASH eating plan for a 2,000-kcal diet.

The results of the original NIH study showed that eating the DASH diet can dramatically improve blood lipids and lower blood pressure. These changes occurred within the first 2 weeks of eating the DASH diet and were maintained throughout the duration of the study. Researchers estimated that if all Americans followed the DASH diet plan and experienced reductions in blood pressure similar to this study, then CHD would be reduced by 15% and the incidence of strokes would be reduced by 27%.

A subsequent study of the DASH diet found that blood pressure decreases even more as sodium intake is reduced below 3,000 mg per day. In the study, participants ate a DASH diet that provided 3,300 mg, 2,300 mg, or 1,500 mg of sodium each day.[21] After 1 month

> For DASH diet recipes, visit the Mayo Clinic at www.mayo.org. From the home page, type "DASH diet" in the search bar, then click on "DASH Diet Recipes" and get cooking!

DASH diet The diet developed in response to research into hypertension funded by the National Institutes of Health: DASH stands for "Dietary Approaches to Stop Hypertension."

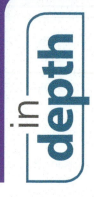

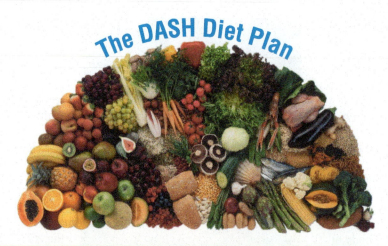

The DASH Diet Plan

Food Group	Daily Servings	Serving Size
Grains and grain products	7–8	1 slice bread 1 cup ready-to-eat cereal* ½ cup cooked rice, pasta, or cereal
Vegetables	4–5	1 cup raw leafy vegetables ½ cup cooked vegetable 6 fl. oz vegetable juice
Fruits	4–5	1 medium fruit ¼ cup dried fruit ½ cup fresh, frozen, or canned fruit 6 fl. oz fruit juice
Low-fat or fat-free dairy foods	2–3	8 fl. oz milk 1 cup yogurt 1½ oz cheese
Lean meats, poultry, and fish	2 or less	3 oz cooked lean meats, skinless poultry, or fish
Nuts, seeds, and dry beans	4–5 per week	⅓ cup or 1½ oz nuts 1 tbsp. or ½ oz seeds ½ cup cooked dry beans
Fats and oils†	2–3	1 tsp. soft margarine 1 tbsp. low-fat mayonnaise 2 tbsp. light salad dressing 1 tsp. vegetable oil
Sweets	5 per week	1 tbsp. sugar 1 tbsp. jelly or jam ½ oz jelly beans 8 fl. oz lemonade

*Serving sizes vary between ½ and 1¼ cups. Check the product's nutrition label.

†Fat content changes serving counts for fats and oils: for example, 1 tablespoon of regular salad dressing equals 1 serving; 1 tablespoon of a low-fat dressing equals ½ serving; 1 tablespoon of a fat-free dressing equals 0 servings.

🔺 **FIGURE 4** The DASH diet plan.

Note: This example is based on 2,000-kcal/day. Your number of servings in a food group may differ from the number listed, depending on your own energy needs.
Data adapted from: Healthier Eating with DASH. The National Institutes of Health (NIH).

that if you combine the DASH diet with physical activity and weight loss (of approximately 20 pounds), not only blood pressure, but blood lipids and other markers of CVD improve.[22]

Prescription Medications Can Improve Blood Lipids and Blood Pressure

For some individuals, lifestyle changes are not completely effective in normalizing blood lipids and blood pressure. When this is the case, a variety of medications can be prescribed. Some inhibit the body's production of cholesterol. These types of drugs, typically called *statins*, block an enzyme in the cholesterol synthesis pathway, which can help to lower blood levels of LDL-cholesterol and VLDL-cholesterol.[2] Other medications prevent the reabsorption of bile in the gastrointestinal (GI) tract. Because bile is made from cholesterol, blocking its reabsorption and promoting its excretion in feces reduces the total cholesterol pool, which means the liver must draw on body cholesterol stores to make new bile acids. Diuretics may also be prescribed to flush excess water and sodium from the body, reducing blood volume and thus blood pressure. Other hypertension medications work to relax the blood vessel walls, allowing more room for blood flow. People taking such medications should also continue to practice the lifestyle changes listed earlier in this section because these changes will continue to benefit their long-term health.

on this diet, all the participants experienced a significant decrease in their blood pressure; however, those who ate the lowest-sodium version of the DASH diet experienced the largest decrease. Even more recent research shows

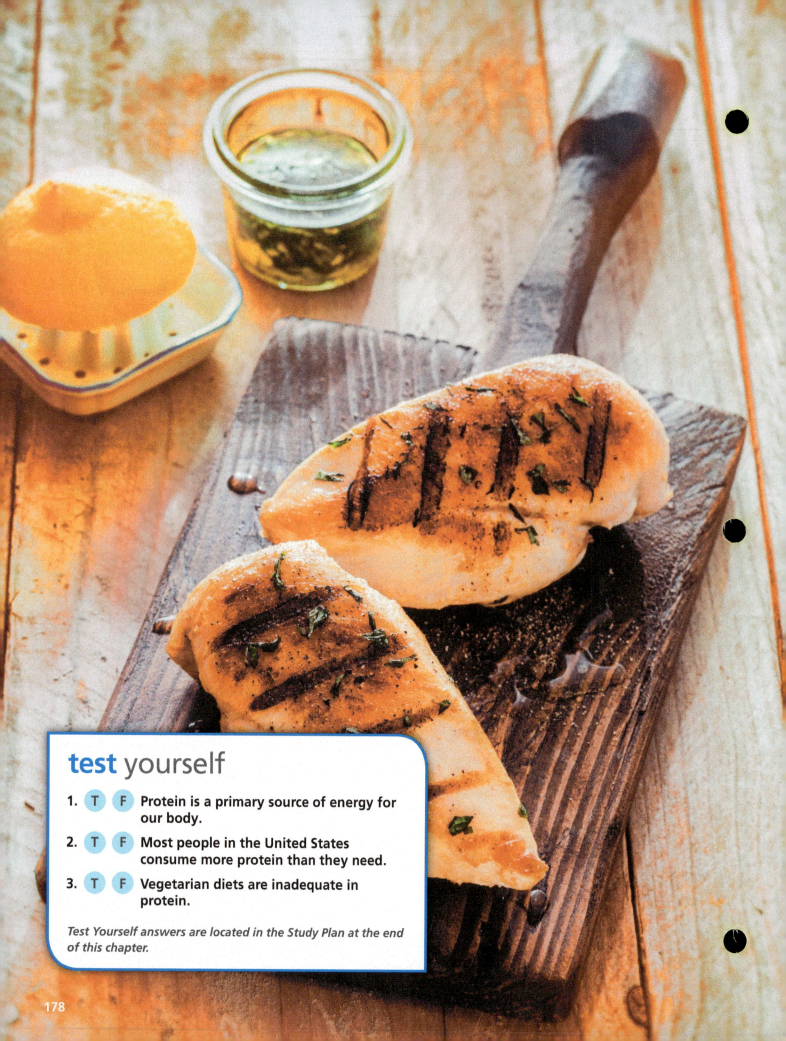

test yourself

1. T F Protein is a primary source of energy for our body.

2. T F Most people in the United States consume more protein than they need.

3. T F Vegetarian diets are inadequate in protein.

Test Yourself answers are located in the Study Plan at the end of this chapter.

6 Proteins
Crucial components of all body tissues

In their three years studying environmental sciences together at their small liberal arts college, Tamir, Kate, and Jian have built a strong friendship—strong enough to withstand disagreements, which they often have over food choices in the campus dining hall: Tamir is a passionate vegan—no animal-based foods of any kind, not even eggs or cheese. He insists that everyone should adopt a vegetarian diet to preserve the environment and protect their own health. Kate takes a more nuanced view. She cites studies pointing out the benefits of fish consumption twice a week, and also eats poultry, eggs, and cheese. She believes that a diet higher in protein helps her maintain a healthful weight and that Tamir's diet would leave her exhausted. Jian is a meat eater: He knows that red meat consumption is linked to climate change and certain health risks, but says if he didn't eat it several times a week, he'd lose muscle mass and wouldn't be able to keep up his workouts at the gym. So who's right? Is there any one approach to protein intake that's best for most people?

It seems as if everybody has an opinion about protein, both how much you should consume and from what sources. In this chapter, we discuss the importance of protein in the diet and dispel common myths about this crucial nutrient.

LO 1 Describe the chemical structure of proteins.

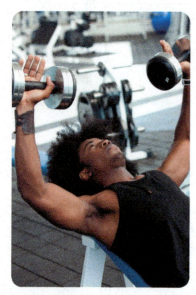

↖ Proteins are an integral part of our body tissues, including our muscle tissue.

proteins Large, complex molecules made up of amino acids and found as essential components of all living cells.

amino acids Nitrogen-containing molecules that combine to form proteins.

essential amino acids Amino acids not produced by the body that must be obtained from food.

What are proteins?

Proteins are large, complex molecules found in the cells of all living things. Although proteins are best known as a part of our muscle mass, they are, in fact, critical components of all the tissues of the human body, including bones, blood, and skin. Proteins also function in metabolism, immunity, fluid balance, and nutrient transport, and in certain circumstances they can provide energy. The functions of proteins will be discussed in detail later in this chapter.

The Building Blocks of Proteins Are Amino Acids

Like carbohydrates and lipids, proteins are macronutrients, but their chemical structure differs. In addition to the carbon, hydrogen, and oxygen also found in carbohydrates and lipids, proteins contain a special form of nitrogen that our body can readily use. Our body is able to break down the proteins in foods and utilize this nitrogen for many important processes. Carbohydrates and lipids do not provide nitrogen.

The proteins in our body are assembled according to instructions provided by our genetic material, or DNA, from building blocks called **amino acids**. These compounds are made up of a central carbon atom connected to four other groups: an amine group, an acid group, a hydrogen atom, and a side chain **(FIGURE 6.1a)**. The word *amine* means "nitrogen-containing," and nitrogen is indeed the essential component of the amine portion of the molecule.

As shown in Figure 6.1b, the portion of the amino acid that makes each unique is its side chain. The amine group, acid group, and carbon and hydrogen atoms do not vary. Variations in the structure of the side chain give each amino acid its distinct properties.

The singular term *protein* is misleading because there are potentially an infinite number of unique types of proteins in living organisms. Most of the proteins in our body are made from combinations of just 20 amino acids, identified in **TABLE 6.1**. Two of the 20 amino acids listed in Table 6.1, cysteine and methionine, are unique in that, in addition to the components present in the other amino acids, they contain sulfur. By combining a few dozen to more than 300 of these 20 amino acids in various sequences, our body synthesizes an estimated 10,000 to 50,000 unique proteins.

Nine Amino Acids Are Essential

Of the 20 amino acids in our body, nine are classified as essential. This does not mean that they are more important than the others. Instead, an **essential amino acid**

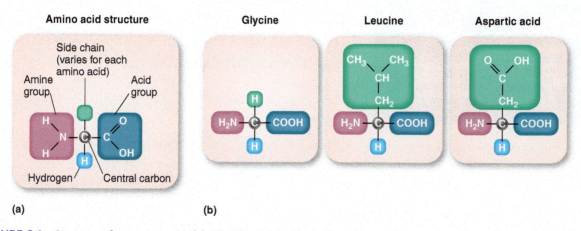

(a)   **(b)**

↖ **FIGURE 6.1** Structure of an amino acid. **(a)** All amino acids contain five parts: a central carbon atom; an amine group that contains nitrogen; an acid group; a hydrogen atom; and a side chain. **(b)** Only the side chain differs for each of the 20 amino acids, giving each its unique properties.

Transamination

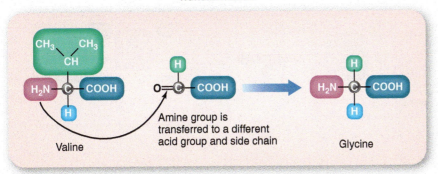

FIGURE 6.2 Transamination. Our body can make nonessential amino acids by transferring the amine group from an essential amino acid to a different acid group and side chain.

TABLE 6.1 Amino Acids of the Human Body

Essential Amino Acids	Nonessential Amino Acids
These amino acids must be consumed in the diet.	*These amino acids can be manufactured by the body.*
Histidine	Alanine
Isoleucine	Arginine
Leucine	Asparagine
Lysine	Aspartic acid
Methionine	Cysteine
Phenylalanine	Glutamic acid
Threonine	Glutamine
Tryptophan	Glycine
Valine	Proline
	Serine
	Tyrosine

is one that our body cannot produce at all or cannot produce in sufficient quantities to meet our physiologic needs. Thus, we must obtain essential amino acids from food. Without an adequate supply of essential amino acids in our body, we lose our ability to make the proteins and other nitrogen-containing compounds we need.

Nonessential amino acids are just as important to our body as essential amino acids, but our body can synthesize them in sufficient quantities, so we do not need to consume them in our diet. We make nonessential amino acids by transferring the amine group from other amino acids to a different acid group and side chain. This process is called **transamination** (FIGURE 6.2). The acid groups and side chains can be donated by amino acids, or they can be made from the breakdown products of carbohydrates and fats.

Under some conditions, a nonessential amino acid can become an essential amino acid. In this case, the amino acid is called a **conditionally essential amino acid**. Consider the disease known as phenylketonuria (PKU), in which the body cannot metabolize phenylalanine (an essential amino acid). In an infant with undiagnosed PKU, phenylalanine builds up in the blood to toxic levels that can cause irreversible brain damage. Moreover, because the body normally breaks down phenylalanine to produce the nonessential amino acid tyrosine, an inability to metabolize phenylalanine results in failure to make tyrosine, which then becomes a conditionally essential amino acid that must be provided by the diet. Other conditionally essential amino acids include arginine, cysteine, and glutamine.

To learn more about amino acids, go to www.johnkyrk.com, and click on "Amino Acids and Proteins."

nonessential amino acids Amino acids that can be manufactured by the body in sufficient quantities and therefore do not need to be consumed regularly in our diet.

transamination The process of transferring the amine group from one amino acid to another in order to manufacture a new amino acid.

conditionally essential amino acids Amino acids that are normally considered nonessential but become essential under certain circumstances when the body's need for them exceeds the ability to produce them.

recap Proteins are critical components of all the tissues of the human body. They contain carbon, hydrogen, oxygen, and nitrogen, and some contain sulfur. Their precise structure is dictated by DNA. The building blocks of proteins are amino acids. The amine group of the amino acid contains nitrogen. The portion of the amino acid that changes, giving each amino acid its distinct identity, is the side chain. Our body cannot make essential amino acids, so we must obtain them from our diet. Our body can make nonessential amino acids from parts of other amino acids, carbohydrates, and fats.

How are proteins made?

Cells synthesize proteins by selecting the needed amino acids from the pool of all amino acids available at any given time. Let's look more closely at how this occurs.

LO 2 Discuss protein synthesis, degradation, and organization, including the role of mutual supplementation.

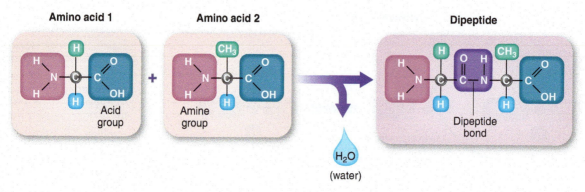

FIGURE 6.3 Amino acid bonding. Two amino acids join together to form a dipeptide. By combining multiple amino acids, proteins are made.

Amino Acids Bond to Form a Variety of Peptides

FIGURE 6.3 shows that, when two amino acids join together, the amine group of one binds to the acid group of another in a unique type of chemical bond called a **peptide bond**. In the process, a molecule of water is released as a by-product.

Two amino acids joined together form a *dipeptide*, and three amino acids joined together are called a *tripeptide*. The term *oligopeptide* is used to identify a string of four to nine amino acids, whereas a *polypeptide* is 10 or more amino acids bonded together. As a polypeptide chain grows longer, it begins to fold into any of a variety of complex shapes that give proteins their sophisticated structure.

Genes Regulate Amino Acid Binding

Each of us is unique because we inherited a specific "genetic code" that integrates the code from each of our parents. Each person's genetic code dictates minor differences in amino acid sequences, which in turn lead to differences in our body's individual proteins. These differences in proteins result in the unique physical and physiologic characteristics each one of us possesses.

A *gene* is a segment of deoxyribonucleic acid (DNA) that serves as a template for the synthesis—or expression—of a particular protein. That is, **gene expression** is the process by which cells use genes to make proteins.

Proteins are actually manufactured at the site of ribosomes in the cell's cytoplasm. But DNA never leaves the nucleus. So for gene expression to occur, a gene's DNA has to replicate itself—that is, it must make an exact copy of itself, which can then be carried out to the cytoplasm. DNA replication ensures that the genetic information in the original gene is identical to the genetic information used to build the protein. Through the process of replication, DNA provides the instructions for building every protein in the body.

Cells use a special molecule to copy, or transcribe, the information from DNA and carry it to the ribosomes. This molecule is *messenger RNA* (*messenger ribonucleic acid*, or *mRNA*). During **transcription**, mRNA copies the genetic information from DNA in the nucleus (**FOCUS FIGURE 6.4, step 1**). Then, mRNA detaches from the DNA and leaves the nucleus, carrying its genetic "message" to the ribosomes in the cytoplasm (Focus Figure 6.4, step 2).

Once the genetic information reaches the ribosomes, **translation** occurs; that is, the language of the mRNA genetic information is translated into the language of amino acid sequences. At the ribosomes, mRNA binds with ribosomal RNA (rRNA) and its genetic information is distributed to molecules of transfer RNA (tRNA) (Focus Figure 6.4, step 3). Now the tRNA molecules roam the cytoplasm until they succeed in binding with the specific amino acid that matches their genetic information. They then transfer their amino acid to the ribosome, which assembles the amino acids into proteins (Focus Figure 6.4, step 4).

Once the amino acids are loaded onto the ribosome, tRNA works to maneuver each amino acid into its proper position (Focus Figure 6.4, step 5). When synthesis

peptide bond Unique type of chemical bond in which the amine group of one amino acid binds to the acid group of another in order to manufacture dipeptides and all larger peptide molecules.

gene expression The process of using a gene to make a protein.

transcription The process through which messenger RNA copies genetic information from DNA in the nucleus.

translation The process that occurs when the genetic information carried by messenger RNA is translated into a chain of amino acids at the ribosome.

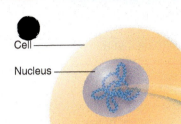

Cell ——
Nucleus ——

In the nucleus, genetic information from DNA is transcribed by messenger RNA (mRNA), which then carries it to ribosomes in the cytoplasm, where this genetic information is translated into a chain of amino acids that eventually make a protein.

1 Part of the DNA unwinds, and a section of its genetic code is transcribed to the mRNA inside the nucleus.

2 The mRNA leaves the nucleus via a nuclear pore and travels to the cytoplasm.

3 Once the mRNA reaches the cytoplasm, it binds to a ribosome via ribosomal RNA (rRNA). The code on the mRNA is translated into the instructions for a specific order of amino acids.

4 The transfer RNA (tRNA) binds with specific amino acids in the cytoplasm and transfers the amino acids to the ribosome as dictated by the mRNA code.

5 The amino acid is added to the growing amino acid chain, and the tRNA returns to the cytoplasm.

6 Once the synthesis of the protein is complete, the protein is released from the ribosome. The protein may go through further modifications in the cell or can be functional in its current state.

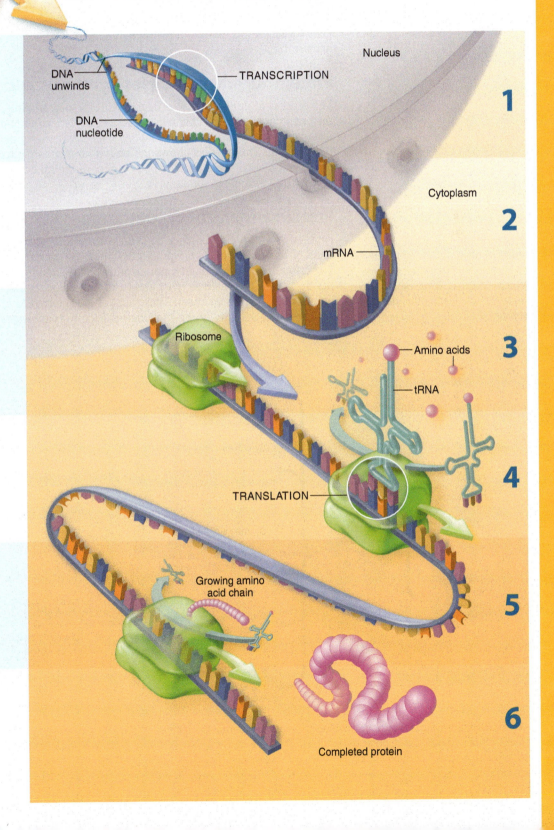

Nucleus

DNA unwinds

TRANSCRIPTION

DNA nucleotide

1

Cytoplasm

2

mRNA

Ribosome

Amino acids

3

tRNA

TRANSLATION

4

Growing amino acid chain

5

Completed protein

6

of the new protein is completed, it is released from the ribosome and can either go through further modification in the cell or can be functional in its current state (Focus Figure 6.4, step 6).

Although the DNA for making every protein in our body is contained within each cell nucleus, not all genes are expressed, and each cell does not make every type of protein. For example, each cell contains the DNA to manufacture the hormone insulin. However, only the beta cells of the pancreas *express* the insulin gene to produce insulin. Our physiologic needs alter gene expression, as do various nutrients. For instance, a cut in the skin that causes bleeding will prompt the production of various proteins that clot the blood. Or if we consume more dietary iron than we need, the gene for ferritin (a protein that stores iron) will be expressed, so that we can store this extra iron.

Protein Turnover Involves Synthesis and Degradation

The process of *protein turnover* begins with the degradation of proteins from food or the breakdown of cells. This releases amino acids into the body's *amino acid pool*, from which cells select the amino acids needed for the synthesis of new proteins **(FIGURE 6.5)**. This process allows the body to replace the proteins in worn-out cells and functional compounds. The body's pool of amino acids is also used to produce glucose, fat, and other compounds.

Protein Organization Determines Function

denaturation The process by which proteins uncoil and lose their shape and function when they are exposed to heat, acids, bases, heavy metals, alcohol, and other damaging substances.

Four levels of protein structure have been identified **(FIGURE 6.6)**. The sequential order of the amino acids in a protein is called the *primary structure* of the protein. The different amino acids in a polypeptide chain possess unique chemical characteristics that cause the chain to twist and turn into a characteristic spiral shape, or to fold into a so-called pleated sheet. These shapes are referred to as the protein's *secondary structure*. The stability of the secondary structure is achieved by hydrogen bonds that

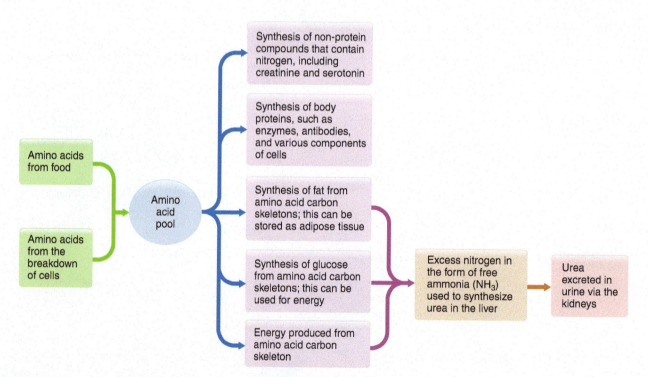

◆ **FIGURE 6.5** Protein turnover involves the synthesis of new proteins and breakdown of existing proteins to provide building blocks for new proteins. Amino acids are drawn from the body's amino acid pool and can be used to build proteins, fat, glucose, and nonprotein, nitrogen-containing compounds. Urea is produced as a waste product from any excess nitrogen, which is then excreted by the kidneys.

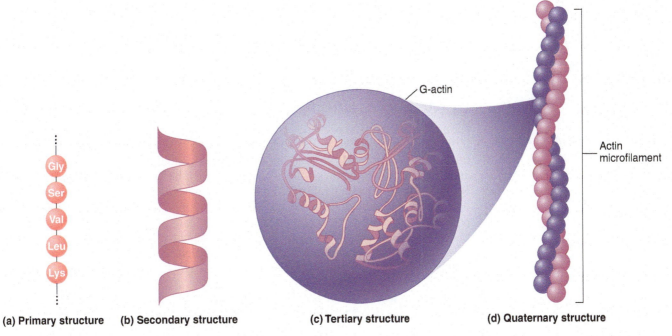

(a) Primary structure   **(b) Secondary structure**   **(c) Tertiary structure**   **(d) Quaternary structure**

G-actin

Actin microfilament

🔺 **FIGURE 6.6**   Levels of protein structure. **(a)** The primary structure of a protein is the sequential order of amino acids. **(b)** The secondary structure of a protein is the twisting or folding of the amino acid chain. **(c)** The tertiary structure is a further folding that results in the three-dimensional shape of the protein. **(d)** In proteins with a quaternary structure, two or more polypeptides interact, forming a larger protein, such as the actin molecule illustrated here. In muscle tissue, strands of actin molecules intertwine to form contractile elements involved in generating muscle contractions.

create a bridge between two protein strands or two parts of the same strand of protein. The spiral or pleated sheet of the secondary structure further folds into a unique three-dimensional shape, referred to as the protein's *tertiary structure*. Bonds between hydrogen atoms and between sulfur atoms, if any, maintain the tertiary shape, which is critical because it determines each protein's function in the body.

Many large proteins have a fourth level of organization. This *quaternary structure* forms when two or more identical or different polypeptides bond. The resulting larger protein may be *globular* or *fibrous*.

The importance of the shape of a protein to its function cannot be overemphasized. For example, the protein strands in muscle fibers are much longer than they are wide (see Figure 6.6d). This structure plays an essential role in enabling muscle contraction and relaxation. In contrast, the proteins that form red blood cells are globular in shape, and they result in the red blood cells being shaped like flattened discs with depressed centers, similar to a miniature doughnut **(FIGURE 6.7)**. This structure and the flexibility of the proteins in the red blood cells permit them to change shape and flow freely through even the tiniest capillaries to deliver oxygen and still return to their original shape.

Protein Denaturation Affects Shape and Function

Proteins can uncoil and lose their shape when they are exposed to heat, acids, bases, heavy metals, alcohol, and other damaging substances. The term used to describe this change in the shape of proteins is **denaturation**. Everyday examples of protein denaturation are the stiffening of egg whites when they are whipped, the curdling of milk when lemon juice or another acid is added, and the solidifying of eggs as they cook.

Denaturation does not affect the primary structure of proteins. However, when a protein is denatured, its function is lost. For instance, denaturation of critical body proteins on exposure to heat or acidity is harmful, because it prevents them from performing their functions. This type of denaturation can occur during times of high

To view a video showing a protein developing from primary to quaternary structure, go to www.dnatube.com, click on "Watch Videos," and then type "aminoacids" (as one word) into the search box. Click on the video titled "How bunch of aminoacids organise to form functional protein."

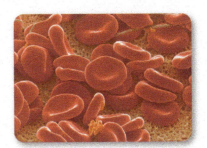

🔺 **FIGURE 6.7**   Protein shape determines function. The globular shape of protein in red blood cells contributes to the flexible-disk shape of the cells. This in turn enables their passage through the tiniest blood vessels of the body.

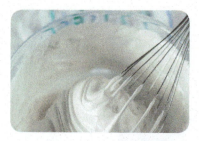

⬆ Stiffening egg whites adds air through the beating action, which denatures some of the proteins within them.

fever or when blood pH is out of the normal range. In some cases, however, denaturation is helpful. For instance, denaturation of proteins during the digestive process allows for their breakdown into amino acids and the absorption of these amino acids from the digestive tract into the bloodstream.

Protein Synthesis Can Be Limited by Missing Amino Acids

For protein synthesis to occur, all essential amino acids must be available to the cell. If this is not the case, the amino acid that is missing or in the smallest supply is called the **limiting amino acid**. Without the proper combination and quantity of essential amino acids, protein synthesis slows to the point at which proteins cannot be generated. For instance, the protein hemoglobin contains the essential amino acid histidine. If we do not consume enough histidine, it becomes the limiting amino acid in hemoglobin production. Because no other amino acid can be substituted, our body becomes unable to make adequate hemoglobin, and we lose the ability to transport oxygen to our cells.

Inadequate energy consumption also limits protein synthesis. If there is not enough energy available from our diets, our body will use any accessible proteins for energy, thus preventing them from being used to build new proteins.

A protein that does not contain all of the essential amino acids in sufficient quantities to support growth and health is called an **incomplete** (*low-quality*) **protein**. A protein that has all nine of the essential amino acids is considered a **complete** (*high-quality*) **protein**. The most complete protein sources are foods derived from animals and include egg whites, meat, poultry, fish, and milk. Soybeans and a pseudo-grain called quinoa (pronounced keen-wah) are the most complete sources of plant protein. In general, the typical American diet is very high in complete proteins because we consume proteins from a variety of food sources.

Protein Synthesis Can Be Enhanced by Mutual Supplementation

We also obtain complete proteins by combining foods. Consider a meal of red beans and rice. Red beans are low in the amino acids methionine and cysteine but have adequate amounts of isoleucine and lysine. Rice is low in isoleucine and lysine but contains sufficient methionine and cysteine. Combining red beans and rice creates a complete protein.

Mutual supplementation is the process of combining two or more incomplete protein sources to make a complete protein. The two foods involved are called complementary foods; these foods provide **complementary proteins (FIGURE 6.8)**, which, when combined, provide all nine essential amino acids.

It is not necessary to eat complementary proteins at the same meal. Recall that we maintain a free pool of amino acids in the blood; these amino acids come from food and sloughed-off cells. When we eat one complementary protein, its amino acids join those in the free amino acid pool. These free amino acids can then combine to synthesize complete proteins. However, it is wise to eat complementary-protein foods during the same day because partially completed proteins cannot be stored and saved for a later time. Mutual supplementation is important for people eating a vegetarian diet, particularly if they consume no animal products whatsoever.

limiting amino acid The essential amino acid that is missing or in the smallest supply in the amino acid pool and is thus responsible for slowing or halting protein synthesis.

incomplete protein Food that does not contain all of the essential amino acids in sufficient amounts to support growth and health.

complete protein Food that contains sufficient amounts of all nine essential amino acids to support growth and health.

mutual supplementation The process of combining two or more incomplete protein sources to make a complete protein.

complementary proteins Two or more foods that together contain all nine essential amino acids necessary for a complete protein. It is not necessary to eat complementary proteins at the same meal.

recap Amino acids bind together to form proteins. Genes regulate the amino acid sequence, and thus the structure, of all proteins. The shape of a protein determines its function. When a protein is denatured by damaging substances, such as heat and acids, it loses its shape and its function. When a particular essential amino acid is unavailable, protein synthesis cannot occur. A complete protein provides all nine essential amino acids. Mutual supplementation combines two complementary-protein sources to make a complete protein.

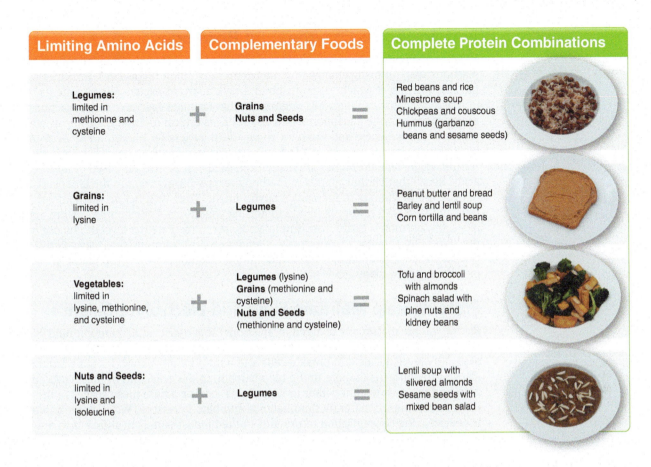

Limiting Amino Acids		Complementary Foods		Complete Protein Combinations
Legumes: limited in methionine and cysteine	+	**Grains** **Nuts and Seeds**	=	Red beans and rice Minestrone soup Chickpeas and couscous Hummus (garbanzo beans and sesame seeds)
Grains: limited in lysine	+	**Legumes**	=	Peanut butter and bread Barley and lentil soup Corn tortilla and beans
Vegetables: limited in lysine, methionine, and cysteine	+	**Legumes** (lysine) **Grains** (methionine and cysteine) **Nuts and Seeds** (methionine and cysteine)	=	Tofu and broccoli with almonds Spinach salad with pine nuts and kidney beans
Nuts and Seeds: limited in lysine and isoleucine	+	**Legumes**	=	Lentil soup with slivered almonds Sesame seeds with mixed bean salad

▲ **FIGURE 6.8** Complementary food combinations.

Why do we need proteins?

The functions of proteins in the body are so numerous that only a few can be described in detail in this chapter. Note that proteins function most effectively when we also consume adequate amounts of energy as carbohydrates and fat. When there is not enough energy available, the body uses proteins as an energy source, limiting their availability for the functions described in this section.

LO 3 List eight functions of proteins in the body.

Proteins Contribute to Cell Growth, Repair, and Maintenance

We've noted that the proteins in our body are constantly being broken down, repaired, and replaced. Think about all of the new proteins that are needed to allow an embryo to develop into a fetus and grow into a newborn baby with more than 10 trillion body cells. This growth continues, of course, throughout childhood, but even in adulthood, our cells are constantly turning over, as damaged or worn-out cells are broken down and their components are used to create new cells. Our red blood cells live for only 3 to 4 months and then are replaced by new cells that are produced in bone marrow. The cells lining our intestinal tract are replaced every 3 to 6 days. The "old" intestinal cells are treated just like the proteins in food; they are digested and the amino acids absorbed back into the body. The constant turnover of proteins from our diet is essential for such cell growth, repair, and maintenance.

Proteins Act as Enzymes and Hormones

Recall that enzymes are compounds—usually proteins—that speed up chemical reactions without being changed by the chemical reaction themselves. Enzymes can increase the rate at which reactants bond, break apart, or exchange components.

Each cell contains thousands of enzymes that facilitate specific cellular reactions. For example, the enzyme phosphofructokinase (PFK) is critical to driving the rate at which we break down glucose and use it for energy during exercise. Without PFK, we would be unable to generate energy at a fast enough rate to allow us to be physically active.

Although some hormones are made from lipids, most are composed of amino acids. Recall that various glands in the body release hormones into the bloodstream in response to changes in the body's environment. They then act on the body's cells and tissues to restore the body to normal conditions. For example, insulin and glucagon, hormones made from amino acids, act to regulate the level of glucose in the blood (see Chapter 4). *Melatonin* is an amino-acid hormone that plays a critical role in the regulation of sleep. Other amino-acid hormones help regulate growth, metabolism, and many other processes.

Proteins Help Maintain Fluid and Electrolyte Balance

Electrolytes are electrically charged atoms (ions) that assist in maintaining fluid balance. For our body to function properly, fluids and electrolytes must be maintained at healthy levels inside and outside cells and within blood vessels. Proteins attract fluids, and the proteins that are in the bloodstream, in the cells, and in the spaces surrounding the cells work together to keep fluids moving across these spaces in the proper quantities to maintain fluid balance and blood pressure. When protein intake is deficient, the concentration of proteins in the bloodstream is insufficient to draw fluid from the tissues and across the blood vessel walls; fluid then collects in the tissues, causing **edema (FIGURE 6.9)**. In addition to being uncomfortable, edema can lead to serious medical problems.

Sodium (Na^+) and potassium (K^+) are examples of common electrolytes. Under normal conditions, Na^+ is more concentrated outside the cell, and K^+ is more concentrated inside the cell. This proper balance of Na^+ and K^+ is accomplished by the action of **transport proteins** located within the cell membrane. **FIGURE 6.10** (page 190) shows how these transport proteins work to pump Na^+ outside and K^+ inside of the cell. The conduction of nerve signals and contraction of muscles depend on a proper balance of electrolytes. If protein intake is deficient, we lose our ability to maintain these functions, resulting in potentially fatal changes in the rhythm of the heart. Other consequences of chronically low protein intakes include muscle weakness and spasms, kidney failure, and, if conditions are severe enough, death.

Proteins Help Maintain Acid–Base Balance

The body's cellular processes result in the constant production of acids and bases. Recall that acids are fluids containing a level of hydrogen ions higher than that of pure water, whereas bases (alkaline fluids) have fewer hydrogen ions than pure water. Acids and bases are transported in the blood to be excreted through the kidneys and the lungs. The body goes into a state called **acidosis** when the blood becomes too acidic. **Alkalosis** results if the blood becomes too basic (alkaline). Both acidosis and alkalosis can be caused by respiratory or metabolic problems, and both can cause coma and death by denaturing body proteins.

You can appreciate, then, why the body maintains very tight control over the pH, or the acid–base balance, of the blood. It does this by means of several mechanisms, including **buffers**, compounds that help return acidic and alkaline fluids closer to neutral. Proteins are excellent buffers because their side chains have negative charges that can bind hydrogen ions when the blood becomes acidic, neutralizing their detrimental effects on the body. Proteins can also release the hydrogen ions when the blood becomes too basic. By buffering acids and bases, proteins maintain acid–base balance and blood pH.

edema A disorder in which fluids build up in the tissue spaces of the body, causing fluid imbalances and a swollen appearance.

transport proteins Protein molecules that help transport substances throughout the body and across cell membranes.

acidosis A disorder in which the blood becomes acidic; that is, the level of hydrogen in the blood is excessive. It can be caused by respiratory or metabolic problems.

alkalosis A disorder in which the blood becomes basic; that is, the level of hydrogen in the blood is deficient. It can be caused by respiratory or metabolic problems.

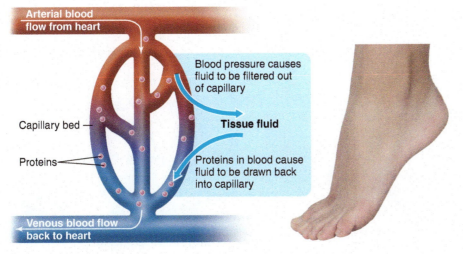

(a) Normal fluid balance

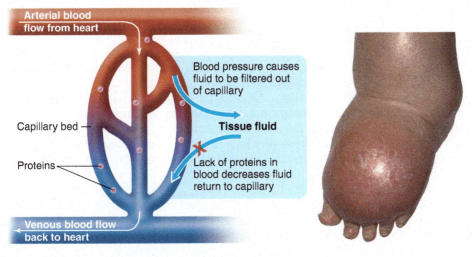

(b) Edema caused by insufficient protein in bloodstream

◀ **FIGURE 6.9** The role of proteins in maintaining fluid balance. The heartbeat exerts pressure that continually pushes fluids in the bloodstream through the arterial walls and out into the tissue spaces. By the time blood reaches the veins, the pressure of the heartbeat has greatly decreased. In this environment, proteins in the blood are able to draw fluids out of the tissues and back into the bloodstream. **(a)** This healthy (nonswollen) tissue suggests that body fluids in the bloodstream and in the tissue spaces are in balance. **(b)** When the level of proteins in the blood is insufficient to draw fluids out of the tissues, edema can result. This foot with edema is swollen due to fluid imbalance.

Proteins Help Maintain a Strong Immune System

Antibodies are special proteins that are critical to immune function. When a foreign substance attacks the body, the immune system produces antibodies to defend against it. Bacteria, viruses, toxins, and allergens (substances that cause allergic reactions) are examples of antigens that can trigger antibody production. (An *antigen* is any substance—but typically a protein—that our body recognizes as foreign and that triggers an immune response.)

Each antibody is designed to destroy one specific invader. When that substance invades the body, antibodies are produced to neutralize or target the specific antigen so that it can be destroyed. Once antibodies have been made, the body "remembers" this process and can respond more quickly the next time that particular invader appears. *Immunity* refers to the development of the molecular memory to produce antibodies quickly upon subsequent invasions.

Adequate protein is necessary to support the increased production of antibodies that occurs in response to a cold, flu, or an allergic reaction. If we do not consume enough protein, our resistance to illnesses and disease is weakened. On the other hand, eating more protein than we need does not improve immune function.

buffers Proteins that help maintain proper acid–base balance by attaching to, or releasing, hydrogen ions as conditions change in the body.

antibodies Defensive proteins of the immune system. Their production is prompted by the presence of bacteria, viruses, toxins, allergens, and other antigens.

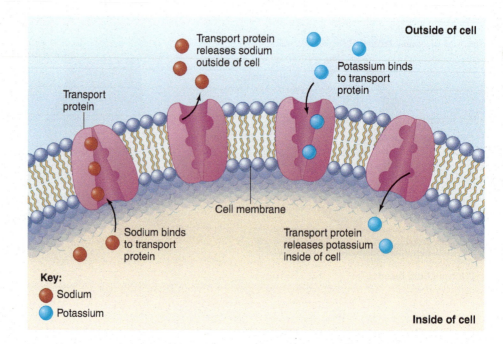

Proteins Serve as an Energy Source

The body's primary energy sources are carbohydrate and fat. Remember that both carbohydrate and fat have specialized storage forms that can be used for energy: glycogen for carbohydrate and triglycerides for fat. Proteins do not have a specialized storage form for energy. This means that, when proteins need to be used for energy, they are taken from the blood, liver, skeletal muscle, and other body tissues. In healthy people, proteins contribute very little to energy needs. Because we are efficient at recycling amino acids, protein needs are relatively low as compared to needs for carbohydrate and fat.

To use proteins for energy, the liver removes the amine group from the amino acids in a process called **deamination**. The nitrogen bonds with hydrogen, creating ammonia, which is a toxic compound that can upset acid–base balance. This is avoided, however, because the liver quickly converts ammonia to *urea*. The urea is then transported to the kidneys, where it is filtered out of the blood and is subsequently excreted in the urine. The remaining fragments of the amino acid contain carbon, hydrogen, and oxygen. The body can use these fragments to generate energy or to build carbohydrates. Certain amino acids can be converted into glucose via gluconeogenesis. This is a critical process during times of low carbohydrate intake or starvation. Fat cannot be converted into glucose, but body proteins can be broken down and converted into glucose to provide needed energy to the brain.

To protect the proteins in our body tissues, it is important that we regularly eat an amount of carbohydrate and fat sufficient to meet our energy needs. We also need to consume enough dietary protein to meet our physiologic needs and spare the proteins in blood and other body tissues. Again, our body cannot store excess dietary protein. As a consequence, eating too much protein results in the removal and excretion of the nitrogen in the urine and the use of the remaining components for energy. Any remaining components not used for energy are converted to fatty acids and stores as triglycerides in body fat.

deamination The process by which an amine group is removed from an amino acid. The nitrogen is then transported to the kidneys for excretion in the urine, while the carbon and other components are metabolized for energy or used to make other compounds.

Proteins Assist in the Transport and Storage of Nutrients

Proteins act as carriers for many important nutrients in the body. As you've learned, lipoproteins contain lipids bound to proteins, which allows the transport of hydrophobic lipids through the watery medium of blood (see Chapter 5). Another example of a transport protein is transferrin, which carries iron in the blood. Ferritin, in contrast, is an example of a storage protein: it is the compound in which iron is stored in the liver.

We've also said that transport proteins located in cell membranes allow the proper transport of many nutrients into and out of the cell. These transport proteins also help in the maintenance of fluid and electrolyte balance and conduction of nerve impulses.

Proteins Are Critical to Nerve Function, Blood Clotting, and Wound Healing

The amino acids from proteins can also be used to make **neurotransmitters**, chemicals that transmit messages from one nerve cell to another. Examples of neurotransmitters include epinephrine and norepinephrine, both of which stimulate the sympathetic nervous system; and serotonin, which is important for the functioning of the central nervous system and the enteric nervous system of the gastrointestinal (GI) tract.

Proteins are also critical in blood clotting. The watery portion of blood, called plasma, contains clotting factors, proteins that initiate a chain of reactions that convert another plasma protein, fibrinogen, to a fibrous protein called *fibrin*. Strands of fibrin form a mesh that helps to temporarily seal a broken blood vessel. The scar tissue that is formed to heal wounds comprises another protein, *collagen*, which is also a key component of bone, tendons, skin, and many other tissues.

To learn more about how blood clots and wounds heal, go to www.medlineplus.gov, click on "Videos and Tools," then "Health Videos," and then click "blood clotting."

recap Proteins serve eight broad functions in the body. They (1) enable growth, repair, and maintenance of body tissues; (2) act as enzymes and hormones; (3) help maintain fluid and electrolyte balance; (4) contribute to acid–base balance; (5) make antibodies, which are essential to immune function; (6) provide energy when carbohydrate and fat intake are inadequate; (7) transport and store nutrients; and (8) are components of neurotransmitters, clotting proteins, and collagen. Proteins function best when adequate amounts of carbohydrate and fat are consumed.

How does the body process proteins?

LO 4 Explain how proteins are digested and absorbed.

Again, our body does not directly use proteins from the diet to make the proteins we need. Dietary proteins are first digested into amino acids, which are absorbed and transported to the cells. In this section, we will review this process. Refer to **FOCUS FIGURE 6.11** (page 192) for a visual overview of protein digestion.

Stomach Acids and Enzymes Break Proteins into Short Polypeptides

Virtually no enzymatic digestion of proteins occurs in the mouth. As shown in Focus Figure 6.11, proteins in food are chewed, crushed, and moistened with saliva to ease swallowing and to increase the surface area of the protein for more efficient digestion. There is no further digestive action on proteins in the mouth.

When proteins reach the stomach, hydrochloric acid denatures the protein strands. It also converts the inactive enzyme, *pepsinogen*, into its active form, **pepsin**, which is a protein-digesting enzyme. Although pepsin is itself a protein, it is not denatured by the acid in the stomach because it has evolved to work optimally in an acidic environment. The hormone *gastrin* controls both the production of hydrochloric acid and the release of pepsin; thinking about food or actually chewing food stimulates the gastrin-producing cells in the stomach. Pepsin begins breaking proteins into single amino acids and shorter polypeptides; these amino acids and polypeptides then travel to the small intestine for further digestion and absorption.

Enzymes in the Small Intestine Break Polypeptides into Single Amino Acids

As the polypeptides reach the small intestine, the pancreas and the small intestine secrete enzymes that digest them into oligopeptides, tripeptides, dipeptides, and single

neurotransmitters Chemical compounds that transmit messages from one nerve cell to another.

pepsin An enzyme in the stomach that begins the breakdown of proteins into shorter polypeptide chains and single amino acids.

Digestion of dietary proteins into single amino acids occurs primarily in the stomach and small intestine. The single amino acids are then transported to the liver, where they may be converted to glucose or fat, used for energy or to build new proteins, or transported to cells as needed.

ORGANS OF THE GI TRACT

ACCESSORY ORGANS

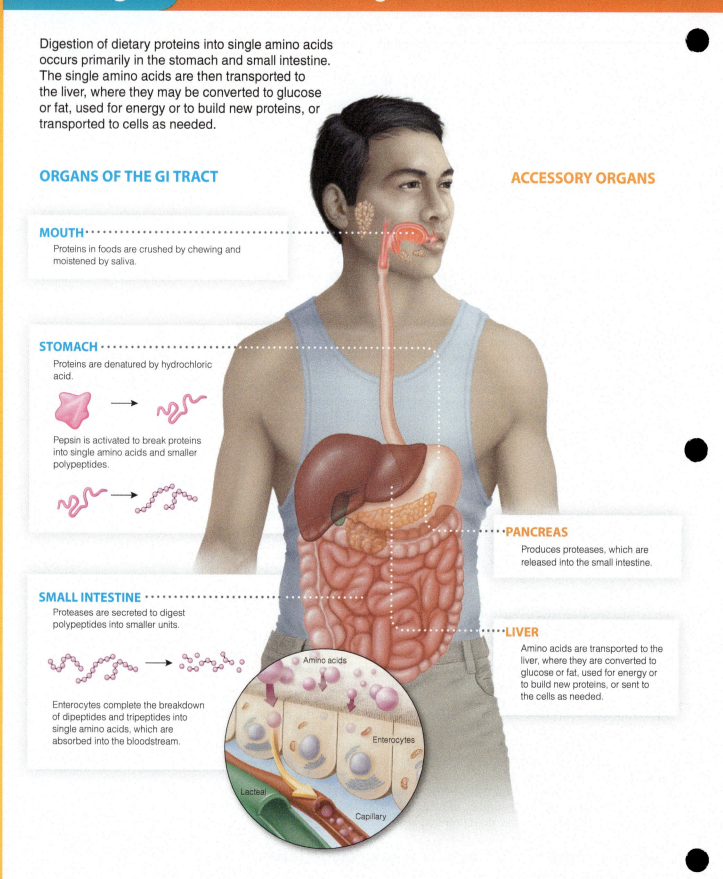

MOUTH

Proteins in foods are crushed by chewing and moistened by saliva.

STOMACH

Proteins are denatured by hydrochloric acid.

Pepsin is activated to break proteins into single amino acids and smaller polypeptides.

PANCREAS

Produces proteases, which are released into the small intestine.

SMALL INTESTINE

Proteases are secreted to digest polypeptides into smaller units.

Enterocytes complete the breakdown of dipeptides and tripeptides into single amino acids, which are absorbed into the bloodstream.

LIVER

Amino acids are transported to the liver, where they are converted to glucose or fat, used for energy or to build new proteins, or sent to the cells as needed.

Amino acids

Enterocytes

Lacteal

Capillary

amino acids (see Focus Figure 6.11). The enzymes that digest proteins in the small intestine are called **proteases**.

The enterocytes of the small intestine then absorb the single amino acids, dipeptides, and tripeptides. Peptidases, enzymes located in the enterocytes, break the dipeptides and tripeptides into single amino acids. The amino acids are then transported via the portal vein into the liver. Once in the liver, amino acids may be converted to glucose or fat, combined to build new proteins, used for energy, or released into the bloodstream and transported to other cells as needed.

The cells of the small intestine have different sites that specialize in transporting certain types of amino acids, dipeptides, and tripeptides. This fact has implications for users of amino acid supplements. When very large doses of supplements containing single amino acids are taken on an empty stomach, they typically compete for the same absorption sites. This competition can block the absorption of other amino acids and could in theory lead to deficiencies. In reality, people rarely take such large doses of single amino acids on an empty stomach.

Protein Digestibility Affects Protein Quality

Earlier in this chapter, we discussed how various protein sources differ in quality of protein. The quantity of essential amino acids in a protein determines its quality: higher-protein-quality foods are those that contain more of the essential amino acids in sufficient quantities needed to build proteins, and lower-quality-protein foods contain fewer essential amino acids. Another factor in protein quality is *digestibility*. Animal protein sources, such as meat and dairy products, are highly digestible, as are many soy products; we can absorb more than 90% of the amino acids in these protein sources. Legumes are also highly digestible (about 70% to 80%). Grains and many vegetable proteins are less digestible, ranging from 60% to 90%.

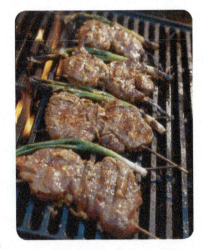

▲ Meats are highly digestible sources of dietary protein.

recap In the stomach, hydrochloric acid denatures proteins and converts pepsinogen to pepsin; pepsin breaks proteins into polypeptides and individual amino acids. In the small intestine, proteases break polypeptides into smaller fragments and single amino acids. Enzymes in the enterocytes break the smaller peptide fragments into single amino acids, which are then absorbed into the bloodstream and transported to the liver for distribution to body cells. Protein digestibility and the provision of essential amino acids influence protein quality.

How much protein should you eat?

Consuming adequate protein is a major concern of many people. In fact, one of the most common concerns among active people and athletes is that their diets are deficient in protein. This concern about dietary protein is generally unnecessary because we can easily consume the protein our body needs by eating an adequate and varied diet.

LO 5 Identify your recommended daily protein intake, healthful sources of protein, and consequences of high intake and deficiency.

Nitrogen Balance Is a Method Used to Determine Protein Needs

A highly specialized procedure referred to as *nitrogen balance* is used to determine a person's protein needs. Nitrogen is excreted through the body's processes of recycling or using proteins; thus, the balance can be used to estimate whether protein intake is adequate to meet protein needs.

Typically performed only in experimental laboratories, nitrogen balance involves measuring both nitrogen intake and nitrogen excretion over a 2-week period. A standardized diet, the nitrogen content of which has been measured and recorded, is fed to the study participant. The person is required to consume all of the foods provided. Because the majority of nitrogen is excreted in the urine and feces, laboratory technicians directly measure the nitrogen content of the subject's urine and fecal samples. Small amounts of nitrogen are excreted in the skin, hair, and body fluids such as mucus and semen, but, because of the complexity of collecting nitrogen excreted via these routes, the measurements are estimated. Then, technicians add the estimated

proteases Enzymes that continue the breakdown of polypeptides in the small intestine.

nitrogen losses to the nitrogen measured in the subject's urine and feces. Nitrogen balance is then calculated as the difference between nitrogen intake and nitrogen excretion.

People who consume more nitrogen than is excreted are considered to be in positive nitrogen balance **(FIGURE 6.12)**. This state indicates that the body is retaining or adding protein, and it occurs during periods of growth, pregnancy, or recovery from illness or a protein deficiency. People who excrete more nitrogen than they consume are in negative nitrogen balance. This situation indicates that the body is losing protein, and it occurs during starvation or when people are consuming very-low-energy diets. This is because, when energy intake is too low to meet energy demands over

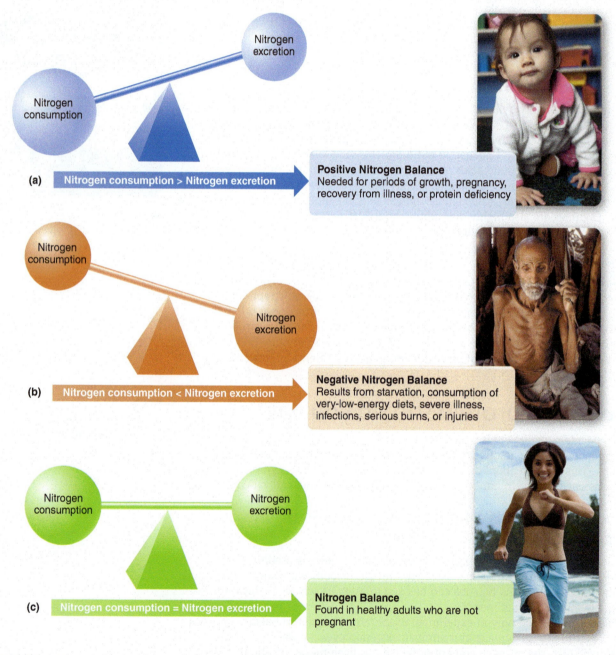

(a) Nitrogen consumption > Nitrogen excretion

Positive Nitrogen Balance
Needed for periods of growth, pregnancy, recovery from illness, or protein deficiency

(b) Nitrogen consumption < Nitrogen excretion

Negative Nitrogen Balance
Results from starvation, consumption of very-low-energy diets, severe illness, infections, serious burns, or injuries

(c) Nitrogen consumption = Nitrogen excretion

Nitrogen Balance
Found in healthy adults who are not pregnant

◆ **FIGURE 6.12** Nitrogen balance describes the relationship between how much nitrogen (protein) we consume and how much we excrete each day. **(a)** Positive nitrogen balance occurs when nitrogen consumption is greater than excretion. **(b)** Negative nitrogen balance occurs when nitrogen consumption is less than excretion. **(c)** Nitrogen balance is maintained when nitrogen consumption equals excretion.

Calculating Your Protein Needs

Theo wants to know how much protein he needs each day. During the off-season, he works out three times a week at a gym and practices basketball with friends every Friday night. He is not a vegetarian. Although Theo exercises regularly, he would not be considered an endurance athlete or a strength athlete during the off-season. At this level of physical activity, Theo's requirement for protein probably ranges from the RDA of 0.8 up to 1.0 g per kg body weight per day. To calculate the total number of grams of protein Theo should eat each day:

1. Convert Theo's weight from pounds to kilograms. Theo presently weighs 200 pounds. To convert this value to kilograms, divide by 2.2:

   200 pounds ÷ 2.2 pounds/kg = 91 kg

2. Multiply Theo's weight in kilograms by his RDA for protein, like so:

   91 kg × 0.8 g/kg = 72.8 grams of protein per day
   91 kg × 1.0 g/kg = 91 grams of protein per day

What happens during basketball season, when Theo practices, lifts weights, and has games 5 or 6 days a week? This will probably raise his protein needs to approximately 1.2 to 1.7 g per kg body weight per day. How much more protein should he eat? See below:

   91 kg × 1.2 g/kg = 109.2 grams of protein per day
   91 kg × 1.7 g/kg = 154.7 grams of protein per day

Now calculate your own recommended protein intake based on your activity level.

Answers will vary depending upon body weight and individual activity levels.

a prolonged period, the body metabolizes body proteins for energy. The nitrogen from these proteins is excreted in the urine and feces. Negative nitrogen balance also occurs during severe illness, infections, high fever, serious burns, or injuries that cause significant blood loss. People in these situations require increased dietary protein. A person is in nitrogen balance when nitrogen intake equals nitrogen excretion. This indicates that protein intake is sufficient to cover protein needs. Healthy adults who are not pregnant are in nitrogen balance.

Although nitrogen balance has been used for many years as a method to estimate protein needs in humans, it has been criticized because it is so time- and labor-intensive for both research participants and scientists. In addition, because it is not possible to collect and measure all of the nitrogen excreted each day, this method is recognized as underestimating protein needs.[1]

Recommended Dietary Allowance for Protein

The RDA for protein for sedentary people is 0.8 g per kg body weight per day. The recommended percentage of energy that should come from protein is 10% to 35% of total energy intake. Protein needs are higher for children, adolescents, and pregnant/lactating women because more protein is needed during times of growth and development (see Chapters 14 and 15). Protein needs can also be higher for active people, older adults, and vegetarians. For example, recent evidence indicates that the dietary intake needed to promote the needs of active people ranges from 1.2 to 2.0 g per kg body weight per day.[2] To learn more about the evidence surrounding increased protein needs for various groups, refer to the **Nutrition Debate** at the end of this chapter.

How can you convert the RDA into the total grams of protein your need per day? See the **You Do the Math** box on this page to calculate Theo's protein requirements, and then calculate your own.

Most Americans Meet or Exceed the RDA for Protein

Surveys indicate that Americans eat almost 16% of their total daily energy intake as protein,[3] averaging about 78 to 87 g per day.[4] Putting these values into perspective, let's assume that the average man weighs 75 kg (165 pounds) and the average woman weighs 65 kg (143 pounds). Their protein requirements (assuming they are sedentary) are 60 g and 52 g per day, respectively. As you can see, many adults in the United States eat more than the RDA for protein.

As previously discussed, active individuals have higher protein needs than people who are inactive. Does this mean you should add more protein to your diet if you are active? Not necessarily. You need to assess your current level of protein intake to determine if it is within the current recommendations of 1.2 to 2 g per kg body weight per day for active people. It is important to note that certain groups of athletes are at risk for low protein intakes. Athletes who consume inadequate energy and limit food choices, such as some distance runners, figure skaters, female gymnasts, wrestlers, and body builders who are dieting, are all at risk for inadequate protein intakes or increased protein needs due to low energy intakes. Unlike people who consume adequate energy, individuals who are restricting their total energy intake (kilocalories) need to pay close attention to their protein intake.

Protein Sources Include Much More Than Meat!

Although some people think that the only good sources of protein are meats (beef, pork, poultry, seafood), many other foods are rich in proteins. These include dairy products (milk, cheese, yogurt, etc.), eggs, legumes (including soy products), whole grains, and nuts. Fruits and many vegetables are not particularly high in protein; however, these foods are excellent sources of carbohydrates and energy, so eating them can enable your body to use proteins for building and maintaining tissues. Lean sources of protein recommended by the *2015–2020 Dietary Guidelines for Americans* include lean meats and poultry, fish, processed soy products, legumes, and nuts and seeds.[5] These foods are high in nutrient density. To compare the protein and energy content of a day's meals, see **MEAL FOCUS FIGURE 6.13**.

TABLE 6.2 (page 198) compares the protein content of a variety of foods. After reviewing this table, you might wonder how much protein you eat in a typical day—and whether or not you're meeting your needs. See the **Nutrition Label Activity** (page 199) to find out.

Legumes

Legumes include foods such as soybeans, kidney beans, pinto beans, black beans, garbanzo beans (chickpeas), green peas, black-eyed peas, dal, and lentils. Would you be surprised to learn that the quality of the protein in some of these legumes is almost equal to that of meat? It's true! The quality of soybean protein is also nearly identical to that of meat. It's available as soy milk, tofu, textured vegetable protein, and tempeh, a firm cake that is made by cooking and fermenting whole soybeans. The protein quality of other legumes is also relatively high. In addition to being excellent sources of protein, legumes are high in fiber, iron, calcium, and many of the B-vitamins. They are also low in saturated fat and cholesterol.

Eating legumes regularly, including foods made from soybeans, may help reduce the risk for heart disease by lowering blood cholesterol levels. Diets high in legumes and soy products are also associated with lower rates of some cancers. Legumes are not nutritionally complete, however, because they do not contain vitamins B_{12}, C, or A. Most are also deficient in methionine, an essential amino acid; however, combining them with grains, nuts, or seeds gives you a complete protein.

Considering their nutrient profile, satiety value, and good taste, it's no wonder that many experts consider legumes an almost perfect food. From main dishes to snacks, the **Quick Tips** feature (page 200) offers simple ways to add legumes to your daily diet.

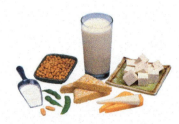

◄ Soy products are a good source of dietary protein.

a day of meals

about **16%** of energy from protein

BREAKFAST

2 fried eggs
3 slices bacon, fried
2 slices of white toast with
  1 tbsp. of butter
8 fl. oz whole milk

about **21%** of energy from protein

1 cup granola (with oats, wheat and raisins)
1 tbsp slivered almonds
1 cup soy milk

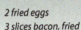

LUNCH

2 slices pepperoni pizza
  (14" pizza, hand-tossed crust)
1 medium banana
24 fl. oz cola beverage

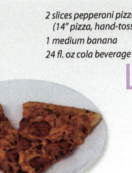

½ fillet broiled salmon
Spinach salad:
  2 cups fresh spinach
  ½ cup raw carrots, sliced
  3 cherry tomatoes
  1 tbsp. chopped green onions
  ¼ cup kidney beans
  2 tbsp. fat-free Caesar dressing
1 medium banana
24 fl. oz iced tea

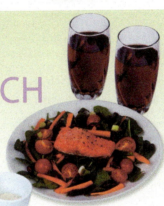

DINNER

Fried chicken, 1 drumstick and
  1 breast (with skin)
1 cup mashed potatoes with
  ¼ cup gravy
½ cup yellow sweet corn
8 fl. oz whole milk
1 slice chocolate cake with
  chocolate frosting
  (1/12 of cake)

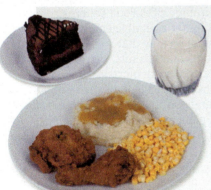

½ chicken breast, roasted
  without skin
1 cup mashed potatoes with
  ¼ cup gravy
1 cup steamed broccoli
24 fl. oz ice water with slice of
  lemon
1 cup fresh blueberries with

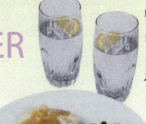
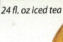

nutrient analysis

3,552 kcal
40.4% of energy from carbohydrates
43.2% of energy from fat
16.3% of energy from saturated fat
146 grams of protein
18.2 grams of dietary fiber
6,246 milligrams of sodium

Saves 1,653 calories!

nutrient analysis

1,899 kcal
54% of energy from carbohydrates
25.5% of energy from fat
6% of energy from saturated fat
100 grams of protein
33.3 grams of dietary fiber
2,402 milligrams of sodium

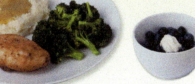
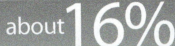

TABLE 6.2 **Protein Content of Commonly Consumed Foods**

Food	Serving Amount	Protein (g)	Food	Serving Amount	Protein (g)
Beef			**Dairy**		
Ground, lean, broiled (15% fat)	3 oz	22	Whole milk (3.25% fat)	8 fl. oz	7.7
			Skim milk	8 fl. oz	8.8
Beef tenderloin steak, broiled (1/8-in. fat)	3 oz	24.7	Low-fat, plain yogurt	8 fl. oz	12
Top sirloin, broiled (1/8-in. fat)	3 oz	23	Cottage cheese, low-fat (2%)	1 cup	23.6
Poultry			**Soy Products**		
Chicken breast, broiled, no skin (bone removed)	1/2 breast	27	Tofu, firm	1/2 cup	10
			Tempeh, cooked	3 oz	5.5
Chicken thigh, bone and skin removed	1 thigh	28	Soy milk beverage	1 cup	8
Turkey breast, roasted, luncheon meat	3 oz	18.7	**Beans**		
			Refried	1/2 cup	6.4
Seafood			Kidney, red	1/2 cup	6.7
Salmon, Chinook, baked	3 oz	22	Black	1/2 cup	7.2
Shrimp, cooked	3 oz	20.4	**Nuts**		
Tuna, in water, drained	3 oz	16.5	Peanuts, dry roasted	1 oz	6.9
Pork			Peanut butter, creamy	2 tbsp.	7
Pork loin chop, broiled	3 oz	22	Almonds, blanched	1 oz	6
Ham, roasted, extra lean (5% fat)	3 oz	18.7			

Source: Data from U.S. Department of Agriculture, Agricultural Research Service. 2015. USDA National Nutrient Database for Standard Reference, Release 28.

Nuts

Nuts are another healthful high-protein food. In fact, the USDA Food Patterns counts one-third cup of nuts or two tablespoons of peanut butter as equivalent to 1 ounce—about one-third of a serving—of meat! Moreover, studies show that consuming about 2 to 5 oz of nuts per week, in particular walnuts and peanuts, significantly reduces people's risk for cardiovascular disease and premature mortality from a range of causes.[6-8] Although the exact mechanism behind this is not known, nuts contain many nutrients and other substances that are associated with health benefits, including fiber, unsaturated fats, potassium, folate, plant sterols, and *antioxidants*, substances that can protect body cells (see Chapter 8).

"New" Foods

A new source of nonmeat protein that is available on the market is *quorn*, a protein product derived from fermented fungus. It is mixed with a variety of other foods to produce various types of meat substitutes. Other "new" foods high in protein include some very ancient grains! For instance, earlier we mentioned quinoa, a pseudo-grain that provides all nine essential amino acids. Quinoa is highly digestible and was so essential to the diet of the ancient Incas that they considered it sacred. Cooked much like rice, quinoa provides 8 g of protein in a 1-cup serving. A similar pseudo-grain, called amaranth, also provides complete protein. Teff, millet, and sorghum are grains long cultivated in Africa as rich sources of protein. They are now widely available in the United States. Although these three grains are low in the essential amino acid lysine, combining them with legumes produces a complete-protein meal.

How Much Protein Do You Eat?

One way to find out if your diet contains enough protein is to keep a food diary. Record everything you eat and drink for at least 3 days, and the grams of protein each item provides. To determine the grams of protein for packaged foods, use the Nutrition Facts panel, and make sure to adjust for the amount you actually consume. For products without labels, check Table 6.3 (on page 203), or use the diet analysis tools that accompany this text, or visit the U.S. Department of Agriculture National Nutrient Database for Standard Reference to find the energy and nutrient content of thousands of foods (see **Web Links**).

Below is an example, using Theo's food choices for 1 day. Do you think he's meeting his protein needs?

As calculated in the **You Do the Math** box (on page 195), Theo's RDA is 72.8 to 91 g of protein. He is consuming 2.3 to 2.8 times that amount! You can see that he does not need to use amino acid or protein supplements because he has more than adequate amounts of protein to build lean tissue.

Now calculate your own protein intake using food labels and a diet analysis program. Do you obtain more protein from animal or nonanimal sources? If you consume mostly nonanimal sources, are you eating soy products and complementary foods throughout the day? If you eat animal-based products on a regular basis, notice how much protein you consume from even small servings of meat and dairy products.

Foods Consumed	Protein Content (g)
Breakfast:	
Brewed coffee (2 cups) with 2 tbsp. cream	1.4
1 large bagel (5-in. diameter)	13
Low-fat cream cheese (2 tbsp.)	1.6
Mid-morning snack:	
Cola beverage (32 fl. oz)	0
Low-fat strawberry yogurt (1 cup)	10
Fruit and nut granola bar (2; 37 g each)	5.7
Lunch:	
Ham and cheese sandwich:	
Whole-wheat bread (2 slices)	4
Mayonnaise (1.5 tbsp.)	0.2
Extra lean ham (4 oz)	24
Swiss cheese (2 oz)	15
Iceberg lettuce (2 leaves)	0.3
Sliced tomato (3 slices)	0.5
Banana (1 large)	1.5
Wheat Thin crackers (20)	3.6
Bottled water (20 fl. oz)	0.0

Foods Consumed	Protein Content (g)
Dinner:	
Cheeseburger:	
Broiled ground beef (1/2 lb cooked)	52
American cheese (1 oz)	5
Seeded bun (1 large)	8
Ketchup (2 tbsp.)	0.5
Mustard (1 tbsp.)	0.7
Shredded lettuce (1/2 cup)	0.3
Sliced tomato (3 slices)	0.5
French fries (30; 2- to 3-in. strips)	5
Baked beans (2 cups)	24
2% low-fat milk (2 cups)	16
Evening snack:	
Chocolate chip cookies (4; 3-in. diameter)	3
2% low-fat milk (1 cup)	8
Total Protein Intake for the Day:	**203.8 g**

The Health Effects of High Protein Intake Are Unclear

Although protein deficiency is known to be life-threatening, the effect of high protein intakes on health risks is unclear. Three disorders linked in some research to high protein intakes are bone loss, kidney disease, and coronary heart disease.

Although high-protein diets can increase calcium excretion, current evidence does not support that this leads to bone loss. In fact, eating too *little* protein causes bone loss, which increases the risk for fractures and osteoporosis. Higher intakes of animal and soy protein have been shown to protect bone in middle-aged and older women. A recent systematic review concluded that there is no evidence to support

QuickTips

Adding Legumes to Your Daily Diet

Breakfast

✓ Instead of cereal, eggs, or a doughnut, microwave a frozen bean burrito for a quick, portable breakfast.

✓ Make your pancakes with soy milk, or pour soy milk on your cereal.

✓ If you normally have a side of bacon, ham, or sausage with your eggs, have a side of black beans instead.

Lunch and Dinner

✓ Try a sandwich made with hummus (a garbanzo bean spread), cucumbers, tomato, avocado, and/or lettuce on whole-wheat bread or in a whole-wheat pocket.

✓ Use deli "meats" made with soy in your sandwich. Also try soy hot dogs, burgers, and "chicken" nuggets.

✓ Add garbanzo beans, kidney beans, or fresh peas to tossed salads, or make a three-bean salad with kidney beans, green beans, and garbanzo beans.

✓ Make a side dish using legumes such as peas with pearl onions; succotash (lima beans, corn, and tomatoes); or homemade chili with kidney beans and tofu instead of meat.

✓ Make black bean soup, lentil soup, pea soup, minestrone soup, or a batch of dal (a type of yellow lentil used in Indian cuisine) and serve over brown rice. Top with plain yogurt, a traditional accompaniment in many Asian cuisines.

✓ Use soy "crumbles" in any recipe calling for ground beef.

✓ Make burritos with black or pinto beans instead of shredded meat.

✓ To stir-fried vegetables, add cubes of tofu or strips of tempeh.

✓ Make a "meatloaf" using cooked, mashed lentils instead of ground beef.

✓ For fast food at home, keep canned beans on hand. Serve over rice, couscous, or quinoa with a salad for a quick, complete, and hearty meal.

Snacks

✓ Instead of potato chips or pretzels, try one of the new bean chips.

✓ Dip fresh vegetables in bean dip.

✓ Serve hummus on wedges of pita bread.

✓ Spread peanut butter on celery sticks, apple slices, or whole-grain rice cakes.

✓ Add roasted soy "nuts" to your trail mix.

✓ Stock up on microwavable pouches of edamame (soybeans in pods). They're in the frozen foods section of most markets.

✓ Keep frozen tofu desserts, such as tofu ice cream, in your freezer.

the contention that high-protein diets lead to bone loss, except in people consuming inadequate calcium.[9]

A high-protein diet can increase the risk of acquiring kidney disease in people who are susceptible. Because people with diabetes have higher rates of kidney disease, it was previously assumed that they would benefit from a lower-protein diet. However, the evidence is inconclusive regarding the optimal amount of protein that people with diabetes should consume. The American Diabetes Association does not recommend a reduction in protein intake even in people with diabetes-related kidney disease.[10] In addition, there is no evidence that eating more protein causes kidney disease in healthy people. In fact, a recent review emphasizes that high protein intakes have no deleterious effects in athletes with normal renal function.[11] Thus, experts agree that eating as much as 2 g of protein per kilogram of body weight each day is safe for healthy people.

High-protein diets composed of predominantly animal sources have long been associated with higher blood cholesterol levels and an increased risk for coronary heart disease. These effects were assumed to be due to the saturated fat in animal products. As discussed in Chapter 5, although a recent review study found that eating more saturated fat was *not* associated with an increased risk for heart disease,[12] this topic is highly contentious as other studies have not supported the conclusions of this review.[13] So until we reach consensus on the optimal AMDR and sources of protein, nutrition experts recommend limiting your saturated fat intake and replacing it with healthful polyunsaturated fats from foods such as nuts, avocados, fish, whole grains, and olive oil.

Protein Deficiency Can Result in Severe Illness and Death

Consuming too little protein can cause severe debility, increased risk for infection, and death. Typically, this occurs when people do not consume enough total energy, and the result is **protein-energy malnutrition** (also called *protein-Calorie malnutrition*). Two diseases that can follow are marasmus and kwashiorkor **(FIGURE 6.14)**.

Protein Deficiency and Marasmus

Marasmus is a disease that results from a grossly inadequate intake of total energy, especially protein. Essentially, people with marasmus slowly starve to death. It is most common in young children (6 to 18 months of age) living in impoverished conditions who are severely undernourished. People suffering from marasmus have a look of "skin and bones" because their body fat and tissues are wasting (see Figure 6.14a). The consequences of marasmus include:

- Wasting and weakening of muscles, including the heart muscle.
- Stunted brain development and learning impairment.

protein-energy malnutrition A disorder caused by inadequate consumption of protein. It is characterized by severe wasting.

marasmus A form of protein-energy malnutrition that results from grossly inadequate intake of energy and protein and other nutrients and is characterized by extreme tissue wasting and stunted growth and development.

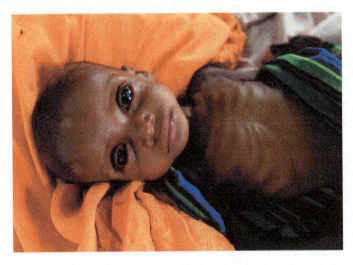

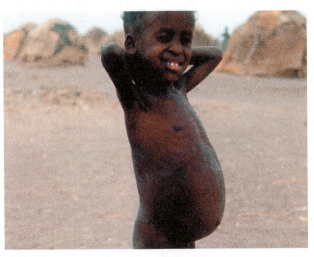

(a) (b)

🔺 **FIGURE 6.14** Two forms of protein-energy malnutrition: **(a)** marasmus and **(b)** kwashiorkor.

- Depressed metabolism and little insulation from body fat, causing a dangerously low body temperature.
- Stunted physical growth and development.
- Deterioration of the intestinal lining, which further inhibits the absorption of nutrients.
- *Anemia* (abnormally low levels of hemoglobin in the blood).
- Severely weakened immune system.
- Fluid and electrolyte imbalances.

If marasmus is left untreated, death from dehydration, heart failure, or infection will result. Treating marasmus involves carefully correcting fluid and electrolyte imbalances. Protein and carbohydrates are provided once the body's condition has stabilized. Fat is introduced much later, as the protein levels in the blood must improve to the point at which the body can use them to carry fat, so that it can be safely metabolized by the body.

Protein Deficiency and Kwashiorkor

Kwashiorkor often occurs in developing countries where infants are weaned early due to the arrival of a subsequent baby. This deficiency disease is typically seen in young children (1 to 3 years of age) who no longer drink breast milk. Instead, they often are fed a low-protein, starchy cereal. Recent research suggests that dysfunctional GI flora combined with a low-protein diet interact to contribute to the development of kwashiorkor.[14] Unlike marasmus, kwashiorkor often develops quickly and causes edema, particularly in the belly (see Figure 6.14b). This is because the low protein content of the blood is inadequate to keep fluids from seeping into the tissue spaces. The following are other signs and symptoms of kwashiorkor:

- Some weight loss and muscle wasting, with some retention of body fat.
- Retarded growth and development but less severe than that seen with marasmus.
- Fatty degeneration of the liver.
- Loss of appetite, sadness, irritability, apathy.
- Development of sores and other skin problems; skin pigmentation changes.
- Dry, brittle hair that changes color, straightens, and falls out easily.

Kwashiorkor can be reversed if adequate protein and energy are given in time. Because of their severely weakened immune systems, many individuals with kwashiorkor die from infections they contract in their weakened state. Of those who are treated, many return home to the same impoverished conditions, only to develop this deficiency again.

Many people think that only children in developing countries suffer from these diseases. However, protein-energy malnutrition occurs in all countries and affects both children and adults. In the United States, poor people living in inner cities and isolated rural areas are especially affected. Others at risk include the elderly, the homeless, people with eating disorders, those addicted to alcohol and other drugs, and individuals with wasting diseases, such as AIDS or cancer.

recap The RDA for protein for most nonpregnant, nonlactating, nonvegetarian adults is 0.8 g per kg body weight. Children, pregnant women, nursing mothers, vegetarians, and active people need more. Most people who eat enough kilocalories and carbohydrates have no problem meeting their RDA for protein. Good sources of protein include meats, eggs, dairy products, legumes, nuts, quorn, and certain "ancient grains." The health effects of a high protein intake are unclear; however, eating too much protein from animal sources may increase a person's risk for coronary heart disease. Protein-energy malnutrition can lead to marasmus and kwashiorkor. These diseases primarily affect impoverished children in developing nations. However, elderly, impoverished, and critically ill people in developed countries are also at risk.

kwashiorkor A form of protein-energy malnutrition that is typically seen in malnourished infants and toddlers and is characterized by wasting, edema, and other signs of protein deficiency.

Can a vegetarian diet provide adequate protein?

LO 6 List the benefits and potential challenges of consuming a vegetarian diet.

Vegetarianism is the practice of restricting the diet to food substances of plant origin, including vegetables, fruits, grains, and nuts. In a 2015 nationwide poll, 3.4% of all U.S. adults reported that they are vegetarian (never eat meat, poultry, or fish), and another 10% said that more than half of their meals are vegetarian.[15] And in 2014 a national poll found that 4% of youth age 8 to 18 are vegetarians.[16] Although precise statistics of vegetarianism among college students aren't available, moving away from home and taking responsibility for one's eating habits appears to influence many college students to try vegetarianism.

There Are Many Types of Vegetarian Diets

There are almost as many types of vegetarian diets as there are vegetarians. Some people who consider themselves vegetarians regularly eat poultry and fish. Others avoid the flesh of animals but consume eggs, milk, and cheese liberally. Still others strictly avoid all products of animal origin, including milk and eggs, and even by-products such as candies and puddings made with gelatin.

TABLE 6.3 identifies the various types of vegetarian diets, ranging from the most inclusive to the most restrictive. Notice that, the more restrictive the diet, the more challenging it becomes to achieve an adequate protein intake.

One type of "vegetarian" diet receiving significant media attention recently is the **plant-based diet**: it consists mostly of plant foods, as well as eggs, dairy, and occasionally red meat, poultry, and/or fish. A plant-based diet is consistent with the healthy eating pattern recommended in the *2015–2020 Dietary Guidelines for Americans*.[5]

TABLE 6.3 Terms and Definitions of a Vegetarian Diet

Type of Diet	Foods Consumed	Comments
Semivegetarian (also called flexitarian or plant-based diet)	Vegetables, grains, nuts, fruits, legumes; sometimes meat, seafood, poultry, eggs, and dairy products	Typically exclude or limit red meat; may also avoid other meats
Pescovegetarian	Similar to semivegetarian but excludes poultry	*Pesco* means "fish," the only animal source of protein in this diet
Lacto-ovovegetarian	Vegetables, grains, nuts, fruits, legumes, dairy products (*lacto*), and eggs (*ovo*)	Excludes animal flesh and seafood
Lacto-vegetarian	Similar to lacto-ovovegetarian but excludes eggs	Relies on milk and cheese for animal sources of protein
Ovovegetarian	Vegetables, grains, nuts, fruits, legumes, and eggs	Excludes dairy, flesh, and seafood products
Vegan (also called strict vegetarian)	Only plant-based foods (vegetables, grains, nuts, seeds, fruits, legumes)	May not provide adequate vitamin B_{12}, zinc, iron, or calcium
Macrobiotic diet	Vegan-type diet; becomes progressively more strict until almost all foods are eliminated; at the extreme, only brown rice and small amounts of water or herbal tea	Taken to the extreme, can cause malnutrition and death
Fruitarian	Only raw or dried fruit, seeds, nuts, honey, and vegetable oil	Very restrictive diet; deficient in protein, calcium, zinc, iron, vitamin B_{12}, riboflavin, and other nutrients

vegetarianism The practice of restricting the diet to foods and food substances of plant origin, including vegetables, fruits, grains, nuts, and seeds.

plant-based diet A diet consisting mostly of plant sources of foods, especially whole foods, with only limited amounts, if any, of animal-based and processed foods.

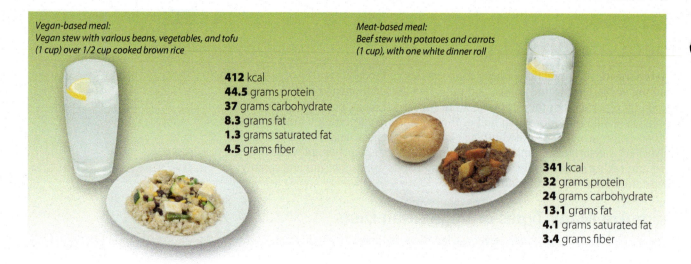

Vegan-based meal:
Vegan stew with various beans, vegetables, and tofu
(1 cup) over 1/2 cup cooked brown rice

412 kcal
44.5 grams protein
37 grams carbohydrate
8.3 grams fat
1.3 grams saturated fat
4.5 grams fiber

Meat-based meal:
Beef stew with potatoes and carrots
(1 cup), with one white dinner roll

341 kcal
32 grams protein
24 grams carbohydrate
13.1 grams fat
4.1 grams saturated fat
3.4 grams fiber

FIGURE 6.15 A comparison of the energy and macronutrient content of a vegan meal and a meat-based meal. Note that the amount and quality of protein in a vegan meal is comparable to that of a meat-based meal when the vegan meal combines a variety of vegetables, whole grain, and legumes.

Vegan diets have also attracted a great deal of attention in recent years. People who are vegans who do not eat meat, fish, or poultry, or foods considered to be animal products or by-products such as eggs and dairy products.[17] Some vegans also restrict the consumption of honey and the use of leather, fur, silk, wool, cosmetics, and soaps that have been derived from animal products. It is estimated that almost 15% of people who identify as vegetarians in the U.S. are vegans.[15] Although a vegan diet is more restrictive than some forms of vegetarianism, if carefully planned with a variety of foods, including fortified foods, it can be as nutritionally sound as an eating plan that includes animal products. **FIGURE 6.15** compares the macronutrient content of a vegan meal to that of a meat-based meal. As illustrated in this figure, a meal of vegan stew served with brown rice can provide more protein and fiber, and less fat and saturated fat, than a beef stew with potatoes and carrots served with a dinner roll.

People Choose Vegetarianism for Many Different Reasons

When discussing vegetarianism, one of the most often asked questions is why people would make this food choice. The most common responses are included here.

Religious, Ethical, and Food-Safety Reasons

Some make the choice for religious or spiritual reasons. Several religions prohibit or restrict the consumption of animal flesh; however, generalizations can be misleading. For example, whereas certain sects within Hinduism forbid the consumption of meat, perusing the menu at any Indian restaurant will reveal that many other Hindus regularly consume small quantities of meat, poultry, and fish. Many Buddhists are vegetarians, as are some Christians, including Seventh-Day Adventists.

Many vegetarians are guided by their personal philosophy to choose vegetarianism. These people feel that it is morally and ethically wrong to consume animals and, in the case of veganism, any products from animals (such as dairy or egg products), usually because they view the practices in the modern animal industries as inhumane. If vegetarians do consume milk and eggs, they may choose to purchase them only from family farms where they feel animals are treated humanely.

There is also a great deal of concern about meat handling practices, because contaminated meat has occasionally made its way into our food supply. Many outbreaks of severe illness, sometimes resulting in permanent disability and even death, have

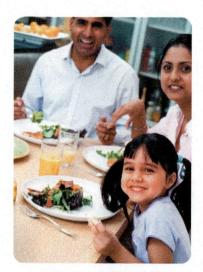

People who follow certain sects of Hinduism refrain from eating meat.

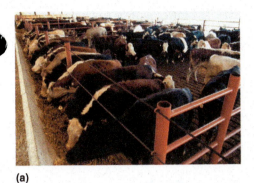
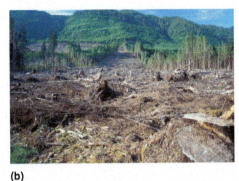

(a)   **(b)**

⬥ Some people choose vegetarianism out of concern for the environmental effects of meat production. For example, livestock production **(a)** and aggressive deforestation that clears land for grazing **(b)** both contribute to increased greenhouse gas emissions.

been traced to hamburgers and other meat items served at fast-food restaurants and meats sold in markets and consumed at home.

Ecological Benefits

Many people choose vegetarianism because of their concerns about the effect of meat production on the global environment. The growing global population and rising standard of living has increased the demand for meat in developed and developing nations. As a result, meat production has evolved from small family farming operations to the larger system of agribusiness. Critics point to the environmental costs of agribusiness: massive uses of natural resources to support animals; release of methane and other greenhouse gases produced by the animals; pollution of water and soils; and deforestation for land use to support livestock. For an in-depth discussion of this complex and often emotionally charged topic, refer to Chapter 13.

Health Benefits

Still others practice vegetarianism because of its health benefits. Research over several years has consistently shown that a varied and balanced vegetarian diet can reduce the risk for many chronic diseases. Its health benefits include the following:

- Reduced intake of fat and total energy, which reduces the risk for obesity. This may in turn lower a person's risk for type 2 diabetes.
- Lower blood pressure, which may be due to a higher intake of fruits and vegetables. However, people who eat vegetarian diets tend to be nonsmokers, to drink alcohol in moderation if at all, and to exercise regularly, all of which are also factors known to reduce blood pressure.
- Reduced risk for heart disease, which may be due to lower saturated fat intake and a higher consumption of dietary fiber and *antioxidant vitamins, minerals, and phytochemicals.* As noted earlier, antioxidants (discussed in detail in Chapter 8) help protect our cells. They are abundant in fruits and vegetables.
- Fewer digestive problems such as constipation and diverticular disease, perhaps due to the higher fiber content of vegetarian diets. Diverticular disease (discussed in Chapter 4) occurs when the wall of the large intestine pouches and becomes inflamed.
- Reduced risk for some cancers. Research shows that vegetarians may have lower rates of cancer, particularly colorectal cancer. Many components of a vegetarian diet could contribute to reducing cancer risks, including antioxidants, fiber, no intake of red meats and processed meats (which increase the risk for colorectal cancer), and lower consumption of *carcinogens* (cancer-causing agents) that are formed when cooking meat.[18]

- Reduced risk for kidney stones and gallstones. The lower protein contents of vegetarian diets, plus the higher intake of legumes and vegetable proteins such as soy, may be protective against these conditions.

A recent review of the evidence from three prospective cohort studies of Seventh-Day Adventists in North America confirmed that vegetarian diets conferred greater health benefits as highlighted above.[19] In addition, this review stated that consuming a vegan-type eating pattern appeared to provide additional benefits of reduced obesity, hypertension, type 2 diabetes, and premature mortality from cardiovascular disease as compared to a lacto-ovovegetarian eating pattern.[19]

A Vegetarian Diet Can Present Some Challenges

Although a vegetarian diet can be healthful, it also presents some challenges. Limiting the consumption of flesh and dairy products introduces the potential for inadequate intakes of certain nutrients, especially for people consuming a vegan, macrobiotic, or fruitarian diet. TABLE 6.4 lists the nutrients that can be deficient in a vegan type of diet plan and describes good nonanimal sources that can provide these nutrients. Vegetarians who consume dairy and/or egg products obtain these nutrients more easily.

Research indicates that individuals with a history of disordered eating are more likely to switch to a vegetarian diet.[20] Instead of eating a healthful variety of non-animal foods, people with disordered eating problems may use vegetarianism as an excuse to restrict many foods from their diet. To learn more about disordered eating, refer to In Depth 11.5.

Can a vegetarian diet provide enough protein? In developed countries, where high-quality nonmeat protein sources are easy to obtain, the answer is yes. In fact, the Academy of Nutrition and Dietetics endorses an appropriately planned vegetarian diet as healthful, nutritionally adequate, and beneficial in reducing and preventing various diseases. Like any diet, however, a vegetarian diet should be *balanced* and *adequate*; thus, it is important for vegetarians to eat complementary proteins and obtain enough energy from other macronutrients to spare protein from being used as an energy

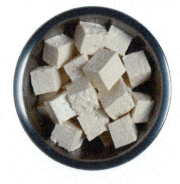

▲ Vegetarians should eat two to three servings of beans, nuts, seeds, eggs, or meat substitutes (such as tofu) daily.

TABLE 6.4 Nutrients of Concern in a Vegan Diet

Nutrient	Functions	Nonmeat/Nondairy Food Sources
Vitamin B$_{12}$	Assists with DNA synthesis; protection and growth of nerve fibers	Vitamin B$_{12}$–fortified cereals, yeast, soy products, and other meat analogs; vitamin B$_{12}$ supplements
Vitamin D	Promotes bone growth	Vitamin D–fortified cereals, margarines, and soy products; adequate exposure to sunlight; supplementation may be necessary for those who do not get adequate exposure to sunlight
Riboflavin (vitamin B$_2$)	Promotes release of energy; supports normal vision and skin health	Whole and enriched grains, green leafy vegetables, mushrooms, beans, nuts, and seeds
Iron	Assists with oxygen transport; involved in making amino acids and hormones	Whole-grain products, prune juice, dried fruits, beans, nuts, seeds, and leafy vegetables (such as spinach)
Calcium	Maintains bone health; assists with muscle contraction, blood pressure, and nerve transmission	Fortified soy milk and tofu, almonds, dry beans, leafy vegetables, calcium-fortified juices, and fortified breakfast cereals
Zinc	Assists with DNA and RNA synthesis, immune function, and growth	Whole-grain products, wheat germ, beans, nuts, and seeds

nutri-case | THEO

"No way would I ever become a vegetarian! The only way to build up muscle is to eat meat. I read in a bodybuilding magazine about some guy who doesn't eat anything from animals, not even milk or eggs, and he did look pretty buff . . . but I don't buy it. They can do anything to pictures these days. Besides, after a game I just crave red meat. If I don't have it, I feel sort of like my batteries don't get recharged. It's just not natural for a competitive athlete to go without meat!" What claims does Theo make here about the role of red meat in his diet? Do you think his claims are valid? Why or why not? Without trying to convert Theo to vegetarianism, what facts might you offer him about the nature of plant and animal proteins?

source. Although the digestibility of a vegetarian diet is potentially lower than that of an animal-based diet, there is no separate protein recommendation for vegetarians who consume complementary plant proteins.[21]

MyPlate Can Help You Plan a Vegetarian Diet

Although the USDA has not designed a version of MyPlate specifically for people following a vegetarian diet, healthy eating tips for vegetarians are available at MyPlate online (see the **Web Links** at the end of this chapter). For example, to meet their needs for protein and calcium, lacto-vegetarians can consume low-fat or nonfat dairy products. Vegans and ovovegetarians can consume calcium-fortified soy milk or one of the many protein bars fortified with calcium.

Vegans need to consume vitamin B_{12} either from fortified foods or supplements because this vitamin is found naturally only in foods derived from animals. They should also pay special attention to consuming foods high in vitamin D, riboflavin (B_2), and the minerals zinc and iron. Supplementation of these micronutrients may be necessary for some people if they do not consume adequate amounts in their diet.

> If you're interested in trying a vegetarian diet but don't know where to begin, check out the website of the Physicians Committee for Responsible Medicine at www.pcrm.org. Click on "Health and Nutrition," and then select "Vegetarian and Vegan Diets." Scroll down until you see the "Vegetarian Starter Kit."

recap Vegetarian diets vary from vegan diets, which include no animal-based foods or ingredients of any kind, to plant-based diets, which may include eggs, dairy, and even limited amounts of meat, poultry, and fish. A balanced vegetarian diet may reduce the risk for obesity, type 2 diabetes, hypertension and heart disease, digestive problems, some cancers, kidney stones, and gallstones. Whereas varied vegetarian diets can provide enough protein, vegans need to make sure they consume adequate plant sources of complementary proteins and foods fortified with vitamin B_{12}. They also need to ensure their diet provides adequate vitamin D, riboflavin, iron, calcium, and zinc.

In 2005, the Institute of Medicine (IOM, which is now the Health and Medicine Division of the National Academies of Sciences, Engineering, and Medicine) concluded that a protein intake of 0.8 gram per kilogram body weight is sufficient to maintain nitrogen balance in healthy adults no matter what their activity level.[21] However, there is now increasing evidence that the current RDA may not be sufficient to support optimal health and function for various groups, and experts are calling for a critical reexamination of the RDA to determine whether or not it should be increased.[22]

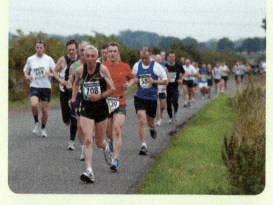

A growing body of research suggests that the current RDA for protein is not high enough to support the needs of athletes or older adults.

Specifically, experts working with athletes and highly active people have argued for a number of years that ample evidence indicates that the protein needs of these groups are higher than the current RDA.[2] Although the IOM states there is insufficient evidence to support this contention,[21] these experts point to several factors that increase athletes' protein requirements:

- Regular exercise increases the transport of oxygen to body tissues, requiring changes in the oxygen-carrying capacity of the blood. To carry more oxygen, we need to produce more of the protein that carries oxygen in the blood (that is, hemoglobin, which is a protein).

- During intense exercise, we use a small amount of protein directly for energy.

- We also use protein to make glucose to prevent hypoglycemia (low blood sugar) during exercise.

- Regular exercise stimulates tissue growth and causes tissue damage, which must be repaired by additional proteins.

As a result of these increased demands for protein, the American College of Sports Medicine has concluded that athletes need 1.2 to 2 grams of protein per kilogram body weight per day, which is equivalent to 1.8 to 2.5 times more protein than the current RDA. They state that there should no longer be a distinction made between strength and endurance athletes, as protein needs vary based on training, personal performance goals, energy and nutrient needs, and a person's food choices.[2] Based on this evidence, protein intake recommendations should be flexible and individualized.

Research examining protein needs in adults older than 65 years of age and children suggests that the protein needs

for these populations—to meet optimal growth, tissue repair, and regeneration, function, and health—also are higher than the current RDA.[23-26] For instance, some researchers suggest that, to preserve lean body tissue and physical function, older adults may need 1.0 to 1.5 grams of protein per kilogram of body weight, which is 1.25 to 1.88 times the current RDA. Children's protein needs may be 1.63 to 1.71 higher than the current RDA.

What could be contributing to this discrepancy between recent research findings and the evidence used to set the RDAs for protein? One factor may be that the current RDAs are based on evidence determined by the nitrogen balance method, which is known to underestimate protein needs. In contrast, a relatively new method, referred to as the *indicator amino acid technique* (*IAAO*), appears to overestimate protein needs.[21] A second factor in the discrepancy may be a lack of correspondence between nitrogen balance and health; that is, we don't currently know whether or not consuming enough protein to meet nitrogen balance optimizes health and functioning. As such, there is clearly a need for research that critically examines the methods used to measure protein needs, and the amounts needed to support health.

Should you worry about your protein intake? As discussed earlier in this chapter, most Americans, no matter what their activity level, already consume more than twice the RDA for protein. Thus, even if the RDA were increased, it is highly likely that you are already meeting or exceeding it.

CRITICAL THINKING QUESTIONS

1. Before taking this course, did you feel you would benefit from consuming more protein? Why or why not?

2. Based on your estimate of your current protein intake in the Nutrition Label Activity, do you already meet or exceed the suggested protein intake for athletes indicated above?

3. Using an Internet search, identify at least two adverse effects to people's health, and two adverse effects on the environment, that could result from increasing the current RDA for protein. How would your answer differ if people increased their protein exclusively through consuming plant-based sources?

TEST YOURSELF | ANSWERS

1 F Although protein can be used for energy in certain circumstances, fats and carbohydrates are the primary sources of energy for our body.

2 T Most people in the United States consume up to two times more protein than they need.

3 F Vegetarian diets can meet and even exceed an individual's protein needs, assuming that adequate energy-yielding macronutrients, a variety of protein sources, and complementary protein sources are consumed.

review questions

LO 1 **1.** Proteins contain
a. carbon, nitrogen, and aluminum.
b. hydrogen, oxygen, and nitrates.
c. hydrogen, carbon, oxygen, and nitrogen.
d. helium, carbon, oxygen, and ammonia.

LO 2 **2.** Which of the following statements about protein synthesis is true?
a. Protein synthesis occurs in the nucleus of the cell.
b. Messenger RNA carries amino acids to ribosomes for assembly into proteins.
c. In the process of transcription, transfer RNA transfers its DNA onto a ribosome.
d. None of the above is true.

LO 2 **3.** The process of combining peanut butter and whole-wheat bread to make a complete protein is called
a. deamination.
b. vegetarianism.
c. transamination.
d. mutual supplementation.

LO 3 **4.** Proteins in the blood
a. exert pressure that draws fluid out of tissue spaces, preventing edema.
b. can bind to excessive hydrogen ions, preventing alkalosis.
c. can be converted to urea, which can then be used as energy.
d. all of the above.

LO 4 **5.** The enzyme that helps break down polypeptides in the small intestine is called
a. hydrochloric acid.
b. pepsin.
c. protease.
d. bile.

LO 5 **6.** Which of the following statements about the RDA for protein is true?
a. Athletes typically require about three times as much protein as nonathletes.
b. The RDA for protein is higher for men than for women.
c. The RDA for protein is higher for children and adolescents than for adults.
d. Most Americans eat about three times the RDA for protein.

LO 5 **7.** In treating protein-energy malnutrition, why is protein intake restored before feeding the patient fats?
a. Protein is a more readily available source of energy than fats.
b. Protein levels in the blood must be adequate to transport fat.
c. Protein is made up of DNA, which directs the metabolism of fats.
d. Protein is the primary component of bile, which is required to emulsify fats.

LO 6 8. Which of the following meals is typical of a vegan diet?

    a. Rice, pinto beans, acorn squash, soy butter, and almond milk

    b. Veggie dog, bun, and a banana blended with yogurt

    c. Brown rice and green tea

    d. Egg salad on whole-wheat toast, broccoli, carrot sticks, and soy milk

LO 4 9. **True or false?** After leaving the small intestine, amino acids are transported to the liver and stored for later use.

LO 5 10. **True or false?** The only sources of complete proteins are foods derived from animals.

math review

LO 5 11. Barry is concerned he is not eating enough protein. After reading this chapter, he recorded his diet each day for 1 week to calculate how much protein he is eating. Barry's average protein intake for the week is equal to 190 g, his body weight is 75 kg, and his daily energy intake averages 3,000 kcal. Based on your calculations, is Barry (a) meeting or exceeding the AMDR for protein and (b) meeting or exceeding the RDA for protein?

Answers to Review Questions and Math Review are located at the back of this text and in the MasteringNutrition Study area.

web links

www.eatright.org

Academy of Nutrition and Dietetics

Search for "vegetarian diets" to learn more about vegetarian lifestyles, types of vegetarianism, and how to plan healthful meat-free meals.

ndb.nal.usda.gov

USDA National Nutrient Database for Standard Reference

Click on "Start your search here" to find a searchable database of the nutrient values of many foods.

www.who.int/nutrition/en/

World Health Organization Nutrition

Visit this site to find out more about the worldwide scope of protein–deficiency diseases and related topics, in their nutrition topics.

www.vrg.org

The Vegetarian Resource Group

Visit this site for additional information on how to build a balanced vegetarian diet, or to download their vegan MyPlate.

www.choosemyplate.gov

The USDA's MyPlate Website

The MyPlate website contains useful, healthy eating tips for vegetarians. Enter "vegetarian" in the search box, then click on "Tips for Vegetarians."

www.meatlessmonday.com

Meatless Monday Campaign

Find out how to start going meatless one day a week with this innovative campaign's website.

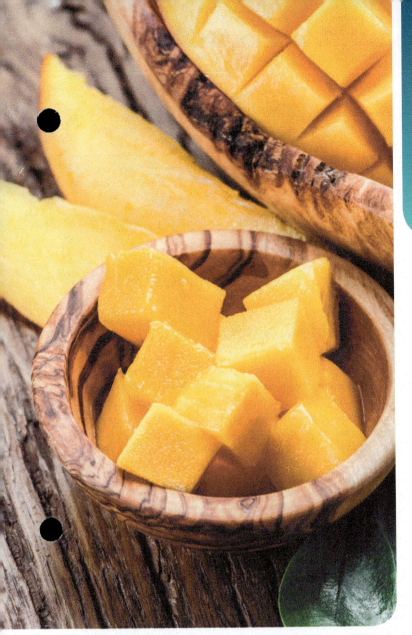

Vitamins and Minerals: Micronutrients with Macro Powers

learning outcomes

After studying this In Depth, you should be able to:

1 Identify some observations that led to the discovery of micronutrients, p. 212.

2 Distinguish between fat-soluble and water-soluble vitamins, pp. 212–214.

3 Describe the differences between major, trace, and ultra-trace minerals, pp. 214–218.

4 Explain why the amount of a micronutrient we consume differs from the amount our body absorbs and uses, p. 218.

5 Discuss three controversial topics in micronutrient research, pp. 218–221.

Have you ever heard about the college student on a junk-food diet who developed scurvy, a disease caused by inadequate intake of vitamin C? This urban legend seems to circulate on many college campuses every year, but that might be because there's some truth behind it. Away from their families, many college students adopt diets that are deficient in one or more micronutrients. For instance, some students adopt a vegan diet with insufficient iron, while others neglect foods rich in calcium and vitamin D. Why is it important to consume adequate levels of the micronutrients, and exactly what constitutes a micronutrient, anyway? This **In Depth** essay explores the discovery of micronutrients, their classification and naming, and their impact on our health.

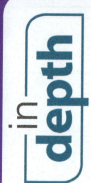
How were the micronutrients discovered?

LO 1 Identify some observations that led to the discovery of micronutrients.

Recall that the macronutrients carbohydrates, fats, and proteins provide energy; thus, we need to consume them in relatively large amounts. In contrast, the micronutrients, vitamins and minerals, are needed in very small amounts. They are nevertheless essential to our survival, assisting critical body functions such as energy metabolism and the formation and maintenance of healthy cells and tissues.

Much of our knowledge of vitamins and minerals comes from accidental observations of animals and humans. For instance, in the 1890s, a Dutch physician named C. Eijkman noticed that chickens fed polished rice developed paralysis, which could be reversed by feeding them whole-grain rice. Noting the high incidence of *beriberi*—a disease that results in extensive nerve damage—among hospital patients fed polished rice, Eijkman hypothesized that a highly refined diet was the primary cause of beriberi. We now know that whole-grain rice, with its nutrient-rich bran layer, contains the vitamin thiamin and that thiamin deficiency results in beriberi.

Similarly, in the early 1900s, it was observed that Japanese children living in fishing villages rarely developed a type of blindness that was common among Japanese children who did not eat fish. Experiments soon showed that cod liver oil, chicken liver, and eel fat prevented the disorder. We now know that each of these foods contains vitamin A, which is essential for healthy vision.

Such observations were followed by years of laboratory research before nutritionists came to fully accept the idea that very small amounts of substances present in food are critical to good health. In 1906, English scientist F. G. Hopkins coined the term *accessory factors* for those substances; we now call them vitamins and minerals.

How are vitamins classified?

LO 2 Distinguish between fat-soluble and water-soluble vitamins.

Vitamins are organic compounds that regulate a wide range of body processes. Of the 13 vitamins recognized as essential, humans can synthesize only small amounts of vitamins D and K and niacin (a B vitamin), so we must consume virtually all of the vitamins in our diet. Most people who eat a varied and healthful diet can readily meet their vitamin needs from foods alone. The exceptions to this will be discussed shortly.

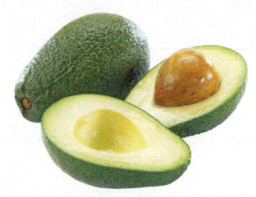

Avocados are a source of fat-soluble vitamins.

Fat-Soluble Vitamins

Vitamins A, D, E, and K are fat-soluble vitamins (TABLE 1). They are found in the fatty portions of foods (butterfat, cod liver oil, corn oil, etc.) and are absorbed along with dietary fat. Fat-containing meats, dairy products, nuts, seeds, vegetable oils, and avocados are all sources of one or more fat-soluble vitamins.

In general, the fat-soluble vitamins are readily stored in the body's adipose tissue; thus, we don't need to consume them every day. While this may simplify day-to-day menu planning, there is also a disadvantage to our ability to store these nutrients. When we consume more of them than we can use, they build up in the adipose tissue, liver, and other tissues and can reach toxic levels. Symptoms of fat-soluble vitamin toxicity, described in Table 1, include damage to our hair, skin, bones, eyes, and nervous system. Overconsumption of vitamin supplements is the most common cause of vitamin toxicity in the United States; rarely do our dietary choices lead to toxicity. Of the four fat-soluble vitamins, vitamins A and D are the most toxic; **megadosing** with 10 or more times the recommended intake of either can result in irreversible organ damage and even death.

Even though we can store the fat-soluble vitamins, deficiencies can occur, especially in people who have a malabsorption disorder, such as celiac disease, that reduces their ability to absorb dietary fat. In addition, people who eat very little dietary fat are at risk for a deficiency due to low intake and poor absorption. The consequences of fat-soluble vitamin deficiencies, described in Table 1, include osteoporosis, the loss of night vision, and even death in the most severe cases.

Water-Soluble Vitamins

Vitamin C (ascorbic acid) and the B-vitamins (thiamin, riboflavin, niacin, vitamin B$_6$, vitamin B$_{12}$, folate, pantothenic acid, and biotin) are all water-soluble vitamins

---

megadosing Taking a dose of a nutrient that is 10 or more times greater than the recommended amount.

TABLE 1   Fat-Soluble Vitamins

Vitamin Name	Primary Functions	Recommended Intake*	Reliable Food Sources	Toxicity/Deficiency Symptoms
A (retinol, retinal, retinoic acid)	Required for ability of eyes to adjust to changes in light Protects color vision Assists cell differentiation Required for sperm production in men and fertilization in women Contributes to healthy bone Contributes to healthy immune system	RDA: Men: 900 μg/day Women: 700 μg/day UL: 3,000 μg/day	Preformed retinol: beef and chicken liver, egg yolks, milk Carotenoid precursors: spinach, carrots, mango, apricots, cantaloupe, pumpkin, yams	*Toxicity:* Fatigue, bone and joint pain, spontaneous abortion and birth defects of fetuses in pregnant women, nausea and diarrhea, liver damage, nervous system damage, blurred vision, hair loss, skin disorders *Deficiency:* Night blindness and xerophthalmia; impaired growth, immunity, and reproductive function
D (cholecalciferol)	Regulates blood calcium levels Maintains bone health Assists cell differentiation	RDA: Adults aged 19–70: 15μg/day Adults aged >70: 20 μg/day UL 100 μg/day	Canned salmon and mackerel, milk, fortified cereals	*Toxicity:* Hypercalcemia *Deficiency:* Rickets in children, osteomalacia and/or osteoporosis in adults
E (tocopherol)	As a powerful antioxidant, protects cell membranes, polyunsaturated fatty acids, and vitamin A from oxidation Protects white blood cells Enhances immune function Improves absorption of vitamin A	RDA: Men: 15 mg/day Women: 15 mg/day UL: 1,000 mg/day	Sunflower seeds, almonds, vegetable oils, fortified cereals	*Toxicity:* Rare *Deficiency:* Hemolytic anemia; impairment of nerve, muscle, and immune function
K (phylloquinone, menaquinone, menadione)	Serves as a coenzyme during production of specific proteins that assist in blood coagulation and bone metabolism	AI: Men: 120 μg/day Women: 90 μg/day	Kale, spinach, turnip greens, brussels sprouts	*Toxicity:* None known *Deficiency:* Impaired blood clotting, possible effect on bone health

*RDA: Recommended Dietary Allowance; UL: upper limit; AI: Adequate Intake.

(TABLE 2) (see page 215). They are found in a wide variety of foods, including whole grains, fruits, vegetables, meats, and dairy products. In general, they are easily absorbed through the intestinal tract directly into the bloodstream, where they then travel to target cells.

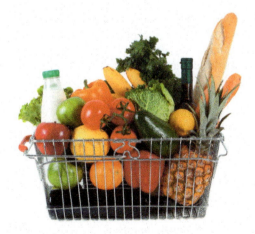

Water-soluble vitamins can be found in a variety of foods.

With the exception of vitamin B$_{12}$, we do not store large amounts of water-soluble vitamins. Instead, our kidneys filter from our bloodstream any excess, which is excreted in urine. Because our tissues don't store these vitamins, toxicity is rare. When it does occur, however, it is often from the overuse of high-potency vitamin supplements. Toxicity can cause nerve damage and skin lesions.

Because most water-soluble vitamins are not stored in large amounts, they need to be consumed on a daily or weekly basis. Deficiency symptoms, including serious disorders, can arise fairly quickly, especially during fetal development and in growing infants and children. The signs of water-soluble vitamin deficiency vary widely and are identified in Table 2.

Same Vitamin, Different Names and Forms

Food and supplement labels, magazine articles, and even nutrition textbooks often use simple, alphabetic (A, D, E, K, etc.) names for the fat-soluble vitamins. The letters reflect their order of discovery: vitamin A was discovered in 1916, whereas vitamin K was not isolated until 1939. These lay terms, however, are more appropriately viewed as "umbrellas" that unify a small cluster of chemically related compounds. For example, the term *vitamin A* refers to the specific compounds retinol, retinal, and retinoic acid. Similarly, *vitamin E* occurs naturally in eight forms, known as tocopherols, of which the primary form is alpha-tocopherol. Compounds with *vitamin D* activity include cholecalciferol and ergocalciferol, and the *vitamin K* "umbrella" includes phylloquinone and menaquinone. As you can see, most of the individual compounds making up a fat-soluble vitamin cluster have similar chemical designations (tocopherols, calciferols, and so on). Table 1 lists both the alphabetic and the chemical terms for the fat-soluble vitamins.

Similarly, there are both alphabetic and chemical designations for water-soluble vitamins. In some cases,

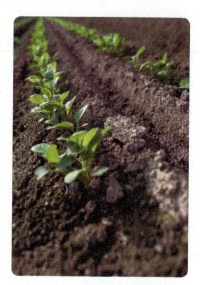

Plants absorb minerals from soil and water.

such as *vitamin C* and *ascorbic acid*, you may be familiar with both terms. But few people would recognize *cobalamin* as *vitamin B$_{12}$*. Some of the water-soluble vitamins, such as niacin and vitamin B$_6$, mimic the "umbrella" clustering seen with vitamins A, E, D, and K: the term *vitamin B$_6$* includes pyridoxal, pyridoxine, and pyridoxamine. If you read any of these three terms on a supplement label, you'll know it refers to vitamin B$_6$.

The vitamins pantothenic acid and biotin exist in only one form. There are no other related chemical compounds linked to either vitamin. Table 2 lists both the alphabetic and chemical terms for the water-soluble vitamins.

Since all vitamins are organic compounds, they are all more or less vulnerable to degradation from exposure to heat, oxygen, or other factors. For tips on preserving the vitamins in the foods you eat, see the nearby **Quick Tips**.

How are minerals classified?

LO 3 Describe the differences between major, trace, and ultra-trace minerals.

Minerals—such as calcium, iron, and zinc—are crystalline elements; that is, you'll find them on the periodic table. Because they are already in the simplest chemical form possible, the body does not digest or break them down prior to absorption. For the same reason, they cannot be degraded on exposure to heat or any other natural process, so the minerals in foods remain intact during storage and cooking. Furthermore, unlike vitamins, they cannot be synthesized in the laboratory or by any plant or animal, including humans. Minerals are the same wherever they are found—in soil, a car part, or the human body. The minerals in our foods ultimately come from the environment; for example, the selenium in soil and water is taken up into plants and then incorporated into the animals that eat the plants. Whether we eat the plant foods directly or the animal products, we consume the minerals.

Minerals are classified according to the intake required and the amount present in the body. The three groups include major, trace, and ultra-trace minerals.

Major Minerals

Major minerals are those the body requires in amounts of at least 100 mg per day. In addition, these minerals are found in the body in amounts of 5 g (5,000 mg) or higher. There are seven major minerals: sodium, potassium, phosphorus, chloride, calcium, magnesium, and sulfur.

TABLE 2 **Water-Soluble Vitamins**

Vitamin Name	Primary Functions	Recommended Intake*	Reliable Food Sources	Toxicity/Deficiency Symptoms
Thiamin (vitamin B_1)	Required as enzyme cofactor for carbohydrate and amino acid metabolism	RDA: Men: 1.2 mg/day Women: 1.1 mg/day	Pork, fortified cereals, enriched rice and pasta, peas, tuna, legumes	*Toxicity:* None known *Deficiency:* Beriberi; fatigue, apathy, decreased memory, confusion, irritability, muscle weakness
Riboflavin (vitamin B_2)	Required as enzyme cofactor for carbohydrate and fat metabolism	RDA: Men: 1.3 mg/day Women: 1.1 mg/day	Beef liver, shrimp, milk and other dairy foods, fortified cereals, enriched breads and grains	*Toxicity:* None known *Deficiency:* Ariboflavinosis; swollen mouth and throat; seborrheic dermatitis; anemia
Niacin, nicotinamide, nicotinic acid	Required for carbohydrate and fat metabolism Plays a role in DNA replication and repair and cell differentiation	RDA: Men: 16 mg/day Women: 14 mg/day UL: 35 mg/day	Beef liver, most cuts of meat/fish/poultry, fortified cereals, enriched breads and grains, canned tomato products	*Toxicity:* Flushing, liver damage, glucose intolerance, blurred vision *Deficiency:* Pellagra; vomiting, constipation, or diarrhea; apathy
Pyridoxine, pyridoxal, pyridoxamine (vitamin B_6)	Required as enzyme cofactor for carbohydrate and amino acid metabolism Assists synthesis of blood cells	RDA: Men and women aged 19–50: 1.3 mg/day Men aged >50: 1.7 mg/day Women aged >50: 1.5 mg/day UL: 100 mg/day	Chickpeas (garbanzo beans), most cuts of meat/fish/poultry, fortified cereals, white potatoes	*Toxicity:* Nerve damage, skin lesions *Deficiency:* Anemia; seborrheic dermatitis; depression, confusion, and convulsions
Folate (folic acid)	Required as enzyme cofactor for amino acid metabolism Required for DNA synthesis Involved in metabolism of homocysteine	RDA: Men: 400 µg/day Women: 400 µg/day UL: 1,000 µg/day	Fortified cereals, enriched breads and grains, spinach, legumes (lentils, chickpeas, pinto beans), greens (spinach, romaine lettuce), liver	*Toxicity:* Masks symptoms of vitamin B_{12} deficiency, specifically signs of nerve damage *Deficiency:* Macrocytic anemia, neural tube defects in a developing fetus, elevated homocysteine levels
Cobalamin (vitamin B_{12})	Assists with formation of blood cells Required for healthy nervous system function Involved as enzyme cofactor in metabolism of homocysteine	RDA: Men: 2.4 µg/day Women: 2.4 µg/day	Shellfish, all cuts of meat/fish/poultry, milk and other dairy foods, fortified cereals	*Toxicity:* None known *Deficiency:* Pernicious anemia; tingling and numbness of extremities; nerve damage; memory loss, disorientation, and dementia
Pantothenic acid	Assists with fat metabolism	AI: Men: 5 mg/day Women: 5 mg/day	Meat/fish/poultry, shiitake mushrooms, fortified cereals, egg yolk	*Toxicity:* None known *Deficiency:* Rare
Biotin	Involved as enzyme cofactor in carbohydrate, fat, and protein metabolism	RDA: Men: 30 µg/day Women: 30 µg/day	Nuts, egg yolk	*Toxicity:* None known *Deficiency:* Rare
Ascorbic acid (vitamin C)	Antioxidant in extracellular fluid and lungs Regenerates oxidized vitamin E Assists with collagen synthesis Enhances immune function Assists in synthesis of hormones, neurotransmitters, and DNA Enhances iron absorption	RDA: Men: 90 mg/day Women: 75 mg/day Smokers: 35 mg more per day than RDA UL: 2,000 mg	Sweet peppers, citrus fruits and juices, broccoli, strawberries, kiwi	*Toxicity:* Nausea and diarrhea, nosebleeds, increased oxidative damage, increased formation of kidney stones in people with kidney disease *Deficiency:* Scurvy, bone pain and fractures, depression, anemia

*RDA: Recommended Dietary Allowance; UL: upper limit; AI: Adequate Intake.

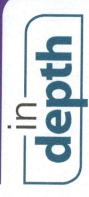
TABLE 3 summarizes the primary functions, recommended intakes, food sources, and toxicity/deficiency symptoms of these minerals.

Trace and Ultra-Trace Minerals

Trace minerals are those we need to consume in amounts of less than 100 mg per day. They are found in the human body in amounts of less than 5 g (5,000 mg). Four trace minerals have an established RDA or AI: fluoride, iron, manganese, and zinc.[1] **TABLE 4** identifies the primary functions, recommended intakes, food sources, and toxicity/deficiency symptoms of these minerals.

A subset of trace minerals is a group known as *ultra-trace minerals* because they are required in amounts less than 1 mg per day. The DRI Committee has established an RDA or AI guideline for five ultra-trace minerals: chromium, copper, iodine, molybdenum, and selenium.[1]

TABLE 3 Major Minerals

Mineral Name	Primary Functions	Recommended Intake*	Reliable Food Sources	Toxicity/Deficiency Symptoms
Sodium	Fluid balance Acid–base balance Transmission of nerve impulses Muscle contraction	AI: Adults: 1.5 g/day (1,500 mg/day)	Table salt, pickles, most canned soups, snack foods, cured luncheon meats, canned tomato products	*Toxicity:* Water retention, high blood pressure in some populations, loss of calcium in urine *Deficiency:* Muscle cramps, dizziness, fatigue, nausea, vomiting, mental confusion
Potassium	Fluid balance Transmission of nerve impulses Muscle contraction	AI: Adults: 4.7 g/day (4,700 mg/day)	Most fresh fruits and vegetables: potatoes, bananas, tomato juice, orange juice, melons	*Toxicity:* Muscle weakness, vomiting, irregular heartbeat *Deficiency:* Muscle weakness, paralysis, mental confusion, irregular heartbeat
Phosphorus	Fluid balance Bone formation Component of ATP, which provides energy for our body	RDA: Adults: 700 mg/day	Milk/cheese/yogurt, soy milk and tofu, legumes (lentils, black beans), nuts (almonds, peanuts and peanut butter), poultry	*Toxicity:* Muscle spasms, convulsions, low blood calcium *Deficiency:* Muscle weakness, muscle damage, bone pain, dizziness
Chloride	Fluid balance Transmission of nerve impulses Component of stomach acid (HCl) Antibacterial	AI: Adults: 2.3 g/day (2,300 mg/day)	Table salt	*Toxicity:* None known *Deficiency:* dangerous blood acid–base imbalances, irregular heartbeat
Calcium	Primary component of bone Acid–base balance Transmission of nerve impulses Muscle contraction	RDA: Adults aged 19–50 and men aged 51–70: 1,000 mg/day Women aged 51–70 and adults aged >70: 1,200 mg/day UL for adults 19–50: 2,500 mg/day UL for adults aged 51 and above: 2,000 mg/day	Milk/yogurt/cheese (best-absorbed form of calcium), sardines, collard greens and spinach, calcium-fortified juices	*Toxicity:* Mineral imbalances, shock, kidney failure, fatigue, mental confusion *Deficiency:* Osteoporosis, convulsions, heart failure
Magnesium	Component of bone Muscle contraction Assists more than 300 enzyme systems	RDA: Men aged 19–30: 400 mg/day Men aged >30: 420 mg/day Women aged 19–30: 310 mg/day Women aged >30: 320 mg/day UL: 350 mg/day	Greens (spinach, kale, collard greens), whole grains, seeds, nuts, legumes (navy and black beans)	*Toxicity:* None known *Deficiency:* Low blood calcium, muscle spasms or seizures, nausea, weakness, increased risk for chronic diseases (such as heart disease, hypertension, osteoporosis, and type 2 diabetes)
Sulfur	Component of certain B-vitamins and amino acids Acid–base balance Detoxification in liver	No DRI	Protein-rich foods	*Toxicity:* None known *Deficiency:* None known

*RDA: Recommended Dietary Allowance; UL: upper limit; AI: Adequate Intake; DRI: Dietary Reference Intake.

TABLE 4 Trace and Ultra-Trace Minerals

Mineral Name	Primary Functions	Recommended Intake*	Reliable Food Sources	Toxicity/Deficiency Symptoms
Trace Minerals				
Fluoride	Development and maintenance of healthy teeth and bones	RDA: Men: 4 mg/day Women: 3 mg/day UL: 2.2 mg/day for children aged 4–8; 10 mg/day for children aged >8	Fish, seafood, legumes, whole grains, drinking water (variable)	*Toxicity:* Fluorosis of teeth and bones *Deficiency:* Dental caries, low bone density
Iron	Component of hemoglobin in blood cells Component of myoglobin in muscle cells Assists many enzyme systems	RDA: Adult men: 8 mg/day Women aged 19–50: 18 mg/day Women aged >50: 8 mg/day	Meat/fish/poultry (best-absorbed form of iron), fortified cereals, legumes, spinach	*Toxicity:* Nausea, vomiting, and diarrhea; dizziness and confusion; rapid heartbeat; organ damage; death *Deficiency:* Iron-deficiency microcytic anemia (small red blood cells), hypochromic anemia
Manganese	Assists many enzyme systems Synthesis of protein found in bone and cartilage	AI: Men: 2.3 mg/day Women: 1.8 mg/day UL: 11 mg/day for adults	Whole grains, nuts, leafy vegetables, tea	*Toxicity:* Impairment of neuromuscular system *Deficiency:* Impaired growth and reproductive function, reduced bone density, impaired glucose and lipid metabolism, skin rash
Zinc	Assists more than 100 enzyme systems Immune system function Growth and sexual maturation Gene regulation	RDA: Men: 11 mg/day Women: 8 mg/day UL: 40 mg/day	Meat/fish/poultry (best-absorbed form of zinc), fortified cereals, legumes	*Toxicity:* Nausea, vomiting, and diarrhea; headaches; depressed immune function; reduced absorption of copper *Deficiency:* Growth retardation, delayed sexual maturation, eye and skin lesions, hair loss, increased incidence of illness and infection
Ultra-Trace Minerals				
Chromium	Glucose transport Metabolism of DNA and RNA Immune function and growth	AI: Men aged 19–50: 35 μg/day Men aged >50: 30 μg/day Women aged 19–50: 25 μg/day Women aged >50: 20 μg/day	Whole grains, brewers yeast	*Toxicity:* None known *Deficiency:* Elevated blood glucose and blood lipids, damage to brain and nervous system
Copper	Assists many enzyme systems Iron transport	RDA: Adults: 900 μg/day UL: 10 mg/day	Shellfish, organ meats, nuts, legumes	*Toxicity:* Nausea, vomiting, and diarrhea; liver damage *Deficiency:* Anemia, reduced levels of white blood cells, osteoporosis in infants and growing children
Iodine	Synthesis of thyroid hormones Temperature regulation Reproduction and growth	RDA: Adults: 150 μg/day UL: 1,100 μg/day	Iodized salt, saltwater seafood	*Toxicity:* Goiter *Deficiency:* Goiter, hypothyroidism, cretinism in infant of mother who is iodine deficient
Molybdenum	Assists many enzyme systems	RDA: Adults: 45 μg/day UL: 2 mg/day	Legumes, nuts, grains	*Toxicity:* Symptoms not well defined in humans *Deficiency:* Abnormal metabolism of sulfur containing compounds
Selenium	Required for carbohydrate and fat metabolism	RDA: Adults: 55 μg/day UL: 400 μg/day	Nuts, shellfish, meat/fish/poultry, whole grains	*Toxicity:* Brittle hair and nails, skin rashes, nausea and vomiting, weakness, liver disease *Deficiency:* Specific forms of heart disease and arthritis, impaired immune function, muscle pain and wasting, depression, hostility

*RDA: Recommended Dietary Allowance; UL: upper limit; AI: Adequate Intake.

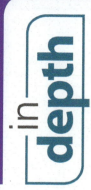

These are included in Table 4. Other ultra-trace minerals such as arsenic, nickel, and vanadium are thought to be important or essential for human health, but there is not yet enough research to establish an RDA or AI guideline.[1] As research into these ultra-trace minerals continue, scientists may soon be able to define a DRI value.

Same Mineral, Different Forms

Unlike vitamins, most of which can be identified by either alphabetic designations or their chemical name, minerals are simply referred to by their chemical name. Minerals in foods and supplements are often bound to other chemicals in compounds called salts; for example, a supplement label might identify calcium as calcium lactate, calcium gluconate, or calcium citrate. As we will discuss shortly, these different salts, while all containing the same elemental mineral, may differ in their ability to be absorbed by the body.

How does our body use micronutrients?

LO 4 Explain why the amount of a micronutrient we consume differs from the amount our body absorbs and uses.

The micronutrients found in foods and supplements are not always in a chemical form that our cells can use. This discussion will highlight some of the ways in which our body modifies the food forms of vitamins and minerals to maximize their absorption and utilization.

What We Eat Differs from What We Absorb

The most healthful diet is of no value unless the body can absorb its nutrients and transport them to the cells that need them. Unlike carbohydrates, fats, and proteins, which are efficiently absorbed (85–99% of what is eaten makes it into the blood), some micronutrients are so poorly absorbed that only 3–10% of what is eaten ever enters the bloodstream.

The absorption of many vitamins and minerals depends on their chemical form. Dietary iron, for example, can be in the form of *heme iron* (found only in meats, fish, and poultry) or *non-heme iron* (found in plant and animal foods, as well as iron-fortified foods and supplements). Healthy adults absorb heme iron more readily than non-heme iron.

In addition, the presence of other factors within the same food influences mineral absorption. For example, approximately 30% to 45% of the calcium found in milk and dairy products is absorbed, but the calcium in spinach, Swiss chard, seeds, and nuts is absorbed at a much lower rate because factors in these foods bind the calcium and prevent its absorption.

Some micronutrients actually compete with one another for absorption. Several minerals, for example, use the same protein carriers to move across the enterocytes for release into the bloodstream. Iron and zinc compete for intestinal absorption, as do iron and copper.

The absorption of many vitamins and minerals is also influenced by other foods within the meal. For example, the fat-soluble vitamins are much better absorbed when the meal contains some dietary fat. Calcium absorption is increased by the presence of lactose, found in milk, and non-heme iron absorption can be doubled if the meal includes vitamin C–rich foods, such as red peppers, oranges, or tomatoes. On the other hand, high-fiber foods, such as whole grains, and foods high in oxalic acid, such as tea, spinach, and rhubarb, can decrease the absorption of zinc and iron. It may seem an impossible task to correctly balance your food choices to optimize micronutrient absorption, but the best approach, as always, is to eat a variety of healthful foods every day. See an example in **MEAL FOCUS FIGURE 1**, which compares a day's meals high and low in micronutrients.

What We Eat Differs from What Our Cells Use

Many vitamins undergo one or more chemical transformations after they are eaten and absorbed into our body. For example, before they can go to work for our body, thiamin and vitamin B_6 must combine with phosphate groups, and vitamin D must have two hydroxyl (OH) groups added to its structure. These transformations activate the vitamin; because the reactions don't occur randomly, but only when the active vitamin is needed, they help the body maintain control over its metabolic pathways.

While the basic nature of minerals does not change, they can undergo minor modifications that change their atomic structure. Iron (Fe) may alternate between Fe^{2+} (ferrous) and Fe^{3+} (ferric); copper (Cu) may exist as Cu^{1+} or Cu^{2+}. These are just two examples of many modifications that help the body make the best use of dietary micronutrients.

What are some controversies in micronutrient research?

LO 5 Discuss three controversial topics in micronutrient research.

The science of nutrition continues to evolve, and our current understanding of vitamins and minerals will no doubt change over the next several years or decades. While some people interpret the term *controversy* as negative, nutrition controversies are exciting developments, proof of new information, and a sign of continued growth in the field.

a day of meals

low in MICRONUTRIENTS

high in MICRONUTRIENTS

BREAKFAST

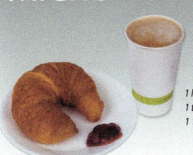

1 large butter croissant
1 tbsp. strawberry jam
1 16 fl. oz latte with whole milk

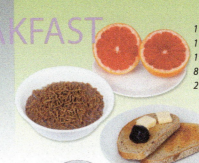

1 cup All-Bran cereal
1 cup skim milk
1 grapefruit
8 fl. oz low-fat plain yogurt
2 slices rye toast with 2 tsp. butter and 1 tbsp. blackberry preserves

LUNCH

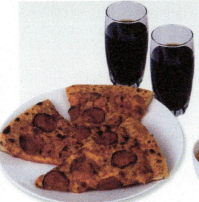

3 slices pepperoni pizza (14-inch pizza)
1.5 oz potato chips
24 fl. oz cola beverage

1 chicken breast, boneless, skinless, grilled

Spinach salad
2 cups spinach leaves
1 boiled egg
1 tbsp. chopped green onions
4 cherry tomatoes
½ medium carrot, chopped
1 tbsp. pine nuts
2 tbsp. Ranch dressing (reduced fat)
2 falafels (2-¼ inch diameter) with 2 tbsp. hummus

DINNER

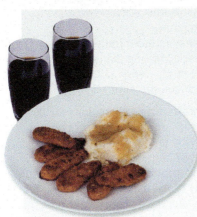

6 fried chicken tenders
1 cup mashed potatoes with ½ cup chicken gravy
24 fl. oz diet cola beverage
1 yogurt and fruit parfait

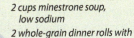
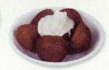

2 cups minestrone soup, low sodium
2 whole-grain dinner rolls with 2 tsp. margarine
2 pork loin chops, roasted
1 cup mixed vegetables, cooked
8 fl. oz skim milk
1 cup fresh strawberries (sliced) with 1 tbsp. low-fat whipped cream

nutrient analysis

2,789 kcal
46 milligrams of vitamin C
28.6 milligrams of niacin
929 milligrams of calcium
13.4 milligrams of iron
490 mcg of folate
5,792 milligrams of sodium

nutrient analysis

2,528 kcal
255 milligrams of vitamin C
42.8 milligrams of niacin
1,780 milligrams of calcium
27.5 milligrams of iron
1,335 mcg of folate
2,832 milligrams of sodium

Provides more nutrients!

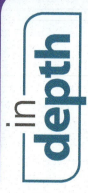

Are Supplements Healthful Sources of Micronutrients?

For millions of years, humans relied solely on natural foodstuffs as their source of nutrients. Only within the past 75 years or so has a second option become available: purified supplemental nutrients, including those added to fortified foods. We discuss the effects and safety of dietary supplements in In Depth 12.5. For now, consider these differences between micronutrients from foods and from supplements:

- In general, it is much easier to develop a toxic overload of nutrients from supplements than it is from foods. It is very difficult, if not impossible, to develop a vitamin or mineral toxicity through food alone.
- Consumption of certain micronutrient supplements appears to be harmful. For example, recent research has shown that the use of antioxidant supplements, including beta-carotene, vitamin A, and vitamin E, may actually increase mortality.[2] There is also some evidence that a high intake of vitamin A, including supplement use, increases the risk for osteoporosis and bone fractures in older women with low intakes of vitamin D.[3]
- Most minerals are better absorbed from animal food sources than they are from supplements or fortified foods. The one exception might be calcium citrate-malate, used in calcium-fortified juices. The body uses this form as effectively as the calcium from milk or yogurt.
- Enriching a low-nutrient food with a few vitamins and/or minerals does not turn it into a healthful food. For example, soda that has been fortified with selected micronutrients is still a sugary drink.
- Eating a variety of healthful foods provides you with many more nutrients, phytochemicals, and other dietary factors than supplements alone. Nutritionists are not even sure they have identified all the essential nutrients; it is possible that the list will expand in the future. Supplements provide only those nutrients that the manufacturer puts in; foods provide the nutrients that have been identified as well as yet-unknown factors, which likely work in concert with one another to maintain health and functioning.

Can Micronutrients Prevent or Treat Chronic Disease?

Researchers continue to investigate the links between macronutrients such as dietary fat and carbohydrate and the prevention and/or treatment of chronic diseases such as heart disease and diabetes. For example, there is strong agreement that *trans* fats increase the risk of heart disease and that high-fiber diets help regulate blood

glucose levels. Less clear, however, are the links between individual vitamins and minerals and certain chronic diseases.

A number of research studies have suggested, but not proven, links between the following micronutrients and disease states. In each case, adequate intake of the nutrient has been associated with a reduced risk for the condition.

- Vitamin D and colon cancer
- Vitamin E and complications of diabetes
- Vitamin K and osteoporosis
- Calcium and pregnancy-induced hypertension
- Magnesium and muscle wasting (sarcopenia) in older adults
- Potassium and high blood pressure

The DRIs identify intake recommendations for large population groups; however, another subject of controversy is the question, "What is the optimal intake of each micronutrient for any given individual?" Contemporary research suggests that the answer to this question should take into account aspects of the individual's genetic profile. For example, researchers have identified genetic variations in certain populations that modify their need for dietary folate.[4] Future studies may identify other examples of how our genetic profile may influence our need for vitamins and minerals.

Again, it's important to critically evaluate any claim about the protective or disease-preventing ability of a specific vitamin or mineral. Supplements that provide megadoses of micronutrients are potentially harmful and should be avoided unless prescribed by your healthcare provider.

Do More Essential Micronutrients Exist?

Nutrition researchers continue to explore the potential of a variety of substances to qualify as essential micronutrients. Vitamin-like factors such as carnitine and trace minerals such as boron, nickel, and silicon seem to have beneficial roles in human health, yet additional information is needed to fully define their metabolic roles. Until more research is done, such substances can't be classified as essential micronutrients.

As the science of nutrition continues to evolve, the next 50 years will be an exciting time for micronutrient research. Consult the Office of Dietary Supplements at the National Institutes of Health for updates on the research into micronutrients.

Before you purchase a dietary supplement, check out this one-minute video from the Office of Dietary Supplements (ODS) at http://ods.od.nih.gov. From the home page, search for "ODS Videos" and choose "Thinking About Taking a Dietary Supplement?"

web links

www.fda.gov/food/dietarysupplements/default.htm
U.S. Food and Drug Administration

Select "Using Dietary Supplements" for information about the advantages and potential risks of supplement use.

fnic.nal.usda.gov/dietary-supplements
Food and Nutrition Information Center

Click on "General Information and Resources" to obtain information on vitamin and mineral supplements.

www.ods.od.nih.gov
Office of Dietary Supplements

This site provides summaries of current research results and helpful information about the use of dietary supplements.

lpi.oregonstate.edu
Linus Pauling Institute of Oregon State University

This site provides information on vitamins and minerals that promote health and lower disease risk. You can search for individual nutrients (for example, vitamin C) as well as types of nutrients (e.g., antioxidants).

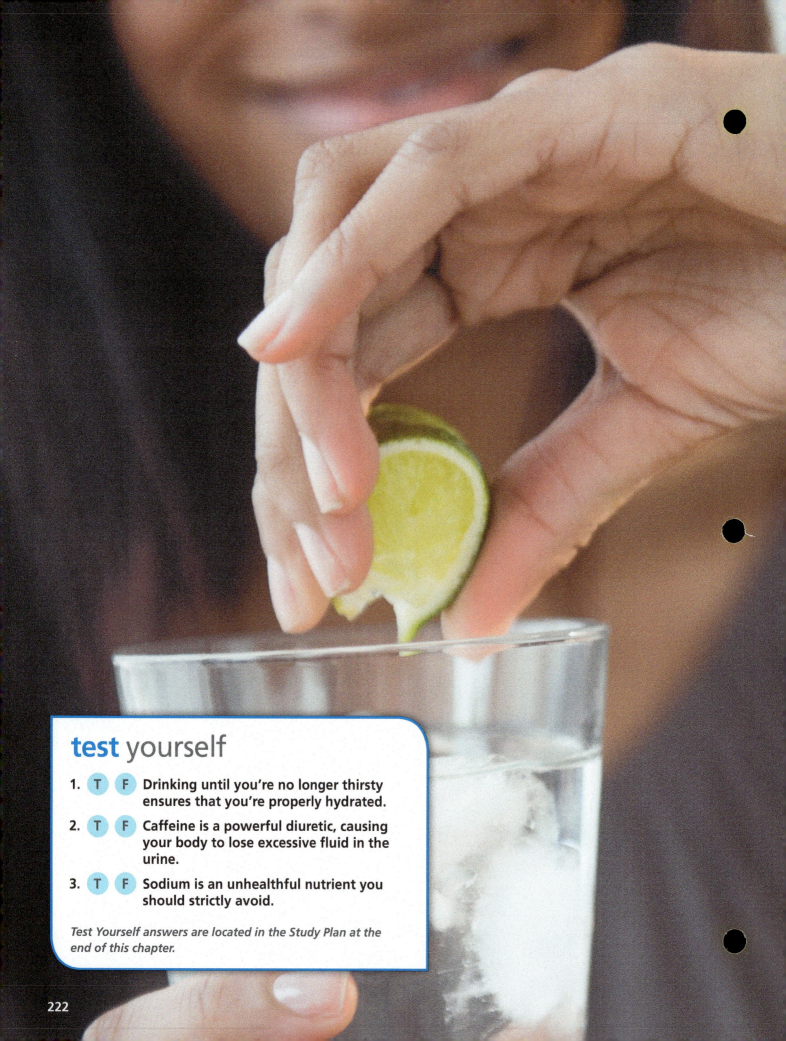

test yourself

1. T F Drinking until you're no longer thirsty ensures that you're properly hydrated.

2. T F Caffeine is a powerful diuretic, causing your body to lose excessive fluid in the urine.

3. T F Sodium is an unhealthful nutrient you should strictly avoid.

Test Yourself answers are located in the Study Plan at the end of this chapter.

7

Nutrients Essential to Fluid and Electrolyte Balance

learning outcomes

After studying this chapter you should be able to:

1 Describe the location and composition of body fluid, pp. 224–225.

2 Identify the critical contributions of water and electrolytes to human functioning, pp. 226–230.

3 Discuss the mechanisms by which the body gains or loses fluids, pp. 230–232.

4 Identify the DRIs for water and compare the nutritional quality of several common beverages, pp. 233–237.

5 Identify the functions, DRIs, and common dietary sources of sodium, potassium, chloride, and phosphorus, pp. 237–243.

6 Discuss several disorders related to fluid and electrolyte balance, pp. 243–245.

Vani used to buy her favorite energy drink by the case. She'd gulp one on the way to her first class, another before working out at the gym, and a couple more to get through a long night of studying. Then, alone in her dorm room one night, she was hit with a wave of nausea. Her heart began to beat erratically, and she broke out in a sweat. A premed student, she knew it was unlikely she was having a heart attack. Had she overdosed on caffeine? Her hands shaking, she logged on to her favorite medical website. The symptoms fit exactly. Now Vani lets herself buy just one can of her favorite energy drink a day. And even though she pays more per can, she still saves money, because the rest of her day's fluid intake is water.

Energy drinks are increasingly popular among teens and young adults despite their known health risks.[1] In 2013, the U.S. Food and Drug Administration (FDA) released records of nearly 150 adverse events between 2004 and 2012 that were linked to energy drinks. The reports included incidents of vomiting, difficulty breathing, seizures, cardiac arrests, miscarriages, and at least 18 deaths. Since 2012, 17 additional deaths have been linked to these products.[2]

In this chapter, we'll review the health and nutritional profile of energy drinks, sugary drinks, sports drinks, and many other popular beverages. But first, we'll explain the role of fluids and electrolytes in keeping the body properly hydrated and maintaining nerve and muscle function. We'll also discuss some disorders related to fluid and electrolyte balance. Immediately following this chapter, we'll take an **In Depth** look at the health benefits and concerns related to consumption of alcohol.

MasteringNutrition™

Go online for chapter quizzes, pre-tests, interactive activities, and more!

LO 1 Describe the location and composition of body fluid.

What is body fluid?

Of course, you know that orange juice, blood, and shampoo are all fluids, but what makes them so? A **fluid** is characterized by its ability to move freely, adapting to the shape of the container that holds it. This might not seem very important, but as you'll learn in this chapter, the fluid composition of your cells and tissues is critical to your body's ability to function.

Body Fluid Is the Liquid Portion of Our Cells and Tissues

Between 50% and 70% of a healthy adult's body weight is fluid. When we cut a finger, we can see some of this fluid dripping out as blood, but the fluid in the blood-stream can't account for such a large percentage. So where is all this fluid hiding?

About two-thirds of an adult's body fluid is held within the walls of cells and is therefore called **intracellular fluid** (FIGURE 7.1a). Every cell in our body contains fluid. When our cells lose their fluid, they quickly shrink and die. On the other hand, when

fluid A substance composed of molecules that move past one another freely. Fluids are characterized by their ability to conform to the shape of whatever container holds them.

intracellular fluid The fluid held at any given time within the walls of the body's cells.

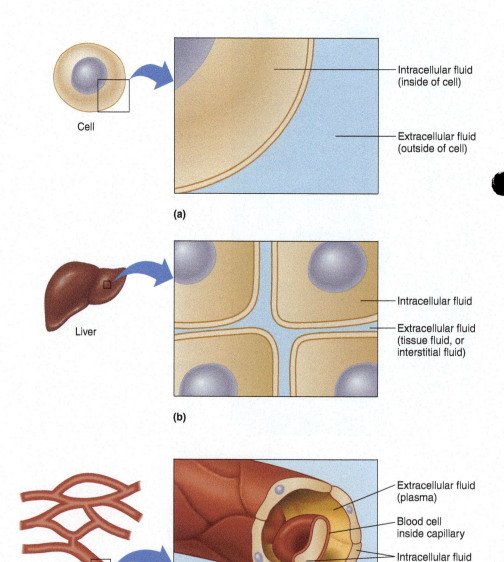

▶ **FIGURE 7.1** The components of body fluid. **(a)** Intracellular fluid is contained inside the cells that make up body tissues. **(b)** Extracellular fluid is external to cells. Tissue fluid is external to tissue cells. **(c)** Another form of extracellular fluid is intravascular fluid—that is, fluid contained within vessels. Plasma is the fluid in blood vessels and is external to blood cells.

cells take in too much fluid, they swell and burst apart. This is why appropriate fluid balance—which we'll discuss throughout this chapter—is so critical to life.

The remaining third of body fluid is referred to as **extracellular fluid** because it flows outside our cells (Figure 7.1a). There are two types of extracellular fluid:

1. *Tissue fluid* (sometimes called *interstitial fluid*) flows between the cells that make up a particular tissue, such as muscle or liver tissue (Figure 7.1b). Other extracellular fluids, such as cerebrospinal fluid, mucus, and synovial fluid within joints, are also considered tissue fluid.
2. *Intravascular fluid* is found within blood and lymphatic vessels. Plasma is the fluid portion of blood that transports blood cells through blood vessels. Plasma also contains proteins that are too large to leak out of blood vessels into the surrounding tissue fluid. As you learned (in Chapter 6), protein concentration plays a major role in regulating the movement of fluids into and out of the bloodstream (Figure 7.1c).

Not every tissue contains the same amount of fluid. Lean tissues, such as muscle, are more than 70% fluid by weight, whereas fat tissue is only between 10% and 20% fluid. This is not surprising, considering the water-repellant nature of lipids (see Chapter 5).

Body fluid levels also vary according to gender and age. Compared to females, males have more lean tissue and thus a higher percentage of body weight as fluid. The amount of body fluid as a percentage of total weight decreases with age. About 75% of an infant's body weight is water, whereas the total body water of an elderly person is generally less than 50% of body weight. This decrease in total body water is the result of the loss of lean tissue that typically occurs as people age.

▲ As we age, our body's water content decreases: approximately 75% of an infant's body weight is composed of water, whereas an elderly adult's body weight is only 50% water (or less).

Body Fluid Is Composed of Water and Electrolytes

Water is made up of molecules consisting of two hydrogen atoms bound to one oxygen atom (H_2O). You might think that pure water would be healthful, but we would quickly die if our cell and tissue fluids contained only pure water. Instead, body fluids contain a variety of dissolved substances (called *solutes*) critical to life. These include six major minerals: sodium, potassium, chloride, phosphorus, calcium, and magnesium. We consume these minerals in compounds called *salts*, including table salt, which is made of sodium and chloride.

These mineral salts are called **electrolytes** because when they dissolve in water, the two component minerals separate and form charged particles called **ions**, which can carry an electrical current and themselves are also commonly referred to as electrolytes. An ion's electrical charge, which can be positive or negative, is the "spark" that stimulates the transmission of nerve impulses and causes muscles to contract, making electrolytes critical to body functioning.

Of the six major minerals just mentioned, sodium and potassium are positively charged, whereas chloride and phosphorus (in the form of hydrogen phosphate) are negatively charged. Calcium and magnesium, because they play critical roles in bone health, are discussed in Chapter 9. In the intracellular fluid, potassium and phosphate are the predominant ions. In the extracellular fluid, sodium and chloride predominate. There is a slight difference in electrical charge on either side of the cell's membrane that is needed in order for the cell to perform its normal functions.

extracellular fluid The fluid outside the body's cells, either in the body's tissues or as the liquid portion of blood or lymph.

electrolyte A substance that disassociates in solution into positively and negatively charged ions and is thus capable of carrying an electrical current; the ions in such a solution.

ion Any electrically charged particle, either positively or negatively charged.

recap Between 50% and 70% of a healthy adult's body weight is fluid. About two-thirds is intracellular fluid and the remaining third is extracellular fluid; that is, either tissue fluid or intravascular fluid. Body fluid consists of water plus a variety of solutes (dissolved substances), including six major minerals called electrolytes because they can carry an electrical current. Electrolytes are critical to the body's fluid balance, nerve-impulse transmission, and muscle contraction.

LO 2 Identify the critical contributions of water and electrolytes to human functioning.

Why do we need water and electrolytes?

The functions of water and electrolytes are interrelated and their levels in the body delicately balanced.

Water Performs Functions Critical to Life

Water not only quenches our thirst; it also performs functions critical to life.

Solubility and Transport

Water is an excellent **solvent**; that is, it's capable of dissolving a wide variety of substances. The chemical reactions upon which life depends would not be possible without water. Because blood is mostly water, it's able to transport a variety of solutes—such as water-soluble nutrients and medications—to body cells. In contrast, fats do not dissolve in water. To overcome this chemical incompatibility, lipids and fat-soluble vitamins are either attached to or surrounded by water-soluble proteins, so that they, too, can be transported in the blood to the cells.

Blood Volume and Blood Pressure

Blood volume is the amount of fluid in blood; thus, appropriate fluid levels are essential to maintaining healthful blood volume. When blood volume rises inappropriately, blood pressure increases; when blood volume decreases inappropriately, blood pressure decreases. Hypertension is an important risk factor for heart attacks and strokes. (For more information, see the **In Depth** essay following Chapter 5.) In contrast, low blood pressure can cause people to feel tired, confused, or dizzy.

Body Temperature

Just as overheating is disastrous to a car engine, a high internal temperature can impair body functioning. Fluids are vital to the body's ability to maintain its temperature within a safe range. Two factors account for the ability of fluids to keep us cool. First, water has a relatively high capacity for heat: in other words, it takes a lot of energy to raise its temperature. Because the body contains a lot of water, only prolonged exposure to high heat can increase body temperature.

Second, body fluids are our primary coolant **(FIGURE 7.2)**. When heat needs to be released from the body, there is an increase in blood flow from the warm body core to the vessels lying just under the skin. This action transports heat from the body core out to the periphery, where it can be released from the skin. At the same time, sweat

> Would the proteins in your body tissues "cook" at the same temperature that would fry an egg? For a short, fun video on an experiment that answers this question, go to www.npr.org and type in the search bar "How Much Heat Can You Take?"

solvent A substance that is capable of mixing with and breaking apart a variety of compounds. Water is an excellent solvent.

blood volume The amount of fluid in blood.

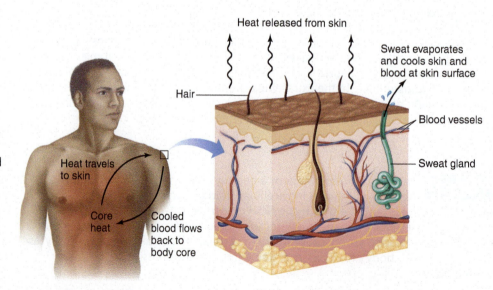

▶ **FIGURE 7.2** Evaporative cooling occurs when heat is transported from the body core through the bloodstream to the surface of the skin. The water evaporates into the air and carries away heat. This cools the blood, which circulates back to the body core, reducing body temperature.

Heat released from skin

Sweat evaporates and cools skin and blood at skin surface

Hair

Blood vessels

Sweat gland

Heat travels to skin

Core heat

Cooled blood flows back to body core

glands secrete more sweat from the skin. As this sweat evaporates off the skin's surface, heat is released and the skin and underlying blood are cooled. This cooler blood
flows back to the body's core and reduces internal body temperature.

Tissue Protection and Lubrication

Water is a major part of the fluids that protect and lubricate tissues. The cerebrospinal fluid that surrounds the brain and spinal cord protects them from damage, and
a fetus in a mother's womb is protected by amniotic fluid. Synovial fluid lubricates
joints, and tears cleanse and lubricate the eyes. Saliva moistens the food we eat and
the mucus lining the walls of the gastrointestinal (GI) tract eases the movement of
food. Finally, pleural fluid covering the lungs allows their friction-free expansion and
retraction within the chest cavity.

Electrolytes Support Many Body Functions

Now that you know why fluid is so essential to the body's functioning, we're ready to
explore the critical roles of electrolytes.

Fluid Balance

Cell membranes are *permeable* to water, meaning water flows easily through them.
Cells cannot voluntarily regulate this flow of water and thus have no active control
over the balance of fluid between the intracellular and extracellular environments.
In contrast, cell membranes are *not* freely permeable to electrolytes. Sodium, potassium, and the other electrolytes stay where they are, either inside or outside a cell,
unless they are actively transported across the cell membrane by special transport
proteins. So how do electrolytes help cells maintain their fluid balance? To answer this
question, a short review of chemistry is needed.

  Imagine that you have a special filter with the same properties as cell membranes; in other words, this filter is freely permeable to water but not permeable to
electrolytes. Now imagine that you insert this filter into a glass of dilute salt water
to divide the glass into two separate chambers **(FIGURE 7.3a)**. Of course, the water
levels on both sides of the filter would be identical because the filter is freely permeable to water. Now imagine that you add a teaspoon of salt (which would immediately dissolve into sodium and chloride ions) to the water on only one side of the

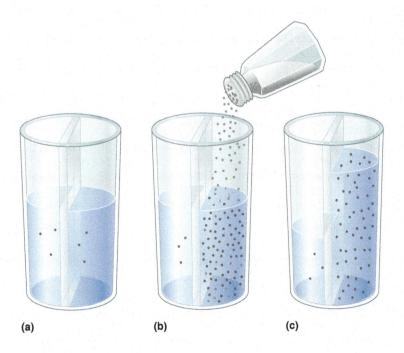

(a)   (b)   (c)

FIGURE 7.3 Osmosis. **(a)** A filter that is freely permeable to water but not permeable to sol-utes is placed in a glass of dilute salt water. **(b)** Additional salt is sprinkled on one side of the glass only. **(c)** Drawn by the high concentration of electrolytes, water flows to the "saltier" side of the filter. This flow of water into the more concentrated solution will continue until the concentration of electrolytes on both sides of the membrane is equal.

filter (Figure 7.3b). Immediately, you would see the water on the "dilute salt water" side of the glass begin to flow through the filter to the "saltier" side of the glass (Figure 7.3c).

Why would this movement of water occur? It is because water always moves from areas where solutes, such as sodium and chloride, are low in concentration (or completely absent) to areas where they are high in concentration. To put it another way, solutes *attract* water toward areas where they are more concentrated. This movement of water toward solutes, called **osmosis**, continues until the concentration of solutes is equal on both sides of the cell membrane.

Osmosis governs the movement of fluid into and out of cells. Recall that cells can regulate the balance of fluids between their cytoplasm and the extracellular environment by using special transport proteins to actively pump electrolytes across the cell membrane (see Chapter 6). The health of the body's cells depends on maintaining an appropriate balance of fluid and electrolytes between the intracellular and extracellular environments. If the concentration of electrolytes is much higher inside cells as compared to outside, water will flow into the cells in such large amounts that the cells can burst. On the other hand, if the extracellular environment contains too high a concentration of electrolytes, water flows out of the cells, and they can dry up. **FOCUS FIGURE 7.4** provides an illustration of how an imbalance between fluid and electrolyte intake during strenuous exercise can affect the balance of fluid and electrolytes between the intracellular and extracellular environments. Keep in mind that when you exercise, what and how much you should drink depends on multiple factors, including how strenuously you are exercising, how long the exercise session is, and how warm or humid the environment is.

Certain illnesses can threaten the delicate balance of fluid inside and outside the cells. You may have heard of someone being hospitalized because of excessive diarrhea and/or vomiting. When this happens, the body loses a great deal of fluid from the intestinal tract and extracellular fluid compartment. This causes the loss of both water and electrolytes. In some cases, the relative loss of water is greater than the loss of electrolytes, and the body's extracellular electrolyte concentration then becomes very high. In response, a great deal of fluid flows out of body cells. These imbalances in fluid and electrolytes change the flow of electrical impulses through the heart, causing an irregular heart rate that can be fatal if left untreated. Severe food poisoning and eating disorders involving repeated vomiting and diarrhea can result in death from life-threatening fluid and electrolyte imbalances.

Nerve Impulse Conduction

In addition to their role in maintaining fluid balance, electrolytes are critical in allowing our nerves to respond to stimuli **(FIGURE 7.5)** (page 230). Nerve impulses are initiated at the membrane of a nerve cell in response to a stimulus—for example, the touch of a hand or the clanging of a bell. Stimuli prompt changes in membranes that allow an influx of sodium into the nerve cell, causing the cell to become slightly less negatively charged. This is called *depolarization*. If enough sodium enters the cell, an electrical impulse is generated along the cell membrane (Figure 7.5b).

Once this impulse has been transmitted, the cell membrane returns to its normal electrical state through the release of potassium to the outside of the cell (Figure 7.5c). This return to the initial electrical state is termed *repolarization*. Thus, both sodium and potassium play critical roles in ensuring that nerve impulses are generated, transmitted, and completed.

Muscle Contraction

Muscles contract in response to a series of complex physiological changes that we will not describe in detail here. Simply stated, muscle contraction occurs in response to stimulation of nerve cells. As described earlier, sodium and potassium play a key role in the generation of nerve impulses, or electrical signals. Stimulation from an electrical signal causes changes in the muscle cell membrane that lead to an increased flow of calcium from their storage site in the muscle cell. This movement

osmosis The movement of water (or any solvent) through a semipermeable membrane from an area where solutes are less concentrated to areas where solutes are highly concentrated.

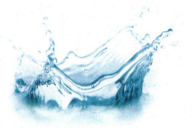

The health of our body's cells depends on maintaining the proper balance of fluids and electrolytes on both sides of the cell membrane, both at rest and during exercise. Let's examine how this balance can be altered under various conditions of exercise and fluid intake.

MODERATE EXERCISE

When you are appropriately hydrated, engaged in moderate exercise, and not too hot, the concentration of electrolytes is likely to be the same on both sides of cell membranes. You will be in fluid balance.

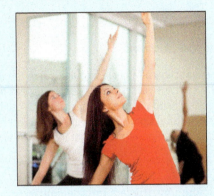

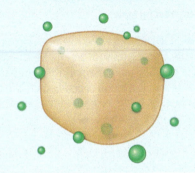

Concentration of electrolytes about equal inside and outside cell

STRENUOUS EXERCISE WITH RAPID AND HIGH WATER INTAKE

If a person drinks a great deal of water quickly during intense, prolonged exercise, the extracellular fluid becomes diluted. This results in the concentration of electrolytes being greater inside the cells, which causes water to enter the cells, making them swell. Drinking moderate amounts of water or sports drinks more slowly will replace lost fluids and restore fluid balance.

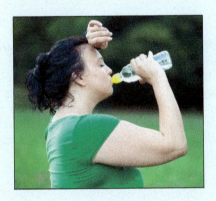

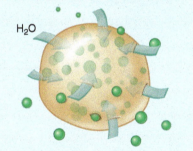

Lower concentration of electrolytes outside

H_2O

Higher concentration of electrolytes inside

STRENUOUS EXERCISE WITH INADEQUATE FLUID INTAKE

If a person does not consume adequate amounts of fluid during strenuous exercise of long duration, the concentration of electrolytes becomes greater outside the cells, drawing water away from the inside of the cells and making them shrink. Consuming sports drinks will replace lost fluids and electrolytes.

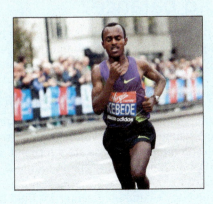

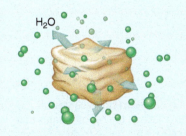

Higher concentration of electrolytes outside

H_2O

Lower concentration of electrolytes inside

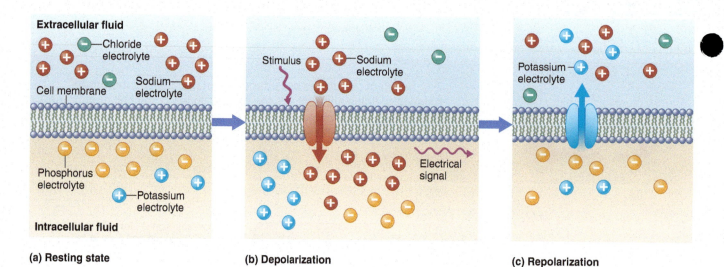

▲ FIGURE 7.5 The role of electrolytes in conduction of a nerve impulse. **(a)** In the resting state, the intracellular fluid has slightly more electrolytes with a negative charge. **(b)** A stimulus causes changes to occur that prompt the influx of sodium into the interior of the cell. Sodium has a positive charge so when this happens, the charge inside the cell becomes slightly positive. This is called depolarization. If enough sodium enters the cell, an electrical signal is transmitted to adjacent regions of the cell membrane. **(c)** Release of potassium to the exterior of the cell allows the first portion of the membrane almost immediately to return to the resting state. This is called repolarization.

of calcium ions triggers muscle contraction. The muscle cell can relax after a contraction once the electrical signal is complete and calcium has been pumped back into its storage site.

recap Water serves many important functions in the body, including dissolving and transporting substances, accounting for blood volume and thereby influencing to blood pressure, regulating body temperature, and protecting and lubricating body tissues. Via the process of osmosis, electrolytes help regulate fluid balance by controlling the movement of fluid into and out of cells. Electrolytes, specifically sodium and potassium, play a key role in the generation and transmission of nerve impulses in response to stimuli. Calcium is an electrolyte essential to muscle contraction.

LO 3 Discuss the mechanisms by which the body gains and loses fluids.

How does the body maintain fluid balance?

The proper balance of fluid is maintained in the body by a series of mechanisms that prompt us to drink and retain fluid when we are dehydrated and to excrete fluid as urine when we consume more than we need.

The Hypothalamus Regulates Thirst

Imagine that, at lunch, you ate a ham sandwich and a bag of salted potato chips. Now it's almost time for your afternoon seminar to end and you are very thirsty. The last 5 minutes of class are a torment, and when the instructor ends the session you dash to the nearest drinking fountain. What prompted you to suddenly feel so thirsty?

The body's command center for fluid intake is a cluster of nerve cells in the same part of the brain we studied in relation to food intake; that is, the *hypothalamus*. Within the hypothalamus is a group of cells, collectively referred

thirst mechanism A cluster of nerve cells in the hypothalamus that stimulate the desire to drink fluids in response to an increase in the concentration of blood solutes or a decrease in blood pressure and blood volume.

to as the **thirst mechanism**, which causes you to consciously desire fluids. The thirst mechanism prompts us to feel thirsty whenever it is stimulated by the following:

- An increased concentration of salt and other dissolved substances in our blood. Remember that ham sandwich and those potato chips? Both of these foods are salty, and eating them increased the blood's sodium concentration.
- A reduction in blood volume and blood pressure. This can occur when fluids are lost because of profuse sweating, blood loss, vomiting, or diarrhea, or simply when fluid intake is too low.
- Dryness in the tissues of the mouth and throat. Tissue dryness reflects a lower amount of fluid in the bloodstream, which causes a reduced production of saliva.

Once the hypothalamus detects such changes, it stimulates the release of a hormone called ADH (for *antidiuretic hormone*) from the pituitary gland, which signals the kidneys to reabsorb more water, thereby returning more water to the bloodstream and reducing the volume of urine **(FIGURE 7.6)**. The kidneys also secrete an enzyme that triggers the retention of water. Water is drawn out of the salivary glands, for example, diluting the concentration of blood solutes; this causes the mouth and throat to become even more dry, and we feel the sensation of thirst. Together, these mechanisms prevent a further loss of body fluid and help the body avoid dehydration.

We Gain Fluids Through Intake and Metabolism

Typically, when we experience thirst, we drink. Water and other beverages are our primary fluid sources. However, fluid intake alone is not always sufficient: We tend to drink until we're no longer thirsty, but the amount of fluid we consume may not be enough to achieve fluid balance. This is particularly true when body water is lost rapidly, such as during intense exercise in the heat. Because the thirst mechanism has some limitations, it's important to drink regularly throughout the day, especially when you're active.

You can clearly see that beverages are mostly water, but foods are another source of water intake. For example, iceberg lettuce is almost 99% water, and even almonds contain a small amount of water **(FIGURE 7.7)**.

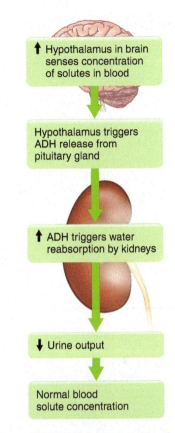

↑ Hypothalamus in brain senses concentration of solutes in blood

Hypothalamus triggers ADH release from pituitary gland

↑ ADH triggers water reabsorption by kidneys

↓ Urine output

Normal blood solute concentration

◆ **FIGURE 7.6** Regulation of blood volume and blood pressure by the brain and kidneys. The hypothalamus senses increased concentration of solutes in the blood, triggering the release of ADH from the pituitary gland. ADH signals the kidneys to increase water reabsorption.

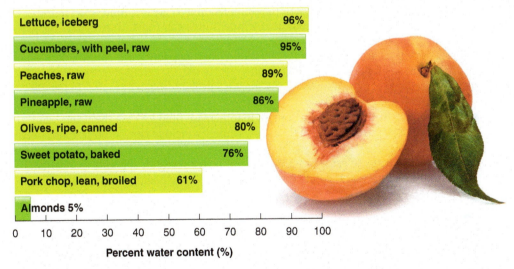

Lettuce, iceberg — 96%
Cucumbers, with peel, raw — 95%
Peaches, raw — 89%
Pineapple, raw — 86%
Olives, ripe, canned — 80%
Sweet potato, baked — 76%
Pork chop, lean, broiled — 61%
Almonds 5%

Percent water content (%)

◆ **FIGURE 7.7** Water content of different foods. Much of your daily water intake comes from the foods you eat.

Data from: U.S. Department of Agriculture, Agricultural Research Service, Nutrient Data Laboratory. USDA National Nutrient Database for Standard Reference, Release 28. Version Current: September 2015. Internet: http://www.ars.usda.gov/nea/bhnrc/ndl

Metabolic water is the water formed from the body's metabolic reactions such as the breakdown of carbohydrates, fats, and proteins. This water contributes about 10% to 14% of the water the body needs each day.

We Lose Fluids Through Urine, Sweat, Evaporation, Exhalation, and Feces

We can perceive—or sense—water loss through urine output and sweating, so we refer to this as **sensible water loss**. Most of the water we consume is excreted through the kidneys in the form of urine. When we consume more water than we need, the kidneys process and excrete the excess in the form of dilute urine.

The second type of sensible water loss is via sweat. Our sweat glands produce more sweat during exercise or when we are in a hot environment. The evaporation of sweat from the skin releases heat, which cools the skin and reduces the body's core temperature.

Water is continuously evaporated from the skin, even when a person is not visibly sweating, and water is continuously exhaled from the lungs during breathing. Water loss through these routes is known as **insensible water loss** because we do not perceive it. Under normal resting conditions, insensible water loss is less than 1 liter (L) of fluid each day; during heavy exercise or in hot weather, a person can lose up to 2 L of water per hour from insensible water loss.

On average, only about 150 to 200 ml of water is lost each day in feces. The GI tract typically absorbs most of the fluid that passes through it, unless a person is experiencing diarrhea.

In addition to these five common routes of fluid loss, certain situations can cause a significant loss of fluid from our body:

- Illnesses that involve fever, coughing, vomiting, diarrhea, and a runny nose significantly increase fluid loss. This is one reason that doctors advise people to drink plenty of fluids when they are ill.
- Traumatic injury, internal bleeding, blood donation, and surgery also increase loss of fluid because of the blood loss involved.
- Exercise increases fluid loss via sweat and respiration; although urine production typically decreases during exercise, fluid losses increase through the skin and lungs.
- Environmental conditions that increase fluid loss include high altitudes, cold and hot temperatures, and low humidity, such as in a desert or an airplane. Because the water content of these environments is low, water from the body more easily evaporates into the surrounding air. We also breathe faster at high altitudes to compensate for the lower oxygen pressure, leading to greater fluid loss via the lungs. We sweat in the heat, but cold temperatures can trigger hormonal changes that also increase fluid loss.
- Pregnancy increases fluid loss for the mother because fluids are continually diverted to the fetus and amniotic fluid.
- Breastfeeding requires a tremendous increase in fluid intake to make up for the loss of fluid as breast milk.
- Consumption of **diuretics**—substances that increase fluid loss via the urine—can result in dangerously excessive fluid loss. Diuretics include certain prescription medications, alcohol, and many over-the-counter weight loss remedies. In the past, it was believed that caffeine acted as a diuretic, but recent research suggests that caffeinated drinks do not significantly influence fluid status in healthy adults.[3,4]

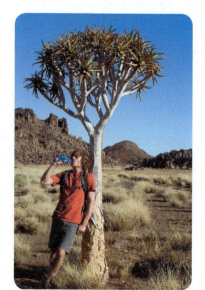

▲ Fluid losses increase in hot, dry environments.

metabolic water The water formed as a by-product of our body's metabolic reactions.

sensible water loss Water loss that is noticed by a person, such as through urine output and visible sweating.

insensible water loss The loss of water not noticeable by a person, such as through evaporation from the skin and exhalation from the lungs during breathing.

diuretic A substance that increases fluid loss via the urine.

recap A healthful fluid level is maintained by balancing intake and excretion. The thirst mechanism in the hypothalamus prompts us to feel thirsty whenever it is stimulated by a high concentration of blood solutes, reduction in blood volume and blood pressure, or dryness of the mouth and throat. The primary sources of fluids are intake of water, other beverages, and foods, and the production of metabolic water. Fluid losses occur through urination, sweating, the feces, exhalation from the lungs, and insensible evaporation from the skin.

How much water should you drink?

Water is essential for life. Although we can live weeks without food, we can survive only a few days without water, depending on the environmental temperature. The human body does not have the capacity to store water, so we must continuously replace the water lost each day.

Our Requirements for Water Are Individualized

The DRI for water for adult men aged 19 to 50 years is 3.7 L of total water per day. This includes approximately 3.0 L (about 13 cups) as beverages, including water and 0.7 L (about 3 cups) from foods. The DRI for adult women aged 19 to 50 years is 2.7 L of total water per day, including about 2.2 L (about 9 cups) as beverages and 0.5 L (about 2 cups) from foods.[5]

FIGURE 7.8 shows the amount and sources of water intake and output for a woman expending 2,500 kcal per day. This woman loses about 3,000 ml (3 L) of fluid per day, which she replaces with beverages (2,200 ml), food (500 ml), and metabolism (300 ml).

An 8-oz glass of fluid is equal to 240 ml. In this example, the woman would need to drink nine glasses of fluid to meet her needs. Although you may have heard the recommendation to drink eight glasses of fluid each day, this is a myth. Fluid requirements are highly individualized, and even the DRIs are only a general guideline. For example, athletes and other people who are active, especially those working in very hot environments, require more fluid than people working a desk job in an air-conditioned office. In fact, a recent study reported that competitive athletes can lose up to 2 liters of sweat per hour when they are intensely exercising in the heat.[6] Thus, these individuals need to drink more to replace the fluid they lose. Dehydration and other disorders related to fluid imbalances are discussed later in this chapter.

Tap Water Is as Healthful as Bottled Water

In 2016, the FBI joined a criminal investigation of lead-contaminated tap water in Flint, Michigan. Does this suggest that municipal water supplies are unsafe? Is bottled water better? Let's have a look.

Millions of Americans routinely consume the tap water found in homes and public places, which generally comes from two sources: surface water comes from lakes, rivers, and reservoirs, and groundwater is from underground rock formations called

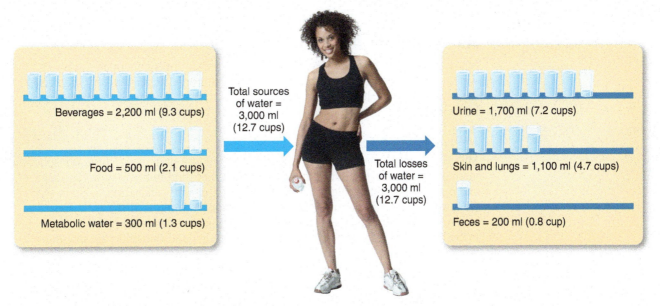

Beverages = 2,200 ml (9.3 cups)

Food = 500 ml (2.1 cups)

Metabolic water = 300 ml (1.3 cups)

Total sources of water = 3,000 ml (12.7 cups)

Total losses of water = 3,000 ml (12.7 cups)

Urine = 1,700 ml (7.2 cups)

Skin and lungs = 1,100 ml (4.7 cups)

Feces = 200 ml (0.8 cup)

FIGURE 7.8 Amount and sources of water intake and output for a woman expending 2,500 kcal/day.

aquifers. The Environmental Protection Agency (EPA) sets and monitors the standards for public water systems. The most common chemical used to treat and purify public water supplies is *chlorine*, which is effective in killing many microorganisms. Water treatment plants also routinely check water supplies for hazardous chemicals, including toxic minerals such as lead (which damages the nervous system). Because of these efforts, the United States has one of the safest water systems in the world. The criminal investigation in Flint, Michigan, can be seen as evidence of federal commitment to safe public water supplies.

Many people who live in rural areas depend on groundwater pumped from a well as their water source. The EPA does not monitor water from private wells, but it publishes recommendations for well owners to help them maintain a safe water supply. For more information on drinking water safety, go to the EPA website (see the **Web Links** at the end of this chapter).

Decades before the crisis in Flint, a major shift in consumption from tap water to bottled water began. Americans now drink about 34 gallons of bottled water per person, per year, totaling more than 11 billion gallons![7] The meteoric rise in bottled water production and consumption is most likely due to the convenience of drinking bottled water, the health messages related to drinking more water, and the public's fears related to the safety of tap water. Even with this growth, however, bottled water represents only a small fraction of the over 1 billion gallons of tap water the U.S. public water systems supply every hour of every day.[7] Recent environmental concerns related to the disposal of water bottles has begun to limit the growth of bottled water, and the industry has responded by using smaller bottle caps, thinner bottles, and a higher proportion of recyclable materials.

The FDA is responsible for the regulation of bottled water. Like tap water, bottled water is taken from either surface water or groundwater sources. But it is often treated and filtered differently. Although this treatment may make bottled water taste better than tap water, it doesn't necessarily make it any safer to drink. Also, although some types of bottled water contain more minerals than tap water, there are no other additional nutritional benefits of drinking bottled water. How can you tell what's in your favorite brand of bottled water? See the **Nutrition Label Activity** to find out!

Many types of bottled water are available in the United States. Carbonated water (seltzer water) contains carbon dioxide gas that either occurs naturally or is added to the water. Mineral waters contain various levels of minerals and offer a unique taste. Some brands, however, contain high amounts of sodium and should be avoided by people who are trying to reduce their sodium intake. Distilled water is mineral free but has a "flat" taste. For more information on bottled water, go to www.bottledwater.org.

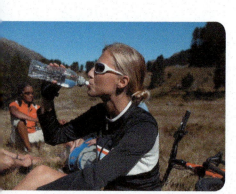

▲ Drinking bottled water is convenient, but costly to your budget and the environment.

All Beverages Are Not Created Equal

Many commercial beverages contain several important nutrients in addition to their water content, whereas others provide water and refined sugar but very little else. Let's review the health benefits and potential concerns of some of the most popular beverages on the market.

Milk and Milk Alternatives

Milk is a healthful beverage choice because it provides protein, calcium, phosphorus, vitamin D, and, usually, vitamin A. Many brands of fluid milk are now "specialized" and provide additional calcium, vitamin E, essential fatty acids, and/or plant sterols (to lower serum cholesterol). Kefir, a blended yogurt drink, is also a good source of most of these nutrients. Calcium-fortified soy milk provides protein and calcium, and many brands provide vitamin D. In contrast, almond and rice milks are low in protein, with only 1 gram per cup.

When purchasing flavored milk, kefir, or milk alternatives, check the Nutrition Facts panel for the sugar content. Some brands of chocolate milk, for example, can contain 6 or more teaspoons of sugar in a single cup!

Is Bottled Water Better Than Tap?

The next time you reach for a bottle of water, check the label! If it doesn't identify a specific water source, the bottle may actually contain tap water with minerals added to improve the taste. To avoid paying a high price for bottled tap water, make sure the label includes the phrase "Bottled at the source." Water that comes from a protected groundwater source is less likely to have contaminants, such as disease-causing microbes. If the label doesn't identify the water's source, it should at least provide contact information, such as a phone number or website of the bottled water company, so that you can track down the source.

Although many labels lack information about treatment methods, you might use the company's website to find out how their bottled water was treated. There are several ways of treating water, but what you're looking for is either of the following two methods, which have been proven to be most effective against the most common waterborne disease-causing microorganisms:

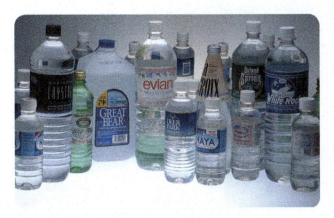

◆ Numerous varieties of drinking water are available to consumers.

- *Micron filtration,* which is a process whereby water is filtered through screens with various-sized microscopic holes. High-quality micron filtration can eliminate most chemical contaminants and microbes.

- *Reverse osmosis,* which is a process often referred to as *ultrafiltration* because it uses a membrane with microscopic openings that allow water to pass through but not larger compounds. Reverse osmosis membranes also utilize electrical charges to reject harmful chemicals.

If the label on your bottle of water says that the water was purified using any of the following methods, you might want to consider switching brands: filtered, carbon-filtered, particle-filtered, ozonated or ozone-treated, ultraviolet light, ion exchange, or deionized. These methods have not been proven to be effective against the most common waterborne disease-causing microorganisms.

It is also a good idea to check the nutrient content on the water bottle label. Ideally, water should be high in magnesium (at least 20 mg per 8 fl. oz serving) and calcium but low in sodium (less than 5 mg per 8 fl. oz serving). Avoid bottled waters with sweeteners because their "empty Calories" can contribute significantly to your energy intake. These products are often promoted as healthful beverage choices with names including words such as *vitamins, herbs, nature,* and *life,* but they are essentially "liquid candy." Check the Nutrition Facts panel and don't be fooled.

Hot Beverages Containing Caffeine

Coffee made without cream or nondairy creamer can be a healthful beverage choice if consumed in moderation. As mentioned earlier, recent research suggests that its caffeine content does not significantly decrease the body's hydration status, and the calcium in coffee drinks made with milk, such as café con leche and café latte, can be significant. Coffee is also known to provide several types of phytochemicals that may lower risk of certain chronic diseases such as type 2 diabetes, liver disease, heart disease, and stroke.[8] The 2015 Dietary Guidelines Advisory Committee reported that intake of 1 cup of coffee per day was associated with a 3% to 4% decrease in risk of total mortality.[9]

Tea is second only to water as the most commonly consumed beverage in the world. With the exception of red tea and herbal teas, which do not contain caffeine, all forms of tea come from the same plant, *Camellia sinesis,* and all contain caffeine. However, the level is typically about half that of the same amount of brewed coffee. Black tea is the most highly processed (the tea leaves are fully fermented). Oolong tea leaves are only partially fermented, and both green and white tea leaves have been dried but not fermented. As compared to black and oolong teas, green

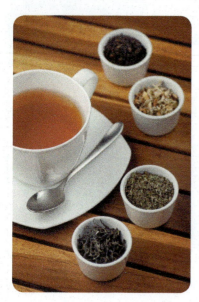

After water, tea is the most commonly consumed beverage in the world.

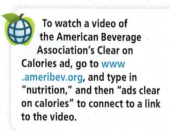

To watch a video of the American Beverage Association's Clear on Calories ad, go to www.ameribev.org, and type in "nutrition," and then "ads clear on calories" to connect to a link to the video.

and white teas are higher in phytochemicals. Consumption of green tea decreases the risk of cardiovascular disease, including strokes.[10] Research has also shown that green tea mouthwash has an effective antiplaque effect.[11] If consumed without added sugar, tea is an excellent source of fluid that may have unexpected long-term health benefits.

Hot chocolate also provides caffeine, although the levels are much lower than those found in coffee or tea. Dark chocolate is rich in phytochemicals known as flavanols, which may reduce the risk of heart attacks and strokes[12] and the onset of age-related cognitive decline.[13] Hot chocolate made with dark cocoa powder and skim or low-fat milk is a nutritious and satisfying drink.

Energy Drinks

Energy drinks represent another popular beverage option, with over $10 billion in U.S. sales in 2015. About 30% of teenagers and 65% of Millennials drink them on a regular basis, even though public health experts have raised significant concerns over their harmful effects.[14] Many energy drinks contain more than three times the amount of caffeine in a comparable serving of cola, and some also contain guarana seed extract, which is a potent source of additional caffeine. Moreover, unlike hot coffee, which is sipped slowly, the drinks are typically downed in a few minutes. Some are even packaged as a "shot." This sudden surge of caffeine can cause a dramatic rise in blood pressure and heart rate. Seizures, miscarriage, mood swings, insomnia, dehydration, and other health problems, as well as over 20,000 emergency department visits, have been linked to consumption of energy drinks. Although the FDA limits the amount of caffeine in soft drinks, it has no legal authority to regulate the ingredients, including caffeine, in energy drinks because they are classified as dietary supplements, not food. In contrast, Canada now caps caffeine levels in energy drinks, and Mexico is proposing to ban their sale to adolescents.

Energy drinks are also a source of significant added sugars. For example, a 16-oz bottle of Rockstar Original contains 62 grams—more than 15 teaspoons—of added sugars. In short, as a source of fluid, energy drinks should be avoided by children and adolescents and used sparingly by adults.

Beverages with Added Sugars

Soft drinks, juice drinks, flavored waters, and bottled teas and coffee drinks made with added sugars are referred to as *sugary drinks*. Whether they are sweetened with high fructose corn syrup (HFCS), honey, cane sugar, or fruit juice concentrate is unimportant: all forms of sugar provide the same number of Calories per gram, no matter their molecular structure. Even 100% fruit juice with no added sugar is high in Calories. For instance, an 8-oz carton of a popular brand of premium orange juice provides 110 Calories.

As we've discussed (see Chapters 4 and 5), added sugars contribute not only to obesity, but also to chronic disease. Research data has linked diets high in added sugars to increased risk of cardiovascular disease and overall mortality due to chronic diseases.[15,16]

In the past, very few people realized how many Calories were in the beverages they drank. Recently, however, public health agencies have been raising awareness of the empty Calorie content of sugary drinks. Some are advocating that a first step in any weight loss program should be to entirely eliminate these products from the diet. The city of Berkeley, California, recently became the first community to impose a sales tax on sugary drinks, and the FDA's proposed changes to the Nutrition Facts panel will identify added sugars separately from total sugars. In addition, the American Beverage Association's "Clear on Calories" campaign now puts Calorie information per package on the front of the product. Thus, when buying a 20-oz bottle of sweetened tea, consumers will know they'll be consuming, for example, 250 Calories if they drink the whole bottle. Some beverage companies have reduced the average Calorie content of their products by introducing a variety of smaller cans and bottles. Most consumer advocates, however, view these efforts simply as a marketing ploy.

Specialty Waters

Specialty waters are made with added nutrients, herbs, or a higher pH. The labels claim they enhance memory, delay aging, boost energy levels, or strengthen the immune response. Notice, however, that these claims are accompanied by a disclaimer such as, "This statement has not been evaluated by the FDA. This product is not intended to diagnose, treat, cure, or prevent any disease." The FDA requires this disclaimer whenever a food manufacturer makes a structure-function claim (see Chapter 2). It acknowledges that the statement made on the label is not based on research!

In fact, the amounts of nutrients, phytochemicals, or other substances added to these waters are usually so low, compared to what can be obtained from foods, that they rarely make much of an impact on the consumer's health. In contrast, some of these designer waters can add more than 300 Calories to the day's intake, and they are expensive.

Sports Beverages and Coconut Water

Because of the potential for fluid and electrolyte imbalances during rigorous exercise, many endurance athletes drink sports beverages, which provide water, electrolytes, and a source of carbohydrate, before, during, and after workouts. Others are turning to coconut water, marketed as a good source of electrolytes and "natural sugars." Recently, these beverages have become popular with nonathletes, including children and adolescents.[17] However, as a general rule, only people who exercise or do manual labor vigorously for 60 minutes or more benefit from drinking either sports beverages or coconut water. (Fluid requirements for physical activity are discussed in detail in Chapter 11.)

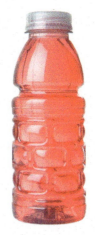

◄ Sports beverages can help meet the nutrient needs of athletes, but are unnecessary for most consumers.

recap According to the DRIs, adult males need to drink about 13 cups of beverages each day, and females need about 9 cups. However, fluid intake needs are highly variable and depend on body size, age, physical activity, health status, and environmental conditions. All beverages provide water, and some, such as milk and milk alternatives, provide other important nutrients as well. Coffee and tea provide phytochemicals and are considered healthful if consumed in moderation. Energy drinks typically release more caffeine more quickly into the bloodstream, and can be harmful. Sugary drinks can contribute substantially to weight gain and an increased risk for chronic disease. Most nonathletes do not need to consume sports beverages or coconut water.

How do four major minerals contribute to fluid balance?

LO 5 Identify the functions, DRIs, and common dietary sources of sodium, potassium, chloride, and phosphorus.

The micronutrients involved in maintaining hydration and neuromuscular function are the major minerals sodium, potassium, chloride, and phosphorus (TABLE 7.1). Calcium and magnesium also function as electrolytes and influence the body's fluid

TABLE 7.1   Overview of Minerals Involved in Hydration and Neuromuscular Function

To see the full profile of all micronutrients, turn to the **In Depth** essay following Chapter 6, Vitamins and Minerals: Micronutrients with Macro Powers (pages 211–221).

Nutrient	Recommended Intake
Sodium	AI for 19 to 50 years of age: 1.5 g/day
Potassium	AI for 19 years of age and older: 4.7 g/day
Chloride	AI for 19 to 50 years of age: 2.3 g/day
Phosphorus	RDA for 19 years of age and older: 700 mg/day

balance and neuromuscular function; however, because of their critical importance to bone health, they are discussed in Chapter 9.

Sodium Is a Positively Charged Extracellular Electrolyte

Over the last 20 years, researchers have linked high sodium intake to an increased risk for hypertension among some groups of individuals. Because of this link, many people have come to believe that sodium is harmful to the body. This oversimplification, however, is just not true: sodium is essential for survival.

Functions of Sodium

Sodium is the major positively charged electrolyte in the extracellular fluid. Its exchange with potassium across cell membranes allows cells to maintain proper fluid balance. Moreover, the kidneys' excretion and reabsorption of sodium contribute to blood pressure regulation. Sodium also assists with the initiation and transmission of nerve signals. The stimulation of muscles by nerve impulses provides the impetus for muscle contraction.

Recommended Intakes and Food Sources of Sodium

The AI for sodium is listed in Table 7.1. Most people in the United States consume two to four times the AI daily. Several national guidelines, including the *2015–2020 Dietary Guidelines for Americans* (DGAs) recommend a daily sodium intake of no more than 2,300 mg per day. The DGAs specifically recommend that persons who have prehypertension or hypertension limit their daily sodium intake to no more than 1,500 mg.[18]

Sodium is found naturally in many whole foods, but most dietary sodium comes from processed foods and restaurant foods, which typically contain large amounts of added sodium. Try to guess which of the following foods contains the most sodium: 1 cup of tomato juice, 1 oz of potato chips, or 4 saltine crackers. Now look at **TABLE 7.2** to find the answer. This table shows foods that are high in sodium and gives lower-sodium alternatives. Are you surprised to find out that, of all of these food items, the tomato juice has the most sodium?

Because sodium is so abundant, it's easy to overdo it. See the **Quick Tips** feature for ways to reduce your sodium intake. For more help curbing your sodium intake, try the DASH diet (see the **In Depth** essay on cardiovascular disease following Chapter 5).

TABLE 7.2   High-Sodium Foods and Lower-Sodium Alternatives

High-Sodium Food	Sodium (mg)	Lower-Sodium Food	Sodium (mg)
Dill pickle (1 large, 4 in.)	1,731	Low-sodium dill pickle (1 large, 4 in.)	23
Ham, cured, roasted (3 oz)	1,023	Pork, loin roast (3 oz)	54
Turkey pastrami (3 oz)	915	Roasted turkey, cooked (3 oz)	54
Tomato juice, regular (1 cup)	877	Tomato juice, lower sodium (1 cup)	24
Macaroni and cheese (1 cup)	800	Spanish rice (1 cup)	5
Ramen noodle soup (chicken flavor) (1 package [85 g])	1,960	Ramen noodle soup made with sodium-free chicken bouillon (1 cup)	0
Teriyaki chicken (1 cup)	3,210	Stir-fried pork/rice/vegetables (1 cup)	575
Tomato sauce, canned (1/2 cup)	741	Fresh tomato (1 medium)	11
Creamed corn, canned (1 cup)	730	Cooked corn, fresh (1 cup)	28
Tomato soup, canned (1 cup)	695	Lower-sodium tomato soup, canned (1 cup)	480
Potato chips, salted (1 oz)	168	Baked potato, unsalted (1 medium)	14
Saltine crackers (4 crackers)	156	Saltine crackers, unsalted (4 crackers)	100

Data from: U.S. Department of Agriculture. 2011. USDA Nutrient Database for Standard Reference, Release 24.

QuickTips

Reducing the Sodium in Your Diet

✔ Put away the salt shaker—keep it off the table and train your taste buds to prefer foods with less salt.

✔ Follow the DASH diet plan (see page 176), which is high in fruits, vegetables, whole grains, and lean protein foods. The more you include fresh, whole foods in your diet, the less sodium you will be eating.

✔ Look for the words *low sodium* or *no added salt* when buying processed foods. Use the Nutrition Facts panel to find foods that contain 5% or less of the daily value for sodium or less than 200 mg per serving.

✔ Look for *hidden* salt content on food labels; for example, both monosodium glutamate and sodium benzoate are forms of sodium.

✔ Choose fresh or frozen vegetables (without added sauces) because they are usually much lower in sodium than canned vegetables. Alternatively, choose salt-free canned vegetables.

✔ Stay away from prepared stews, canned and dried soups, gravies, and pasta sauces as well as packaged pasta, rice, and potato dishes that are high in sodium.

✔ Choose low-sodium versions of pickles, olives, three-bean salad, salad dressings, smoked meats and fish, and nuts.

✔ Snack on fruits and vegetables instead of salty pretzels, chips, and other snack items.

✔ When cooking, experiment with herbs, spices, lemon juice, chutneys, salsas, and cooking wine to flavor your food. Products that end in the word *salt,* such as garlic salt or celery salt, are high in sodium and should be avoided.

✔ Rinse canned legumes, such as black, navy, garbanzo, or kidney beans, with cold water to lower the sodium content before heating and consuming them.

✔ Limit the amounts of condiments you use. Condiments such as ketchup, mustard, pickle relish, and soy sauce can add a considerable amount of sodium to your foods.

✔ When eating out, look for entrées labeled "heart healthy" or "lower in sodium"; if nutrition information is provided, compare foods to select those with lower amounts of sodium.

✔ Check the labels of the beverages you consume as well; fluids are often a "hidden" source of dietary sodium.

✔ Also check your medications. Some are high in sodium.

Sodium Toxicity and Deficiency

Hypertension is typically more common in people who consume high-sodium diets, especially if potassium intake is low. This strong relationship has prompted many health organizations to recommend lowering sodium intakes. Whether high-sodium diets actually cause hypertension is a matter of continuing debate; many researchers believe that a high-sodium/low-potassium dietary pattern is the greatest risk factor. Researchers also debate the effect of high-sodium intake on bone loss: some studies suggest high-sodium intakes have a negative effect on bone density, whereas other research has shown no impact on bone density.

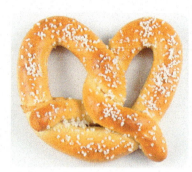

⬅ Many popular snack foods are high in sodium.

Hypernatremia refers to an abnormally high blood sodium concentration. Although theoretically it could be caused by a rapid intake of high amounts of sodium—for instance, if a shipwrecked sailor resorted to drinking seawater—consuming too much sodium does not usually cause hypernatremia in a healthy person because the kidneys are able to excrete excess sodium in the urine. But people with congestive heart failure or kidney disease are not able to excrete sodium effectively, making them more prone to the condition. Hypernatremia is dangerous because it causes an abnormally high blood volume, again, by pulling water from the intracellular environment to dilute the sodium in the extracellular tissue spaces and vessels. This leads to edema (swelling) of tissues and elevation of blood pressure to harmful levels.

Because the dietary intake of sodium is so high among Americans, deficiencies of sodium are extremely rare. Nevertheless, certain conditions can cause **hyponatremia**, abnormally low blood sodium levels.

Hyponatremia can occur during periods of intense physical activity, such as a marathon or day-long hike in warm weather, when people drink large volumes of water and fail to replace sodium. Severe diarrhea, vomiting, or excessive, prolonged sweating can also cause hyponatremia. Symptoms include headaches, dizziness, fatigue, nausea, vomiting, and muscle cramps.

If hyponatremia is left untreated, it can progress to seizures, coma, and death. Treatment includes careful sodium replacement, such as the intravenous administration of an electrolyte-rich solution.

Potassium Is a Positively Charged Intracellular Electrolyte

As we discussed previously, potassium is the major positively charged electrolyte in the intracellular fluid. It is a major constituent of all living cells and is found in both plants and animals.

Functions of Potassium

Potassium and sodium work together to maintain proper fluid balance and regulate the transmission of nerve impulses and the contraction of muscles. And in contrast to a high-sodium diet, a diet high in potassium actually helps maintain a lower blood pressure.

Recommended Intakes and Food Sources of Potassium

Potassium is found in abundance in many fresh foods, especially fresh fruits and vegetables. Processed foods generally have less potassium than fresh foods.

The AI for potassium is listed in Table 7.1. Just as most Americans' sodium intake exceeds the recommended limits, the average potassium intake of Americans falls well below the recommended amount. Many researchers think that this sodium–potassium imbalance is a major factor contributing to the increased incidence of hypertension in the United States. By avoiding processed foods and eating more fresh fruits, legumes and other vegetables, whole grains, and dairy foods, you'll increase your potassium intake and decrease your sodium intake, achieving a more healthful diet. **FIGURE 7.9** identifies foods that are high in potassium. See the **Quick Tips** for suggestions on how to increase your dietary potassium.

Potassium Toxicity and Deficiency

People with healthy kidneys are able to excrete excess potassium effectively. However, people with kidney disease are not able to regulate their blood potassium levels. **Hyperkalemia**, or high blood potassium levels, occurs when potassium is not excreted efficiently from the body. Because of potassium's role in cardiac muscle contraction, severe hyperkalemia can alter the normal rhythm of the heart, resulting in heart attack and death. People with kidney failure must monitor their potassium intake very carefully. Individuals at risk for hyperkalemia should avoid consuming salt substitutes because these products are high in potassium.

Because potassium is widespread in many foods, a dietary potassium deficiency is rare. However, potassium deficiency, called **hypokalemia**, is not uncommon among

hypernatremia A condition in which blood sodium levels are dangerously high.

hyponatremia A condition in which blood sodium levels are dangerously low.

hyperkalemia A condition in which blood potassium levels are dangerously high.

hypokalemia A condition in which blood potassium levels are dangerously low.

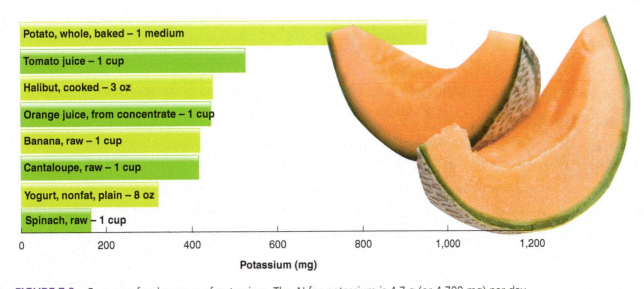

FIGURE 7.9 Common food sources of potassium. The AI for potassium is 4.7 g (or 4,700 mg) per day.

Data from: U.S. Department of Agriculture, Agricultural Research Service, Nutrient Data Laboratory. USDA National Nutrient Database for Standard Reference, Release 28. Version Current: September 2015. Internet: http://www.ars.usda.gov/nea/bhnrc/ndl

people who have serious medical disorders. In addition, people with hypertension who are prescribed diuretic medications are at risk. Diuretics promote the excretion of fluid as urine through the kidneys. Whereas some diuretics spare potassium, others increase the excretion of potassium. People who are taking diuretic medications therefore require close medical monitoring.

Extreme dehydration, vomiting, diarrhea, alcohol abuse, and laxative abuse increase the risk for hypokalemia. Symptoms include confusion, loss of appetite,

Quick Tips

Increasing Your Potassium Intake

✔ Avoid processed foods that are high in sodium and low in potassium. Check the Nutrition Facts panel of the food before you buy it!

✔ For breakfast, look for cereals containing bran and/or wheat germ, or add wheat germ to homemade bran muffins.

✔ Sprinkle wheat germ on yogurt and top with banana slices.

✔ Drink milk! If you don't like milk, try kefir. Many brands of soy milk are also good sources of potassium.

✔ Make a smoothie by blending ice cubes and yogurt with a banana.

✔ Pack a can of low-sodium vegetable or tomato juice in your lunch in place of a soft drink.

✔ Serve avocado or bean dip with veggie slices.

✔ Replace the meat in your sandwich with thin slices of avocado or marinated tofu.

✔ Replace the meat in tacos and burritos with black or pinto beans.

✔ For a healthful alternative to french fries, toss slices of sweet potato in olive oil, place on a cookie sheet, and oven bake at 400°F for 10–15 minutes.

✔ Toss a banana, some dried apricots, or a bag of sunflower seeds into your lunch bag.

✔ Make a fruit salad with apricots, bananas, cantaloupe, honeydew melon, mango, or papaya.

✔ Bake and enjoy a fresh pumpkin pie!

and muscle weakness. Severe cases result in fatal changes in heart rate; many deaths attributed to extreme dehydration or eating disorders are caused by abnormal heart rhythms due to hypokalemia.

Chloride Is a Negatively Charged Extracellular Electrolyte

Chloride should not be confused with *chlorine*, which is a poisonous gas used to kill bacteria and other germs in our water supply. Chloride is a negatively charged ion that is obtained almost exclusively in our diet from sodium chloride, or table salt.

Coupled with sodium in the extracellular fluid, chloride assists with the maintenance of fluid balance. Chloride is also a part of hydrochloric acid in the stomach, which aids in preparing food for further digestion (see Chapter 3). Chloride works with the white blood cells of our body during an immune response to help kill bacteria, and it assists in the transmission of nerve impulses.

The AI for chloride is listed in Table 7.1. Our primary dietary source of chloride is the sodium chloride in the salt in our foods. Chloride is also found in some fruits and vegetables. As you've learned, consuming excess amounts of salt over a prolonged period leads to hypertension in salt-sensitive individuals. There is no other known toxicity symptom for chloride. Moreover, because of the relatively high salt intake in the United States, chloride deficiency is rare, even when a person consumes a low-sodium diet. A chloride deficiency can occur, however, during conditions of severe dehydration and frequent vomiting, including in people with eating disorders who vomit after food intake.

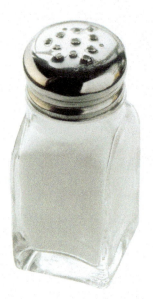

⬆ Almost all chloride is consumed through table salt.

Phosphorus Is a Negatively Charged Intracellular Electrolyte

Phosphorus is the major intracellular negatively charged electrolyte. In the body, phosphorus is most commonly found in the form of phosphate. Phosphorus is an essential constituent of all cells and is found in both plants and animals.

Phosphorus works with potassium inside cells to maintain proper fluid balance. It also plays a critical role in bone formation because it is part of the mineral complex of bone. In fact, about 85% of our body's phosphorus is stored in our bones.

As a primary component of adenosine triphosphate (ATP), phosphorus plays a key role in the conversion of food to energy. It also helps regulate many other chemical reactions by activating and deactivating enzymes. Phosphorus is a part of deoxyribonucleic acid (DNA) and ribonucleic acid (RNA), and it is a component in cell membranes (as phospholipids) and lipoproteins.

The RDA for phosphorus is listed in Table 7.1. The average U.S. adult consumes about twice this amount each day; thus, phosphorus deficiencies are rare. Phosphorus is widespread in many foods; high-protein foods such as milk, meats, and eggs are good sources. **FIGURE 7.10** shows the phosphorus content of various foods. Phosphorus is absorbed more readily from animal sources than from plant sources. Another beneficial role of the GI flora is to help release the phosphorus in plant foods, allowing more of it to be absorbed.

People suffering from kidney disease, who cannot efficiently excrete phosphorus; people consuming excessive amounts of supplemental vitamin D, which tends to increase absorption and retention of phosphorus; and people taking too many phosphorus-containing antacids can suffer from high blood phosphorus levels. Severely high levels of blood phosphorus cause muscle spasms and convulsions. Deficiencies of phosphorus are rare except in people with very poor diets, vitamin D deficiency, or oversecretion of parathyroid hormone. People who overuse antacids that bind with phosphorus may also have low blood phosphorus levels.

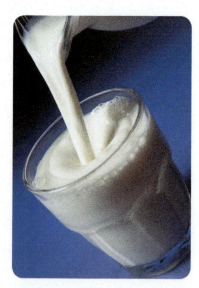

⬆ Milk is a good source of phosphorus.

recap The four electrolytes critical for hydration and neuromuscular function are sodium, potassium, chloride, and phosphorus. Sodium and potassium are positively charged electrolytes. Most Americans consume more than the recommended 2,300 mg of sodium per day, and many consume too little potassium.

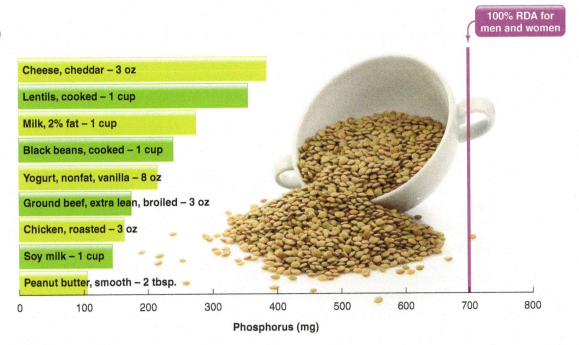

100% RDA for men and women

Cheese, cheddar – 3 oz

Lentils, cooked – 1 cup

Milk, 2% fat – 1 cup

Black beans, cooked – 1 cup

Yogurt, nonfat, vanilla – 8 oz

Ground beef, extra lean, broiled – 3 oz

Chicken, roasted – 3 oz

Soy milk – 1 cup

Peanut butter, smooth – 2 tbsp.

| 0 | 100 | 200 | 300 | 400 | 500 | 600 | 700 | 800 |

Phosphorus (mg)

🔺 **FIGURE 7.10** Common food sources of phosphorus. The RDA for phosphorus is 700 mg/day.

Data from: U.S. Department of Agriculture, Agricultural Research Service, Nutrient Data Laboratory. USDA National Nutrient Database for Standard Reference, Release 28. Version Current: September 2015. Internet: http://www.ars.usda.gov/nea/bhnrc/ndl

This imbalance, which tends to reflect Americans' high intake of processed foods and low intake of fresh fruits and vegetables, has been associated with an increased risk for cardiovascular disease. Intakes of the negatively charged electrolytes chloride and phosphorus are almost always adequate, except in people with very poor diets or serious disorders. Toxicities are also rare. Electrolyte imbalances can result in heart failure, seizures, and death.

What disorders are related to fluid and electrolyte balance?

LO 6 Discuss several disorders related to fluid and electrolyte balance.

A number of serious, and potentially fatal, disorders, including dehydration and heat illnesses, are related to fluid and electrolytes imbalances. We review some of these here.

Dehydration Develops as Fluid Loss Exceeds Fluid Intake

Dehydration is a serious condition that develops when fluid losses exceed fluid intake. It is classified in terms of the percentage of weight loss that is exclusively due to the loss of fluid (**TABLE 7.3**) (page 244).

Dehydration most commonly develops as a result of heavy exercise or hard physical labor in high environmental temperatures, when the body loses significant amounts of water through increased sweating and breathing. However, elderly people and infants can get dehydrated even when inactive, as their risk for dehydration is much higher than that of healthy young and middle-aged adults. The elderly are at increased risk because they have a lower total amount of body fluid and their thirst mechanism is less effective than that of a younger person; they are therefore less likely to meet their fluid needs. Infants, on the other hand, excrete urine at a higher rate, cannot tell us when they are thirsty, and have a greater ratio of body surface area to body core, causing them to respond more dramatically to heat and cold and to lose more body water than an older child. Finally, extended bouts of diarrhea, vomiting, or fever can also lead to dehydration.

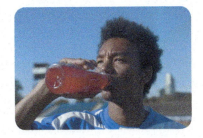

🔺 Adequate fluid replacement during and after physical activity is critical in preventing dehydration.

dehydration The depletion of body fluid. It results when fluid excretion exceeds fluid intake.

TABLE 7.3 Percentages of Body Fluid Loss Correlated with Weight Loss and Symptoms

Body Water Loss (%)	Weight Lost If You Weigh 160 lb	Weight Lost If You Weigh 130 lb	Symptoms
1–2	1.6–3.2 lb	1.3–2.6 lb	Strong thirst, loss of appetite, feeling uncomfortable
3–5	4.8–8.0 lb	3.9–6.5 lb	Dry mouth, reduced urine output, greater difficulty working and concentrating, flushed skin, tingling extremities, impatience, sleepiness, nausea, emotional instability
6–8	9.6–12.8 lb	7.8–10.4 lb	Increased body temperature that doesn't decrease, increased heart rate and breathing rate, dizziness, difficulty breathing, slurred speech, mental confusion, muscle weakness, blue lips
9–11	14.4–17.6 lb	11.7–14.3 lb	Muscle spasms, delirium, swollen tongue, poor balance and circulation, kidney failure, decreased blood volume and blood pressure

Data from: *Nutrition and Aerobic Exercise*, edited by D. K. Layman. © 1986 American Chemical Society.

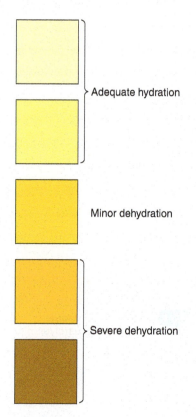

Adequate hydration

Minor dehydration

Severe dehydration

◄ FIGURE 7.11 Urine color chart. Color variations indicate levels of hydration.

overhydration The dilution of body fluid. It results when water retention or intake is excessive.

heat cramps Involuntary, spasmodic, and painful muscle contractions that are caused by electrolyte imbalances occurring as a result of strenuous physical activity in high environmental heat.

Adequate fluid replacement is the most important factor in preventing dehydration. If you're physically active, how can you tell whether you are drinking enough fluid before, during, and after your exercise or training sessions? First, you can hop on the scale before and after each session, ideally when unclothed or just wearing underclothes. If you weighed in at 160 pounds before basketball practice, and immediately afterwards you weighed 158 pounds, then you would have lost 2 pounds of body weight, virtually all as fluid. This is equal to 1.3% of your body weight prior to practice. As you can see in Table 7.3, you would most likely experience strong thirst and diminished appetite, and you might even feel generally uncomfortable.

If you find you have lost weight during a session of physical activity, what should you do about it? Your goal is to consume enough water and other fluids to replace 1 1/2 times as much fluid as was lost—and to do this prior to your next exercise session. Fortunately, this isn't difficult. Every 1 pound of weight loss equals about 2 cups of fluid, which you would need to replace by drinking 3 cups of fluid (2 multiplied by 1.5 equals 3). In general, by following the daily fluid intake recommendations discussed earlier, plus replacing fluids lost during sessions of physical activity, you should be able to avoid becoming dehydrated.

If you don't have time to weigh yourself before and after every workout, don't despair! A simpler method of monitoring your fluid levels is to observe the color of your urine. If you are properly hydrated, your urine should be clear to pale yellow in color, similar to diluted lemonade (**FIGURE 7.11**). Urine that is medium to dark yellow in color, similar to apple juice, indicates an inadequate fluid intake. Very dark or brown urine, such as the color of a cola beverage, is a sign of severe dehydration and indicates potential muscle breakdown and kidney damage. Your goal should be to maintain a urine color that is clear or pale yellow.

Water Intoxication Can Be Fatal

Overhydration, or water intoxication, generally occurs only in people with disorders that cause the kidneys to retain too much water, diluting blood sodium and leading to hyponatremia, as discussed earlier. However, individuals have died of overhydration while following a fad diet or participating in a hazing ritual or competition involving excessive water intake. Thus, no one should ever be encouraged to drink excessive amounts of water.

Heat Illnesses Are Linked to Dehydration

Three common types of heat illness are closely linked to dehydration: in order of severity, these are heat cramps, heat exhaustion, and heat stroke.

Heat Cramps

Heat cramps are painful muscle cramps, usually in the abdomen, arms, or legs, that develop during sessions of vigorous physical activity in the heat. The spasms can last for several seconds or even minutes and are caused by a fluid and electrolyte imbalance.

nutri-case | GUSTAVO

"Something is going on with me this week. Every day, at work, I've been feeling weak and like I'm going to be sick to my stomach. It's been really hot, over a hundred degrees out in the fields, but I'm used to that, and besides, I've been drinking lots of water. It's probably just my high blood pressure acting up again."

What do you think might be affecting Gustavo? If you learned that he was following a low-sodium diet to manage his hypertension, would this information argue for or against your assumptions about the source of his discomfort? Why or why not? What would you advise Gustavo to do differently at work tomorrow?

If you ever experience muscle cramps during a workout or athletic event, stop your activity immediately. Go to a cool place, rest, and sip a sports beverage, juice, or—if these are not available—plain water. You can also sprinkle a dash of salt into a full glass of water. If the cramps don't subside within an hour, seek medical attention.

Heat Exhaustion

Like heat cramps, **heat exhaustion** typically occurs when people are engaging in vigorous physical activity in a hot environment. It can also develop after several days in high temperatures when fluid intake is inadequate.

Signs and symptoms typically include increased thirst; weakness; muscle cramps; nausea and vomiting; dizziness and possibly fainting; and possibly elevated blood pressure and pulse. In a person with heat exhaustion, the sweat mechanism still functions; in fact, the person is typically sweating heavily. Immediate cooling and fluid intake are essential to avoid heat stroke.

Heat Stroke

Heat stroke is a potentially fatal heat illness characterized by failure of the body's heat-regulating mechanisms. Thus, the person's skin is hot and dry, not sweaty. Other signs and symptoms include rapid pulse; high core body temperature; rapid, shallow breathing; and disorientation or loss of consciousness.

Recall that evaporative cooling is less efficient in a humid environment because the sweat is less able to evaporate. Therefore, athletes who work out in hot, humid weather are particularly vulnerable to heat stroke. Heat-related deaths occur among high school, collegiate, and professional athletes. The deaths are more common in overweight or obese athletes for two reasons: Significant muscle mass produces a lot of body heat, whereas excess body fat adds an extra layer of insulation that makes it more difficult to dissipate that heat. In football players, tight-fitting uniforms and helmets also trap warm air and blunt the ability of the body to cool itself.

If you are active in a hot environment and begin to feel dizzy, light-headed, disoriented, or nauseated, stop exercising at once. Get into a cool environment, such as a cool shower or a bath. Drink a sports beverage. If you are working out with someone who exhibits the symptoms of heat stroke, call 911 immediately.

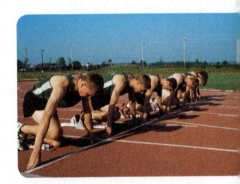

◂ Athletes who train or compete in hot weather are vulnerable to heat stroke.

recap Dehydration is the depletion of body fluid, and occurs when fluid losses exceed fluid intake. If you are properly hydrated, your urine should be clear to pale yellow in color. Overhydration is dilution of body fluid, whether because of a medical disorder or excessive water intake. Heat cramps develop during sessions of vigorous physical activity in the heat, and are caused by fluid and electrolyte imbalances. Heat exhaustion is a more serious condition that develops with inadequate fluid intake in a hot environment. If not addressed, it can lead to heat stroke, a medical emergency characterized by failure of the body's heat-regulating mechanisms.

heat exhaustion A serious condition, characterized by heavy sweating and moderately elevated body temperature, that develops from dehydration in high heat.

heat stroke A potentially fatal response to high temperature characterized by failure of the body's heat-regulating mechanisms; also commonly called *sunstroke*.

Low-Sodium Diets: Fit for All or Just a Few?

For decades, U.S. and international public health organizations recommended a low-sodium diet to prevent and treat hypertension (HTN) and reduce the risk for cardiovascular disease. Many still do.[18] Yet recently, some organizations have modified their sodium-intake recommendations in response to research suggesting that a low intake of sodium may not benefit the population as a whole and may even increase health risks for some. So who should reduce their sodium intake? Should you? Keeping in mind that nutrition research is always providing new information, let's explore our current understanding of this issue.

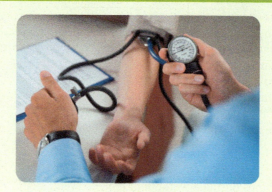

The influence of sodium intake on blood pressure is the subject of ongoing research.

How Have Sodium Intake Recommendations Evolved Over Time?

Prior to 2005, the *Dietary Guidelines for Americans* used only descriptive phrases, not specific numerical targets, for their sodium intake recommendations. For example, the 1990 recommendation was to "Use salt and sodium only in moderation."[19] In contrast, the 2005, 2010, and 2015–2020 DGAs all recommended a specific sodium intake of less than 2,300 mg per day. The 2015–2020 Guidelines also advise people with prehypertension and HTN to limit their sodium intake to 1,500 mg per day and follow the DASH diet.[18] These recommendations were based on a careful review of available research, including epidemiologic studies, double-blind clinical trials, and community-based interventions.

In 2009 and 2012, however, some public health organizations released recommendations that were lower than those of the DGAs: In 2009, the American Heart Association (AHA) proposed "no more than 1,500 mg of sodium per day" for everyone.[20] In 2012, the World Health Organization (WHO) recommended a target intake of 2,000 mg per day—300 mg per day lower than the DGA guideline.[21] Then a 2014 meta-analysis of 25 studies found that a sodium intake between 2,645 and 4,945 mg/day was associated with the lowest mortality risk. The researchers concluded that a sodium intake both lower and higher than these levels was associated with premature mortality.[22] As new research becomes available each year, the controversy over sodium guidelines is likely to continue!

Should You Reduce Your Sodium Intake?

Given the uncertainty regarding what level of sodium intake is the most healthful, should you take steps to reduce your sodium intake?

- First, recognize that lifestyle interventions, including food choices, are low-risk, low-cost approaches to preventing chronic diseases and, for people already affected by disease, can be effective treatments. Because most Americans currently consume well above recommended levels, almost everyone would do well to reduce their current intake of sodium by at least 1,000 mg per day.

- Second, the most practical approach is to follow a healthful dietary pattern. Following the DASH diet or Mediterranean diet can greatly reduce your sodium intake without your having to monitor your milligrams of sodium. These diets have no known health risks; moreover, they will increase your potassium intake, which is known to lower your risk of HTN.

- Third, limit your choice of highly processed foods. Choose fresh foods as much as possible.

- Fourth, remember that the cardiovascular benefits of reducing your sodium intake will be even stronger if you also participate in regular physical activity, maintain a healthful weight, avoid smoking, and drink alcohol only in moderation if you drink at all.[18]

- Finally, focus on gradual change. A modest increase in fruit and vegetable intake and regular physical activity along with fewer restaurant and packaged meals can make a significant and lasting impact.

In addition to the steps just described, if you have been diagnosed with HTN and/or have a family history of cardiovascular disease, consult your health care team, including a Registered Dietitian Nutritionist (RDN), for help designing a dietary pattern for your needs.

CRITICAL THINKING QUESTIONS

1. Has reading about the sodium controversy inspired you to try to reduce your sodium intake? Why or why not?
2. The DASH diet recommends increasing your fruit and vegetable intake to 10 servings a day. Would this fit into your current lifestyle? Why or why not?
3. Visit the CDC's "How to Reduce Sodium" web page at http://www.cdc.gov/salt/reduce_sodium_tips.htm. Check out the tips for shopping and eating out. How many of these behaviors do you practice? Which seem practical for you to begin following, and why?

TEST YOURSELF | ANSWERS

1 F Although your thirst mechanism signals that you need to drink, it is not sufficient to ensure that you're completely hydrated.

2 F Recent research suggests that caffeine intake has virtually no effect on fluid balance.

3 F Sodium is a nutrient critical to human functioning; however, the Dietary Guidelines for Americans advise us to keep our intake below 2,300 milligrams per day.

review questions

LO 1 **1.** Plasma is one example of
a. extracellular fluid.
b. intracellular fluid.
c. tissue fluid.
d. metabolic water.

LO 2 **2.** Which of the following is a critical function of water?
a. It dissolves fat-soluble vitamins.
b. Its relatively low capacity for heat keeps the body warm.
c. It provides protection for the brain and spinal cord.
d. All of the above are true.

LO 2 **3.** Which of the following is true of the cell membrane?
a. It is freely permeable to electrolytes but not to water.
b. It is freely permeable to water but not to electrolytes.
c. It is freely permeable to both water and electrolytes.
d. It is freely permeable to neither water nor electrolytes.

LO 3 **4.** We lose fluids through
a. sweat.
b. breath.
c. feces.
d. all of the above.

LO 4 **5.** Which of the following is the most healthful beverage for most people most of the time?
a. tap water
b. vitamin water sweetened with honey
c. tomato or other vegetable juice
d. black coffee with non-Caloric sweetener

LO 5 **6.** Which of the following statements about sodium is true?
a. One serving of ramen noodle soup provides nearly half the AI for sodium.
b. High-sodium diets are the primary cause of hypertension.
c. The kidney's excretion and reabsorption of sodium contribute to blood pressure regulation.
d. Sodium intake should be kept to an absolute minimum.

LO 5 **7.** Which of the following is a characteristic of potassium?
a. It is the major positively charged electrolyte in the extracellular fluid.
b. It can be found in fresh fruits and vegetables.
c. It is a critical component of the mineral complex of bone.
d. It is found only in plants, not in animals.

LO 6 **8.** Which of the following factors commonly contributes to dehydration?
a. drinking too much plain water while active in a hot environment
b. sweating and breathing heavily while active in a hot environment
c. failure of the body's heat-regulating mechanisms
d. failure of the kidneys to excrete sufficient water

LO 4 **9.** **True or false?** The chemical most commonly used to treat and purify public water supplies is chlorine.

LO 5 **10.** **True or false?** Chloride's only important body function is to help maintain fluid balance.

math review

LO 6 **11.** Theo comes home after basketball practice, weighs himself, and discovers he has lost 3 pounds. Knowing that 1 pound of body weight loss represents the loss of 2 cups of fluid, how much fluid should he consume over the next few hours in order to fully rehydrate?

Answers to Review Questions and Math Review are located at the back of this text and in the MasteringNutrition Study Area.

web links

www.epa.gov
U.S. Environmental Protection Agency: Water
Go to the EPA's water website, then enter "your drinking water" into the search bar to find the link to information about drinking water quality, standards, and safety.

www.bottledwater.org
International Bottled Water Association
Find current information about bottled water from this trade association, which represents the bottled water industry.

www.mayoclinic.org
Mayo Clinic
Search for "hyponatremia" to learn more about this potentially fatal condition.

www.nhlbi.nih.gov
National Heart, Lung, and Blood Institute
Go to this site to learn more about cardiovascular disease, including how to reduce your risk for high blood pressure by following the DASH diet.

www.heart.org
American Heart Association
The American Heart Association provides plenty of tips on how to lower your blood pressure.

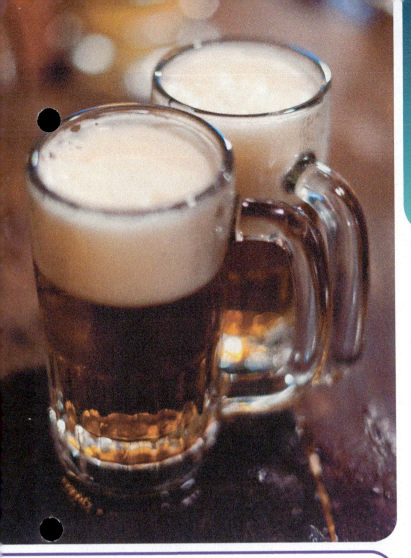

Alcohol

learning outcomes

After reading this In Depth, you should be able to:

1 Explain what happens to alcohol in the body, pp. 250–251.

2 Identify some potential benefits and concerns related to moderate drinking, pp. 251–252.

3 Distinguish two types of alcohol use disorders and discuss their health effects, pp. 252–257.

4 Identify at least three strategies for limiting your drinking and three signs of an alcohol use disorder, pp. 257–258.

5 Explain how to talk to someone about an alcohol use disorder, p. 258.

No one should have to spend his 21st birthday in an emergency room, but that's what happened to Todd the night he turned 21. His friends took him off campus to celebrate, and, with their encouragement, he attempted to drink 21 shots before the bar closed at 2 AM. Fortunately for Todd, when he passed out and couldn't be roused, his best friend noticed his cold, clammy skin and erratic breathing and drove him to the local emergency room. There, his stomach was pumped and he was treated for alcohol poisoning. He regained consciousness but felt sick and shaky for several more hours.

Not everyone is so lucky. Alcohol poisoning, which occurs when people consume more alcohol than their liver can metabolize, impairs essential body functions, including breathing, heart rate, and the transmission of nerve signals in the brain. In the United States, 2,200 people die of alcohol poisoning each year. That's about six deaths every day.[1]

What makes excessive alcohol intake so dangerous, and why is moderate alcohol consumption often considered healthful? How can you tell if someone is struggling with problem drinking, and what can you do to help? What if that someone is you? We explore these questions **In Depth** here.

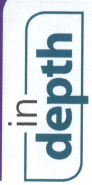

Alcohol is a chemical compound structurally similar to carbohydrates. *Ethanol* is the specific type of alcohol found in beer, wine, and distilled spirits such as whiskey and vodka. Throughout this discussion, the common term *alcohol* will be used to represent the specific compound *ethanol*.

Alcohol intake is usually described as "drinks per day." A **drink** is defined as the amount of a beverage that provides ½ fluid ounce of pure alcohol. For example, 12 oz of beer, 10 oz of a wine cooler, 4 to 5 oz of wine, and 1½ oz of 80-**proof** whiskey, scotch, gin, or vodka are each equivalent to one drink (FIGURE 1). The term "proof" reflects the alcohol content of distilled spirits: 100-proof liquor is 50% alcohol whereas 80-proof liquor is 40% alcohol.

What happens to alcohol in the body?

LO 1 Explain what happens to alcohol in the body.

Alcohol is absorbed directly from both the stomach and the small intestine; it does not require digestion prior to absorption. Consuming foods with some fat, protein, and fiber slows the absorption of alcohol and can reduce blood alcohol concentration (BAC) by as much as 50% compared to peak BAC when drinking on an empty stomach. Carbonated alcoholic beverages are absorbed very rapidly, which explains why champagne and sparkling wines are so quick to generate an alcoholic "buzz." Women typically absorb 30% to 35% more of a given alcohol intake compared to a man of the same size, which may explain why women often show a greater response to alcohol compared to men.

Once absorbed, most alcohol is oxidized, or broken down, in the liver at a fairly steady rate. However, a small amount is oxidized in the stomach before it has even been absorbed. Cells in both the stomach and the liver secrete

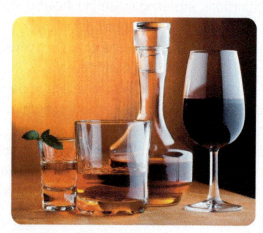

FIGURE 1 What does one drink look like? A drink is equivalent to 1½ oz of distilled spirits, 4 to 5 oz of wine, 10 oz of wine cooler, or 12 oz of beer.

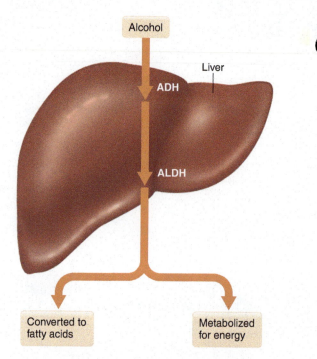

FIGURE 2 Metabolism of alcohol.

the enzyme alcohol dehydrogenase (ADH), which triggers the first step in alcohol degradation, while aldehyde dehydrogenase (ALDH) takes the breakdown process one step further (FIGURE 2). In women, ADH in the stomach is less active than in men; thus, women do not oxidize as much alcohol in their stomach, leaving up to 30% to 35% more intact alcohol to be absorbed.

On average, a healthy adult metabolizes the equivalent of one drink per hour. If someone has more than one drink in an hour, the excess alcohol is released back into the bloodstream, where it elevates BAC and triggers a range of behavioral and metabolic reactions. Through the blood, alcohol is quickly and completely distributed throughout all body fluids, exposing every tissue in your body—including your brain—to its toxic effects.

Despite what you may have heard, there is no effective intervention to speed up the

> To find out how many Calories are in your favorite drink, go to http://rethinkingdrinking.niaaa.nih.gov/. From the "Tools" tab, click the "Calculators" link and select "Alcohol Calorie calculator."

alcohol Chemically, a compound characterized by the presence of a hydroxyl group; in common usage, a beverage made from fermented fruits, vegetables, or grains and containing ethanol.

drink The amount of an alcoholic beverage that provides approximately 0.5 fl. oz of pure ethanol.

proof A measure of the alcohol content of a liquid; 100-proof liquor is 50% alcohol by volume, 80-proof liquor is 40% alcohol by volume, and so on.

TABLE 1 Myths about Alcohol Metabolism

The Claim	The Reality
Physical activity, such as walking around, will speed up the breakdown of alcohol.	Muscles don't metabolize alcohol; the liver does.
Drinking a lot of coffee will keep you from getting drunk.	Coffee intake simply leaves you both wired and drunk.
Using a sauna or steam room will force the alcohol out of your body.	Very little alcohol is lost in sweat; the alcohol will remain in your bloodstream.
Herbal and nutritional products are available that speed up the breakdown of alcohol.	No commercial supplement is effective in increasing the rate of alcohol metabolism.

breakdown of alcohol (TABLE 1). The key to keeping your BAC low is to drink alcoholic beverages while eating a meal or large snack, to drink very slowly, to have no more than one drink per hour, and to limit your total consumption of alcohol on any one occasion.

A person who steadily increases his or her alcohol consumption over time becomes more tolerant of a given intake of alcohol. Chronic drinkers experience *metabolic tolerance,* a condition in which the liver becomes more efficient in its breakdown of alcohol. This means that the person's BAC rises more slowly after consuming a certain number of drinks. In addition, chronic drinkers develop what is called *functional tolerance,* meaning they show few, if any, signs of impairment or intoxication, even at high BACs. As a result, these individuals may consume twice as much alcohol as when they first started drinking before they reach the same state of euphoria.

What do we know about moderate drinking?

LO 2 Identify some potential benefits and concerns related to moderate drinking.

The *2015–2020 Dietary Guidelines for Americans* (DGAs) advise "If alcohol is consumed, it should be consumed in moderation and only by adults of legal drinking age."[2] The definition of **moderate drinking** is based on a maximal daily intake of up to one drink per day for women and two drinks per day for men. A person who does not drink any alcohol on weekdays but downs a six-pack of beer most Saturday nights would *not* be classified as a "moderate drinker"! The DGAs also identify groups of individuals who should not consume alcohol at all, including women who are or may become pregnant and women who are breastfeeding.

The DGAs do not recommend that anyone begin consuming alcohol or drink more often in order to achieve certain health benefits because, as we discuss here, moderate alcohol intake is associated with both benefits and

risks. When deciding whether or how much alcohol to drink, you need to weigh the pros and cons of alcohol consumption against your own personal health history.

Moderate Drinking Has Certain Health Benefits

In most people, moderate alcohol intake offers some psychological benefits, reducing stress and anxiety. Moderate use of alcohol can also improve appetite, especially for savory foods high in protein.[3] This can be of great value to the elderly and people with a chronic disease that suppresses appetite.

In addition, light/moderate alcohol consumption appears to lower the risk of subsequent age-related dementia compared to those who abstain from alcohol and those who consume increasingly greater amounts.[4] It has also been linked to lower rates of cardiovascular disease, especially in older adults and in people already at risk, such as those with type 2 diabetes. Consumption of a moderate amount of alcohol in any form (wine, beer, or distilled spirits) increases levels of the "good" type of cholesterol (HDL) while decreasing the concentration of "bad" cholesterol (LDL); it also reduces the risk of abnormal clot formation in the blood vessels.[5]

Recently, there has been a great deal of interest in *resveratrol,* a phytochemical found in red wines, grapes, and other plant foods. Some researchers are proposing that resveratrol may be able to reduce the risk for certain chronic diseases. However, the amount of resveratrol in a glass of red wine may be too small to provide a meaningful health benefit for most individuals.[6]

Moderate Drinking Is Associated with Certain Risks

Not everyone responds to alcohol in the same manner. A person's age, genetic makeup, state of health, and use of medications can influence both immediate and long-term responses to alcohol intake, even at moderate levels. For example, women consuming low to moderate amounts of alcohol appear to have a slightly increased risk for breast cancer.[7] In some studies, moderate drinking has been linked to a higher risk of bleeding in the brain (*hemorrhagic stroke*); however, other research has not found this association.[8]

Another concern is the effect of alcohol on our waistlines! As we pointed out in Chapter 1, alcohol is not classified as a nutrient because it does not serve any unique metabolic role in humans. It does, however, provide energy: 7 Calories per gram. Only fat has more Calories per gram. As illustrated in FIGURE 3 on page 252, if you're watching your weight, it makes sense to strictly limit your consumption of alcohol to stay within your daily energy needs.

---

moderate drinking Alcohol consumption of up to one drink per day for women and up to two drinks per day for men.

Alcohol intake may also increase your *food* intake, because alcoholic beverages enhance appetite, particularly during social events, leading some people to overeat. Both current and lifelong intakes of alcohol increase the risk for obesity in both males and females, particularly for those who binge drink.[9]

Because the liver detoxifies both alcohol and medications, harmful drug–alcohol interactions are common. Many medications carry a warning label advising consumers to avoid alcohol while taking the drug. Alcohol magnifies the effect of certain pain relievers, sleeping pills, antidepressants, and antianxiety medications and can lead to loss of consciousness. It also increases the risk for gastrointestinal bleeding in people taking aspirin, as well as the risk for both bleeding and liver damage in people taking ibuprofen or acetaminophen.[10] In diabetics using insulin or oral medications to lower blood glucose, alcohol can exaggerate the drug's effect, leading to an inappropriately low level of blood glucose.

As you can see, there are risks to moderate alcohol consumption. Although moderate drinkers at low risk for alcohol addiction or medication interaction can safely continue their current level of use, individuals who have a personal or family history of alcoholism or fall into any other risk category should consider abstaining.

What do we know about alcohol use disorders?

LO 3 Distinguish two types of alcohol use disorders and discuss their health effects.

Problem drinking that has become severe is medically diagnosed as an **alcohol use disorder (AUD)**.[11]

Alcohol Use Disorders Include Abuse and Dependence

The National Institute on Alcohol Abuse and Alcoholism (NIAAA) recognizes two general types of AUD: alcohol abuse and alcohol dependence, commonly known as alcoholism. In the United States, about 17 million adults have an AUD.[11]

Alcohol abuse is a pattern of alcohol consumption, whether chronic or occasional, that results in distress,

alcohol use disorder (AUD) Medical diagnosis for problem drinking that has become severe and is characterized by either abuse or dependence.

alcohol abuse A pattern of alcohol consumption, whether chronic or occasional, that results in harm to one's health, functioning, or interpersonal relationships.

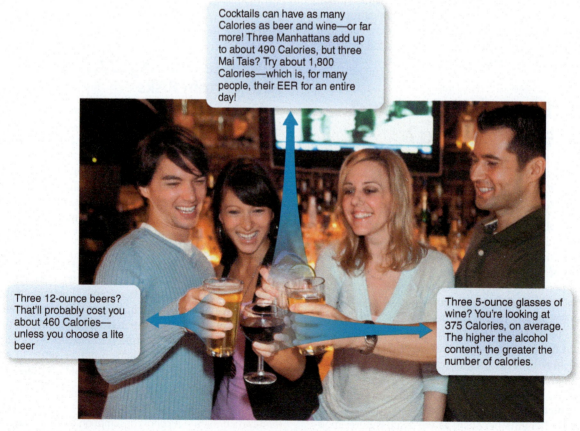

Cocktails can have as many Calories as beer and wine—or far more! Three Manhattans add up to about 490 Calories, but three Mai Tais? Try about 1,800 Calories—which is, for many people, their EER for an entire day!

Three 12-ounce beers? That'll probably cost you about 460 Calories—unless you choose a lite beer

Three 5-ounce glasses of wine? You're looking at 375 Calories, on average. The higher the alcohol content, the greater the number of calories.

FIGURE 3 Going out for a few drinks? You might want to stick to just one—Calories in alcoholic beverages really add up!

danger, or harm to one's health, functioning, or interpersonal relationships. Both chronic and occasional alcohol abuse can eventually lead to alcoholism.

Binge drinking is a form of alcohol abuse defined as the consumption of five or more alcoholic drinks on one occasion by a man or four or more drinks for a woman. In a recent survey, nearly 25% of people ages 18 or older reported binge drinking within the previous month.[11] People who binge-drink report engaging in about four episodes a month.[12]

Among the many consequences of binge drinking is an increased risk for potentially fatal falls, drownings, and automobile accidents. Acts of physical violence, including vandalism and physical and sexual assault, are also associated with binge drinking. The consequences also carry over beyond a particular episode: binge drinking impairs cognition, planning, problem solving, memory, and inhibition, leading to significant social, educational, and employment problems. About 25% of college students who binge-drink report academic consequences of their drinking, from missed classes to a low GPA.[13] Finally, hangovers, which are discussed shortly, are practically inevitable, given the amount of alcohol consumed during a binge.

Alcohol dependence, commonly known as *alcoholism,* is a disease characterized by:

- *Craving:* a strong need or urge to drink alcoholic beverages.
- *Loss of control:* the inability to stop once drinking has begun.
- *Physical dependence:* the presence of nausea, sweating, shakiness, and other signs of withdrawal after stopping alcohol intake.
- *Tolerance:* the need to drink larger and larger amounts of alcohol to get the same "high," or pleasurable sensations, associated with alcohol intake.

Alcohol Use Disorders Have Toxic Effects

Alcohol is a drug. It exerts a narcotic effect on virtually every part of the brain, acting as a sedative and depressant. Alcohol also has the potential to act as a direct toxin; in high concentrations, it can damage or destroy cell membranes and internal cell structures. As shown in **FIGURE 4**, an alcohol intake between 1/2 and 1 drink per day is associated with the lowest risk of mortality for both men and women. The risk of death increases sharply as alcohol intake increases above 2 drinks per day for women, and 3½ drinks per day for men. These increased mortality risks are related to alcohol's damaging effects on the brain, the liver, and other organs, as well as its role in motor vehicle accidents and other traumatic injuries.

Alcohol Hangovers

Alcohol hangover is an extremely unpleasant consequence of drinking too much alcohol. It lasts up

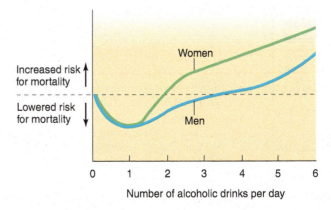

FIGURE 4 The effect of alcohol consumption on mortality risk. Consuming 1/2 to 1 drink per day is associated with the lowest mortality risk for all adults. The risk of death increases sharply at levels of alcohol intake above 2 drinks per day for women and above 3½ drinks per day for men.

to 24 hours, and its symptoms include headache, fatigue, dizziness, muscle aches, nausea and vomiting, sensitivity to light and sound, and extreme thirst. Some people also experience depression, anxiety, irritability, and other mood disturbances. While some aspects of a hangover may be due to nonalcoholic compounds known as *congeners* (found in red wines, brandy, and whiskey, for example), most of the consequences are directly related to the alcohol itself. These include the following:

- *Fluid and electrolyte imbalance:* Alcohol's diuretic effect increases urine output, leading to an excessive loss of fluid and electrolytes and contributing to dizziness and lightheadedness.
- *Irritation and inflammation:* Alcohol irritates the lining of the stomach, causing inflammation (gastritis), increasing gastric acid production, and triggering abdominal pain, nausea, and vomiting.
- *Metabolic disturbances:* Alcohol disrupts normal metabolism, leading to low levels of blood glucose and elevated levels of lactic acid, and resulting in fatigue, weakness, and mood changes.
- *Biological disturbances:* Alcohol disrupts various biological rhythms, such as sleep patterns, leading to an effect similar to that of jet lag.

While many folk remedies, including various herbal products, claim to prevent or reduce hangover effects, few have proven effective. Drinking water or other

binge drinking The consumption of five or more alcoholic drinks on one occasion for a man, or four or more drinks for a woman.

alcohol dependence A disease state characterized by alcohol craving, loss of control, physical dependence, and tolerance.

alcohol hangover A cluster of signs and symptoms, including headache, nausea, and vomiting, that occurs as a consequence of drinking too much alcohol.

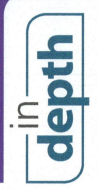
nonalcoholic beverages will minimize the risk for dehydration, and toast or dry cereal is effective in bringing blood glucose levels back to normal. Getting adequate sleep can counteract the fatigue, and the use of antacids can help reduce nausea and abdominal pain. While aspirin, ibuprofen, and acetaminophen might be useful for headaches, they are not safe for treating hangovers. As noted earlier, all three drugs can cause gastrointestinal bleeding, and interactions between alcohol and either acetaminophen or ibuprofen can cause liver damage.[10]

Reduced Brain Function

Alcohol is known for its ability to alter behavior, mainly through its effects on the brain. Even a low BAC impairs reasoning and judgment (FIGURE 5). Alcohol also interferes with normal sleep patterns, alters sight and speech, and leads to loss of both fine and gross motor skills such as handwriting, hand–eye coordination, and balance. Many people who drink experience unexpected mood swings, intense anger, or unreasonable irritation. Others react in the opposite direction, becoming sad, withdrawn, and lethargic. When teens or young adults chronically consume excessive amounts of alcohol, they may permanently alter brain structure and function.[14] Intellectual functioning and memory can be lost or compromised. In addition, early exposure to alcohol increases the risk for

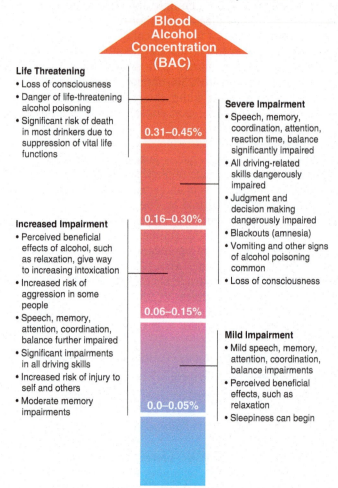

As BAC Increases, So Does Impairment

Blood Alcohol Concentration (BAC)

Life Threatening
- Loss of consciousness
- Danger of life-threatening alcohol poisoning
- Significant risk of death in most drinkers due to suppression of vital life functions

0.31–0.45%

Severe Impairment
- Speech, memory, coordination, attention, reaction time, balance significantly impaired
- All driving-related skills dangerously impaired
- Judgment and decision making dangerously impaired
- Blackouts (amnesia)
- Vomiting and other signs of alcohol poisoning common
- Loss of consciousness

0.16–0.30%

Increased Impairment
- Perceived beneficial effects of alcohol, such as relaxation, give way to increasing intoxication
- Increased risk of aggression in some people
- Speech, memory, attention, coordination, balance further impaired
- Significant impairments in all driving skills
- Increased risk of injury to self and others
- Moderate memory impairments

0.06–0.15%

Mild Impairment
- Mild speech, memory, attention, coordination, balance impairments
- Perceived beneficial effects, such as relaxation
- Sleepiness can begin

0.0–0.05%

▲ **FIGURE 5** Effects of increasing blood alcohol concentration on brain function. The first brain region affected is the cerebral cortex, which governs reasoning and judgment. At increasing levels of impairment, the cerebellum, which controls and coordinates movement, the hippocampus, which is involved in memory storage, and the brain stem, which regulates consciousness, breathing, and other essential functions, may become involved.

future alcohol addiction and may contribute to lifelong deficits in learning-related behaviors.[15]

Alcohol Poisoning

As shown in Figure 5, as BAC increases, the person is at increasing risk for **alcohol poisoning**, a metabolic state in which the respiratory center of the brain is depressed. This reduces the level of oxygen reaching the brain and increases the risk for fatal respiratory or cardiac failure.

Like Todd in our opening story, many binge drinkers lose consciousness, but their BAC can continue to rise as the alcohol in their GI tract is absorbed and released into

alcohol poisoning A potentially fatal condition in which an overdose of alcohol results in cardiac and/or respiratory failure.

nutri-case | THEO

"I was driving home from a post-game party last night when I was pulled over by the police. The officer said I seemed to be driving 'erratically' and asked me how many drinks I'd had. I told him I'd only had three beers and explained that I was pretty tired from the game. Then, just to prove I was fine, I offered to count backward from a hundred, but I must have sounded sober, because he didn't make me do it. I can't believe he thought I was driving drunk! Still, maybe three beers after a game really is too much."

Do you think it is physiologically possible that Theo's driving had been impaired after consuming three beers? To answer, you'll need to consider both Theo's body weight and the effect of playing a long basketball game. What other factors that influence the rate of alcohol absorption or breakdown could have affected Theo's BAC? How could all of these factors influence a decision about whether "three beers after a game really is too much"?

the bloodstream. Moreover, alcohol irritates the GI tract, and vomiting—even while unconscious—is common. The person can choke on their vomit and suffocate. For these reasons, if someone passes out after a night of hard drinking, he or she should never be left alone to "sleep it off." If the person has cold and clammy skin, a bluish tint to the skin, or slow or irregular breathing, or if the person exhibits confusion or stupor, or cannot be roused, seek emergency health care immediately.

Reduced Liver Function

The liver performs an astonishing number and variety of body functions, including nutrient metabolism, glycogen storage, the synthesis of many essential compounds, and the detoxification of medications and other potential poisons. As noted earlier, it is the main site of alcohol metabolism. When an individual's rate of alcohol intake exceeds the rate at which the liver can break down the alcohol, liver cells are damaged or destroyed. The longer the alcohol abuse continues, the greater the damage to the liver.

Fatty liver, a condition in which abnormal amounts of fat build up in the liver, is an early yet reversible sign of liver damage commonly linked to alcohol abuse. Once alcohol intake stops and a healthful diet is maintained, the liver is able to heal and resume normal function.

Alcoholic hepatitis is a more severe condition, resulting in loss of appetite, nausea and vomiting, abdominal pain, and jaundice (a yellowing of the skin and eyes, reflecting reduced liver function). Mental confusion and impaired immune response often occur with alcoholic hepatitis. While avoidance of alcohol and a healthful diet often result in full recovery, many people experience lifelong complications from alcoholic hepatitis.

Cirrhosis of the liver is often the result of long-term alcohol abuse; liver cells are scarred, blood flow through the liver is impaired, and liver function declines (FIGURE 6). This condition almost always results in irreversible damage to the liver and can be life-threatening. Blood pressure increases dramatically, large amounts of fluid are retained in the abdominal cavity, and metabolic wastes accumulate. In some cases, liver function fails completely, resulting in the need for a liver transplant or the likelihood of death.

Increased Risk for Chronic Disease

While moderate drinking may provide some health benefits, it is clear that chronically high intakes of alcohol damage a number of body organs and systems, increasing a person's risk for chronic disease and death:[16]

- *Bone health:* Men and women who are alcohol dependent experience abnormal vitamin D and calcium metabolism with the result that up to 40% of alcoholics have osteoporosis.
- *Pancreatic injury and diabetes:* Alcohol damages the pancreas, which produces insulin, and decreases the body's ability to properly respond to insulin. The result is chronically elevated blood glucose levels and an increased risk for diabetes.
- *Cancer:* Research has most strongly linked alcohol consumption, particularly at high intakes, to increased risk for cancer of the mouth and throat, esophagus, stomach, liver, colon, and female breast.[17]

Malnutrition

As alcohol intake increases to 30% or more of total energy intake, appetite is lost and intake of healthful foods declines. Over time, the diet becomes deficient in protein, fats, carbohydrates, vitamins A and C, and minerals such as iron, zinc, and calcium (FIGURE 7) (page 256).

Even if food intake is maintained, long-term exposure to alcohol damages the stomach, small intestine, and pancreas. As a result, the digestion of foods and absorption of

---

fatty liver An abnormal accumulation of fat in the liver that develops in people who abuse alcohol.

alcoholic hepatitis A serious condition of inflammation of the liver caused by alcohol abuse.

cirrhosis of the liver End-stage liver disease characterized by significant abnormalities in liver structure and function; may lead to complete liver failure.

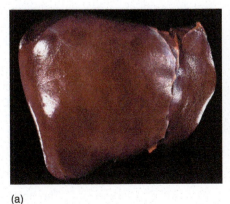 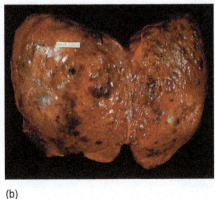

(a)   (b)

FIGURE 6 Cirrhosis of the liver is often caused by chronic alcohol abuse. **(a)** A healthy liver; **(b)** a liver damaged by cirrhosis.

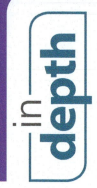
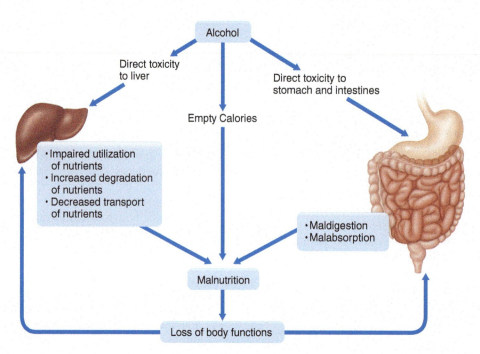

Alcohol

Direct toxicity
to liver

Direct toxicity to
stomach and intestines

Empty Calories

- Impaired utilization
  of nutrients
- Increased degradation
  of nutrients
- Decreased transport
  of nutrients

- Maldigestion
- Malabsorption

Malnutrition

Loss of body functions

▲ **FIGURE 7** Alcohol-related malnutrition. Excess alcohol consumption contributes directly and indirectly to widespread nutrient deficiencies.

nutrients become inadequate, leading to malnutrition and inappropriate weight loss. Finally, alcohol interferes with the ability of cells to utilize nutrients.

Increased Risk for Traumatic Injury

Excessive alcohol intake is the third leading preventable, lifestyle-related cause of death for Americans of all ages, contributing to nearly 80,000 deaths per year.[18] It has been estimated that nearly 2,000 young Americans die each year from alcohol-related unintentional injuries, including motor vehicle accidents, falls, and drownings. An additional 600,000 college-age students are seriously injured while under the influence of alcohol.[19] Rates of physical

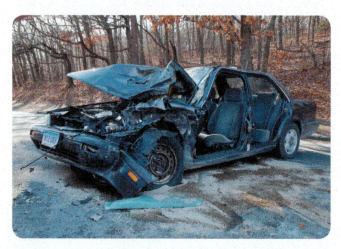

Excessive alcohol intake greatly increases the risk for car accidents and other traumatic injuries.

and sexual assaults and vandalism also increase when people are under the influence of alcohol.

Fetal and Infant Health Problems

Alcohol is a known **teratogen** (a substance that causes fetal harm). It readily enters the fetal bloodstream and, because the fetal liver cannot effectively break it down, accumulates in the fetal blood and tissues, increasing the risk for various birth defects. The effects of maternal alcohol intake are dose-related: the more the mother drinks, the greater the potential harm to the fetus. Drinking early in pregnancy—even before the woman realizes she is pregnant—is particularly harmful. However, no level of alcohol consumption at any time during pregnancy is safe. Women who are or think they may be pregnant should entirely abstain. Despite the fact that this advice is widely publicized, nearly 8% of women report consuming alcohol during their pregnancy and over 17% of these women report binge drinking.[20] It is estimated that more than 40,000 U.S. infants are born each year with some type of alcohol-related defect.

Fetal alcohol syndrome (FAS) is the most severe consequence of maternal alcohol consumption and is characterized by malformations of the face, limbs, heart, and nervous system. The characteristic facial features

---

teratogen Any substance known to have the potential to harm a developing embryo or fetus.

fetal alcohol syndrome (FAS) The most severe consequence of maternal alcohol consumption; characterized by physical malformations and emotional, behavioral, and learning problems.

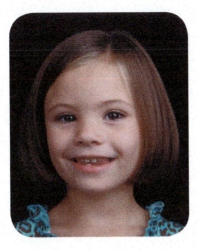

▲ **FIGURE 8** A child with fetal alcohol syndrome (FAS). The facial features typical of children with FAS include a short nose with a low, wide bridge; drooping eyes with an extra skinfold; and a flat, thin upper lip. These external traits are typically accompanied by behavioral problems and learning disorders. The effects of FAS are irreversible.

of a child with FAS persist throughout life **(FIGURE 8)**. Newborn and infant death rates are abnormally high, and those who do survive may suffer from lifelong emotional, behavioral, social, learning, and developmental problems. FAS is one of the most common causes of mental retardation in the United States, despite the fact that it is completely preventable.

Fetal alcohol effects (FAE) are a more subtle set of consequences related to maternal alcohol intake. Although usually not diagnosed at birth, FAE often becomes evident when the child enters preschool or kindergarten. The child may exhibit hyperactivity, attention deficit disorders, or impaired learning abilities. It is estimated that the incidence of FAE may be 10 times greater than that of FAS.

The only way to prevent these disorders is for sexually active women not using reliable contraception to abstain from all alcoholic beverages. In addition, women who are pregnant should entirely abstain from alcohol consumption. Although some pregnant women do have an occasional alcoholic drink with no apparent ill effects, FAE can occur with light to moderate alcohol intake; thus, the best advice is to abstain throughout pregnancy.

Women who are breastfeeding should also abstain from alcohol because it easily passes into the breast milk at levels equal to blood alcohol concentrations. If consumed by the infant, the alcohol in breast milk can slow motor development and depress the central nervous system. Alcohol also has a diuretic effect. The normal fluid losses experienced by a breastfeeding woman are therefore exacerbated with alcohol intake, leaving her at risk for dehydration, and reducing her ability to produce milk, putting the infant at risk for malnutrition.

Should you be concerned about your alcohol intake?

LO 4 Identify at least three strategies for limiting your drinking and three signs of an alcohol use disorder.

Knowing that a moderate intake of alcohol may provide some health benefits and that excessive intake causes a wide range of problems, what can you do to control your drinking? Check out the **Quick Tips** for practical strategies

QuickTips

Taking Control of Your Alcohol Intake

✔ Think about *why* you are planning to drink. Is it to relax and socialize, or are you using alcohol to release stress? If the latter, try some stress-reduction techniques that don't involve alcohol, such as working out or talking with a friend.

✔ Decide in advance what your alcohol intake will be, and plan some strategies for sticking to your limit. If you are going to a bar, for example, take only a small amount of cash and leave your credit card at home. At a party, stay occupied dancing, sampling the food, and talking with friends.

✔ Make sure you have a protein-containing meal or snack before your first alcoholic drink. Having food in the stomach delays its emptying, allowing time for more of the alcohol to be broken down. As a result, less will be absorbed into the bloodstream.

✔ "Pace and Space" your drinks. Before your first alcoholic drink, have something nonalcoholic. Once your thirst has been satisfied, your rate of fluid intake will drop. After that, rotate between alcoholic and nonalcoholic drinks. Remember, pure orange juice doesn't look any different from orange juice laced with vodka, so no one will even know what you are—or are not—drinking.

✔ Dilute hard liquor with large amounts of diet soda, sparkling water, or juice. Diluted beverages are lower in Calories, too.

✔ Whether or not your drink is diluted, sip slowly to allow your liver time to keep up with your alcohol intake.

✔ If your friends pressure you to drink and you'd rather not, volunteer to be the designated driver. You'll have a "free pass" for the night in terms of saying no to alcohol.

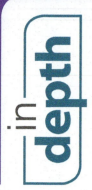

that can help you avoid the negative consequences of excessive alcohol consumption.

If you have trouble keeping your drinking moderate, for example, by practicing the Quick Tips, then even if you're not dependent on alcohol, you may be experiencing an alcohol use disorder. In addition to the amount you drink, you should be concerned if you drink at inappropriate times. This includes, for example, before or while driving a car, while at work/school, when you need to deal with negative emotions, or if you are or might be pregnant.

If you answer "yes" to one or more of the following questions, provided by the NIAAA, you may have an AUD:

- Have you ever felt you should cut down on your drinking?
- Have people annoyed you by criticizing your drinking?
- Have you ever felt bad or guilty about your drinking?
- Do you drink alone when you feel angry or sad?
- Has your drinking ever made you late for school or work?
- Have you ever had a drink first thing in the morning to steady your nerves or get rid of a hangover?
- Do you ever drink after promising yourself you won't?

If you need help taking control of your drinking, talk with a trusted friend, relative, coach, teacher, or health-care provider. Many campuses have support groups that can help.

How can you talk to someone about an alcohol use disorder?

LO 5 Explain how to talk to someone about an alcohol use disorder.

You may suspect that a close friend or relative might be one of the nearly 17 million Americans with an AUD. If your friend or relative uses alcohol to calm down, cheer up, or relax, that may be a sign of alcohol dependency. The appearance of tremors or other signs of withdrawal as well as the initiation of secretive behaviors when consuming alcohol are other indications that alcohol has become a serious problem.

Many people become defensive or hostile when asked about their use of alcohol; denial is very common. The single hardest step toward sobriety is often the first: accepting the fact that help is needed. Some people respond well when confronted by a single person, while others benefit more from a group intervention. There should be no blaming or shaming: AUD is a medical disorder with a genetic component. The NIAAA suggests the following approaches when trying to get a friend or relative into treatment:

- *Stop "covering" and making excuses:* Often, family and friends will make excuses to others to protect the person from the results of his or her drinking. It is important, however, to stop covering for that person so he or she can experience the full consequences of inappropriate alcohol consumption.
- *Intervene at a vulnerable time:* The best time to talk to someone about problem drinking is shortly after an alcohol-related incident, such as a DUI arrest, an alcohol-related traffic accident, or a public scene. Wait until the person is sober and everyone is relatively calm.
- *Be specific:* Tell the person exactly why you are concerned; use examples of specific problems associated with his or her drinking habits (e.g., poor school or work performance; legal problems; inappropriate behaviors). Explain what will happen if the person chooses not to get help—for example, no longer going out with the person if alcohol will be available, no longer riding with him or her in motor vehicles, moving out of a shared home, and so on.
- *Get help:* Professional help is available from a wide variety of agencies and providers. Several contacts are listed in the **Web Links**. If the person indicates a willingness to get help, take him or her to a treatment center immediately. The longer the delay, the more likely it is that the person won't go.
- *Enlist the support of others:* Whether or not the person agrees to get help, calling upon other friends and relatives can often be effective, especially if one of these people has battled an AUD.

Treatment for AUDs works for many, but not all, individuals. Success is measured in small steps, and relapses are common. Research suggests that most people with an AUD cannot just "cut down"; they need to completely abstain from alcohol consumption if they are to achieve full and ongoing recovery.

web links

www.aa.org
Alcoholics Anonymous

This site provides both links to local AA groups and information on the AA program.

www.al-anon.alateen.org
Al-Anon Family Group Headquarters

This site provides links to local Al-Anon and Alateen groups, which offer support to spouses, children, and other loved ones of people addicted to alcohol.

www.niaaa.nih.gov
National Institute on Alcohol Abuse and Alcoholism

Visit this website for information on the prevalence, consequences, and treatments of alcohol-related disorders.

www.collegedrinkingprevention.gov
College Drinking: Changing the Culture

The NIAAA developed this website for college students seeking information and advice on the subject of college drinking.

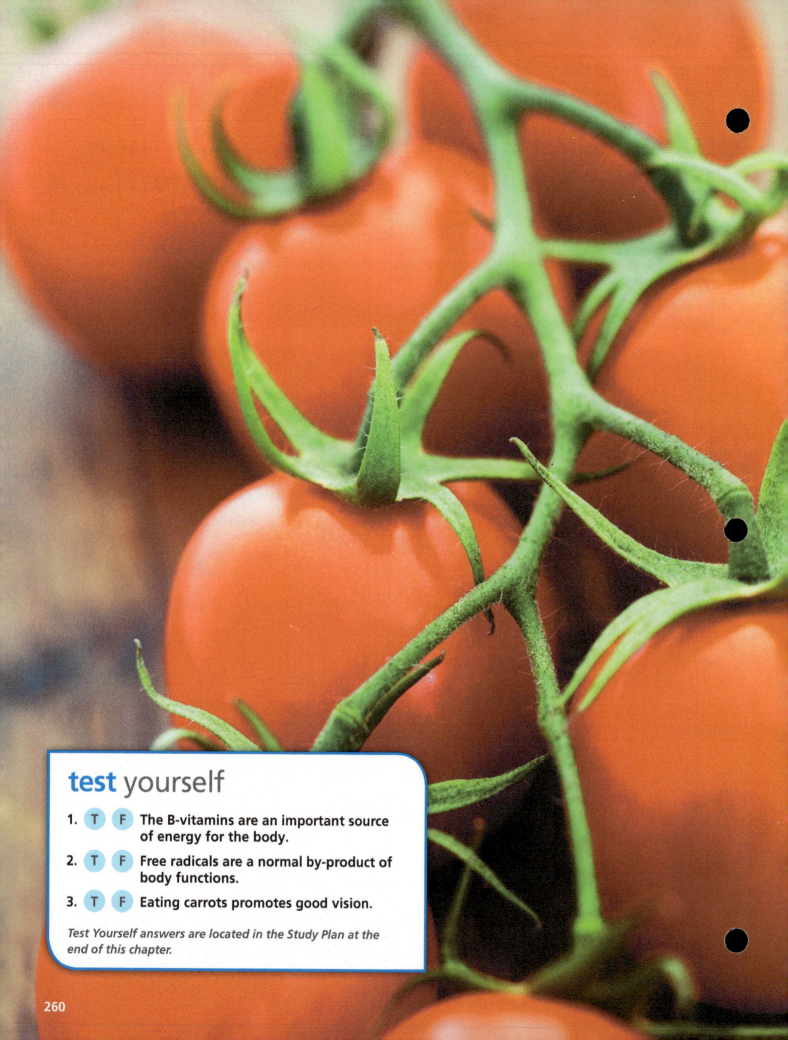

test yourself

1. **T** **F** The B-vitamins are an important source of energy for the body.

2. **T** **F** Free radicals are a normal by-product of body functions.

3. **T** **F** Eating carrots promotes good vision.

Test Yourself answers are located in the Study Plan at the end of this chapter.

8 Nutrients Essential to Key Body Functions

learning outcomes

After studying this chapter you should be able to:

1 Explain how the body regulates energy metabolism, pp. 262–264.

2 Identify the contributions of each of the eight B-vitamins to energy metabolism, pp. 264–273.

3 Discuss the contributions of choline and four minerals to energy metabolism, pp. 273–275.

4 Describe the process by which oxidation can damage cells and the role of antioxidants in opposing this damage, pp. 275–277.

5 Identify the antioxidant functions of key micronutrients and carotenoids, pp. 278–283.

6 Discuss the contribution of vitamin A to vision, cell differentiation, and growth and reproduction, pp. 283–288.

Bailey and her brother Miles both enjoy distance running, and are always looking for ways to stay hydrated and maintain their stamina. So when Miles came back to their apartment from a trip to the mall with a 12-pack of bottles of *Energy-boosting vitamin water!*, Bailey was intrigued. Then she read the ingredients list on the label. It indicated simply that each bottle provided 100% of the Daily Value (DV) for a handful of vitamins and minerals, along with some caffeine. When she asked her brother why he had "wasted good money for stuff he was already getting from food and a cup of coffee," he looked annoyed. "It's not stuff! The sales clerk told me the ingredients in this vitamin water boost your energy!"

Bailey shrugged. "What else did you expect a sales clerk to say? But go ahead and drink it and see what happens. In the meantime, I'll be getting my energy from food and my water from the tap!"

Over the last century, scientists have come to recognize the many critical roles of micronutrients in body functioning. But are certain vitamins and minerals really "energy-boosting"? In this chapter we explore the role of micronutrients in the metabolism of carbohydrates, fats, and proteins, and answer that question. We also explain how micronutrients act as antioxidants and support healthy vision.

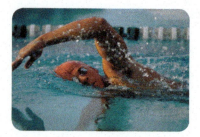

⬆ Vitamins do not provide energy directly, but the B-vitamins help our body create the energy we need from the foods we eat.

How does the body regulate energy metabolism?

Vitamins and minerals do not contain Calories, so don't provide energy directly, but we're unable to generate energy from the macronutrients without them. The B-vitamins are particularly important to energy metabolism. They include thiamin (vitamin B_1), riboflavin (vitamin B_2), niacin (nicotinamide and nicotinic acid), vitamin B_6 (pyridoxine), folate (folic acid), vitamin B_{12} (cobalamin), pantothenic acid, and biotin.

The primary role of the B-vitamins is to act as coenzymes. Recall that an *enzyme* is a compound, usually a protein, that accelerates the rate of chemical reactions but is not used up or changed during the reaction. A **coenzyme** is a molecule that combines with an enzyme to activate it and help it do its job. **FIGURE 8.1** illustrates how coenzymes work. Without coenzymes, we would be unable to produce the energy necessary for sustaining life.

FIGURE 8.2 shows how some of the B-vitamins act as coenzymes to promote energy metabolism. For instance, thiamin is part of the coenzyme thiamin pyrophosphate (TPP), which assists in the breakdown of glucose. Riboflavin is a part of two coenzymes, flavin mononucleotide (FMN) and flavin adenine dinucleotide (FAD), which help break down glucose and fatty acids. The specific functions of each B-vitamin are described in detail shortly.

Certain minerals play roles in energy metabolism, too. These include iodine, chromium, manganese, and sulfur. For instance, iodine is necessary for the synthesis of thyroid hormones, which regulate our metabolic rate and promote growth and development, and chromium helps improve glucose uptake into cells. The minerals involved in energy metabolism are discussed in a later section, along with a vitamin-like substance called choline, which is involved in fat metabolism. For a list of recommended intakes of all of the micronutrients involved in energy metabolism, see **TABLE 8.1**.

recap Vitamins and minerals are not direct sources of energy, but they help generate energy from carbohydrates, fats, and proteins. Acting as coenzymes, the B-vitamins assist enzymes in metabolizing nutrients to produce energy. Certain minerals also play roles in energy metabolism.

coenzyme A molecule that combines with an enzyme to activate it and help it do its job.

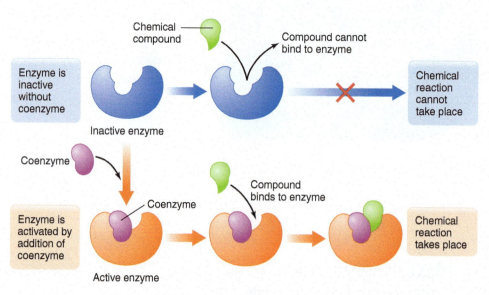

⬆ **FIGURE 8.1** Coenzymes combine with enzymes to activate them, ensuring that the chemical reactions that depend on these enzymes can occur.

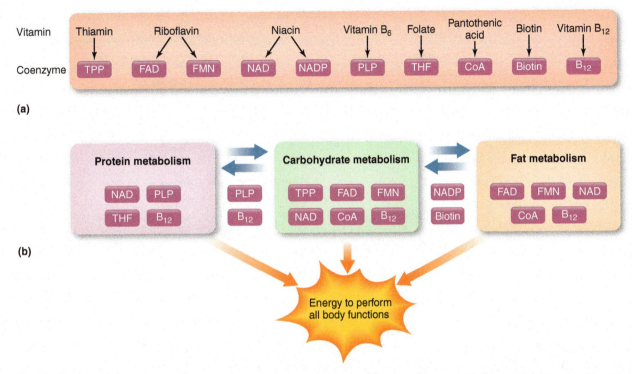

(a)

(b)

⬅ **FIGURE 8.2** The B-vitamins play many important roles in the reactions involved in energy metabolism. **(a)** B-vitamins and the coenzymes they are a part of. **(b)** This chart illustrates many of the coenzymes essential for various metabolic functions; however, this is only a small sample of the thousands of roles that the B-vitamins serve in our body.

TABLE 8.1   Overview of Nutrients Involved in Energy Metabolism

To see the full profile of all micronutrients, turn to the **In Depth** essay following Chapter 6, Vitamins and Minerals: Micronutrients with Macro Powers (pages 211–221).

Nutrient	Recommended Intake
Thiamin (vitamin B_1)	RDA for 19 years of age and older: Women = 1.1 mg/day Men = 1.2 mg/day
Riboflavin (vitamin B_2)	RDA for 19 years of age and older: Women = 1.1 mg/day Men = 1.3 mg/day
Niacin (nicotinamide and nicotinic acid)	RDA for 19 years of age and older: Women = 14 mg/day Men = 16 mg/day
Vitamin B_6 (pyridoxine)	RDA for 19 to 50 years of age: 1.3 mg/day RDA for 51 years of age and older: Women = 1.5 mg/day Men = 1.7 mg/day
Folate (folic acid)	RDA for 19 years of age and older: 400 µg/day
Vitamin B_{12} (cobalamin)	RDA for 19 years of age and older: 2.4 µg/day
Pantothenic acid	AI for 19 years of age and older: 5 mg/day
Biotin	AI for 19 years of age and older: 30 µg/day

(continued)

TABLE 8.1 Overview of Nutrients Involved in Energy Metabolism (continued)

Nutrient	Recommended Intake
Choline	AI for 19 years of age and older: Women = 425 mg/day Men = 550 mg/day
Iodine	RDA for 19 years of age and older: 150 μg/day
Chromium	RDA for 19 to 50 years of age: Women = 25 μg/day Men = 35 μg/day RDA for 51 years of age and older: Women = 20 μg/day Men = 30 μg/day
Manganese	AI for 19 years of age and older: Women = 1.8 mg/day Men = 2.3 mg/day
Sulfur	No DRI.

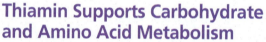

LO 2 Identify the key contributions of each of the eight B-vitamins to energy metabolism.

How do the B-vitamins function in energy metabolism?

This section identifies the key contributions of each of the eight B-vitamins to energy metabolism. Three of these vitamins—vitamin B_6 (pyridoxine), folate (folic acid), and vitamin B_{12} (cobalamin)—play key roles in blood health, and folate is also critical for proper formation of the brain and spinal cord during fetal development. The tissue-supporting functions of these three B-vitamins are discussed in Chapter 9.

Thiamin Supports Carbohydrate and Amino Acid Metabolism

Thiamin deficiency results in a disease called **beriberi**, which became widespread in the 19th century when steam-powered mills began removing the outer layer of grains—the bran—to improve their acceptability to consumers. What wasn't known was that the bran contained the highest concentrations of B-vitamins, including thiamin,[1] which were being removed and discarded. In 1890, two doctors described how they caused beriberi in chickens by feeding them polished rice and cured them by feeding them rice bran.[1,2] In 1911, Polish chemist Casimir Funk was able to isolate the water-soluble nitrogen-containing compound in rice bran that cured beriberi. He referred to this compound as a "vital amine" and called it thiamin. Because it was the first B-vitamin discovered, it is designated vitamin B_1.[1]

Thiamin is part of the coenzyme thiamin pyrophosphate, which plays a critical role in the metabolism of glucose and the essential amino acids leucine, isoleucine, and valine (referred to as the *branched-chain amino acids*). These amino acids are metabolized primarily in the muscle and can be used to produce glucose if necessary. TPP also assists in producing DNA and RNA and plays a role in the synthesis of *neurotransmitters,* chemicals important in the transmission of messages throughout the nervous system.

Good food sources of thiamin include enriched and whole-grain products, wheat germ and yeast extracts, pork products, and some green vegetables, including peas, asparagus, and okra **(FIGURE 8.3)**. Overall, whole grains are some of the best sources of thiamin, whereas processed foods are the poorest sources.

Because thiamin is involved in energy-generating processes, the symptoms of beriberi include a combination of fatigue, apathy, muscle weakness, and reduced cognitive function. The body's inability to metabolize energy or synthesize neurotransmitters also leads to muscle wasting, nerve damage, and paralysis. The heart muscle may also be affected, and the patient may die of heart failure.

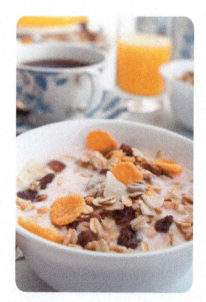

▲ Whole-grain or enriched ready-to-eat cereals are a good source of thiamin.

beriberi A disease of muscle wasting and nerve damage caused by thiamin deficiency.

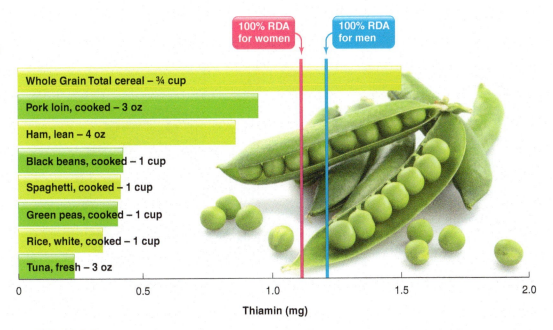

100% RDA for women

100% RDA for men

Whole Grain Total cereal – ¾ cup

Pork loin, cooked – 3 oz

Ham, lean – 4 oz

Black beans, cooked – 1 cup

Spaghetti, cooked – 1 cup

Green peas, cooked – 1 cup

Rice, white, cooked – 1 cup

Tuna, fresh – 3 oz

0   0.5   1.0   1.5   2.0

Thiamin (mg)

FIGURE 8.3 Common food sources of thiamin. The RDA for thiamin is 1.2 mg/day for men and 1.1 mg/day for women 19 years and older.

Source: Data from U.S. Department of Agriculture, Agricultural Research Service. 2015. USDA Nutrient Database for Standard Reference, Release 28.

Beriberi still occurs in refugee camps and other settlements dependent on poor-quality food supplies. It is also seen in people with heavy alcohol consumption and limited food intake. Chronic alcohol abuse is associated with a host of neurologic symptoms, collectively called Wernicke-Korsakoff syndrome, in which thiamin intake is decreased and absorption and utilization impaired.[1] There are no known adverse effects from consuming excess amounts of thiamin; thus, the Health and Medicine Division of the National Academies of Science has not been able to set a tolerable upper intake level (UL).[3]

Riboflavin Supports the Metabolism of Carbohydrates and Fats

In 1917, researchers found that there were at least two vitamins in the extracts of rice polishing, one that cured beriberi and another that stimulated growth. The latter substance was first called vitamin B₂ and then named riboflavin for its ribose-like side chain and the yellow color it produced in water (*flavus* means "yellow" in Latin).[4]

Riboflavin is an important component of the coenzymes flavin mononucleotide (FMN) and flavin adenine dinucleotide (FAD), which are involved in the metabolism of carbohydrates and fat. Riboflavin is also a part of the antioxidant enzyme glutathione peroxidase. Antioxidants are discussed later in this chapter.

Milk is a good source of riboflavin. Because riboflavin is destroyed when it is exposed to light, milk is generally stored in opaque containers. In the United States, meat and meat products, including poultry, fish, eggs, and milk and other dairy products, are the most significant sources of dietary riboflavin.[4] However, green vegetables, such as broccoli, asparagus, and spinach, are also good sources. Finally, although whole grains are relatively low in riboflavin, fortification and enrichment of grains have increased the intake of riboflavin from these sources, especially ready-to-eat cereals and energy bars, which can provide 25% to 100% of the DV for riboflavin in one serving **(FIGURE 8.4)** (page 266).

There are no known adverse effects from consuming excess amounts of riboflavin. Because coenzymes derived from riboflavin are so widely distributed in metabolism, riboflavin deficiency, referred to as **ariboflavinosis**, lacks the specificity seen with other vitamins. However, riboflavin deficiency can have profound effects on energy

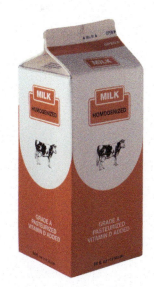

Milk is a good source of riboflavin and is stored in opaque containers to prevent the destruction of riboflavin by light.

ariboflavinosis A condition caused by riboflavin deficiency.

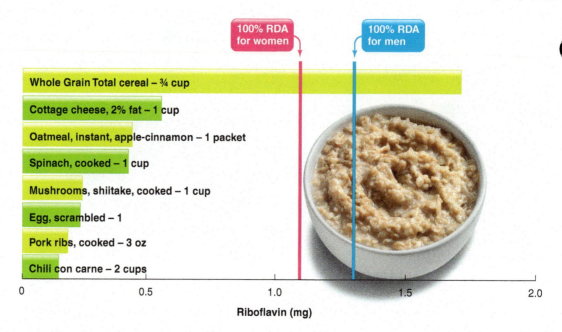

100% RDA for women

100% RDA for men

Whole Grain Total cereal – ¾ cup

Cottage cheese, 2% fat – 1 cup

Oatmeal, instant, apple-cinnamon – 1 packet

Spinach, cooked – 1 cup

Mushrooms, shiitake, cooked – 1 cup

Egg, scrambled – 1

Pork ribs, cooked – 3 oz

Chili con carne – 2 cups

| 0 | 0.5 | 1.0 | 1.5 | 2.0 |

Riboflavin (mg)

▲ **FIGURE 8.4** Common food sources of riboflavin. The RDA for riboflavin is 1.3 mg/day for men and 1.1 mg/day for women 19 years and older.

Source: Data from U.S. Department of Agriculture, Agricultural Research Service, 2015. USDA Nutrient Database for Standard Reference, Release 28.

production, which result in "nondescript" symptoms such as fatigue and muscle weakness. More advanced riboflavin deficiency can result in irritation, inflammation, and ulceration of body tissues, changes in the cornea of the eyes, and anemia.[4] Severe riboflavin deficiency can also impair the metabolism of vitamin B_6 and niacin.[3] Thus, a deficiency in riboflavin can affect a number of body systems.

Niacin Supports Metabolism, DNA Replication, and Cell Differentiation

Whole grains are rich not only in thiamin, but also in niacin; thus, it's not surprising that the niacin-deficiency disease **pellagra** also first emerged with the refining of grains.[5] The body can convert the amino acid tryptophan to niacin, but diets that are low in both tryptophan and niacin—such as traditional corn-based diets, increase the risk for pellagra.

The term *pellagra* literally means "angry skin."[5] The four characteristic symptoms—dermatitis, diarrhea, dementia, and death—are referred to as the *four Ds*. At the present time, pellagra is rarely seen in industrialized countries, except in cases of chronic alcoholism. However, it is still found in impoverished areas of some developing nations.

The two forms of niacin, nicotinamide and nicotinic acid, are converted to active coenzymes that assist in the metabolism of carbohydrates and fatty acids. Niacin also plays an important role in DNA replication and repair and in the process of cell differentiation. A deficiency of niacin can therefore disrupt many body systems.

Niacin is widely distributed in foods, with good sources being meat, poultry, and fish, and whole grain or enriched bread products **(FIGURE 8.5)**. Other foods such as milk, leafy vegetables, coffee, and some teas can also add appreciable amounts of niacin to the diet.[5]

Niacin can cause toxicity symptoms when taken in supplement form. These symptoms include *flushing*, which is defined as burning, tingling, and itching sensations accompanied by a reddened flush primarily on the face, arms, and chest. Liver damage, glucose intolerance, blurred vision, and edema of the eyes can be seen with very large doses of niacin taken over long periods.

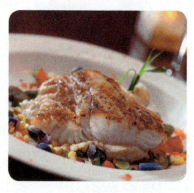

▲ Halibut is a good source of niacin.

pellagra A disease that results from severe niacin deficiency.

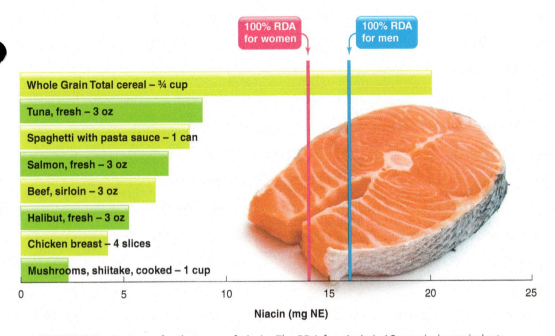

Niacin (mg NE)

⬥ **FIGURE 8.5** Common food sources of niacin. The RDA for niacin is 16 mg niacin equivalents (NE)/day for men and 14 mg NE/day for women 19 years and older.

Source: Data from U.S. Department of Agriculture, Agricultural Research Service, 2015. USDA Nutrient Database for Standard Reference, Release 28.

Vitamin B_6 Is a Coenzyme for Over 100 Enzymes

Researchers discovered vitamin B_6 by ruling out a deficiency of other B-vitamins as the cause of a scaly dermatitis in rats.[6] They then discovered that B_6 deficiency was associated with convulsions in birds and later that infants fed formulas lacking B_6 also had convulsions and dermatitis.[6]

Functions of Vitamin B_6

The term *vitamin B_6* can actually refer to any of six related compounds: pyridoxine (PN), pyridoxal (PL), pyridoxamine (PM), and the phosphate forms of these three compounds. A coenzyme for more than 100 enzymes, vitamin B_6 is involved in many metabolic processes, including the following:

- **Amino acid metabolism.** Vitamin B_6 is important for the metabolism of amino acids because it plays a critical role in transamination, which is a key process in making nonessential amino acids (see Chapter 6 for more details). Without adequate vitamin B_6, all amino acids become essential because our body cannot make them in sufficient quantities.
- **Neurotransmitter synthesis.** Vitamin B_6 is required for enzymes involved in the synthesis of several neurotransmitters, which is also a transamination process. Because of this, vitamin B_6 is important in cognitive function and normal brain activity. Abnormal brain waves have been observed in both infants and adults in vitamin B_6–deficient states.[6]
- **Carbohydrate metabolism.** Vitamin B_6 is required for an enzyme that breaks down stored glycogen to glucose. Thus, vitamin B_6 plays an important role in maintaining blood glucose during exercise. It is also important for the conversion of amino acids to glucose.
- **Heme synthesis.** Vitamin B_6 is necessary for the body to synthesize heme, a component of hemoglobin, the iron-containing protein that transports oxygen in red blood cells. Chronic vitamin B_6 deficiency can lead to small red blood cells with inadequate amounts of hemoglobin.[6]
- **Immune function.** Vitamin B_6 plays a role in maintaining the health and activity of immune cells called lymphocytes and in producing adequate levels of antibodies in response to an immune challenge. The depression of immune

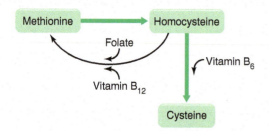

◆ **FIGURE 8.6** The body metabolizes methionine, an essential amino acid, to homocysteine. Notice, however, that homocysteine can then be converted back to methionine through a vitamin B_{12}– and folate-dependent reaction or to cysteine through a vitamin B_6–dependent reaction. Cysteine is a nonessential amino acid important for making other biological compounds. Without these B-vitamins, blood levels of homocysteine can increase. High levels of homocysteine are a risk factor for cardiovascular disease.

homocysteine An amino acid that requires adequate levels of folate, vitamin B_6, and vitamin B_{12} for its metabolism. High levels of homocysteine in the blood are associated with an increased risk for vascular diseases, such as cardiovascular disease.

function seen in vitamin B_6 deficiency may also be due to a reduction in the vitamin B_6–dependent enzymes involved in DNA synthesis.

- **Metabolism of other nutrients.** Vitamin B_6 also plays a role in the metabolism of other nutrients, including niacin and folate.[6]
- **Reduction in cardiovascular disease (CVD) risk.** Vitamin B_6, folate, and vitamin B_{12} are closely interrelated in some metabolic functions, including the metabolism of methionine, an essential amino acid. The body metabolizes methionine to another amino acid called **homocysteine**. In the presence of sufficient levels of vitamin B_6, homocysteine can then be converted to the nonessential amino acid cysteine **(FIGURE 8.6)**. In the presence of sufficient levels of folate and vitamin B_{12}, homocysteine can also be converted back to methionine if the body's level of methionine becomes deficient. If these nutrients are not available, these conversion reactions cannot occur and homocysteine will accumulate in the blood. High levels of homocysteine have been associated with an increased risk of CVD.[6]

Recommended Intakes and Food Sources of Vitamin B_6

The recommended intakes for vitamin B_6 are listed in Table 8.1. Rich sources are meats, fish, poultry, eggs, dairy products, and peanut butter **(FIGURE 8.7)**. Many vegetables, such as asparagus, potatoes, and carrots; fruits, especially bananas; and whole-grain cereals are also good sources of vitamin B_6. As with the other B-vitamins discussed in this chapter, fortified or enriched grains, cereals, and energy bars can provide 25% to 100% of the DV in one serving. Little vitamin B_6 is lost in the storage or handling of foods, except the milling of grains; however, vitamin B_6 is sensitive to both heat and light, so it can easily be lost in cooking.

Vitamin B_6 Toxicity and Deficiency

Whereas consuming excess vitamin B_6 from food sources does not cause toxicity, excess B_6 from supplements can result in nerve damage and lesions of the skin. A condition called *sensory neuropathy* (damage to the sensory nerves) has been documented in individuals taking high-dose B_6 supplements. The symptoms of sensory

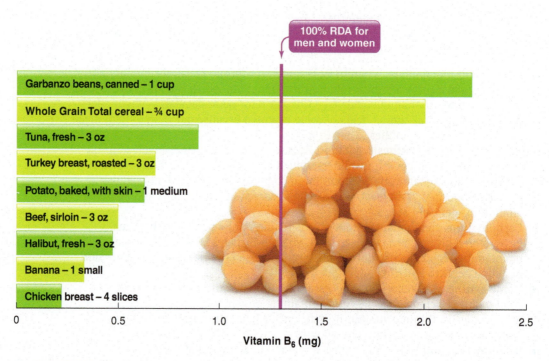

◆ **FIGURE 8.7** Common food sources of vitamin B_6. The RDA for vitamin B_6 is 1.3 mg/day for men and women 19–50 years.

Source: Data from U.S. Department of Agriculture, Agricultural Research Service, 2015. USDA Nutrient Database for Standard Reference, Release 28.

neuropathy include numbness and tingling involving the face, neck, hands, and feet, with difficulty manipulating objects and walking.

The symptoms of vitamin B_6 deficiency include anemia, convulsions, depression, confusion, and inflamed, irritated patches on the skin. As just discussed, deficiency of vitamin B_6, folate, or vitamin B_{12} has also been associated with an increased risk for CVD.

The Most Basic Cellular Functions Require Folate

Reports of the symptoms we now recognize as folate deficiency go back two centuries. By the late 1800s, a disorder associated with large red blood cells had been characterized, but it wasn't until the 1970s that researchers understood the relationship between this blood abnormality and a deficiency of folate, a substance found in many foods, especially leafy green vegetables. The name *folate* originated from the fact the vitamin is abundant in "foliage."[7]

Functions of Folate

Folate-requiring reactions in the body are collectively called *1-C metabolism*. This means folate is involved in adding "one-carbon units" to other organic compounds during the synthesis of new compounds or the modification of existing ones. Thus, the most basic cellular functions require folate. The following are some of these functions.

- **Nucleotide synthesis.** Folate is required for DNA synthesis and cell division. Adequate intake is especially critical during the first few weeks of pregnancy, when the combined sperm–egg cell multiplies rapidly to form the primitive tissues and structures of the human embryo.
- **Amino acid metabolism.** Folate is involved in the metabolism of many of the amino acids and is required, like vitamins B_6 and B_{12}, for the metabolism of methionine.
- **Red blood cell synthesis**. Without adequate folate, the synthesis of normal red blood cells is impaired. (This is discussed in Chapter 9.)

Recommended Intakes and Food Sources of Folate

The recommended intakes for folate are listed in Table 8.1. The critical role of folate during the first few weeks of pregnancy and the fact that many women of childbearing age do not consume adequate amounts led to the mandatory fortification of grain products with folic acid—the form of folate used in fortification and supplements—in 1998. Because of fortification, the primary sources of folate in the American diet are ready-to-eat cereals, breads, pasta, and other grain products. Other good food sources include eggs; oatmeal and whole grain foods; meats, especially liver; fruits and fruit juices; and vegetables **(FIGURE 8.8)** (page 270).

Because folate is sensitive to heat, it can be lost when foods are cooked. It can also leach out into cooking water, which may then be discarded.

Folate Toxicity and Deficiency

There have been no studies suggesting toxic effects of consuming high amounts of folate in food; however, toxicity can occur when taking supplements.[8] Folate toxicity can mask a simultaneous vitamin B_{12} deficiency, which can severely damage the nervous system.[9] There do not appear to be any clear symptoms of folate toxicity independent from this interaction.

Folate deficiency can impair DNA synthesis, which decreases the ability of blood cells to divide. (This is discussed further in Chapter 9.) Another significant concern with folate deficiency is an increased risk for *neural tube defects*. In a folate-deficient environment, the embryonic neural tube may fail to fold and close properly. As a result, the newborn will be born with a birth defect involving the spinal cord or brain. Neural tube defects occur very early in a woman's pregnancy, almost always before she knows she is pregnant. Thus, all sexually active women of childbearing age, whether or not they intend to become pregnant, are advised to consume 400 µg of folate daily from supplements or fortified foods.[3] (Neural tube defects are described in more detail in Chapter 14.)

How much do you know about folic acid? Take the quiz at http://www.cdc.gov/ncbddd/folicacid/quiz.html

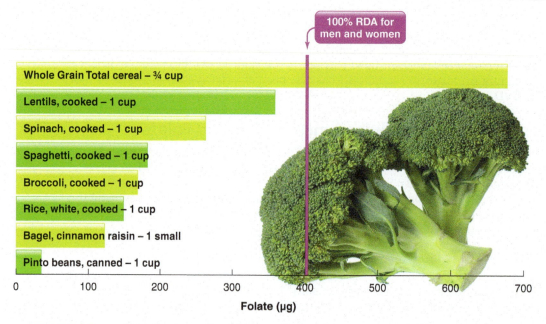

100% RDA for men and women

Whole Grain Total cereal – ¾ cup

Lentils, cooked – 1 cup

Spinach, cooked – 1 cup

Spaghetti, cooked – 1 cup

Broccoli, cooked – 1 cup

Rice, white, cooked – 1 cup

Bagel, cinnamon raisin – 1 small

Pinto beans, canned – 1 cup

0   100   200   300   400   500   600   700

Folate (µg)

🔺 **FIGURE 8.8** Common food sources of folate and folic acid. The RDA for folate is 400 µg/day for men and women.

Source: Data from U.S. Department of Agriculture, Agricultural Research Service, 2015. USDA Nutrient Database for Standard Reference, Release 28.

Folate is also required for homocysteine metabolism (see Figure 8.6), but there is insufficient research to support recommending folate supplementation to reduce CVD risk. However, research does show that adequate levels of vitamins B$_6$, folate, and B$_{12}$ are protective.[10,11,12]

Vitamin B$_{12}$ Participates in Amino Acid and Homocysteine Metabolism

In 1855, a clinician named Thomas Addison described a strange form of anemia in patients that left them feeling weak and exhausted.[9,13] To our knowledge, this is the first report describing the often fatal course of vitamin B$_{12}$ deficiency, later called pernicious anemia (the word *pernicious* means "causing great harm"). Studies over the next 100 years eventually revealed that some special "extrinsic factor" in animal proteins, when combined with an "intrinsic factor" in the stomach, prevented pernicious anemia. When both of these factors were provided to patients with pernicious anemia, they recovered. The final step in the identification of vitamin B$_{12}$ as the extrinsic factor and in determining its structure was done by Dr. Dorothy Crowfoot Hodgkin, who was awarded the Nobel Prize for Chemistry in 1964.[13]

Functions of Vitamin B$_{12}$

Vitamin B$_{12}$ is important for the metabolism of some essential amino acids and the breakdown of certain abnormal fatty acids. It also helps maintain the myelin sheath that coats nerve fibers. When this sheath is damaged or absent, the conduction of nervous signals is slowed, causing numerous neurologic problems.[9] It is not known how vitamin B$_{12}$ deficiency disrupts the myelin sheath, but one hypothesis is that it is due to abnormal fatty acid metabolism.[13]

As noted earlier, adequate levels of folate, vitamin B$_6$, and vitamin B$_{12}$ are necessary to prevent the buildup of homocysteine, which may be important in reducing the risk of CVD.[12] Moreover, the metabolic pathway involved in the metabolism of methionine also converts folate to its active form. This process depends on vitamin B$_{12}$; without adequate B$_{12}$, folate becomes "trapped" in an inactive form and folate deficiency symptoms develop, even though adequate amounts of folate may be present in the diet. Finally, vitamin B$_{12}$ is essential for the formation of healthy red blood cells, and as noted above, deficiency leads to a unique form of anemia (discussed in Chapter 9).

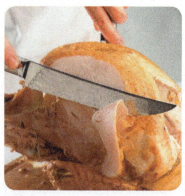

🔺 Vitamin B$_{12}$ is available only from animal-based foods, such as turkey, and fortified foods.

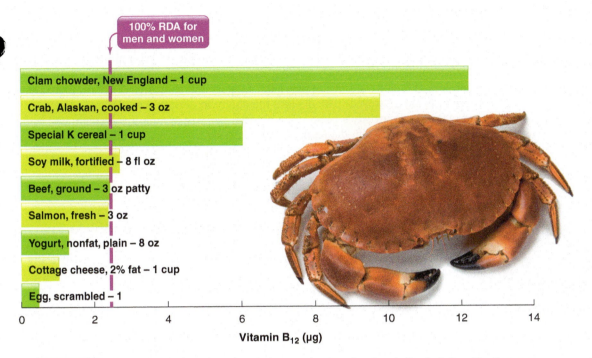

100% RDA for men and women

Clam chowder, New England – 1 cup

Crab, Alaskan, cooked – 3 oz

Special K cereal – 1 cup

Soy milk, fortified – 8 fl oz

Beef, ground – 3 oz patty

Salmon, fresh – 3 oz

Yogurt, nonfat, plain – 8 oz

Cottage cheese, 2% fat – 1 cup

Egg, scrambled – 1

Vitamin B$_{12}$ (µg)

FIGURE 8.9 Common food sources of vitamin B$_{12}$. The RDA for vitamin B$_{12}$ is 2.4 µg/day for men and women.

Source: Data from U.S. Department of Agriculture, Agricultural Research Service, 2015. USDA Nutrient Database for Standard Reference, Release 28.

Recommended Intakes and Food Sources of Vitamin B$_{12}$

The recommended intakes for vitamin B$_{12}$ are listed in Table 8.1. Vitamin B$_{12}$ is found primarily in animal products, such as meats, fish, poultry, dairy products, and eggs, and in fortified soy milk and cereal products, such as ready-to-eat cereals **(FIGURE 8.9)**. Individuals consuming a vegan diet need to eat foods that are fortified with vitamin B$_{12}$ or take vitamin B$_{12}$ supplements or injections to ensure that they maintain adequate blood levels of this nutrient.

Vitamin B$_{12}$ Toxicity and Deficiency

There are no known adverse effects from consuming excess amounts of vitamin B$_{12}$ as either food or supplements.[3]

The two primary causes of vitamin B$_{12}$ deficiency are insufficient intake and malabsorption. Insufficient vitamin B$_{12}$ intake typically occurs in people who follow a strict vegan diet and fail to consume adequate amounts of fortified foods, take supplements, or receive injections. Again, vitamin B$_{12}$ is available only from animal-based foods and fortified foods.

Malabsorption of vitamin B$_{12}$ can be due to either atrophic gastritis or *pernicious anemia, both of which are more common as we age:*

- **Atrophic gastritis**, which results in low stomach acid secretion, occurs in an estimated 10% to 30% of adults older than 50 years of age.[3] Atrophic gastritis is most commonly caused by infection with *H. pylori,* the same bacterium implicated in ulcers (see Chapter 3), or by an autoimmune disorder. Because stomach acid separates food-bound vitamin B$_{12}$ from dietary proteins, if the stomach pH is too high, then too little vitamin B$_{12}$ will be freed up from food. People over 50 years of age are advised to consume foods fortified with vitamin B$_{12}$, take a vitamin B$_{12}$–containing supplement, or have periodic B$_{12}$ injections.

- As just discussed, **pernicious anemia** is due to inadequate production of a protein called *intrinsic factor* that normally is secreted by parietal cells in the stomach. Intrinsic factor binds to vitamin B$_{12}$ and aids its absorption in the small intestine. When not bound to intrinsic factor, vitamin B$_{12}$ is not recognized and absorbed by the enterocytes. Like atrophic gastritis, inadequate production of intrinsic factor

atrophic gastritis A condition in which chronic inflammation of the stomach lining erodes gastric glands, reducing stomach acid secretion and thus absorption of vitamin B$_{12}$ from foods.

pernicious anemia A vitamin B$_{12}$ deficiency disease that occurs when immune destruction of parietal cells in the stomach reduces production of intrinsic factor, thereby limiting vitamin B$_{12}$ absorption.

occurs more commonly in older people. Individuals who lack intrinsic factor may receive periodic vitamin B_{12} injections.

Vitamin B_{12} deficiency is also commonly seen in people with more generalized malabsorption disorders, such as celiac disease. Symptoms of vitamin B_{12} deficiency, regardless of the cause, include pale skin, fatigue, and shortness of breath. Because nerve cells are destroyed, patients lose the ability to perform coordinated movements and maintain their body's positioning. Central nervous system involvement can lead to irritability, confusion, depression, and dementia that even with treatment can be only partially reversed.

Pantothenic Acid and Biotin Are Required for All Energy Pathways

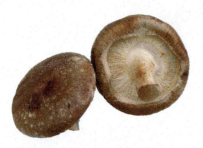

↥ Shiitake mushrooms contain pantothenic acid.

Pantothenic acid was named after the Greek word meaning "from everywhere" because the vitamin is widespread in the food supply.[14] It is a component of a coenzyme required for all the energy-producing metabolic pathways. It is especially important for the breakdown and synthesis of fatty acids. Thus, pantothenic acid ensures that the foods we eat can be used for energy and that the excess energy we consume can be stored as fat.

The recommended intakes for pantothenic acid are listed in Table 8.1. Again, it is widespread in the food supply; however, particularly good food sources include chicken, beef, egg yolks, potatoes, oat cereals, tomato products, whole grains, organ meats, and yeast. There are no known adverse effects from consuming excess amounts of pantothenic acid. Deficiencies of pantothenic acid are very rare.

Biotin is a coenzyme for five enzymes that are critical in the metabolism of carbohydrate, fat, and protein. It also plays an important role in gluconeogenesis. The recommended intakes for biotin are listed in Table 8.1. The biotin content has been determined for very few foods, and these values are not reported in food composition tables or dietary analysis programs. Biotin appears to be widespread in foods but is especially high in liver, egg yolks, and cooked cereals. Biotin is also produced by the GI flora, but its availability for absorption appears low.

There are no known adverse effects from consuming excess amounts of biotin. Biotin deficiencies are typically seen only in people who consume a large number of raw egg whites over long periods. This is because raw egg whites contain a protein called avidin, which binds biotin in the gastrointestinal tract and prevents its absorption. Symptoms of deficiency include thinning of hair; loss of hair color; development of a red, scaly rash around the eyes, nose, and mouth; depression; lethargy; and hallucinations.

recap Thiamin plays critical roles in the metabolism of glucose and the branched-chain amino acids. Thiamin-deficiency disease is called beriberi. Riboflavin is an important coenzyme involved in the metabolism of carbohydrates and fat. Riboflavin-deficiency disease is called ariboflavinosis. Niacin assists in the metabolism of carbohydrates and fatty acids. It also plays an important role in DNA replication and repair and in cell differentiation. Niacin-deficiency disease is called pellagra. Vitamin B_6 is a coenzyme for more than 100 enzymes involved in processes such as the metabolism of amino acids and carbohydrates and the synthesis of neurotransmitters. Folate is required for the most basic cellular functions, such as the synthesis of DNA as well as cell differentiation, and deficiency can lead to neural tube defects in a developing embryo. Vitamin B_{12} is essential for the metabolism of certain essential amino acids, normal maturation of blood cells, and maintenance of the myelin sheath that coats nerve fibers. Deficiency of vitamin B_6, folate, or vitamin B_{12} may increase the risk for CVD by elevating blood homocysteine levels. Pantothenic acid is especially important for the breakdown and synthesis of fatty acids, whereas biotin is a coenzyme for enzymes that are critical in the metabolism of carbohydrate, fat, and protein.

nutri-case | JUDY

"Ever since my doctor put me on this crazy diet, I've been feeling hungry and exhausted. This morning I'm sitting in the lunch room on my break, and I actually doze off and start dreaming about food! Maureen, one of the girls I work with, comes in and has to wake me up! I told her what's been going on with me, and she thinks I should start taking some B-vitamins so I stay healthy while I'm on the diet. She says B-vitamins are the most important because they give you energy. Maybe after work I'll stop off at the drugstore and buy some. If they give you energy, maybe they'll make it easier to stick to my diet, too."

Is Judy's coworker correct when she asserts that B-vitamins "give you energy"? Either way, do you think it's likely that Judy needs to take B-vitamin supplements to ensure that she "stays healthy" while she is on her prescribed diet? Why or why not? Finally, could taking B-vitamins help Judy stick to her diet?

How do choline and four minerals function in energy metabolism?

LO 3 Discuss the contributions of choline and four minerals to energy metabolism.

As noted earlier, vitamins aren't alone in assisting energy metabolism. A vitamin-like compound called choline and the minerals iodine, chromium, manganese, and sulfur also play key roles in this and other body functions.

Choline Is a Vitamin-Like Nutrient

Choline is an essential nutrient important in metabolism. Although not a vitamin, it is typically grouped with the B-vitamins because of its role in the metabolism and transport of fats and cholesterol and in homocysteine metabolism. Choline also accelerates the synthesis and release of **acetylcholine**, a neurotransmitter that is involved in many functions, including muscle movement and memory storage. In addition, choline is necessary for the synthesis of phospholipids and other components of cell membranes; thus, choline plays a critical role in the structural integrity of cells.

The recommended intakes for choline are listed in Table 8.1. The choline content of foods is not typically reported in nutrient databases. However, we do know that choline is widespread in foods, especially milk, liver, eggs, and peanuts. Inadequate intakes of choline can lead to increased fat accumulation in the liver, which eventually leads to liver damage. Excessive intake of supplemental choline results in various toxicity symptoms, including diarrhea, vomiting, and low blood pressure.

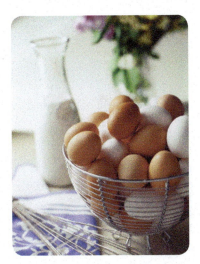

◀ Choline is widespread in foods and can be found in eggs and milk.

Iodine Is Required for the Synthesis of Thyroid Hormones

Iodine is a trace mineral responsible for just one function within the body, the synthesis of thyroid hormones. Our body requires thyroid hormones to regulate body temperature, maintain resting metabolic rate, and support reproduction and growth.

We need relatively small amounts of iodine to maintain good health (see Table 8.1). However, the iodine content of foods and beverages depends on the level of inorganic iodide in the environment, such as the soil in which crops are grown and the water and fertilizers used. Saltwater fish and shrimp tend to have higher amounts because marine animals concentrate iodine from seawater. Because iodine is added to

acetylcholine A neurotransmitter that is involved in many functions, including muscle movement and memory storage.

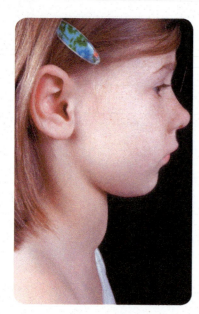

▲ **FIGURE 8.10** Goiter, or enlargement of the thyroid gland, most commonly develops as a result of iodine deficiency.

dairy cattle feed and used in sanitizing solutions in the dairy industry, milk and other dairy foods are an important source.

In addition, iodized salt and white and whole-wheat breads made with iodized salt and bread conditioners are an important source of iodine. The United States began adding iodine to table salt in 1924. Today, a majority of households worldwide use iodized salt, and for many people, it is their only source of iodine. Approximately one-half teaspoon meets the full adult RDA for iodine. When you buy salt, check the package label: Most specialty salts, such as kosher salt or sea salt, do not have iodine added. People who strictly limit their salt intake to help reduce their blood pressure also limit the primary source of iodine in their diet. These people need to add other sources of iodine to their diet.

Iodine toxicity, which generally occurs only with excessive supplementation, impairs the synthesis of thyroid hormones, as does iodine deficiency. Either toxicity or deficiency will cause the thyroid to attempt to produce more hormones. It may therefore enlarge, a condition known as **goiter** (FIGURE 8.10). Iodine deficiency is the primary cause of goiter worldwide.

A low level of circulating thyroid hormones is known as *hypothyroidism*. In addition to goiter, symptoms of hypothyroidism include decreased body temperature, inability to tolerate cold environmental temperatures, weight gain, fatigue, and sluggishness.

If a woman experiences iodine deficiency during pregnancy, her infant has a high risk of being born with a form of mental impairment referred to as **cretinism**, which is also characterized by stunted growth, deafness, and muteness. The World Health Organization (WHO) considers iodine deficiency the greatest single cause of preventable brain damage and mental impairment in the world.[15]

Chromium Is Important in Carbohydrate Metabolism

Chromium is a trace mineral that plays an important role in carbohydrate metabolism. You may be interested to learn that the chromium in your body is the same metal used in the chrome plating for cars.

Chromium enhances the ability of insulin to transport glucose from the bloodstream into cells.[16] It also plays important roles in the metabolism of RNA and DNA, in immune function, and in growth. We have only very small amounts of chromium in our body. Whether the U.S. diet provides adequate chromium is controversial; our body appears to store less as we age.

The recommended intakes for chromium are listed in Table 8.1. Food sources include mushrooms, prunes, dark chocolate, nuts, whole grains, cereals, asparagus, brewer's yeast, some beers, and red wine.

There appears to be no toxicity related to consuming chromium naturally found in the diet or in supplements. Chromium deficiency appears to be uncommon in the United States. When induced in a research setting, chromium deficiency inhibits the uptake of glucose by the cells, causing a rise in blood glucose and insulin levels. Chromium deficiency can also result in elevated blood lipid levels and in damage to the nervous system.

Manganese Assists in Energy Metabolism and Bone Health

A trace mineral, manganese assists enzymes involved in energy metabolism and in the formation of urea, the primary component of urine. It also assists in the synthesis of the protein matrix found in bone tissue and of cartilage, a tissue that supports joints. Manganese is also an integral component of an antioxidant enzyme system (discussed later in this chapter).

The recommended intakes for manganese are listed in Table 8.1. Manganese requirements are easily met because this mineral is widespread in a varied diet. Whole-grain foods, such as oat bran, wheat flour, whole-wheat spaghetti, and brown rice, are especially good sources of manganese, as are pineapple, raspberries, okra, spinach, garbanzo beans, and pine nuts.

goiter Enlargement of the thyroid gland; can be caused by iodine toxicity or deficiency.

cretinism A form of mental impairment that occurs in children whose mothers experienced iodine deficiency during pregnancy.

antioxidant A compound that has the ability to prevent or repair the damage caused by oxidation.

nucleus The positively charged, central core of an atom. It is made up of two types of particles—protons and neutrons—bound tightly together. The nucleus of an atom contains essentially all of its atomic mass.

electron A negatively charged particle orbiting the nucleus of an atom.

oxidation A chemical reaction in which molecules of a substance are broken down into their component atoms. During oxidation, the atoms involved lose electrons.

Manganese toxicity, which affects the nervous system, can occur in occupational environments in which people inhale manganese dust; it can also result from drinking water high in manganese. Manganese deficiency is rare in humans.

Sulfur Is a Component of Thiamin, Biotin, and Two Amino Acids

Sulfur is a major mineral and a component of the B-vitamins thiamin and biotin. In addition, as part of the amino acids methionine and cysteine, sulfur helps stabilize the three-dimensional shapes of proteins. The liver requires sulfur to assist in the detoxification of alcohol and various drugs, and sulfur helps the body maintain acid–base balance.

The body is able to obtain ample amounts of sulfur from our consumption of protein-containing foods; as a result, there is no DRI specifically for sulfur. There are no known toxicity or deficiency symptoms associated with sulfur.

recap Choline is a vitamin-like nutrient that assists in homocysteine metabolism and the production of acetylcholine. Iodine is necessary for the synthesis of thyroid hormones, which regulate metabolic rate and body temperature. Chromium promotes glucose transport, metabolism of RNA and DNA, and immune function and growth. Manganese is involved in energy metabolism, urea formation, synthesis of bone and cartilage, and protection against free radicals. Sulfur is part of thiamin and biotin and the amino acids methionine and cysteine.

What are antioxidants, and how do they protect our cells?

LO 4 Describe the process by which oxidation can damage cells and the role of antioxidants in opposing this damage.

Antioxidants are compounds that protect our cells from the damage caused by oxidation. *Anti* means "against," and antioxidants work *against* oxidation. But what is oxidation, and why is it potentially harmful?

Oxidation Is a Chemical Reaction in Which Atoms Lose Electrons

The body is made up of atoms, tiny units of matter that join together to form molecules (see Chapter 3). Some molecules, such as hydrogen gas (H_2), contain only one type of atom—in this case, hydrogen. Most molecules, however, are *compounds*—they contain two or more different types of atoms (such as water, H_2O). Our body is constantly breaking down compounds of food, water, and air into their component atoms, then rearranging these freed atoms to build new substances.

Although atoms cannot be broken down by natural means, during the 20th century, physicists learned how to split atoms into their component *particles*. As shown in **FIGURE 8.11**, all atoms have a central core, called a **nucleus**, which is positively charged. Orbiting around this nucleus are one or more **electrons**, which are negatively charged. The opposite attraction between the positive nucleus and the negative electrons keeps an atom together by making it stable, so that its electrons remain with it and don't veer off toward other atoms.

As they participate in the chemical reactions that constitute metabolism, atoms may lose electrons **(FIGURE 8.12a)**. We call this loss of electrons **oxidation**, because it is fueled by oxygen. Atoms are capable of gaining electrons during metabolism as well. We call this process *reduction* (Figure 8.12b). A chemical reaction involving this loss and gain of electrons typically results in an even exchange of electrons, and is known as an *exchange reaction*.

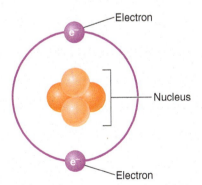

FIGURE 8.11 An atom consists of a central nucleus and orbiting electrons. The nucleus exerts a positive charge, which keeps the negatively charged electrons in its vicinity. Notice that this atom has an even number of electrons in orbit around the nucleus. This pairing of electrons results in the atom being chemically stable.

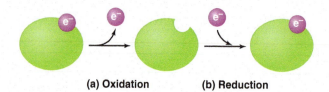

(a) Oxidation   **(b) Reduction**

◀ **FIGURE 8.12** Exchange reactions consist of two parts. **(a)** During oxidation, atoms *lose* electrons. **(b)** In the second part of the reaction, atoms *gain* electrons, which is called reduction.

Oxidation Sometimes Results in the Formation of Free Radicals

Stable atoms have an even number of electrons orbiting in pairs at successive distances (called *shells*) from the nucleus. When a stable atom loses an electron during oxidation, it is left with an odd number of electrons in its outermost shell. In other words, it now has an *unpaired electron*. Also during metabolism, oxygen sometimes gains the single electron that was released during oxidation. As a result, the oxygen atom now has an unpaired electron **(FIGURE 8.13)**. In most exchange reactions, unpaired electrons immediately pair up with other unpaired electrons, making newly stabilized atoms, but in some cases, an atom's unpaired electrons remain unpaired. Such atoms are highly unstable and are called **free radicals**.

Free radicals are also formed from other physiologic processes, such as when the immune system produces inflammation to fight allergens or infections. Other factors that cause free radical formation include exposure to tobacco smoke and other types of air pollution, ultraviolet (UV) rays from the sun, and industrial chemicals. Continual exposure leads to uncontrollable free radical formation, cell damage, and disease, as discussed next.

Free Radicals Can Destabilize Other Molecules and Damage Our Cells

We are concerned with the formation of free radicals because of their destabilizing power. If you were to think of paired electrons as a married couple, a free radical would be an extremely seductive outsider. Its unpaired electron exerts a powerful attraction toward the stable molecules around it. In an attempt to stabilize itself, a free radical will "steal" an electron from these molecules, in turn generating more unstable free radicals. This is a dangerous chain reaction because the free radicals generated can damage or destroy cells.

One of the most significant sites of free radical damage is the cell membrane. As shown in **FIGURE 8.14a**, free radicals that form within the phospholipid bilayer of cell membranes steal electrons from the stable lipid heads. Recall that lipids are insoluble in water, so a stable lineup of lipid heads allows cell membranes to keep water out. When these lipid heads are destroyed, the cell membrane can no longer repel water, and, its ability to regulate the movement of fluids and nutrients into and out of the cell is lost. This loss of cell integrity damages the cell and all systems affected by the cell.

Other sites of free radical damage include low-density lipoproteins (LDLs), cell proteins, and DNA. Damage to LDLs disrupts the transport of substances into and out of cells; damage to cell proteins alters cell function; and damage to DNA

free radical A highly unstable atom with an unpaired electron in its outermost shell.

▶ **FIGURE 8.13** Normally, an oxygen atom contains eight electrons. Occasionally, oxygen will accept an unpaired electron during the oxidation process. This acceptance of a single electron causes oxygen to become an unstable atom called a free radical.

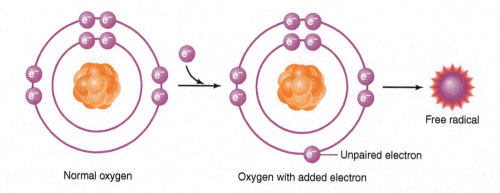

Normal oxygen   Oxygen with added electron

Unpaired electron

Free radical

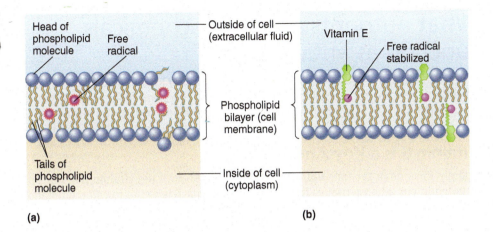

Head of phospholipid molecule
Free radical
Outside of cell (extracellular fluid)
Tails of phospholipid molecule
Phospholipid bilayer (cell membrane)
Inside of cell (cytoplasm)

(a)

Vitamin E
Free radical stabilized

(b)

◀ **FIGURE 8.14** **(a)** The formation of free radicals in the lipid portion of our cell membranes can cause a dangerous chain reaction that damages the integrity of the membrane and can cause cell death. **(b)** Vitamin E is stored in the lipid portion of our cell membranes. By donating an electron to free radicals, it protects the lipid molecules in our cell membranes from being oxidized and stops the chain reaction of oxidative damage.

results in faulty protein synthesis. These changes can also cause harmful changes (mutations) in cells or prompt cells to die prematurely. Free radicals also promote blood vessel inflammation and the formation of clots, both of which are risk factors for CVD (see In Depth 5.5). Other diseases linked with free radical production include cancer, type 2 diabetes, arthritis, cataracts, and Alzheimer's and Parkinson's diseases.

Antioxidants Work by Stabilizing Free Radicals or Opposing Oxidation

Antioxidant vitamins, minerals, and phytochemicals fight free radicals and repair the damage they cause:

1. Antioxidant vitamins work independently by donating their electrons or hydrogen atoms to stabilize free radicals (Figure 8.14b).
2. Antioxidant minerals act as **cofactors**, substances required to activate enzymes so that they can do their work. These minerals function within complex *antioxidant enzyme systems* that convert free radicals to less damaging substances that our body then excretes. They also work to break down fatty acids that have become oxidized, thereby destroying the free radicals associated with them. They also make more antioxidant vitamins available to fight other free radicals. Examples of antioxidant enzyme systems are superoxide dismutase, catalase, and glutathione peroxidase.
3. Antioxidant phytochemicals such as beta-carotene and other carotenoids may inhibit the oxidation of lipids or donate electrons to help stabilize free radicals.

In summary, free radical formation is generally kept safely under control by certain vitamins, minerals working within antioxidant enzyme systems, and phytochemicals. Next, we take a look at the specific antioxidants involved.

recap During metabolism, molecules break apart and their atoms gain, lose, or exchange electrons; loss of electrons is called oxidation. Free radicals are highly unstable atoms with an unpaired electron in their outermost shell. A normal by-product of oxidation reactions, they can damage the cell membrane, cell proteins, and DNA and are associated with many diseases. Antioxidant vitamins and phytochemicals such as the carotenoids donate electrons to stabilize free radicals and reduce oxidative damage. Antioxidant minerals are part of antioxidant enzyme systems that convert free radicals to less damaging substances.

cofactor A mineral or non-protein compound that is needed to allow enzymes to function properly.

LO 5 Identify the antioxidant functions of key micronutrients and carotenoids.

What nutrients and phytochemicals function as antioxidants?

Micronutrients that play a role in stabilizing free radicals include vitamins E, C, and possibly A, and the minerals selenium, copper, iron, zinc, and manganese (TABLE 8.2). Carotenoids such as beta-carotene also appear to have antioxidant properties.

Vitamin E Is a Key Antioxidant

Vitamin E is one of the fat-soluble vitamins. About 90% of the vitamin E in our body is stored in our adipose tissue. The remaining vitamin E is found in cell membranes.

The most potent form of vitamin E found in food and supplements is *alpha-tocopherol*. The RDA for vitamin E is expressed as alpha-tocopherol in milligrams per day. Food and supplements labels may express vitamin E in units of alpha-tocopherol equivalents (α-TE), in milligrams, or as International Units (IU). The following can be used for conversion purposes:

- In food, 1 α-TE is equal to 1 mg of active vitamin E.
- In supplements containing a natural form of vitamin E, 1 IU is equal to 0.67 mg α-TE.
- In supplements containing a synthetic form of vitamin E, 1 IU is equal to 0.45 mg α-TE.

Functions of Vitamin E

The primary function of vitamin E is as an antioxidant: it donates an electron to free radicals, stabilizing them and preventing them from destabilizing other molecules. Once vitamin E is oxidized, it is either excreted from the body or recycled back into active vitamin E through the help of other antioxidant nutrients, such as vitamin C.

Vitamin E acts specifically to protect fatty components of our cells and cell membranes from being oxidized (see Figure 8.14b). It also protects LDLs from being oxidized, thereby reducing our risk for CVD. Vitamin E protects the membranes of our red blood cells from oxidation and protects the white blood cells of our immune system, thereby helping the body defend against disease. It also protects lung cells, which are constantly exposed to oxygen and the potentially damaging effects of oxidation. Vitamin E is critical for normal nerve and muscle development and function. Finally, it boosts absorption of vitamin A if dietary intake of vitamin A is low.

TABLE 8.2 Overview of Nutrients Essential to Antioxidant Function and Vision

To see the full profile of all micronutrients, turn to the **In Depth** essay following Chapter 6, Vitamins and Minerals: Micronutrients with Macro Powers (pages 211–221).

Nutrient	Recommended Intake
Vitamin E (fat soluble)	RDA for 19 years of age and older: 15 mg alpha-tocopherol
Vitamin C (water soluble)	RDA for 19 years of age and older: Women = 75 mg Men = 90 mg Smokers = 35 mg more per day than RDA
Selenium (trace mineral)	RDA for 19 years of age and older: 55 μg
Beta-carotene (fat soluble; provitamin for vitamin A)	No DRI
Vitamin A (fat soluble)	RDA for 19 years of age and older: Women = 700 μg Men = 900 μg

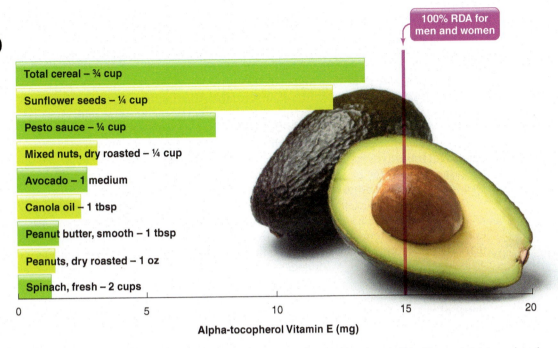

100% RDA for men and women

Total cereal – ¾ cup	
Sunflower seeds – ¼ cup	
Pesto sauce – ¼ cup	
Mixed nuts, dry roasted – ¼ cup	
Avocado – 1 medium	
Canola oil – 1 tbsp	
Peanut butter, smooth – 1 tbsp	
Peanuts, dry roasted – 1 oz	
Spinach, fresh – 2 cups	

Alpha-tocopherol Vitamin E (mg)

▲ **FIGURE 8.15** Common food sources of vitamin E. The RDA for vitamin E is 15 mg alpha-tocopherol per day for men and women.

Source: Data from U.S. Department of Agriculture, Agricultural Research Service, 2015. USDA Nutrient Database for Standard Reference, Release 28.

Recommended Intakes and Food Sources of Vitamin E

Despite its importance to health, the RDA for vitamin E is modest: 15 mg alpha-tocopherol per day (see Table 8.2).[17] The UL is 1,000 mg alpha-tocopherol per day. Vitamin E is widespread in foods from plant sources **(FIGURE 8.15)**, including vegetable oils and spreads, salad dressings, and mayonnaise made from vegetable oils. Nuts, seeds, soybeans, and some vegetables—including spinach, broccoli, and avocados—also provide vitamin E. Cereals are often fortified with vitamin E, and other grain products contribute modest amounts to our diet.

Vitamin E is destroyed by exposure to oxygen, metals, ultraviolet light, and heat. Although raw (uncooked) vegetable oils contain vitamin E, heating these oils destroys vitamin E. Thus, fried foods contain little vitamin E; this includes most fast foods. See the nearby **Quick Tips** for increasing your intake of vitamin E.

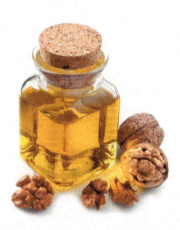

▲ Vegetable oils, nuts, and seeds are good sources of vitamin E.

QuickTips

Eating More Vitamin E

✔ Eat cereals high in vitamin E for breakfast or as a snack.

✔ Add sunflower seeds to salads and trail mixes, or just have them as a snack.

✔ Add sliced almonds to salads, granola, and trail mixes to boost vitamin E intake.

✔ Pack a peanut butter sandwich for lunch.

✔ Eat veggies throughout the day—for snacks, for sides, and in main dishes.

✔ When dressing a salad, use vitamin E–rich oils, such as sunflower, safflower, or canola.

✔ Enjoy some fresh, homemade guacamole: mash a ripe avocado with a squeeze of lime juice and a sprinkle of garlic salt.

Vitamin E Toxicity and Deficiency

Nausea, intestinal distress, and diarrhea have been reported with vitamin E supplementation. Moreover, research has shown that vitamin E supplementation above the RDA can increase the risk of prostate cancer in men and the risk for premature mortality in women and men.[18,19]

Vitamin E is a mild *anticoagulant,* a substance that inhibits blood clotting. Thus, vitamin E supplements can augment the action of medications with anticoagulant effects. These include the prescription drug Coumadin, as well as over-the-counter pain relievers such as aspirin and ibuprofen. Increased anticoagulant activity can lead to uncontrollable bleeding. In addition, evidence suggests that in some people, long-term use of standard vitamin E supplements may lead to a *hemorrhagic stroke.*[17]

True vitamin E deficiencies are uncommon in humans. This is primarily because vitamin E is fat soluble, so we typically store adequate amounts in our fatty tissues, even when our current intakes are low. Deficiencies usually result from diseases that cause malabsorption of fat, such as those that affect the small intestine, liver, gallbladder, and pancreas. With poor fat absorption, the fat-soluble vitamins also cannot be absorbed.

One vitamin E deficiency symptom is *erythrocyte hemolysis,* or the rupturing (*lysis*) of red blood cells (*erythrocytes*). This rupturing of red blood cells leads to *anemia* (a condition discussed in Chapter 9). Vitamin E deficiency can also cause loss of muscle coordination and reflexes and impair immune function, especially when body stores of the mineral selenium are low.

Vitamin C Is a Water-Soluble Antioxidant

Because it is water soluble, vitamin C is an important antioxidant in the extracellular fluid. Like vitamin E, it donates electrons to free radicals, thus preventing damage to cells and tissues. It also protects LDL-cholesterol from oxidation, which may reduce the risk for CVD. Vitamin C acts as an important antioxidant in the lungs, helping to protect cells from inhaled air pollutants such as cigarette smoke. It also enhances immune function by protecting white blood cells from the oxidative damage that occurs in response to fighting infection. But contrary to popular belief, it is not a miracle cure: vitamin C supplementation has not been shown to ward off colds, although it may reduce the duration of symptoms.[20] In the stomach, vitamin C reduces the formation of *nitrosamines,* cancer-causing agents found in foods such as cured and processed meats.

Vitamin C also regenerates vitamin E after it has been oxidized. It does this by donating electrons to vitamin E radicals, thereby enabling vitamin E to continue to protect our cell membranes and body tissues.

Vitamin C also helps ensure appropriate levels of thyroid hormones, which support metabolism and help maintain body temperature, as discussed earlier. It also plays a key role in synthesizing other hormones, bile, neurotransmitters, and other functional chemicals. Finally, vitamin C is critical to the synthesis and maintenance of collagen, the most abundant tissue in the body. We discuss this function of vitamin C in more detail, along with its DRI and food sources, in Chapter 9.

Selenium Is a Key Antioxidant Mineral

We have learned only recently about the critical role of selenium as a nutrient in human health. In 1979, a heart disorder called **Keshan disease** was linked to selenium deficiency, which occurs in children in the Keshan province of China, where the soil is depleted of selenium.

Most of the selenium in our body is contained in amino acids: *selenomethionine* is the storage form for selenium, whereas *selenocysteine* is the active form. Selenocysteine is a critical component of the glutathione peroxidase antioxidant enzyme system.

Like vitamin C, selenium is needed for the production of thyroid hormones and appears to play a role in immune function. Poor selenium status is associated with higher rates of some forms of cancer.

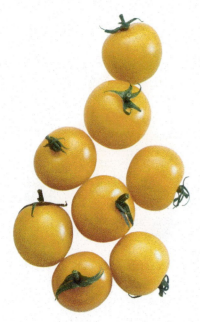

◄ Many fruits and vegetables, like these yellow tomatoes, are high in vitamin C.

Keshan disease A heart disorder caused by selenium deficiency. It was first identified in children in the Keshan province of China.

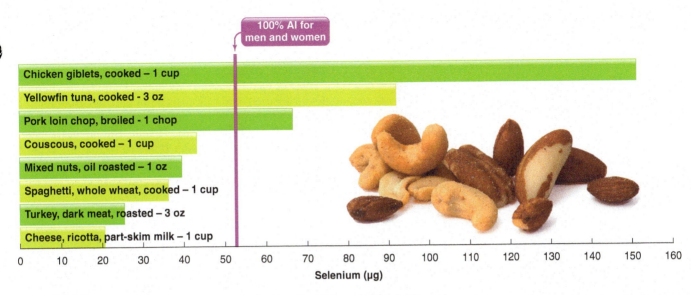

100% AI for men and women

Chicken giblets, cooked – 1 cup

Yellowfin tuna, cooked - 3 oz

Pork loin chop, broiled - 1 chop

Couscous, cooked – 1 cup

Mixed nuts, oil roasted – 1 oz

Spaghetti, whole wheat, cooked – 1 cup

Turkey, dark meat, roasted – 3 oz

Cheese, ricotta, part-skim milk – 1 cup

0 10 20 30 40 50 60 70 80 90 100 110 120 130 140 150 160

Selenium (µg)

◀ **FIGURE 8.16** Common food sources of selenium. The AI for selenium is 55 µg/day.
Source: Data from U.S. Department of Agriculture, Agricultural Research Service, 2015. USDA Nutrient Database for Standard Reference, Release 28.

A trace mineral, selenium is required in only minute amounts to maintain health. The RDA is identified in Table 8.2. Because it is stored in the tissues of animals, selenium is found in reliably consistent amounts in animal foods. Organ meats, such as liver and kidneys, as well as pork and fish, are particularly good sources **(FIGURE 8.16)**. In contrast, the amount of selenium in plants varies according to the selenium content of the soil in which the plant is grown. Although the selenium content of soil varies greatly across North America, we obtain our food from a variety of geographic locations, which means that few people in the United States suffer from selenium deficiency.

Selenium toxicity does not result from eating foods high in selenium, but supplementation can cause toxicity. Toxicity symptoms include brittle hair and nails, skin rashes, nausea, vomiting, weakness, and cirrhosis of the liver.

In addition to Keshan disease, selenium deficiency can cause *a deforming arthritis*, impaired immune responses, infertility, depression, hostility, impaired cognitive function, and muscle pain and wasting. Deficiency in pregnant women can cause a form of *cretinism* in the infant similar to that seen with iodine deficiency.

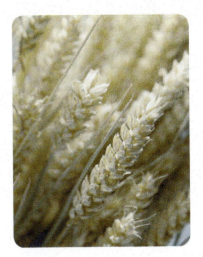

◀ Wheat is a rich source of selenium.

Manganese, Copper, Iron, and Zinc Assist in Antioxidant Function

Manganese, copper, and zinc are part of the superoxide dismutase antioxidant enzyme system, and iron is a component of catalase. In addition to their antioxidant roles, these minerals are essential to the optimal functioning of many other important enzymes. The role of manganese in carbohydrate metabolism was discussed earlier in this chapter. Copper, iron, and zinc contribute to metabolism and to healthy tissues, such as blood. They are discussed in detail in Chapter 9.

Carotenoids Like Beta-Carotene Have Antioxidant Properties

Recall from In Depth 1.5 that **carotenoids** are plant pigments that are the basis for the red, orange, and deep-yellow colors of many fruits and vegetables. (Even dark-green leafy vegetables contain plenty of carotenoids, but the green pigment, chlorophyll, masks their color.) Many carotenoids are known to have antioxidant properties, and researchers are beginning to explore other potential functions of carotenoids and their effects on human health.

Although beta-carotene is considered a phytochemical, not an essential nutrient, it acts as a **provitamin**, an inactive form of a vitamin that the body cannot use until it is

carotenoid A fat-soluble plant pigment that the body stores in the liver and adipose tissues. The body is able to convert certain carotenoids to vitamin A.

provitamin An inactive form of a vitamin that the body can convert to an active form. An example is beta-carotene.

converted to its active form. Our body converts beta-carotene to the active form of vitamin A, *retinol;* thus, beta-carotene is a precursor of retinol.

Although one molecule of beta-carotene splits to form two molecules of active vitamin A, 12 units of beta-carotene are considered equivalent to one unit of vitamin A. Several factors account for this. For example, our body doesn't convert to vitamin A all of the beta-carotene that we consume, and our absorption of beta-carotene is not as efficient as our absorption of vitamin A. Nutritionists express the units of beta-carotene in a food as Retinol Activity Equivalents (RAE). This measurement indicates how much active vitamin A is available to the body after it has converted the beta-carotene in the food.

Functions of Beta-Carotene

Beta-carotene and some other carotenoids, such as lycopene and lutein, are recognized to have antioxidant properties. Like vitamin E, they are fat-soluble and fight the harmful effects of oxidation in the lipid portions of our cell membranes and in LDLs.

Through their antioxidant actions, carotenoids also enhance immune function, protect the skin from the sun's ultraviolet rays, and protect our eyes from oxidative damage, preventing or delaying age-related vision impairment. Carotenoids are also associated with a decreased risk for certain types of cancer. (We discuss the roles of antioxidants in cancer **In Depth** following this chapter.)

Recommended Intakes and Food Sources of Beta-Carotene

Because beta-carotene and other carotenoids are not considered essential nutrients, no RDA for these compounds has been established. Eating the recommended five servings of fruits and vegetables each day provides approximately 6 to 8 mg of beta-carotene, which is thought to be an adequate intake.[21]

Supplements containing beta-carotene have become popular, but before you try one, read the **Nutrition Debate** at the end of this chapter, which discusses the serious risks of antioxidant supplementation.

Fruits and vegetables that are red, orange, yellow, and deep green are generally high in beta-carotene and other carotenoids, such as lutein and lycopene. Tomatoes, sweet potatoes, kale, spinach, apricots, and pumpkin are good sources **(FIGURE 8.17)**.

We generally absorb only between 20% and 40% of the carotenoids present in the foods we eat. Carotenoids are better absorbed from cooked foods, as they are bound in the cells of plants, and the process of lightly cooking these plants breaks chemical bonds and can rupture cell walls, which humans don't digest. These actions result in more of the carotenoids being released from the plant. The **Quick Tips** feature suggests ways to increase your intake of beta-carotene.

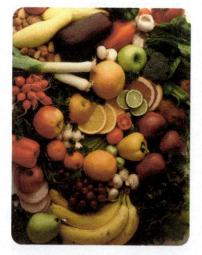

⬅ Foods that are high in carotenoids are easy to recognize by their bright colors.

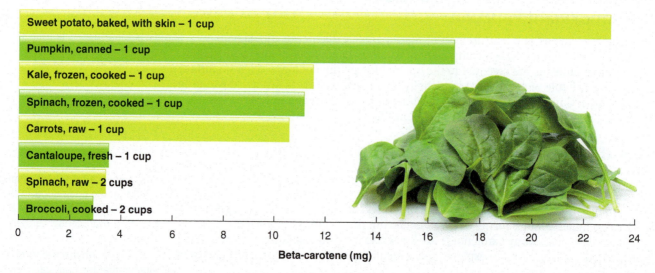

⬆ **FIGURE 8.17** Common food sources of beta-carotene. There is no RDA for beta-carotene.

Source: Data from U.S. Department of Agriculture, Agricultural Research Service, 2015. USDA Nutrient Database for Standard Reference, Release 28.

QuickTips

Boosting Your Beta-Carotene

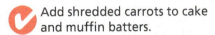

Start your day with an orange, grapefruit, a pear, a banana, an apple, or a slice of cantaloupe. All are good sources of beta-carotene.

Pack a zip-lock bag of carrot slices or dried apricots in your lunch.

Instead of french fries, think orange! Slice raw sweet potatoes, toss the slices in olive or canola oil, and bake.

Add veggies to homemade pizza.

Add shredded carrots to cake and muffin batters.

Taking dessert to a potluck? Make a pumpkin pie! It's easy if you use canned pumpkin and follow the recipe on the can.

Go green, too! The next time you have a salad, go for the dark-green leafy vegetables instead of iceberg lettuce.

Add raw spinach or other green leafy vegetables to wraps and sandwiches.

Beta-Carotene Toxicity and Deficiency

Consuming large amounts of beta-carotene or other carotenoids in foods does not appear to cause toxic symptoms. However, it can cause your skin to turn yellow or orange. This condition appears to be both reversible and harmless. Again, taking beta-carotene supplements is not recommended.

There are no known deficiency symptoms for beta-carotene or other carotenoids apart from beta-carotene's function as a precursor for vitamin A.

recap Vitamin E protects cell membranes from oxidation, enhances immune function, and improves our absorption of vitamin A if dietary intake is low. It is found primarily in vegetable oils and nuts and seeds. Toxicity is uncommon, but taking high doses can cause excessive bleeding. Deficiency is rare. Vitamin C scavenges free radicals and regenerates vitamin E after it has been oxidized. Selenium is part of the glutathione peroxidase antioxidant enzyme system. It indirectly spares vitamin E from oxidative damage, and it assists with immune function and the production of thyroid hormones. Organ meats, pork, and seafood are good sources of selenium, as are nuts, wheat, and rice. Copper, zinc, manganese, and iron are cofactors for the antioxidant enzyme systems. Beta-carotene is a provitamin of vitamin A and one of the carotenoid phytochemicals. Its antioxidant activities protect the lipid portions of cell membranes, enhance immune function, and protect vision. There is no RDA for beta-carotene. Orange, red, and deep-green fruits and vegetables are good sources.

What is the role of vitamin A in vision and other functions?

LO 6 Discuss the contribution of vitamin A to vision, cell differentiation, and growth and reproduction.

As early as AD 30, the Roman writer Aulus Cornelius Celsus described in his medical encyclopedia, *De Medicina*, a condition called night blindness and recommended as a cure the consumption of liver. We now know that night blindness is due to a deficiency of vitamin A, a fat-soluble vitamin stored primarily in the liver of animals. When we consume vitamin A, we store 90% in our liver, and the remainder in our adipose tissue, kidneys, and lungs.

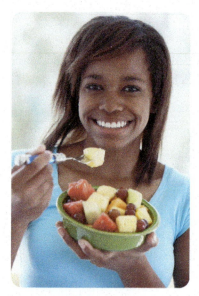

⬆ Eating plenty of fruits and vegetables can help prevent vitamin A deficiency.

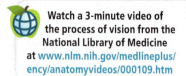

Watch a 3-minute video of the process of vision from the National Library of Medicine at www.nlm.nih.gov/medlineplus/ency/anatomyvideos/000109.htm

retinol An active, alcohol form of vitamin A that plays an important role in healthy vision and immune function.

retinal An active, aldehyde form of vitamin A that plays an important role in healthy vision and immune function.

retinoic acid An active, acid form of vitamin A that plays an important role in cell growth and immune function.

retina The delicate, light-sensitive membrane lining the inner eyeball and connected to the optic nerve. It contains retinal.

rhodopsin A light-sensitive pigment found in the rod cells that is formed by retinal and opsin.

night blindness A vitamin A deficiency disorder that results in loss of the ability to see in dim light.

cell differentiation The process by which immature, undifferentiated stem cells develop into highly specialized functional cells of discrete organs and tissues.

There Are Several Forms of Vitamin A

There are three active forms of vitamin A in our body: **retinol** is the alcohol form, **retinal** is the aldehyde form, and **retinoic acid** is the acid form. These three forms are collectively referred to as the *retinoids*. Of the three, retinol has the starring role in maintaining our body's physiologic functions. Remember from the previous section that beta-carotene is a precursor to vitamin A. When we eat foods that contain beta-carotene, it is converted to retinol in the wall of our small intestine.

The unit of expression for vitamin A is Retinol Activity Equivalents. You may still see the expression Retinol Equivalents (RE) or International Units for vitamin A on food labels and dietary supplements.

Vitamin A Is Essential to Sight

Vitamin A enables our eyes to react to changes in the brightness of light, and to distinguish between various wavelengths of light—in other words, to see different colors. Let's take a closer look at this process.

Light enters our eyes through the cornea, travels through the lens, and then hits the **retina**, which is a delicate membrane lining the back of the inner eyeball **(FOCUS FIGURE 8.18)**. You might already have guessed how *retinal* got its name: it is found in—and is integral to—the retina. In the retina, retinal combines with a protein called *opsin* to form **rhodopsin**, a light-sensitive pigment. Rhodopsin is found in the *rod cells*, which are cells that react to dim light and interpret black-and-white images.

When light hits the retina, the rod cells go through a *bleaching process*. In this reaction, rhodopsin is split into retinal and opsin, and the rod cells lose their color. The retinal and opsin components also change shape, an event that generates a nerve impulse that travels to the brain, resulting in the perception of a black-and-white image. Most of the retinal is then converted back to its original form and binds with opsin to regenerate rhodopsin, allowing the visual cycle to begin again. However, some of the retinal is lost with each cycle and must be replaced by retinol from the bloodstream. This visual cycle goes on continually, allowing our eyes to adjust to subtle changes in our surroundings or in the level of light.

When levels of vitamin A are deficient, people suffer from **night blindness**, a condition in which the eyes are unable to adjust to dim light. It can also result in the failure to regain sight quickly after a bright flash of light **(FIGURE 8.19)** (page 286).

At the same time we are interpreting black-and-white images, the *cone cells* of the retina, which are only effective in bright light, use retinal to interpret different wavelengths of light as different colors. The pigment involved in color vision, *iodopsin*, experiences similar changes during the color vision cycle as rhodopsin does during the black-and-white vision cycle. As with the rod cells, the cone cells can also be affected by a deficiency of vitamin A, resulting in color blindness.

Vitamin A Supports Cell Differentiation, Reproduction, and Bone Growth

Vitamin A also contributes to **cell differentiation**, the process by which stem cells mature into highly specialized cells that perform unique functions. It begins when the retinoic acid form of vitamin A interacts with receptor sites on a cell's DNA. This interaction influences gene expression and the type of cells that the stem cells eventually become. Obviously, this process is critical to the development of healthy tissues, organs, and body systems.

For example, vitamin A is necessary for differentiation of epithelial cells such as skin cells and the mucus-producing cells lining the lungs, eyes, bladder, and other organs. The mucus that epithelial cells produce lubricates the tissue and helps us eliminate microbes and irritants (e.g., when we cough up secretions or empty our bladder). When vitamin A levels are insufficient, the epithelial cells fail to differentiate appropriately, and we lose these protective barriers against infectious microbes and irritants. Vitamin A is also critical to the differentiation of specialized immune

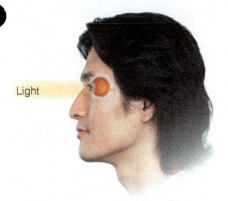

Light

Vitamin A is a component of two light-sensitive proteins, rhodopsin and iodopsin, that are essential for vision. Here we examine rhodopsin's role in vision. Although the breakdown of iodopsin is similar, rhodopsin is more sensitive to light than iodopsin and is more likely to become bleached.

EYE STRUCTURE

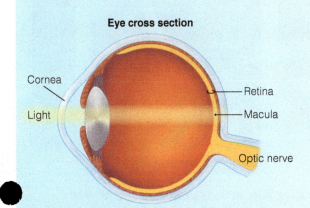

Eye cross section

Cornea

Light

Retina

Macula

Optic nerve

1 After light enters your eye through the cornea, it travels to the back of your eye to the macula, which is located in the retina. The macula allows you to see fine details and things that are straight in front of you.

Rod and cone cells in retina

Rod

Cone

Rhodopsin protein in rod cell membrane

Rhodopsin

Retinal (Vitamin A)

2 Inside the retina are two types of light-absorbing cells, rods and cones. Rods contain the protein rhodopsin, while cones contain the protein iodopsin.

EFFECT OF LIGHT ON RHODOPSIN

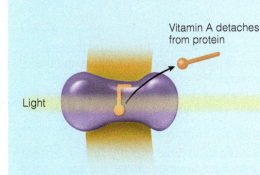

Vitamin A detaches from protein

Light

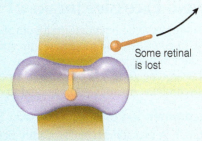

Some retinal is lost

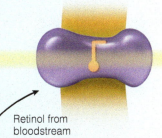

Retinol from bloodstream

1 As rhodopsin absorbs incoming light, the shape of vitamin A is altered, and it detaches from the rhodopsin.

2 This process, called bleaching, causes a cascade of events that transmits visual messages through your optic nerve to your brain. After bleaching, some retinal is lost.

3 Retinol from the blood is converted to retinal to replenish what is lost. The vitamin A returns to its original shape and becomes part of rhodopsin again, regenerating the eye's light-absorbing capabilities. This regeneration can take a few moments.

▶ **FIGURE 8.19** A deficiency of vitamin A can result in night blindness. This condition results in **(a)** diminished side vision and overall poor night vision and **(b)** difficulty in adjusting from bright light to dim light.

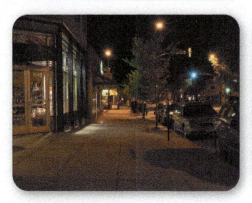 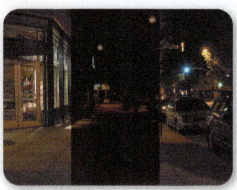

(a) Normal night vision   **Poor night vision**

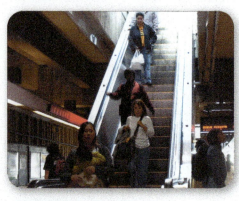 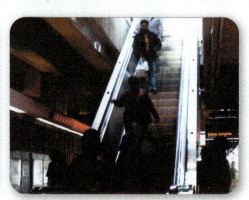

(b) Normal light adjustment   **Slow light adjustment**

cells called *T-cells*, which assist in fighting infections. You can therefore see why vitamin A deficiency significantly increases the risk of infectious disease.

Vitamin A is also involved in reproduction. Although its exact role is unclear, it appears necessary for sperm production and for fertilization. It also contributes to healthy bone growth by assisting in breaking down old bone, so that new, longer, and stronger bone can develop. As a result of a vitamin A deficiency, children suffer from stunted growth and wasting.

Some research has indicated that vitamin A may act as an antioxidant by scavenging free radicals and protecting LDLs from oxidation. However, it is unclear if vitamin A makes some minimal contribution to antioxidant function.

Avoid Excessive Intake of Vitamin A

Vitamin A can be obtained from both plant and animal sources. To calculate the total RAE in your diet, you must take into consideration both the amount of retinol and the amount of provitamin A beta-carotene you consume. For example, because 12 μg of beta-carotene yields 1 μg of RAE, if a person consumes 400 μg retinol and 1,200 μg of beta-carotene, the total RAE is equal to 400 μg + (1,200 μg ÷ 12), or 500 μg RAE.

Recommended Intakes and Food Sources of Vitamin A

Vitamin A toxicity can occur readily because it is a fat-soluble vitamin, so it is important to consume only the amount recommended for your gender and age range (see Table 8.1). The UL is 3,000 μg per day of preformed vitamin A in women (including those pregnant and lactating) and men.

The most abundant natural sources of dietary preformed vitamin A are animal foods, such as beef liver, chicken liver, eggs, and whole-fat dairy products. Vitamin A is also found in fortified reduced-fat milks, margarine, and some breakfast cereals **(FIGURE 8.20)**.

Other good sources of vitamin A are foods high in beta-carotene and other carotenoids that can be converted to vitamin A. Carrots, spinach, mango, cantaloupe, and tomato juice are examples.

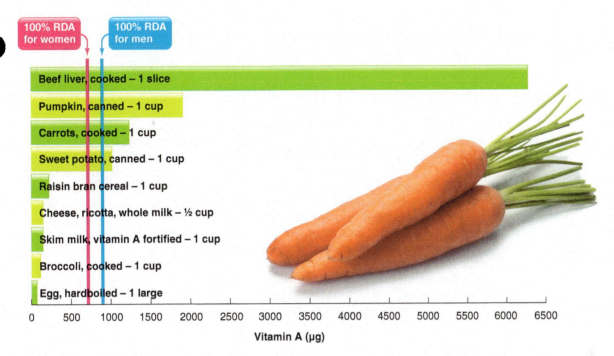

◄ **FIGURE 8.20** Common food sources of vitamin A. The RDA for vitamin A is 900 μg/day for men and 700 μg/day for women.

Source: Data from U.S. Department of Agriculture, Agricultural Research Service, 2015. USDA Nutrient Database for Standard Reference, Release 28.

Vitamin A Toxicity and Deficiency

Vitamin A is highly toxic, and toxicity symptoms develop after consuming only three to four times the RDA. Toxicity rarely results from food sources, but vitamin A supplementation is known to have caused severe illness and even death. In pregnant women, it can cause serious birth defects and spontaneous abortion. Other toxicity symptoms include fatigue, loss of appetite, blurred vision, hair loss, skin disorders, diarrhea, and damage to the liver and nervous system. If caught in time, many of these symptoms are reversible once vitamin A supplementation is stopped. However, permanent damage can occur to the liver, eyes, and other organs. Because liver contains such a high amount of vitamin A, children and pregnant women should not consume liver on a daily or weekly basis.

Although not common among people of developed nations, vitamin A deficiency is a severe public health concern in developing nations. According to the World Health Organization, approximately 250 million preschool children worldwide suffer from vitamin A deficiency,[22] which can result in irreversible blindness. This occurs because lack of vitamin A causes the epithelial cells of the cornea (the transparent membrane covering the front of the eye) to lose their ability to produce mucus, causing drying, hardening, and an increased risk for damage and infection.

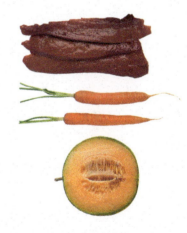

◄ Liver, carrots, and cantaloupe all contain vitamin A.

Vitamin A deficiency can also lead to follicular *hyperkeratosis*, a condition in which a protein called keratin clogs hair follicles, and the skin becomes dry, thick, rough, and bumpy. Other deficiency symptoms include impaired immunity, increased risk for illness and infections, reproductive system disorders, and failure of normal growth. Individuals who are at risk for vitamin A deficiency include newborn or premature infants (due to low liver stores of vitamin A), and people with poor diets. Any condition that results in fat malabsorption can also lead to vitamin A deficiency.

Vitamin A Derivatives Are Effective in Treating Acne

Acne is a skin disorder affecting approximately 50 million Americans.[23] The characteristic lesions form when an oily substance called sebum accumulates in hair follicles, typically on the face and upper torso. The deposits can become infected, resulting in painful cysts that sometimes leave scars.

Vitamin A is commonly identified on the Internet as an effective treatment for acne. However, there are no well-conducted studies linking vitamin A intake or status directly with acne, and vitamin A supplements are not recommended in acne treatment. In contrast, synthetic derivatives of vitamin A are effective treatments. These drugs, which are classified as retinoids, work by affecting the body's rate of replacement of skin cells. Retinoids are available by prescription and over-the-counter (OTC).

Prescription retinoids include Retin-A (or tretinoin) and isotretinoin. Retin-A is a cream applied to the skin. It may cause skin redness, irritation, and worsening of acne in the initial weeks of use, as well as increased sensitivity to the sun. Retin-A is absorbed from the skin into body tissues, and its use during pregnancy is not recommended. Isotretinoin is taken orally. It also typically causes a temporary worsening of acne in the initial weeks of use, as well as dry lips, dry skin, and increased risk of sunburn. Because of the high risk for severe birth defects associated with its use, isotretinoin is prescribed in women only as part of a special procedure, including pregnancy testing and mandatory use of effective contraceptives. The drug is also associated with a variety of other complications, from vision disorders to inflammatory bowel disease. In 2009, lawsuits stemming from complications of the drug caused one pharmaceutical company to remove their version of the drug (called Accutane) from the U.S. market.

In 2016, the U.S. Food and Drug Administration (FDA) approved an OTC topical retinoid called Differin Gel 0.1% (adapalene) for treatment of acne. It is the only OTC retinoid approved for acne. Although there is inadequate research on Differin Gel in pregnant women, absorption of the drug is limited, and there is no evidence that its use causes birth defects.[23]

recap Vitamin A is critical for maintaining our vision. It is also necessary for cell differentiation, reproduction, and growth. The role of vitamin A as an antioxidant is still under investigation. Animal liver, dairy products, and eggs are good animal sources of vitamin A; fruits and vegetables are high in beta-carotene, a pro-vitamin for vitamin A. Supplementation can be dangerous because toxicity is reached at levels of only three to four times the RDA. Toxicity can cause birth defects, spontaneous abortion, organ damage, and other disorders. Deficiency symptoms include night blindness, hyperkeratosis, impaired immune function, and growth failure. Vitamin A supplements are not effective in treating acne; however, a class of retinoid medications can provide effective treatment.

Antioxidants: From Foods or Supplements?

Although antioxidants from a nourishing diet play an important role in reducing the risk for chronic diseases such as cancer and cardiovascular disease (CVD), research studies into the effects of antioxidant supplements on cancer and CVD risk are troubling. The results of two large, randomized, controlled trials—the Alpha-Tocopherol Beta-Carotene (ATBC) Cancer Prevention Study and the Beta-Carotene and Retinol Efficacy Trial (CARET)—were particularly surprising.[24,25]

The ATBC Cancer Prevention Study was conducted in Finland from 1985 to 1993 to determine the effects of beta-carotene and vitamin E supplements on lung and other forms of cancer among nearly 30,000 male smokers 50 to 69 years of age. Contrary to expectations, the male smokers who took beta-carotene supplements experienced *higher* rates of prostate and stomach cancers and an *increased* number of deaths from lung cancer and CVD.

CARET began as a pilot study in the United States in 1985 and included more than 18,000 men and women who were smokers, former smokers, or workers who had been exposed to asbestos. During the 4-year study period, the incidence of lung cancer was 28% *higher* among those taking a beta-carotene and vitamin A supplement than among those taking a placebo. This finding prompted researchers to end the CARET study early.[25]

A 2010 systematic review of the available published studies reported that beta-carotene supplementation has no effect on the incidence of most cancers; however, the incidence of lung and stomach cancers was significantly increased in those taking high doses (20–30 mg per day) of beta-carotene as well as in smokers and asbestos workers.[26]

As discussed earlier in this chapter, more recent studies indicate that vitamin E supplementation increases the risk of prostate cancer in men, and is associated with an increased risk for premature mortality in women and men.[18,19]

Studies of antioxidants and CVD also show inconsistent results. Two large-scale surveys conducted in the United States show that men and women who eat more fruits and vegetables have a significantly reduced risk of CVD.[27,28] And in the ATBC Cancer Prevention Study, vitamin E supplements were found to lower the number of deaths due to heart disease, but had no effect on the risk for stroke.[29] Other large intervention studies have shown no reductions in major cardiovascular events in adults taking vitamins E or C.[30,31] Thus, the evidence indicates that antioxidant supplements do not reduce our risk for CVD.

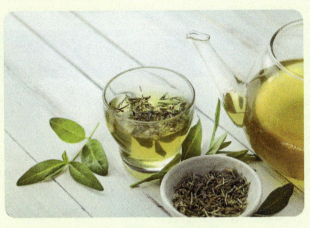

The flavonoids in tea might reduce the risk for CVD.

Why might foods high in antioxidants reduce our risks for cancer and CVD, whereas supplements do not—and may even be harmful? First, as with any other chemicals, antioxidants may be beneficial at lower, appropriate doses—such as we consume in plant foods—but may become toxic at the higher doses present in a supplement. Second, other compounds (besides antioxidants) found in fruits, vegetables, and whole grains can reduce our risk for cancer and CVD. Here are just a few examples:

- Dietary fiber has been shown to reduce the risk for colorectal cancer, decrease blood pressure, lower total cholesterol levels, and improve blood glucose and insulin levels.

- Folate, which is found in many vegetables, is known to reduce blood levels of the amino acid homocysteine, and a high concentration of homocysteine is a known risk factor for CVD.

- Flavonoids are a group of phytochemicals found in berries, nuts, soybeans, and many other plant foods, including tea and coffee. Recent studies have shown that Japanese adults who consumed at least two cups of coffee or green tea per day had a lower risk for CVD than those who consumed lower amounts,[32] while premature mortality was reduced in a multiethnic group of U.S. adults consuming any amount of coffee or tea (all types) compared to those who did not consume coffee or tea.[33]

Thus, it appears that any number of nutrients and other components in plant-based foods may be protective against cancer and CVD. As you can see, there is still much to learn about how people respond to foods high in antioxidants as compared to antioxidant supplements.

CRITICAL THINKING QUESTIONS

1. With everything you've learned in this chapter, how do you plan to ensure that you regularly consume appropriate levels of antioxidants?

2. If a friend or family member decided to take antioxidant supplements as "health insurance," what advice might you give them about this decision?

3. Go to your local drugstore and research various brands of vitamin C, vitamin E, and beta-carotene supplements, recording the amount of each nutrient in the recommended dose. Estimate if, and how much, the recommended dose exceeds the RDA for each nutrient.

TEST YOURSELF | *ANSWERS*

1 F B-vitamins do not directly provide energy. However, they play critical roles in ensuring that the body is able to generate energy from carbohydrates, fats, and proteins.

2 T Free radicals are highly unstable atoms that can destabilize neighboring atoms or molecules and harm body cells; however, they are produced as a normal by-product of human physiology.

3 T Carrots are an excellent source of beta-carotene, a precursor for vitamin A, which is essential for good vision.

review questions

LO 1 **1.** A coenzyme is
  a. an inactive enzyme.
  b. any enzyme containing a B vitamin.
  c. a molecule that combines with and activates an enzyme.
  d. a molecule such as a B-vitamin that is released as a by-product of enzymatic reactions.

LO 2 **2.** The B-vitamin most important for the synthesis of nonessential amino acids is
  a. thiamin.
  b. riboflavin.
  c. niacin.
  d. vitamin B_6.

LO 2 **3.** Although a good source of many B-vitamins, a meal of brown rice, red beans, and fresh vegetables does not provide
  a. thiamin.
  b. vitamin B_6.
  c. folate.
  d. vitamin B_{12}.

LO 3 **4.** A trace mineral critical for the synthesis of thyroid hormones is
  a. iodine.
  b. chromium.
  c. manganese.
  d. sulfur.

LO 4 **5.** Oxidation is a chemical reaction during which
  a. radiation causes a mutation in a cell's DNA.
  b. an atom loses an electron.
  c. an element loses an atom of oxygen.
  d. a compound loses a molecule of water.

LO 5 **6.** Which of the following is a role of both vitamin E and vitamin C?
  a. Both vitamins spare vitamin A.
  b. Both vitamins donate electrons to free radicals.
  c. Both vitamins are critical cofactors in antioxidant enzyme systems.
  d. All of the above are true.

LO 5 **7.** Which of the following statements about beta-carotene is true?
  a. Beta-carotene is a provitamin precursor of vitamin A.
  b. Beta-carotene is a water-soluble form of vitamin A.
  c. The RDA for beta-carotene is 12 times the RDA for vitamin A.
  d. We absorb a greater percentage of beta-carotene from fruits and vegetables consumed raw than from fruits and vegetables that have been cooked.

LO 6 **8.** The light-sensitive pigment rhodopsin
  a. is a form of vitamin A that regenerates iodopsin.
  b. is found in the cone cells of the retina.
  c. transmits visual messages from the retina to the brain.
  d. is regenerated by a form of vitamin A.

LO 2 **9.** **True or false?** Pantothenic acid is found only in foods of animal origin.

LO 4 **10.** **True or false?** Free radical formation can occur as a result of normal cellular metabolism.

math review

LO 5   **11.** Joey is home visiting his parents for the weekend, and he finds a bottle of vitamin E supplements in the medicine cabinet. He asks his parents about these, and his mother says that she is worried about having a weak immune system and read on the Internet that vitamin E can boost immunity. Because Joey's mother eats plenty of plant foods and oils that are good sources of vitamin E, he is worried she may be consuming too much by adding these supplements to her diet. Each supplement capsule contains 400 IU of synthetic α-TE, and she takes one capsule each day. Answer the following questions:

a. How much vitamin E in mg is Joey's mother consuming each day from these supplements?
b. What percentage of the RDA for vitamin E do these supplements provide?
c. Based on what you've learned in this chapter about vitamin E, should Joey's mother be worried about vitamin E toxicity? Would your answer be different if you learned that she is taking aspirin each day as prescribed by her doctor?

Answers to Review Questions and Math Review are located at the back of this text and in the MasteringNutrition Study Area.

web links

www.ars.usda.gov
Nutrient Data Laboratory Home Page
Start by entering "nutrient data laboratory home page" in the search box. Then, click on "Reports for Single Nutrients" to find reports listing food sources for selected nutrients.

www.cancer.org
American Cancer Society
Visit this site for an overview of micronutrients and phytochemicals, with functions, food sources, and research into their use in disease prevention.

www.who.int
World Health Organization
Click on "Health Topics" and select "nutrition disorders" and then "Nutrition: micronutrients" to find out more about vitamin and mineral deficiencies around the world.

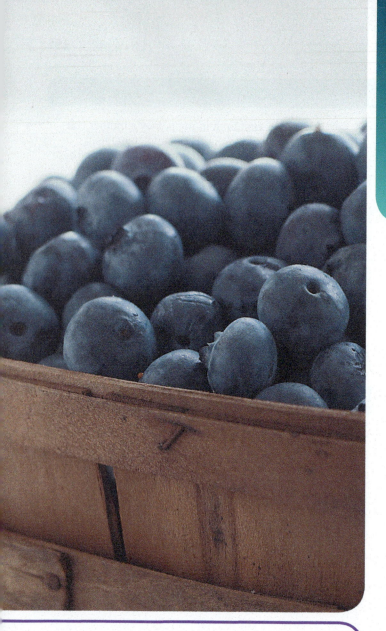

in depth

8.5

Cancer

learning outcomes

After studying this In Depth, you should be able to:

1 Describe the three stages of cancer development, p. 293.

2 Discuss the factors that influence our risk for cancer, pp. 293–296.

3 Explain how cancer is diagnosed and treated, pp. 296–297.

4 Describe ways in which we can prevent, or reduce our risks for, cancer, pp. 297–299.

The American Cancer Society (ACS) estimates that about 1,630 Americans die of cancer every day. Although the five-year survival rate is now 69%, cancer accounts for one out of every four deaths in the United States, making it the second most common cause of death, exceeded only by heart disease.[1]

With such alarming statistics, it's not surprising that television commercials, Internet sites, and health and fitness publications are filled with product claims promising to reduce your risk of developing cancer. Many of these claims tout the benefits of antioxidants. Others say that eating or avoiding certain foods, drinking special types of juices or waters, following a certain diet, or taking certain supplements can reduce cancer risk. In opposition to these claims, some research evidence suggests that taking antioxidant supplements may actually increase the risk of cancer for certain people (refer to the Nutrition Debate in Chapter 8, page 289).

In this **In Depth** essay, we'll explore how cancer begins and spreads. We'll then identify the factors that current research evidence indicates might most significantly influence cancer risk. We'll also review what is currently known about the role of antioxidant nutrients in cancer and identify other strategies for reducing your risk.

What is cancer and how does it arise?

LO 1 Describe the three stages of cancer development.

Cancer is a group of diseases that are all characterized by cells that grow "out of control." By this we mean that cancer cells reproduce spontaneously and independently, and they are not inhibited by the boundaries of tissues and organs. Thus, they can aggressively invade tissues and organs far away from those in which they originally formed.

Most forms of cancer result in one or more **tumors**, which are newly formed masses of undifferentiated cells that are immature and have no physiologic function. Although the word *tumor* sounds frightening, it is important to note that not every tumor is *malignant*, or cancerous. Many are *benign* (not harmful to us) and are made up of cells that will not spread widely.

FIGURE 1 (page 294) shows how changes to normal cells prompt a series of other changes that can lead to cancer. There are three primary stages of cancer development: initiation, promotion, and progression. They occur as follows:

1. *Initiation.* The initiation of cancer occurs when a cell's DNA is *mutated* (changed). This mutation may be random, inherited, or due to environmental factors, such as exposure to the chemicals in tobacco smoke, UV radiation, or certain viruses. Cells with mutated DNA may engage in self-repair or self-destruction, or they may be destroyed by the body's immune system; if they escape destruction, they can develop characteristics that enable their promotion.

2. *Promotion.* During this stage, the genetically altered cell is stimulated to divide. A single mutated cell divides in two, and these double to four, and so on. The mutated DNA is locked into each new cell's genetic instructions. Because the enzymes that normally work to repair damaged cells cannot detect alterations in the DNA, the cells can continue to divide uninhibited. Typically, it takes many years for a mutated cell to double repeatedly into a tumor mass large enough to be detectable (about the size of a grape), and promotion is the longest stage in cancer development.

3. *Progression.* During this stage, the cancerous cells grow out of control. They grow their own blood vessels, which supply them with oxygen and nutrients, and invade adjacent tissues. In the early stage of progression, the immune system can sometimes detect these cancerous cells and destroy them. However, if the cells continue to grow, they develop into malignant tumors, disrupting body functioning at their primary site and invading the circulatory and lymphatic systems to *metastasize* (spread) to distant sites in the body.

Although cancer is often fatal, over 14 million Americans who have been diagnosed with cancer are still alive today.[1] Of course, cancers can be more or less aggressive, some are more readily detectable than others, and some tissues and organs are more vulnerable to cancer. All these factors influence the patient's *prognosis*, the clinical estimate of the expected course of the disease. The type of cancer with the highest mortality rate is lung cancer, with almost 160,000 deaths projected for 2016. Cancer of the colon and rectum ranks second (slightly fewer than 50,000 deaths projected for 2016), pancreatic cancer ranks third (almost 42,000 deaths), and breast cancer ranks fourth (slightly more than 40,000 deaths).[1] Pancreatic cancer has received a great deal of attention in recent years because death rates from this form of cancer have increased slowly in men and women over the past decade, whereas death rates from other major cancers (such as female breast, colon and rectum, and prostate) have been slowly declining over this same period. Pancreatic cancer is one of the deadliest types, with most people dying within the first year of diagnosis and only 7% surviving 5 years following diagnosis.[1]

Watch a video providing a basic overview of cancer on www.youtube.com. Enter "what is cancer?" into the search box, then scroll down to the link to the video titled, "M D Anderson Answer the Question, 'What is Cancer?'" from the MD Anderson Cancer Center.

What factors influence cancer risk?

LO 2 Discuss the factors that influence our risk for cancer.

Researchers estimate that about half of all men and one-third of all women will develop cancer during their lifetimes.[1] Are you and your loved ones at risk? The answer depends on several factors, including your family history of cancer, your exposure to environmental agents, and various lifestyle choices.

Nonmodifiable Factors Play a Role

The ACS states that, for most types of cancer, risk is higher when there is a family history. Two mechanisms are thought to contribute to this increased risk. First, inherited "cancer genes," such as the *BRC* genes for breast

---

cancer A group of diseases characterized by cells that reproduce spontaneously and independently and may invade other tissues and organs.

tumor Any newly formed mass of undifferentiated cells.

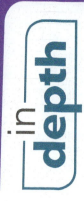

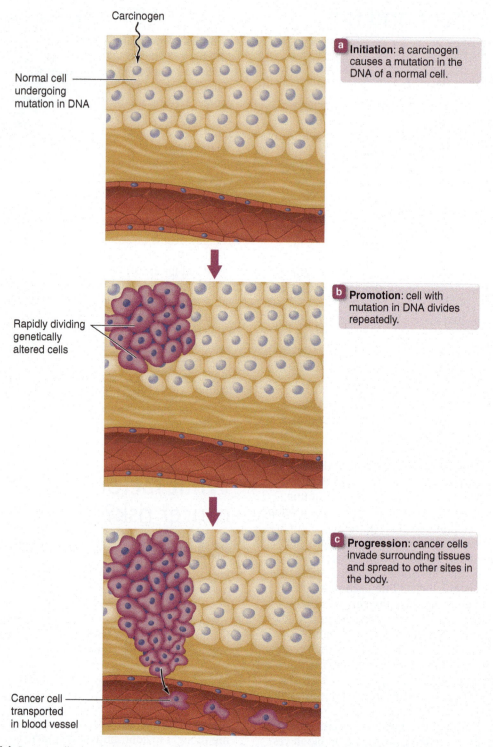

Carcinogen

Normal cell undergoing mutation in DNA

a **Initiation**: a carcinogen causes a mutation in the DNA of a normal cell.

Rapidly dividing genetically altered cells

b **Promotion**: cell with mutation in DNA divides repeatedly.

c **Progression**: cancer cells invade surrounding tissues and spread to other sites in the body.

Cancer cell transported in blood vessel

FIGURE 1 **(a)** Cancer cells develop as a result of a genetic mutation in the DNA of a normal cell. **(b)** The mutated cell replicates uncontrollably, eventually resulting in a tumor. **(c)** If not destroyed or removed, the cancerous tumor grows its own blood supply, invades nearby tissues, and often metastasizes to other parts of the body.

cancer, increase the risk that an individual with those genes will develop cancer. Such genes do not directly cause cancer; rather, they impair mechanisms that—in people without these genetic variants—would suppress the progression of tumors. Second, many familial cancers appear to arise from interactions between common genetic variants and lifestyle and environmental factors. The ACS emphasizes, however, that even given these two mechanisms, only a small proportion of all cancers are strongly hereditary.[1]

In addition, it's important to bear in mind that a family history of cancer does not guarantee you will get cancer, too. It just means that you are at an increased risk and should take all preventive actions available to you. Although some risk factors are out of your control, others are modifiable, which means that you can take positive steps to reduce your risk.

Many Risk Factors Are Modifiable

The ACS identifies six modifiable risk factors that have been shown to have the greatest impact on an individual's cancer risk; each is discussed next.[1]

Tobacco Use

More than 40 compounds in tobacco and tobacco smoke are **carcinogens**, or substances that can cause cancer. Smoking accounts for at least 32% of all cancer deaths and 80% of lung cancer deaths, and it increases the risk for acute myeloid leukemia and cancers of the nasopharynx, nasal cavity, paranasal sinus, lip, oral cavity, pharynx, larynx, esophagus, pancreas, uterine cervix, ovaries, kidney, bladder, stomach, and colorectum (FIGURE 2).[1] Smoking can also cause heart disease, stroke, and emphysema. Overall, tobacco use is responsible for almost 6 million deaths per year, 80% of which are in low- and middle-income countries.[1] The positive news is that tobacco use is a modifiable risk factor. If you smoke or use smokeless tobacco, you can reduce your risk for cancer considerably by quitting.

Weight, Diet, and Physical Activity

It is estimated that about 20% of cancers that occur in the United States are due to the combined effects of overweight or obesity, poor nutrition, physical inactivity, and excess alcohol consumption, and thus could be prevented.[1] Nutritional factors that are protective against cancer include the consumption of foods rich in antioxidant micronutrients and phytochemicals, and fiber. Diets

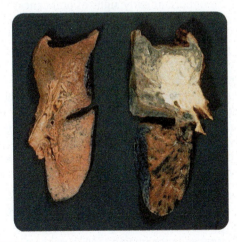

FIGURE 2 Cigarette smoking significantly increases our risk for lung and other types of cancer. Smoking causes 83% of lung cancer deaths among men and 76% of lung cancer deaths among women. **(a)** A normal, healthy lung; **(b)** the lung of a smoker. Notice the deposits of tar as well as the areas of tumor growth.

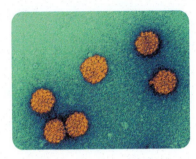

FIGURE 3 *Human papillomavirus (HPV)* is an infectious agent that can cause cancer.

high in saturated fats and low in fruits and vegetables increase the risk for cancers of the esophagus, colon, breast, and prostate. Consumption of alcohol and compounds found in cured, charbroiled, red, and processed meats can also increase the risk for cancer.

A sedentary lifestyle increases the risk for colon cancer and possibly other forms of cancer. There is convincing evidence that regular physical activity decreases the risk for colon cancer as well as probable evidence of a protective effect for endometrial cancer and postmenopausal breast cancer. There is limited evidence that suggests physical activity may also be protective against cancers of the lung, pancreas, and breast (premenopausal). Exercise may also reduce risks for various forms of cancer because of its role in helping people maintain a healthy weight, improving energy metabolism, and reducing circulation of various hormones that are linked with cancer risk (such as estrogen, insulin, and insulin-like growth factors).[1] These findings have prompted the ACS and the National Cancer Institute to promote increased physical activity as a way to reduce our risk for cancer.

Infectious Agents

Infectious agents account for 15% to 20% of cancers worldwide.[2] For example, persistent infection of the female cervix with certain strains of the sexually transmitted virus *Human papillomavirus* (HPV) is a known cause of cervical cancer (FIGURE 3), and infection with HIV (human immunodeficiency virus) can cause many cancers. The bacterium *Helicobacter pylori* is linked not only to ulcers but also to stomach cancer. Certain parasites are also linked to specific cancers. As microbial research advances, it is thought that more cancers will be linked to infectious agents.

Ultraviolet Radiation

Skin cancer is the most common form of cancer in the United States. Most skin cancer cases are linked to

---

carcinogen Any substance capable of causing the cellular mutations that lead to cancer.

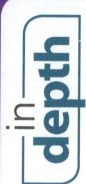

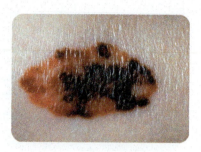

FIGURE 4 A lesion associated with malignant melanoma is characterized by five qualities known by the acronym ABCDE: asymmetry; borders that are uneven or blurred; colors that are mixtures of tan, brown, black, and sometimes red or blue; a diameter larger than a pencil eraser (6 mm); and evolution—that is, the lesion tends to change over time.

personal or family history of skin cancer, presence of atypical, large, or numerous (more than 50) moles, and high exposure to ultraviolet (UV) rays from the sun and indoor tanning beds.[1] UV rays damage the DNA of immature skin cells, which then reproduce uncontrollably. Even though a person's risk for skin cancer is higher with repeated sunburns, your risk for skin cancer still increases with UV exposure even if you do not get sunburned. Recent studies confirm the association between use of tanning beds and skin cancer, with more than 400,000 cases of skin cancer in the United States related to indoor tanning.[3,4] Contrary to popular belief, newer models of tanning beds are no safer than older models.[3]

Skin cancer includes the nonmelanoma cancers (basal cell and squamous cell cancers), which are not typically invasive, and malignant melanoma, which is one of the most deadly of all types of cancer (FIGURE 4). Limiting exposure to sunlight to no more than 20 minutes between 10 AM and 4 PM can help reduce your risk for skin cancer while allowing your body to synthesize adequate vitamin D. After that, wear sunscreen with at least a 15 SPF (sun protection factor) rating and protective clothing.

How is cancer diagnosed and treated?

LO 3 Explain how cancer is diagnosed and treated.

Cancer is sometimes diagnosed before it has produced any signs or symptoms, typically as a result of a **screening test** such as mammography or colonoscopy. In many cases, however, a variety of signs and symptoms cause a person to seek a diagnosis.

The signs and symptoms of cancer vary according to the structures affected, how large the tumor is, and how widely it has metastasized. Here, we discuss the most common signs and symptoms that people diagnosed with

cancer typically report. However, it's important to bear in mind that these also occur with many other illnesses and even nonillness conditions. Also, having just one or two of these symptoms rarely means that a person has cancer. Still, the ACS suggests that people who experience these symptoms for a long time see their primary healthcare provider.[5]

- *Unexplained weight loss.* Most people with cancer lose weight, so an unexplained weight loss of 10 pounds or more may be a first sign of cancer.
- *Fever.* Fever is very common with cancer, but it often happens when the cancer has metastasized or affects the blood.
- *Fatigue.* Extreme tiredness that isn't relieved with rest may be an important symptom of cancer. The blood loss that occurs with some cancers, such as colon and stomach cancers, can also cause fatigue.
- *Pain.* Headache, back pain, or bone pain that does not go away or respond to treatment can be an early symptom of certain types of cancer.
- *Skin changes.* Along with cancers of the skin, some other cancers can cause skin changes, including a darkened pigmentation, jaundice (yellowish skin tone), redness, excessive hair growth, and itching. Sores that don't heal and recent changes in a wart or mole should also be checked by a healthcare provider.
- *Change in bowel habits or bladder function.* Long-term constipation, diarrhea, painful urination, or the need to pass urine more or less frequently may signal cancer.
- *Indigestion or trouble swallowing.* Although these are most often caused by other disorders, if they persist, they should be evaluated by a healthcare provider.
- *White patches inside the mouth or on the tongue.* Especially in people who smoke or chew tobacco, these are important early signs of oral cancer.
- *Unusual bleeding or discharge.* Blood in the urine or stool, abnormal vaginal bleeding, a bloody discharge from the nipple, and bloody sputum (phlegm) can all occur in early or advanced cancer.
- *Any thickening or lump.* Many cancers can be felt through the skin, especially those involving the breast, testicle, or lymph nodes.
- *Nagging cough or hoarseness.* A cough that doesn't resolve can be a sign of lung cancer, whereas hoarseness can be a sign of cancer of the larynx (voice box) or thyroid gland.

Physicians typically evaluate signs and symptoms of cancer using a variety of blood tests and diagnostic scans, such as ultrasound, computed tomography (CT), and magnetic resonance imaging (MRI) scans. Once a diagnosis is made, the patient is often referred to the care

screening test Clinical exam performed on a large population to detect early evidence of disease.

of an oncologist, a physician who specializes in cancer treatment (*onco-* means "tumor").

As noted earlier, the 5-year survival rate for cancer now stands at 69%, an increase from just 49% in 1975 to 1977.[1] Both earlier diagnosis and improvements in cancer treatment have contributed to this increased survival.[1] Cancer treatment varies according to the location of the cancer, the cell type, whether or not it has metastasized, and, if so, how much. Other factors, such as the patient's general health, extent of weight loss, age, and personal preferences, as well as the type, scope, and quality of healthcare insurance coverage, may also come into play.

The three major types of cancer treatment are surgery, radiation, and chemotherapy. Surgery is most effective when it can entirely remove the mass. Radiation therapy delivers high-energy X-rays, gamma rays, electron beams, or photons to tumor cells to kill them outright or damage their DNA so that they can no longer reproduce. Chemotherapy is drug therapy, and any of more than 100 different drugs can be combined for different patient needs. For cancers that are localized—that is, confined to a limited area, with no metastasis—surgery may be the only treatment advised. Other cancers may require surgery followed by radiation and/or chemotherapy. Diffuse cancers, such as blood cancers, and tumors in locations that cannot be accessed safely with surgery, such as head and neck tumors, may be considered inoperable, and radiation and/or chemotherapy may be prescribed. In some cases, a large tumor is first radiated with the goal of shrinking it prior to surgery.

Can cancer be prevented?

LO 4 Describe ways in which we can prevent or reduce our risks for cancer.

Some types of cancer can be prevented. For instance, vaccines, the appropriate use of antibiotics, and behavioral changes can prevent certain cancers known to be caused by infectious agents. Most cancers, however, are multifactorial—we cannot link them to only one cause. This means that there is no way to guarantee that you—or anyone else—won't get cancer. Still, if you consider the population of the United States, more than half of all cancer deaths could be prevented if no one used tobacco and everyone took certain key steps to improve his or her health.[1] These steps can be summarized into four key cancer-prevention behaviors: check, quit, move, and nourish.

Check

Regular screening examinations can allow for the detection and removal of precancerous tissues. For instance, a test called a Pap smear can detect subtle changes in the cells lining a woman's cervix (the entrance to the uterus) that, if allowed to progress, could result in cervical cancer. Women with a Pap smear indicating these changes typically return to their physician for a quick outpatient procedure in which the layer of precancerous cells is removed. Similarly,

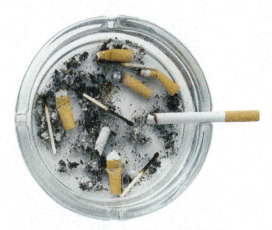

Using tobacco is a risk factor for cancer.

colonoscopies allow for the detection and removal of precancerous polyps. And regular skin checks allow for suspicious lesions to be removed—and cell samples sent to a lab—to evaluate for skin cancer. Screening can also allow for detection at an early stage, when cancer is most treatable. For example, a mammogram may be able to detect a breast mass that is too small for the woman to feel.

Quit

As noted earlier, tobacco use is a risk factor in the development of a wide variety of cancers, but all cancers caused by long-term tobacco use are entirely preventable. In fact, about one-third of all cancer deaths could be prevented if everyone followed the ACS recommendation to quit smoking.[1]

> Want to see how much money you or someone you know has spent on cigarettes in the past, and how much they could cost in the future? Check out the Health Status website at www.healthstatus.com/calculate/smc, and enter the information as requested.

Alcohol abuse is also a factor in cancer. Excessive drinking is linked with an increased risk for cancers of the esophagus, pharynx, and mouth and may increase the risk for cancers of the liver, breast, colon, and rectum. Alcohol may also impair cells' ability to repair damaged DNA, increasing the possibility of cancer initiation.

Move

Regular physical activity can significantly lower your lifetime risk for cancer. The ACS recommends that we engage in at least 150 minutes (2 hours and 30 minutes) of moderate or 75 minutes (1 hour and 15 minutes) of vigorous physical activity throughout each week. The amount of activity can be spread across the day and does not have to be done all at once. For example, on busy days, try to work in 10 minutes of activity three times a day, perhaps by taking a 10-minute walk at lunch then again between your afternoon classes and, when you get home, cycling for 10 minutes. Short activity sessions like these can quickly add up to 30 minutes.

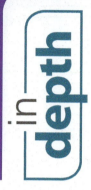

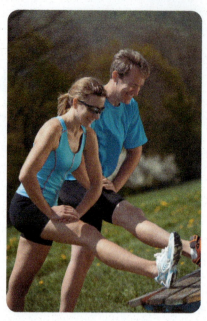

Staying physically active may help reduce the risk for some cancers.

Nourish

One of the smartest ways to reduce your risk for cancer is to maintain a healthful weight and a healthful diet. The ACS emphasizes reading food labels to increase your awareness of portion sizes and the Calorie content of food.[6] Consuming smaller portions of foods high in Calories and saturated fat is suggested, as is reducing your intake of beverages high in added sugars such as soft drinks and fruit drinks. See the **Quick Tips** box for additional nutrition-related tips.

Antioxidants Play a Role in Preventing Cancer

A large and growing body of evidence suggests that antioxidant micronutrients and phytochemicals consumed in food play an important role in cancer prevention, but how? The following are some proposed mechanisms.

- Enhancing the immune system, which assists in the destruction and removal of precancerous cells from the body.

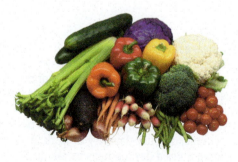

These vegetables provide antioxidant nutrients, fiber, and phytochemicals, all of which reduce the risk for some cancers.

QuickTips

Reducing Your Cancer Risk

✓ Lose weight or maintain your current healthful weight. Obesity appears to increase the risk for at least a dozen cancers, possibly as a result of hormonal changes associated with fat cells.

✓ Avoid heterocyclic amines in cooked meat. These carcinogenic chemicals are formed when meat is cooked at high temperatures, such as during broiling, barbecuing, and frying.

✓ Avoid nitrites and nitrates in cured meats. These compounds, which are found in some sausages, hams, bacon, and lunch meats, bind with amino acids to form nitrosamines, which are potent carcinogens.

✓ Eat a diet low in saturated fat. Diets high in saturated fat have been associated with increased risk for many cancers, including prostate and breast cancers. However, not all studies support this association.

✓ Eat a diet rich in vegetables and fruits. Consuming at least 2 1/2 cups cups of vegetables and fruit each day is recommended. These foods are high in antioxidants and in fiber, which some studies link to a reduced risk for certain cancers.

✓ When choosing fruits and vegetables, select versions that have more intense colors or flavors: purple potatoes instead of white, for example, and arugula instead of iceberg lettuce. These foods tend to be higher in antioxidant phytochemicals than lighter-colored or milder-tasting counterparts.

✓ Select foods containing phytoestrogens (plant estrogens). These compounds, found in soy-based foods and some vegetables and grains, may decrease the risk for breast, endometrial, and prostate cancers.

✓ Choose whole-grain breads, cereals, pasta, and brown rice instead of products made from refined grains (see Chapter 4).

✓ Make sure to consume adequate omega-3 fatty acids (see Chapter 5). Consuming foods high in omega-3 fatty acids is associated with reduced rates of breast, colon, and rectal cancers.

- Preventing oxidative damage to the cells' DNA by scavenging free radicals and stopping the formation and subsequent chain reaction of oxidized molecules.
- Inhibiting the growth of cancer cells and tumors.
- Inhibiting the capacity of cancer cells to avoid aging and apoptosis (programmed cell death).

"Last night, there was this actress on TV talking about having colon cancer and saying that everybody over 50 should get tested. It brought back memories of my father's cancer, how thin and weak he got before he went to the doctor, so that by the time they found the cancer it had already spread too far. But I don't think I'm at risk. I only eat red meat two or three times a week, and I eat a piece of fruit or a vegetable at every meal. I don't smoke, and I get plenty of exercise, sunshine, and fresh air working in the vineyard."

Which lifestyle factors reduce Gustavo's risk for cancer? What factors increase his risk? Would you recommend he increase his consumption of fruits and vegetables? Why or why not? If Gustavo were your father, would you urge him to have the screening test for colon cancer?

Eating whole foods—especially fruits, vegetables, and whole grains—that are high in antioxidant phytochemicals is linked with probable evidence of decreased risk for various cancers. (See the In Depth essay following Chapter 1 on pages 29–35 for a detailed look at phytochemicals.) For example, several recent studies have suggested that consuming fruits, vegetables, spices, and teas high in a phytochemical called apigenin, a type of flavonoid, might alter gene regulation in cancer cells in a way that impairs their ability to avoid aging and apoptosis.[7,8]

Another group of flavonoids, anthocyanins, are plant pigments thought to have antioxidant and anti-inflammatory properties. Produce with intense colors, such as blue corn and blackberries, has higher levels of anthocyanin pigments. Finally, glucosinolates, a group of phytochemicals found in cruciferous vegetables like Brussels sprouts and broccoli, as well as in bitter greens such as arugula, inhibit cell division and stimulate apoptosis in tumor cells.[9]

In addition, population studies associate diets low in antioxidant micronutrients with a higher risk for cancer. These studies do not, of course, prove cause and effect. Nutrition experts agree that interactions between antioxidant nutrients and phytochemicals, fiber, and other substances in foods probably work together to reduce cancer risk. Studies are now being conducted to determine whether eating foods high in antioxidants directly causes lower rates of cancer.

As noted previously, growing evidence over the past 20 years indicates that antioxidant supplementation does not reduce cancer risk; in fact, it may increase risks for various cancers and other chronic diseases.[10] It has been speculated that this effect occurs because antioxidants taken in supplement form may in some situations act as prooxidants, whereas antioxidants consumed in foods may be more balanced.

Thus, it appears that the best ways to reduce our risks for cancer are to eat a diet with ample fruits and vegetables; maintain a healthful body weight; engage in regular physical activity; quit smoking if applicable; avoid alcohol abuse; and avoid exposure to infectious agents and UV radiation. Many studies are currently examining the impact of whole foods on the risk for various forms of cancer. The results of these studies will provide important insights into the link between whole foods and cancer.

web links

www.cancer.org
American Cancer Society

Get ACS recommendations for nutrition and physical activity for cancer prevention.

www.cancer.gov
The National Cancer Institute

Learn more about the nutritional and other factors that can influence your risk for cancer.

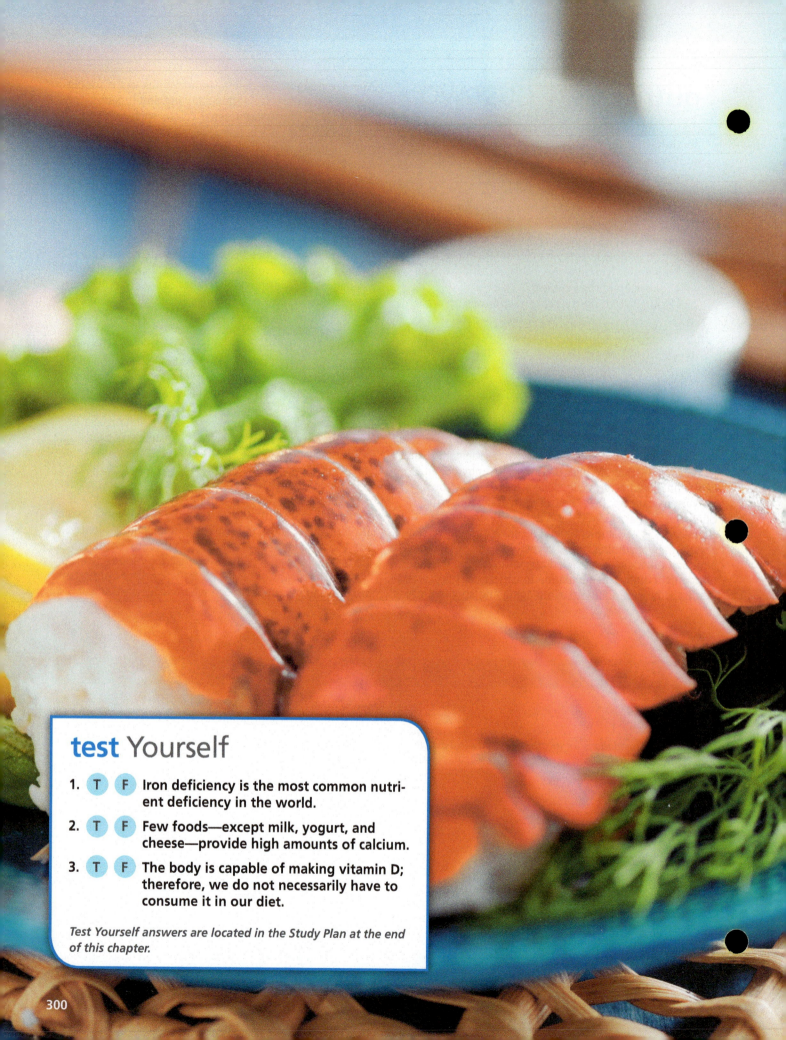

test Yourself

1. T F Iron deficiency is the most common nutrient deficiency in the world.

2. T F Few foods—except milk, yogurt, and cheese—provide high amounts of calcium.

3. T F The body is capable of making vitamin D; therefore, we do not necessarily have to consume it in our diet.

Test Yourself answers are located in the Study Plan at the end of this chapter.

9

Nutrients Essential to Healthy Tissues

When Cassie started college, she began following a strict vegan diet: whole oats for breakfast, salads for lunch, and rice and vegetables for most of her evening meals. Then, halfway through her second semester, she began to feel exhausted and "fuzzy." She explained to the nurse practitioner at her campus health center, "It's like I just can't think straight." He asked Cassie some questions about her diet, then ran some blood tests. At Cassie's follow-up appointment, he told her that she had iron-deficiency anemia and suggested she see a registered dietitian for nutrition counseling.

When the registered dietitian analyzed Cassie's diet, she determined that it was deficient in iron, and low in protein, zinc, calcium, and vitamins B_{12} and D. She explained the importance of these nutrients to the health of Cassie's blood, bone, and other body tissues, and helped Cassie design a healthful vegan diet.

Recall (from Chapter 3) that groups of body cells make up tissues, which in turn make up all of the larger structures of the body, including internal organs, nerves, muscles, bones, and blood. The most abundant tissue in the body is *connective tissue,* a type in which the cells are somewhat separated from one another by a surrounding substance called a *matrix.* Two of the body's connective tissues, blood and bone, require protein and certain key micronutrients (identified in **TABLE 9.1** on page 302) for their structure and functions, as you'll discover in this chapter. We'll also explore the role of vitamin C in the synthesis of collagen, a protein present in the matrix of connective tissues throughout the body.

TABLE 9.1 Overview of Nutrients Essential to Healthy Tissues

To see the full profile of all micronutrients, turn to the **In Depth** essay following Chapter 6, Vitamins and Minerals: Micronutrients with Macro Powers (pages 211–221).

Nutrient	Recommended Intake
Iron	RDA for 19 to 50 years of age: Women = 18 mg/day Men = 8 mg/day
Zinc	RDA for 19 to 50 years of age: Women = 8 mg/day Men = 11 mg/day
Copper	RDA for 19 to 50 years of age: 90 µg/day
Vitamin B$_6$ (pyridoxine)	RDA for 19 to 50 years of age: 1.3 mg/day RDA for 51 years of age and older: Women = 1.5 mg/day Men = 1.7 mg/day
Folate (folic acid)	RDA for 19 years of age and older: 400 µg/day
Vitamin B$_{12}$ (cobalamin)	RDA for 19 years of age and older: 2.4 µg/day
Vitamin K	AI for 19 to 50 years of age: Women = 90 µg/day Men = 120 µg/day
Vitamin C	RDA for 19 years of age and older: Women = 75 mg/day Men = 90 mg/day Smokers = 35 mg more per day than RDA
Calcium	RDA for 19 to 50 years of age: 1,000 mg/day Women 51 years of age and older = 1,200 mg/day Men 51 to 70 years of age = 1,000 mg/day; 70 years of age and older = 1,200 mg/day
Phosphorus	RDA for 19 years of age and older: 700 mg/day
Magnesium	RDA for 19 to 30 years of age: Women = 310 mg/day Men = 400 mg/day RDA for 31 years of age and older: Women = 320 mg/day Men = 420 mg/day
Fluoride	RDA for 19 years of age and older: Women = 3 mg/day Men = 4 mg/day
Vitamin D	RDA for 19 to 70 years of age:* 600 IU/day RDA for 71 years of age and older: 800 IU/day

*Based on the assumption that a person does not get adequate sun exposure.

LO 1 Identify and discuss the contributions of three trace minerals to blood health.

How do three trace minerals help maintain healthy blood?

Like all connective tissue, blood has cellular components and a matrix. The three cellular components are as follows (**FIGURE 9.1**):

- **Erythrocytes**, or red blood cells, are the cells that transport oxygen.
- **Leukocytes**, or white blood cells, are the key to our immune function. They defend against infection and the progression of cancer.
- **Platelets** are cell fragments that assist in the formation of blood clots and help stop bleeding.

erythrocytes The red blood cells, which are the cells that transport oxygen in our blood.

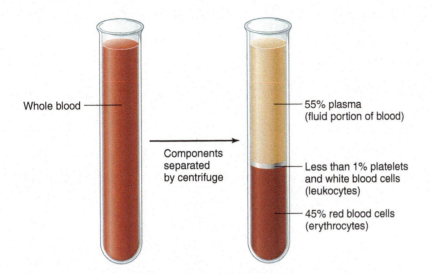

Whole blood

Components separated by centrifuge

55% plasma (fluid portion of blood)

Less than 1% platelets and white blood cells (leukocytes)

45% red blood cells (erythrocytes)

◀ **FIGURE 9.1** Blood has four components, which are visible when the blood is drawn into a test tube and spun in a centrifuge. The bottom layer is the erythrocytes, or red blood cells. The milky layer above the erythrocytes contains the leukocytes and platelets. The yellow fluid on top is the plasma.

Plasma is the watery matrix of blood in which the cells and platelets flow. The circulation of blood is critical to life because it transports oxygen and nutrients to our cells, and removes carbon dioxide and other waste products generated from metabolism. Among the micronutrients required for healthy blood, the trace mineral iron plays the leading role in enabling blood cells to transport oxygen.

Watch a video of red blood cell production from the National Library of Medicine at www.nlm.nih.gov/medlineplus/ency/anatomyvideos/000104.htm.

Iron Is a Component of the Oxygen-Carrying Proteins in Blood and Muscle

A trace mineral, iron is needed in very small amounts, yet the World Health Organization lists iron deficiency as the most common nutrient deficiency in the world.[1]

Functions of Iron

Iron is a component of numerous proteins in the body. Almost two-thirds of all the iron in the body is found in **hemoglobin**, the oxygen-carrying protein in our red blood cells. As shown in **FIGURE 9.2** on page 304, the hemoglobin molecule has four polypeptide chains, each with an iron-containing **heme** group. Because you cannot survive for longer than a few minutes without oxygen, the ability to transport oxygen throughout the body is critical to life. In the bloodstream, iron acts as a shuttle, picking up oxygen inhaled into the lungs, binding it during its transport in red blood cells, and then dropping it off again in body tissues.

Iron is also a component of **myoglobin**, a protein similar to hemoglobin but found in muscle cells. As a part of myoglobin, iron assists in the transport of oxygen into muscle cells.

Iron is also found in enzymes called *cytochromes* that are active in the metabolism of carbohydrates, fats, and proteins. In the mitochondria alone, more than 12 of these iron-requiring enzymes help produce energy.[2] Iron is also necessary for the enzymes involved in DNA synthesis, and plays an important role in cognitive development and immune health.[3,4] Finally, iron is part of an antioxidant enzyme system that assists in fighting free radicals. Interestingly, excess iron can also act as a **prooxidant** and promote the production of free radicals.

Iron Storage and Recycling

Our body contains relatively little iron; men have 500 to 1,500 mg of iron in their body, while women have 300 to 1,000 mg. Excess iron can be stored in the liver, bone marrow, intestinal mucosa, and spleen. These stores can provide us with iron when our diets are inadequate.

As aging cells, including red blood cells, break down, their iron is released and recycled. The liver and spleen are responsible for this iron-recycling program, which

leukocytes The white blood cells, which protect us from infection and illness.

platelets Cell fragments that assist in the formation of blood clots and help stop bleeding.

plasma The fluid portion of the blood; needed to maintain adequate blood volume so that the blood can flow easily throughout our body.

hemoglobin The oxygen-carrying protein found in our red blood cells; almost two-thirds of all the iron in our body is found in hemoglobin.

heme The iron-containing molecule found in hemoglobin.

myoglobin An iron-containing protein similar to hemoglobin except that it is found in muscle cells.

prooxidant A substance that promotes oxidation and oxidative cell and tissue damage.

▶ **FIGURE 9.2** Iron is contained in the heme portion of hemoglobin and myoglobin.

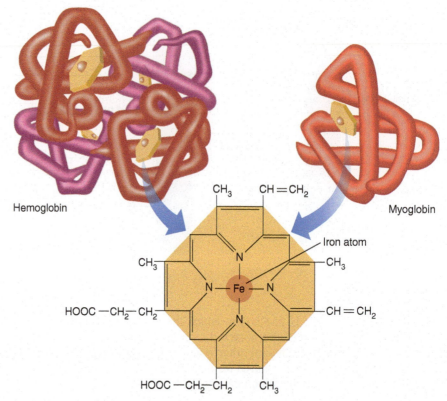

Heme portion containing iron (Fe)

greatly reduces the body's reliance on dietary iron. Each day, about 85% of the iron released from hemoglobin breakdown is reused by the body.

Iron Absorption

A person's ability to absorb iron from the diet is influenced by the following factors.

■ **Iron status.** When iron stores are high, the amount of iron absorbed in the diet is low; however, iron absorption rates are higher in people with poor iron status, such as those with iron deficiency, pregnant women, or people who have recently experienced blood loss (including via menstruation).

■ **Stomach acid.** Adequate amounts of stomach acid are necessary for iron absorption. People with low levels of stomach acid have a decreased ability to absorb iron. This population includes many older adults and people who take medications that inhibit stomach acid production.

■ **The amount of iron in the diet.** People who consume low levels of dietary iron absorb more iron from their foods than people with higher dietary iron intakes.

■ **The type of iron in the foods you eat.** Foods have two types of iron: **Heme iron** is a part of hemoglobin and myoglobin and is found only in animal-based foods, such as meat, fish, and poultry. **Non-heme iron**, which is not a part of hemoglobin or myoglobin, is found in both plant-based and animal-based foods. Heme iron is more absorbable than non-heme iron. Since the iron in animal-based foods is about 40% heme iron and 60% non-heme iron, animal-based foods are good sources of absorbable iron. Meat, fish, and poultry also contain a special **meat factor**, which enhances the absorption of non-heme iron. In contrast, all of the iron found in plant-based foods is non-heme iron, and no absorption-enhancing factor is present. However, any vitamin C (ascorbic acid) in the food itself or in accompanying foods or beverages will enhance the absorption of non-heme iron.

■ **Other dietary factors.** Iron absorption is reduced from foods containing phytates, including legumes, rice, and whole grains. Polyphenols in tea, coffee, and red wine also reduce iron absorption, as do soybean protein and calcium. Because these dietary factors alter the amount of iron absorbed, it is estimated that the

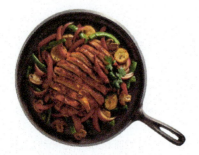

◆ Cooking foods in cast-iron pans significantly increases their iron content.

heme iron Iron that is a part of hemoglobin and myoglobin; found only in animal-based foods, such as meat, fish, and poultry.

non-heme iron The form of iron that is not a part of hemoglobin or myoglobin; found in animal- and plant-based foods.

meat factor A special factor found in meat, fish, and poultry that enhances the absorption of non-heme iron.

Calculating Daily Iron Intake

Determining whether or not you're getting the iron your body needs each day can be tricky because the amount you consume may not be the amount that is absorbed. Food combinations, fortified foods, and supplements all make a difference. Determine the amount of iron available for absorption in the following food choices for one day for Hannah, who is menstruating normally:

Foods with heme iron (15% available):

- Turkey, light meat (3 oz): 1.1 mg
- Tuna, light canned (3 oz): 1.3 mg

Foods with non-heme iron (5% available):

- Oatmeal, 1 instant packet: 11 mg
- Spinach, 1 cup raw: 6.4 mg
- Bread, whole wheat 2 slices: 1.4 mg

Multivitamin/mineral supplement with 18 mg of Fe (5% available). This is the amount of iron in a typical 1-day multivitamin/mineral supplement designed for menstruating women.

What is the total available iron for absorption (mg/d)? Does it cover the amount of iron lost each day? If Hannah were not taking a daily supplement, would she still be getting adequate iron?

Answers can be found in the MasteringNutrition Study Area.

---

bioavailability of iron from a vegan diet is approximately 1% to 10%, whereas it averages 18% for a mixed Western diet.[5]

A number of special circumstances can significantly affect iron status. These are identified in TABLE 9.2.

Recommended Intakes and Food Sources of Iron

When scientists established the DRIs for iron (see Table 9.1), they accounted for the range of iron availability from food sources. The higher iron requirement for younger women is due to the excess iron and blood lost during menstruation. See the **You Do the Math** box on this page to learn how to calculate your iron intake.

Good food sources of heme iron are meats, poultry, and fish (FIGURE 9.3). Many breakfast cereals and breads are also enriched with iron; although this is non-heme iron and less absorbable, it adds significant iron to the diet because we eat so many of

TABLE 9.2 Circumstances Affecting Iron Status

Circumstances That Improve Iron Status	Circumstances That Diminish Iron Status
• Use of oral contraceptives—reduces menstrual blood loss in women. • Breastfeeding—delays resumption of menstruation in new mothers and thereby reduces menstrual blood loss. It is therefore an important health measure, especially in developing nations. • Consumption of iron-containing foods and supplements.	• Use of hormone replacement therapy—can cause uterine bleeding. • Eating a vegetarian diet—reduces or eliminates sources of heme iron. • Intestinal parasitic infection—causes intestinal bleeding. Iron-deficiency anemia is common in people with intestinal parasitic infection. • Blood donation—reduces iron stores; people who donate frequently, particularly premenopausal women, may require iron supplementation. • Intense endurance exercise training—appears to increase risk for inflammation, suboptimal iron intake, increased iron loss due to rupture of red blood cells, and losses in sweat and feces.

Source: Data from Dietary Reference Intakes for Vitamin A, Vitamin K, Arsenic, Boron, Chromium, Copper, Iodine, Manganese, Molybdenum, Nickel, Silicon, Vanadium, and Zinc © 2002 by the National Academy of Sciences, National Academies Press.

bioavailability The degree to which the body can absorb and utilize any given nutrient.

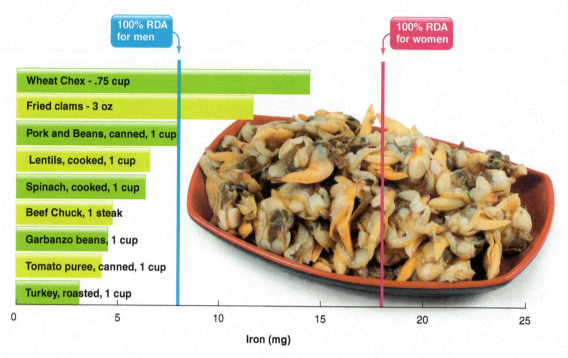

100% RDA for men

100% RDA for women

Wheat Chex - .75 cup

Fried clams - 3 oz

Pork and Beans, canned, 1 cup

Lentils, cooked, 1 cup

Spinach, cooked, 1 cup

Beef Chuck, 1 steak

Garbanzo beans, 1 cup

Tomato puree, canned, 1 cup

Turkey, roasted, 1 cup

0   5   10   15   20   25

Iron (mg)

FIGURE 9.3 Common food sources of iron. The RDA for iron is 8 mg/day for men and 18 mg/day for women aged 19 to 50 years.

Source: Data from U.S. Department of Agriculture, Agricultural Research Service, 2015. USDA Nutrient Database for Standard Reference, Release 28.

these foods. Some legumes and green, leafy vegetables are also good sources of iron, and the absorption of their non-heme iron can be enhanced by eating them with even a small amount of meat, fish, or poultry, or with vitamin C–rich foods, such as citrus fruits, red and green peppers, and tomatoes. See the **Quick Tips** for more ways to increase your iron intake.

Iron Toxicity

In the United States, accidental iron overdose is the most common cause of poisoning deaths in children 6 years and younger.[6] Thus, dietary supplements need to be stored well out of the reach of children. Symptoms of iron toxicity include nausea, vomiting, diarrhea, dizziness, confusion, and rapid heartbeat. If iron toxicity is not treated quickly, significant damage to the heart, central nervous system, liver, and kidneys can result in death.

Adults who take iron supplements even at low doses commonly experience constipation and gastrointestinal (GI) distress, such as nausea, vomiting, and diarrhea.[4] Taking iron supplements with food can reduce these adverse effects in most, but not all, people.

In the United States, 1 in 200 to 500 people suffer from a hereditary disorder called hemochromatosis, which causes excessive dietary iron absorption.[7] Because the body has no mechanism for eliminating excess iron, iron accumulates in body tissues, causing organ damage and other diseases. Treatment includes restricting dietary iron intake, avoiding high intakes of vitamin C, and occasionally withdrawing blood.

Iron Deficiency

Populations at particularly high risk for iron deficiency include infants and young children, adolescent girls, menstruating women, and pregnant women. Iron deficiency progresses in stages, beginning with depletion of iron *stores*. During this first stage, there are generally no physical symptoms because hemoglobin levels are not yet affected. The second stage of iron deficiency causes a decrease in the *transport* of iron and the production of heme, leading to symptoms of reduced work capacity.

QuickTips

Increasing Your Iron Intake

✓ Shop for iron-fortified breads and breakfast cereals. Check the Nutrition Facts panel!

✓ Consume a food or beverage that is high in vitamin C along with plant or animal sources of iron. For instance, drink a glass of orange juice with your morning toast to increase the absorption of the non-heme iron in the bread. Or add chopped tomatoes to beans or lentils. Or sprinkle lemon juice on fish.

✓ Add small amounts of meat, poultry, or fish to baked beans, vegetable soups, stir-fried vegetables, or salads to enhance the absorption of the non-heme iron in the plant-based foods.

✓ Cook foods in cast-iron pans to significantly increase their iron content. The iron in the pan will be absorbed into the food during the cooking process.

✓ Avoid drinking red wine, coffee, or tea when eating iron-rich foods because the polyphenols in these beverages will reduce iron absorption.

✓ Avoid drinking cow's milk or soy milk with iron-rich foods because both calcium and soybean protein inhibit iron absorption.

✓ Avoid taking calcium supplements or zinc supplements with iron-rich foods because these minerals decrease iron absorption.

The final stage of iron deficiency is true anemia. The term *anemia* literally means "without blood"; it is used to refer to any condition in which hemoglobin levels are low. Some anemias are inherited disorders. For instance, *sickle cell anemia* is a genetic disorder in which the red blood cells have a sickle or "half-moon" shape, and *thalassemia* is a genetic disorder in which red blood cells are small and short-lived. *Hemorrhagic anemias* result from blood loss. Other anemias are due to micronutrient deficiencies. These can be classified according to the general way they alter the size and shape of the red blood cells. Low iron, copper, and vitamin B_6 cause *microcytic anemia* (small red blood cells; *micro* means "small," and *cyte* means "cell"). In contrast, inadequate intakes of folate or vitamin B_{12} cause *macrocytic anemia*. These processes are shown in Figure 9.6 on page 311.

In **iron-deficiency anemia**, the red blood cells produced are smaller than normal, with low hemoglobin, and therefore cannot transport adequate oxygen. As a result, the body produces less energy, and the classic symptoms of iron-deficiency anemia occur. These include impaired work performance and neurological function, general fatigue, pale skin, and depressed immune function. Pregnant women with severe anemia are at higher risk for low-birth-weight infants, premature delivery, increased infant mortality, and postpartum hemorrhage (excessive bleeding immediately following childbirth).[8]

Zinc Contributes to Hemoglobin

Zinc is a trace mineral that has multiple functions within nearly every body system.

Functions of Zinc

The functions of zinc can be grouped into three general categories: enzymatic, structural, and regulatory.

- **Enzymatic functions.** Zinc is required for more than 300 different enzymes in the body. Without zinc, these enzymes cannot function. For example, we require

iron-deficiency anemia A form of anemia that results from severe iron deficiency.

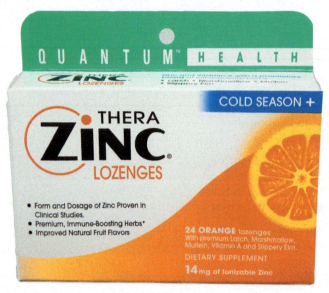

Research suggests that zinc lozenges may be modestly helpful in treating the common cold.

zinc for digestion and metabolism, and to synthesize the heme structure of hemoglobin. In this way, zinc contributes to the maintenance of blood health.

- **Structural functions.** If proteins lose their shape, they lose their function. Zinc helps to stabilize the structure of proteins involved in gene expression, vision, antioxidant enzyme systems, and immune function. In fact, zinc has received so much attention for its contribution to immune health that zinc lozenges have been formulated to fight the common cold. Research suggests that these lozenges may be at least modestly effective.[9,10]

- **Regulatory functions.** Zinc helps regulate gene expression and thus the body functions that these genes control. For example, without zinc, certain genes that help regulate cell division during fetal development are not expressed. After the child is born, growth is stunted.

A number of biological actions require zinc in all three of the functions above. A key example is normal growth. In fact, zinc deficiency was discovered in the early 1960s when researchers were trying to determine the cause of severe growth retardation in a group of Middle Eastern men.

Recommended Intakes and Food Sources of Zinc

Overall, zinc absorption is similar to that of iron, ranging from 10% to 35% of dietary zinc. People with poor zinc status absorb more zinc than individuals with optimal zinc status, and zinc absorption is increased during pregnancy, childhood, and adolescence.

Several dietary factors influence zinc absorption. High non-heme iron intakes can inhibit zinc absorption, which is a primary concern with iron supplements (which are non-heme), particularly during pregnancy and lactation. High intakes of heme iron appear to have no effect on zinc absorption. The phytates and fiber found in whole grains and beans strongly inhibit zinc absorption. In contrast, dietary protein, especially animal-based protein, enhances zinc absorption. It's not surprising, then, that the primary cause of the zinc deficiency in the Middle Eastern men just mentioned was their low consumption of meat and high consumption of beans and flat breads (unleavened breads) high in phytates. The yeast added to leavened breads reduces the phytate content.

The recommended intakes for zinc are listed in Table 9.1. Good food sources include meat, fish, and poultry and enriched grains and cereals **(FIGURE 9.4)**. As zinc is significantly more absorbable from animal-based foods, zinc deficiency is a concern for people eating a vegan diet.

Zinc Toxicity and Deficiency

Consuming a diet high in zinc does not appear to lead to toxicity; however, toxicity can occur from consuming zinc supplements. Toxicity symptoms include GI pain and dysfunction, headaches, and depressed immune function. High intakes of zinc also interfere with copper absorption and thus can reduce copper status.

Zinc deficiency is uncommon in the United States, but does occur in countries in which people consume predominantly grain-based foods. Symptoms include growth retardation, delayed sexual maturation and impotence, impaired appetite, and other problems. As zinc is critical to a healthy immune system, zinc deficiency also results in increased incidence of infections.

Copper Is Critical for Iron Transport

Copper is a trace mineral that plays an important role in blood health because it is a component of *ceruloplasmin*, a protein that is important for iron transport.[4] If ceruloplasmin levels are inadequate, iron accumulates, causing symptoms similar to those described with the genetic disorder hemochromatosis.

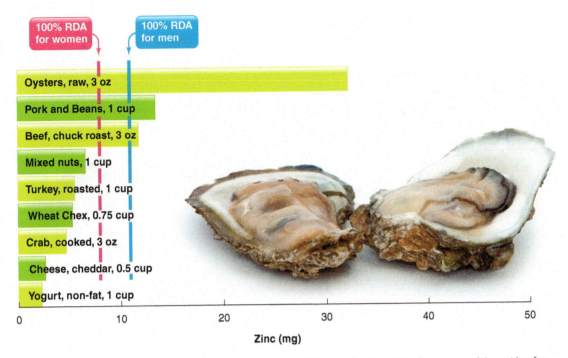

100% RDA for women

100% RDA for men

Oysters, raw, 3 oz

Pork and Beans, 1 cup

Beef, chuck roast, 3 oz

Mixed nuts, 1 cup

Turkey, roasted, 1 cup

Wheat Chex, 0.75 cup

Crab, cooked, 3 oz

Cheese, cheddar, 0.5 cup

Yogurt, non-fat, 1 cup

0   10   20   30   40   50

Zinc (mg)

FIGURE 9.4 Common food sources of zinc. The RDA for zinc is 11 mg/day for men and 8 mg/day for women.

Source: Data from U.S. Department of Agriculture, Agricultural Research Service, 2015. USDA Nutrient Database for Standard Reference, Release 28.

Copper also functions in energy metabolism, in the synthesis of the connective-tissue proteins collagen and elastin, and in the superoxide dismutase antioxidant enzyme system. Copper is also necessary for the regulation of certain neurotransmitters, especially serotonin, important to nervous system function.

As you can see in Table 9.1, our need for copper is small. Copper is widely distributed in foods, and people who eat a varied diet can easily meet their requirements **(FIGURE 9.5)** (page 310). Good food sources of copper include organ meats, seafood, nuts, and seeds. Whole-grain foods are also relatively good sources.

As with iron and zinc, people with low dietary copper intakes absorb more copper than people with high dietary intakes. Also recall that high zinc intakes can reduce copper absorption and, subsequently, copper status. In fact, zinc supplementation is used to treat a rare disorder called Wilson's disease, in which copper toxicity occurs.

The long-term effects of copper toxicity are not well studied in humans. Copper deficiency is rare; however, low copper status can inhibit the synthesis of hemoglobin, as a result of inadequate iron utilization, and trigger microcytic anemia.[4]

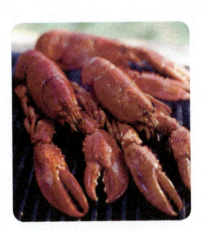

Lobster is a food that contains copper.

recap Blood is a fluid connective tissue composed of erythrocytes, leukocytes, platelets, and plasma. It transports nutrients and oxygen to our cells and removes metabolic wastes. Iron is a trace mineral that, as part of hemoglobin, is required for oxygen transport. Iron is also a coenzyme in many pathways involved in energy metabolism. Meat, fish, and poultry are good sources of heme iron, which is more absorbable than non-heme iron, which is available from animal- and plant-based foods. Iron toxicity can cause organ damage, whereas iron deficiency can lead to a type of microcytic anemia. Zinc is a trace mineral that is a part of more than 300 enzymes that impact virtually every body system. It plays a critical role in hemoglobin synthesis, physical growth and sexual maturation, and immune function, and assists in fighting oxidative damage. Copper is a trace mineral that functions in the metabolic pathways that produce energy, in the production of connective tissues, and as part of an antioxidant enzyme system. It is also a component of ceruloplasmin, a protein that is critical for the transport of iron, and thus hemoglobin synthesis.

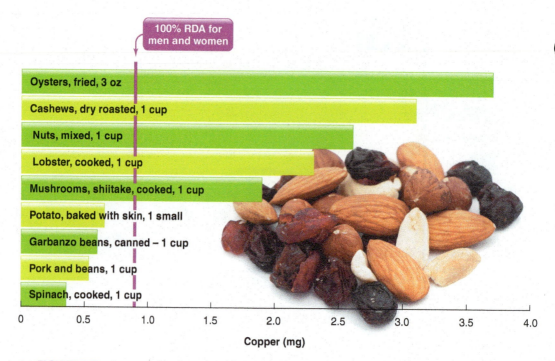

100% RDA for men and women

- Oysters, fried, 3 oz
- Cashews, dry roasted, 1 cup
- Nuts, mixed, 1 cup
- Lobster, cooked, 1 cup
- Mushrooms, shiitake, cooked, 1 cup
- Potato, baked with skin, 1 small
- Garbanzo beans, canned – 1 cup
- Pork and beans, 1 cup
- Spinach, cooked, 1 cup

0   0.5   1.0   1.5   2.0   2.5   3.0   3.5   4.0

Copper (mg)

FIGURE 9.5 Common food sources of copper. The RDA for copper is 900 μg/day for men and women.

Source: Data from U.S. Department of Agriculture, Agricultural Research Service, 2015. USDA Nutrient Database for Standard Reference, Release 28.

LO 2 Name four vitamins that help maintain healthy blood and explain their roles.

How do four vitamins promote healthy blood?

Three water-soluble B vitamins and the fat-soluble vitamin K all contribute to healthy blood.

Vitamin B₆, Folate, and Vitamin B₁₂ Are Required for the Healthy Development of Red Blood Cells

We've said that deficiency of iron, copper, or vitamin B_6 can impair hemoglobin synthesis and lead to forms of microcytic anemia. Specifically, vitamin B_6 is required for the first step of heme synthesis, in which the heme porphyrin ring that surrounds iron is formed.[11] (See Figure 9.2 on page 304.) Without vitamin B_6, heme synthesis is impaired, just as it is with iron or copper deficiency. Thus, vitamin B_6 deficiency can contribute to microcytic hypochromic anemia, just as iron does. This is shown in the top portion of **FIGURE 9.6**. See Chapter 8 for more details about vitamin B_6 requirements and food sources.

In contrast, deficiency of either folate or vitamin B_{12} can impair DNA synthesis, which decreases the ability of blood cells to divide. If they cannot divide, differentiate, and mature, the cells remain large and immature precursors to red blood cells, known as *megaloblasts* (from *megalo*, meaning "large," and *blast*, meaning "a precursor cell"). (See the bottom portion of Figure 9.6.) The resulting condition is sometimes referred to as *megaloblastic anemia* but is more commonly called **macrocytic anemia** (from *macro*, meaning "large," and *cyte*, meaning "cell").

Megaloblasts contain inadequate hemoglobin; thus, their ability to transport oxygen is diminished. Symptoms of macrocytic anemia are therefore similar to those of other types of anemia, and include weakness, fatigue, difficulty concentrating, irritability, headache, shortness of breath, and reduced exercise tolerance.

macrocytic anemia A form of anemia manifested as the production of larger than normal red blood cells containing insufficient hemoglobin; also called megaloblastic anemia.

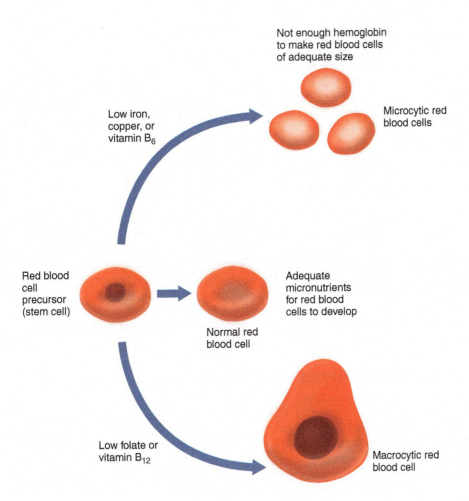

Not enough hemoglobin to make red blood cells of adequate size

Low iron, copper, or vitamin B_6

Microcytic red blood cells

Red blood cell precursor (stem cell)

Normal red blood cell

Adequate micronutrients for red blood cells to develop

Low folate or vitamin B_{12}

Macrocytic red blood cell

◀ **FIGURE 9.6** Development of healthy red blood cells versus anemias. When iron, copper, or vitamin B_6 is inadequate, microcytic anemia develops because there is not enough hemoglobin synthesis to make normal red blood cells. When folate or vitamin B_{12} is inadequate, macrocytic anemia develops because the red blood cells cannot mature and divide appropriately.

Vitamin K Supports Blood Clotting

Vitamin K is a fat-soluble vitamin important for a number of metabolic functions, including functions involved in blood and bone health. Research has also revealed roles for vitamin K in inflammation, hormone regulation, and defense against cancer.[12] Its role in the synthesis of proteins involved in maintaining bone density is discussed shortly.

Vitamin K supports blood health by acting as a coenzyme that assists in the synthesis of a number of proteins that are involved in the coagulation (clotting) of blood, including *prothrombin* and several proteins called *procoagulants*. Without adequate vitamin K, blood does not clot properly: clotting time can be delayed or may even fail to occur. The failure of blood to clot can lead to increased bleeding from even minor wounds as well as internal hemorrhaging.

The AI for vitamin K is listed in Table 9.1. Although it is relatively low, many Americans fail to meet it because vitamin K is found in few foods.[12] Green, leafy vegetables such as broccoli, turnip greens, brussels sprouts, and cabbage are good sources, as are soybean and canola oils. The GI flora in the large intestine produce vitamin K, providing us with an important nondietary source. Newborns are typically given an injection of vitamin K at birth because they lack the mature flora necessary to produce this nutrient.

There are no known side effects associated with consuming large amounts of vitamin K from supplements or from food, and no upper limit (UL) has been established for vitamin K at this time.[4] As just noted, vitamin K deficiency inhibits the blood's ability to clot, resulting in excessive bleeding. Although vitamin K deficiency is rare in humans, people with diseases that cause malabsorption of fat, such as celiac disease, Crohn's disease, and cystic fibrosis, can suffer secondarily from a deficiency of vitamin K.

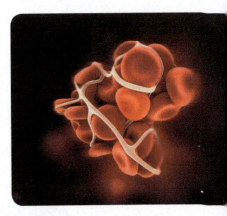

▲ Without enough vitamin K, blood will not clot properly.

LO 3 Describe the role of vitamin C in maintaining healthy collagen.

How does vitamin C help maintain healthy collagen?

Collagen is a fibrous protein present in the matrix of connective tissues. The most abundant protein in the body, it provides structure to bone, teeth, skin, tendons, blood vessels, and many other tissues and organs. Collagen has a helical structure and acts like a scaffold, helping to hold the tissue together and giving it strength and flexibility. It also helps prevent bruises, and it supports wound healing because it is a component of scar tissue and of the tissue that mends broken bones.

Collagen cannot be formed and maintained without adequate vitamin C. In severe vitamin C deficiency, the body tissues essentially fall apart. This disorder is known as scurvy.

Vitamin C Is Required for the Synthesis of Collagen

Scurvy is thought to have caused more than half of the deaths that occurred on long sea voyages centuries ago. In fact, the name for one of the active forms of vitamin C, *ascorbic acid,* is derived from the combined Latin terms *a* (meaning "not") and *scorbic* (meaning "having scurvy"). During long sea voyages, the crew ate all of the fruits and vegetables—rich sources of vitamin C—early in the trip, then had only grain and animal products available until they reached land to resupply. In 1740 in England, Dr. James Lind discovered that citrus fruits can prevent scurvy. We now know that this is due to their high vitamin C content. Decades after Lind's discovery, the British Navy began requiring all ships to provide daily lemon or lime juice rations for sailors, earning them the nickname "limeys." It wasn't until 1930 that vitamin C was discovered and identified as a nutrient.

Adequate intake of vitamin C prevents scurvy because it is critical to the synthesis of collagen. Vitamin C acts as a coenzyme to specific enzymes that are required to convert collagen's precursor, procollagen, to collagen. Recall from Chapter 8 that a coenzyme is a compound that is needed for an enzyme to be active. If a person is deficient in vitamin C, then the necessary synthesis reactions cannot occur; as a result, the collagen chains that are produced cannot link and twist into thick strands and fibers **(FIGURE 9.7)**. Instead, they are weak and quickly destroyed.

collagen A protein that forms strong fibers in the matrix of bone, blood vessels, and other connective tissues.

scurvy Vitamin C deficiency disease caused by failure of collagen synthesis.

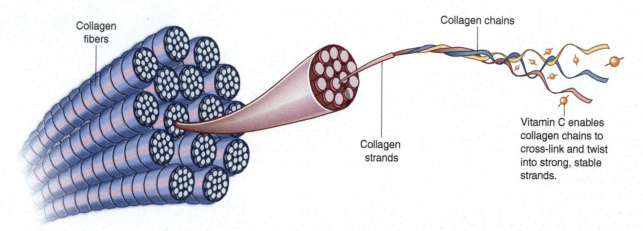

Collagen fibers

Collagen chains

Collagen strands

Vitamin C enables collagen chains to cross-link and twist into strong, stable strands.

FIGURE 9.7 Vitamin C is essential for the healthy cross-linking of the chains that make up collagen strands.

Because the body cannot form collagen without adequate vitamin C, tissue hemorrhage, or bleeding, occurs. The symptoms of scurvy appear after about 1 month of a vitamin C–deficient diet and include bleeding gums **(FIGURE 9.8)**, loose teeth, wounds that fail to heal, swollen ankles and wrists, bone pain and fractures, diarrhea, weakness, and depression. Vitamin C may also be involved in the synthesis of other components of connective tissues, such as elastin and bone matrix.

Vitamin C Has Many Other Roles in the Body

In addition to connective tissues, vitamin C assists in the synthesis of DNA, bile, neurotransmitters such as serotonin (which helps regulate mood), and carnitine, which transports long-chain fatty acids from the cytosol into the mitochondria for energy production. In addition, many hormones are synthesized with assistance from vitamin C, including epinephrine, norepinephrine, thyroid hormones, and steroid hormones, and vitamin C is important for a healthy immune system.

As you learned (in Chapter 8), vitamin C also acts as a water-soluble antioxidant in the extracellular fluid and regenerates vitamin E after it has been oxidized. Finally, vitamin C enhances the absorption of iron. It is recommended that people with low iron stores consume foods rich in vitamin C along with iron sources to improve absorption.

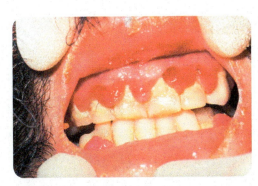

▲ **FIGURE 9.8** Bleeding gums are one symptom of scurvy, the most common vitamin C-deficiency disease.

The RDA for Vitamin C Is Easily Obtained

Most animals can make their own vitamin C from glucose. Humans and guinea pigs are two groups that cannot synthesize their own vitamin C and must consume it in the diet. As vitamin C is a water-soluble vitamin, we must consume it on a regular basis because any excess is excreted (primarily in our urine) rather than stored.

Recommended Intakes and Food Sources of Vitamin C

The recommended intakes for vitamin C are listed in Table 9.1. Notice that smoking increases a person's need for vitamin C; thus, the RDA for smokers is higher. Other high-stress situations that may increase the need for vitamin C include healing from a traumatic injury, surgery, or burns and the use of oral contraceptives among women; there is no consensus on how much extra vitamin C is needed in these circumstances.

Although many people believe that vitamin C can prevent the common cold, a recent review found that people taking vitamin C supplements regularly to ward off the common cold experienced as many colds as people taking a placebo.[13] However, the duration of colds was modestly reduced—by 8% in adults and 14% in children. Timing appears to be important, as those who took vitamin C after the onset of cold symptoms did not reduce either the duration or severity of the cold.

Fruits and vegetables are the best sources of vitamin C **(FIGURE 9.9)** (page 214). Because heat and oxygen destroy vitamin C, fresh sources of these foods have the highest content. Cooking foods, especially boiling them, leaches their vitamin C, which is then lost when we strain them. The forms of cooking that are least likely to compromise the vitamin C content of foods are steaming, microwaving, and stir-frying. See the **Quick Tips** on page 315 for help increasing your intake of vitamin C.

Vitamin C Toxicity and Deficiency

Because vitamin C is water soluble, we usually excrete any excess. Consuming excess amounts in food sources does not lead to toxicity, and only supplements can lead to

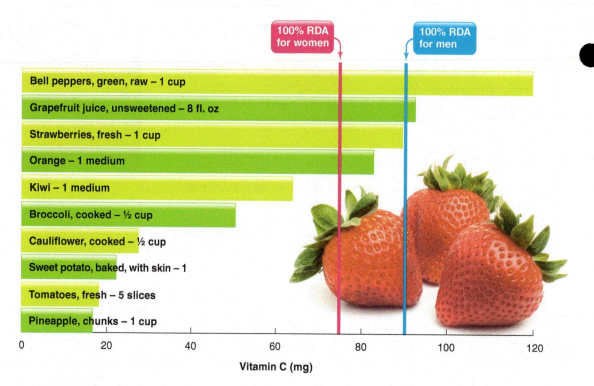

FIGURE 9.9 Common food sources of vitamin C. The RDA for vitamin C is 90 mg/day for men and 75 mg/day for women.

Source: Data from U.S. Department of Agriculture, Agricultural Research Service, 2015. USDA Nutrient Database for Standard Reference, Release 28.

toxic doses. Taking a **megadose** of vitamin C is not fatally harmful. However, side effects of doses exceeding 2,000 mg/day for a prolonged period include nausea, diarrhea, nosebleeds, and abdominal cramps.

There are rare instances in which consuming even moderately excessive doses of vitamin C can be harmful. As mentioned earlier, vitamin C enhances the absorption of iron. This action is beneficial to people who need to increase iron absorption. It can be harmful, however, to people with a disease called *hemochromatosis,* which causes an excess accumulation of iron in the body and leads to tissue damage and a heart attack. In people who have preexisting kidney disease, taking excess vitamin C can lead to the formation of kidney stones. This does not appear to occur in healthy individuals.

Vitamin C deficiencies are rare in developed countries but can occur in developing countries. Scurvy is the most common vitamin C–deficiency disease. Anemia can also result from vitamin C deficiency. People most at risk are those who eat few fruits and vegetables, including impoverished or homebound individuals, and people who abuse alcohol and drugs.

megadose A nutrient dose that is 10 or more times greater than the recommended amount.

recap Collagen is a structural protein present in the matrix of connective tissues, including blood vessels and bone. Vitamin C is required for the synthesis of collagen, and deficiency results in scurvy. Vitamin C also assists in the synthesis of various hormones, neurotransmitters, and DNA, enhances iron absorption, and regenerates vitamin E after it has been oxidized. Many fruits and vegetables are high in vitamin C. Toxicity is uncommon with dietary intake; symptoms include nausea, diarrhea, and nosebleeds. Deficiency symptoms include scurvy, anemia, diarrhea, and depression.

QuickTips

Selecting Foods High in Vitamin C

✅ Mix strawberries, kiwi fruit, cantaloupe, and oranges for a tasty fruit salad loaded with vitamin C.

✅ Include tomatoes on salads, wraps, and sandwiches for more vitamin C.

✅ Make your own fresh-squeezed orange or grapefruit juice.

✅ Add your favorite vitamin C–rich fruits, such as strawberries, to smoothies.

✅ Buy ready-to-eat vegetables, such as baby carrots and cherry tomatoes, and toss some in a zip-lock bag to take to school or work.

✅ Put a few slices of romaine lettuce on your sandwich.

✅ Throw a small container of orange slices, fresh pineapple chunks, or berries into your backpack for an afternoon snack.

✅ Store some juice boxes in your freezer to pack with your lunch. They'll thaw slowly, keeping the rest of your lunch cool, and many brands contain a full day's supply of vitamin C in just 6 oz.

✅ Enjoy raw bell peppers with low-fat dip for a crunchy snack.

✅ Serve reduced-salt corn chips with fresh salsa.

What are the components and activities of healthy bone?

LO 4 Describe the composition and activities of healthy bone.

Bones are living organs that contain connective tissue, cartilage, and two types of bone tissue. Nerves and blood vessels run within channels in bone tissue, supporting its activities. Bones have many important functions in our body (TABLE 9.3). Bone health is achieved through complex interactions among nutrients, hormones, and environmental factors.

The Composition of Bone Provides Strength and Flexibility

Bones are not totally rigid—they need to be both strong and flexible so that they can withstand the compression, stretching, and twisting that occur through daily activity. Fortunately, the composition of bone is ideally suited for its complex job: about 65% of bone tissue is made up of an assortment of minerals (mostly calcium and phosphorus) that provide hardness, but the remaining 35% is a mixture of organic substances, including collagen, that provide strength, durability, and flexibility. Within our bones, the minerals form tiny crystals (called *hydroxyapatite*) that cluster around the collagen fibers. This design enables bones to bear weight while responding to our demands for movement.

TABLE 9.3 Functions of Bone in the Human Body

Functions Related to Structure and Support	Functions Related to Metabolic Processes
• Bones provide physical support for organs and body segments. • Bones protect vital organs; for example, the rib cage protects the lungs, the skull protects the brain, and the vertebrae of the spine protect the spinal cord. • Bones work with muscles and tendons to allow movement—muscles attach to bones via tendons, and their contraction produces movement at the body's joints.	• Bone tissue acts as a storage reservoir for many minerals, including calcium, phosphorus, and fluoride. The body draws upon such deposits when these minerals are needed for various body processes; however, this can reduce bone mass. • Most blood cells are produced in the bone marrow.

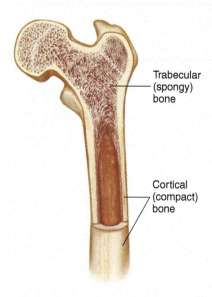

Trabecular (spongy) bone

Cortical (compact) bone

◄ FIGURE 9.10 The structure of bone. Notice the difference in density between the trabecular (spongy) bone and the cortical (compact) bone.

cortical bone (compact bone) A dense bone tissue that makes up the outer surface of all bones as well as the entirety of most small bones of the body.

trabecular bone (spongy bone) A porous bone tissue that makes up only 20% of our skeletons and is found within the ends of the long bones, inside the spinal vertebrae, inside the flat bones (sternum, ribs, and most bones of the skull), and inside the bones of the pelvis.

bone density The degree of compactness of bone tissue, reflecting the strength of the bones. *Peak bone density* is the point at which a bone is strongest.

remodeling The two-step process by which bone tissue is recycled; includes the breakdown of existing bone and the formation of new bone.

resorption The process by which the surface of bone is broken down by cells called osteoclasts.

osteoclasts Cells that erode the surface of bones by secreting enzymes and acids that dig grooves into the bone matrix.

If you examine a bone very closely, you will notice two distinct types of tissue (FIGURE 9.10): cortical bone and trabecular bone. **Cortical bone**, also called *compact bone*, is very dense. It constitutes approximately 80% of the skeleton. The outer surface of all bones is cortical; plus, many small bones of the body, such as the bones of the wrists, hands, and feet, are made entirely of cortical bone.

Trabecular bone makes up 20% of the skeleton. It is found within the ends of the long bones (such as the bones of the arms and legs), the spinal vertebrae, the sternum (breastbone), the ribs, most bones of the skull, and the pelvis. Trabecular bone is sometimes referred to as *spongy bone* because to the naked eye it looks like a sponge, with cavities and no clear organization. The microscope reveals that trabecular bone is, in fact, aligned in a precise network of columns that protects the bone from stress. You can think of trabecular bone as the scaffolding inside the bone that supports the outer cortical bone.

The Constant Activity of Bone Tissue Promotes Bone Health

Bones develop through a series of three processes: bone growth, bone modeling, and bone remodeling.

Bone Growth and Modeling

Through the process of *bone growth*, the size of bones increases. The first period of rapid bone growth is from birth to age 2, but growth continues in spurts throughout childhood and into adolescence. Most girls reach their full adult height by about age 18, with most boys continuing to grow up to the age of 21. Some loss in height usually occurs in the later decades of life because of decreased bone density in the spine.

Bone modeling is the process by which the shape of our bones is determined, from the round "pebble" bones that make up our wrists, to the uniquely shaped bones of our face, to the long bones of our arms and legs. Although the size and shape of our bones do not change significantly after puberty, our **bone density**, or the compactness of our bones, continues to develop into early adulthood. *Peak bone density* is the point at which our bones are strongest because they are at their highest density. The following factors are associated with a lower peak bone density:[14]

- Late pubertal age in boys and late onset of menstruation in girls
- Inadequate calcium intake
- Low body weight
- Physical inactivity during adolescence

About 90% of a woman's bone density has been built by 17 years of age, whereas the majority of a man's has been built by his 20s. Before we reach the age of 30, our body reaches peak bone mass, and we can no longer significantly add to our bone density. In our 30s, our bone density remains relatively stable, but by age 40, it has begun its irreversible decline.

Bone Remodeling

Bone **remodeling**, the breakdown of older bone tissue and the formation of new bone tissue, occurs throughout adulthood. Remodeling also occurs during fracture repair, and it strengthens bone regions that are exposed to higher physical stress. Cortical and trabecular bones differ in their rate of remodeling: trabecular bone has a faster turnover rate than cortical bone. This makes trabecular bone more sensitive to fluctuations in hormones and nutritional deficiencies. It also accounts for the much higher rate of age-related fractures in the spine and pelvis (including the hip)—both of which contain a significant amount of trabecular bone.

The process of remodeling involves two steps: resorption and formation. Bone is broken down through **resorption** (FIGURE 9.11a). During resorption, cells called **osteoclasts** erode the bone surface by secreting enzymes and acids that dig grooves into the bone matrix. One of the primary reasons the body regularly breaks down bone is to release calcium into the bloodstream. As discussed in more detail later in

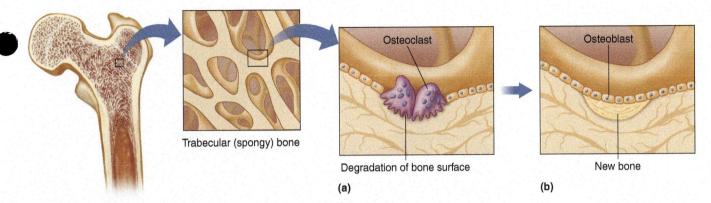

Trabecular (spongy) bone

Osteoclast

Degradation of bone surface

(a)

Osteoblast

New bone

(b)

◀ **FIGURE 9.11** Bone remodeling involves resorption and formation. **(a)** Osteoclasts erode the bone surface by degrading its components, including calcium, other minerals, and collagen; these components are then transported to the bloodstream. **(b)** Osteoblasts work to build new bone by filling the pit formed by the resorption process with new bone.

this chapter, calcium is critical for many physiologic processes, and bone is an important calcium reservoir. The body also resorbs bone at the site of a fracture, smoothing the rough edges created by the break. Bone may also be resorbed in areas away from the fracture site to obtain the minerals that are needed to repair the damage. Regardless of the reason, once bone is broken down, the resulting products are transported into the bloodstream and used for various body functions.

New bone is formed through the action of cells called **osteoblasts**, or "bone builders" (see Figure 9.11b). These cells work to synthesize new bone matrix by laying down the collagen-containing organic component of bone. Within this substance, the hydroxyapatite crystallizes and packs together to create new bone where it is needed.

In young, healthy adults, the processes of bone resorption and formation are equal so that just as much bone is broken down as is built, maintaining bone mass. Around 40 years of age, bone resorption begins to occur more rapidly than bone formation, and this imbalance results in an overall loss in bone density. Because this affects the vertebrae of the spine, people tend to lose height as they age. As discussed shortly, achieving a high peak bone mass through proper nutrition and exercise when we are young provides us with a stronger skeleton before the loss of bone begins. It can therefore reduce our risk for *osteoporosis*, a disorder characterized by low-density bones that fracture easily. Osteoporosis is discussed **In Depth** in the essay following this chapter (on pages 334–341).

> To learn more about bone biology, watch any of the several videos at www .bonebiology.amgen.com.
>
>

Bone Density Is Assessed with a DXA Test

Dual-energy x-ray absorptiometry (DXA or DEXA) is considered the most accurate assessment tool for measuring bone density. This method can measure the density of the bone mass over the entire body. Software is also available that provides an estimation of percentage body fat.

The DXA procedure is simple, painless, and noninvasive, and it is considered to be of minimal risk. It takes just 15 to 30 minutes to complete. The person participating in the test is scanned fully clothed through the use of a very low level of x-ray **(FIGURE 9.12)** (page 318).

DXA is a very important tool in determining a person's risk for osteoporosis. It generates a bone density score, which is compared to the average peak bone density of a healthy 30-year-old. Doctors use this comparison, which is known as a **T-score**, to assess the risk for fracture and determine whether the person has osteoporosis. T-scores are interpreted as follows:

- A T-score between +1 and −1 means that the individual's bone density is normal.
- A T-score between −1 and −2.5 indicates low bone mass and an increased risk for fractures.
- A T-score more negative than −2.5 indicates that the person has osteoporosis.

osteoblasts Cells that prompt the formation of new bone matrix by laying down the collagen-containing component of bone, which is then mineralized.

dual-energy x-ray absorptiometry (DXA or DEXA) Currently, the most accurate tool for measuring bone density.

T-score A comparison of an individual's bone density to the average peak bone density of a 30-year-old healthy adult.

▶ **FIGURE 9.12** Dual-energy x-ray absorptiometry is a safe and simple procedure that assesses bone density.

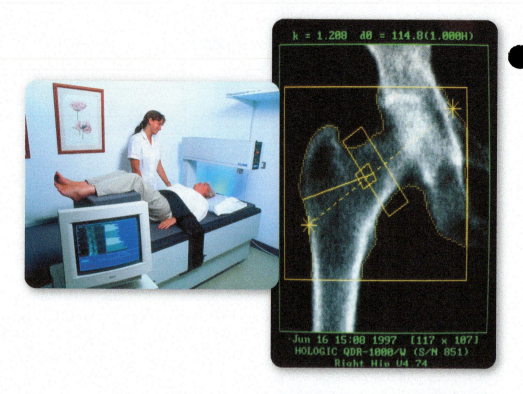

Take a closer look at a DXA scan at www.webmd.com. Type "dr siris bone density test" into the search bar, and then select the Bone Density Summary link.

DXA tests are generally recommended for postmenopausal women because they are at highest risk for osteoporosis and fracture. Men and younger women may also be recommended for a DXA test if they have significant risk factors for osteoporosis (see the **In Depth** essay on osteoporosis immediately following this chapter).

recap Bones are organs that contain metabolically active tissues composed primarily of minerals and collagen. Of the two types of bone, cortical bone is more dense and trabecular bone is more porous. Trabecular bone is also more sensitive to hormonal and nutritional factors and turns over more rapidly than cortical bone. The three types of bone activity are growth, modeling, and remodeling. Bones reach their peak bone mass by the late teenage years into the 20s; bone mass begins to decline around age 40. Dual-energy x-ray absorptiometry (DXA or DEXA) is the gold standard measurement of bone mass. The result of a DXA is a T-score, which is a comparison of a person's bone density with that of a healthy 30-year-old. A T-score more negative than −2.5 indicates osteoporosis.

LO 5 Identify and discuss the contributions of three major minerals and one trace mineral to bone health.

How do four minerals help maintain healthy bone?

Calcium is the most recognized nutrient associated with bone health; however, phosphorus, magnesium, and fluoride are also essential for strong bones, as are vitamins D and K.

Calcium Is the Major Mineral Component of Bone

Recall from Chapter 1 that the major minerals are those required in our diets in amounts greater than 100 mg per day. Calcium is by far the most abundant major mineral in our body, comprising about 2% of our entire body weight. Not surprisingly, it plays many critical roles in maintaining overall function and health.

Functions of Calcium

One of the primary functions of calcium is to provide structure to our bones and teeth. About 99% of the calcium found in our body is stored in the hydroxyapatite crystals built up on the collagen foundation of bone. The remaining 1% of calcium in our body is found in the blood and soft tissues. Calcium is alkaline, or basic, and plays a critical role in assisting with acid–base balance. We cannot survive for long if our blood calcium level rises above or falls below a very narrow range; therefore, our body maintains the appropriate blood calcium level at all costs.

FOCUS FIGURE 9.13 on page 320 illustrates how various organ systems and hormones work together to maintain blood calcium levels. When blood calcium levels fall, the parathyroid glands are stimulated to produce **parathyroid hormone (PTH)**. PTH stimulates the activation of vitamin D. PTH increases absorption of calcium in the kidneys, while PTH and vitamin D stimulate osteoclasts to break down bone, releasing more calcium into the bloodstream. In addition, vitamin D increases the absorption of calcium from the intestines. Through these mechanisms, blood calcium levels increase.

When blood calcium levels are too high, the secretion of PTH is inhibited. This suppresses the synthesis of vitamin D, thereby leading to decreased reabsorption of calcium by the kidneys, decreased calcium absorption from the intestines, and inhibition of osteoclasts, which decreases the breakdown of bone.

As just noted, the body must maintain blood calcium levels within a very narrow range. Thus, when an individual does not consume or absorb enough calcium from the diet, osteoclasts erode bone so that calcium can be released into the blood. To maintain healthy bone density, we need to consume and absorb enough calcium to balance the calcium taken from our bones.

Calcium is also critical for the normal transmission of nerve impulses. Calcium flows into nerve cells and stimulates the release of molecules called neurotransmitters, which transfer the nerve impulses from one nerve cell (neuron) to another. Without adequate calcium, our nerves' ability to transmit messages is inhibited. When blood calcium levels fall dangerously low, a person can experience convulsions.

A fourth role of calcium is to assist in muscle contraction, which is initiated when calcium is released from storage areas in muscle cells. Conversely, muscles relax when calcium is pumped back into these storage sites. If calcium levels are inadequate, normal muscle contraction and relaxation are inhibited, and the person may suffer from twitching and spasms. High levels of blood calcium can prevent the muscles from relaxing, which leads to a hardening or stiffening of the muscles. These problems affect the function not only of skeletal muscles but also of heart muscle and can cause heart failure.

Other functions of calcium include the maintenance of healthy blood pressure, the initiation of blood clotting, and the regulation of various hormones and enzymes.

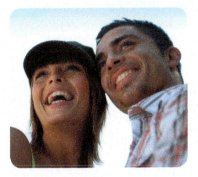

◆ One major role of calcium is to form and maintain bones and teeth.

Recommended Intakes and Food Sources of Calcium

The recommended intakes for calcium are listed in Table 9.1. Bioavailability depends in part on age and calcium need. For example, infants, children, and adolescents can absorb more than 60% of the calcium they consume because calcium needs are very high during these stages of life. In addition, pregnant and lactating women can absorb about 50% of dietary calcium. In contrast, healthy young adults absorb only about 30% of the calcium they consume. When our calcium needs are high, the body can generally increase its level of absorption from the small intestine. Although older adults have a high need for calcium, their ability to absorb calcium from the small intestine diminishes with age and can be as low as 25%. These variations in bioavailability and absorption capacity were taken into account when calcium recommendations were determined.

The bioavailability of calcium also depends on how much calcium we consume throughout the day or at any one time. When our diets are generally high in calcium, absorption of calcium is reduced. In addition, our body cannot absorb more than 500 mg of calcium at any one time, and as the amount of calcium in a single meal or supplement goes up, the fraction that is absorbed goes down. This explains why it is critical to consume calcium-rich foods throughout the day rather than relying on a single, high-dose supplement. Conversely, when dietary intake of calcium is low, the absorption of calcium is increased.

Dietary factors can also affect our absorption of calcium. Binding factors, such as phytates and oxalates, occur naturally in some calcium-rich seeds, nuts, grains, and vegetables, such as spinach and Swiss chard. Such factors bind to the calcium

parathyroid hormone (PTH) A hormone secreted by the parathyroid gland when blood calcium levels fall. It increases blood calcium levels by stimulating the activation of vitamin D, increasing reabsorption of calcium from the kidneys, and stimulating osteoclasts to break down bone.

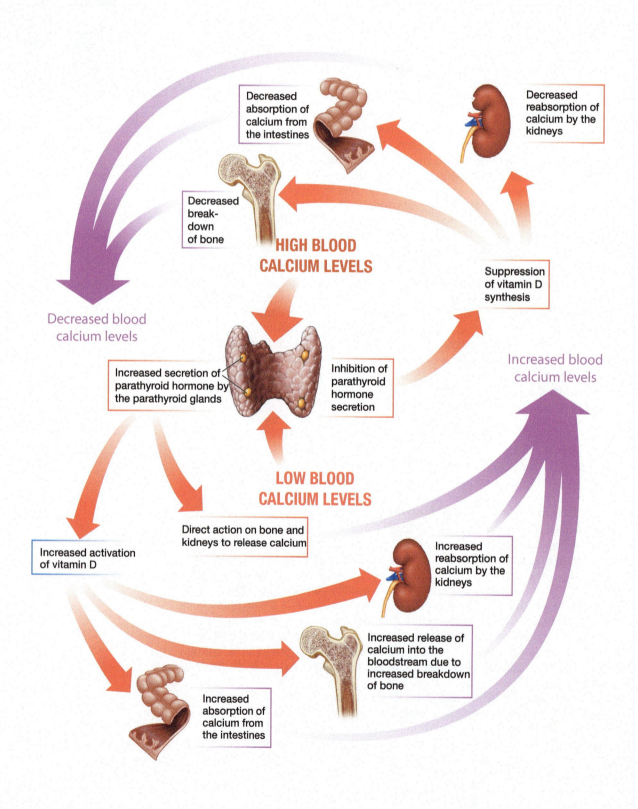

Decreased absorption of calcium from the intestines

Decreased reabsorption of calcium by the kidneys

Decreased break-down of bone

HIGH BLOOD CALCIUM LEVELS

Suppression of vitamin D synthesis

Decreased blood calcium levels

Increased secretion of parathyroid hormone by the parathyroid glands

Inhibition of parathyroid hormone secretion

Increased blood calcium levels

LOW BLOOD CALCIUM LEVELS

Direct action on bone and kidneys to release calcium

Increased activation of vitamin D

Increased reabsorption of calcium by the kidneys

Increased release of calcium into the bloodstream due to increased breakdown of bone

Increased absorption of calcium from the intestines

in these foods and reduce its absorption from the small intestine. Additionally, consuming calcium with iron, zinc, magnesium, or phosphorus can interfere with the absorption and utilization of all these minerals. Despite these potential interactions, the Health and Medicine Division of the National Academies of Sciences, Engineering, and Medicine (formerly the Institute of Medicine, or IOM) has concluded that there is not sufficient evidence to suggest that these interactions cause deficiencies of calcium or other minerals in healthy individuals.[15]

Finally, because vitamin D is necessary for the absorption of calcium, a lack of vitamin D severely limits the bioavailability of calcium. We'll discuss this and other contributions of vitamin D to bone health shortly.

Dairy products are among the most common sources of calcium in the U.S. diet. Skim milk, low-fat cheeses, and nonfat yogurt are nutritious sources **(FIGURE 9.14)**. Greek yogurts have also become very popular and are a good source of calcium, but their calcium content is lower than that of regular yogurt (1 cup of Greek yogurt has about 270 mg calcium, compared to 448 mg in a cup of regular yogurt). This is due to some calcium being lost in the straining process of Greek yogurt. Ice cream, regular cheese, and whole milk also contain a relatively high amount of calcium, but these foods should be eaten in moderation because of their high fat and energy content.

Other good nondairy sources of calcium are green leafy vegetables, such as kale, collard greens, turnip greens, broccoli, cauliflower, green cabbage, brussels sprouts, and Chinese cabbage (bok choy). The bioavailability of the calcium in these vegetables is relatively high compared to spinach because these vegetables contain low levels of oxalates. Many processed foods are now fortified with calcium. For example, you can buy calcium-fortified orange juice, soymilk and other milk alternatives, and tofu processed with calcium. Some dairies have even boosted the amount of calcium in their brand of milk!

Although many foods are good sources of calcium, many Americans do not have adequate intakes (AIs) because they consume few dairy-based foods and calcium-rich nondairy sources such as green leafy vegetables. Recent results from the National Health and Nutrition Examination Survey (NHANES) indicate that on average, adult

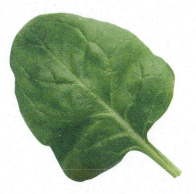

◄ Although spinach contains high levels of calcium, binding factors in the plant prevent much of its absorption in the body.

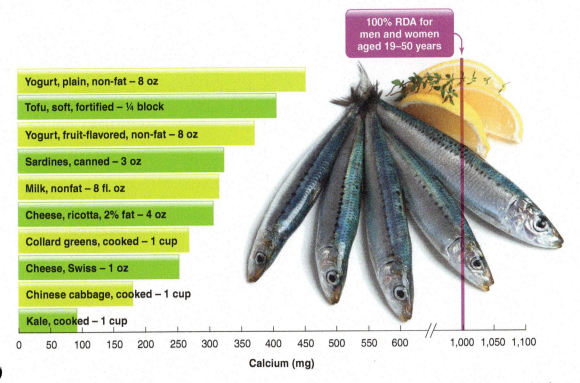

◄ **FIGURE 9.14** Common food sources of calcium. The RDA for calcium is 1,000 mg of calcium per day for men and women aged 19 to 50.

Source: Data from U.S. Department of Agriculture, Agricultural Research Service. 2015. USDA Nutrient Database for Standard Reference, Release 28.

QuickTips

Capitalizing on Calcium

✓ At the grocery store, stock up on calcium-fortified juices and milk alternatives. Look for single-serving portable "juice boxes" with milk, soymilk, or calcium-fortified juice.

✓ Purchase breakfast cereals and breads that are fortified with calcium.

✓ For quick snacks, purchase single-serving cups of no-sugar-added yogurts, individually wrapped "cheese sticks," or calcium-fortified protein bars.

✓ Choose kale, broccoli, and other leafy green vegetables high in calcium at least once every day.

✓ Keep on hand shredded parmesan or any other hard cheese, and sprinkle it on hot soups, chili, salads, pasta, and other dishes.

✓ In any recipe, replace sour cream or mayonnaise with nonfat plain yogurt.

✓ Add nonfat dry milk powder to hot cereals, soups, chili, recipes for baked goods, coffee, and hot cocoa. One-third of a cup of nonfat dry milk powder provides the same amount of calcium as a whole cup of nonfat milk.

✓ Make a yogurt smoothie by blending nonfat plain or flavored yogurt with fresh or frozen fruit.

✓ For a "guilt-free" dessert, try half a cup of plain nonfat Greek yogurt with a drizzle of maple syrup.

✓ At your favorite cafe, instead of black coffee, order a skim milk latte. Instead of black tea, order a cup of chai—spiced Indian tea brewed with milk.

✓ At home, brew a cup of strong coffee; then add half a cup of warm milk for a café au lait.

> To find out if you are getting enough calcium in your diet, take the calcium quiz at www.healthyeating.org. Type "healthy eating tools calcium quiz" into the search box, then click on the top link.

men between the ages of 20 to 59 years exceed the RDA for calcium. However, adult women across all age groups, and men 60 years and older, fail to consume the RDA for calcium.[16]

A variety of quick, simple tools are available on the Internet to help you determine your daily calcium intake. Refer to the Nutrition Online link (in the margin) to access one of these tools. For more help in capitalizing on calcium, see the **Quick Tips** box on this page.

Calcium Toxicity and Deficiency

In general, consuming too much calcium from foods does not lead to toxicity in healthy individuals. Much of the excess calcium we consume is excreted in the feces. However, an excessive intake of calcium from supplements can lead to health problems. Consuming too much calcium can interfere with the absorption of other minerals, including iron, zinc, and magnesium and lead to various mineral imbalances. This may only be of major concern in individuals vulnerable to mineral imbalance, such as the elderly and people who consume very low amounts of minerals in their diets. Another potential problem is kidney stone formation: calcium from foods does not increase the risk for kidney stones, but taking calcium supplements can.[17]

Various diseases and metabolic disorders can alter our ability to regulate blood calcium. **Hypercalcemia** is a condition in which blood calcium levels reach abnormally high concentrations. It can be caused by cancer and by the overproduction of PTH. Symptoms include fatigue, loss of appetite, constipation, and mental confusion, and it can lead to liver and kidney failure, coma, and possibly death.

There are no short-term symptoms associated with consuming too little calcium. Even when we do not consume enough dietary calcium, our body continues to

hypercalcemia A condition marked by an abnormally high concentration of calcium in the blood.

tightly regulate blood calcium levels by taking the calcium from bone. A long-term repercussion of inadequate calcium intake is osteoporosis, discussed **In Depth** immediately following this chapter.

Hypocalcemia is an abnormally low level of calcium in the blood. Hypocalcemia does not result from consuming too little dietary calcium but is caused by various diseases, including kidney disease, vitamin D deficiency, and diseases that inhibit the production of PTH. Symptoms of hypocalcemia include muscle spasms and convulsions.

Phosphorus Combines with Calcium in Hydroxyapatite Crystals

In the body, phosphorus is most commonly found combined with oxygen in the form of phosphate. About 85% of our body's phosphorus is stored in our bones, where it combines with calcium to form hydroxyapatite crystals, which provide the hardness of bone. In addition, phosphorus is the major intracellular negatively charged electrolyte (as discussed in Chapter 7). Phosphorus also helps activate and deactivate enzymes, and it is a component of lipoproteins, cell membranes, DNA and RNA, and several energy molecules, including adenosine triphosphate (ATP).

The RDA for phosphorus is listed in Table 9.1. In general, phosphorus is widespread in many foods and is found in high amounts in foods that contain protein. Milk, meats, and eggs are good sources. (The details of phosphorus recommendations, food sources, and deficiency and toxicity symptoms are covered in Chapter 7.)

Phosphorus is also found in many processed foods as a food additive, where it enhances smoothness, binding, and moisture retention. Moreover, in the form of phosphoric acid, it is added to soft drinks to give them a sharper, or more tart, flavor and to slow the growth of molds and bacteria. Our society has increased its consumption of phosphorus during the past 30 years in processed foods and soft drinks. This could be detrimental to our health, as a recent study found that high phosphorus intake is associated with increased risk of premature mortality in healthy adults.[18]

People with kidney disease and those who take too many vitamin D supplements or too many phosphorus-containing antacids can suffer from high blood phosphorus levels (as discussed in Chapter 7). Severely high levels of blood phosphorus can cause muscle spasms and convulsions.

Phosphorus deficiencies are rare but can occur in people who abuse alcohol, in premature infants, and in elderly people with poor diets. People with vitamin D deficiency, people with hyperparathyroidism (oversecretion of parathyroid hormone), and those who overuse antacids that bind with phosphorus may also have low blood phosphorus levels.

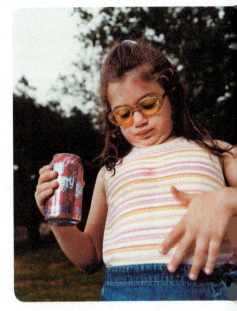

▲ Phosphorus, in the form of phosphoric acid, is a major component of soft drinks.

Magnesium Is a Component of Bone and Helps Regulate Bone Status

Magnesium is a major mineral. Our total body magnesium content is approximately 25g, about 50% to 60% of which is found in our bones. Magnesium is also important in the regulation of bone and mineral status. Specifically, magnesium influences the formation of hydroxyapatite crystals through its regulation of calcium balance and its interactions with vitamin D and PTH.

Magnesium is a critical cofactor for more than 300 enzyme systems. It is necessary for the production of ATP, and it plays an important role in DNA and protein synthesis and repair. Magnesium supplementation has been shown to improve insulin sensitivity, and there is epidemiological evidence that a high magnesium intake is associated with a decrease in the risk for colorectal cancer.[19] Magnesium supports normal vitamin D metabolism and action and is necessary for normal muscle contraction and blood clotting.

The RDA for magnesium is identified in Table 9.1. Magnesium is found in green leafy vegetables, such as spinach; whole grains; seeds; and nuts. Other good sources include seafood and beans **(FIGURE 9.15)** (page 324). Because magnesium is found in a wide variety of foods, people who regularly consume foods high in magnesium and who are adequately nourished should be consuming enough magnesium in their diets.

hypocalcemia A condition characterized by an abnormally low concentration of calcium in the blood.

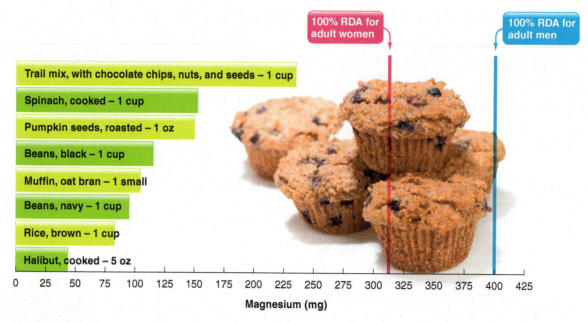

⬥ FIGURE 9.15 Common food sources of magnesium. For adult men 19 to 30 years of age, the RDA for magnesium is 400 mg per day; the RDA increases to 420 mg per day for men 31 years of age and older. For adult women 19 to 30 years of age, the RDA for magnesium is 310 mg per day; this value increases to 320 mg per day for women 31 years of age and older.

Source: Data from U.S. Department of Agriculture, Agricultural Research Service. 2015. USDA Nutrient Database for Standard Reference, Release 28.

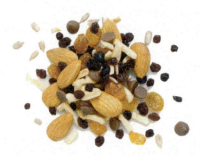

⬥ Trail mix with chocolate chips, nuts, and seeds is a common food source of magnesium.

hypermagnesemia A condition marked by an abnormally high concentration of magnesium in the blood.

hypomagnesemia A condition characterized by an abnormally low concentration of magnesium in the blood.

The ability of the small intestine to absorb magnesium is reduced when one consumes a diet that is extremely high in fiber and phytates because these substances bind with magnesium. Even though seeds and nuts are relatively high in fiber, they are excellent sources of absorbable magnesium. Overall, our absorption of magnesium should be sufficient if we consume the recommended amount of fiber each day (20 to 35 g per day). In contrast, higher dietary protein intakes enhance the absorption and retention of magnesium.

There are no known toxicity symptoms related to consuming excess magnesium in the diet. The toxicity symptoms that result from pharmacologic use of magnesium include diarrhea, nausea, and abdominal cramps. In extreme cases, large doses can result in acid–base imbalances, massive dehydration, cardiac arrest, and death. High blood magnesium levels, or **hypermagnesemia**, occur in individuals with impaired kidney function who consume large amounts of nondietary magnesium, such as antacids. Side effects include the impairment of nerve, muscle, and heart function.

Hypomagnesemia, or low blood magnesium, results from magnesium deficiency. This condition may develop secondary to kidney disease, chronic diarrhea, or chronic alcohol abuse, or as a result of low dietary intake of magnesium. Low blood calcium levels are a side effect of hypomagnesemia.

Symptoms of magnesium deficiency include muscle cramps, spasms or seizures, nausea, weakness, irritability, and confusion. Long-term magnesium deficiency is associated with osteoporosis, as well as many other chronic diseases, including heart disease, high blood pressure, and type 2 diabetes.

Fluoride Is Found in Teeth and Bones

Fluoride, a trace mineral, is the ionic form of the element fluorine. About 99% of the fluoride in our body is stored in our teeth and bones. During the development of both baby and permanent teeth, fluoride combines with calcium and phosphorus to form *fluorohydroxyapatite*, which is more resistant to destruction by acids and bacteria than is hydroxyapatite. Even after all of our permanent teeth are in, treating them

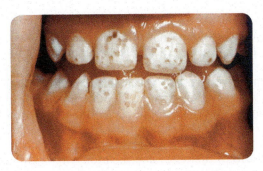

⬥ **FIGURE 9.16** Consuming too much fluoride causes fluorosis, leading to staining and pitting of the teeth.

with fluoride, whether at the dentist's office or by using fluoridated toothpaste, gives them more protection against dental caries (cavities) than teeth that have not been treated. That's because fluoride enhances tooth mineralization, decreases and reverses tooth demineralization, and inhibits the metabolism of the acid-producing bacteria that cause tooth decay.

Our need for fluoride is relatively small. The AI for fluoride is listed in Table 9.1. Fluoride is readily available in many communities in the United States through fluoridated water and dental products. In the mouth, fluoride is absorbed directly into the teeth and gums, and it can be absorbed from the GI tract once it has been ingested.

There are concerns that individuals who consume bottled water exclusively may be getting too little fluoride and increasing their risk for dental caries because most bottled waters do not contain fluoride. However, these individuals may still consume fluoride through other beverages that contain fluoridated water and through fluoridated dental products. Toothpastes and mouthwashes that contain fluoride are widely marketed and used by the majority of consumers in the United States, and these products can contribute as much, if not more, fluoride to our diets than fluoridated water. Fluoride supplements are available only by prescription, and they are generally given only to children who do not have access to fluoridated water. Incidentally, tea is a good source of fluoride: one 8-oz cup provides about 20% to 25% of the AI.

Consuming too much fluoride increases the protein content of tooth enamel, resulting in a condition called **fluorosis**. Because increased protein makes the enamel more porous, the teeth become stained and pitted **(FIGURE 9.16)**. Teeth seem to be at highest risk for fluorosis during the first 8 years of life, when the permanent teeth are developing. To reduce the risk for fluorosis, children should not swallow oral care products that are meant for topical use only, and children under the age of 6 years should be supervised while using fluoride-containing products. Mild fluorosis generally causes white patches on the teeth, but it has no effect on tooth function. Although moderate and severe fluorosis cause greater discoloration of the teeth, there appears to be no adverse effect on tooth function.

Excess consumption of fluoride can also cause fluorosis of our skeletons. Mild skeletal fluorosis results in an increased bone mass and stiffness and pain in the joints. Moderate and severe skeletal fluorosis can be crippling, but it is extremely rare in the United States.

The primary result of fluoride deficiency is dental caries. Adequate fluoride intake appears necessary at an early age and throughout our adult life to reduce our risk for tooth decay.

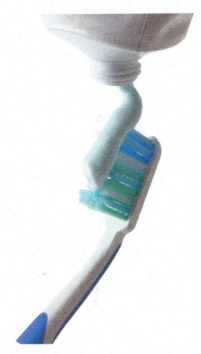

⬥ Fluoride is readily available in many communities in the United States through fluoridated water and dental products.

recap Calcium is the most abundant mineral in the human body and a significant component of our bones. It is also necessary for normal nerve and muscle function. Blood calcium is maintained within a very narrow range, and bone calcium is used to maintain normal blood calcium if dietary intake is inadequate. Dairy products, canned fish with bones, and some green

fluorosis A condition, marked by staining and pitting of the teeth, caused by an abnormally high intake of fluoride.

leafy vegetables are good sources of calcium. The most common long-term effect of inadequate calcium consumption is osteoporosis. Phosphorus is part of the hydroxyapatite crystals of bone. It also helps maintain fluid balance, assists in regulating chemical reactions, and is a primary component of ATP, DNA, and RNA. Phosphorus is commonly found in high-protein foods. Magnesium is important for bone health, energy production, and muscle function. It is found in fresh foods, including spinach, nuts, seeds, whole grains, and seafood. Fluoride is a trace mineral whose primary function is to support the health of teeth and bones. Primary sources of fluoride are fluoridated dental products and fluoridated water. Fluoride toxicity causes fluorosis of the teeth and skeleton, whereas fluoride deficiency causes an increase in tooth decay.

LO 6 Name two fat-soluble vitamins that support bone health and explain their roles.

How do two fat-soluble vitamins support healthy bone?

The fat-soluble vitamins D and K play very different roles in supporting bone health.

Vitamin D Regulates Calcium

Vitamin D is like other fat-soluble vitamins in that we store excess amounts in our liver and adipose tissue. But vitamin D is different from other nutrients in two ways. First, vitamin D does not always need to come from the diet. This is because our body can synthesize vitamin D using energy from exposure to sunlight. However, when we do not get enough sunlight, we must consume vitamin D in foods or supplements. Second, in addition to being a nutrient, vitamin D is considered a *hormone* because it is made in one part of the body yet regulates various activities in other parts of the body.

FIGURE 9.17 illustrates how our body synthesizes vitamin D. When the ultraviolet rays of the sun hit the skin, they react with 7-dehydrocholesterol. This compound is converted into **cholecalciferol**, which is also called provitamin D_3. This inactive form is then converted to calcidiol in the liver, where it is stored. When needed, calcidiol travels to the kidneys, where it is converted into **calcitriol**, which is considered the primary active form of vitamin D in our body. Calcitriol then circulates to various parts of the body, performing its many functions. Excess calcitriol can also be stored in adipose tissue for later use.

Functions of Vitamin D

As illustrated in Focus Figure 9.13, vitamin D and PTH work together continuously to regulate blood calcium levels. They do this by regulating the absorption of calcium and phosphorus from the small intestine, causing more to be absorbed when our needs for them are higher and less when our needs are lower. They also decrease or increase blood calcium levels by signaling the kidneys to excrete more or less calcium in our urine. Finally, vitamin D works with PTH to stimulate osteoclasts to break down bone when calcium is needed elsewhere in the body.

Vitamin D is also necessary for the normal calcification of bone. This means it assists the process by which minerals such as calcium and phosphorus are crystallized. Vitamin D may also play a role in decreasing the formation of some cancerous tumors, as it can prevent certain types of malignant cells from growing out of control. Also, like vitamin A, vitamin D appears to play a role in cell differentiation in various tissues.

Recommended Intakes and Food Sources of Vitamin D

If your exposure to the sun is adequate, then you do not need to consume any vitamin D in your diet. But how do you know whether you are getting enough sun?

Of the many factors that affect your ability to synthesize vitamin D from sunlight, latitude and time of year are the most significant. People living in very sunny climates relatively close to the equator, such as the southern United States and Mexico, may

cholecalciferol Vitamin D_3, a form of vitamin D found in animal foods and the form we synthesize from the sun.

calcitriol The primary active form of vitamin D in the body.

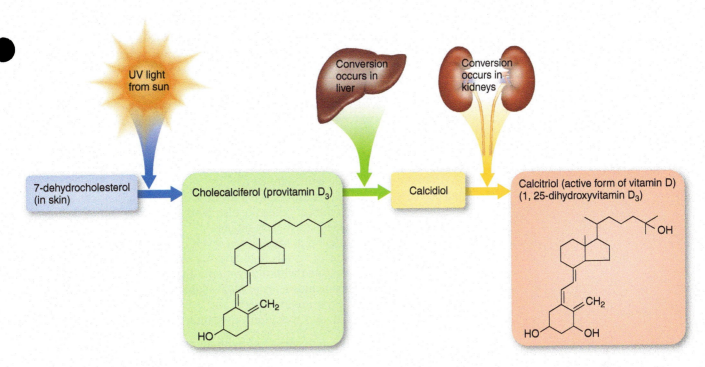

FIGURE 9.17 The process of converting sunlight into vitamin D in our skin. When the ultraviolet rays of the sun hit our skin, they react with 7-dehydrocholesterol. This compound is converted to cholecalciferol, an inactive form of vitamin D also called provitamin D_3. Cholecalciferol is then converted to calcidiol in the liver. Calcidiol travels to the kidneys, where it is converted into calcitriol, which is considered the primary active form of vitamin D in our body.

synthesize enough vitamin D from the sun to meet their needs throughout the year—as long as they spend time outdoors. However, vitamin D synthesis from the sun is not possible during most of the winter months for people living in places located at a latitude of more than 37°N or more than 37°S. At these latitudes in winter the sun never rises high enough in the sky to provide the amount of direct sunlight needed. The 37°N latitude runs like a belt across the United States from northern Virginia in the east to northern California in the west (**FIGURE 9.18**). In addition, entire countries,

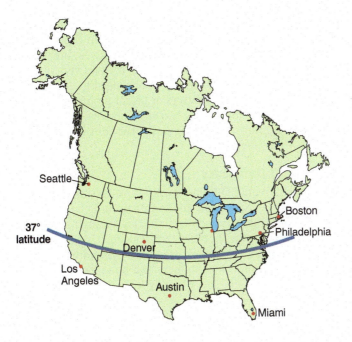

FIGURE 9.18 This map illustrates the geographical location of 37° latitude in the United States. In southern cities below 37° latitude, such as Los Angeles, Austin, and Miami, the sunlight is strong enough to allow for vitamin D synthesis throughout the year. In northern cities above 37° latitude, such as Seattle, Chicago, and Boston, the sunlight is too weak from about mid-October to mid-March to allow for adequate vitamin D synthesis.

such as Canada and the United Kingdom, are affected, as are countries in the far southern hemisphere. Thus, many people around the world need to consume vitamin D in their diets, particularly during the winter months.

Other factors influencing vitamin D synthesis are time of day, skin color, age, and body weight status.

- More vitamin D can be synthesized during the time of day when the sun's rays are strongest, generally between 10 AM and 3 PM. Vitamin D synthesis is severely limited or may be nonexistent on overcast days.
- Darker skin contains more melanin pigment, which reduces the penetration of sunlight. Thus, people with dark skin have a more difficult time synthesizing vitamin D from the sun than do light-skinned people.
- People 65 years of age or older experience a fourfold decrease in their capacity to synthesize vitamin D from the sun; they are also more likely to spend more time indoors and may have inadequate dietary intakes.[20]
- Obesity has recently been found to cause lower levels of circulating vitamin D.[21] Although the exact mechanism for this finding is not clear, this study implicates variations in the genes associated with the synthesis and breakdown of vitamin D. Other possible contributors include a lower bioavailability of cholecalciferol from adipose tissue, decreased exposure to sunlight due to limited mobility or time spent outdoors with skin exposed, and alterations in vitamin D metabolism in the liver.

Wearing protective clothing and sunscreen (with an SPF greater than 8) limits sun exposure, so it is suggested that we expose our hands, face, and arms to the sun two or three times per week for a period of time that is one-third to one-half of the amount needed to get sunburned. This means that, if you normally sunburn in 1 hour, you should expose yourself to the sun for 20 to 30 minutes two or three times per week to synthesize adequate amounts of vitamin D. Again, this guideline does not apply to people living in more northern climates during the winter months; they can get enough vitamin D only by consuming it in their diet.

The recommended intakes of vitamin D are identified in Table 9.1. The current RDA is based on the assumption that an individual does not get adequate sun exposure. Recent evidence suggests that the RDA might not be sufficient to maintain optimal bone health and reduce the risks for diseases such as cancer; the controversy surrounding vitamin D recommendations is discussed in more detail in the **Nutrition Debate** at the end of this chapter.

Most foods naturally contain little vitamin D. The few exceptions are cod liver oil and fatty fish (such as salmon, mackerel, tuna, and sardines), foods that few Americans consume in adequate amounts. Eggs, butter, some margarines, and liver also provide very small amounts of vitamin D.

Thus, the primary sources of vitamin D in the diet are fortified foods **(FIGURE 9.19)**. In the United States, milk is fortified with 100 IU of vitamin D per cup.[20] Additional foods fortified with vitamin D include some milk alternatives, breakfast cereals, margarine, orange juice, and yogurt. Because plants contain very little vitamin D, vegetarians who consume no fortified dairy products need to obtain their vitamin D from sun exposure, fortified milk alternatives or cereal products, or supplements. When reading the labels of fortified foods and supplements, you will see the amount of vitamin D expressed in units of either μg or IU. For conversion purposes, 1 μg of vitamin D is equal to 40 IU of vitamin D.

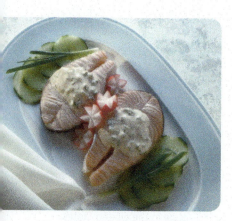

▲ Fatty fish contain vitamin D.

Vitamin D Toxicity and Deficiency

We cannot get too much vitamin D from sun exposure because our skin has the ability to limit its production. As just noted, foods contain little natural vitamin D. Thus, the only way we can consume too much vitamin D is through supplementation.

Consuming too much vitamin D causes hypercalcemia, or high blood calcium concentrations. See the section on calcium for signs and symptoms of hypercalcemia. In addition, toxic levels of vitamin D lead to increased bone loss because calcium is then pulled from the bones and excreted more readily from the kidneys.

The primary deficiency associated with inadequate vitamin D is loss of bone mass. In fact, when vitamin D levels are inadequate, our small intestine can absorb only

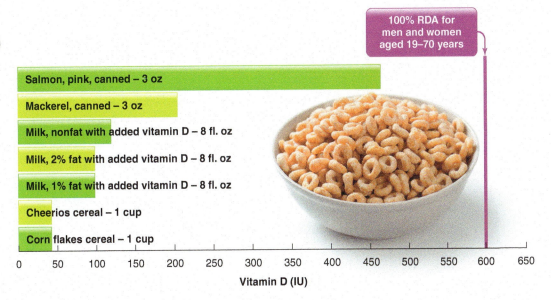

100% RDA for men and women aged 19–70 years

Salmon, pink, canned – 3 oz

Mackerel, canned – 3 oz

Milk, nonfat with added vitamin D – 8 fl. oz

Milk, 2% fat with added vitamin D – 8 fl. oz

Milk, 1% fat with added vitamin D – 8 fl. oz

Cheerios cereal – 1 cup

Corn flakes cereal – 1 cup

0   50   100   150   200   250   300   350   400   450   500   550   600   650

Vitamin D (IU)

🔺 **FIGURE 9.19**   Common food sources of vitamin D. For men and women aged 19 to 70 years, the RDA for vitamin D is 600 IU per day. The RDA increases to 800 IU per day for adults over the age of 70 years.

Source: Data from U.S. Department of Agriculture, Agricultural Research Service. 2015. USDA Nutrient Database for Standard Reference, Release 28.

10% to 15% of the calcium we consume. Vitamin D deficiencies occur most often in individuals who have diseases that cause intestinal malabsorption of fat and thus the fat-soluble vitamins. People with liver disease, kidney disease, Crohn's disease, celiac disease, cystic fibrosis, or Whipple's disease may suffer from vitamin D deficiency and require supplements.

Vitamin D deficiency disease in children, called **rickets**, is caused by inadequate mineralization or demineralization of the skeleton. The classic sign of rickets is deformity of the skeleton, such as bowed legs and knocked knees **(FIGURE 9.20)**. However, severe cases can be fatal. Rickets is not common in the United States because of the fortification of milk products with vitamin D, but children with illnesses that cause fat malabsorption, or who drink no milk and get limited sun exposure, are at increased risk. There is no national surveillance program for rickets, and thus it is not clear what the prevalence of rickets is in the United States. However, a recent study conducted in Minnesota found an increase in cases of rickets in children 3 years of age and younger from 0 in 1970 to 24 per 100,000 in 2000. Increased risk in these children was associated with having darker skin (because the need for adequate sun exposure is higher than for light-skinned children) and breastfeeding (because breast milk contains little vitamin D).[22] None of the breast-fed children were reported to have received vitamin D supplementation before being diagnosed. Other contributing factors included poor feeding, limited sun exposure, limited milk intake, a predominantly vegetarian diet, and being born prematurely.

Vitamin D–deficiency disease in adults is called **osteomalacia**, a term meaning "soft bones." With osteomalacia, bones become weak and prone to fractures. Osteoporosis (discussed **In Depth** on pages 334–341) can also result from a vitamin D deficiency.

Vitamin D deficiencies have recently been found to be more common among American adults than previously thought. This may be partly due to jobs and lifestyle choices that keep people indoors for most of the day. Not surprisingly, the population at greatest risk is older institutionalized individuals who get little or no sun exposure.

Various medications can also alter the metabolism and activity of vitamin D. For instance, glucocorticoids, which are medications used to reduce inflammation, can cause bone loss by inhibiting the ability to absorb calcium through the actions of vitamin D. Antiseizure medications can also alter vitamin D metabolism. Thus, people who are taking such medications may need to increase their vitamin D intake.

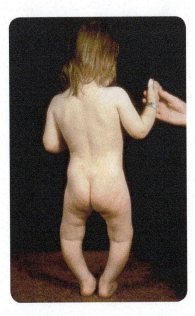

🔺 **FIGURE 9.20**   A vitamin D deficiency causes a bone-deforming disease in children called rickets.

rickets A vitamin D–deficiency disease in children. Signs include deformities of the skeleton, such as bowed legs and knocked knees. Severe rickets can be fatal.

osteomalacia A vitamin D–deficiency disease in adults, in which bones become weak and prone to fractures.

nutri-case | THEO

"The health center here on campus is running a study on vitamin D levels among students, and the instructor in my nutrition class encouraged everyone to participate. I don't think I need to be worried about it, though, 'cause I exercise outdoors a lot—at least, whenever Wisconsin weather allows it! It's true I don't drink much milk, and I hate fish, but otherwise I eat right, and besides, I'm a guy, so I don't have to worry about my bone density."

Should Theo have his vitamin D levels checked? Why or why not? Before you answer, take another look back at the information in this section. Also, consider Theo's assertion that because he is male he doesn't have to worry about his bone density. Is he right? And is calcium regulation the only significant role of vitamin D?

Vitamin K Assists in Remodeling of Bone

The role of fat-soluble vitamin K in blood clotting was discussed earlier in this chapter. Vitamin K also assists in the production of osteocalcin, a protein involved in bone remodeling.

We can obtain vitamin K from our diets, and we absorb the vitamin K produced by bacteria in our large intestine. These two sources usually provide adequate amounts of this nutrient to maintain health, and there is no RDA or UL for vitamin K. The AI is listed in Table 9.1.

Only a few foods contribute substantially to our dietary intake of vitamin K. Green leafy vegetables, including kale, spinach, collard greens, turnip greens, and lettuce, are good sources, as are broccoli, brussels sprouts, and cabbage. Vegetable oils, such as soybean oil and canola oil, are also good sources.

Based on our current knowledge, for healthy individuals there appear to be no side effects associated with consuming large amounts of vitamin K. This appears to be true for both supplements and food sources.

Vitamin K deficiency is associated with a reduced ability to form blood clots, leading to excessive bleeding; however, primary vitamin K deficiency is rare except in people with malabsorption diseases. Long-term use of antibiotics, which typically reduce bacterial populations in the colon, combined with limited dietary intake of vitamin K–rich food sources, can also lead to vitamin K deficiency.

The effect of vitamin K on bone health is controversial. As recently described, the effect of vitamin K on bone mineral density appears to be modest, and studies report inconsistent results.[23] Thus, there is not enough scientific evidence to support the contention that vitamin K deficiency directly causes osteoporosis. In fact, there is no significant impact on overall bone density in people who take anticoagulant medications that result in a relative state of vitamin K deficiency.

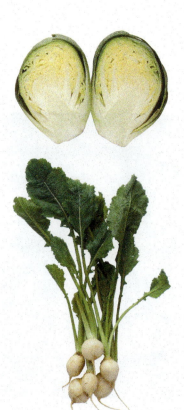

▲ Green leafy vegetables, including brussels sprouts and turnip greens, are good sources of vitamin K.

recap Vitamin D is a fat-soluble vitamin and a hormone. It can be made in the skin using energy from sunlight. Vitamin D regulates blood calcium levels and maintains bone health. Foods contain little vitamin D, with fortified milk being the primary source. Vitamin D toxicity causes hypercalcemia. Vitamin D deficiency can result in osteoporosis; rickets is vitamin D deficiency in children, whereas osteomalacia is vitamin D deficiency in adults. Vitamin K is a fat-soluble vitamin and coenzyme that is important for blood clotting and bone remodeling. We obtain vitamin K largely from bacteria in our large intestine. Green leafy vegetables and vegetable oils contain vitamin K.

nutrition debate

Vitamin D Deficiency: Why the Surge, and What Can Be Done?

No doubt about it: unless you live at a latitude within 37° of the equator and spend time outdoors without sunscreen, it's tough to get enough vitamin D. That's because, as you learned in this chapter, there are very few natural food sources of vitamin D, and even fortified food sources are limited to milk and a handful of other products. But if meeting the National Academy of Science's current RDA for vitamin D is already posing a challenge to many Americans, why are some researchers calling for an even higher intake recommendation?

Measurements of vitamin D status in a variety of population studies in recent years have led to a growing concern about widespread vitamin D deficiency and its associated diseases, including rickets in children and osteomalacia and osteoporosis in adults. The most recently published analysis of vitamin D deficiency in U.S. adults indicates an overall prevalence of 42%, with 82% of Blacks and 69% of Hispanics estimated to be vitamin D deficient.[24] Although the National Academy of Science emphasizes the role of vitamin D in optimizing bone and musculoskeletal health exclusively,[20] the potential role of vitamin D in decreasing the risk for type 2 diabetes and reducing premature mortality suggest a need to further explore whether vitamin D recommendations should be reexamined.[25-27]

What is contributing to the dramatic increase in vitamin D deficiency? Researchers have proposed the following three causative factors:[28]

- A downward trend in the consumption of vitamin D–fortified milk products
- A significant increase in sun avoidance and the use of sun protection products, such as sunscreen
- An increased rate of obesity because obesity appears to alter the metabolism and storage of vitamin D such that vitamin D deficiency is more likely to occur

To address the first factor, people can increase their intake of vitamin D–fortified milk products; however, it is difficult to meet even the current RDA from consumption of milk alone. For instance, children and teens would have to drink a full quart each day to meet the recommendation! As a result, the use of vitamin D supplements is gaining wide support. Recently published clinical practice guidelines state that children and adolescents aged 1 to 18 years who are vitamin D deficient should be treated

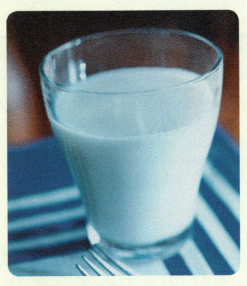

It is difficult to meet the current RDA for vitamin D through the consumption of fortified milk alone.

with 2,000 IU of vitamin D per day for at least 6 weeks, followed by a maintenance supplement of 600 to 1,000 IU per day.[28] Additionally, it is recommended that all adults who are vitamin D deficient should be treated with 6,000 IU of vitamin D per day for 8 weeks, followed by a maintenance supplement of 1,500 to 2,000 IU per day.[28] Supplementation with vitamin D is efficient, inexpensive, and effective. Used correctly, it is also very safe. Although vitamin D toxicity is rare, supplementation should be monitored to ensure both a safe and sufficient intake.

What about the second factor—lack of sufficient exposure to sunlight? Responsible, safe exposure to sunlight offers many advantages: it will never lead to vitamin D toxicity, it is easy and virtually cost-free, and sun exposure may offer benefits beyond that of improved vitamin D status. That's why many healthcare professionals advocate moderate sun exposure. They suggest that public health authorities soften the "sun avoidance" campaigns of recent years; they would like to see "well-balanced" recommendations that promote brief (15 minutes or so) periods of sun exposure without sunscreen or sun-blocking clothing two or three times a week, with avoidance of midday sun during summer months.[29]

To address the third factor in vitamin D deficiency—obesity—the only solution is to maintain a healthful weight. That means losing weight if you are overweight or obese. By doing so, you'll reduce your risk not only for vitamin D deficiency but also for cardiovascular disease, type 2 diabetes, and many forms of cancer.

CRITICAL THINKING QUESTIONS

1. Go online and find the latitude of your geographic area. Do you live in a region where your body can synthesize vitamin D from sunlight all year long, or only from late spring to early fall? In mid-summer, how much sun exposure would you need per week to synthesize adequate vitamin D?
2. Do you think you would benefit from vitamin D supplementation? Why or why not?
3. Would you prefer to try to increase your circulating levels of vitamin D through natural foods, fortified foods, supplements, or increased sun exposure? State your reasoning.

TEST YOURSELF | ANSWERS

1 **T** This deficiency is particularly common in infants, children, and women of childbearing age.

2 **F** Besides milk, yogurt, and cheese, good sources of calcium include green, leafy vegetables such as broccoli and kale, as well as many fortified beverages such as soymilk.

3 **T** When exposed to sunlight, the body can convert a cholesterol compound in the skin into vitamin D.

review questions

LO 1 1. Which of the following statements about iron is true?

a. Iron picks up oxygen in the lungs, binds it to cytochromes in red blood cells, and exchanges it for carbon dioxide in the liver.

b. About two-thirds of the body's iron is found in hemoglobin, the oxygen-carrying compound in red blood cells.

c. Heme iron is available only from animal-based foods, and non-heme iron is available only from plant-based foods.

d. The primary cause of iron toxicity is overconsumption of red meat.

LO 1 2. Abnormally small red blood cells are characteristic of

a. iron-deficiency anemia.
b. sickle cell anemia.
c. pernicious anemia.
d. megaloblastic anemia.

LO 2 3. The micronutrient most closely associated with blood clotting is

a. folate.
b. vitamin K.
c. vitamin B_6.
d. vitamin B_{12}.

LO 3 4. Which of the following is a function of vitamin C?

a. Helps regulate blood calcium levels.
b. Acts as a coenzyme in the synthesis of ascorbic acid.
c. Acts as a coenzyme in the synthesis of procoagulant proteins.
d. Is essential for the synthesis of collagen.

LO 4 5. Which of the following statements about trabecular bone is true?

a. It accounts for about 80% of the skeleton.
b. It is also called compact bone.
c. It has a faster turnover rate than cortical bone.
d. It is not subject to remodeling.

LO 5 6. Calcium is necessary for several body functions, including

a. demineralization of bone, nerve impulse transmission, and immune responses.
b. structure of collagen and cartilage, nerve impulse transmission, and muscle contraction.
c. structure of bone, nerve, and muscle tissue; immune responses; and muscle contraction.
d. structure of bone, nerve impulse transmission, muscle contraction, and blood clotting.

LO 6 7. Which of the following is a function of vitamin D and parathyroid hormone (PTH)?

a. They regulate the absorption of calcium and phosphorus from the small intestine.
b. They regulate the liver's reabsorption of calcium.
c. They stimulate the release of thyroid hormones from the thyroid gland.
d. They stimulate the activity of osteoclasts when blood calcium levels become excessively high.

LO 6 8. Which of the following individuals is most likely to require vitamin D supplements?

a. a dark-skinned child living and playing outdoors in Hawaii.
b. a fair-skinned construction worker living in Florida.
c. a fair-skinned retired teacher living in a nursing home in Ohio.
d. None of the above individuals is likely to require vitamin D supplements.

LO 1 9. **True or false?** Copper deficiency can result in accumulation of iron in the body.

LO 6 10. **True or false?** Our body can absorb vitamin D from sunlight.

math review

LO 1 11. About 2 g of zinc are stored in the body of an average adult. An adult male consumes 20 mg of zinc each day. He thereby replaces his total body store of zinc every 100 days. Is this statement true or false? Why?

Answers to Review Questions and Math Review are located at the back of this text and in the MasteringNutrition Study Area.

web links

www.womenshealth.gov
Office on Women's Health Anemia Fact Sheet
To locate this fact sheet providing information about iron-deficiency anemia, type "Anemia Fact Sheet" into the search box on the home page.

www.ars.usda.gov
Nutrient Data Laboratory Home Page
Start by entering "nutrient data laboratory home page" in the search box. Then, click on "Reports for Single Nutrients" to find reports listing food sources for selected nutrients.

www.medlineplus.gov
MEDLINE Plus Health Information
Search for "rickets" or "osteomalacia" to learn more about these vitamin D–deficiency diseases.

www.ada.org
American Dental Association
Look under "Public Programs" and select "Advocating for the Public" to learn more about the fluoridation of community water supplies and the use of fluoride-containing products.

ods.od.nih.gov
Office of Dietary Supplements, National Institutes of Health
Search for "calcium supplements" and "vitamin D supplements" to learn more about the supplementation in promoting bone health.

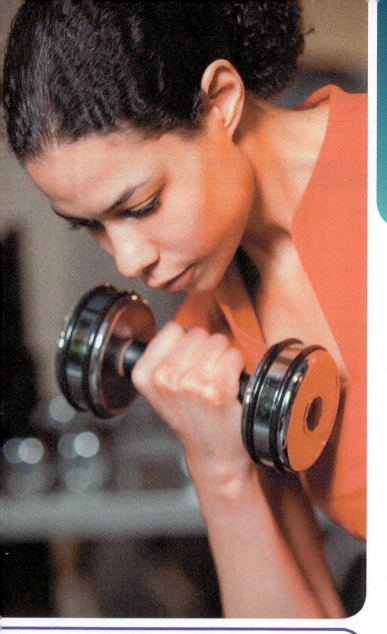

Osteoporosis

A college junior majoring in elementary education, Chloe plans to pursue a teaching career just like her mother. What she hopes she won't share with her mom is her medical history: Chloe's mother is only 53 years old, but after a fall in which she broke her wrist and forearm, her physician told her that she has osteoporosis, a disease characterized by abnormally fragile, "porous" bone. Chloe has been researching osteoporosis, and knows that the condition can cause frequent fractures as well as a disfiguring curvature of the spine. Maintaining a slender and youthful appearance has always been important to Chloe's mother, so Chloe worries how the disease might affect her mother emotionally as well as physically. In the meantime, every time she looks in the mirror she wonders—is she, too, at risk?

In this **In Depth**, we'll take a closer look at osteoporosis. We'll explore its impact on health and longevity and identify the most significant risk factors. We'll also review what is currently known about the role of prescription medications in treating osteoporosis, and the role of lifestyle choices in prevention.

learning outcomes

After studying this In Depth, you should be able to:

1 Define osteoporosis and discuss its impact on a person's health and longevity, p. 335.

2 Discuss the factors that influence our risk for osteoporosis, pp. 335–339.

3 Describe medical treatments and lifestyle changes used to manage osteoporosis, p. 339.

4 Explain how we can prevent, or reduce our risks for, osteoporosis, pp. 339–341.

What is osteoporosis?

Of the many disorders associated with poor bone health, the most prevalent in the United States is **osteoporosis**, a disease characterized by low bone mass. The bone tissue of a person with osteoporosis deteriorates over time, becoming thinner and more porous than that of a person with healthy bone. These structural changes weaken the bone, leading to a significantly reduced ability of the bone to bear weight **(FIGURE 1)**. This greatly increases the person's risk for a fracture (a broken bone). In the United States, more than 2 million fractures each year are attributed to osteoporosis.[1]

Because the hip and the vertebrae of the spinal column are common sites of osteoporosis, it is not surprising that osteoporosis is the single most important cause of fractures of the hip and spine in older adults **(FIGURE 2)**. These fractures are extremely painful and can be debilitating, with many individuals requiring nursing home care.

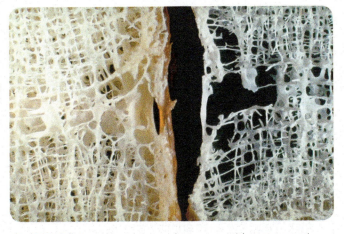

⬆ **FIGURE 1** The vertebrae of a person with osteoporosis (right) are thinner and more collapsed than the vertebrae of a healthy person (left), in which the bone is more dense and uniform.

In addition, they increase the person's risk for infection and other related illnesses, which can lead to premature death. In fact, about 20% of older adults who suffer a hip fracture die within 1 year after the fracture occurs, and because men are typically older at the time of fracture, death rates are higher for men than for women.[1,2]

Osteoporosis of the spine also causes a generalized loss of height and can be disfiguring and painful: gradual compression fractures in the vertebrae of the upper back lead to a shortening and hunching of the spine called *kyphosis,* commonly referred to as *dowager's hump* **(FIGURE 3**, page 336). The changes that kyphosis causes in the structure of the rib cage can impair breathing; moreover, back pain from collapsed or fractured vertebrae can be severe. However, especially in the early stages, osteoporosis can be a silent disease: the person may have no awareness of the condition until a fracture occurs.

Osteoporosis is a common disease: worldwide, one in three women and one in five men over the age of 50 will experience an osteoporotic fracture. In the United States, more than 54 million people have been diagnosed with either osteoporosis or low bone density that can lead to osteoporosis, and half of all women and one in four men over the age of 50 will suffer an osteoporosis-related fracture in their lifetime.[1,2]

What influences osteoporosis risk?

The factors that influence the risk for osteoporosis are age, gender, genetics, substance use, nutrition, and physical activity **(TABLE 1)** (page 336).

osteoporosis A disease characterized by low bone mass and deterioration of bone tissue, leading to increased bone fragility and fracture risk.

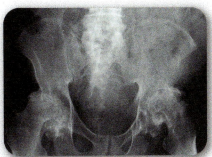
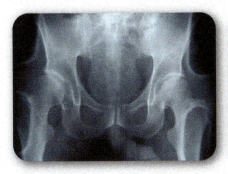
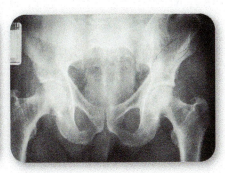

(a) Healthy hip bone   **(b) Osteoporotic hip bone**   **(c) Fractured hip bone**

⬆ **FIGURE 2** These x-rays reveal the progression of osteoporosis in hip bones. **(a)** Healthy bone. **(b)** A hip bone weakened by osteoporosis. **(c)** An osteoporotic bone that has fractured.

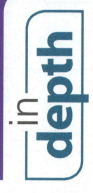

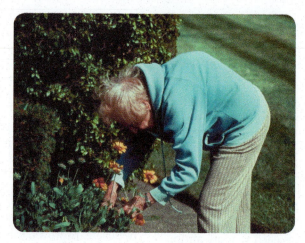

⬥ **FIGURE 3** Gradual compression of the vertebrae in the upper back causes a shortening and rounding of the spine called *kyphosis*.

Aging Increases Osteoporosis Risk

Because bone density declines with age, low bone mass and osteoporosis are significant health concerns for older adults. The prevalence of osteoporosis and low bone mass are predicted to increase in the United States during the next 20 years, primarily because of increased longevity; as the U.S. population ages, more people will live long enough to suffer from osteoporosis.

For a helpful video overview of osteoporosis, go to www .methodisthealthsystem.org. Type "osteoporosis animation" in the search bar, then click on "Osteoporosis."

Hormonal changes that occur with aging have a significant impact on bone loss. Average bone loss is approximately 0.3% to 0.5% per year after 30 years of age; however, during menopause in women, levels of the hormone estrogen decrease dramatically and cause bone loss to increase to about 3% per year during the first 5 years of menopause **(FIGURE 4)**. Both estrogen and testosterone play important roles in promoting the deposition of new bone and limiting the activity of osteoclasts. Thus, age-related decreases in testosterone can contribute to osteoporosis in men. In addition, a decreased ability to metabolize vitamin D with age exacerbates the hormone-related bone loss in both sexes.

Gender and Genetics Affect Osteoporosis Risk

Approximately 80% of Americans with osteoporosis are women. There are three primary reasons for this:

- Women have a lower absolute bone density than men. From birth through puberty, bone mass is the same in girls as in boys. But during puberty, bone mass increases more in boys, probably because of their prolonged period of accelerated growth. This means that, when bone loss begins around age 40, women have less bone stored in their skeleton; thus, the loss of bone that occurs with aging causes osteoporosis sooner and to a greater extent in women.
- The hormonal changes that occur in men as they age do not have as dramatic an effect on bone density as those in women.
- On average, women live longer than men, and because risk increases with age, more elderly women suffer from this disease.

A secondary factor that is gender-specific is the social pressure on girls to be thin. Extreme dieting is particularly harmful in adolescence, when bone mass is building and an adequate consumption of calcium and other nutrients

TABLE 1 Risk Factors for Osteoporosis

Modifiable Risk Factors	Nonmodifiable Risk Factors
Smoking	Older age (elderly)
Low body weight	Caucasian or Asian race
Low calcium intake	History of fractures as an adult
Low sun exposure	Family history of osteoporosis
Alcohol abuse	Gender (female)
History of amenorrhea (failure to menstruate) in women with inadequate nutrition	History of amenorrhea (failure to menstruate) in women with no recognizable cause
Estrogen deficiency (females)	
Testosterone deficiency (males)	
Repeated falls	
Sedentary lifestyle	

Source: Information adapted from the National Osteoporosis Society. 2014. Factors that increase your risk of osteoporosis and fracture. https://www .nos.org.uk/healthy-bones-and-risks/are-you-at-risk

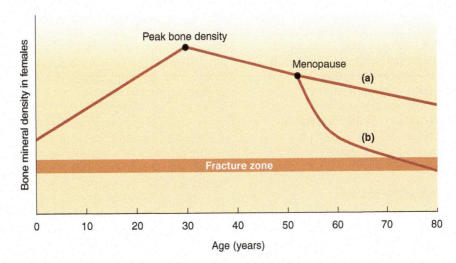

FIGURE 4 Bone mineral density in women tends to decline with aging. **(a)** A healthful lifestyle, an optimal diet, physical activity, and possible use of medication slow loss of bone. **(b)** The rapid loss of estrogen with menopause can cause a decrease in bone density and increased risk for bone fracture for women who do not adhere to a regimen of healthful lifestyle, diet, physical activity, and possibly medication.

is critical. In many girls, weight loss causes both a loss of estrogen and reduced weight-bearing stress on the bones. In contrast, boys experience pressure to "bulk up," typically by lifting weights. This puts healthful stress on the bones, resulting in increased density.

Some individuals have a family history of osteoporosis, which increases their risk for this disease. Particularly at risk are Caucasian women of low body weight who have a first-degree relative (such as a mother or sister) with osteoporosis. Asian women are at higher risk than other non-Caucasian groups. Studies examining families indicate a strong genetic component in bone mineral density, with a recent study identifying an assortment of genes that appear to influence postmenopausal estrogen levels and bone resorption rates, thereby affecting osteoporosis risk.[3] Although we cannot change our gender or genetics, we can modify the lifestyle factors that affect our risk for osteoporosis.

Tobacco, Alcohol, and Caffeine Influence Osteoporosis Risk

Cigarette smoking is known to decrease bone density because of its effects on the hormones that influence bone formation and resorption. For this reason, cigarette smoking increases the risk for osteoporosis and resulting fractures.[4]

Chronic alcohol abuse is detrimental to bone health and is associated with high rates of fractures. In contrast, a recent review has reported that bone density may be higher in people who are *light* or *moderate* drinkers, but the findings differ depending upon a person's age, gender, and the form of alcohol consumed.[5] Although light-to-moderate alcohol intake may be protective for bone, the dangers of alcohol abuse for overall health warrant caution in considering any dietary recommendations. As

is consistent with the alcohol intake recommendations related to heart disease, people should not start drinking if they are nondrinkers, and people who do drink should do so in moderation. That means no more than two drinks per day for men and one drink per day for women.

Some researchers consider excess caffeine consumption to be detrimental to bone health. Caffeine is known to increase calcium loss in the urine, at least over a brief period. Younger people are able to compensate for this calcium loss by increasing absorption of calcium from the intestine; however, some researchers contend that older people are not capable of compensating to the same degree. In contrast to these views, a recent study following

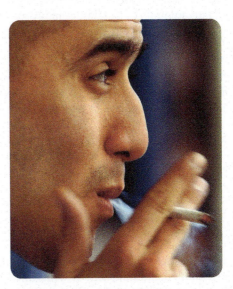

Smoking increases the risk for osteoporosis and resulting fractures.

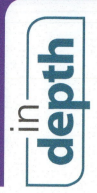
more than 61,000 women in Sweden found that, although a high coffee intake (greater than or equal to 4 cups daily) was associated with a 2% to 4% lower bone density as compared to a low coffee intake (less than 1 cup daily), this did not result in a higher risk for osteoporosis or fractures.[6] Thus, it may be that higher caffeine intakes result in a slight reduction in bone density, but this reduction may not be clinically significant.

Nutritional Factors Influence Osteoporosis Risk

In addition to their role in reducing the risk for heart disease and cancer, diets high in fruits and vegetables are also associated with improved bone health.[7,8] This is most likely due to the fact that many fruits and vegetables are good sources of micronutrients that play a role in bone and collagen health, including calcium, magnesium, vitamin C, and vitamin K. Ahead, we discuss the effects of protein, calcium, vitamin D, and sodium on bone health, as these have been the subject of extensive research.

Protein

Protein is a critical component of bone tissue and is necessary for bone health; however, high protein intakes increase calcium loss. Thus, adequate calcium intake is key. Early research on this topic illustrated that older adults taking calcium and vitamin D supplements and eating higher-protein diets were able to significantly increase bone mass over a 3-year period, whereas those eating more protein and not taking supplements lost bone mass over the same time period.[9] More recent research indicates that adequate intakes of both protein and calcium are necessary to maximize bone mass and prevent fractures in adolescents and older adults.[10] Thus, there appears to be an interaction between dietary calcium and protein, in that adequate amounts of each nutrient are needed together to support bone health.

Calcium and Vitamin D

Of the many nutrients that help maintain bone health, calcium and vitamin D have received the most attention for their role in the prevention of osteoporosis. It is clear that consuming adequate amounts of both nutrients in our diets is critical because people who do not consume enough of these two nutrients over a prolonged period have a lower bone density and thus a higher risk for fractures.

However, whether taking calcium and vitamin D supplements is effective in preventing osteoporosis is somewhat controversial. The U.S. Preventive Services Task Force (USPSTF) recently commissioned two systematic reviews and a meta-analysis to examine the impact of vitamin D supplementation with or without calcium on bone health in community-dwelling adults who did not have a history of fractures.[11] Based on these reviews, the USPSTF has concluded that although appropriate intake of calcium and vitamin D are essential to promoting health, the current evidence is insufficient to draw any conclusions about the benefits and harms of vitamin D and calcium supplementation in preventing fractures in premenopausal women, men, or non-institutionalized postmenopausal women.[11] As such, they recommend against daily supplementation.

Because bones reach peak density when people are young, it is very important to emphasize that children and adolescents should consume a high-quality diet that contains the proper balance of calcium, vitamin D, protein, and other nutrients to allow for optimal bone growth. Adults also require a proper balance of these nutrients to maintain bone mass.

Sodium

Although there is some evidence that high intakes of sodium are associated with increased urinary calcium excretion,[12] there is no direct evidence that a high-sodium diet causes osteoporosis. At this time, the National Academy of Science states that there is insufficient evidence to warrant different calcium recommendations based on dietary salt intake.[13]

Regular Physical Activity Reduces Osteoporosis Risk

Regular exercise is consistently reported to be highly protective against bone loss and osteoporosis. Athletes are consistently shown to have more dense bones than non-athletes, and health professionals and bone health organizations support the contention that regular participation in weight-bearing exercises (such as walking, jogging,

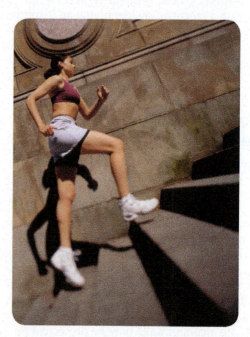

Regularly engaging in weight-bearing exercises, such as jogging, can help increase and maintain your bone mass.

skipping rope, tennis, and strength training) can help increase and maintain bone mass.

How might exercise reduce our risk for osteoporosis? When we exercise, our muscles contract and pull on our bones; this stresses bone tissue in a healthful way that stimulates increases in bone density. In addition, carrying weight during activities such as walking and jogging stresses the bones of the legs, hips, and lower back, resulting in a healthier bone mass in these areas. It appears that people of all ages can improve and maintain bone health through consistent physical activity.

Although a number of studies of the effect of exercise in adults may show relatively small increases or even no change in bone density,[14,15] bone health and fracture risk are not simply a matter of bone density. Factors contributing to a person's risk for fractures include the strength of muscles, joints, and bones, of which bone density is only a part. Based on the current evidence, leading bone health organizations are consistent in maintaining the position that regular weight-bearing exercise such as walking, jogging, and resistance exercises are critical to promoting bone health and reducing a person's risks for falls and fractures.[16]

Can exercise ever be detrimental to bone health? Yes, exercise can be harmful when the body is not receiving the nutrients it needs to rebuild the hydroxyapatite and collagen broken down in response to physical activity. Thus, active people who are chronically malnourished, including people who are impoverished and those who suffer from eating disorders, are at increased fracture risk. Research has confirmed this association in a potentially serious condition called *relative energy deficiency in sport* (RED-S). This syndrome occurs in women and men, and has a negative impact not only on bone health, but also on growth and development, immunity, and many other body functions. A form of RED-S specific to girls and women is the *female athlete triad,* a condition characterized by low energy availability, menstrual dysfunction, and low bone density. This condition is discussed **In Depth** in the essay following Chapter 11 (pages 413–423).

Want to calculate your risk for osteoporosis? Take the International Osteoporosis Foundation's One-Minute Osteoporosis risk quiz at http://www.iofbonehealth.org/. Type "one-minute osteoporosis risk quiz" in the search bar, and then click on the link to the quiz.

How is osteoporosis treated?

LO 3 Describe medical treatments and lifestyle changes used to manage osteoporosis.

Although there is no cure for osteoporosis, a variety of lifestyle changes and medical therapies can slow and even reverse bone loss. First, individuals with osteoporosis are encouraged to consume a diet providing adequate calcium and vitamin D and to exercise regularly. Studies have shown that the most effective exercise programs include impact-loading exercises (such as jogging, jumping, and stair climbing), and resistance training.[17–19]

In addition, several medications are available:

- *Bisphosphonates,* such as alendronate (brand name Fosamax), which decrease bone loss and can increase bone density and reduce the risk for spinal and nonspinal fractures. However, they do not appear to reduce risk for a postmenopausal woman's first osteoporotic fracture, suggesting these medications may not be effective for primary prevention of fractures in postmenopausal women.[20]
- *Selective estrogen receptor modulators,* such as raloxifene (brand name Evista), which have an estrogen-like effect on bone tissue, slowing the rate of bone loss and prompting some increase in bone mass
- *Calcitonin* (brand name Calcimar or Miacalcin), a pharmacologic preparation of a hormone produced by the thyroid gland, which can reduce the rate of bone loss
- *Hormone replacement therapy* (HRT), which combines estrogen with a hormone called progestin and can reduce bone loss, increase bone density, and reduce the risk for hip and spinal fractures.
- *Teriparatide,* which is a synthetic form of parathyroid hormone and is used only in severe cases of osteoporosis, particularly in people with spinal fractures or people with very low bone density, or when other treatments have not been effective. It helps new bone to form.

All of these drugs can prompt side effects, some of which are significant, and therefore the patient should weigh the risks and benefits with their healthcare provider.[21–23]

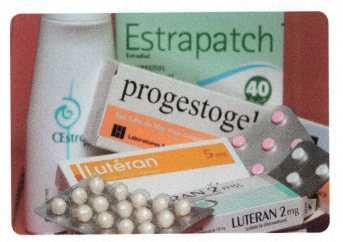

Hormone replacement medications come in a variety of forms.

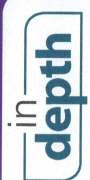

Can osteoporosis be prevented?

LO 4 Explain how we can prevent, or reduce our risks for, osteoporosis.

Although some risk factors for osteoporosis cannot be changed, such as age, gender, race, and family history, there is a great deal you can do to try to prevent osteoporosis.

Some People Might Benefit from Supplements

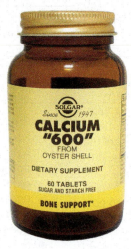

Calcium supplements derived from oyster shell may be high in lead.

As discussed earlier in this chapter, the USP-STF has concluded that the current evidence is insufficient to promote calcium and vitamin D supplementation in community-dwelling older adults who are not at risk for falls. However, some people who have inadequate dietary intakes of these nutrients may benefit from supplementation. These include small, inactive, or elderly people who are not able to consume enough food to provide adequate amounts of these nutrients in their daily diet. In these circumstances, supplements may be warranted.

Calcium

Numerous calcium supplements are available to consumers, but which are best? Most supplements come in the form of calcium carbonate, calcium citrate, calcium lactate, or calcium phosphate. Our body is able to absorb about 30% of the calcium from these various forms. Calcium citrate malate, which is the form of calcium used in fortified juices, is slightly more absorbable, at 35%. Many antacids are also good sources of calcium, and it appears that they are safe to take, as long as you consume only enough to get the recommended level of calcium.

What is the most cost-effective form of calcium? In general, supplements that contain calcium carbonate tend to have more calcium per pill than other types. Thus, you are getting more calcium for your money when you buy this type. However, be sure to read the label of any calcium supplement you are considering taking to determine just how much calcium it contains. Some very expensive calcium supplements do not contain a lot of calcium per pill, and you could be wasting your money.

The lead content of calcium supplements is an important public health concern. Those made from "natural" sources, such as oyster shell, bone meal, and dolomite, are known to be higher in lead, and some of these products can contain dangerously high levels. The Food and Drug Administration (FDA) has set an upper limit of 7.5 μg of lead per 1,000 mg calcium, but currently calcium supplements are not tested for lead content, and it

is the manufacturer's responsibility to ensure that its supplements meet FDA standards. To avoid taking supplements that contain too much lead, look for supplements claiming to be lead-free, and make sure the word *purified* is on the label, in addition to the U.S. Pharmacopeia (USP) symbol.

Evidence has emerged in recent years that taking calcium supplements might increase the risk for a myocardial infarction (MI)—a heart attack. Analyses based on the prospective observational data from the Women's Health Initiative study, in which almost 37,000 postmenopausal women were prescribed a calcium-vitamin D supplement or placebo over an average of 7 years, showed that the supplementation significantly increased total and hip bone density. However, there was no change in risk for fractures, and evidence suggested that taking these supplements could increase the risk for MI.[24] A subsequent analysis of the study data found that among those women who were not already taking calcium or vitamin D supplements before the trial began, the supplement reduced the risk of hip fractures, and did not increase the risk of MI.[25] Even more recently, however, researchers have proposed a mechanism by which an increased load of supplemental calcium in the bloodstream might promote the formation of calcium deposits in the coronary arteries and thereby increase MI risk.[26] Thus, this topic is contentious, and it currently is not known whether or not there is an interaction between calcium supplementation and cardiovascular health.

nutri-case | GUSTAVO

"When my wife, Antonia, fell and broke her hip, I was shocked. See, the same thing happened to her mother, but she was an old lady by then. Antonia's only 68, and she still seems young and beautiful—at least to me! As soon as she's better, her doctor wants to do some kind of scan to see how thick her bones are. But I don't think she has that disease everyone talks about. She's always watched her weight and keeps active with our kids and grandkids. It's true she likes her coffee and diet colas, and doesn't drink milk, but that's not enough to make a person's bones fall apart, is it?"

Take another look at Table 1 in this chapter. What risk factors do *not* apply to Antonia? What risk factors do? Given what Gustavo has said about his wife's nutrition and lifestyle, would you suggest he encourage her to have a bone density scan? Why or why not?

If you decide to use a calcium supplement, how should you take it? Remember that the body cannot absorb more than 500 mg of calcium at one time. Thus, taking a supplement that contains 1,000 mg of calcium is no more effective than taking one that contains 500 mg. If at all possible, try to consume calcium supplements in small doses throughout the day. In addition, calcium is absorbed better with meals, because the calcium stays in the intestinal tract longer during a meal and more can be absorbed.

Vitamin D

As discussed in the Nutrition Debate in Chapter 9, there has been an increase in vitamin D deficiency in the United States. The only way to know if you are vitamin D deficient is to have your blood levels of vitamin D assessed by a qualified healthcare provider. If you are deficient, your healthcare provider may advise you to take vitamin D supplements, which the Office of Dietary Supplements at the National Institutes of Health states appear to be effective in raising and maintaining blood levels of vitamin D.[27] Make sure the word *purified* is on the label, in addition to the U.S. Pharmacopeia (USP) symbol. Because vitamin D is a fat-soluble vitamin, it is important to stay below the UL of 4,000 IU (for adults) per day.

Physical Activity and Other Lifestyle Choices Can Help

Another important strategy for preventing osteoporosis is engaging in regular physical activity throughout life. It's especially important to participate in weight-bearing and impact-loading activities. Examples include brisk walking, dancing, jogging, step-aerobics, hiking, tennis, tai chi, yoga, jumping rope, and resistance training. All of these activities help strengthen muscles and joints and improve balance, and resistance training may help to preserve bone density.

It's also important to avoid becoming underweight. Appropriate body weight stresses the bones, and an adequate, balanced diet provides the nutrients to keep them healthy. In short, maintaining a healthy body weight is essential for preventing osteoporosis.

Other preventive measures include avoiding smoking and alcohol abuse. Finally, increasing sun exposure safely will allow your body to synthesize adequate vitamin D and help prevent osteoporosis.

web links

www.nof.org
National Osteoporosis Foundation

Learn more about the causes, prevention, detection, and treatment of osteoporosis.

http://www.iofbonehealth.org/
International Osteoporosis Foundation

Find out more about this foundation and its mission to increase awareness and understanding of osteoporosis worldwide.

www.niams.nih.gov
National Institutes of Health, National Institute of Arthritis and Musculoskeletal and Skin Diseases

Access this site for additional resources and information on metabolic bone diseases, including osteoporosis. Enter "bone health" into the search box, and then click on the top link to get started.

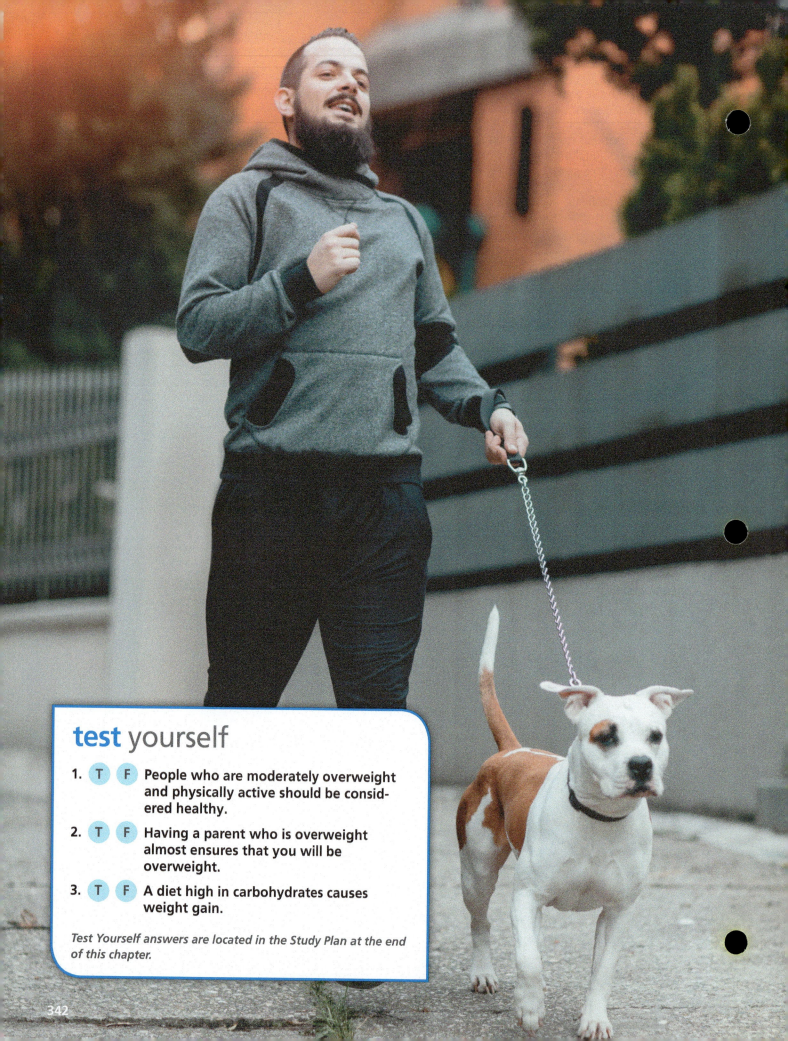

test yourself

1. **T F** People who are moderately overweight and physically active should be considered healthy.

2. **T F** Having a parent who is overweight almost ensures that you will be overweight.

3. **T F** A diet high in carbohydrates causes weight gain.

Test Yourself answers are located in the Study Plan at the end of this chapter.

10

Achieving and Maintaining a Healthful Body Weight

learning outcomes

After studying this chapter you should be able to:

1 Explain what is meant by a healthful body weight, p. 344.

2 Distinguish five categories of body weight and three methods you can use to evaluate your body weight, pp. 344–349.

3 Discuss the concept of energy balance and the limitations of the energy balance equation, pp. 349–355.

4 Identify several biological, cultural, economic, and social influences on body weight, pp. 355–360.

5 Develop a diet, exercise, and behavioral plan for healthful weight loss, pp. 360–367.

6 Identify four key strategies for gaining weight safely and effectively, pp. 367–368.

Tristan has been a mathematics whiz since grade school, winning scholarships, awards, and internships and maintaining high honors in his classes throughout his academic career. Yet his peers are far less likely to acknowledge his talents and achievements than to fault him for his weight. Tristan admits he's "heavy," but he limits his consumption of junk food and alcohol, walks the 2 miles to and from campus each day, and joins his brother in the weight room at the local gym on Saturdays. Sometimes the negative comments about his weight bother him, especially when he compares himself with the athletes on campus. That's when he knows it's time to visit his grandfather. A "big man" all his life, he takes no medications, enjoys the vegetables he grows in his garden, and still coaches a community soccer team—at age 85!

Are you happy with your weight, shape, body composition, and fitness level? If not, what needs to change—your diet, your level of physical activity, or maybe just your attitude? How much of your body size and shape is due to genetics, and what factors can you control? And if you decide that you do need to lose weight, what's the best way to do it? In this chapter, we explore these questions and provide some answers.

LO 1 Explain what is meant by a healthful body weight.

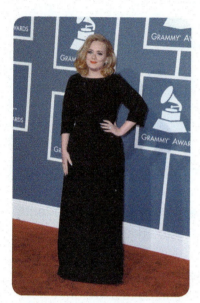

⬆ What constitutes a healthful body weight varies for each individual. British singer Adele is comfortable with her body weight.

What is a healthful body weight?

Throughout history, our standards of physical attraction, especially regarding body shape and weight, have changed. In the 1600s, the full-figured females and muscular males of Flemish Baroque painter Peter Paul Rubens were considered ideal. Fast-forward to the 1960s, when skinny stars such as Twiggy and Mick Jagger were the rage. These ideals shifted again in the 1980s, when physically fit bodies were in style for both women and men, and again in the 1990s, when the emaciated look of "heroin chic" was touted as beautiful for women, whereas the ideal man had broad shoulders and "six-pack abs." There are also cultural differences in body shape and weight standards; in many cultures, being larger is associated with possessing greater wealth, health, fertility, and sexual desirability. These examples illustrate that standards for body shape and weight are influenced by social and cultural norms, fashion, and personal preferences, but they are not necessarily consistent with a body weight that is healthful.

As you begin to think about achieving and maintaining a healthful weight, it's important to make sure you understand what that actually means. We can define a *healthful weight* as all of the following:

- A weight that is appropriate for your age and physical development
- A weight that you can achieve and sustain without severely curtailing your food intake or constantly dieting
- A weight that is compatible with normal blood pressure, lipid levels, and glucose tolerance
- A weight that is based on your genetic background and family history of body shape and weight
- A weight that is supported by good eating habits and regular physical activity
- A weight that is acceptable to you

As you can see, a healthful weight is one at which you don't have to be extremely thin or overly muscular. In addition, there is no *one* body type that can be defined as *healthful*. Thus, achieving a healthful body weight should not be dictated by the latest fad or current societal expectations of what is acceptable.

recap Standards of ideal body weight have changed over the course of human history, and vary from one culture to another. A healthful body weight is appropriate for your age, physical development, genetics, and family history; achievable without constant dieting; compatible with normal blood pressure, lipids, and glucose; supported by good eating and regular physical activity habits; and acceptable to you.

LO 2 Distinguish five categories of body weight and three methods you can use to evaluate your body weight.

body mass index (BMI) A measurement representing the ratio of a person's body weight to his or her height (kg/m²).

underweight Having too little body fat to maintain health, causing a person to have a weight that is below an acceptable defined standard for a given height; a BMI less than 18.5 kg/m².

normal weight Having an adequate but not excessive level of body fat for health.

How can you evaluate your body weight?

Various methods are available to help you determine whether you are currently maintaining a healthful body weight. Let's review a few of these methods.

Determine Your Body Mass Index

Body mass index (BMI), or *Quetelet's index*, is a commonly used index representing the ratio of a person's body weight to the square of his or her height. A person's BMI can be calculated using the following equation:

$$\text{BMI (kg/m}^2) = \text{weight (kg)/height (m)}^2$$

For those less familiar with the metric system, there is an equation to calculate BMI using weight in pounds and height in inches:

$$\text{BMI (kg/m}^2) = [\text{weight (lb)/height (inches)}^2] \times 703$$

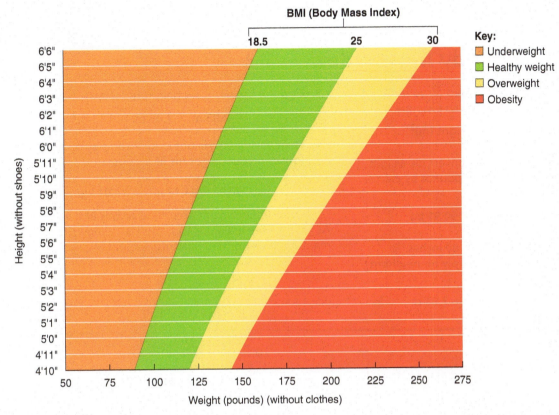

BMI (Body Mass Index)

18.5   25   30

Key:
- ■ Underweight
- ■ Healthy weight
- ■ Overweight
- ■ Obesity

Height (without shoes): 6'6", 6'5", 6'4", 6'3", 6'2", 6'1", 6'0", 5'11", 5'10", 5'9", 5'8", 5'7", 5'6", 5'5", 5'4", 5'3", 5'2", 5'1", 5'0", 4'11", 4'10"

Weight (pounds) (without clothes): 50 75 100 125 150 175 200 225 250 275

◆ **FIGURE 10.1** Estimate your body mass index (BMI) using this graph. To determine your BMI, find the value for your height on the left and follow this line to the right until it intersects with the value for your weight on the bottom axis. The area on the graph where these two lines intersect is your BMI.

A less exact but practical method is to use the graph in **FIGURE 10.1**, which shows approximate BMIs for a person's height and weight and whether a given BMI is in a healthful range.

Why Is BMI Important?

BMI provides an important clue to a person's overall health because it is associated with one of five weight categories, each of which involves a certain level of health risk:

- **Underweight** is defined as having a BMI less than 18.5 kg/m². This weight is below an acceptably defined standard for a given height. A person who is underweight has too little body fat to maintain health and therefore has an increased risk for many health problems.
- **Normal weight** ranges from 18.5 to 24.9 kg/m². This weight is associated with the lowest disease risk.
- **Overweight** is a BMI between 25 and 29.9 kg/m². It is defined as having a moderate amount of excess body fat, resulting in a person having a weight that is greater than some accepted standard for a given height but is not considered obese.
- **Obesity** is a BMI value between 30 and 39.9 kg/m². Clinicians define obesity as having an excess of body fat that adversely affects health, resulting in a person having a weight that is substantially greater than some accepted standard for a given height. Research studies show that a person's risk for type 2 diabetes, cardiovascular disease, and many other diseases increases significantly when BMI is above a value of 30.
- **Morbid obesity** (or extreme obesity) is defined as a BMI greater than or equal to 40 kg/m²; in this case, the person's body weight exceeds 100% of normal, putting him or her at very high risk for serious health consequences.

You can also calculate your BMI more precisely on the Internet using the BMI calculator from the U.S. Centers for Disease Control. Just enter "CDC BMI calculator" into your Internet browser and click on Adult BMI Calculator. Enter your data and the program will calculate your BMI.

overweight Having a moderate amount of excess body fat, resulting in a person having a weight that is greater than some accepted standard for a given height but is not considered obese; a BMI of 25 to 29.9 kg/m².

obesity Having an excess of body fat that adversely affects health, resulting in a person having a weight that is substantially greater than some accepted standard for a given height; a BMI of 30 to 39.9 kg/m².

you do the math

Calculating Your Body Mass Index

Calculate your personal BMI value based on your height and weight. Let's use Theo's values as an example:

$$BMI = weight\ (kg)/height\ (m)^2$$

1. Theo's weight is 200 pounds. To convert his weight to kilograms, divide his weight in pounds by 2.2 pounds per kilogram:

$$200\ lb/2.2\ lb\ per\ kg = 90.91\ kg$$

2. Theo's height is 6 feet 8 inches, or 80 inches. To convert his height to meters, multiply his height in inches by 0.0254 meters/inch:

$$80\ in. \times 0.0254\ m/in. = 2.03\ m$$

3. Find the square of his height in meters:

$$2.03\ m \times 2.03\ m = 4.13\ m^2$$

4. Then, divide his weight in kilograms by his height in square meters to get his BMI value:

$$90.91\ kg/4.13\ m^2 = 22.01\ kg/m^2$$

Is Theo underweight according to this BMI value? No. As you can see in Figure 10.1, this value shows that he is maintaining a normal, healthful weight.

Until recently, data from national surveys have indicated that having a BMI value within the healthful range means that your risk of dying prematurely is within the expected average. Thus, if your BMI value fell outside this range, either higher or lower, your risk of dying prematurely was considered greater than the average risk. However, a 2013 analysis of 97 previously published studies found that people who are overweight (BMI of 25 to 29.99 kg/m^2) but not obese have a 6% *lower* risk of dying prematurely than those with a normal BMI.[1]

These findings created a firestorm of controversy among health professionals and prompted numerous scientists to question the study.[2] Most notably, Dr. Walter Willett of the Harvard School of Public Health called the findings "rubbish" and warned that they would confuse health care providers and discourage overweight and obese people from losing weight. In contrast, an editorial published in the journal *Nature* questioned the motives and views of these critics, emphasizing that the topic is highly complex, and concluding that "a bit of extra weight" does appear to be protective for people who are middle-aged or older or who are already sick.[3] This controversy has drawn international attention to *how* research findings are reported in the media, leading to questions such as: Is it acceptable to reject major research findings when they don't agree? Do we risk misleading the public when we oversimplify our public health messages and fail to report the complexities of an issue such as obesity? Until future research findings clarify the relationship between body weight and risk for chronic disease and premature death, this topic will continue to be controversial.

Knowing how to calculate our BMI is important because we can't always predict our category of body weight based on our appearance. For example, Theo always worries about being too thin, and he wonders if he is underweight. Theo calculates his BMI (see the calculations in the **You Do the Math** box on this page) and is surprised to find that it is 22 kg/m^2 and falls within the normal range.

Limitations of BMI

Although calculating your BMI can be very helpful in estimating your health risk, the method has a number of limitations. BMI cannot tell us how much of a person's body mass is composed of fat, nor can it give us an indication of where on the body excess fat is stored. As we'll discuss shortly, upper-body fat stores increase the risk for chronic disease more than fat stores in the lower body. A person's age affects his or her BMI; BMI does not give a fair indication of overweight or obesity in people over the age of 65 years, as the BMI standards are based on data from younger people, and

morbid obesity A condition in which a person's body weight exceeds 100% of normal, putting him or her at very high risk for serious health consequences; a BMI = 40 kg/m^2.

BMI does not accurately reflect the differential rates of bone and muscle loss in older people. BMI also cannot reflect differences in bone and muscle growth in children. BMI is also more strongly associated with height in young people; thus, taller children are more likely to be identified as overweight or obese, even though they may not have higher levels of body fat.

BMI also does not take into account physical and metabolic differences between people of different ethnic backgrounds. At the same BMI, people from different ethnic backgrounds will have different levels of body fat. For instance, African American and Polynesian people have less body fat than Caucasians at the same BMI value, while Indonesian, Thai, and Ethiopian people have more body fat than Caucasians at the same BMI value. There is also evidence that, even at the same BMI level, Asian, Hispanic, and people of African or Caribbean heritage have a higher risk for diabetes than Caucasians.[4,5]

Finally, BMI is limited when used with pregnant and lactating women, and with people who have a disproportionately higher muscle mass for a given height, such as certain types of athletes. For example, one of Theo's friends, Randy, is a 23-year-old weight lifter who is 5 feet 7 inches and weighs 210 pounds. According to our BMI calculations, Randy's BMI is 32.9, placing him in the obese category. Is Randy really obese? In cases such as his, an assessment of body composition is necessary.

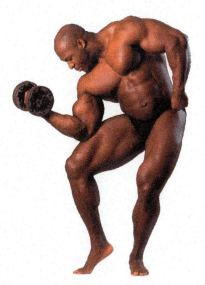

⬥ BMI is not an accurate indicator of overweight for certain populations, including heavily muscled people.

Measure Your Body Composition

There are many methods available to assess your **body composition**, or the amount of **body fat mass** (*adipose tissue*) and **lean body mass** (*lean tissue*) you have. **FIGURE 10.2** (page 348) lists and describes some of the more common methods. It is important to remember that measuring body composition provides only an *estimate* of your body fat and lean body mass; it cannot determine your exact level of these tissues. Because the range of error of these methods can be from 3% to more than 20%, body composition results should not be used as the only indicator of health status.

Let's return to Randy, whose BMI of 32.9 kg/m² places him in the obese category. Is he obese? Randy trains with weights 4 days per week, rides the exercise bike for about 30 minutes per session three times per week, and does not take drugs, smoke cigarettes, or drink alcohol. Through his local gym, Randy contacted a trained technician who assesses body composition. The results of his skinfold measurements show that his body fat is 9%. This value is within the healthful range for men. Randy is an example of a person whose BMI appears very high but who is not actually obese.

Assess Your Fat Distribution Patterns

To evaluate the health of your current body weight, it is also helpful to consider the way fat is distributed throughout your body. This is because your fat distribution pattern is known to affect your risk for various diseases. **FIGURE 10.3** on page 349 shows two types of fat patterning. *Apple-shaped fat patterning*, or upper-body obesity, is known to significantly increase a person's risk for many chronic diseases, such as type 2 diabetes and cardiovascular disease. Apple-shaped patterning causes problems with the metabolism of fat and carbohydrate, leading to unhealthful changes in blood cholesterol, insulin, glucose, and blood pressure. In contrast, *pear-shaped fat patterning*, or lower-body obesity, does not seem to significantly increase your risk for chronic diseases.

You can use the following three-step method to determine your type of fat patterning:

1. Ask a friend to measure the circumference of your natural waist, that is, the narrowest part of your torso as observed from the front (**FIGURE 10.4a**) (page 349).
2. Then, have that friend measure your hip circumference at the maximal width of the buttocks as observed from the side (Figure 10.4b).
3. Then, divide the waist value by the hip value. This measurement is called your *waist-to-hip ratio*. For example, if your natural waist is 30 inches and your hips are 40 inches, then your waist-to-hip ratio is 30 divided by 40, which equals 0.75.

body composition The ratio of a person's body fat to lean body mass.
body fat mass The amount of body fat, or adipose tissue, a person has.
lean body mass The amount of fat-free tissue, or bone, muscle, and internal organs, a person has.

Method		Limitations
Underwater weighing: Considered the most accurate method. Estimates body fat within a 2–3% margin of error. This means that if your underwater weighing test shows you have 20% body fat, this value could be no lower than 17% and no higher than 23%. Used primarily for research purposes.	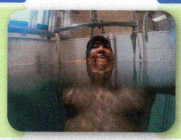	• Subject must be comfortable in water. • Requires trained technician and specialized equipment. • May not work well with extremely obese people. • Must abstain from food for at least 8 hours and from exercise for at least 12 hours prior to testing.
Skinfolds: Involves "pinching" a person's fold of skin (with its underlying layer of fat) at various locations of the body. The fold is measured using a specially designed caliper. When performed by a skilled technician, it can estimate body fat with an error of 3–4%. This means that if your skinfold test shows you have 20% body fat, your actual value could be as low as 16% or as high as 24%.	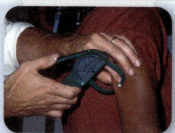	• Less accurate unless technician is well trained. • Proper prediction equation must be used to improve accuracy. • Person being measured may not want to be touched or to expose their skin. • Cannot be used to measure obese people, as their skinfolds are too large for the caliper.
Bioelectrical impedance analysis (BIA): Involves sending a very low level of electrical current through a person's body. As water is a good conductor of electricity and lean body mass is made up of mostly water, the rate at which the electricity is conducted gives an indication of a person's lean body mass and body fat. This method can be done while lying down, with electrodes attached to the feet, hands, and the BIA machine. Hand-held and standing models (which look like bathroom scales) are now available. Under the best of circumstances, BIA can estimate body fat with an error of 3–4%.	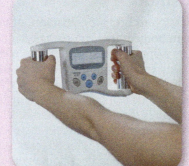	• Less accurate. • Body fluid levels must be normal. • Proper prediction equation must be used to improve accuracy. • Should not eat for 4 hours and should not exercise for 12 hours prior to the test. • No alcohol should be consumed within 48 hours of the test. • Females should not be measured if they are retaining water due to menstrual cycle changes.
Dual-energy x-ray absorptiometry (DXA): The technology is based on using very-low-level x-rays to differentiate among bone tissue, soft (or lean) tissue, and fat (or adipose) tissue. It involves lying for about 30 minutes on a specialized bed fully clothed, with all metal objects removed. The margin of error for predicting body fat ranges from 2% to 4%.	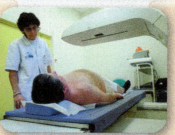	• Expensive; requires trained technician with specialized equipment. • Cannot be used to measure extremely tall, short, or obese people, as they do not fit properly within the scanning area.
Bod Pod: A machine that uses air displacement to measure body composition. This machine is a large, egg-shaped chamber made from fiberglass. The person being measured sits inside, wearing a swimsuit. The door is closed and the machine measures how much air is displaced. This value is used to calculate body composition. It appears promising as an easier and equally accurate alternative to underwater weighing in many populations, but it may overestimate body fat in some African American men.	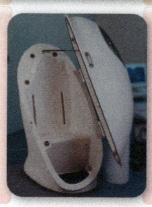	• Expensive. • Less accurate in some populations.

◄ **FIGURE 10.2** Overview of various body composition assessment methods.

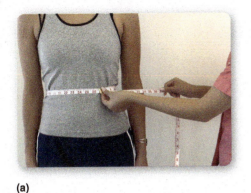
(a)

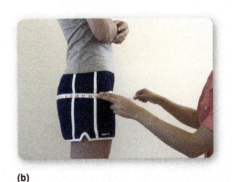
(b)

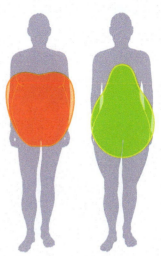
(a) Apple-shaped
fat patterning

(b) Pear-shaped
fat patterning

⬆ **FIGURE 10.4** Determining your type of fat patterning. **(a)** Measure the circumference of your natural waist. **(b)** Measure the circumference of your hips at the maximal width of the buttocks as observed from the side. Dividing the waist value by the hip value gives you your waist-to-hip ratio.

⬆ **FIGURE 10.3** Fat distribution patterns. **(a)** An apple-shaped fat distribution pattern increases an individual's risk for many chronic diseases. **(b)** A pear-shaped fat distribution pattern does not seem to be associated with an increased risk for chronic disease.

Once you figure out your ratio, how do you interpret it? An increased risk for chronic disease is associated with the following waist-to-hip ratios:

- In men, a ratio higher than 0.90
- In women, a ratio higher than 0.80

These ratios suggest an apple-shaped fat distribution pattern. In addition, waist circumference alone can indicate your risk for chronic disease. For males, your risk of chronic disease is increased if your waist circumference is above 40 inches (102 cm). For females, your risk is increased at measurements above 35 inches (88 cm).

recap Body mass index, body composition, and the waist-to-hip ratio and waist circumference are tools that can help you evaluate the health of your current body weight. Body mass index represents the ratio of a person's body weight to the square of his or her height. A BMI in the normal weight category ranges from 18.5 to 24.9 kg/m². Body composition measurements help you estimate your fat-to-lean tissue mass. A waist-to-hip ratio higher than 0.90 for males and 0.80 for females is associated with an apple-shaped fat distribution pattern, which increases your risk for several chronic diseases. None of these methods is completely accurate, but most may be used appropriately as general health indicators.

How does energy balance influence body weight?

LO 3 Discuss the concept of energy balance and the limitations of the energy balance equation.

Have you ever wondered why some people are thin and others are overweight, even though they seem to eat about the same diet? If so, you're not alone. For hundreds of years, researchers have puzzled over what makes us gain and lose weight. In this section, we explore some information and current theories that may shed light on this complex question.

Fluctuations in body weight are a result of changes in **energy intake** (the food and beverages consumed) and **energy expenditure** (the amount of energy expended at rest and during physical activity). This relationship between what we eat and what we do is defined by the energy balance equation:

Energy balance occurs when *energy intake = energy expenditure*

Although the concept of energy balance appears simple, it is a dynamic process.[6] This means that, over time, factors that impact the energy intake side of the equation (including total energy consumed and the macronutrient composition of this energy) need to balance with the factors that impact the energy expenditure side of the equation. **FOCUS FIGURE 10.5** on page 350 is a simplistic representation of how our weight

energy intake The amount of energy a person consumes; in other words, the number of kcal consumed from food and beverages.

energy expenditure The energy the body expends to maintain its basic functions and to perform all levels of movement and activity.

focus figure 10.5 Energy Balance

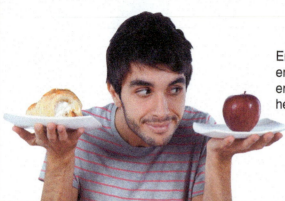

Energy balance is the relationship between the food we eat and the energy we expend each day. Finding the proper balance between energy intake and energy expenditure allows us to maintain a healthy body weight.

ENERGY INTAKE < ENERGY EXPENDITURE = WEIGHT LOSS

ENERGY DEFICIT

When you consume fewer Calories than you expend, your body will draw upon your stored energy to meet its needs. You will lose weight. When you are in a state of energy deficit the body can become more metabolically efficient, which can slow weight loss based on predicted changes.

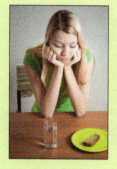

Calories in   Calories out

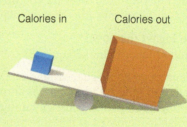

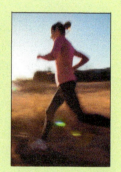

ENERGY INTAKE = ENERGY EXPENDITURE = WEIGHT MAINTENANCE

ENERGY BALANCE

When the Calories you consume meet your needs, you are in energy balance. Your weight will be stable.

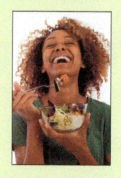

Calories in   Calories out

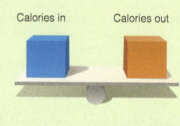

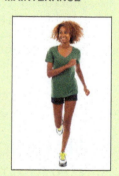

ENERGY INTAKE > ENERGY EXPENDITURE = WEIGHT GAIN

ENERGY EXCESS

When you take in more Calories than you need, the surplus Calories will be stored as fat. You will gain weight. However, when some people consume excess energy their body may attempt to increase energy expenditure through heat to slow weight gain. These people have a hard time gaining weight.

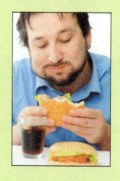

Calories in   Calories out

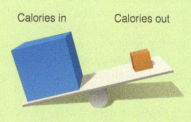

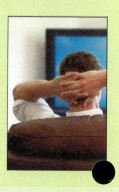

changes when either side of this equation is altered. From this figure, you can see that, in order to lose body weight, we must expend more energy than we consume. In contrast, to gain weight, we must consume more energy than we expend. Unless we purposefully change one side of the equation, weight change is typically gradual and occurs over an extended period of time. Finding the proper balance between energy intake and expenditure allows someone to maintain a healthful body weight over time.

Energy Intake Is the Kilocalories We Consume Each Day

Energy intake is equal to the amount of energy in the foods and beverages we consume each day. Daily energy intake is expressed as *kilocalories per day* (*kcal/day*, or *kcal/d*). Energy intake can be estimated manually by using food composition tables or computerized dietary analysis programs. Remember (from Chapter 1) that the energy value of carbohydrate and protein is 4 kcal/g and the energy value of fat is 9 kcal/g. The energy value of alcohol is 7 kcal/g. By multiplying the energy value (in kcal/g) by the amount of the nutrient (in g), you can calculate how much energy is in a particular food. For instance, 1 cup of quick oatmeal has an energy value of 142 kcal, because it contains 6 g of protein, 25 g of carbohydrate, and 2 g of fat.

Over a period of time, when someone's total daily energy intake exceeds the amount of energy that person expends, then weight gain results. Without exercise, this gain will likely be mostly fat. How many Calories are in a pound of fat?

- First, it is important to remember that there are 454 g in 1 pound and that the energy value of fat is 9 kcal/g.
- Second, you need to know that adipose tissue contains 87% fat (the remainder is water).
- Finally, to calculate the amount of kcal that will result in a gain of 1 pound (454 g), you need to multiply the amount of weight, 454 g, by the proportion of fat in adipose tissue (87%, or 0.87) and then multiply this value by the energy value of fat (9 kcal/g):

$$454 \text{ g} \times 0.87 = 395 \text{ g of fat}$$

$$395 \text{ g} \times 9 \text{ kcal/g} = 3{,}555 \text{ kcal (which, for simplicity, is rounded to 3,500 kcal)}$$

Energy Expenditure Includes More Than Just Physical Activity

Energy expenditure (also known as *energy output*) is the energy the body expends to maintain its basic functions and to perform all levels of movement and activity. Total 24-hour energy expenditure is calculated by estimating the energy used during rest and as a result of physical activity. There are three components of energy expenditure: basal metabolic rate (BMR), thermic effect of food (TEF), and energy cost of physical activity and activities of daily living **(FIGURE 10.6)**.

Basal Metabolic Rate

Basal metabolic rate (BMR) is the energy expended just to maintain the body's *basal*, or *resting*, functions. These functions include respiration, circulation, body temperature, synthesis of new cells and tissues, secretion of hormones, and nervous system activity. The majority of our energy output each day (about 60% to 75%) is a result of our BMR. This means that 60% to 75% of our energy output goes to fuel the basic activities of staying alive, aside from any physical activity.

BMR varies widely among people. The primary determinant is the amount of lean body mass we have. People with a higher lean body mass have a higher BMR, as lean body mass is more metabolically active than body fat. Thus, it takes more energy to support this active tissue. One common assumption is that obese people have a depressed BMR. This is usually not the case. Most studies of obese people show that the amount of energy they expend for every kilogram of lean body mass is similar to

To determine how much energy you consumed in one meal or on one day, log on to ChooseMyPlate at www .choosemyplate.gov. Click on the tab for SuperTracker, then get started!

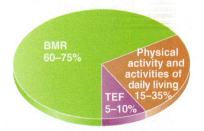

Components of energy expenditure

◄ **FIGURE 10.6** The components of energy expenditure are basal metabolic rate (BMR), the thermic effect of food (TEF), and the energy cost of physical activity and activities of daily living. BMR accounts for 60% to 75% of our total energy output, whereas TEF and physical activity together account for 25% to 40%.

basal metabolic rate (BMR) The energy the body expends to maintain its fundamental physiologic functions.

that of a nonobese person. Moreover, people who weigh more also have more lean body mass and consequently have a *higher* BMR.

BMR decreases with age, approximately 3% to 5% per decade after age 30. This age-related decrease results partly from hormonal changes, but much of this change is due to the loss of lean body mass resulting from physical inactivity. Thus, a large proportion of this decrease may be prevented with regular physical activity. Of the many other factors that can affect a person's BMR, some of the most common are listed in **TABLE 10.1**.

How can you estimate the amount of energy you expend for your BMR? One of the simplest methods is to multiply your body weight in kilograms by 1.0 kcal per kilogram of body weight per hour for men or by 0.9 kcal per kilogram of body weight per hour for women. A little later in this chapter, you will have an opportunity to calculate your BMR and determine your total daily energy needs.

The Thermic Effect of Food

The **thermic effect of food (TEF)** is the energy we expend to digest, absorb, transport, metabolize, and store the nutrients we need. The TEF is equal to about 5% to 10% of the energy content of a meal, a relatively small amount. Thus, if a meal contains 500 kcal, the thermic effect of that meal is about 25 to 50 kcal, depending on how processed the foods contained in the meal happen to be. These values apply to eating what is referred to as a mixed diet, or a diet containing carbohydrate, fat, and protein. Individually, the processing of each nutrient takes a different amount of energy. Whereas fat requires very little energy to digest, transport, and store in our cells, protein and carbohydrate require relatively more energy to process. Finally, the more processed a food is prior to consumption, the less energy it takes to digest this food. For example, it requires more energy to digest an orange than it does to digest orange juice.

The Energy Cost of Physical Activity

The **energy cost of physical activity** represents about 15% to 35% of our total energy output each day. This is the energy we expend in any movement or work above basal levels.

Non-exercise activity thermogenesis (NEAT) is a term used to refer to the energy we expend to do all activities above BMR and TMF, but excluding volitional sporting activities. It includes *spontaneous physical activity,* which in turn includes subconscious activities such as fidgeting and shifting in one's seat. The amount of energy expended through NEAT can vary by as much as 2,000 kcal per day between two individuals of similar size.[7] Because many people are not highly physically active, it has been proposed that NEAT makes a major contribution to overweight and obesity.[7]

The energy cost of physical activity also includes the energy we expend participating in higher-intensity activities such as running, skiing, and bicycling. One of the most obvious ways to increase how much energy we expend as a result of physical

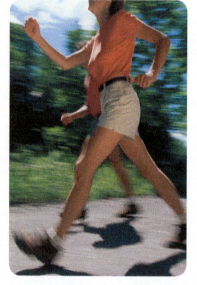

▲ Brisk walking expends energy.

thermic effect of food (TEF) The energy expended as a result of processing food consumed.

energy cost of physical activity The energy that is expended on body movement and muscular work above basal levels.

non-exercise activity thermogenesis (NEAT) The energy that is expended to do all activities above BMR and TMF, but excluding volitional sporting activities.

TABLE 10.1 Factors Affecting Basal Metabolic Rate (BMR)

Factors That Increase BMR	Factors That Decrease BMR
Higher lean body mass	Lower lean body mass
Greater height (more surface area)	Lower height
Younger age	Older age
Elevated levels of thyroid hormone	Depressed levels of thyroid hormone
Stress, fever, illness	Starvation, fasting or very-low-Calorie diets
Male gender	Female gender due to decreased lean tissue
Pregnancy and lactation	
Certain drugs, such as stimulants, caffeine, and tobacco	

TABLE 10.2 Energy Costs of Various Physical Activities

Activity	Intensity	Energy Cost (kcal/kg body weight/min)
Sitting, studying (including reading or writing)	Light	0.022
Cooking or food preparation (sitting or standing)	Light	0.033
Walking (e.g., to neighbor's house)	Light	0.042
Stretching—Hatha yoga	Moderate	0.042
Cleaning (dusting, straightening up, vacuuming, changing linen, carrying out trash)	Moderate	0.058
Weight lifting (free weights, Nautilus, or universal type)	Light or moderate	0.050
Bicycling, 10 mph	Leisure (work or pleasure)	0.067
Walking, 4 mph (brisk pace)	Moderate	0.083
Aerobics	Low impact	0.083
Weight lifting (free weights, Nautilus, or universal type)	Vigorous	0.100
Bicycling, 12 to 13.9 mph	Moderate	0.133
Running, 5 mph (12 minutes per mile)	Moderate	0.138
Running, 6 mph (10 minutes per mile)	Moderate	0.163
Running, 8.6 mph (7 minutes per mile)	Vigorous	0.205

Source: Data from the Compendium of Physical Activities Tracking Guide. Healthy Lifestyles Research Center, College of Nursing and Health Innovation, Arizona State University.

activity is to do more activities for a longer period of time. For example, the energy cost of physical activity in a highly trained athlete may represent 50% of their total energy expenditure, compared to lower values for those who are not as active.

TABLE 10.2 lists the energy costs for certain activities. As you can see, activities such as running, swimming, and cross-country skiing, which involve moving our larger muscle groups (or more parts of the body) require more energy. The amount of energy we expend during activities is also affected by our body size, the intensity of the activity, and how long we perform the activity. This is why the values in Table 10.2 are expressed as kcal of energy per kilogram of body weight per minute.

Using the energy value for running at 6 miles per hour (a 10-minute-per-mile running pace) for 30 minutes, let's calculate how much energy Theo would expend doing this activity:

- Theo's body weight (in kg) = 200 lb/2.2 lb/kg = 90.91 kg
- Energy cost of running at 6 mph = 0.163 kcal/kg body weight/min
- At Theo's weight, the energy cost of running per minute = 0.163 kcal/kg body weight/min × 90.91 kg = 14.82 kcal/min
- If Theo runs at this pace for 30 minutes, his total energy output = 14.82 kcal/min × 30 min = 445 kcal

Given everything we've discussed so far, you're probably asking yourself, "How many kcal do I need each day to maintain my current weight?" This question is not easy to answer, as our energy needs fluctuate from day to day according to our activity level, environmental conditions, and other factors, such as the amount and type of food we eat and our intake of caffeine, which temporarily increases our BMR. However, you can get a general estimate of how much energy your body needs to maintain your present weight. The **You Do the Math** box (on page 354) explains how to estimate your total daily energy needs.

you do the math

Calculating BMR and Total Daily Energy Needs

One potential way to estimate how much energy you need each day is to record your total food and beverage intake for a defined period of time, such as 3 or 7 days. You can then use a food composition table or computer dietary assessment program to estimate the amount of energy you eat each day. Assuming that your body weight is stable over this period of time, your average daily energy intake should represent how much energy you need to maintain your present weight.

Unfortunately, many studies of energy intake in humans have shown that dietary records estimating energy needs are not very accurate. Most studies show that humans underestimate the amount of energy they eat by 10% to 30%. Overweight people tend to underestimate by an even higher margin, at the same time overestimating the amount of activity they do. This means that someone who really eats about 2,000 kcal/day may record eating only 1,400 to 1,800 kcal/day. So one reason many people are confused about their ability to lose weight is that they are eating more than they realize.

A simpler and more accurate way to estimate your total daily energy needs is to calculate your BMR, then add the amount of energy you expend as a result of your activity level. Refer to the following example to learn how to do this. As the energy cost for the thermic effect of food is very small, you don't need to include it in your calculations.

1. *Calculate your BMR.* If you are a man, you will need to multiply your body weight in kilograms by 1 kcal per kilogram of body weight per hour. Assuming you weigh 175 pounds, your body weight in kilograms would be 175 lb/2.2 lb/kg $\times$ 79.5 kg. Next, multiply your weight in kilograms by 1 kcal per kilogram body weight per hour:

$$1 \text{ kcal/kg body weight/hour} \times 79.5 \text{ kg}$$
$$= 79.5 \text{ kcal/hour}$$

Calculate your BMR for the total day (or 24 hours):

$$79.5 \text{ kcal/hour} \times 24 \text{ hours/day} = 1,909 \text{ kcal/day}$$

If you are a woman, multiply your body weight in kg by 0.9 kcal/kg body weight/hour.

2. *Estimate your activity level by selecting the description that most closely fits your general lifestyle.* The energy cost of activities is expressed as a percentage of your BMR. Refer to the values in the following table when estimating your own energy output.

3. *Multiply your BMR by the decimal equivalent of the lower and higher percentage values for your activity level.* Let's use the man referred to in step 1. He is a college student who lives on campus. He walks

to classes located throughout campus, carries his book bag, and spends most of his time reading and writing. He does not exercise on a regular basis. His lifestyle would be defined as lightly active, meaning he expends 50% to 70% of his BMR each day in activities. You want to calculate how much energy he expends at both ends of this activity level. How many kcal does this equal?

$$1,909 \text{ kcal/day} \times 0.50 = 955 \text{ kcal/day}$$
$$1,909 \text{ kcal/day} \times 0.70 = 1,336 \text{ kcal/day}$$

These calculations show that this man expends about 955 to 1,336 kcal/day doing daily activities.

4. *Calculate total daily energy output by adding together BMR and the energy needed to perform daily activities.* In this man's case, his total daily energy output is

$$1,909 \text{ kcal/day} + 955 \text{ kcal/day} = 2,864 \text{ kcal/day}$$

or

$$1,909 \text{ kcal/day} + 1,336 \text{ kcal/day} = 3,245 \text{ kcal/day}$$

Assuming this man is maintaining his present weight, he requires between 2,864 and 3,245 kcal/day to stay in energy balance.

	Men	Women
Sedentary/Inactive Involves mostly sitting, driving, or very low levels of activity	25–40%	25–35%
Lightly Active Involves a lot of sitting; may also involve some walking, moving around, and light lifting	50–70%	40–60%
Moderately Active Involves work plus intentional exercise, such as an hour of walking or walking 4 to 5 days per week; may have a job requiring some physical labor	65–80%	50–70%
Heavily Active Involves a great deal of physical labor, such as roofing, carpentry work, and/or regular heavy lifting and digging	90–120%	80–100%
Exceptionally Active Involves a lot of physical activities for work and intentional exercise; also applies to athletes who train for many hours each day, such as triathletes and marathon runners or other competitive athletes performing heavy, regular training	130–145%	110–130%

Research Suggests Limitations of the Energy Balance Equation

As researchers have learned more about the factors that regulate body weight, the accuracy and usefulness of the classic energy balance equation illustrated in Focus Figure 10.5 has been called into question. Many researchers point out that the equation in its current form is static and can only be applied when one is weight stable—meaning it does not account for many factors that can alter energy intake and expenditure when one side of the equation is changed, nor does it help explain why people gain and lose weight differently.

For example, if you were to consume an additional 100 kcal (the energy content of 8 fl oz of a cola beverage) each day above the energy you expended for 10 years, you would consume an extra intake of 365,000 kcal! Based on the static energy balance equation, and assuming that no other changes occur in energy expenditure, you should gain 104 pounds. However, the static energy balance calculation does not take into account the increase in energy expenditure that would occur, including increased BMR and increased cost of moving a larger body, as weight increased. Thus, after a short period of positive energy balance, your body weight would increase, resulting in an increase in energy expenditure that would eventually balance the increased energy intake. You would then achieve energy balance and become weight stable at a higher body weight. Thus, the extra 100 kcal/day would actually result in a more realistic weight gain of a few pounds. To maintain this larger body size you would need to continue to eat these additional kcal.

The inadequacy of the classic energy balance equation to explain individual differences in weight loss or weight gain has prompted experts to propose a dynamic equation of energy balance that takes into account the rates of energy intake and expenditure and their effect on rate of change of energy stores (including fat and lean tissues) in the body, not simply on body weight overall.[6]

> Predict a realistic time course for weight loss or weight gain using the Body Weight Planner at www.niddk.nih.gov/health-information/health-topics/weight-control/body-weight-planner/Pages/bwp.aspx.

recap The energy balance equation states that energy balance occurs when energy intake equals energy expenditure. Over time, consuming more energy than you expend causes weight gain, while consuming less energy than you expend causes weight loss. The three components of energy expenditure are basal metabolic rate, which is the energy expended to maintain basic physiologic functions; the thermic effect of food, which is the energy expended to process food; and the energy cost of physical activity, which is the energy expended in movement above basal levels. Research has called into question the accuracy and usefulness of the classic energy balance equation because it fails to account for many factors that can alter energy intake and expenditure or to explain why people gain and lose weight differently.

What factors influence body weight?

A variety of types of research studies over many decades suggest that the greatest influence on body weight is our genetic inheritance. However, many nongenetic factors also contribute.

> **LO 4** Identify several biological, cultural, economic, and social influences on body weight.

Genes May Influence Body Weight in Different Ways

Our genetic inheritance influences our height, weight, body shape, and metabolic rate. Research indicates that approximately 46% of children with overweight or obese parents are also overweight or obese, whereas only 14% of children with normal-weight parents are overweight or obese.[8] Does this mean that we are destined to be overweight or obese if our parents are? Not necessarily. It is estimated that 50% to 70% of our BMI can be accounted for by genetic influences.[9] This means that 30% to 50% of our BMI is accounted for by nongenetic, environmental factors and lifestyle choices, such as exposure to cheap, high-energy food and low levels of physical activity.

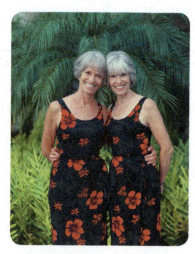

⬆ Genetic factors do influence body weight. Identical twins, for example, tend to maintain a similar weight throughout life.

Exactly how do genetic factors influence body weight? We discuss here some hypotheses attempting to explain this link.

The FTO Gene

The existing evidence on genetics and obesity indicates that there is no one single "obesity gene." Instead, 97 genes currently are thought to be associated with an increased risk for obesity.[10] Nevertheless, one gene that has received a great deal of attention is the fat mass and obesity (FTO)–associated gene. This gene is relatively common: Approximately 44% to 65% of people are estimated to have at least one copy. The gene is associated with higher levels of hunger and increased intake of foods high in fat and refined starches, and increased depressive symptoms.[11] Thus, it's not surprising that people who carry the gene weigh more, on average, than people who do not.

The Thrifty Gene Hypothesis

The **thrifty gene hypothesis** suggests that some people possess a gene (or genes) that causes them to be energetically thrifty. This means that at rest and even during active times these individuals expend less energy than people who do not possess this gene. The proposed purpose of this gene is to protect a person from starving to death during times of extreme food shortages. This hypothesis has been applied to some Native American tribes, as these societies were exposed to centuries of feast and famine. Those with a thrifty metabolism survived when little food was available, and this trait was passed on to future generations. Although an actual thrifty gene (or genes) has not yet been identified, researchers continue to study this explanation as a potential cause of obesity.

If this hypothesis is true, think about how people who possess this thrifty gene might respond to today's environment. Low levels of physical activity, inexpensive food sources that are high in fat and energy, and excessively large serving sizes are the norm. People with a thrifty metabolism would experience a great amount of weight gain, and their body would be more resistant to weight loss.

The Set-Point Hypothesis

The **set-point hypothesis** suggests that our body is designed to maintain our weight within a narrow range, or at a "set point." When we dramatically reduce energy intake (such as with fasting or strict diets), the body responds with physiologic changes that cause BMR to drop. This results in a significant slowing of our energy output. In addition, being physically active while fasting or starving is difficult, because a person just doesn't have the energy for it. These two mechanisms of energy conservation may contribute to some of the rebound weight gain many dieters experience after they quit dieting.

Conversely, overeating in some people may cause an increase in BMR, thought to be due to an increased TEF and increase in spontaneous physical activity. This in turn increases energy output and prevents weight gain. These changes may help to explain the limitations of the classic energy balance equation, mentioned earlier, in predicting how much weight people will gain from eating excess food.

A recent study examined people who participated in a televised weight loss competition *The Biggest Loser* and reported findings supportive of the set-point theory.[12] The average body weight of the participants before they started the competition was just over 327 pounds, and they lost an average of 128 pounds over 30 weeks. As would be expected from this large weight loss, their BMR decreased by 610 kcal/day. When these individuals were followed up 6 years later, all but one had regained some of the weight they had lost—on average, 90 pounds. Despite this increase in body weight, their BMR was now decreased by 704 kcal/day. Moreover, those who were most successful at long-term weight loss were also more likely to experience an ongoing slowing of their BMR. The authors of this study concluded that these individuals were experiencing a persistent metabolic adaptation that worked against their attempts to lose weight and favored maintaining their weight at their original set point.

thrifty gene hypothesis A hypothesis suggesting that some people possess a gene (or genes) that causes them to be energetically thrifty, resulting in their expending less energy at rest and during physical activity.

set-point hypothesis A hypothesis suggesting that the body raises or lowers energy expenditure in response to increased and decreased food intake and physical activity. This action maintains an individual's body weight within a narrow range.

The Protein Leverage Hypothesis

The **protein leverage hypothesis** suggests that humans have evolved to have a fixed daily dietary protein target that must be reached to optimize physiologic functioning, and that we overeat because modern diets contain more foods that are proportionally higher in carbohydrates and fats and lower in protein.[13] That is, we eat more of these foods because our body is trying to meet our genetically programmed protein target.

For example, if you eat two slices of white toast with 1 tablespoon of grape jelly, you would consume approximately 12 grams of protein and 200 kcal. Compare this to 3 ounces of roasted chicken breast, which has about 27 grams of protein and 142 kcal. You would have to eat more than double the amount of toast and jelly to consume the same amount of protein as in the chicken breast, which would lead to you consuming 450 kcal. A review of 38 experimental studies found that the lower the percentage of protein in the diet, the higher the total energy intake in normal, overweight, and obese adults, providing evidence to support the protein leverage hypothesis.[14]

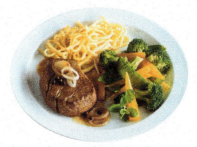

According to the protein-leverage hypothesis, we may be less likely to overeat when our meals provide ample protein.

The Drifty Gene Hypothesis

The **drifty gene hypothesis** suggests an explanation for the observation that, in the current food environment, some people become obese, but others do not. It proposes that the effect is due to random mutation and drift in the genes that control the upper limit of body fatness.[13] This hypothesis states that most mutations in the genes that predispose us to obesity are neutral and have been drifting over evolutionary time. People without these mutations have genetic mechanisms that control the upper limit of body weight and resist obesity, whereas people with "drifty genes" lack this control and therefore are prone to obesity in our current climate of ample, high-energy food and reduced physical activity.

Metabolic Factors Influence Weight Loss and Gain

Six metabolic factors are thought to be predictive of a person's risk for weight gain and resistance to weight loss. These factors are:

- *Relatively low metabolic rate.* At any given size, people vary in their relative BMR—it can be high, normal, or low. People who have a relatively low BMR are more at risk for weight gain and more resistant to weight loss.
- *Low level of spontaneous physical activity.* People who exhibit less spontaneous physical activity are at increased risk for weight gain.
- *Low sympathetic nervous system activity.* The sympathetic nervous system plays an important role in regulating all components of energy expenditure, and people with lower rates of sympathetic nervous system activity are more prone to obesity and more resistant to weight loss.
- *Low rate of the use of fat for energy.* Some people use relatively more carbohydrate for energy, which means that less fat will be used for energy. Thus, relatively more fat will be stored in adipose tissue, so these people are more prone to weight gain. People who use relatively more fat for energy are more resistant to weight gain and are more successful at maintaining weight loss.
- *An abnormally low level of thyroid hormone,* or an elevated level of the hormone cortisol, both of which play roles in metabolism, can lead to weight gain and obesity. A physician can check a patient's blood for levels of these hormones.
- *Certain prescription medications,* including steroids used for asthma and other disorders, seizure medications, and some antidepressants, can slow basal metabolic rate or stimulate appetite, leading to weight gain.[15]

Physiologic Factors Influence Body Weight

Numerous physiologic factors, including hypothalamic regulation of hunger and satiety, specific hormones, and others, contribute to the complexities of weight regulation.

Hypothalamic Cells

After a meal, cells in the hypothalamic *satiety center* are triggered, and the desire to eat is reduced. Some people may have an insufficient satiety mechanism, which

protein leverage hypothesis A hypothesis suggesting that the body has a fixed daily dietary protein target, and because our current diets are proportionally higher in carbohydrates and fats and lower in protein, we overeat to meet this target.

drifty gene hypothesis A hypothesis suggesting that random mutation and drift in the genes that control the upper limit of body fatness can help explain why some people become obese and others do not.

prevents them from feeling full after a meal, allowing them to overeat. Of course, people with a sufficient satiety mechanism can and do override these signals and overeat even when they are not hungry.

Energy-Regulating Hormones

Leptin is a protein hormone produced by adipose cells. First discovered in mice, leptin acts to reduce food intake and to cause a decrease in body weight and body fat. Obese people tend to have very high amounts of leptin in their body but are insensitive to its effects. Researchers are currently studying the role of leptin in starvation and overeating.

Ghrelin, a protein hormone synthesized in the stomach, stimulates appetite and increases the amount of food one eats. Ghrelin levels appear to increase after weight loss, and researchers speculate that this factor could help explain why people who have lost weight have difficulty keeping it off.[16]

Peptide YY (PYY) is a protein hormone produced in the gastrointestinal tract. It is released after a meal in amounts proportional to the energy content of the meal. In contrast with ghrelin, PYY decreases appetite and inhibits food intake. Interestingly, obese individuals have lower levels of PYY when they are fasting and show less of an increase in PYY after a meal, compared with nonobese individuals, which suggests that PYY may be important in the manifestation and maintenance of obesity.[17]

Other Physiologic Factors

The following other physiologic factors are known to increase satiety (or decrease food intake):

- The hormones serotonin and cholecystokinin (CCK); serotonin is made from the amino acid tryptophan, and CCK is produced by the intestinal cells and stimulates the gallbladder to secrete bile
- An increase in blood glucose levels, such as that normally seen after the consumption of a meal
- Stomach expansion
- Nutrient absorption from the small intestine

The following other physiologic factors can decrease satiety (or increase food intake):

- Beta-endorphins, which are hormones that enhance a sense of pleasure while eating, increasing food intake
- Neuropeptide Y, an amino-acid-containing compound produced in the hypothalamus; neuropeptide Y stimulates appetite
- Decreased blood glucose levels, such as the decrease that occurs after an overnight fast

Sociocultural Factors Affect Food Choices and Body Weight

Sociocultural factors can influence food choices, eating patterns, and engagement in physical activity, and thereby contribute to obesity.

Sociocultural Factors and Overeating

Learned food preferences, religious practices, and cultural customs influence the timing, size, and content of meals and snacks. Pressure from family and friends to eat the way they do can encourage people to overeat. For example, the pressure to overeat on special occasions is high, as family members or friends offer an array of favorite foods and may follow a large meal with a rich dessert.

Americans also have numerous opportunities to overeat because of easy access throughout the day to high-energy convenience and fast foods. Vending machines selling junk foods are everywhere, and city streets and shopping malls are filled with fast-food restaurants where inexpensive, high-energy meals are the norm. Fast-food

leptin A hormone, produced by body fat, that acts to reduce food intake and to decrease body weight and body fat.

ghrelin A protein synthesized in the stomach that acts as a hormone and plays an important role in appetite regulation by stimulating appetite.

peptide YY (PYY) A protein produced in the gastrointestinal tract that is released after a meal in amounts proportional to the energy content of the meal; it decreases appetite and inhibits food intake.

franchises are offering meal items in ever-larger sizes: Hardee's ½ lb Frisco Thick-burger® El Diablo packs 1,060 kcal—which is about 50% of the energy intake recommended for an average adult for an entire day! As both parents now work outside the home in most American families, more people are embracing this "fast-food culture," eating high-energy meals from restaurants and grocery stores rather than lower-kcal, home-cooked meals.

In addition to producing ever-larger fast-food meals, the food industry has been manufacturing foods with ever-lower nutrient density. Foods that used to be considered healthful, such as peanut butter, breads and rolls, canned soups, or yogurt, are now made with added sugars, typically high-fructose corn syrup. Over time, the empty Calories from these added sugars contribute to weight gain.

Sociocultural Factors and Inactivity

Coinciding with these influences on food intake are sociocultural factors that promote inactivity. These include the shift from manual labor to more sedentary jobs and increased access to laborsaving devices in all areas of our lives. For instance, many people don't expend energy preparing food anymore, choosing foods that are ready-to-serve or require a few minutes to cook in a microwave oven. Even seemingly minor changes—such as texting someone in your dorm instead of walking down the hall to chat or walking through an automated door instead of pushing a door open—add up to a lower expenditure of energy by the end of the day.

Research with sedentary ethnic minority women indicates that other common barriers to increasing physical activity include lack of time due to placing family responsibilities first, lack of confidence to be physically active, no physically active role models to emulate, acceptance of larger body size, exercise being considered culturally unacceptable, and fear for personal safety.[18,19] In short, cultural factors influence both food consumption and levels of physical activity and can contribute to weight gain.

Economic status is known to be related to health status, particularly in developed countries, such as the United States: people of lower economic status have higher rates of obesity and related chronic diseases than people of higher incomes.[20] Income influences not only eating patterns, but also activity levels, stress levels, and aspects of the environment thought to influence body weight. For example, lower-income populations are more likely to live in areas with higher levels of traffic, and higher levels of pollution from vehicular exhaust have been found to be associated with a higher BMI in children 5 to 11 years of age.[21] Researchers speculate that various factors could contribute to this association, including:

- Reduced levels of physical activity and active travel due to pollution and perceived safety risks;
- Increased stress levels due to higher noise and vibration levels and feeling less safe, which disrupt sleep and increase energy intake; and
- Potential direct effects of pollution itself on hormone regulation and insulin resistance, which could affect appetite and basal metabolic rate.

(For more information on the association between poverty and obesity, see the **In Depth** essay following Chapter 13 on pages 480–485.)

Certainly, social factors are contributing to decreased physical activity among children. There was a time when children played outdoors regularly and physical education was offered daily in school. Today, many children cannot play outdoors due to safety concerns and lack of recreational facilities, and few schools have the resources to regularly offer physical education to children.

Another social factor promoting inactivity in both children and adults is the increasing dominance of technology in our choices of entertainment. Instead of participating in sports or gathering for a dance at the community hall, we go to the movies or stay at home, watching television, surfing the Internet, and playing with video games, smartphones, and other hand-held devices. By reducing energy expenditure, these behaviors contribute to weight gain. For instance, television watching in adults has been shown to be associated with weight gain over a 4-year period.[22]

> Portion sizes have grown over the last few decades. To find out how much, take the Portion Distortion quiz from the National Institutes of Health at www.nhlbi.nih.gov/health/educational/wecan/eat-right/portion-distortion.htm.

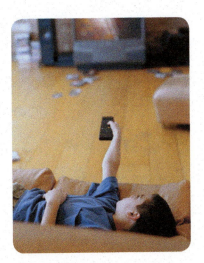

▲ Behaviors learned as a child can affect adult weight and physical activity patterns.

Social Pressures, Overweight, and Underweight

On the other hand, social pressures to maintain a lean body are great enough to encourage many people to undereat or to avoid foods that are perceived as "bad." Our society ridicules and often ostracizes overweight people, many of whom face discrimination in housing, employment, and other areas of their lives. A recent study found that children who are obese are up to 2.7 times more likely to experience bullying than children of normal weight.[23] Moreover, media images of waiflike fashion models and men in tight jeans with muscular chests and abdomens encourage many people—especially adolescents and young adults—to severely restrict their food intake and exercise obsessively to achieve an unrealistic and unattainable weight goal. (See the **In Depth** essay following Chapter 11 on pages 413–423 for information on the consequences of these behaviors.)

It should be clear that how a person gains, loses, and maintains body weight is a complex matter. Most people who are overweight have tried several diet programs but have been unsuccessful in maintaining their weight loss. A significant number of these people have consequently given up all weight-loss attempts. Some even suffer from severe depression related to their body weight. Should we condemn these people as failures and continue to pressure them to lose weight? Should people who are overweight but otherwise healthy (e.g., low blood pressure, cholesterol, triglycerides, and glucose levels) be advised to lose weight? As we continue to search for ways to help people achieve and maintain a healthful body weight, our society must take measures to reduce the social pressures facing people who are overweight or obese.

recap Many factors affect our ability to gain and lose weight. Our genetic background influences our height, weight, body shape, and metabolic rate. The FTO gene variant appears to prompt overeating and weight gain. The thrifty gene hypothesis suggests that some people possess a gene or set of genes that makes their body metabolically thrifty. The set-point hypothesis suggests that our body is designed to maintain weight within a narrow range, also called a set point. The protein-leverage hypothesis suggests that our modern diet, which provides a higher ratio of carbohydrate and fat and a lower ratio of protein, prompts us to overeat. The drifty gene hypothesis suggests that the variation in a people's tendency to maintain a normal weight or to gain weight is due to random mutation and drift in the genes that control the upper limit of body fatness. Metabolic factors, such as low relative resting metabolic rate, low spontaneous physical activity, and low sympathetic nervous system activity, increase the risk for weight gain. Physiologic factors, such as various energy-regulating hormones, impact body weight by their effects on hunger, satiety, appetite, and energy expenditure. Sociocultural factors can significantly influence the amounts and types of food we eat and our engagement in physical activity. These include, for example, the ready availability of large portions of high-energy foods and the dominance of technology in our leisure time. Social pressures on those who are overweight can drive people to use harmful methods to achieve an unrealistic body weight.

LO 5 Develop a diet, exercise, and behavioral plan for healthful weight loss.

How can you lose weight safely and keep it off?

Achieving and maintaining a healthful body weight involve three primary strategies:

- Reasonable reductions in energy intake
- Incorporation of regular and appropriate physical activity
- Application of behavior modification techniques

In this section, we first discuss popular diet plans, which may or may not incorporate these strategies. We then explain how to design a personalized weight-loss plan that includes all three of them.

nutri-case | HANNAH

"I wonder what it would be like to be able to look in the mirror and not feel fat. Like my friend Kristi—she's been skinny since we were kids. I'm just the opposite: I've felt bad about my weight ever since I can remember. One of my worst memories is from the YMCA swim camp the summer I was 10 years old. Of course, we had to wear a swimsuit, and the other kids picked on me so bad I'll never forget it. One of the boys called me 'fatso,' and the girls were even meaner, especially when I was changing in the locker room. That was the last year I was in the swim camp, and I've never owned a swimsuit since."

Think back to your own childhood. Were you ever teased for some aspect of yourself that you felt unable to change? How might organizations that work with children, such as schools, YMCAs, scout troops, and church-based groups, increase their leaders' awareness of social stigmatization of overweight children and reduce incidents of teasing, bullying, and other insensitivity?

Avoid Fad Diets

If you'd like to lose weight and feel more comfortable following an established plan, many are available. How can you know whether or not it is based on sound dietary principles, and whether its promise of long-term weight loss will prove true for *you*? Look to the three strategies just identified: Does the plan promote gradual reductions in energy intake? Does it advocate increased physical activity? Does it include strategies for modifying your eating and activity-related behaviors? Reputable diet plans incorporate all of these strategies. Unfortunately, many dieters are drawn to fad diets, which do not.

Fad diets are simply what their name implies—fads that do not result in long-term, healthful weight changes. To be precise, fad diets are programs that enjoy short-term popularity and are sold based on a marketing gimmick that appeals to the public's desires and fears. The goal of the person or company designing and marketing a fad diet is to make money.

How can you tell if the program you are interested in qualifies as a fad diet? Here are some pointers to help you:

- The promoters of the diet claim that the program is new, improved, or based on some new discovery; however, no scientific data are available to support these claims.
- The program is touted for its ability to promote rapid weight loss or body fat loss, usually more than 2 pounds per week, and may include the claim that weight loss can be achieved with little or no physical exercise.
- Common recommendations for these diets include avoiding certain foods, eating only a special combination of certain foods, and including foods in the diet that are said to "burn fat" and "speed up metabolism."
- The diet may include a rigid menu that must be followed daily or may limit participants to eating a few select foods each day. Variety and balance are discouraged.
- The diet includes special foods and supplements, many of which are expensive and/or difficult to find or can be purchased only from the diet promoter, but are described as critical to the success of the diet. The promoters may also claim that these products can cure or prevent a variety of illnesses or stop the aging process.

In a world where many of us feel we have to meet a certain physical standard to be attractive and "good enough," fad diets flourish, with millions of people trying one each year.[24] Unfortunately, the only people who usually benefit from them are their marketers, who can become very wealthy promoting programs that are highly ineffectual.

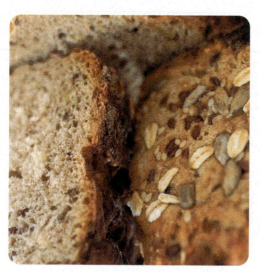

▲ Higher-carbohydrate diets encourage consumption of foods rich in fiber.

Many Diets Focus on Macronutrient Composition

The three main types of weight-loss diets that have been most seriously and comprehensively researched all encourage increased consumption of certain macronutrients and restrict the consumption of others. Provided here is a brief review of these diets and their general effects on weight loss and health parameters.

Diets High in Carbohydrate and Moderate in Fat and Protein

The DASH diet, the USDA Food Guide, Weight Watchers, and Jenny Craig are nutritionally balanced diets that typically contain 55% to 60% of total energy intake as carbohydrate, 20% to 30% as fat, and 15% to 20% as protein. Typical energy deficits are between 500 and 1,000 kcal/day. Although a substantial amount of high-quality scientific evidence indicates that these diets may be effective in decreasing body weight and improving blood lipids and blood pressure, at least initially, other studies have found that these diets do not result in significant long-term weight loss or reduce the risk for cardiovascular disease.[25–28] Is it possible that diets high in carbohydrate and moderate in fat and protein are not as effective as we'd come to believe? Refer to the **Nutrition Debate** essay at the end of this chapter (page 369) to learn more about this controversy.

Diets Low in Carbohydrate and High in Fat and Protein

Low-carbohydrate, high-fat and protein diets generally contain about 55% to 65% of total energy intake as fat and most of the remaining balance of daily energy intake as protein. Examples include Dr. Atkins' Diet Revolution, Sugar Busters!, and the paleo diet. Instead of advising participants to restrict energy intake, they advise restricting carbohydrate intake, proposing that carbohydrates are addictive and cause overeating, insulin surges leading to excessive fat storage, and an overall metabolic imbalance that leads to obesity. The goal is to reduce carbohydrates enough to cause ketosis, which will decrease blood glucose and insulin levels and can reduce appetite.

Countless people claim to have lost substantial weight on these types of diets. The current limited evidence that has examined their effectiveness suggests that individuals following them, in both free-living and experimental conditions, do lose weight and improve their metabolic risk factors (such as blood lipid levels) for a period of at least 6 months.[29] However, the long-term health benefits of this type of a diet are unknown at this time.

If You Design Your Own Diet Plan, Include the Three Strategies

As we noted earlier, a healthful and effective weight-loss plan involves implementing a modest reduction in energy intake, incorporating physical activity into each day, and practicing changes in behavior that can assist you in reducing your energy intake and increasing your energy expenditure. If you'd like to lose weight, the following guidelines can help you design your own personalized diet plan that incorporates these strategies.

Set Realistic Goals

The first key to safe and effective weight loss is setting realistic, achievable goals related to how much weight to lose and how quickly to lose it. A fair expectation for weight loss is gradual: experts recommend a pace of about 0.5 to 2 pounds per week. Unless you are under a physician's supervision your weight-loss plan shouldn't provide less than 1,200 kcal/day, which would be less than the energy needed to cover most individuals' BMR. Your weight-loss goals should also take into consideration any health-related concerns you have. After checking with your physician, you may decide initially to set a goal of simply maintaining your current weight and preventing additional weight gain. After your weight has remained stable for several weeks, you might then write down realistic goals for weight loss.

Goals that are more likely to be realistic and achievable share the following characteristics:

- *They are specific.* Telling yourself "I will eat less this week" is not helpful because the goal is not specific. An example of a specific goal is "I will eat only half of my restaurant entrée tonight and take the rest home and eat it tomorrow for lunch."
- *They are reasonable.* If you are not presently physically active, it would be unreasonable to set a goal of exercising for 30 minutes every day. A more reasonable goal would be to exercise for 15 minutes per day, 3 days per week. Once you've achieved that goal, you can increase the frequency, intensity, and time of exercise according to the improvements in fitness that you have experienced.
- *They are measurable.* Effective goals are ones you can measure. An example is "I will lose at least 1 pound by May 1."

Recording and monitoring your goals will help you better determine whether you are achieving them or whether you need to revise them based on accomplishments or challenges that arise.

Eat Smaller Portions of Nutrient-Dense Foods

The portion sizes of foods and beverages offered and sold in restaurants and grocery stores in the United States have expanded considerably over the past 40 years. Studies associate these larger portion sizes with a corresponding increase in the average energy consumption of American children and adults.[30,31] Thus, reducing the portion size of the foods and beverages you consume may be a highly effective weight-loss strategy. Refer to the **Quick Tips** box to learn more about how to control your portion sizes.

In addition to controlling portion sizes, try to increase the number of times each day that you choose foods that are relatively low in energy density. This includes salads (with low-Calorie dressings), whole fruits and vegetables, whole grains, low-fat and nonfat dairy products, lean meats, and broth-based soups. Research indicates that

Quick Tips

Controlling Portion Sizes

To help increase your understanding of the portion sizes of packaged foods, measure out the amount of food that is identified as 1 serving on the Nutrition Facts panel, and eat it from a plate or bowl instead of straight out of the box or bag.

Try using smaller dishes, bowls, and glasses. This will make your portion appear larger, and you'll be eating or drinking less.

When cooking at home, put a serving of the entrée on your plate; then freeze any leftovers in single-serving containers. This way, you won't be tempted to eat the whole batch before the food goes bad, and you'll have ready-made servings for future meals.

To fill up, take second helpings of plain vegetables. That way, dessert may not seem so tempting!

When buying snacks, go for single-serving, prepackaged items. If you buy larger bags or boxes, divide the snack into single-serving bags.

When you have a treat, such as ice cream, measure out 1/2 cup, eat it slowly, and enjoy it!

To test your understanding of what exactly constitutes a serving size, take the "Portion Distortion" interactive quiz from the National Institutes of Health. (See **Web Links** at the end of this chapter.)

eating a diet low in energy density improves weight loss and weight maintenance.[32] Because low energy-dense foods are relatively high in water and fiber than more energy-dense foods, they have a greater volume and occupy more space in the stomach, helping a person to feel full. In addition, low energy-dense foods are just as satiating as those higher in energy density, but they are lower in energy for every gram of food consumed. Thus, the energy content of an energy-dense eating plan is lower but equally as satisfying.

MEAL FOCUS FIGURE 10.7 illustrates two sets of meals, one higher in energy density and one lower. You can see from this figure that simple changes to a meal, such as choosing leaner meats, skipping the cookies, and reducing portion sizes, can reduce energy intake without sacrificing taste, pleasure, or nutritional quality!

Participate in Regular Physical Activity

The *Dietary Guidelines for Americans* emphasize the role of physical activity in maintaining a healthful weight. Why? Of course, we expend extra energy during physical activity, but there's more to it than that, because exercise alone (without a reduction of energy intake) does not result in dramatic weight loss. Instead, one of the most important reasons for being regularly active is that it helps us maintain or increase our lean body mass and our BMR. In contrast, energy restriction alone causes us to lose lean body mass. As you've learned, the more lean body mass we have, the more energy we expend over the long term.

Although very few weight-loss studies have documented long-term maintenance of weight loss, those that have find that only people who are regularly active are able to maintain most of their weight loss. The National Weight Control Registry is an ongoing project documenting the habits of people who have lost at least 30 pounds and kept their weight off for at least 1 year. Of the people studied thus far, the average weight loss was 66 pounds over 5.5 years.[33] Almost all of the people (98%) reported changing their dietary intake to lose weight, and 94% report increasing their physical activity, with walking being the most commonly reported form of activity. These successful "losers" reported doing an average of at least 1 hour of physical activity per day.

In addition to expending energy and maintaining lean body mass and BMR, regular physical activity improves our mood, results in a higher quality of sleep, increases self-esteem, and gives us a sense of accomplishment. All of these changes enhance our ability to engage in long-term healthful lifestyle behaviors.

What specific changes can you make to your level of physical activity? Although plenty of practical suggestions will be offered (in Chapter 11), the **Quick Tips** box (page 366) provides some ideas that can help you to start identifying and overcoming your barriers to an active life.

Incorporate Appropriate Behavior Modifications into Daily Life

Successful weight loss and long-term maintenance of a healthful weight require people to modify their behaviors. Some of the behavior modifications related to food and physical activity were discussed in the previous sections. Here are a few more **Quick Tips** (page 367) on modifying behavior that will assist you in losing weight and maintaining a healthful weight.

Interest has been growing about the effects of applying mindfulness to our eating practices. *Mindfulness* refers to the nonjudgmental awareness of the present moment. **Mindful eating** refers to a nonjudgmental awareness of the emotional and physical sensations one experiences while eating or in a food-related environment. Several recently published pilot studies conducted with small numbers of participants have indicated that mindful eating may help to promote healthy eating practices when eating out; enhance weight loss and psychological well-being in people with obesity; and improve dietary intake and blood glucose control in adults with type 2 diabetes.[34,35]

Interested in exploring mindful eating practices? Here are some tips to help get you started:

mindful eating The nonjudgmental awareness of the emotional and physical sensations one experiences while eating or in a food-related environment.

- *Focus only on eating*: Turn off the television, put away your cell phone, tune out distractions, and focus on your food and the process of eating.
- *Savor each bite*: Take your time, slow down, and chew slowly.

a day of meals

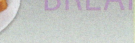
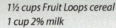
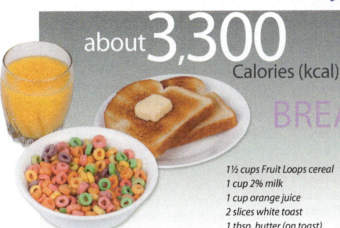

about **3,300**
Calories (kcal)

BREAKFAST

1½ cups Fruit Loops cereal
1 cup 2% milk
1 cup orange juice
2 slices white toast
1 tbsp. butter (on toast)

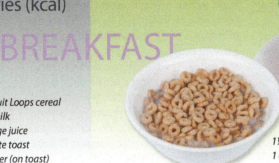
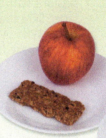

about **1,700**
Calories (kcal)

1½ cups Cheerios cereal
1 cup skim milk
½ fresh pink grapefruit

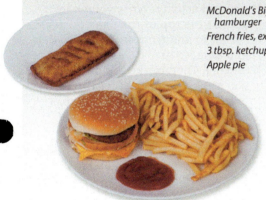

McDonald's Big Mac hamburger
French fries, extra large
3 tbsp. ketchup
Apple pie

LUNCH

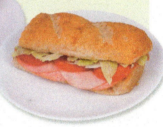

Subway cold-cut trio 6" sandwich
Granola bar, hard, with chocolate chips, 1 bar (24 g)
1 fresh medium apple

DINNER

4.5 oz ground beef (80% lean, crumbled), cooked
2 medium taco shells
2 oz cheddar cheese
2 tbsp. sour cream
4 tbsp. store-bought salsa
1 cup shredded lettuce
½ cup refried beans
6 Oreos

5 oz ground turkey, cooked
2 soft corn tortillas
1 oz low-fat cheddar cheese
4 tbsp. store-bought salsa
1 cup shredded lettuce
1 cup cooked mixed veggies

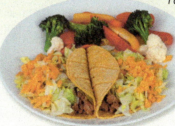

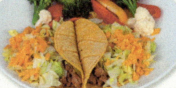

nutrient analysis

3,319 kcal
44.1% of energy from carbohydrates
44.2% of energy from fat
15.6% of energy from saturated fat
12.5% of energy from protein
31.4 grams of dietary fiber
4,752 milligrams of sodium

Saves
1,600
kcal!

nutrient analysis

1,753 kcal
44.6% of energy from carbohydrates
31.5% of energy from fat
10.6% of energy from saturated fat
21% of energy from protein
24.9 grams of dietary fiber
3,161 milligrams of sodium

QuickTips

Overcoming Barriers to Physical Activity

I don't have enough time! An active lifestyle doesn't have to consume all your free time. Try to do a minimum of 30 minutes of moderate activity most—preferably all—days of the week. If you can, do 45 minutes. But remember, you don't have to get in all of your daily activity in one go! Be active for a few minutes at a time throughout your day. Walk from your dorm or apartment to classes, if possible. Instead of meeting friends for lunch, meet them for a lunchtime walk, jog, or workout. Break up study sessions with 3 minutes of jumping jacks. Skip the elevator and take the stairs. When you're talking on the phone, pace instead of sitting still.

I can't manage the details! Bust this excuse by keeping clean clothes, shoes, water, and equipment for physical activity in a convenient place. If time management is an obstacle, enroll in a scheduled fitness class, yoga class, sports activity, walking group, or running club. Put it on your schedule of academic classes and make it part of your weekly routine.

I just don't like to work out! You don't have to! Try dancing, roller blading, walking, hiking, swimming, tennis, or any other activity you enjoy.

I can't stay motivated. Friends can help. Use the "buddy" system by exercising with a friend and calling each other when you need encouragement to stay motivated. Or keep a journal or log of your daily physical activity. Write your week's goal at the top of the page (such as "Walk to and from campus each day, and at least 10 minutes on campus at lunch"). Then track your progress. If you achieve your goal for the week, reward yourself with a massage, a new song for your iPod, or some other nonfood treat.

- *Recruit all of your senses*: Focus your attention on the smell, taste, texture, and even the temperature of your food. Pay attention to any sensations of satisfaction or fullness.
- *Pause and rest between bites*: Take a few breaths, sit back, and relax between each mouthful of food.
- *Try 10 minutes of silence*: If eating with others, try to avoid conversations in order to enhance your ability to be more aware of your food and the experience of eating.

Incorporating mindful eating into your life doesn't have to be a chore. Try practicing mindful eating during one meal each week. With practice, you may be inspired to do it more often!

recap If you would like to lose weight and maintain that weight loss, a first step is to set a realistic, achievable goal. Experts recommend a pace of about 0.5 to 2 pounds of weight loss per week. You can achieve this by making gradual reductions in energy intake, such as by eating smaller portion sizes and choosing foods low in energy density and high in nutrient density. The precise macronutrient composition of the diet is thought to matter less than reduction in your energy intake. Avoid fad diets, programs that enjoy short-term popularity but do not incorporate sensible energy, activity, and behavioral strategies. A second step is to engage in regular physical activity, typically at least 30 minutes a day at least 5 days a week. This will not only burn energy but also help maintain or increase your lean body mass and BMR. Third and finally, apply appropriate behavior modification techniques, such as keeping a food log, avoiding shopping when you're hungry, and engaging in mindful eating.

QuickTips

Modifying Your Behaviors Related to Food

✓ Shop for food only when you're not hungry.

✓ Avoid buying problem foods—that is, foods that you may have difficulty eating in moderate amounts.

✓ Avoid purchasing empty-Calorie foods and beverages from vending machines and convenience stores.

✓ Avoid feelings of deprivation by eating small, regular meals throughout the day.

✓ Always use appropriate utensils.

✓ Eat mindfully, savoring the aromas, tastes, and textures of each food. Do not eat while studying, working, driving, watching television, and so forth.

✓ Eat slowly. Take at least 20 minutes to eat a full meal.

✓ Stop eating if you begin to feel full. Store food for the next meal.

✓ Keep a log of what you eat, when, and why. Try to identify social or emotional cues that cause you to overeat, such as getting a poor grade on an exam or feeling lonely. Then strategize about nonfood-related ways to cope, such as phoning a sympathetic friend.

✓ Save empty-Calorie snack foods (such as ice cream, doughnuts, and cakes) for occasional special treats.

✓ Whether at home or dining out, share food with others.

✓ Prepare healthful snacks to take along with you, so that you won't be tempted by foods from vending machines, fast-food restaurants, and so forth.

✓ Don't punish yourself for deviating from your plan (and you will—everyone does). Ask others to avoid responding to any slips you make.

What if you need to gain weight?

LO 6 Identify four key strategies for gaining weight safely and effectively.

As defined earlier in this chapter, underweight occurs when a person has too little body fat to maintain health. People with a BMI of less than 18.5 kg/m^2 are typically considered underweight. Being underweight can be just as unhealthful as being obese, because it increases the risk for infections and illness and impairs the body's ability to recover. Some people are healthy but underweight because of their genetics and/or because they are very physically active and consume adequate energy to maintain their underweight status, but not enough to gain weight. In others, underweight is due to heavy smoking; an underlying disease, such as cancer or HIV infection; or an eating disorder, such as *anorexia nervosa* (see the **In Depth** essay following Chapter 11).

For Safe and Effective Weight Gain, Choose Nutrient-Dense Foods

With so much emphasis in the United States on obesity and weight loss, some find it surprising that many people are trying to gain weight. People looking to gain weight include those who are underweight to the extent that it is compromising their

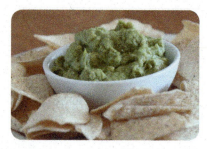

▲ Eating frequent nutrient-dense snacks can help promote weight gain.

health and many athletes who are attempting to increase strength and power for competition.

To gain weight, people must eat more energy than they expend. While overeating large amounts of foods high in saturated fats (such as bacon, sausage, and cheese) can cause weight gain, doing this without exercising is not considered healthful because most of the weight gained is fat, and high-fat diets increase our risks for cardiovascular and other diseases. However, diets that are relatively higher in mono- and polyunsaturated fats, such as a Mediterranean-style diet, can be a healthful approach to weight gain. Recommendations for weight gain include:

- Eat a diet that includes about 500 to 1,000 kcal/day more than is needed to maintain present body weight. Although we don't know exactly how much extra energy is needed to gain 1 pound, estimates range from 3,000 to 3,500 kcal. Thus, eating 500 to 1,000 kcal/day in excess should result in a gain of 1 to 2 pounds of weight each week.
- Eat frequently, including meals and numerous snacks throughout the day. Many underweight people do not take the time to eat often enough.
- Avoid the use of tobacco products, as they depress appetite and increase metabolic rate, and both of these effects oppose weight gain. Tobacco use also causes lung, mouth, esophageal and other cancers and is a factor in cardiovascular disease.
- Exercise regularly and incorporate weight lifting or some other form of resistance training into your exercise routine. This form of exercise is most effective in increasing muscle mass. Performing aerobic exercise (such as walking, running, bicycling, or swimming) at least 30 minutes for 3 days per week will help maintain a healthy cardiovascular system.

The key to gaining weight is to eat frequent meals throughout the day and to select healthful energy-dense foods. For instance, smoothies and milkshakes made with low-fat milk or yogurt are a great way to take in a lot of energy. Eating peanut butter with fruit or celery and including salad dressings on your salad are other ways to increase the energy density of foods. The biggest challenge to weight gain is setting aside time to eat; by packing a lot of foods to take with you throughout the day, you can enhance your opportunities to eat more.

Amino Acid and Protein Supplements Do Not Increase Muscle Mass

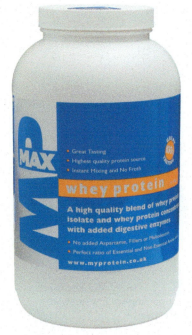

▲ Protein powders or amino acid supplements will not enhance muscle growth or make you stronger.

Many products marketed for weight gain are said to be *anabolic*, that is, to increase muscle mass. The most common of these include amino acid and protein supplements, often powders used to make protein "shakes." However, current evidence indicates that these products are not necessary to increase muscle mass. Instead, adequate intake of energy, protein from high-quality food sources, and resistance training promote healthy increases in muscle mass. Moreover, although they are legal to sell in the United States, all potentially anabolic substances are banned by the National Football League, the National Collegiate Athletic Association, and the International Olympic Committee. We do know that buying these substances can have a substantial slenderizing effect—on your wallet!

recap Weight gain can be achieved by increasing your kcal intake by about 500 to 1,000 kcal/day more than is needed to maintain your present body weight. Focus on eating more nutrient-dense foods. Engage in regular resistance training to build and maintain muscle mass, and aerobic exercise to preserve your cardiovascular fitness. Avoid tobacco use, as it depresses appetite and increases metabolic rate, and is associated with an increased risk of cancer and many other diseases. Protein and amino acid supplements are not necessary to increase muscle mass, as adequate high-quality protein can be easily obtained in the diet. Anabolic substances are banned by major sports governing organizations.

High-Carbohydrate, Moderate-Fat Diets—Have They Been Oversold?

For the past 30 years, dietary fat has been demonized as a cause of obesity, cardiovascular disease, type 2 diabetes, and many types of cancer; thus, national dietary guidelines have encouraged consumption of a moderate-fat, high-carbohydrate diet. Then, in 2006, results from the Women's Health Initiative (WHI) Dietary Modification Trial indicated that, although the more than 48,000 postmenopausal women who participated in the trial lost a modest amount of weight (on average 4.8 pounds), they experienced no significant health benefits. There was no reduction in risk for cardiovascular disease, breast cancer, or colorectal cancer.[36–39]

Moreover, a number of other studies since 2006 have found no significant advantage of high-carbohydrate, moderate-fat diets in promoting weight loss as compared to other types of diets. For example, the Diabetes Excess Weight Loss (DEWL) trial compared weight loss in 419 adults with type 2 diabetes who consumed either a moderate-fat, high-protein diet or a moderate-fat, high-carbohydrate diet.[40] Weight loss over 12 months averaged 4.4 to 6.6 pounds for both diet groups, with a similar number of participants sustaining their weight loss for an additional 12 months. Similarly, in the POUNDS LOST trial, participants consumed one of four diets that differed in levels of fat, protein, and carbohydrate.[41] Weight loss was similar for all groups at 6 months (an average of 13.9 pounds), and maintenance of net weight loss after 2 years was also similar (8.4 pounds).

These studies are part of a growing body of evidence that the key to weight loss is decreasing *total* energy intake—not one particular macronutrient group—sufficiently below energy expenditure, and that the key to reducing chronic disease risks is changing the *types* of dietary fat and carbohydrate consumed, not the relative amounts. Many Americans reduce their intake of all types of dietary fat, including beneficial unsaturated fats, and replace that fat with low-fiber, highly refined carbohydrate foods—often made with added sugars. We now know that this substitution can contribute to weight gain and negative changes in blood lipids and blood glucose.[42]

The detrimental health effects resulting from the overconsumption of processed foods, grains, and grain-fed animals is a key factor driving the popularity of the paleo (or paleolithic) diet, which encourages consumption of only those foods that can be hunted, fished, or gathered. This includes fresh lean meats and fish (ideally wild game and fish), eggs, fruits, some vegetables, nuts and seeds, and olive and

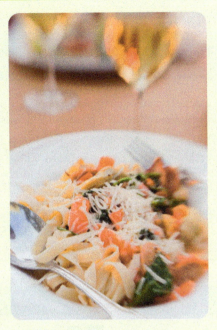

Research findings supporting a high-carbohydrate, moderate-fat diet have been mixed.

coconut oils. All refined foods are prohibited, along with all grains, legumes, dairy, and processed vegetable oils such as canola.

To date, a limited number of research studies have been conducted on the long-term effects of the paleo diet. A recent systematic review found four studies examining the effect of paleo-type diets on the metabolic syndrome and weight loss as compared to control diets based on current dietary recommendations (in three studies) or the Mediterranean diet (in one study).[43] These studies included a small number of participants (17 to 70), and ranged in duration from 2 weeks to 2 years. The findings indicate that the paleo-type diet can promote greater weight loss (almost 6 pounds greater) than the control diets, with greater reductions in waist circumference, triglycerides, and blood pressure. However, the Academy of Nutrition and Dietetics cautions that the paleo diet exceeds the DRIs for saturated fat and protein intake, and is deficient in carbohydrates; moreover, the exclusion of whole grains, legumes, and dairy could lead to deficiencies in micronutrients and dietary fiber.[44]

So what is the most healthful approach to weight loss? Most reputable sources, including the Dietary Guidelines for Americans, recommend reducing total energy intake by 500 to 750 kcal per day, decreasing intake of added sugars and saturated and *trans* fats, increasing intake of foods high in unsaturated fats, and meeting or exceeding the physical activity guidelines for Americans.

CRITICAL THINKING QUESTIONS

1. Do you think that higher-fat diets, such as the paleo diet, are better or worse alternatives to higher-carbohydrate, lower-fat diets? Why or why not?
2. Vegan diets are consistently associated with numerous health benefits. How might both a vegan diet and the paleo diet improve body weight, blood lipids, and other factors associated with the metabolic syndrome?
3. Go to ChooseMyPlate.gov and use the SuperTracker tool to create a one-day food plan for the following diets: (1) high in carbohydrate and moderate in fat and protein; (2) low in carbohydrate and high in fat and protein. Based on your research, which diet do you think would be easier for you to follow long term and provide enough energy and nutrients to maintain your lifestyle, your lean-body mass, and your long-term health?

STUDY PLAN MasteringNutrition™

review questions

LO 1 1. A healthful body weight is a weight that
   a. is very close to that of other members of your immediate family.
   b. you can maintain if you keep your kcal intake no higher than your BMR.
   c. is acceptable to your peers.
   d. None of the above.

LO 2 2. The ratio of a person's body weight to height is represented as his or her
   a. body mass index.
   b. fat distribution pattern.
   c. basal metabolic rate.
   d. fat-to-lean tissue ratio.

LO 3 3. All people gain weight when they
   a. eat a high-fat diet (>35% fat).
   b. take in more energy than they expend.
   c. fail to exercise.
   d. consume more energy, on average, than they did the previous year.

LO 3 4. Energy balance occurs when
   a. energy expended via basal metabolism, the thermic effect of food, and physical activity equals energy intake.
   b. energy expended via basal metabolism, temperature regulation, and exercise is greater than energy intake.
   c. energy expended via the body mass index, basal metabolism, and physical activity equals energy intake.
   d. energy expended via the body mass index, the thermic effect of food, and physical activity is greater than energy intake.

LO 4 5. Which of the following increases appetite?
   a. leptin
   b. ghrelin
   c. an increase in blood glucose
   d. smoking

LO 4 6. Which of the following individuals is most likely to have a BMI over 30?
   a. an investment banker who has time to exercise with a personal trainer twice weekly
   b. a high school home economics teacher who loves to cook and who rides a bicycle to work each day
   c. a low-income single parent who provides child care to other families in their urban apartment block
   d. a college student who smokes and gets no exercise other than walking to and from campus

LO 5 7. A plan for healthful weight loss begins with
   a. a realistic, achievable goal.
   b. behavioral counseling or enrollment in a support group.
   c. a low-fat diet.
   d. a low-carb diet.

LO 6 8. Which of the following would be the most nutritious snack choice for someone who wishes to gain weight healthfully?
   a. a slice of pepperoni pizza with extra cheese
   b. four chocolate-chip cookies
   c. a peanut-butter sandwich on whole-grain bread with an apple
   d. a strawberry shake made by mixing protein powder into strawberry milk

LO 2 9. **True or false?** Pear-shaped fat patterning is known to increase a person's risk for many chronic diseases, including diabetes and heart disease.

LO 3 10. **True or false?** About 60% to 75% of our energy output goes to fuel the basic activities of staying alive.

math review

LO 5 11. Your friend Misty joins you for lunch and confesses that she is discouraged about her weight. She says that she has been trying "really hard" for 3 months to lose weight but that, no matter what she does, she cannot drop below 148 pounds. Based on her height of 5 feet 8 inches, calculate Misty's BMI. Is she overweight? What questions would you suggest she think about? How would you advise her? Misty's level of physical activity would classify her as moderately active. Approximately how many kcal does she need each day to maintain her current body weight?

Answers to Review Questions and Math Review are located at the back of this text, and in the MasteringNutrition Study Area.

web links

www.ftc.gov
Federal Trade Commission
Click on "Tips & Advice" and select "For Consumers" and then "Health and Fitness" to find how to avoid false weight-loss claims.

www.nutrition.gov/weight-management
Nutrition.gov
Visit this site to learn about successful strategies for achieving and maintaining a healthy weight.

www.eatright.org
Academy of Nutrition and Dietetics
Go to this site to learn more about fad diets and nutrition facts.

www.niddk.nih.gov/health-information/Pages/default .aspx
National Institute of Diabetes and Digestive and Kidney Diseases
Find out more about healthy weight loss and how it pertains to diabetes and digestive and kidney diseases.

www.sneb.org
Society for Nutrition Education and Behavior
Click on "Nutrition Resources" and then "Weight Realities Division Resource List" for additional resources related to positive attitudes about body image and healthful alternatives to dieting.

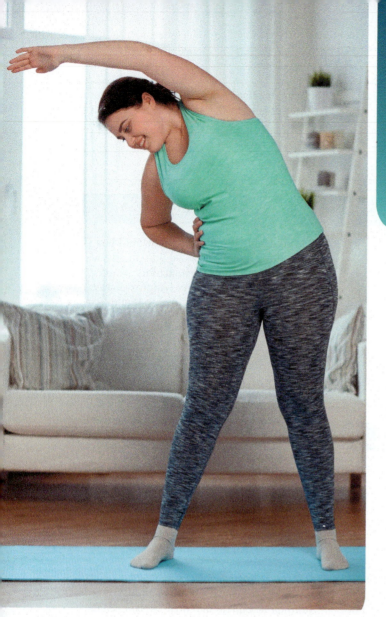

Obesity

Before her weight-loss surgery, Luisa's morbid obesity left her short of breath after climbing a single flight of stairs. Now she begins most days with a brisk walk around her neighborhood, stretches while she listens to the morning news, lifts weights two afternoons a week at her campus fitness center, and joins her friends for a hike, swim, or Frisbee every weekend. Moreover, she follows a healthful eating pattern, choosing nutrient-dense meals rich in dietary fiber that keep her feeling satisfied. As a result, her blood glucose—which formerly had met the criteria for type 2 diabetes—has plummeted, her joints no longer ache, and her breathing isn't labored even after she's climbed two or three flights of stairs.

Luisa's high blood glucose, shortness of breath, aching joints, and other signs and symptoms are not the only consequences of obesity. In this **In Depth** essay, we identify the life-threatening diseases and complications linked to this disorder. We also review the multiple variables that influence energy balance and body weight, and discuss weight-loss surgery and other options for obesity treatment.

learning outcomes

After studying this In Depth, you should be able to:

1 Discuss several chronic diseases and complications linked to obesity, including its association with metabolic syndrome and premature mortality, pp. 373–374.

2 Explain why obesity is considered a multifactorial disease, identifying several contributing factors, pp. 374–375.

3 Describe the effectiveness of lifestyle changes, medications, dietary supplements, and surgery in obesity treatment, pp. 376–379.

Why is obesity harmful?

LO 1 Discuss several chronic diseases and complications linked to obesity, including its association with metabolic syndrome and premature mortality.

Recall from Chapter 10 that obesity is defined as having an excess body fat that adversely affects health, resulting in a person having a weight for a given height that is substantially greater than some accepted standard. People with a BMI between 30 and 39.9 kg/m^2 are considered obese. Morbid obesity occurs when a person's body weight exceeds 100% of normal; people who are morbidly obese have a BMI greater than or equal to 40 kg/m^2.

Obesity rates have increased more than 50% during the past 20 years, and it is now estimated that about 34.9% of adults 20 years and older are obese.[1] This alarming rise in obesity is a major health concern because it is linked to many chronic diseases and complications:

- Hypertension
- Dyslipidemia, including elevated total cholesterol, triglycerides, and LDL-cholesterol and decreased HDL-cholesterol
- Type 2 diabetes
- Heart disease
- Stroke
- Gallbladder disease
- Osteoarthritis
- Sleep apnea
- Certain cancers, such as colon, breast, endometrial, and gallbladder cancer
- Menstrual irregularities and infertility
- Gestational diabetes, premature fetal deaths, neural tube defects, and complications during labor and delivery
- Depression
- Alzheimer's disease, dementia, and cognitive decline

Abdominal obesity is specifically a large amount of visceral fat that is stored deep within the abdomen **(FIGURE 1)**. This stored fat releases excess fatty acids and

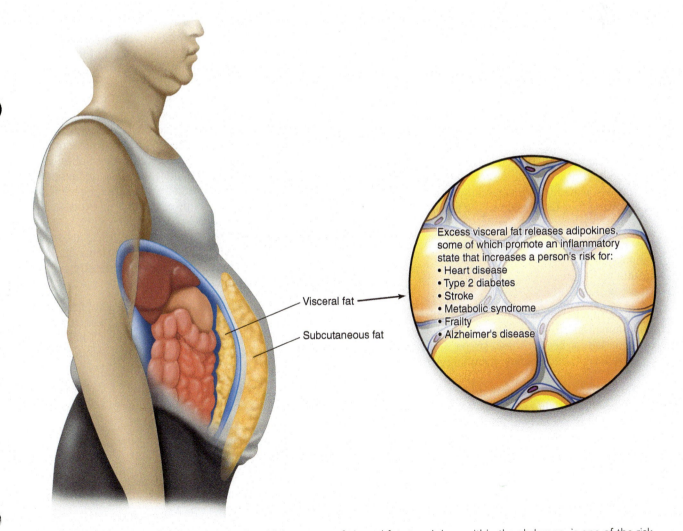

Visceral fat

Subcutaneous fat

Excess visceral fat releases adipokines, some of which promote an inflammatory state that increases a person's risk for:
- Heart disease
- Type 2 diabetes
- Stroke
- Metabolic syndrome
- Frailty
- Alzheimer's disease

FIGURE 1 Abdominal obesity, specifically a high amount of visceral fat stored deep within the abdomen, is one of the risk factors for metabolic syndrome.

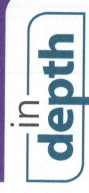
adipokines, cell signaling proteins secreted by adipose tissue. Some adipokines engage in activities that promote an inflammatory state in body tissues, and thus are referred to as *pro-inflammatory*. This inflammatory state increases a person's risk for **metabolic syndrome**, which is diagnosed when a person has three or more of the following five risk factors:[2]

1. Abdominal obesity (defined as a waist circumference greater than or equal to 40 inches for men and 35 inches for women)
2. Higher-than-normal triglyceride levels (greater than or equal to 150 mg/dL)
3. Lower-than-normal HDL-cholesterol levels (less than 40 mg/dL in men and 50 mg/dL in women)
4. Higher-than-normal blood pressure (greater than or equal to 130/85 mm Hg)
5. Fasting blood glucose levels greater than or equal to 100 mg/dL, including people with diabetes

People with metabolic syndrome are twice as likely to develop heart disease and five times as likely to develop type 2 diabetes as people without metabolic syndrome. About 23% of adults in the United States have metabolic syndrome, and rising rates of elevated blood glucose and abdominal obesity are major contributors to the syndrome.[3]

In addition to increasing an individual's risk for heart disease and type 2 diabetes specifically, metabolic syndrome is the major component of an individual's overall cardiometabolic risk—that is, the risk that an individual will develop cardiovascular and metabolic disease. The five factors associated with metabolic syndrome as well as the following four factors contribute to cardiometabolic risk:[3]

elevated LDL-cholesterol (≥ 130 mg/dL)
inflammation
insulin resistance
smoking.

As such, in a person with metabolic syndrome, high-LDL, inflammation, insulin resistance, or smoking further increase the risk for heart disease, stroke, and type 2 diabetes, as well as other disorders, including Alzheimer's disease.[4]

Obesity is also associated with an increased risk for premature death: mortality rates for people with a BMI of 30 kg/m² or higher are 50% to 100% above the rates for those with a BMI between 20 and 25 kg/m². As described in Chapter 1, several of the leading causes of death in the United States are associated with obesity.

To view a detailed interactive graphic of the seven predominant themes highlighted in the Foresight Obesity map, go to www.shiftn.com/obesity/Full-Map.html.

Why does obesity occur?

LO 2 Explain why obesity is considered a multifactorial disease, identifying several contributing factors.

Obesity is a **multifactorial disease**; that is, genetic, metabolic, physiologic, and environmental factors all potentially contribute to the condition. In fact, a landmark report published in 2007 from the Government Office for Science in the United Kingdom revealed that the causes of obesity are embedded within highly complex biological and sociological systems. The authors of this report mapped more than 100 variables that directly or indirectly influence energy balance and body weight **(FOCUS FIGURE 2)**.[5] These variables are grouped into seven predominant themes:

1. *Biology*—including variables such as genetic predisposition to obesity, resting metabolic rate, and levels of certain hormones;
2. *Physical activity environment*—includes variables that can promote or inhibit physical activity such as cost, perceived safety, and reliance on laborsaving devices;
3. *Individual physical activity*—includes variables such as parental modeling of activity, level of fitness, and engagement in recreational or occupational physical activity;
4. *Individual psychology*—includes self-esteem, stress, level of food literacy, pressure to overindulge, and level of parental control over children's diet;
5. *Societal influences*—includes level of education, TV watching, and societal acceptance of obesity;
6. *Food environment*—includes variables related to food production such as industry pressure for growth and marketability, market price of food, and pressure to consume via advertisements; and
7. *Food consumption*—includes variables such as level of food abundance and variety, nutritional quality of food and beverages, and the energy density and portion sizes of foods.

As you can see, obesity is a highly complex problem that cannot be reduced to genetics, overeating, or any other individual factor. This complexity makes the work of obesity prevention and treatment extremely challenging.

---

adipokines Cell signaling proteins secreted by adipose tissue; some promote inflammation.

metabolic syndrome A cluster of five potentially modifiable factors, such as abdominal obesity, that increases the risk for cardiovascular disease and type 2 diabetes.

multifactorial disease A disease that may be attributable to one or more of a variety of causes.

OBESITY SYSTEM

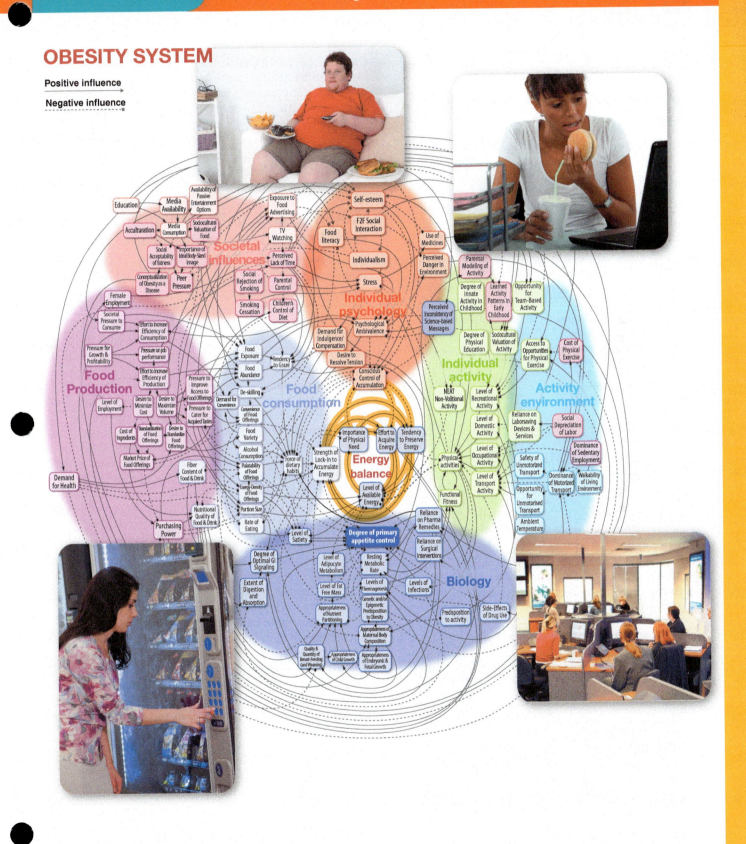

Positive influence →
Negative influence →

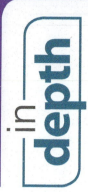
How is obesity treated?

LO 3 Describe the effectiveness of lifestyle changes, medications, dietary supplements, and surgery in obesity treatment.

A recent study found that 63% of obese adults in the United States reported trying to lose weight in the previous year, with 40% losing 5% to 9.9% of body weight, and 20% losing 10% or more of body weight.[6] These results suggest that about 60% of obese people trying to lose weight are successful at least in the short term. In addition, evidence from the National Weight Control Registry (see Chapter 10) indicates that more than 87% of those who joined the registry maintained a weight loss of at least 10% from their maximum weight after 10 years.[7] These individuals lost an average of 68.9 pounds, and maintained an average weight loss of 50.8 pounds after 10 years. Clearly many obese individuals succeed in losing weight and keeping it off. So how do they do it?

> To learn more about the complex factors contributing to the rise in obesity in the United States, go to www.cdc.gov/cdctv/, and type "The Obesity Epidemic" into the search bar. Then select the video of the same name from the list.

Obesity Does Respond to Diet and Exercise

The first line of defense in treating obesity in adults is a low-energy diet and regular physical activity. Overweight and obese individuals should work with their healthcare provider to design and maintain a healthful diet that has a deficit of 500 to 1,000 kcal/day. Physical activity should be increased gradually, so that the person can build a program in which he or she is exercising at least 30 minutes

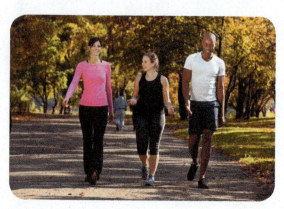

About 90% of the members of the National Weight Control Registry exercise, on average, for 1 hour a day.

per day, five times per week. The Health and Medicine Division of the National Academies of Science, Engineering, and Medicine[8] concurs that 30 minutes a day, five times a week is the minimum amount of physical activity needed, but up to 60 minutes per day may be necessary for many people to lose weight and to sustain a body weight in the healthy range over the long term.

Counseling and support groups, such as Overeaters Anonymous (OA), can help people maintain these dietary and activity changes. Psychotherapy can be particularly helpful in challenging clients to examine the underlying thought patterns, situations, and stressors that may be undermining their efforts at weight loss.

Weight Loss Can Be Enhanced with Prescription Medications

The biggest complaint about the lifestyle recommendations for healthful weight loss is that these behaviors are difficult to maintain. Many people have tried to follow them for years but have not been successful. In response to this challenge, prescription drugs have been developed to assist people with weight loss. These drugs typically act as appetite suppressants and may also increase satiety.

Weight-loss medications should be used only with proper supervision from a physician, and while simultaneously following the diet and physical activity recommendations under which the drugs were tested. Physician involvement is critical because many drugs developed for weight loss have serious side effects. Moreover, the long-term safety of many of these drugs is still being explored.

Nine prescription weight-loss drugs are currently available:[9]

- Diethylpropion (brand name Tenuate), phentermine (brand name Adipex-P or Suprenza), benzphetamine (brand name Didrex), and phendimetrazine (brand name Bontril) are drugs that decrease appetite and increase feelings of fullness. These are approved for only short-term use (typically less than 12 weeks) because of their potential to be abused. Side effects include increased blood pressure and heart rate, nervousness, insomnia, dry mouth, and constipation.
- Lorcaserin (brand name Belviq) also works by decreasing appetite and increasing feelings of fullness. Side effects include increased heart rate, headache, dizziness, and nausea.
- Naltrexone and bupropion extended-release (brand name Contrave) decreases appetite and increases feelings of fullness, with side effects including nausea, constipation, headache, vomiting, and dizziness.
- Liraglutide (brand name Saxenda) slows gastric emptying and increases feelings of fullness. Side effects include nausea, vomiting, and inflammation of the pancreas (or pancreatitis).

- Orlistat (brand name Xenical) is a drug that acts to inhibit the absorption of dietary fat from the intestinal tract. Orlistat is also available in a reduced-strength form (brand name Alli) that is available without a prescription. Side effects include intestinal cramps, gas, diarrhea, and oily spotting. Although rare, liver injury can occur; thus, people taking orlistat should be aware of symptoms of liver injury, which include itching, loss of appetite, yellow eyes or skin, light-colored stools, or brown urine.
- Combination phentermine–topiramate (brand name Qsymia) decreases appetite and increases feelings of fullness. Side effects include increased heart rate, tingling of hands and feet, dry mouth, constipation, anxiety, and birth defects. Because of this increased risk for birth defects, women of childbearing years must avoid getting pregnant while taking this medication. Although it has been approved for long-term use, Qsymia contains phentermine and thus has the potential for abuse.

Although the use of prescribed weight-loss medications is associated with side effects and a certain level of risk, they are justified for people who are obese. That's because the health risks of obesity override the risks of the medications. They are also advised for people who have a BMI greater than or equal to 27 kg/m^2 who also have other significant health risk factors such as heart disease, hypertension, and type 2 diabetes.

Many Supplements Used for Weight Loss Contain Stimulants

The Office of Dietary Supplements (ODS) of the U.S. National Institutes of Health reports that the use of various supplements and alternative treatments for weight loss is common (20.6% among women and 9.7% among men). The most common include bitter orange, chromium, chitosan (derived from the exoskeleton of crustaceans), conjugated linoleic acid, guar gum, raspberry ketone, and yohimbe.[10] The ODS has insufficient evidence of effectiveness for these products, yet they continue their brisk sales to people desperate to lose weight.

Some products marketed for weight loss do indeed increase metabolic rate and decrease appetite; however, they prompt these effects because they contain *stimulants*, substances that speed up physiologic processes. Use of these products may be dangerous because abnormal increases in heart rate and blood pressure can occur. Stimulants commonly found in weight-loss supplements include caffeine, phenylpropanolamine (PPA), and ephedra:

- **Caffeine**. In addition to being a stimulant, caffeine is addictive; nevertheless, it is legal and unregulated in most countries and is considered safe when consumed in moderate amounts (up to the equivalent of three to four cups of coffee a day). Adverse effects of high doses of caffeine include nervousness, irritability,

anxiety, muscle twitching and tremors, headaches, elevated blood pressure, and irregular or rapid heartbeat. Long-term overuse of high doses of caffeine can lead to sleep and anxiety disorders that require clinical attention. Deaths due to caffeine toxicity have been associated primarily with caffeine tablets and energy drinks.
- **Phenylpropanolamine (PPA)**. In the year 2000, in response to several deaths, the U.S. Food and Drug Administration (FDA) banned over-the-counter medications containing PPA, an ingredient that had been used in many cough and cold medications as well as in weight-loss formulas. However, PPA may still be present in dietary supplements marketed for weight loss because these are not required to undergo testing for safety or effectiveness prior to marketing.
- **Ephedra**. The use of ephedra has been associated with dangerous elevations in heart rate, blood pressure, and death. The FDA has banned the manufacture and sale of ephedra in the United States; however, some weight-loss supplements still contain *mahuang*, the so-called herbal ephedra. *Mahuang* is simply the Chinese name for ephedra. Some weight-loss supplements contain a combination of *mahuang*, caffeine, and aspirin.

As you can see, using weight-loss dietary supplements entails serious health risks.

Surgery Can Be Used to Treat Morbid Obesity

For people who are morbidly obese, surgery may be recommended. Generally, **bariatric surgery** (from the Greek word *baros*, meaning "weight") is advised for people with a BMI greater than or equal to 40 kg/m^2 or for people with a BMI greater than or equal to 35 kg/m^2 who have other life-threatening conditions, such as diabetes, hypertension, or elevated cholesterol levels. The three most common types of weight-loss surgery are sleeve gastrectomy, gastric bypass, and gastric banding (**FIGURE 3**, page 378).

Bariatric surgery is considered a last resort for morbidly obese people who have not been able to lose weight with energy restriction, exercise, and medications. This is because the risks of surgery in people with morbid obesity are extremely high. They include an increased rate of infections, formation of blood clots, and adverse reactions to anesthesia.

However, bariatric surgery is not a simple procedure or a guaranteed cure for obesity. As a form of major surgery, associated risks include excessive bleeding, infection, adverse reaction to anesthesia, blood clots, leaking from the gastrointestinal tract, and in relatively rare cases, death. After the surgery, many recipients face a lifetime of

bariatric surgery Surgical alteration of the gastrointestinal tract performed to promote weight loss.

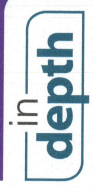

problems with chronic diarrhea, vomiting, intolerance to dairy products and certain other foods, dehydration, and nutritional deficiencies resulting from alterations in nutrient digestion and absorption that occur with bypass procedures. Additional longer-term complications include bowel obstruction, gallstones, hernias, hypoglycemia, ulcers, and perforation of the stomach. Thus, the potential benefits of the procedure must outweigh the risks.

It is critical that each surgery candidate be carefully screened by a trained bariatric surgical team, which includes assessments of physical and psychological readiness for the surgery itself, and also for the lifestyle changes that need to be followed to ensure weight loss and maintenance of weight loss post-surgery. If the immediate threat of serious disease and death is more dangerous than the risks associated with surgery, then the procedure is justified.

About one-third to one-half of people who undergo bariatric surgery lose significant amounts of weight, and the limited research examining longer-term maintenance of weight loss indicates that people are able to maintain their weight loss for 3 to 5 years.[11] They also substantially reduce their risk for type 2 diabetes, and in many cases type 2 diabetes is fully resolved. Hypertension, elevated blood lipids, cardiovascular disease, and sleep apnea are also significantly reduced following the surgery.[11] The reasons that one-half to two-thirds do not experience long-term success include the following:

- Inability to eat less over time, even with a smaller stomach
- Loosening of staples and gastric bands and sleeves and enlargement of the stomach pouch
- Failure to survive the surgery or the postoperative recovery period

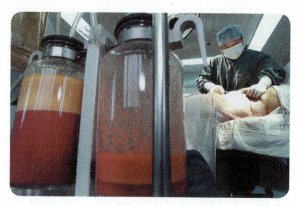

Liposuction removes fat cells from specific areas of the body.

Liposuction is a cosmetic surgical procedure that removes fat cells from localized areas in the body. It is not recommended or typically used to treat obesity or morbid obesity. Instead, it is often used by normal or mildly overweight people to "spot reduce" fat from various areas of the body.

Liposuction is not without risks. Blood clots, skin and nerve damage, adverse drug reactions, and perforation injuries can and do occur as a result of the procedure. It can also cause deformations in the area where the fat is removed.

In addition, liposuction does not contribute to long-term weight loss, because the millions of fat cells that remain in the body after the procedure enlarge if the person continues to overeat. Although liposuction may reduce the fat content of a localized area, it does not reduce a person's risk for the diseases that are more common among overweight or obese people. Only traditional weight loss with diet and exercise can reduce body fat and the risks for chronic diseases.

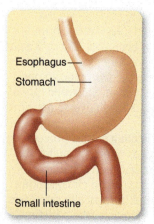

(a) Normal anatomy

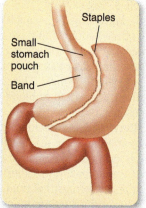

(b) Sleeve gastrectomy

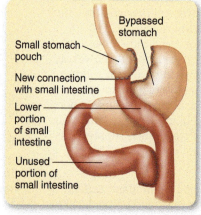

(c) Gastric bypass

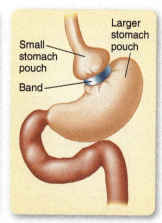

(d) Gastric banding

FIGURE 3 Various forms of bariatric surgery alter the normal anatomy **(a)** of the gastrointestinal tract to result in weight loss. Sleeve gastrectomy **(b)**, gastric bypass **(c)**, and gastric banding **(d)**, are three surgical procedures used to reduce morbid obesity.

www.oa.org
Overeaters Anonymous

Visit this site to learn about ways to reduce compulsive overeating.

www.mayoclinic.org
The Mayo Clinic

To learn more about weight-loss basics, diet plans, diet pills, supplements, and bariatric surgery, click on Patient Care & Health Info, choose Healthy Lifestyle, and then click on Weight Loss.

www.cdc.gov
The Centers for Disease Control and Prevention

Visit this site to investigate the latest statistics on overweight and obesity in the United States. Click on Diseases & Conditions, Select Data & Statistics, then click on Overweight & Obesity.

www.obesityaction.org/
Obesity Action Coalition

Visit this site to learn more about this nonprofit organization dedicated to giving a voice to people with obesity and helping individuals through education, advocacy, and support.

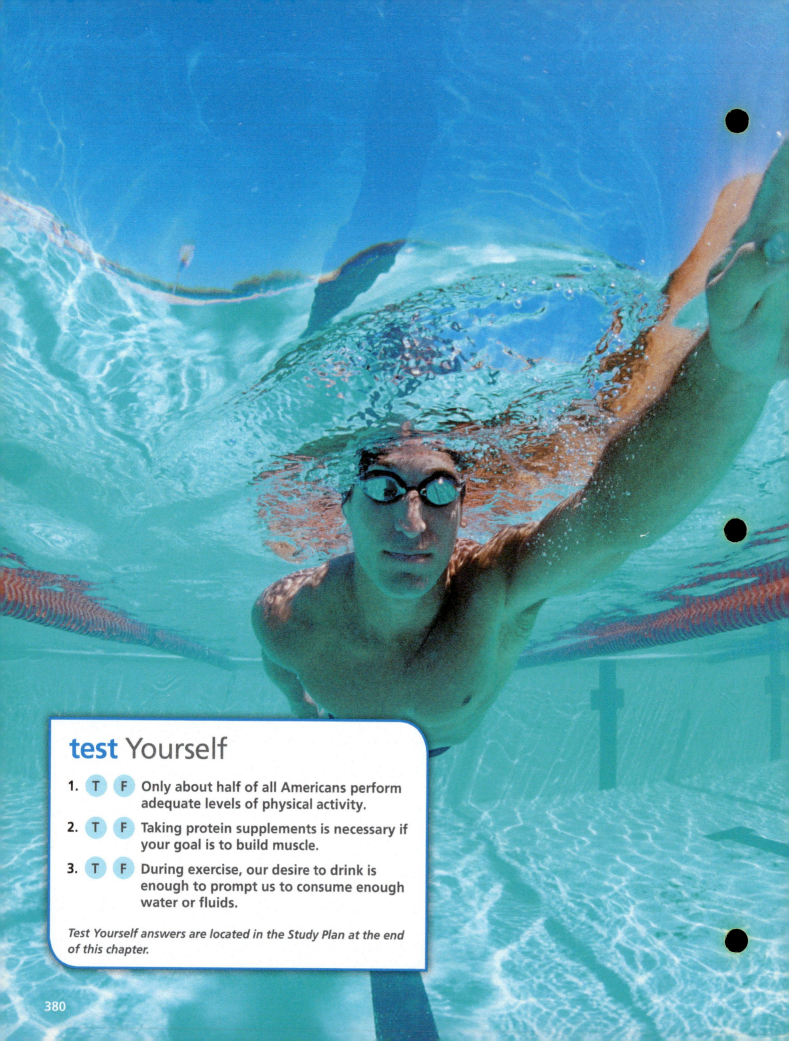

test Yourself

1. T F Only about half of all Americans perform adequate levels of physical activity.

2. T F Taking protein supplements is necessary if your goal is to build muscle.

3. T F During exercise, our desire to drink is enough to prompt us to consume enough water or fluids.

Test Yourself answers are located in the Study Plan at the end of this chapter.

11 Nutrition and Physical Fitness
Keys to good health

In July of 2015, Mary Kay of South Dakota and Harold Bach of North Dakota each took the gold medal for the 100-meter dash in track and field at the National Senior Games. Kay did it in just over 35 seconds, and Bach's time was less than 25 seconds. If these performance times don't amaze you, perhaps they will when you consider these athletes' ages: Kay was 97 years old, and Bach was 95!

There's no doubt about it: regular physical activity dramatically improves strength, stamina, health, and quality of life, and promotes longevity. But what qualifies as "regular physical activity"? In other words, how much and what types of physical activity do we need to do to reap the benefits? And if we do become more active, does our diet have to change, too?

A healthful eating pattern and regular physical activity are like two sides of the same coin, interacting in a variety of ways to improve our strength and stamina and increase our resistance to many acute illnesses and chronic diseases. In this chapter, we'll define physical activity, identify its many benefits, and discuss the nutrients needed to maintain an active life.

LO 1 Identify the key benefits of engaging in physical activity on a regular basis.

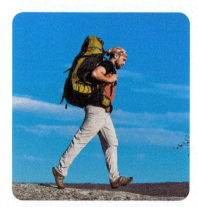

▲ Hiking is a leisure-time physical activity that can contribute to your physical fitness.

physical activity Any movement produced by muscles that increases energy expenditure; includes occupational, household, leisure-time, and transportation activities.

leisure-time physical activity Any activity not related to a person's occupation; includes competitive sports, recreational activities, and planned exercise training.

exercise A subcategory of leisure-time physical activity; any activity that is purposeful, planned, and structured.

physical fitness The ability to carry out daily tasks with vigor and alertness, without undue fatigue, and with ample energy to enjoy leisure-time pursuits and meet unforeseen emergencies.

aerobic exercise Exercise that involves the repetitive movement of large muscle groups, increasing the body's use of oxygen and promoting cardiovascular health.

resistance training Exercise in which our muscles act against resistance.

stretching Exercise in which muscles are gently lengthened using slow, controlled movements.

What are the benefits of physical activity?

The term **physical activity** describes any movement produced by muscles that increases energy expenditure.[1] Different categories of physical activity include occupational, household, leisure-time, and transportation. **Leisure-time physical activity** is any activity not related to a person's occupation and includes competitive sports, planned exercise training, and recreational activities such as hiking, walking, and bicycling. **Exercise** is therefore considered a subcategory of leisure-time physical activity and refers to activity that is purposeful, planned, and structured.[1]

Physical Activity Increases Our Fitness

A lot of people are looking for a "magic pill" that will help them maintain weight loss, reduce their risk for diseases, make them feel better, and improve their quality of sleep. Although they may not be aware of it, regular physical activity is this "magic pill." That's because it promotes **physical fitness**: the ability to carry out daily tasks with vigor and alertness, without undue fatigue, and with ample energy to enjoy leisure-time pursuits and meet unforeseen emergencies.[2]

The four components of physical fitness are cardiorespiratory fitness, which is the ability of the heart, lungs, and circulatory system to efficiently supply oxygen and nutrients to working muscles; musculoskeletal fitness, which is fitness of the muscles and bones; flexibility; and body composition **(TABLE 11.1)**.[3] These are achieved through three types of exercise:

- **Aerobic exercise** involves the repetitive movement of large muscle groups, which increases the body's use of oxygen and promotes cardiovascular health. In your daily life, you get aerobic exercise when you walk to a bus stop or take the stairs to a third-floor classroom.
- **Resistance training** is a form of exercise in which our muscles work against resistance, such as against handheld weights. Carrying grocery bags or books and moving heavy objects are everyday activities that make our muscles work against resistance.
- **Stretching** exercises are those that increase flexibility, as they involve lengthening muscles using slow, controlled movements. You can perform stretching exercises even while you're sitting in a classroom by flexing, extending, and rotating your neck, limbs, and extremities.

Both aerobic and resistance training promote a healthy body composition and body weight. Although stretching exercises don't help build lean tissue or lose weight, they are critical to supporting one's ability to engage in all forms of exercise and activities of daily living.

TABLE 11.1 The Components of Fitness

Fitness Component	Examples of Activities that Improve Fitness in Each Component
Cardiorespiratory	Aerobic-type activities, such as walking, running, swimming, cross-country skiing
Musculoskeletal fitness:	Resistance training, weight lifting, calisthenics, sit-ups, push-ups
Muscular strength	Weight lifting or related activities using heavier weights with few repetitions
Muscular endurance	Weight lifting or related activities using lighter weights with more repetitions
Flexibility	Stretching exercises, yoga
Body composition	Aerobic exercise, resistance training

Physical Activity Reduces Our Risk for Chronic Diseases

In addition to contributing to our fitness, regular physical activity can improve our health right now, and reduce our risk for certain diseases. Specifically, the health benefits of physical activity include (FIGURE 11.1):

- *Reduces our risks for, and complications of, heart disease, stroke, and high blood pressure.* Regular physical activity increases high-density lipoprotein (HDL) cholesterol and lowers triglycerides in the blood, improves the strength of the heart, helps maintain healthy blood pressure, and limits the progression of atherosclerosis, reducing the risk for heart disease and stroke.
- *Reduces our risk for obesity.* Regular physical activity maintains lean body mass and promotes more healthful levels of body fat, may help in appetite control, and increases energy expenditure and the use of fat as an energy source.
- *Reduces our risk for type 2 diabetes.* Regular physical activity enhances the action of insulin, which improves the cells' uptake of glucose from the blood, and it can improve blood glucose control in people with diabetes, which in turn reduces the risk for, or delays the onset of, diabetes-related complications.
- *May reduce our risk for colon cancer.* Although the exact role that physical activity may play in reducing colon cancer risk is still unknown, we do know that regular physical activity enhances gastric motility, which reduces transit time of potential cancer-causing agents through the gut.
- *Reduces our risk for osteoporosis.* Regular physical activity, especially weight-bearing exercise, increases bone density and enhances muscular strength and flexibility, thereby reducing the likelihood of falls and the incidence of fractures and other injuries when falls occur.

Regular physical activity is also known to improve our sleep patterns, increase our lung efficiency and capacity, reduce our risk for upper respiratory infections by improving immune function, and reduce anxiety and mental stress. It also can be effective in treating mild and moderate depression.

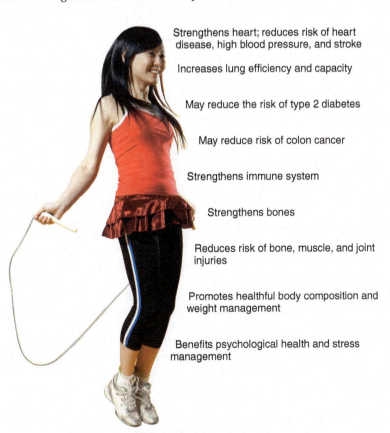

Strengthens heart; reduces risk of heart disease, high blood pressure, and stroke

Increases lung efficiency and capacity

May reduce the risk of type 2 diabetes

May reduce risk of colon cancer

Strengthens immune system

Strengthens bones

Reduces risk of bone, muscle, and joint injuries

Promotes healthful body composition and weight management

Benefits psychological health and stress management

FIGURE 11.1 Health benefits of regular physical activity.

recap Physical activity is any movement produced by muscles that increases energy expenditure. It contributes to physical fitness, the ability to carry out daily tasks with vigor and alertness, without undue fatigue, and with ample energy to enjoy leisure-time pursuits and meet unforeseen emergencies. Physical activity also reduces our risks for obesity, cardiovascular disease, type 2 diabetes, osteoporosis, and musculoskeletal injuries; strengthens our immune system; and helps relieve anxiety, stress, and mild to moderate depression.

LO 2 Explain how to improve your fitness using the FITT principle and calculating your maximal and training heart rate range.

How can you improve your fitness?

For most of our history, humans were very physically active. This was not by choice, but because their survival depended on it. Prior to the industrial age, humans expended a considerable amount of energy each day foraging, hunting, planting, harvesting, and preparing food, as well as securing and maintaining shelter. This lifestyle pattern contrasts considerably with today's, which is characterized by sedentary jobs and few opportunities for occupational or recreational activities. In fact, the Centers for Disease Control and Prevention (CDC) report that only 20.1% of adults in the United States do enough physical activity to meet national recommendations (identified shortly), and 23.7% admit to doing no leisure-time physical activity at all **(FIGURE 11.2)**.[4] These statistics mirror the reported increases in obesity, cardiovascular disease, and type 2 diabetes in industrialized countries.

If you'd like to improve your fitness, you'll find the help you need in this section. Keep in mind that people with heart disease, high blood pressure, diabetes, obesity, osteoporosis, asthma, or arthritis should get approval to exercise from their health-care practitioner prior to starting a fitness program. In addition, a medical evaluation should be conducted before starting an exercise program for an apparently healthy but currently inactive man 40 years or older or woman 50 years or older.

Assess Your Current Level of Fitness

Before beginning any fitness program, it is important to know your initial level of fitness. This information can then be used to help you design a fitness program that meets your goals and is appropriate for you. How can you go about estimating your current fitness level? Check out the **Web Links** at the end of the chapter to take the President's Challenge Adult Fitness test.

Identify Your Personal Fitness Goals

A fitness program that may be ideal for you is not necessarily right for everyone. Before designing or evaluating any program, it is important to define your personal fitness goals. Do you want to prevent osteoporosis, diabetes, or another chronic disease that runs in your family? Do you simply want to increase your energy and stamina? Or do you intend to compete in athletic events? Each of these scenarios requires a unique fitness program. This concept is referred to as the *specificity principle*: specific actions yield specific results.

Training is generally defined as activity leading to skilled behavior. Training is very specific to any activity or goal. For example, if you want to train for athletic competition, a traditional approach that includes planned, purposive exercise sessions under the guidance of a trainer or coach would be beneficial. If you wanted to achieve cardiorespiratory fitness, you might be advised to participate in an aerobics class at least three times per week or jog for at least 20 minutes three times per week.

In contrast, if your goal is to transition from doing no regular physical activity to doing enough physical activity to maintain your overall health, you could follow the minimum recommendations put forth in the 2008 Physical Activity Guidelines for Americans.[5] To gain significant health benefits, including reducing the risk for chronic

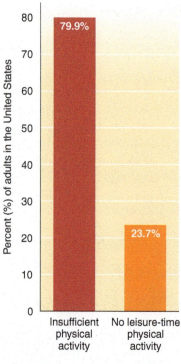

FIGURE 11.2 Rates of physical inactivity in the United States. Almost 80% of the U.S. population does not do enough physical activity to meet national recommendations, and 23.7% report doing no leisure-time physical activity.

Source: Nutrition, Physical Activity and Obesity Data, Trends and Maps website. 2015. U.S. Department of Health and Human Services, Centers for Disease Control and Prevention (CDC), National Center for Chronic Disease Prevention and Health Promotion, Division of Nutrition, Physical Activity and Obesity, Atlanta, GA, 2015. Available at www.cdc.gov/nccd-php/DNPAO/index.html

diseases, you can participate in at least 30 minutes per day of moderate-intensity aerobic physical activity (such as gardening, brisk walking, or basketball). The activity need not be completed in one session. You can divide the amount of physical activity into two or more shorter sessions throughout the day as long as the total cumulative time is achieved (e.g., brisk walking for 10 minutes three times per day). Although these minimum guidelines are appropriate for achieving health benefits, performing physical activities at a higher intensity and for longer duration will confer even greater health benefits.

The promotion of various physical activity guidelines in recent years has led to some confusion among consumers regarding exactly how much physical activity is enough to enhance health and fitness levels. For example, the Health and Medicine Division of the National Academies of Sciences, Engineering, and Medicine published guidelines stating that the minimum amount of physical activity that should be done each day to maintain health and fitness is 60 minutes—not 30 minutes, as stated in the 2008 Physical Activity guidelines.[5,6] Refer to the **Nutrition Debate** at the end of this chapter to learn more about this controversy.

Make Your Program Varied, Consistent, and Fun!

A number of factors motivate us to be active. Some are *intrinsic* factors, which are those done for the satisfaction a person gains from engaging in the activity. Others are *extrinsic*, which are those done to obtain rewards or outcomes that are separate from the behavior itself.[7] Examples of intrinsic factors that motivate us to engage in physical activity include the desire to gain competence, the desire to be challenged by the activity and enhance our skills, and enjoyment. Some of the most common extrinsic factors are desires to improve appearance and to increase fitness. Recently, some employers have been offering financial incentives to log in time at the company's fitness center, another example of an extrinsic factor.

Whether we are more motivated by intrinsic or extrinsic factors is related to the type of activity in which we engage and whether we're a regular or infrequent exerciser. People who are regularly active tend to be more motivated by intrinsic factors, whereas extrinsic factors appear to be more important to people who are not regularly active or are engaging in activity for the first time. Being intrinsically motivated to be physically active has also been shown to positively influence eating behaviors and promote healthy weight control.[8]

An important motivator in maintaining regular physical activity is enjoyment—or fun! People who enjoy being active find it easy to maintain their physical fitness. What activities do you consider fun? If you enjoy the outdoors, hiking, camping, fishing, rock climbing, and gardening are potential activities for you. If you would rather exercise with friends on or near campus, walking, climbing stairs, jogging, roller-blading, or bicycle riding may be more appropriate. Or you may prefer to use the programs and equipment at your campus or community fitness center or purchase your own treadmill and free weights.

Variety is also important to maintaining your fitness and your interest in being regularly active. Although some people enjoy doing similar activities day after day, many get bored with the same fitness routine. Incorporating a variety of activities into your fitness program will help maintain your interest and increase your enjoyment while promoting different types of fitness identified in Table 11.1. Variety can be achieved by:

- Combining aerobic exercise, resistance training, and stretching
- Combining indoor and outdoor activities throughout the week
- Taking different routes when you walk or jog each day
- Watching a movie, reading a book, or listening to music while you ride a stationary bicycle or walk on a treadmill
- Participating in different activities each week, such as walking, dancing, bicycling, yoga, weight lifting, swimming, hiking, and gardening

This "smorgasbord" of activities can increase your fitness without leading to monotony and boredom.

Sitting too long, studying for tomorrow's exam? Stretching can help! Learn some simple stretches by watching the how-to video collection from the Mayo Clinic at www.mayoclinic.org. Enter "health," and then "office stretches" into the search box.

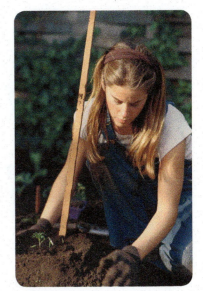

Engaging in an activity you consider fun, such as gardening, can help you maintain your motivation and add variety to your physical activity program.

Appropriately Overload Your Body

To improve your fitness, you must place an extra physical demand on your body. This is referred to as the **overload principle**. A word of caution is in order here: *the overload principle does not advocate subjecting your body to inappropriately high stress,* because this can lead to exhaustion and injuries. In contrast, an appropriate overload on various body systems will result in improvements in fitness. For example, a gain in muscle strength and size that results from repeated work that overloads the muscle is referred to as **hypertrophy**. When muscles are not worked adequately, they **atrophy**, or decrease in size and strength.

To achieve an appropriate overload, four factors should be considered, collectively known as the **FITT principle**: *f*requency, *i*ntensity, *t*ime, and *t*ype of activity. You can use the FITT principle to design either a general physical fitness program or a performance-based exercise program. **FIGURE 11.3** shows how the FITT principle applies to a cardiorespiratory and muscular fitness program. Let's consider each of the FITT principle's four factors in more detail.

overload principle Placing an extra physical demand on your body in order to improve your fitness level.

hypertrophy The increase in strength and size that results from repeated work to a specific muscle or muscle group.

atrophy A decrease in the size and strength of muscles that occurs when they are not worked adequately.

FITT principle The principle used to achieve an appropriate overload for physical training; FITT stands for *f*requency, *i*ntensity, *t*ime, and *t*ype of activity.

frequency Refers to the number of activity sessions per week you perform.

Frequency

Frequency refers to the number of activity sessions per week. Depending on your goals for fitness, the frequency of your activities will vary. The Physical Activity Guidelines for Americans recommend engaging in aerobic (cardiorespiratory) activities for at least 150 minutes a week. To achieve cardiorespiratory fitness, training should be at least 3 to 5 days per week. On the other hand, training more than 6 days per week does not cause significant gains in fitness but can substantially increase the

	Frequency	Intensity	Time and Type
Cardiorespiratory fitness	At least 30 minutes most days of the week	50–70% maximal heart rate for moderate intensity; 70–85% maximal heart rate for vigorous intensity	At least 30 consecutive minutes Choose swimming, walking, running, cycling, dancing, or other aerobic activities
Muscular fitness	2–3 days per week	70–85% maximal weight you can lift	1–3 sets of 8–12 lifts for each set A minimum of 8–10 exercises involving the major muscle groups such as arms, shoulders, chest, abdomen, back, hips, and legs, is recommended.
Flexibility	2–4 days per week	Stretching through full range of motion	For stretching, perform 2–4 repetitions per stretch. Hold each stretch for 15–30 seconds. Or try yoga, tai chi, or other flexibility programs.

FIGURE 11.3 Using the FITT principle to achieve cardiorespiratory and musculoskeletal fitness and flexibility. The recommendations in this figure follow the 2008 Physical Activity Guidelines for Americans (still in effect today).

risks for injury. Training 3 to 6 days per week appears optimal to achieve and maintain cardiorespiratory fitness. In contrast, only 2 to 3 days of training are needed to achieve muscular fitness.

Intensity

Intensity refers to the amount of effort expended or to how difficult the activity is to perform. We describe the intensity of activity as being low, moderate, or vigorous:

- *Low-intensity* activities are those that cause very mild increases in breathing, sweating, and heart rate. Examples include walking at a leisurely pace, fishing, and light house-cleaning.
- *Moderate-intensity* activities cause moderate increases in breathing, sweating, and heart rate. For instance, you can carry on a conversation, but not continuously. Examples include brisk walking, water aerobics, doubles tennis, ballroom dancing, and bicycling slower than 10 miles per hour.
- *Vigorous-intensity* activities produce significant increases in breathing, sweating, and heart rate, so that talking is difficult when exercising. Examples include jogging, running, racewalking, singles tennis, aerobics, bicycling 10 miles per hour or faster, jumping rope, and hiking uphill with a heavy backpack.

Traditionally, heart rate has been used to indicate level of intensity during aerobic activities. You can calculate the range of exercise intensity that is appropriate for you by estimating your **maximal heart rate**, which is the rate at which your heart beats during maximal-intensity exercise. Maximal heart rate is estimated by subtracting your age from 220.

FIGURE 11.4 shows an example of a heart rate training chart, which you can use to estimate the intensity of your own workout. The Centers for Disease Control and Prevention makes the following recommendations:[9]

- To achieve moderate-intensity physical activity, your target heart rate should be 50% to 70% of your estimated maximal heart rate. Older adults and anyone who has been inactive for a long time may want to exercise at the lower end of the moderate-intensity range.

intensity The amount of effort expended during an activity, or how difficult the activity is to perform.

maximal heart rate The rate at which your heart beats during maximal-intensity exercise.

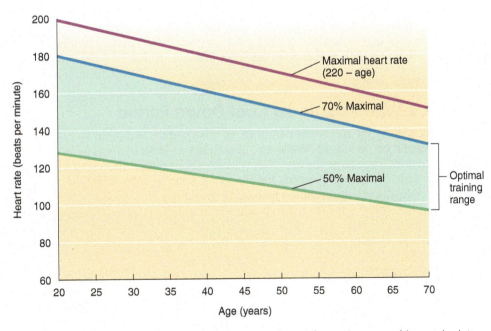

▲ **FIGURE 11.4** This heart rate training chart can be used to estimate aerobic exercise intensity. The top line indicates the predicted maximal heart rate value for a person's age (220 – age). The shaded area represents the heart rate values that fall between 50% and 70% of maximal heart rate, which is the range generally recommended to achieve aerobic fitness.

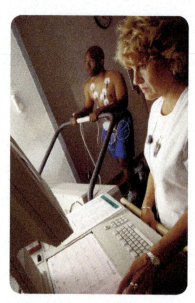

■ To achieve vigorous-intensity physical activity, your target heart rate should be 70% to 85% of your estimated heart rate. Those who are physically fit or are striving for a more rapid improvement in fitness may want to exercise at the higher end of the vigorous-intensity range.

■ Competitive athletes generally train at a higher intensity, around 80% to 95% of their maximal heart rate.

Although the calculation of *220 minus age* has been used extensively for years to predict maximal heart rate, it was never intended to accurately represent everyone's true maximal heart rate or to be used as the standard of aerobic training intensity. The most accurate way to determine your own maximal heart rate is to complete a maximal exercise test in a fitness laboratory; however, this test is not commonly conducted with the general public and can be very expensive. Although not completely accurate, the estimated maximal heart rate method can still be used to give you a general idea of your aerobic training range.

So what is your maximal heart rate and training range? To find out, try the easy calculation in the **You Do the Math** box on the next page.

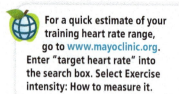

← Testing in a fitness lab is the most accurate way to determine maximal heart rate.

For a quick estimate of your training heart rate range, go to www.mayoclinic.org. Enter "target heart rate" into the search box. Select Exercise intensity: How to measure it.

Time of Activity

Time of activity refers to how long each session lasts. To achieve general health, you can do multiple short bouts of activity that add up to 30 minutes each day. However, to achieve higher levels of cardiovascular fitness, it is important that the activities be done for at least 30 consecutive minutes.

For example, let's say you want to compete in triathlons. To be successful during the running segment of the triathlon, you will need to be able to run quickly for at least 5 miles. Thus, it is appropriate for you to train so that you can complete 5 miles during one session and still have enough energy to swim and bicycle during the race. You will need to consistently train at a distance of 5 miles; you will also benefit from running longer distances.

Type of Activity

Type of activity refers to the range of physical activities a person can engage in to promote health and physical fitness. Many examples of types of physical activities one can engage in are illustrated in Table 11.1 and Figure 11.3. The types of activity you choose to engage in will depend on your goals for health and physical fitness, your personal preferences, and the range of activities available to you.

time of activity How long each exercise session lasts.

type of activity The range of physical activities a person can engage in to promote health and physical fitness.

warm-up Also called preliminary exercise; includes activities that prepare you for an exercise bout, including stretching, calisthenics, and movements specific to the exercise bout.

cool-down Activities done after an exercise session is completed; should be gradual and allow your body to slowly recover from exercise.

Include a Warm-Up and a Cool-Down Period

To properly prepare for and recover from an exercise session, warm-up and cool-down activities should be performed. **Warm-up**, also called preliminary exercise, includes general activities, such as gentle aerobics, calisthenics, and then stretching followed by specific activities that prepare you for the actual activity, such as jogging or swinging a golf club. The warm-up should be brief (5 to 10 minutes), gradual, and sufficient to increase muscle and body temperature. It should not cause fatigue or deplete energy stores.

Warming up prior to exercise is important because it properly prepares your muscles for exertion by increasing blood flow and body temperature. It enhances the body's flexibility and may also help prepare you psychologically for the exercise session or athletic event.

Cool-down activities are done after the exercise session. The cool-down should be gradual, allowing your body to recover slowly. The cool-down should include some of the same activities you performed during the exercise session, but at a low intensity, and should allow ample time for stretching. Cooling down after exercise assists in the prevention of injury and may help reduce muscle soreness.

Calculating Your Maximal and Training Heart Rate Range

Judy's healthcare provider has recommended she begin an exercise program. She plans to begin by either walking on the treadmill or riding the stationary bicycle at the fitness center during her lunch break.

Judy's doctor has recommended that she set her exercise intensity range at the low end of the currently recommended moderate intensity, or 50% to 70% estimated maximal heart rate.

Judy is 38 years old. Let's calculate her maximal heart rate values:

- Maximal heart rate: 220 − age = 220 − 38 = 182 beats per minute (bpm)

- Lower end of intensity range: 50% of 182 bpm = 0.50 × 182 bpm = 91 bpm

- Higher end of intensity range: 70% of 182 bpm = 0.70 × 182 bpm = 127 bpm

Because Judy is a trained nurse's aide, she is skilled at measuring a heart rate, or pulse. To measure your own pulse, take the following steps:

- Place your second (index) and third (middle) fingers on the inside of your wrist, just below the wrist crease and near the thumb. Press lightly to feel your pulse. Don't press too hard, or you will occlude the artery and be unable to feel its pulsation.

- If you can't feel your pulse at your wrist, try the carotid artery at your neck. This is located below your ear, on the side of your neck directly below your jaw. Press lightly against your neck under the jaw bone to find your pulse.

- Begin counting your pulse with the count of "zero"; then count each beat for 15 seconds.

- Multiply that value by 4 to estimate heart rate over 1 minute.

- Do not take your pulse with your thumb because it has its own pulse, which would prevent you from getting an accurate estimate of your heart rate.

As you can see from these calculations, when Judy walks on the treadmill or rides the bicycle, her heart rate should be between 91 and 127 bpm; this will put her in her aerobic training zone and allow her to achieve cardiorespiratory fitness. It will also help her lose weight, assuming she consumes less energy than she expends each day.

Now you do the math. Sam is a recreational runner who is 70 years old and wishes to train to compete in track and field events at the National Senior Games. His doctor has approved him for competition and has advised that Sam train at 75% to 80% of his maximal heart rate. (A) Calculate Sam's maximal heart rate. (B) What is Sam's heart rate training range in bpm?

Answers are located online in the MasteringNutrition Study Area.

Keep It Simple, Take It Slow

There are 1,440 minutes in every day. Spend just 30 of those minutes in physical activity, and you'll be taking an important step toward improving your health. See the **Quick Tips** on the next page for working daily activity into your life.

If you have been inactive for a while, use a sensible approach by starting out slowly. The first month is an initiation phase, which is the time to start to incorporate relatively brief bouts of physical activity into your daily life and reduce the time you spend in sedentary activities. Gradually build up the time you spend doing the activity by adding a few minutes every few days until you reach 30 minutes a day.

The next 4 to 6 months is the improvement phase, in which you can increase the intensity and duration of the activities you engage in. As you become more fit, the 30-minute minimum becomes easier and you'll need to gradually increase either the length of time you spend in activity or the intensity of the activities you choose, or both, to continue to progress toward your fitness goals. Once you've reached your goals and a plateau in your fitness gains, you've entered into the maintenance phase. At this point you can either maintain your current activity levels, or you may choose to reevaluate your goals and alter your training accordingly.

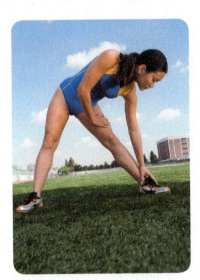

▲ Stretching should be included in the warm-up before and the cool-down after exercise.

QuickTips

Increasing Your Physical Activity

✓ Walk as often and as far as possible: park your car farther away from your dorm, lecture hall, or shops; walk to school or work; go for a brisk walk between classes; get on or off the bus one stop away from your destination. And don't be in such a rush to reach your destination—take the long way and burn a few more Calories.

✓ At every opportunity, take the stairs instead of the escalator or elevator.

✓ When working on the computer for long periods, take a 3- to 5-minute break every hour to stretch, walk to another room, or make a cup of tea.

✓ Exercise while watching television—for example, by doing sit-ups, stretching, or using a treadmill or stationary bike.

✓ While talking on your cell phone, memorizing vocabulary terms, or practicing your choral part, don't stand still—pace!

✓ Turn on some music and dance!

✓ Get an exercise partner: join a friend for walks, hikes, cycling, skating, tennis, or a fitness class.

✓ Take up a group sport.

✓ Register for a class from the physical education department in an activity you've never tried before, maybe yoga or fencing.

✓ Register for a dance class, such as jazz, tap, or ballroom.

✓ Use the pool, track, rock-climbing wall, or other facilities at your campus fitness center or join a health club, gym, or YMCA/YWCA in your community.

✓ Join an activity-based club, such as a skating, tennis, or hiking club.

✓ Play golf without using a golf cart—choose to walk and carry your clubs instead.

✓ Choose a physically active vacation that provides daily activities combined with exploring new surroundings.

✓ Use the pedometer app in your smartphone to keep track of your number of daily steps, working toward a daily goal of at least 10,000 steps per day.

---

recap A sound fitness program must meet your personal fitness goals. It should be fun and include variety and consistency to help you maintain interest and achieve fitness in all components. It must also place an extra physical demand, or an overload, on your body. To achieve appropriate overload, follow the FITT principle: *frequency* refers to the number of activity sessions per week; *intensity* refers to how difficult the activity is to perform; *time* refers to how long each activity session lasts; *type* refers to the range of physical activities one can engage in. Warm-up exercises prepare the muscles for exertion by increasing blood flow and temperature. Cool-down activities help prevent injury and may help reduce muscle soreness.

Want to learn more about the various tools used to measure physical activity levels? Go to the University of Pittsburgh Physical Activity Resource Center for Public Health at www.parcph.org to find out more.

What fuels our activities?

LO 3 List and describe at least three metabolic processes cells use to fuel physical activity.

In order to perform exercise, or muscular work, we must be able to generate energy. The common currency of energy for virtually all cells in the body is **adenosine triphosphate (ATP)**. As you might guess from its name, a molecule of ATP includes an organic compound called adenosine and three phosphate groups **(FIGURE 11.5)**. When one of the phosphates is cleaved, or broken away, from ATP, energy is released. The products remaining after this reaction are adenosine diphosphate (ADP) and an independent inorganic phosphate group (P$_i$). In a mirror image of this reaction, the body regenerates ATP by adding a phosphate group back to ADP. In this way, we continually provide energy to our cells.

The amount of ATP stored in a muscle cell is very limited; it can keep the muscle active for only about 1 to 3 seconds. Thus, we need to generate ATP from other sources to fuel activities for longer time periods. Fortunately, we are able to generate ATP from the breakdown of carbohydrate, fat, and protein, providing our cells with a variety of sources from which to derive energy. The primary energy systems that provide energy for physical activities are the adenosine triphosphate–creatine phosphate (ATP-CP) energy system and the anaerobic and aerobic breakdown of carbohydrates. Our body also generates energy from the breakdown of fats. As you will see, the type, intensity, and duration of the activities performed determine the amount of ATP needed and, therefore, the energy system that is used.

The ATP-CP Energy System Uses Creatine Phosphate to Regenerate ATP

As previously mentioned, muscle cells store only enough ATP to maintain activity for 1 to 3 seconds. When more energy is needed, a high-energy compound called **creatine phosphate (CP)** (also called *phosphocreatine* [*PCr*]) can be broken down to support the regeneration of ATP **(FIGURE 11.6)** (page 392). Because this reaction can occur in the absence of oxygen, it is referred to as an **anaerobic** reaction (meaning "without oxygen").

Muscle tissue contains about four to six times as much CP as ATP, but there is still not enough CP available to fuel long-term activity. CP is used the most during very intense, short bouts of activity, such as lifting, jumping, and sprinting **(FOCUS FIGURE 11.7)** (page 392). Together, our stores of ATP and CP can support a *maximal* physical effort for only about 3 to 15 seconds. We must rely on other energy sources, such as carbohydrate and fat, to support activities of longer duration.

The Breakdown of Carbohydrates Provides Energy for Both Brief and Long-Term Exercise

During activities lasting about 30 seconds to 3 minutes, our body needs an energy source that can be used quickly to produce ATP. The breakdown of carbohydrates, specifically glucose, provides this quick energy in a process called **glycolysis**. The

adenosine triphosphate (ATP) The common currency of energy for virtually all cells of the body.

creatine phosphate (CP) A high-energy compound that can be broken down for energy and used to regenerate ATP.

anaerobic Means "without oxygen"; the term used to refer to metabolic reactions that occur in the absence of oxygen.

glycolysis The breakdown of glucose; yields two ATP molecules and two pyruvic acid molecules for each molecule of glucose.

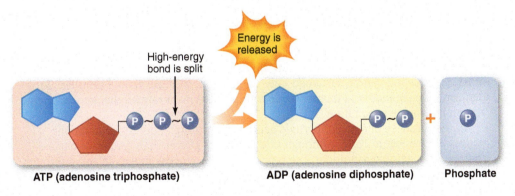

ATP (adenosine triphosphate) **ADP (adenosine diphosphate)** **Phosphate**

◆ **FIGURE 11.5** Structure of adenosine triphosphate (ATP). Energy is produced when ATP is split into adenosine diphosphate (ADP) and inorganic phosphate (P$_i$).

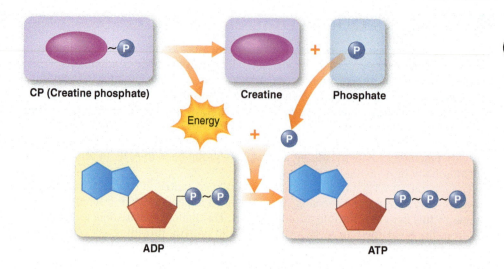

<figure>◀ **FIGURE 11.6** When the compound creatine phosphate (CP) is broken down into a molecule of creatine and an independent phosphate molecule, energy is released. This energy, along with the independent phosphate molecule, can then be used to regenerate ATP.</figure>

CP (Creatine phosphate)   Creatine   Phosphate

Energy

ADP   ATP

most common source of glucose during exercise comes from glycogen stored in the muscles and glucose found in the blood. As shown in **FIGURE 11.8** (page 394), for every glucose molecule that goes through glycolysis, two ATP molecules are produced. The primary end product of glycolysis is **pyruvic acid**.

When oxygen availability is limited in the cell, pyruvic acid is converted to **lactic acid**. For years it was assumed that lactic acid was a useless, even potentially toxic, by-product of high-intensity exercise. We now know that lactic acid is an important intermediate of glucose breakdown and that it plays a critical role in supplying fuel for working muscles, the heart, and resting tissues. But does lactic acid build-up cause muscle fatigue and soreness?

The exact causes of muscle fatigue are not known, and there appear to be many contributing factors. Recent evidence suggests that fatigue may be due not only to the accumulation of many acids and other metabolic by-products, such as inorganic phosphate, but also to the depletion of creatine phosphate and changes in calcium in muscle cells. Depletion of muscle glycogen, liver glycogen, and blood glucose, as well as psychological factors, can all contribute to fatigue.[10]

As with fatigue, many factors probably contribute to muscle soreness. Strenuous exercise causes microscopic tears in the muscle fibers. This damage triggers an inflammatory reaction, which causes an influx of fluid and various chemicals to the damaged tissue area. These substances work to remove damaged tissue and initiate tissue repair, but they may also stimulate pain. However, it appears highly unlikely that lactic acid is an independent cause of muscle soreness.

Recent studies indicate that lactic acid is produced even under aerobic conditions! This means it is produced at rest as well as during exercise at any intensity. The reasons for this constant production of lactic acid are still being studied. We do know that endurance training improves the muscle's ability to use lactic acid for energy. Thus, contrary to being a waste product of glucose metabolism, lactic acid is actually an important fuel for resting tissues, for working cardiac and skeletal muscles, and even for the brain both at rest and during exercise.[11]

Overall, the major advantage of glycolysis is that it is the fastest way that we can regenerate ATP for exercise, other than the ATP-CP system. However, this high rate of ATP production can be sustained only briefly, generally less than 3 minutes. To perform exercise that lasts longer than 3 minutes, we must rely on the aerobic energy system to provide adequate ATP.

In the presence of oxygen, pyruvic acid can go through additional metabolic pathways (see Figure 11.8). Although this process is slower than glycolysis occurring under anaerobic conditions, the breakdown of 1 glucose molecule going through aerobic metabolism yields 36 to 38 ATP molecules for energy, whereas the anaerobic process yields only 2 ATP molecules. Thus, this aerobic process supplies 18 times more energy! Another advantage of the aerobic process is that it does not result in the significant production of acids and other compounds that contribute to muscle

pyruvic acid The primary end product of glycolysis.

lactic acid A compound that results when pyruvic acid is metabolized in the presence of insufficient oxygen.

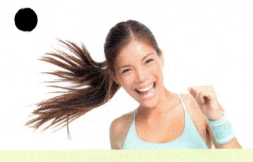

Depending on the duration and intensity of the activity, our body may use ATP-CP, carbohydrate, or fat in various combinations to fuel muscular work. Keep in mind that the amounts and sources shown below can vary based on the person's fitness level and health, how well fed the person is before the activity, and environmental temperatures and conditions.

SPRINT START (0–3 seconds)
A short, intense burst of activity like sprinting is fueled by ATP and creatine phosphate (CP) under anaerobic conditions.

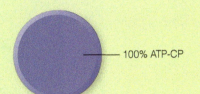

100% ATP-CP

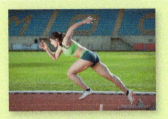

100-M DASH (10–12 seconds)
ATP and CP provide energy for about 10 seconds of quick, intense activity, after which energy is provided as ATP from the breakdown of carbohydrates.

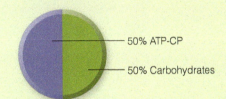

50% ATP-CP

50% Carbohydrates

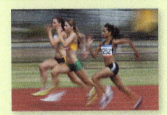

1500-M RACE (4–6 minutes)
Energy derived from ATP and CP is small and would be exhausted after about 10 seconds of the race. At this point, most of the energy is derived from aerobic metabolism of primarily carbohydrates.

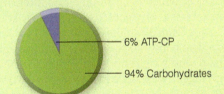

6% ATP-CP

94% Carbohydrates

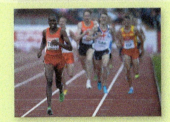

10-KM RACE (30–40 minutes)
During moderately intense activities such as a 10-kilometer race, ATP is provided by fat and carbohydrate metabolism. As the intensity increases, so does the utilization of carbohydrates for energy.

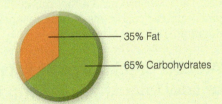

35% Fat

65% Carbohydrates

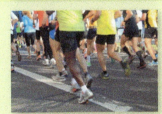

MARATHON (2.5–3 hours)
During endurance events such as marathons, ATP is primarily derived from carbohydrates, and to a lesser extent, fat. A very small amount of energy is provided by the breakdown of amino acids to form glucose.

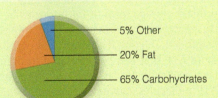

5% Other

20% Fat

65% Carbohydrates

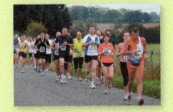

DAY-LONG HIKE (5.5–7 hours)
The primary energy source for events lasting several hours at low intensity is fat (free fatty acids in the bloodstream) which derive from triglycerides stored in fat cells. Carbohydrates contribute a relatively smaller percentage of energy needs.

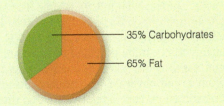

35% Carbohydrates

65% Fat

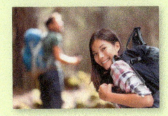

▶ **FIGURE 11.8** The breakdown of one molecule of glucose, or the process of glycolysis, yields two molecules of pyruvic acid and two ATP molecules. The further metabolism of pyruvic acid in the presence of insufficient oxygen (anaerobic process) results in the production of lactic acid. The metabolism of pyruvic acid in the presence of adequate oxygen (aerobic process) yields 36 to 38 molecules of ATP.

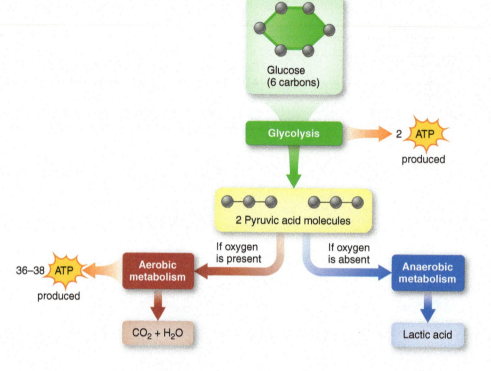

fatigue, which means that a low-intensity activity can be performed for hours. Aerobic metabolism of glucose is the primary source of fuel for our muscles during activities lasting from 3 minutes to 4 hours (see Focus Figure 11.7).

The body can store only a limited amount of glycogen. An average, well-nourished man who weighs about 154 pounds (70 kg) can store about 200 to 500 g of muscle glycogen, which is equal to 800 to 2,000 kcal of energy. Although trained athletes can store more muscle glycogen than the average person, even their body does not have enough stored glycogen to provide an unlimited energy supply for long-term activities. Thus, we also need a fuel source that is very abundant and can be broken down under aerobic conditions, so that it can support activities of lower intensity and longer duration. This fuel source is fat.

Aerobic Breakdown of Fats Supports Exercise of Low Intensity and Long Duration

When we refer to fat as a fuel source, we mean stored triglycerides, which is the primary storage form of fat in our cells. Their fatty acid chains provide much of the energy we need to support long-term activity. Fatty acids are classified by their length—that is, by the number of carbons they contain. The longer the fatty acid, the more ATP that can be generated from its breakdown. For instance, palmitic acid is a fatty acid with 16 carbons. If palmitic acid is broken down completely, it yields 129 ATP molecules. Obviously, far more energy is produced from this one fatty acid molecule than from the aerobic breakdown of a glucose molecule.

There are two major advantages of using fat as a fuel. First, fat is an abundant energy source, even in lean people. For example, a man who weighs 154 pounds (70 kg) who has a body fat level of 10% has approximately 15 pounds of body fat, which is equivalent to more than 50,000 kcal of energy. This is significantly more energy than can be provided by his stored muscle glycogen (800 to 2,000 kcal). Second, fat provides 9 kcal of energy per gram, more than twice as much energy per gram as carbohydrate. The primary disadvantage of using fat as a fuel is that the breakdown process is relatively slow; thus, fat is used predominantly as a fuel source during activities of lower intensity and longer duration. Fat is also our primary energy source during rest, sitting, and standing in place.

What specific activities are fueled primarily by fat? Walking long distances uses fat stores, as do hiking, long-distance cycling, and other low- to moderate-intensity forms of exercise. Fat is also an important fuel source during endurance events such as marathons (26.2 miles) and ultra-marathon races (49.9 miles). Endurance exercise training improves our ability to use fat for energy, which may be one reason that people who exercise regularly tend to have lower body fat levels than people who do not exercise.

It is important to remember that we are almost always using some combination of carbohydrate and fat for energy. At rest, we use very little carbohydrate, relying mostly on fat. During maximal exercise (100% effort), we are using mostly carbohydrate and very little fat. However, most activities we do each day involve some use of both fuels **(FIGURE 11.9a)**.

If you want to decrease your body fat, is it better to exercise at low intensity, or at moderate or high intensity? The answer to this question depends on how long you are able to engage in an activity. Even though fat is the primary fuel source during very low-intensity activities such as sitting and standing, to decrease body fat you would obviously want to do activities of higher intensity to expend additional energy and decrease body fat stores (see Figure 11.9b). If you have a low fitness level and can

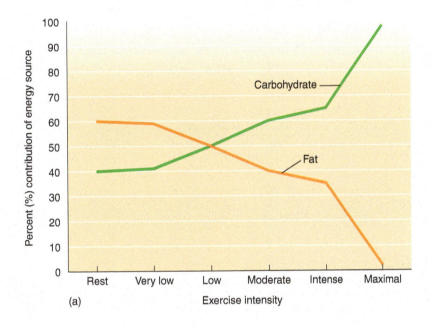

(a)

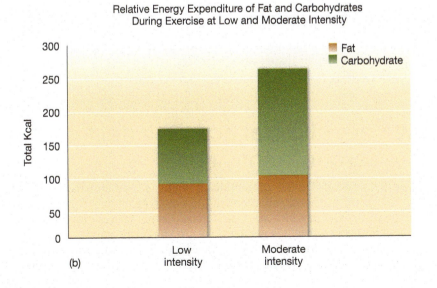

(b)

FIGURE 11.9 (a) For most daily activities, including exercise, we use a mixture of carbohydrate and fat for energy. At lower exercise intensities, we rely more on fat as a fuel source. As exercise intensity increases, we rely more on carbohydrate for energy. (b) If total exercise time is equal, the total amount of energy expended is greater when exercising at a higher intensity. However, note that the relative contribution of fat as a fuel source during low intensity exercise is higher (~50%) than during moderate intensity exercise (~40%).

Source: Data adapted from Brooks, G. A., and J. Mercier. 1994. Balance of carbohydrate and lipid utilization during exercise: The "crossover" concept. *Journal of Applied Physiology* 76(6):2253–2261.

walk for 20 minutes but can only jog for 2 minutes, then the overall amount of fat utilized and energy expended for walking would be higher than for jogging, and walking would be the better choice to decrease body fat in this particular case.

Recent evidence suggests that engaging in *high-intensity interval training* (*HIIT*) is a time-efficient strategy to optimize aerobic fitness and the use of fat as a fuel.[12] HIIT involves engaging in brief (1 to 2 minutes), intermittent bursts of vigorous activity interspersed with bouts of rest or low-intensity exercise. Beneficial changes have been observed with only about 15 total minutes per week of very intense exercise performed over 2 weeks; improvements in aerobic fitness have been observed in people with cardiovascular disease, congestive heart failure, metabolic syndrome, and obesity.[12]

When it comes to eating properly to support regular physical activity or exercise training, the nutrient to focus on is carbohydrate. This is because most people store more than enough fat to support exercise, whereas our storage of carbohydrate is limited. It is especially important that we maintain adequate stores of glycogen for moderate to intense exercise. Dietary recommendations for fat, carbohydrate, and protein are reviewed later in this chapter.

Amino Acids Are Not Major Sources of Fuel During Exercise

Proteins, or more specifically amino acids, can be used directly for energy if necessary, but they are more often used to make glucose to maintain our blood glucose levels during exercise. Amino acids also help build and repair tissues after exercise. Depending on the intensity and duration of the activity, amino acids may contribute about 3% to 6% of the energy needed.

Given this, why is it that so many active people are concerned about their protein intakes? As you learned (in Chapter 6), appropriate physical training combined with an adequate intake of dietary protein is the optimal stimulus for muscles to grow and strengthen. The protein needs of athletes are higher than the needs of nonathletes, but most people eat more than enough protein to support even the highest requirements for competitive athletes! Thus, there is generally no need for recreationally active people or even competitive athletes to consume protein or amino acid supplements.

recap The amount of ATP stored in a muscle cell is limited and can keep a muscle active for only about 1 to 3 seconds. For intense activities lasting about 3 to 15 seconds, creatine phosphate can be broken down to provide energy and support the regeneration of ATP. To support activities that last from 30 seconds to 2 minutes, energy is produced from glycolysis. Fatty acids can be broken down aerobically to support activities of low intensity and longer duration. The two major advantages of using fat as a fuel are that it is an abundant energy source and it provides more than twice the energy per gram as compared with carbohydrate. Amino acids may contribute from 3% to 6% of the energy needed during exercise, depending on the intensity and duration of the activity. Amino acids help build and repair tissues after exercise.

LO 4 Explain how an increase in physical activity or fitness training can affect energy and energy-yielding macronutrient needs.

How does physical activity affect energy and macronutrient needs?

Lots of people wonder, "Do my nutrient needs change if I become more physically active?" The answer to this question depends on the type, intensity, frequency, and duration of the activity in which you participate. It is not necessarily true that our requirement for every nutrient is greater if we are physically active.

People who are performing moderate-intensity daily activities for health can follow the dietary guidelines put forth in the USDA Food Patterns. For smaller or less active

TABLE 11.2 Suggested Intakes of Nutrients to Support Vigorous Exercise

Nutrient	Functions	Suggested Intake
Energy	Supports exercise, activities of daily living, and basic body functions	Depends on body size and the type, intensity, and duration of activity For many female athletes: 1,800 to 3,500 kcal/day For many male athletes: 2,500 to 7,500 kcal/day
Carbohydrate	Provides energy, maintains adequate muscle glycogen and blood glucose; high complex carbohydrate foods provide vitamins and minerals	45–65% of total energy intake Depending on sport and gender, should consume 6–10 g of carbohydrate per kg body weight per day
Fat	Provides energy, fat-soluble vitamins, and essential fatty acids; supports production of hormones and transport of nutrients	20–35% of total energy intake
Protein	Helps build and maintain muscle; provides building material for glucose; energy source during endurance exercise; aids recovery from exercise	10–35% of total energy intake 1.2–2.0 g per kg body weight
Water	Maintains temperature regulation (adequate cooling); maintains blood volume and blood pressure; supports all cell functions	Consume fluid before, during, and after exercise Consume enough to maintain body weight Consume at least 8 cups (64 fl. oz) of water daily to maintain regular health and activity Athletes may need up to 10 liters (170 fl. oz) every day; more is required if exercising in a hot environment
B-vitamins	Critical for energy production from carbohydrate, fat, and protein	May need slightly more (one to two times the RDA) for thiamin, riboflavin, and vitamin B_6
Calcium	Builds and maintains bone mass; assists with nervous system function, muscle contraction, hormone function, and transport of nutrients across cell membrane	Meet the current RDA: 14–18 years: 1,300 mg/day 19–50 years: 1,000 mg/day 51–70 years: 1,000 mg/day (men); 1,200 mg/day (women) 71 and older: 1,200 mg/day
Iron	Primarily responsible for the transport of oxygen in blood to cells; assists with energy production	Consume at least the RDA: Males: 14–18 years: 11 mg/day 19 and older: 8 mg/day Females: 14–18 years: 15 mg/day 19–50 years: 18 mg/day 51 and older: 8 mg/day

people, the lower end of the range of recommendations for each food group may be appropriate. For larger or more active people, the higher end of the range is suggested. Modifications may be necessary for people who exercise vigorously every day, particularly for athletes training for competition. **TABLE 11.2** provides an overview of the nutrients that can be affected by regular, vigorous exercise training. Each of these nutrients is described in more detail in the following section.

Vigorous Exercise Increases Energy Needs

Athletes generally have higher energy needs than moderately physically active or sedentary people. The amount of extra energy needed to support regular training is determined by the type, intensity, and duration of the activity. In addition, the energy needs of male athletes are higher than those of female athletes because male athletes typically weigh more, have more muscle mass, and expend more energy during activity. This is relative, of course: a large woman who trains 3 to 5 hours each day will probably need more energy than a small man who trains 1 hour each day. The energy needs of athletes can range from only 1,500 to 1,800 kcal/day for a small female gymnast to more than 7,500 kcal/day for a male cyclist competing in the Tour de France cross-country cycling race.

MEAL FOCUS FIGURE 11.10 on page 398 shows an example of 1 day's meals and snacks, totaling about 1,800 kcal and 4,000 kcal, with the carbohydrate content of these foods meeting around 60% of total energy intake. As you can see, athletes who require more than 4,000 kcal per day need to consume very large quantities of

a day of meals

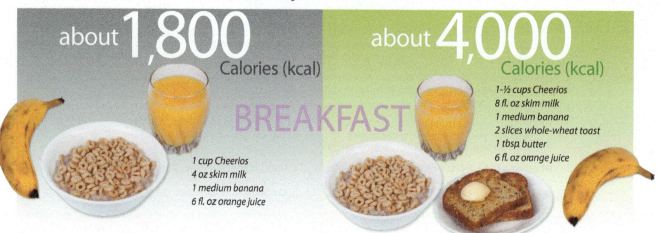

about 1,800 Calories (kcal)

about 4,000 Calories (kcal)

BREAKFAST

1 cup Cheerios
4 oz skim milk
1 medium banana
6 fl. oz orange juice

1-½ cups Cheerios
8 fl. oz skim milk
1 medium banana
2 slices whole-wheat toast
1 tbsp. butter
6 fl. oz orange juice

LUNCH

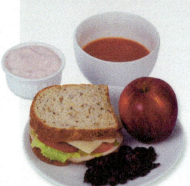

Turkey sandwich:
2 slices whole-wheat bread
3 oz turkey lunch meat
1 oz Swiss cheese slice
1 leaf iceberg lettuce
2 slices tomato
1 cup tomato soup
   (made withwater)
1 large apple
8 oz nonfat fruit yogurt
¼ cup dried sweetened
   cranberries

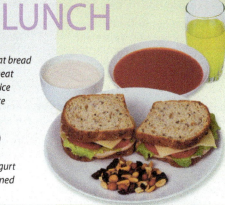

2 turkey sandwiches, each with:
2 slices whole-wheat bread
3 oz turkey lunch meat
1 oz Swiss cheese slice
1 leaf iceberg lettuce
2 slices tomato
2 cups tomato soup
   (made with water)
Two 8 oz containers of low-fat
   fruit yogurt
¼ cup trail mix
12 fl. oz Gatorade

DINNER

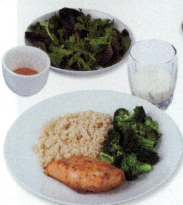

4 oz grilled skinless chicken breast
1-½ cups mixed salad greens
1 tbsp. French salad dressing
1 cup steamed broccoli
½ cup cooked brown rice
4 fl. oz skim milk
1 cup fresh blackberries

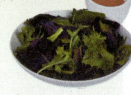

6 oz grilled skinless chicken breast
3 cups mixed salad greens
3 tbsp. French salad dressing
2 cups cooked spaghetti noodles
1 cup spaghetti sauce with meat
8 fl. oz skim milk
1 large apple
2 tbsp. peanut butter

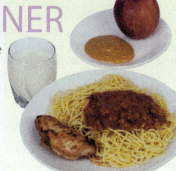

nutrient analysis

1,797 kcal
60.8% of energy from carbohydrates
15.7% of energy from fat
4.7% of energy from saturated fat
23.5% of energy from protein
35 grams of dietary fiber
2,097 milligrams of sodium

More
energy
for activity!

nutrient analysis

3,984 kcal
59.4% of energy from carbohydrates
22.6% of energy from fat
7.0% of energy from saturated fat
18.0% of energy from protein
45.4 grams of dietary fiber
6019 milligrams of sodium

High-carbohydrate (approximately 60% of total energy) meals that contain approximately 1,800 kcal/day (on left) and 4,000 kcal/day (on right). Athletes, particularly those with very high energy needs, must plan their meals carefully to meet energy demands.

food. However, the heavy demands of daily physical training, work, school, and family responsibilities often leave these athletes with little time to eat adequately. Thus, many athletes meet their energy demands by planning regular meals and snacks and **grazing** (eating small meals throughout the day) consistently. They may also take advantage of the energy-dense snack foods and meal replacements specifically designed for athletes participating in vigorous training. These steps help athletes maintain their blood glucose and energy stores.

If an athlete is losing body weight, then his or her energy intake is inadequate. Conversely, weight gain may indicate that energy intake is too high. Weight maintenance is generally recommended to maximize performance. If weight loss is warranted, food intake should be lowered no more than 200 to 500 kcal per day, and athletes should try to lose weight prior to the competitive season, if at all possible. Weight gain may be necessary for some athletes and can usually be accomplished by consuming 500 to 700 kcal/day more than needed for weight maintenance. The extra energy should come from a healthy balance of carbohydrate (45% to 65% of total energy intake), fat (20% to 35% of total energy intake), and protein (10% to 35% of total energy intake).

Many athletes are concerned about their weight. Jockeys, boxers, wrestlers, judo athletes, and others are required to "make weight"—to meet a predefined weight category. Others, such as distance runners, gymnasts, figure skaters, and dancers, are required to maintain a very lean figure for performance and aesthetic reasons. These athletes tend to eat less energy than they need to support vigorous training, which puts them at risk for inadequate intakes of all nutrients. They are also at a higher risk of suffering from a body image or eating disorder (see the **In Depth** essay immediately following this chapter) and from disorders resulting from poor energy and nutrient intake, including osteoporosis, menstrual disturbances (in women), dehydration, heat and physical injuries, and even death.

In addition, athletes should not adopt low-carbohydrate diets in an attempt to lose weight. As we discuss next, carbohydrates are a critical energy source for maintaining exercise performance.

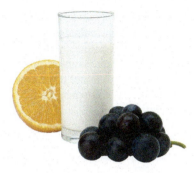

◆ Small snacks can help active people meet their daily energy needs.

Carbohydrate Needs Increase for Many Active People

Carbohydrate (in the form of glucose) is one of the primary sources of energy needed to support exercise. Both endurance athletes and strength athletes require adequate carbohydrate to maintain their glycogen stores and provide quick energy.

DRIs for Carbohydrate for Athletes

Recall (from Chapter 4) that the AMDR for carbohydrates is 45% to 65% of total energy intake. Athletes should consume carbohydrate within this recommended range. Although high-carbohydrate diets (greater than 60% of total energy intake) have been recommended in the past, this percentage value may not be appropriate for all athletes. To optimize muscle glycogen stores, it is recommended that athletes consume a daily carbohydrate intake of approximately 6 to 10 grams of carbohydrate per kilogram body weight. However, the need may be much greater in athletes who train heavily daily, as they have less time to recover and require more carbohydrate to support both training and storage needs.

To illustrate the importance of carbohydrate intake for athletes, let's see what happens to Theo when he participates in a study designed to determine how carbohydrate intake affects glycogen stores during a period of heavy training. Theo was asked to go to the exercise laboratory at the university and ride a stationary bicycle for 2 hours a day for 3 consecutive days at 75% of his maximal heart rate. Before and after each ride, samples of muscle tissue were taken from his thighs to determine the amount of glycogen stored in the working muscles. Theo performed these rides under two different experimental conditions—once when he had eaten a high-carbohydrate diet (80% of total energy intake) and again when he had eaten a moderate-carbohydrate diet (40% of total energy intake). As you can see in **FIGURE 11.11** on page 400, Theo's muscle glycogen levels decreased dramatically after each training session. More important, his muscle glycogen levels did not recover to baseline levels

grazing Consistently eating small meals throughout the day; done by many athletes to meet their high energy demands.

▶ **FIGURE 11.11** The effects of a low-carbohydrate diet on muscle glycogen stores. When a low-carbohydrate diet is consumed, glycogen stores cannot be restored during a period of regular vigorous training.

Source: Data from Costill, D. L., and J. M. Miller. 1980. Nutrition for endurance sport: CHO and fluid balance. *International Journal of Sports Medicine* 1:2–14. Copyright © 1980 Georg Thieme Verlag. Used with permission.

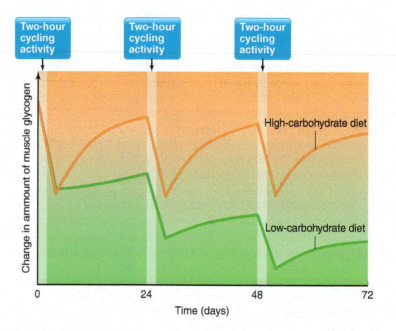

over the 3 days when Theo ate the lower-carbohydrate diet. He was able to maintain his muscle glycogen levels only when he was eating the higher-carbohydrate diet. Theo also told the researchers that completing the 2-hour rides was much more difficult when he had eaten the moderate-carbohydrate diet as compared to when he ate the diet that was higher in carbohydrate.

Timing of Carbohydrate Consumption

It is important for athletes not only to consume enough carbohydrate to maintain glycogen stores but also to time their intake optimally. The body stores glycogen very

nutri-case | JUDY

"I can't remember a time in my life when I wasn't trying to lose weight, but nothing ever works! Last week I had my annual checkup and my doctor confirmed what I already knew—I'm obese! The doctor also said my weight is contributing to my high blood sugar, and my blood pressure is high, too. As a nurse's aide, I see the health problems caused by obesity every day. But knowing how bad it is doesn't help me lose weight and keep it off. So we talked about some 'slow and steady' strategies for losing weight: I promised I'd watch my diet, take my meds, and start working out at the new fitness center here at the hospital. It has a couple of treadmills and stationary bikes right in front of a big TV so you can watch the soaps while you work out. Still, I'm not really sure what I'm supposed to do, or how many times a week, or for how long. I mean, if I only had to lose 5 pounds that would be easy. But I've got to lose 50! And I only get half an hour for lunch!"

Imagine that you were a trainer at the Valley Hospital employee fitness center, and Judy told you about her weight-loss and health goals. Applying the FITT principle, recommend an initial physical activity program that can get Judy started on improving her health that includes an appropriate:

- number of times per 5-day workweek
- intensity
- duration of activity
- variety of activities

rapidly during the first 24 hours of recovery from exercise, with the highest storage rates occurring during the first 4 to 6 hours. Higher carbohydrate intakes during the first 24 hours of recovery from exercise, particularly when consumed with a source high in protein (such as chocolate milk), are associated with higher amounts of glucose being stored as muscle glycogen and enhanced performance.[13]

If an athlete has to perform or participate in training bouts that are scheduled less than 8 hours apart, then he or she should try to consume 1 to 1.2 g of carbohydrate per kg body weight in the first 4 hours following training to allow for ample glycogen storage.[14] However, with a longer recovery time (generally 12 hours or more), the athlete can eat when he or she chooses, and glycogen levels should be restored as long as the total carbohydrate eaten is sufficient. Current evidence indicates that the glycemic index and glycemic load do not influence an athlete's performance if the amount of carbohydrate and energy of the diet are sufficient.[14]

Food Sources of Carbohydrates for Athletes

What are good carbohydrate sources to support vigorous training? In general, fiber-rich, less-processed carbohydrate foods, such as whole grains and cereals, fruits, vegetables, and juices, are excellent sources that also supply fiber, vitamins, and minerals. Dietary guidelines for the general public recommend that intake of simple sugars be less than 10% of total energy intake, but some athletes who require very large energy intakes to support training may need to consume more. Thus, there are advantages to consuming a wide variety of carbohydrate sources.

As a result of time constraints, many athletes have difficulties consuming enough food to meet carbohydrate demands. Sports drinks and energy bars have been designed to help athletes increase their carbohydrate intake. **TABLE 11.3** identifies some energy bars and other simple, inexpensive snacks and meals that contain 50 to 100 grams of carbohydrate.

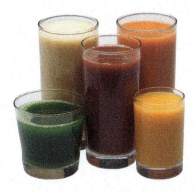

◆ Fruit and vegetable juices can be a good source of carbohydrates.

TABLE 11.3 Carbohydrate and Total Energy in Various Foods

Food	Amount	Carbohydrate (g)	Energy from Carbohydrate (%)	Total Energy (kcal)
Sweetened applesauce	1 cup	50	97	207
Large apple with	1 each	50	82	248
saltine crackers	8 each			
Whole-wheat bread	1-oz slice	50	71	282
with jelly	4 tsp.			
and skim milk	12 fl. oz			
Spaghetti (cooked)	1 cup	50	75	268
with tomato sauce	1/4 cup			
Brown rice (cooked)	1 cup	100	88	450
with mixed vegetables	1/2 cup			
and apple juice	12 fl. oz			
Grape-Nuts cereal	1/2 cup	100	84	473
with raisins	3/8 cup			
and skim milk	8 fl. oz			
Clif Bar (chocolate chip)	2.4 oz	43	75	230
Meta-Rx (fudge brownie)	100 g	41	41	400
Power Bar (chocolate)	1 bar	45	75	240
PR Bar Ironman	50 g	22	44	200

Source: Data adapted from Manore, M. M., N. L. Meyer, and J. L. Thompson. 2009. *Sport Nutrition for Health and Performance,* 2nd ed. Champaign, IL: Human Kinetics.

TABLE 11.4 Recommended Carbohydrate Loading Guidelines for Endurance Athletes

Days Prior to Event	Exercise Duration (in minutes)	Carbohydrate Content of Diet (g per kg body weight)
6	90 (at 70% max effort)	5 (moderate)
5	40 (at 70% max effort)	5 (moderate)
4	40 (at 70% max effort)	5 (moderate)
3	20 (light training)	10–12 (high)
2	20 (light training)	10–12 (high)
1	Rest	10–12 (high)
Day of race	Competition	Precompetition food and fluid

Sources: Current Trends in Performance Nutrition, by Marie Dunford. Copyright © 2005 by Human Kinetics, Champaign, IL. Reprinted with permission; and American College of Sports Medicine, Academy of Nutrition and Dietetics, and Dietitians of Canada. 2016. Nutrition and Athletic Performance. Joint Position Statement. *Medicine and Science in Sports and Exercise* 48(3):543–568.

Carbohydrate Loading

As you know, carbohydrate is a critical energy source to support exercise—particularly endurance-type activities—yet we have a limited capacity to store it. So it's not surprising that discovering ways to maximize carbohydrate storage has been at the forefront of sports nutrition research for many years. The practice of **carbohydrate loading**, also called *glycogen loading,* involves altering both exercise duration and carbohydrate intake such that it maximizes the amount of muscle glycogen. **TABLE 11.4** provides a schedule for carbohydrate loading for an endurance athlete.

Athletes who may benefit from carbohydrate loading are those competing in marathons, ultra-marathons, long-distance swimming, cross-country skiing, and triathlons. Athletes who compete in baseball, American football, 10-kilometer runs, walking, hiking, weight lifting, and most swimming events will not gain any performance benefits from this practice, nor will people who regularly participate in moderately intense physical activities to maintain fitness.

It is important to emphasize that, even in endurance events, carbohydrate loading does not always improve performance. There are many adverse side effects of this practice, including extreme gastrointestinal distress, particularly diarrhea. We store water along with the extra glycogen in the muscles, which leaves many athletes feeling heavy and sluggish. Athletes who want to try carbohydrate loading should experiment prior to competition to determine whether it is an acceptable and beneficial approach for them.

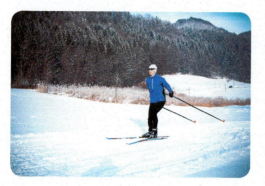

🔺 Carbohydrate loading may benefit endurance athletes, such as cross-country skiers.

Moderate Fat Consumption Is Enough to Support Most Activities

Fat is an important energy source for both moderate physical activity and vigorous endurance training. When athletes reach a physically trained state, they are able to use more fat for energy; in other words, they become better "fat burners." This can also occur in people who are not athletes but who regularly participate in aerobic-type fitness activities. This training effect occurs for a number of reasons, including an increase in the number and activity of various enzymes involved in fat metabolism, improved ability of the muscle to store fat, and improved ability to extract fat from the blood for use during exercise. By using fat as a fuel, athletes can spare carbohydrate, so that they can use it during prolonged, intense training or competition.

Many athletes concerned with body weight and physical appearance believe they should eat less than 15% of their total energy intake as fat, but this is inadequate for vigorous activity. Instead, a fat intake of 20% to 35% of total energy intake is generally recommended for most athletes, with less than 10% of total energy intake as

carbohydrate loading Also known as *glycogen loading*. A process that involves altering training and carbohydrate intake, so that muscle glycogen storage is maximized.

saturated fat. The same recommendations are put forth for nonathletes. Fat provides not only energy but also fat-soluble vitamins and essential fatty acids that are critical to maintaining general health. If fat consumption is too low, inadequate levels of these nutrients can eventually prove detrimental to training and performance. Athletes who have chronic disease risk factors, such as high blood lipids, high blood pressure, or unhealthful blood glucose levels, should work with their physician to adjust their intake of fat and carbohydrate according to their health risks.

Many Athletes Have Increased Protein Needs

The protein intakes suggested for active people range from 1.2 to 2.0 grams per kilograms body weight. Intakes at the lower end of this range are for people who exercise four to five times a week for 30 minutes or less. At the upper end are athletes who train five to seven times a week for more than an hour a day. Higher intakes may be needed for brief periods of time to prevent the loss of lean body mass during periods of intensified training or when restricting energy to promote fat loss.[14]

Most inactive people and many athletes in the United States consume more than enough protein to support their needs. However, some athletes do not consume enough protein, including those with very low energy intakes, vegetarians or vegans who do not consume high-protein food sources, and young athletes who are growing and are not aware of their higher protein needs.

High-quality protein sources include lean meats, poultry, fish, eggs, low-fat dairy products, legumes, and soy products. By following their personalized MyPlate food patterns, people of all fitness levels can consume more than enough protein without the use of supplements or specially formulated foods. Many athletes use protein shakes and other products in an attempt to build muscle mass and strength; some even use ergogenic aids to try to enhance performance. The safety and effectiveness of ergogenic aids is discussed later in this chapter.

recap The type, intensity, and duration of activities a person participates in determine his or her nutrient needs. Carbohydrate needs may increase for some active people. In general, athletes should consume 45% to 65% of their total energy as carbohydrate. Carbohydrate loading involves altering physical training and the diet such that the storage of muscle glycogen is maximized. Active people use more fat than carbohydrates for energy because they experience an increase in the number and activity of the enzymes involved in fat metabolism and they have an improved ability to store fat and extract it from the blood for use during exercise. A dietary fat intake of 20% to 35% is recommended for athletes, with less than 10% of total energy intake as saturated fat. Although protein needs can be higher for active people and athletes, most people in the United States already consume more than twice their daily needs for protein.

How does physical activity affect fluid and micronutrient needs?

LO 5 Explain how an increase in physical activity or fitness training can affect fluid and micronutrient needs.

In this section, we review some of the basic functions of water and its role during exercise. (For a detailed discussion of fluid and electrolyte balance, see Chapter 7.) We also discuss changes in micronutrient needs to support vigorous physical activity.

Dehydration and Heat-Related Illnesses

Heat production can increase by 15 to 20 times during heavy exercise! The primary way in which we dissipate this heat is through evaporative cooling (see Figure 7.2 on page 226). When body temperature rises, more blood (which contains water) flows to the surface of the skin. Heat is carried in this way from the core of our body to the

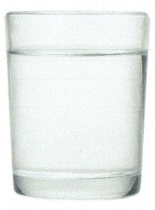

⬆ Water is essential for maintaining fluid balance and preventing dehydration.

surface of our skin. When we sweat, the water (and body heat) leaves our body and the air around us picks up the evaporating water from our skin, cooling our body.

Heat illnesses occur because, when we exercise in the heat, our muscles and skin constantly compete for blood flow. When there is no longer enough blood flow to simultaneously provide adequate blood to both our muscles and our skin, muscle blood flow takes priority and evaporative cooling is inhibited. Exercising in heat plus humidity is especially dangerous; whereas the heat dramatically raises body temperature, the high humidity inhibits evaporative cooling—that is, the environmental air is already so saturated with water that it is unable to absorb the water in sweat. Body temperature becomes dangerously high, and heat illness is likely.

Dehydration significantly increases our risk for heat illnesses. **FIGURE 11.12** identifies the symptoms of dehydration during heavy exercise.

Heat illnesses include heat syncope, heat cramps, heat exhaustion, and heatstroke:

- *Heat syncope* is dizziness that occurs when people stand for too long in the heat and the blood pools in their lower extremities. It can also occur when people stop suddenly after a race or stand suddenly from a lying position.
- *Heat cramps* are muscle spasms that occur during exercise or several hours after strenuous exercise or manual labor in the heat. They are most commonly felt in the legs, arms, or abdomen after a person cools down.
- *Heat exhaustion* and *heatstroke* occur on a continuum, with unchecked heat exhaustion leading to heatstroke. Early signs of heat exhaustion include excessive sweating, cold and clammy skin, rapid but weak pulse, weakness, nausea, dizziness, headache, and difficulty concentrating. Signs that a person is progressing to heatstroke are hot, dry skin; rapid and strong pulse; vomiting; diarrhea; a body temperature greater than or equal to 104°F; hallucinations; and coma. Prompt medical care is essential to save the person's life. (For more information about heat illnesses, see Chapter 7.)

Guidelines for Proper Fluid Replacement

How can we prevent dehydration and heat illnesses? Obviously, adequate fluid intake is critical before, during, and after exercise. Unfortunately, our thirst mechanism cannot be relied on to signal when we need to drink. If we rely only on our feelings of thirst, we will not consume enough fluid to support exercise.

General fluid replacement recommendations are based on maintaining body weight. Athletes who are training and competing in hot environments should weigh themselves before and after the training session or event and should regain the weight

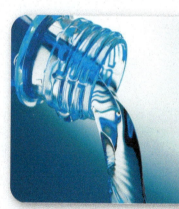

Symptoms of Dehydration During Heavy Exercise:
- Decreased exercise performance
- Increased level in perceived exertion
- Dark yellow or brown urine color
- Increased heart rate at a given exercise intensity
- Decreased appetite
- Decreased ability to concentrate
- Decreased urine output
- Fatigue and weakness
- Headache and dizziness

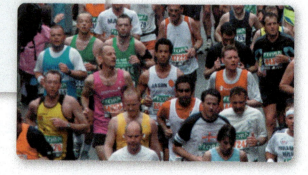

⬆ **FIGURE 11.12** Symptoms of dehydration during heavy exercise.

lost over the subsequent 24-hour period. They should avoid losing more than 2% to 3% of body weight during exercise because performance can be impaired with fluid losses as small as 1% of body weight.

TABLE 11.5 reviews the guidelines for proper fluid replacement. For activities lasting less than 1 hour, plain water is generally adequate to replace fluid losses. However, for training and competition lasting longer than 1 hour in any weather, sports beverages containing carbohydrates and electrolytes are recommended. These beverages are also recommended for people who will not drink enough water because they don't like the taste. If drinking these beverages will guarantee adequate hydration, they are appropriate to use. (For more specific information about sports beverages, refer to Chapter 7, page 237.)

Inadequate Micronutrient Intake Can Diminish Health and Performance

When people train vigorously for athletic events, their requirements for certain vitamins and minerals may be altered. It is essential to eat an adequate, varied, and balanced diet to try to meet the increased micronutrient needs associated with vigorous training.

B-Vitamins

The B-vitamins are directly involved in energy metabolism (see Chapter 8). There is reliable evidence that—as a population—active people may require slightly more thiamin, riboflavin, and vitamin B_6 than the current RDA to support increased production of energy. However, these increased needs are easily met by consuming adequate

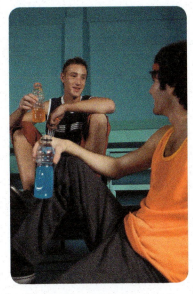

◀ Drinking sports beverages during training and competition lasting more than 1 hour replaces fluid, carbohydrates, and electrolytes.

TABLE 11.5 **Guidelines for Fluid Replacement**

Activity Level	Environment	Fluid Requirements (liters per day)
Sedentary	Cool	2–3
Active	Cool	3–6
Sedentary	Warm	3–5
Active	Warm	5–10

Before Exercise or Competition
- Drink adequate fluids during the 24 hours before event; should be able to maintain body weight.
- Slowly drink about 0.17 to 0.34 fl. oz per kg body weight of water or a sports drink in the 2 to 4 hours prior to exercise or event to achieve urine that is pale yellow in color while allowing sufficient time for excretion of excess fluid prior to exercise.
- Consuming beverages with sodium and/or small amounts of salted snacks at a meal will help stimulate thirst and retain fluids consumed.

During Exercise or Competition
- Amount and rate of fluid replacement depend on individual sweating rate, exercise duration, weather conditions, and opportunities to drink.
- Drink sufficient fluids during exercise to replace sweat losses such that total fluid loss is less than 2% of body weight.

Following Exercise or Competition
- Consume about 3 cups of fluid for each pound of body weight lost.
- Fluids after exercise should contain water to restore hydration status and sodium to support rehydration.
- Consume enough fluid to permit regular urination and to ensure the urine color is very light or light yellow in color; drinking about 125–150% of fluid loss is usually sufficient to ensure complete rehydration.

In General
- Products that contain fructose should be limited, as these may cause gastrointestinal distress.
- Alcohol should be avoided, as it increases urine output and reduces fluid retention.

Source: American College of Sports Medicine, Academy of Nutrition and Dietetics, and Dietitians of Canada. 2016. Nutrition and Athletic Performance. Joint Position Statement. *Medicine and Science in Sports and Exercise* 48(3):543–568.

energy and plenty of fiber-rich carbohydrates. Active people at risk for poor B-vitamin status are those who consume inadequate energy or who consume mostly refined carbohydrate foods, such as soda pop and sugary snacks. Vegan athletes and active individuals may be at risk for inadequate intake of vitamin B_{12}; food sources enriched with this nutrient include soy and cereal products.

Calcium

Calcium supports proper muscle contraction and ensures bone health. Calcium intakes are inadequate for most women in the United States, including both sedentary and active women. This is most likely due to a failure to consume foods that are high in calcium, particularly dairy products. Although vigorous training does not appear to directly increase our need for calcium, we need to consume enough calcium to support bone health. If we do not, stress fractures and severe loss of bone can result.

Some female athletes suffer from a syndrome known as the *female athlete triad* (see **In Depth 11.5** immediately following this chapter). In the female athlete triad, nutritional inadequacies cause irregularities in the menstrual cycle and hormonal disturbances that lead to a significant loss of bone mass. Thus, for female athletes, consuming the recommended amounts of calcium is critical. For female athletes who are physically small and have lower energy intakes, calcium supplementation may be needed to meet current recommendations.

Iron

Iron is a part of the hemoglobin molecule in blood cells and is critical for the transport of oxygen to body cells and working muscles. Iron also is involved in energy production. Active individuals lose more iron in the sweat, feces, and urine than do inactive people, and endurance runners lose iron when their red blood cells break down in their feet as a consequence of the high impact of running. Female athletes and nonathletes lose more iron than male athletes because of menstrual blood losses, and females in general tend to eat less iron in their diet. Vegetarian athletes and active people may also consume less iron. Thus, many athletes and active people are at higher risk for iron deficiency. Depending on its severity, poor iron status can impair athletic performance and our ability to maintain regular physical activity.

A phenomenon known as *sports anemia* was identified in the 1960s. Sports anemia is not true anemia, but rather a transient decrease in iron stores that occurs at the start of an exercise program for some people, and it is seen in athletes who increase their training intensity. Exercise training increases the amount of water in our blood (called *plasma volume*); however, the amount of hemoglobin does not increase until later into the training period. Thus, the iron content in the blood appears to be low but instead is falsely depressed due to increases in plasma volume. Sports anemia, because it is not true anemia, does not affect performance.

In general, it appears that physically active females are at relatively high risk of suffering from the first stage of iron depletion, in which iron stores are low. Because of this, it is suggested that blood tests of iron stores and monitoring of dietary iron intake be done routinely for active people. In some cases, iron needs cannot be met through the diet, and supplementation is necessary. Iron supplementation should be done with a physician's approval and proper medical supervision.

Map your walking, running, or cycling route and share it with friends—or check out dozens of fitness loops right in your neighborhood at www .livestrong.com. Enter "tools" into the search box, then scroll down to select "Tools" under the Livestrong Search Results heading. Then select "Loops" to get underway.

recap Regular exercise increases fluid needs. Fluid is critical to cool our internal body temperature and prevent heat illnesses. Dehydration is a serious threat during exercise in extreme heat and high humidity. Heat illnesses include heat syncope, heat cramps, heat exhaustion, and heat stroke. Active people may need more thiamin, riboflavin, and vitamin B_6 than inactive people. Exercise itself does not increase our calcium needs, but most women, including active women, do not consume enough calcium. Many active individuals require more iron, particularly female athletes and vegetarian athletes.

Are ergogenic aids necessary for active people?

LO 6 Discuss the marketing claims, performance effects, and health risks of several popular ergogenic aids.

Many competitive athletes and even some recreationally active people continually search for that something extra that will enhance their performance. **Ergogenic aids** are substances used to improve exercise and athletic performance. For example, dietary supplements can be classified as ergogenic aids, as can anabolic steroids and other pharmaceuticals. Interestingly, people report using ergogenic aids not only to enhance athletic performance but also to improve their physical appearance, prevent or treat injuries and diseases, and help them cope with stress. Some people even report using them because of peer pressure.

As you have learned in this chapter, adequate nutrition is critical to athletic performance and to regular physical activity, and products such as sports bars and beverages can help athletes maintain their competitive edge. However, as we will explore shortly, many ergogenic aids are not effective, some are dangerous, and most are very expensive. For the average consumer, it is virtually impossible to track the latest research findings for these products. In addition, many have not been adequately studied, and unsubstantiated claims surrounding them are rampant. How can you become a more educated consumer about ergogenic aids?

New ergogenic aids are available virtually every month. It is therefore not possible to discuss every product here. However, a brief review of a number of currently popular ergogenic aids is provided.

Many Ergogenic Aids Are Said to Build Muscle Mass and Strength

Many ergogenic aids are said to be **anabolic**, meaning that they build muscle and increase strength. Most anabolic substances promise to increase testosterone, which is the hormone associated with male sex characteristics and that increases muscle size and strength. Although some anabolic substances are effective, they are generally associated with harmful side effects.

Anabolic Steroids

Anabolic steroids are testosterone-based drugs known to be effective in increasing muscle size, strength, power, and speed. They have been used extensively by strength and power athletes; however, these products are illegal in the United States, and their use is banned by all major collegiate and professional sports organizations, in addition to both the U.S. and the International Olympic Committees. Proven long-term and irreversible effects of steroid use include infertility; early closure of the plates of the long bones, resulting in permanently shortened stature; shriveled testicles, enlarged breast tissue (that can be removed only surgically), and other signs of "feminization" in men; enlarged clitoris, facial hair growth, and other signs of "masculinization" in women; increased risk for certain forms of cancer; liver damage; unhealthful changes in blood lipids; hypertension; severe acne; hair thinning or baldness; and depression, delusions, sleep disturbances, and extreme anger (so-called roid rage).

Androstenedione and Dehydroepiandrosterone

Androstenedione ("andro") and dehydroepiandrosterone (DHEA) are precursors of testosterone. Manufacturers of these products claim that taking them will increase testosterone levels and muscle strength. Androstenedione became very popular around 20 years ago after baseball player Mark McGwire claimed he used it during the time he was breaking home run records. Contrary to popular claims, neither androstenedione nor DHEA increases testosterone levels, and early research on androstenedione has been shown to increase the risk for heart disease in men aged 35 to 65 years.[15] There are no studies that support the products' claims of improving strength and increasing muscle mass.

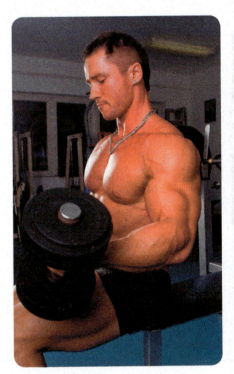

▲ Anabolic substances are often marketed to people striving to increase their muscle mass and strength; however, many cause harmful side effects.

ergogenic aids Substances used to improve exercise and athletic performance.

anabolic The characteristic of a substance that builds muscle and increases strength.

Creatine

Creatine, or creatine phosphate, is found in meat and fish and stored in our muscles. Because cells use creatine phosphate (CP) to regenerate ATP, it is theorized that creatine supplements make more CP available to replenish ATP, which prolongs a person's ability to train and perform in short-term, explosive activities, such as weight lifting and sprinting. Creatine does not seem to enhance performance in aerobic-type events but may increase the work performed and amount of strength gained during resistance exercise and to enhance sprint performance in swimming, running, and cycling. Side effects include acute weight gain and gastrointestinal discomfort.[14]

Some Ergogenic Aids Are Said to Optimize Fuel Use

Certain ergogenic aids are touted as increasing energy levels and improving athletic performance by optimizing the use of fat, carbohydrate, and protein. The products reviewed here are caffeine, ephedrine, carnitine, chromium, and beta-alanine.

Caffeine

Caffeine is a stimulant that makes us feel more alert and energetic, decreasing feelings of fatigue during exercise. In addition, caffeine has been shown to increase the use of fat as a fuel during endurance exercise, thereby sparing muscle glycogen and improving performance. Energy drinks that contain high amounts of caffeine, such as Red Bull, have become popular with athletes and many college students. These drinks should be avoided during exercise, however, because they can prompt severe dehydration due to the combination of fluid loss from exercise and increased fluid excretion from the caffeine. Research also indicates that energy drinks are associated with serious side effects in children, adolescents, and young adults, including irregularities in heart rhythm, seizures, diabetes, and mood disorders.[16] It should be recognized that caffeine is a controlled or restricted drug in the athletic world, and athletes can be banned from Olympic competition if their urine levels are too high. However, the amount of caffeine that is banned is quite high, and athletes would need to consume caffeine in pill form to reach this level. Side effects of caffeine use include increased blood pressure, increased heart rate, dizziness, insomnia, headache, and gastrointestinal distress.

Ephedrine

Ephedrine, also known as ephedra, Chinese ephedra, and *ma huang*, is a strong stimulant marketed as a weight-loss supplement and energy enhancer. In reality, many products sold as Chinese ephedra (or herbal ephedra) contain ephedrine synthesized in a laboratory and other stimulants, such as caffeine. The use of ephedra does not appear to enhance performance, but supplements containing both caffeine and ephedra have been shown to prolong the amount of exercise that can be done until exhaustion is reached. Side effects of ephedra use include headaches, nausea, nervousness, anxiety, irregular heart rate, high blood pressure, and death. It is currently illegal to sell ephedra-containing supplements in the United States.

Carnitine

Carnitine is a compound made from amino acids and is found in the membranes of mitochondria in our cells. Carnitine helps shuttle fatty acids into the mitochondria, so that they can be used for energy. It has been proposed that exercise training depletes our cells of carnitine and that supplementation should restore carnitine levels, thereby enabling us to improve our use of fat as a fuel source. Thus, carnitine is marketed not only as a performance-enhancing substance but also as a "fat burner." Research studies of carnitine supplementation do not support these claims, as neither the transport of fatty acids nor their oxidation appears to be enhanced with supplementation. The use of carnitine supplements has not been associated with significant side effects.

Chromium

Chromium is a trace mineral that enhances insulin's action of increasing the transport of amino acids into the cell. It is found in whole-grain foods, cheese, nuts, mushrooms, and asparagus. It is theorized that many people are chromium deficient and that supplementation will enhance the uptake of amino acids into muscle cells, which will increase muscle growth and strength. Like carnitine, chromium is marketed as a fat burner, with claims that its effect on insulin stimulates the brain to decrease food intake. Chromium supplements are available as chromium picolinate and chromium nicotinate. Early studies of chromium supplementation showed promise, but more recent, better-designed studies do not support any benefit of chromium supplementation on muscle mass, muscle strength, body fat, or exercise performance.

Beta-Alanine

Beta-alanine is a nonessential amino acid that has been identified as the limiting factor in the production of carnosine, which plays a key role in the regulation of pH in the muscle and is thought to buffer acids produced during exercise, thereby enhancing a person's ability to perform short-term, high-intensity activities. Recent evidence suggests that beta-alanine supplementation can increase muscle carnosine levels and delay the onset of muscle fatigue.[17] Additionally, beta-alanine supplementation results in improved exercise performance during single or repeated high-intensity exercise bouts or maximal muscle contractions. It appears that several weeks of supplementation are needed to increase muscle carnosine levels and positively affect performance.

As this review indicates, many ergogenic aids fail to live up to their claims of enhancing athletic performance, strength, or body composition. And many have uncomfortable or even dangerous side effects. Be a savvy consumer. Before purchasing any ergogenic aid, do some homework to make sure you wouldn't be wasting your money or putting your health at risk by using it.

recap Ergogenic aids are substances used to improve exercise and athletic performance. Many claim to be anabolic, meaning that they build muscle and increase strength. Although some anabolic substances are effective, they are generally associated with harmful side effects. Certain ergogenic aids are said to increase energy levels and improving athletic performance by optimizing the use of fat, carbohydrate, and/or protein. Caffeine and beta-alanine appear to improve athletic performance. Studies do not support any ergogenic benefit of carnitine or chromium, and ephedrine is dangerous and cannot be sold in the United States.

The first physical activity recommendations were published in 1996, when a report of the Surgeon General recommended that Americans engage in at least 30 minutes of physical activity on most days of the week.[18] Then, in 2002, the Institute of Medicine (IOM, which is now the Health and Medicine Division of the National Academies of Sciences, Engineering, and Medicine) released a recommendation that Americans be active 60 minutes per day to optimize health.[6] As this amount and frequency of physical activity was significantly higher than the Surgeon General's recommendation, it caused a great deal of confusion and controversy. For most Americans, how much physical activity is enough?

To tackle that question, let's look at the basis for the IOM's more challenging recommendation. It was derived from metabolic studies specifically examining the energy expenditure associated with maintaining a healthful body weight (defined as a BMI of 18.5 to 25 kg/m^2). After reviewing a large number of studies that assessed energy expenditure and BMI, the IOM concluded that participating in about 60 minutes of moderately intense physical activity per day will move people to an active lifestyle and will allow them to maintain a healthful body weight.

The IOM recommendation was not based on evidence supporting the wider range of health benefits that result when a person moves from doing no physical activity to at least some level of physical activity. The growing body of evidence regarding the health benefits of physical activity clearly indicates that doing at least some physical activity is better than doing none, and doing more physical activity is better than doing less.

In 2008, the U.S. Department of Health and Human Services (HHS) released the *Physical Activity Guidelines for Americans*.[5] These include guidelines for children and adolescents, adults, and older adults, with additional information for women who are pregnant; people with disabilities, type 2 diabetes, or osteoarthritis; and people who are cancer survivors. These guidelines build upon the Surgeon General's recommendation of 30 minutes per day on most, if not all, days of the week. Specifically, the 2008 HHS guidelines for adults state the following:

- Inactivity should be avoided. Participating in any amount of physical activity will provide some health benefits.

- To gain substantial health benefits, adults should do a minimum of 150 minutes per week of moderate-intensity activity, or 75 minutes per week of vigorous intensity activity, or an equivalent combination of these two intensities of activity. The activities should be aerobic in nature and performed in episodes of at least 10 minutes' duration, spread throughout the week.

- To gain additional and more extensive health benefits, adults should increase their aerobic activity level to 300 minutes per week of moderate-intensity activity, or 150 minutes per week of vigorous-intensity activity, or an equivalent combination of these two intensities.

- Adults should also participate in muscle-strengthening activities that are moderate or vigorous in intensity and involve all major muscle groups on at least 2 days per week.

Notice that these guidelines promote a *minimum* of 150 minutes per week of moderate-intensity aerobic physical activity, with additional encouragement to increase both the intensity and the duration of activity throughout the week to gain even more health benefits. Two recent studies tracking hundreds of thousands of individuals over several years support these recommendations. They found that those who exercised moderately for at least 150 minutes a week had about a 30% to 47% lower risk of dying during the study period, and that those who exercised longer (up to 450 minutes a week) or more vigorously at least occasionally during the week experienced an even greater reduction in mortality risk.[19,20] This research supports the reliability of the 2008 HHS guidelines while helping to illustrate that the IOM and Surgeon General's recommendations are not really that different after all.

CRITICAL THINKING QUESTIONS

1. How might an overweight person gain substantial health benefits by shifting from doing no physical activity to meeting the minimum recommendation of 30 minutes per day on most days of the week?

2. Conduct a literature search using Google Scholar to identify the various benefits of regular physical activity that are not related to weight loss.

3. Based on the results of this literature search, devise a marketing campaign that could be used to encourage college students to regularly engage in physical activity.

TEST YOURSELF | ANSWERS

1 **T** Almost 80% of Americans do not get enough physical activity. Moreover, nearly 24% of the population report doing no leisure-time physical activity at all.

2 **F** Evidence indicates that adequate protein intake is critical for muscle growth, and active people have higher protein needs than inactive people. However, protein supplements are not required to support muscle growth, as most Americans consume more than adequate protein from food. In contrast, weight-bearing exercise is necessary to appropriately stress the body and increase muscle mass and strength.

3 **F** During exercise, our thirst mechanism cannot be relied upon to signal when we need to drink. If we rely solely on our feelings of thirst, we will not consume enough fluid to support exercise.

review questions

LO 1 **1.** Which of the following is a benefit of regular physical activity?

a. Reduces body cells' uptake of glucose from the blood
b. Reduces the risk of nearly all forms of cancer
c. Reduces anxiety and mental stress
d. All of the above

LO 2 **2.** For achieving and maintaining cardiorespiratory fitness, the intensity range typically recommended is

a. 25% to 50% of your estimated maximal heart rate.
b. 35% to 75% of your estimated maximal heart rate.
c. 50% to 70% of your estimated maximal heart rate.
d. 75% to 95% of your estimated maximal heart rate.

LO 3 **3.** The amount of ATP stored in a muscle cell can keep a muscle active for about

a. 1 to 3 seconds.
b. 10 to 30 seconds.
c. 1 to 3 minutes.
d. 1 to 3 hours.

LO 3 **4.** To support a long afternoon of gardening, the body predominantly uses which nutrient for energy?

a. Carbohydrate
b. Fat
c. Amino acids
d. Lactic acid

LO 4 **5.** Which of the following statements about carbohydrate loading is true?

a. Carbohydrate loading involves altering the duration and intensity of exercise and intake of carbohydrate such that the storage of fat is minimized.
b. Carbohydrate loading results in increased storage of glycogen in muscles and the liver.
c. Carbohydrate loading is beneficial for most athletes prior to most competitive events.
d. All of the above are true.

LO 4 **6.** The recommended protein intake for active people who are not competitive athletes is

a. the same as for sedentary adults, 0.8 g protein per kg body weight.
b. somewhat higher than for sedentary adults, about 1.0 to 1.2 g protein per kg body weight.
c. about twice the recommended intake for sedentary adults; that is, about 1.6 to 1.8 g protein per kg body weight.
d. two to three times the recommended intake for sedentary adults; that is, about 2.0 to 2.4 g protein per kg body weight.

LO 5 7. Athletes participating in an intense athletic competition lasting more than 1 hour should

a. drink caffeinated beverages to improve their performance while maintaining their hydration.

b. drink plain warm water copiously both before and during the event in response to fluid losses from sweating and the desire to drink.

c. drink plain ice water both before and during the event in response to thirst.

d. drink a beverage containing carbohydrate and electrolytes both before and during the event in amounts that balance hydration with energy, carbohydrate, and electrolyte needs.

LO 6 8. Which of the following ergogenic aids has been shown in research studies to improve athletic performance?

a. androstenedione

b. chromium

c. carnitine

d. caffeine

LO 2 9. **True or false?** A sound fitness program overloads the body.

LO 5 10. **True or false?** Sports anemia is a chronic decrease in iron stores that occurs in some athletes who have been training intensely for several months to years.

math review

LO 4 11. Liz is a dance major. She participates in two 90-minute dance classes each day, 5 days a week, plus does a 60-minute strength-training workout during her lunch break twice a week. She is a vegetarian, and her current energy intake is 1,800 kcal per day. She weighs 105 pounds. After referring to Table 6.2 (page 198) she estimates that her protein intake should be 1.5 grams per kilogram of body weight, and she wants to keep her fat intake relatively low at 20% of her total daily energy intake. Based on this information, calculate how many grams of protein, fat, and carbohydrate Liz needs to consume daily to support this activity program. Does Liz's carbohydrate intake fall within the AMDR, which is 45% to 65% of total energy intake?

Answers to Review Questions and Math Review are located at the back of this text and in the MasteringNutrition Study Area.

web links

www.heart.org
American Heart Association
The "Healthy Living" part of this site has sections on healthy eating, physical activity, weight management, and more.

www.acsm.org
American College of Sports Medicine
Click on "Public Information," then select "Brochures and Fact Sheets" to access brochures on why we eat and reducing sedentary behaviors; select the "Newsletters" section to access the ACSM's Fit Society Page newsletter.

www.hhs.gov
U.S. Department of Health and Human Services
Review this site for multiple statistics on health, exercise, and weight, as well as information on supplements, wellness, and more.

www.win.niddk.nih.gov
Weight-Control Information Network
To find out more about tips to help you get active and how to be active at any size, log onto this site and search the "WIN Health Topics A-Z" to explore these and other activity-related topics.

ods.od.nih.gov
NIH Office of Dietary Supplements
Look on this National Institutes of Health site to learn more about the health effects of specific nutritional supplements.

www.fnic.nal.usda.gov
Food and Nutrition Information Center
Visit this site, searching on "ergogenic aids," and "sports nutrition" for links to detailed information about these topics.

www.adultfitnesstest.org
The President's Challenge Adult Fitness test
Go to this site to determine you are healthy enough to exercise by completing the American Heart Association Physical Activity Readiness Questionnaire, and then complete the test to determine your fitness level.

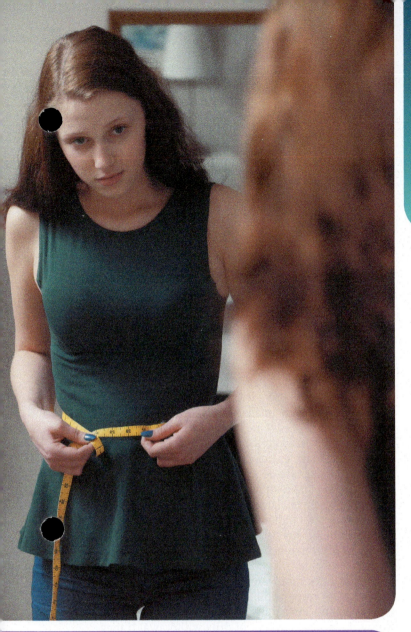

in depth 11.5

Disorders Related to Body Image, Eating, and Exercise

During the last decade, modeling agencies and fashion shows worldwide have increasingly adopted health standards for fashion models, some requiring they meet a certain BMI, and others requiring a doctor's certificate certifying that they are healthy enough to work. At the same time, regulatory groups have been monitoring images printed in magazines and other media. For example, in both 2015 and 2016, the Advertising Standards Authority of Britain denounced advertisements for the fashion brands Yves Saint Laurent and Gucci that showed models who looked emaciated.[1] Both ads were pulled.

Behind these actions are numerous deaths of severely underweight fashion models in recent decades, and longstanding concerns that images glamorizing underweight models promote an unrealistic, even dangerous standard of beauty for girls and women. Is this true? What factors are thought to contribute to body image, eating patterns, and exercise—in both women and men? And how do abnormal eating and exercise behaviors differ from true psychiatric disorders? In the following pages, we explore **In Depth** some answers to these important questions.

learning outcomes

After studying this In Depth, you should be able to:

1 Explain how body image can affect eating and exercise patterns, as well as physical and mental health, pp. 414–416.

2 Identify several factors that contribute to the development of disorders related to body image, eating, and exercise, pp. 416–417.

3 Identify the most common characteristics and health risks of anorexia nervosa, bulimia nervosa, and binge-eating disorder, pp. 417–420.

4 Describe night-eating syndrome and the female athlete triad, pp. 420–422.

5 Discuss treatment for individuals with eating disorders, p. 422–423.

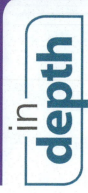

What is body image, and how does it influence health?

LO 1 Explain how body image can affect eating and exercise patterns, as well as physical and mental health.

When you look in the mirror, do you criticize aspects of your appearance—such as your facial features, complexion, body shape, muscle definition, or weight? If you do, you're not alone. Many people experience anxiety about their body image. In a recent national survey, over 25% of college students—including 17% of males and nearly 30% of females—reported that, in the past year, concerns about their personal appearance had been "very difficult to handle" or even "traumatic."[2]

Your **body image** is the way you perceive, feel about, and critique your body. This, in turn, can strongly influence your eating and exercise patterns. A recent study found, for example, that "feeling fat"—not necessarily being overweight according to BMI—increased unhealthful eating behaviors such as skipping meals in both adolescent boys and girls.[3] And another study found an association between feelings of anxiety about being judged by others on one's appearance—known as *social physique anxiety*—and increased risk for engaging in an uncontrollable pattern of excessive exercise.[4] Let's take a closer look at these relationships.

Body Image Influences Eating Behaviors

Body image and eating patterns both occur on a *continuum,* a spectrum that can't be divided neatly into parts. An example is a rainbow—where exactly does the red end and the orange begin? The continuum model can help us understand how a person with a preoccupation with body image can progress from relatively normal eating behaviors to a pattern that is abnormal. For example, in the study just mentioned, the adolescents who "felt fat" typically skipped breakfast, and some also skipped lunch.[3]

Take a moment to study the Eating Issues and Body Image Continuum **(FIGURE 1)**. Which of the five columns best describes your feelings about food and your body? If you find yourself identifying with the statements on the left side of the continuum, you probably have a healthy body image and few issues with food. Most likely you accept your body size and view eating and engaging in regular physical activity as a normal part of maintaining your health. As you progress to the right side of the continuum, where body image is an overriding concern, food restriction and excessive exercise become common. The food restriction can take either of two forms:

- **Disordered eating** is a general term used to describe a variety of atypical eating behaviors that people use

to achieve or maintain a lower body weight. These behaviors may be as simple as going on and off diets or as extreme as refusing to eat any fat. Such behaviors don't usually continue for long enough to make the person seriously ill, nor do they significantly disrupt the person's normal routine.
- An **eating disorder** is a psychiatric condition that involves extreme body dissatisfaction and long-term eating patterns that negatively affect body functioning. Three clinically diagnosed eating disorders are anorexia nervosa, bulimia nervosa, and binge-eating disorder. Whereas anorexia nervosa is characterized by severe food restriction, bulimia nervosa and binge-eating disorder involve extreme overeating. These disorders will be discussed in more detail shortly.

Body Image Influences Exercise Behaviors

Disorders of body image and eating patterns are often associated with excessive exercise, because individuals with a distorted body image related to weight or shape frequently use excessive exercise as a method of purging unwanted Calories from the body.[5] In the research literature, this excessive exercise is sometimes called exercise addiction[6] or exercise dependence.[4]

How does one distinguish between healthful levels of exercise and exercise addiction? Researchers generally agree that an individual who is addicted to exercise will continue to exercise in spite of a physical injury, illness, or personal inconvenience. They will prioritize exercise above other factors in their personal lives, such as relationships, family commitments, academic studies, and work responsibilities. The exercise program also dominates their thinking, and they will experience symptoms similar to those of drug withdrawal if they cannot exercise.[6] Moreover, although exercise is known to help relieve depression and anxiety, individuals who are addicted to exercise are found to have higher levels of depression and anxiety.[7]

Conversely, someone who is committed—but not addicted—to exercise will engage in physical activity for health, enjoyment, and to achieve sport or fitness goals, but they will not suffer withdrawal symptoms when they cannot exercise.[6] These individuals have a sense of "life-balance" around physical activity.

---

body image A person's perception, feelings about, and critique of his or her body's appearance and functioning.

disordered eating A general term used to describe a variety of abnormal or atypical eating behaviors that are used to keep or maintain a lower body weight.

eating disorder A clinically diagnosed psychiatric disorder characterized by severe disturbances in body image and eating behaviors.

FOOD IS NOT AN ISSUE	CONCERNED/WELL	FOOD PREOCCUPIED/ OBSESSED	DISRUPTIVE EATING PATTERNS	EATING DISORDERED
• I am not concerned about what others think regarding what and how much I eat. • When I am upset or depressed I eat whatever I am hungry for without any guilt or shame. • I feel no guilt or shame no matter how much I eat or what I eat. • Food is an important part of my life but only occupies a small part of my time. • I trust my body to tell me what and how much to eat.	• I pay attention to what I eat in order to maintain a healthy body. • I may weigh more than what I like, but I enjoy eating and balance my pleasure with eating with my concern for a healthy body. • I am moderate and flexible in goals for eating well. • I try to follow Dietary Guidelines for healthy eating.	• I think about food a lot. • I feel I don't eat well most of the time. • It's hard for me to enjoy eating with others. • I feel ashamed when I eat more than others or more than what I feel I should be eating. • I am afraid of getting fat. • I wish I could change how much I want to eat and what I am hungry for.	• I have tried diet pills, laxatives, vomiting, or extra time exercising in order to lose or maintain my weight. • I have fasted or avoided eating for long periods of time in order to lose or maintain my weight. • I feel strong when I can restrict how much I eat. • Eating more than I wanted to makes me feel out of control.	• I regularly stuff myself and then exercise, vomit, or use diet pills or laxatives to get rid of the food or Calories. • My friends/family tell me I am too thin. • I am terrified of eating fat. • When I let myself eat, I have a hard time controlling the amount of food I eat. • I am afraid to eat in front of others.

BODY OWNERSHIP	BODY ACCEPTANCE	BODY PREOCCUPIED/ OBSESSED	DISTORTED BODY IMAGE	BODY HATE/ DISASSOCIATION
• Body image is not an issue for me. • My body is beautiful to me. • My feelings about my body are not influenced by society's concept of an ideal body shape. • I know that the significant others in my life will always find me attractive. • I trust my body to find the weight it needs to be at so I can move and feel confident about my physical body.	• I base my body image equally on social norms and my own self-concept. • I pay attention to my body and my appearance because it is important to me, but it only occupies a small part of my day. • I nourish my body so it has the strength and energy to achieve my physical goals. • I am able to assert myself and maintain a healthy body without losing my self-esteem.	• I spend a significant amount time viewing my body in the mirror. • I spend a significant amount of time comparing my body to others. • I have days when I feel fat. • I am preoccupied with my body. • I accept society's ideal body shape and size as the best body shape and size. • I believe that I'd be more attractive if I were thinner, more muscular, etc.	• I spend a significant amount of time exercising and dieting to change my body. • My body shape and size keep me from dating or finding someone who will treat me the way I want to be treated. • I have considered changing or have changed my body shape and size through surgical means so I can accept myself. • I wish I could change the way I look in the mirror.	• I often feel separated and distant from my body—as if it belongs to someone else. • I hate my body and I often isolate myself from others. • I don't see anything positive or even neutral about my body shape and size. • I don't believe others when they tell me I look OK. • I hate the way I look in the mirror.

▲ **FIGURE 1** The Eating Issues and Body Image Continuum. The progression from normal eating (far left) to disordered eating (far right) occurs on a continuum.

Source: Data from Smiley, L., L. King, and H. Avery. University of Arizona Campus Health Service. Original Continuum, C. Shlaalak. Preventive Medicine and Public Health. Copyright © 1997 Arizona Board of Regents.

Body Dysmorphic Disorder Is a Psychiatric Diagnosis

A psychiatric disorder of body image that typically involves disordered eating and excessive exercise is **body dysmorphic disorder (BDD)**. It is estimated to affect as much as 2.4% of the population[8] and is about equally common in males and females.[9] In medicine, a *dysmorphia* is an abnormality of structure; in BDD, the individual obsesses over a perceived defect—real or imaginary—in his or her appearance.

body dysmorphic disorder (BDD) A clinically diagnosed psychiatric disorder characterized by a disabling preoccupation with perceived defects in appearance.

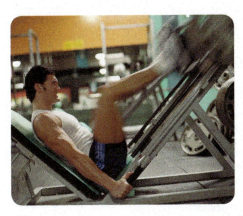

Men are more likely than women to exercise excessively in an effort to control their weight.

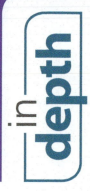

A common form of BDD is *muscle dysmorphia,* a pathological pursuit of increased muscularity that causes individuals—usually men—to engage in highly disordered eating behaviors and excessive exercise, typically strength training. Men with muscle dysmorphia perceive themselves as small and frail even though they may actually be quite large and muscular. As a result, they spend long hours lifting weights and follow a meticulous diet, often consisting of excessive high-protein foods and dietary supplements. They may also abuse anabolic steroids.[9,10]

Muscle dysmorphia shares several characteristics with other body image and eating disorders. For instance, individuals report "feeling fat" and express significant discomfort with the idea of having to expose their body to others (e.g., take off their clothes in the locker room). They also have increased rates of other psychiatric illnesses, including anxiety and depression.[11]

What factors contribute to disorders related to body image, eating, and exercise?

LO 2 Identify several factors that contribute to the development of disorders related to body image, eating, and exercise.

The factors that contribute to the development of body image disorders, excessive exercise, and eating disorders in any particular individual are very complex.

Influence of Genetic Factors

Overall, the diagnosis of BDD and eating disorders is more common in siblings and other blood relatives who also have the diagnosis than in the general population.[12,13] Data derived from studies examining twins estimate that genetic factors account for 43% of the variance in BDD,[12] and 50% to 83% of the variance in eating disorders.[13] These observations might suggest that one or more genes contribute to these disorders; however, it is difficult to separate the contribution of genetic and environmental factors within families.

Think that eating disorders develop only in teenage girls? Or that the individual's mother is always to blame? Guess again. Visit the National Institute of Mental Health at www.nimh.nih.gov and type in the search bar "eating disorders myths" to find a series of short videos busting nine myths about disordered eating.

Influence of Family

Research suggests that the family environment, including high levels of conflict, lack of cohesion, negative communication patterns, inappropriate modeling of attitudes toward weight and shape, poor-quality parent-child relationships, and low family expressiveness can all influence the development and maintenance of an eating disorder.[14] Compared to families without a member with an eating disorder, families of a person with an eating disorder tend to share three traits:[15]

- *Anxiety.* Within families, anxiety can be contagious and can maintain or even exacerbate a pattern of disordered eating. For example, parents may display a high level of anxiety in response to a child's disordered eating behaviors. The child senses this anxiety and responds by intensifying the behavior.
- *Compulsivity.* The families of individuals who develop eating disorders are typically characterized by inflexibility, rigidity, and the need for order. Thus, when the family experiences an unpredictable event, the individual may turn to compulsive behaviors—such as refusing food or obsessively exercising—to adapt.
- *Abnormal eating behavior in one family member.* A pattern of disordered eating may already be present within the family, leading other family members to view this behavior as normal or acceptable.

Influence of Media

Media, including social media, can play an important role in the formation of body image in both males and females, and can create unrealistic expectations for body weight and shape.[9,16,17] Most adults understand that computer-enhanced images of lean, beautiful women and muscular

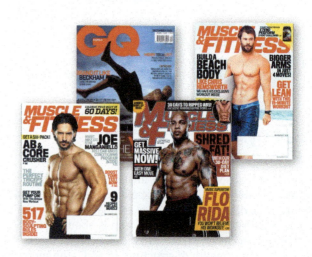

Photos of models and celebrities are routinely airbrushed or altered to "enhance" physical appearance. Unfortunately, many young people believe these portrayals are accurate and, hence, strive to meet unrealistic physical goals.

men are unrealistic, but adolescents, who are still developing a sense of their identity and body image, may lack the same ability to distance themselves from what they see.[18] Because body image influences eating behaviors, it is likely that this barrage of unrealistic media models may contribute to eating disorders.[19,20] However, scientific evidence demonstrating that media *causes* eating disorders does not exist.

Influence of Social and Cultural Values

Eating disorders are significantly more common in white females in Western societies than in other women worldwide.[13] This may be due in part to the white Western culture's association of slenderness with attractiveness, wealth, and high fashion. In contrast, until recently, the prevailing view in developing societies has been that excess body fat is desirable as a sign of health and material abundance.

The members of society with whom we most often interact—our family members, friends, classmates, and coworkers—also influence the way we see ourselves. Their comments related to our appearance can be particularly hurtful—enough so to contribute to BDD[9] or disordered eating.[13] Peer relationships also appear to be highly influential in the development of an eating disorder. Research shows that frequent comparison of one's body to peers can contribute to the developed of body dissatisfaction and disordered eating.[21] For example, a 2011 study from the London School of Economics concluded that anorexia is primarily socially induced. The higher the BMI of one's peers, the lower the risk of developing anorexia.[22]

Comorbidity with Other Psychological Disorders

Individuals with body image or eating disorders often have comorbidity with other psychological disorders such as obsessive-compulsive disorder (OCD).[8,9,23] In one study, over 60% of individuals with BDD were classified as having a lifetime history of anxiety disorder, including OCD.[8] The OCD may manifest, for example, as compulsive checking and counting of foods eaten, Calories, body weight, waist or other measurements, or aspects of their exercise program.[8,9,23]

Eating disorders are also associated with perfectionism, low self-esteem, moodiness, and interpersonal difficulties.[20,24] Individuals with anorexia nervosa may also experience excessive anxiety over unfamiliar or unpredictable situations or events. They have a high need for control; thus, they find it difficult to complete tasks, since nothing is ever quite good enough or done well enough.[25] Conversely, those with bulimia nervosa may demonstrate more impulsivity and respond more negatively or erratically to challenges.[20] These negative moods may trigger overeating.[13,26]

What psychiatric eating disorders are recognized?

LO 3 Identify the most common characteristics and health risks of anorexia nervosa, bulimia nervosa, and binge-eating disorder.

Recall that eating disorders are psychiatric conditions. The clinical manual of the American Psychiatric Association, which is the world's largest psychiatric organization, recognizes three such eating disorders. These are anorexia nervosa, bulimia nervosa, and binge-eating disorder.[24]

All three of these eating disorders occur in males as well as females; however, the signs and symptoms may differ. Females may focus more on the desire to be thin, while males may focus more on muscularity.[27] That is, males may be less concerned with actual body weight (scale weight) and more concerned with body composition (percentage of muscle mass compared to fat mass).[5]

The methods that males and females use to achieve weight loss also appear to differ. Males are more likely to use excessive exercise, whereas females tend to use severe energy restriction, vomiting, and laxative abuse. These differences may stem from sociocultural biases; that is, dieting is considered to be more acceptable for women, whereas the overwhelming sociocultural belief is that eating disorders are "not masculine."[28]

Anorexia Nervosa

Anorexia nervosa is a potentially life-threatening eating disorder that is characterized by an extremely low body weight achieved through self-starvation, which eventually leads to a severe nutrient deficiency. According to the National Eating Disorders Association, 20 million women and 10 million men suffer from a clinically significant eating disorder at some time in their life.[29] Approximately 0.5% to 3.7% of American females develop anorexia, and 20% of these women will die prematurely from complications related to their disorder, including suicide and heart problems.[30] These statistics make anorexia nervosa the most common and most deadly psychiatric disorder diagnosed in women and one of the leading causes of death in females between the ages of 15 and 24.[30] As the statistics indicate, anorexia nervosa also occurs in males, but the prevalence is much lower than it is in females.[27,30]

Signs and Symptoms of Anorexia Nervosa

The classic sign of anorexia nervosa is an extremely restrictive eating pattern that leads to self-starvation. People with this disorder may fast completely, restrict energy intake to only a few kilocalories per day, or eliminate all but one or

---

anorexia nervosa A serious, potentially life-threatening eating disorder that is characterized by self-starvation, which eventually leads to a deficiency in the energy and essential nutrients required by the body to function normally.

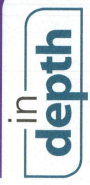

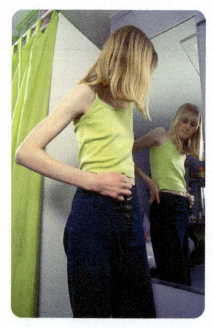

People with anorexia nervosa experience an extreme drive for thinness, resulting in potentially fatal weight loss.

two food groups from their diet. They also have an intense fear of weight gain, and even small amounts (e.g., 1 to 2 pounds) trigger high stress and anxiety.

In females, **amenorrhea** (the condition of having no menstrual periods for at least 3 continuous months) is a common feature of anorexia nervosa. It occurs when a young woman consumes insufficient energy to maintain normal body functions.

The American Psychiatric Association identifies the following conditions of anorexia nervosa.[24,31]

- Refusal to maintain body weight at or above a minimally normal weight for age and height
- Intense fear of gaining weight or becoming fat, even though considered underweight by all medical criteria
- Disturbance in the way in which one's body weight or shape is experienced, undue influence of body weight or shape on self-evaluation, or denial of the seriousness of the current low body weight

Health Risks of Anorexia Nervosa

Left untreated, anorexia nervosa eventually leads to a deficiency in energy and nutrients that are required by the body to function normally **(FIGURE 2)**. The body will then use stored fat and lean tissue (e.g., organ and muscle tissue) as an energy source to maintain brain tissue and vital body functions. The body will also shut down or reduce nonvital body functions to conserve energy. Electrolyte imbalances can lead to heart failure and death. The best chance for recovery is when an individual receives intensive treatment early.

Bulimia Nervosa

Bulimia nervosa is characterized by repeated episodes of binge eating and purging. Unlike individuals with anorexia nervosa, those with bulimia nervosa can be normal weight; however, they either fear gaining weight or are extremely unhappy with their body size and want to lose weight.[30,32] According to the National Institutes of Mental Health (NIMH), the lifetime rate for bulimia nervosa is 0.5% for women and 0.1% for men.[32] Thus, women are at a much higher risk for bulimia nervosa than men.

The following behaviors characterize bulimia nervosa:

- **Binge eating** is usually defined as consumption of a quantity of food that is large for the person and for the amount of time in which it is eaten. For example, a person may eat a dozen brownies with 2 quarts of ice cream in a period of just 30 minutes. While binge eating, the person feels a loss of self-control, including an inability to end the binge once it has started.[24,33] At the same time, the person feels a sense of euphoria not unlike a drug-induced high.
- **Purging** is a compensatory behavior used to prevent weight gain. Methods of purging include vomiting, laxative or diuretic abuse, enemas, fasting, and

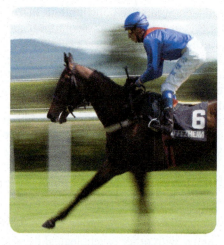

Men who participate in "thin-build" sports, such as jockeys, have a higher risk for bulimia nervosa than men who do not.

amenorrhea The absence of menstruation. In females who had previously been menstruating, it is defined as the absence of menstrual periods for 3 or more continuous months.

bulimia nervosa A serious eating disorder characterized by recurrent episodes of binge eating and recurrent inappropriate compensatory behaviors in order to prevent weight gain, such as self-induced vomiting, fasting, excessive exercise, or misuse of laxatives, diuretics, enemas, or other medications.

binge eating Consumption of a large amount of food in a short period of time, usually accompanied by a feeling of loss of self-control.

purging An attempt to rid the body of unwanted food by vomiting or other compensatory means, such as excessive exercise, fasting, or laxative abuse.

Skin/hair/nails:
- Hair becomes thin, dry, and brittle; hair loss occurs
- Skin is dry, easily bruised, and discolored
- Nails turn brittle

Blood and immune system:
- Anemia
- Compromised immune system increases risk of infection

Kidneys:
- Dehydration
- Electrolyte abnormalities that can be life-threatening
- Chronic renal failure

Reproductive function:
- Disruption of sex hormone production, resulting in menstrual dysfunction and amenorrhea in females
- Infertility

Muscle:
- Loss of muscle tissue as the body uses the muscles as an energy source

Brain:
- Altered levels of serotonin and other neurotransmitters
- Alteration in glucose metabolism
- Mood changes

Thyroid gland:
- Abnormal thyroid levels due to starvation

Heart:
- Low blood pressure and abnormal heart rate contribute to dizziness and fainting
- Abnormal electrocardiogram (ECG)
- Sudden death due to ventricular arrhythmias

Gastrointestinal system:
- Abdominal pain and bloating caused by slowed gastric emptying and intestinal motility
- Acute pancreatitis
- Constipation

Bone:
- Decreased bone mineral density (osteopenia)
- Decreased ability to absorb calcium due to low estrogen levels
- Decreased intake of bone-building nutrients due to starvation
- Increased loss of bone due to elevated cortisol levels

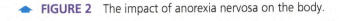

FIGURE 2 The impact of anorexia nervosa on the body.

excessive exercise. For example, after a binge, a runner may increase her daily mileage to equal the "calculated" energy content of the binge.

Signs and Symptoms of Bulimia Nervosa

The American Psychiatric Association has identified the following criteria for diagnosis of bulimia nervosa:[31]

- Recurrent episodes of binge eating (e.g., eating a large amount of food in a short period, such as within 2 hours).
- Recurrent inappropriate compensatory behavior in order to prevent weight gain, such as self-induced vomiting; misuse of laxatives, diuretics, enemas, or other medications; fasting; or excessive exercise.
- Binge eating occurs on average at least twice a week for 3 months.
- Body shape and weight unduly influence self-evaluation.

- The disturbance does not occur exclusively during episodes of anorexia nervosa. Some individuals will have periods of binge eating and then periods of starvation, which makes classification of their disorder difficult.

Moreover, an individual with bulimia nervosa typically purges after most episodes but not necessarily on every occasion. Weight gain as a result of binge eating can therefore be significant.

How can you tell if someone has bulimia nervosa? In addition to the recurrent and frequent binge-eating and purging episodes, the National Institutes of Health have identified the following signs and symptoms:[34]

- Chronically inflamed and sore throat
- Swollen glands in the neck and below the jaw
- Worn tooth enamel and increasingly sensitive and decaying teeth as a result of exposure to stomach acids

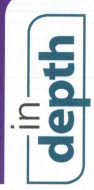
- Gastroesophageal reflux disorder
- Intestinal distress and irritation from laxative abuse
- Kidney problems from diuretic abuse
- Severe dehydration from purging of fluids

Health Risks of Bulimia Nervosa

The destructive behaviors of bulimia nervosa can lead to illness and even death. The most common health consequences associated with bulimia nervosa are:

- *Electrolyte imbalance*: typically caused by dehydration and the loss of potassium and sodium from the body with frequent vomiting. This can lead to irregular heartbeat and even heart failure and death.
- *Gastrointestinal problems*: inflammation, ulceration, and possible rupture of the esophagus and stomach from frequent bingeing and vomiting. Chronic irregular bowel movements and constipation may result in people with bulimia who chronically abuse laxatives.
- *Dental problems*: tooth decay and staining from stomach acids released during frequent vomiting

As with anorexia nervosa, the chance of recovery from bulimia nervosa increases, and the negative effects on health decrease, if the disorder is detected at an early stage. Familiarity with the warning signs of bulimia nervosa can help you identify friends and family members who might be at risk.

Binge-Eating Disorder

When was the last time a friend or relative confessed to you about "going on an eating binge"? Most likely, he or she explained that the behavior followed some sort of stressful event, such as a problem at work, the breakup of a relationship, or a poor grade on an exam. Many people have one or two binge episodes every year or so, in response to stress. But in people with **binge-eating disorder**, the behavior occurs frequently. Because it is not usually followed by purging, the person tends to gain a lot of weight. This lack of compensation for the binge distinguishes binge-eating disorder from bulimia nervosa.

The prevalence of binge-eating disorder is estimated to be 3% to 5% of the adult female and 2% of the adult male population, most of whom are overweight or obese.[30] Our current food environment, which offers an abundance of good-tasting, cheap food any time of the day, makes it difficult for people with binge-eating disorder to avoid food triggers.

Again, the increased energy intake associated with binge eating significantly increases a person's risk of being overweight or obese. In addition, the types of foods typically consumed during a binge episode are high in fat and sugar, which can increase blood lipids. Finally, the stress associated with binge eating can have psychological consequences, such as low self-esteem, avoidance of social contact, depression, and negative thoughts related to body size.

What syndromes of disordered eating are recognized?

LO 4 Describe night-eating syndrome and the female athlete triad.

A *syndrome* is a type of disorder characterized by the presence of two or more distinct health problems that tend to occur together. Two syndromes involving disordered eating behaviors are night-eating syndrome and the female athlete triad.

Night-Eating Syndrome

Night-eating syndrome was first described in a group of patients who were not hungry in the morning but spent the evening and night eating and reported insomnia. Like binge-eating disorder, it is associated with obesity because, although night eaters don't binge, they do consume significant energy in their frequent snacks, and they don't compensate for the excess energy intake.

The distinguishing characteristic of night-eating syndrome is the time during which most of the day's energy intake occurs. Night eaters have a daily pattern of significantly increasing their energy intake in the evening and/or at nighttime and not being hungry at breakfast time. Thus, night-eating syndrome is diagnosed by one or both of the following criteria.[35]

- Eating at least 25% of daily food intake after the evening meal
- Experiencing at least two episodes per week of night eating; that is, getting up to eat after going to bed

Night eating is also characterized by a depressed mood and insomnia.[36] In short, this syndrome combines three unique disorders: an eating disorder, a sleep disorder, and

binge-eating disorder A disorder characterized by binge eating an average of twice a week or more, typically without compensatory purging.

night-eating syndrome Disorder characterized by intake of the majority of the day's energy between 8:00 PM and 6:00 AM. Individuals with this disorder also experience mood and sleep disorders.

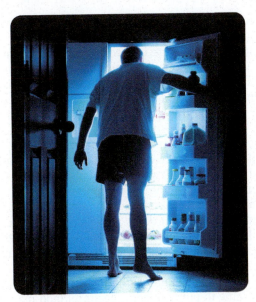

People with night-eating syndrome consume most of their daily energy between 8 PM and 6 AM.

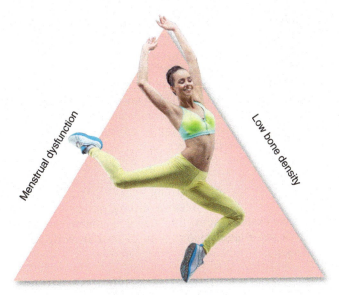

Low energy availability

FIGURE 3 The female athlete triad is a syndrome composed of three coexisting disorders: low energy availability (with or without eating disorders), menstrual dysfunction (such as amenorrhea), and low bone density (such as osteoporosis). Energy availability is defined as dietary energy intake minus exercise energy expenditure.

a mood disorder.[36] Many night eaters are obese, and many experience anxiety or engage in substance abuse. Some engage in other disordered eating behaviors.

Night-eating syndrome is important clinically because of its association with obesity, which increases the risk for several chronic diseases, including heart disease, high blood pressure, stroke, type 2 diabetes, and arthritis. Obesity also increases the risk for sleep apnea, which can further disrupt the night eater's already abnormal sleeping pattern.

The Female Athlete Triad

The **female athlete triad** is part of a larger syndrome called *relative energy deficiency in sport* (*RED-S*), which encompasses numerous health problems associated with inadequate energy consumption to meet the energy needs of active men and women. These health-related issues can impair many aspects of physiological functioning, including BMR, immunity, protein synthesis, and bone, reproductive, and cardiovascular health.[37]

The female athlete triad itself consists of the following three clinical conditions in physically active females (FIGURE 3):[38]

- Low energy availability (such as inadequate energy intake to maintain menstrual function or to cover energy expended in exercise) with or without eating disorders
- Menstrual dysfunction, such as amenorrhea
- Low bone density

Certain sports that strongly emphasize leanness or a thin body build may place a young girl or a woman at risk for the female athlete triad. These sports typically include figure skating, gymnastics, and diving; classical ballet dancers are also at increased risk for the disorder.

Active women experience the general social and cultural demands placed on women to be thin, as well as pressure from their coach, teammates, judges, and/or spectators to meet weight standards or body-size expectations for their sport. Failure to meet these standards can result in severe consequences, such as being cut from the team or losing an athletic scholarship.

As the pressure to be thin mounts, active women may restrict their energy intake, typically by engaging in disordered eating behaviors. Energy restriction combined with high levels of physical activity can disrupt the menstrual cycle and result in amenorrhea. Menstrual dysfunction can also occur in active women who are not dieting and don't have an eating disorder. These women are just not eating enough to cover the energy costs of their exercise training and all the other energy demands of the body and daily living. Female athletes with menstrual dysfunction, regardless of the cause, typically have reduced levels of the reproductive hormones estrogen and progesterone. When estrogen levels in the body

---

female athlete triad A syndrome that consists of three clinical conditions in some physically active females: low energy availability (with or without eating disorders), menstrual dysfunction, and low bone density.

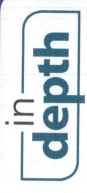

are low, it is difficult for bone to retain calcium, and gradual loss of bone mass occurs. Thus, many female athletes develop premature bone loss (osteoporosis) and are at increased risk for fractures.

Recognition of an athlete with one or more of the components of the female athlete triad can be difficult, especially if the athlete is reluctant to be honest when questioned about her eating behaviors and symptoms. For this reason, familiarity with the early warning signs is critical. These include excessive dieting and/or weight loss, excessive exercise, stress fractures, and comments suggesting that self-esteem appears to be dictated by body weight and shape.

nutri-case | LIZ

"I used to dance with a really cool modern company, where everybody looked sort of healthy and 'real.' No waifs! When they folded after Christmas, I was really bummed, but this spring, I'm planning to audition for the City Ballet. My best friend dances with them, and she told me that they won't even look at anybody over 100 pounds. So I've just put myself on a strict diet. Most days, I come in under 1,200 Calories, though some days I cheat and then I feel so out of control. Last week, my dance teacher stopped me after class and asked me whether or not I was menstruating. I thought that was a pretty weird question, so I just said sure, but then when I thought about it, I realized that I've been so focused and stressed out lately that I really don't know! The audition is only a week away, so I'm going on a juice fast this weekend. I've just got to make it into the City Ballet!"

What factors increase Liz's risk for the female athlete triad? What, if anything, do you think Liz's dance teacher should do? Is intervention even necessary, since the audition is only a week away?

How are eating disorders treated?

LO 5 Discuss treatment for individuals with eating disorders.

As with any health problem, prevention is best: People with concerns about their body image and body weight need help before the issues develop into something more serious.

Patients who are severely underweight, display signs of malnutrition, are medically unstable, or are suicidal may require immediate hospitalization. The goals of nutritional therapies are to restore the individual to a healthy body weight and normal eating patterns, teach the individual to identify hunger and satiety cues, and resolve the nutrition-related health issues.[39] For stable hospitalized patients, the expected weight gain ranges from 2 to 3 pounds per week. For outpatient settings, the expected weight gain is much lower (0.5 to 1 pound/week).

Nutrition counseling is an important aspect of inpatient treatment, especially to deal with the body image issues that occur as weight is regained. Once the patient reaches an acceptable body weight, nutrition counseling will address issues such as the acceptability of certain foods; dealing with food situations, such as family gatherings and eating out; and learning to put together a healthful food plan for weight maintenance.

Patients with an eating disorder who are underweight but medically stable, normal weight, or overweight may be able to enter an outpatient program designed to meet their specific needs. Some outpatient programs are extremely intensive, requiring patients to come in each day for treatment. Others are less rigorous, requiring only weekly visits for nutrition counseling to identify and manage events and feelings that trigger food restriction, binge eating, or purging. Another goal is to establish structured eating behaviors that can enable the patient to maintain a healthful body weight. In addition, nutrition counseling will address factors specific to the individual, such as negative feelings about foods or fears associated with uncontrolled binge eating.

If you're concerned about a friend's eating behaviors, raising the subject can be difficult. Before you do, learn as much as you can about eating disorders. Make sure you know the difference between the facts and myths. Locate a health professional specializing in eating disorders to whom you can refer your friend, and be ready to go with your friend if he or she does not want to go alone. If you are at a university or college, check with your campus health center to see if it has an eating disorder specialist or team or can recommend someone to you.

When it's time to talk, what exactly should you say? The **Quick Tips** on the next page are sensible steps you can take when discussing disordered eating with a friend.

QuickTips

Talking with a Loved One About Disordered Eating

✔ **Set aside a time and place to talk.** Find a private place where you can share your concerns openly and honestly in a caring and supportive way without distractions. Allow enough time—after classes or on the weekend is best.

✔ **Share your observations.** Mention specific times when you felt concerned about your friend's behaviors related to body image, eating, purging, or excessive exercise. Tell your friend that you're mentioning these things because you believe they might indicate that he or she needs professional help.

✔ **Avoid accusing and oversimplifying.** Do not accuse the person of poor behavior or offer simplistic solutions such as, "You just need to eat more." Instead, focus on communicating what you've observed and how it makes you feel. For example, "When you only eat an apple for lunch, I worry about your health."

✔ **Ask your friend to consult the health care professional you've identified as knowledgeable about eating issues.** If you wish, offer to help your friend make an appointment. You could even offer to go with your friend to the appointment.

✔ **Avoid arguments.** If your friend doesn't agree that there is any reason for concern, try repeating your key points, but don't insist on being right.

✔ **Assure your friend that you care.** Say that you're available to listen if he or she would like to talk about it in future.

✔ **Consider your own needs.** Especially if your friend declines your help, consider meeting with a health care professional to share your concerns and get some support.

Source: Adapted from National Eating Disorders Association (NEDA). (2016, September). What Should I Say? www.nationaleatingdisorders.org

web links

www.bddfoundation.org
Body Dysmorphic Disorder Foundation

Visit this site to find information, assessment tools, and support.

www.nimh.nih.gov
National Institute of Mental Health (NIMH) Office of Communications and Public Liaison

Search this site for "disordered eating" or "eating disorders" to find numerous articles on the subject.

www.anad.org
National Association of Anorexia Nervosa and Associated Disorders

Visit this site for information and resources about eating disorders.

www.nationaleatingdisorders.org
National Eating Disorders Association

This site is dedicated to expanding public understanding of eating disorders and promoting access to treatment for those affected and support for their families.

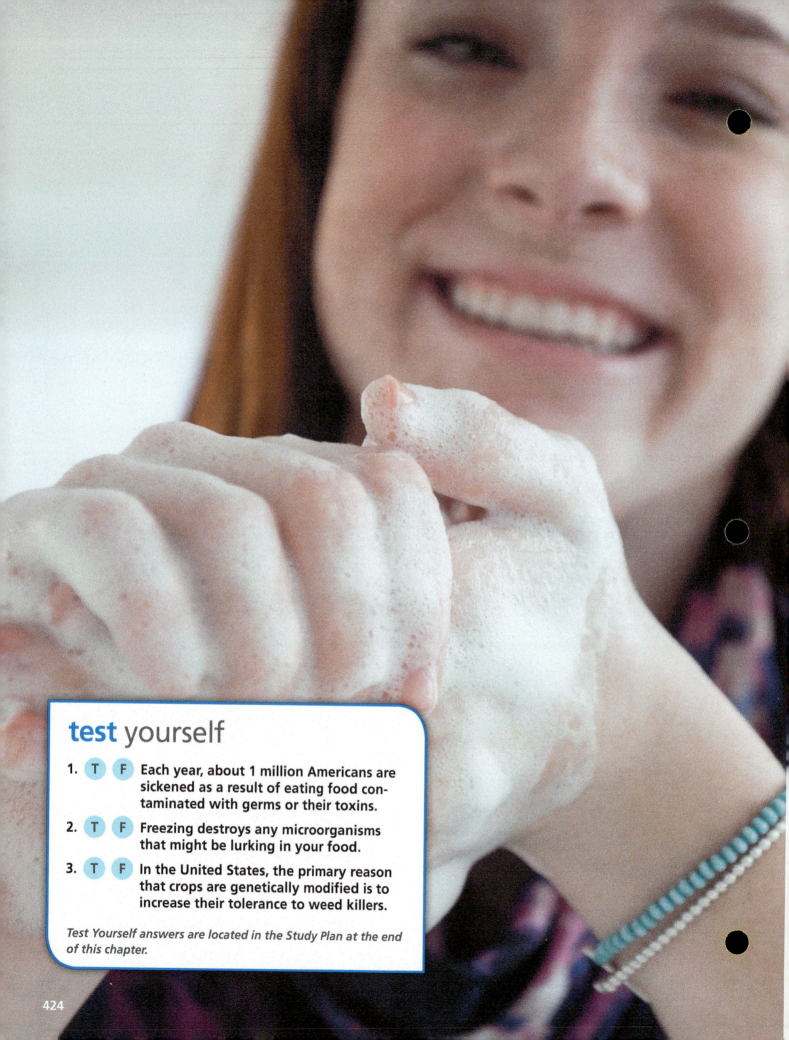

test yourself

1. **T** **F** Each year, about 1 million Americans are sickened as a result of eating food contaminated with germs or their toxins.

2. **T** **F** Freezing destroys any microorganisms that might be lurking in your food.

3. **T** **F** In the United States, the primary reason that crops are genetically modified is to increase their tolerance to weed killers.

Test Yourself answers are located in the Study Plan at the end of this chapter.

12

Food Safety and Technology
Protecting our food

MasteringNutrition™
Go online for chapter quizzes, pre-tests, interactive activities, and more!

In 2015, at least 600 people across the United States became seriously ill and dozens had to be hospitalized after eating at a Chipotle's restaurant. In the weeks following the outbreaks, many food-safety failures were identified, including failing to maintain foods at the proper temperatures to discourage the growth of microbes, and failing to send employees home when they were sick. But astonishingly for a national restaurant chain that promised its customers "food with integrity," some Chipotle's managers also failed to insist on the most fundamental step in food safety: handwashing. Although alarms in the restaurants went off hourly to remind workers to wash their hands, the alarms were routinely ignored. Late in 2015, Chipotle's began implementing a massive new food-safety program. One of its initiatives? Managers must ensure that all employees wash their hands for at least 20 seconds, followed by using a hand sanitizer, at least once an hour.

In the food-illness outbreaks linked to Chipotle's, three different pathogenic (disease-causing) microorganisms (microscopic organisms) were involved: norovirus, which spread from workers to foods, surfaces, and customers; *E. coli*, a bacterium that may have colonized undercooked meats; and *Salmonella*, a bacterium that contaminated fresh produce. These are just 3 of the 31 microorganisms known to cause foodborne illness.[1]

How do pathogenic microorganisms enter foods and beverages, and how can we protect ourselves from them? What makes foods spoil, and what techniques help keep foods fresh longer? And do technologies like genetic modification or the use of pesticides also pose a risk? We explore these and other questions in this chapter.

LO 1 Explain what foodborne illness is and why it is of concern.

What is foodborne illness and why is it a critical concern?

Foodborne illness is a term used to encompass any symptom or disorder that arises from ingesting food or water contaminated with pathogenic microorganisms, their toxic secretions, or pollutants like mercury and other industrial chemicals. It is commonly referred to as *food poisoning*.

Ingestion of Contaminants Prompts Acute Illness

The human immune system has evolved to handle most cases of foodborne illness effectively. Many foodborne contaminants are killed in the mouth by first-line defenses such as antimicrobial enzymes in saliva or hydrochloric acid in the stomach. Any that survive these chemical assaults usually trigger acute vomiting and/or diarrhea as the gastrointestinal tract attempts to expel them. Simultaneously, a defensive response by the white blood cells of the immune system causes nausea, fatigue, fever, and muscle aches.

The U.S. Centers for Disease Control and Prevention (CDC) estimates that, each year, about 48 million Americans—one in six—experience symptoms of foodborne illness.[1] Most cases resolve within hours or days as vomiting and diarrhea rid the body of the offending agent and the immune response ends. However, depending on the status of one's health, the pathogen involved, and the "dose" ingested, symptoms can be severe. Each year, an estimated 128,000 Americans are hospitalized with foodborne illness, and 3,000 die.[1] At highest risk for hospitalization or death are people with reduced immunity, including:

- Developing fetuses, infants, and young children, as their immune system is immature.
- People with compromised immunity, including pregnant women, the very old, the very ill, and people with acquired immunodeficiency syndrome (AIDS).
- People who are receiving immune system–suppressing drugs, such as transplant recipients and cancer patients.

Reducing Foodborne Illness Is a Challenge

Foodborne illness has emerged as a major public health threat in recent years. A key reason is that federal oversight of food safety reflects at least 30 different laws administered among 15 different agencies.[2] One of the most important of these is the CDC, mentioned earlier, which monitors reports from state public health agencies for indications of outbreaks of foodborne illness and assists in investigating and controlling such outbreaks.

The two agencies primarily responsible for preventing foodborne illness are the Food Safety and Inspection Service (FSIS) of the United States Department of Agriculture (USDA) and the Food and Drug Administration (FDA). These agencies require certain food producers to follow a multistep protocol called the Hazard Analysis Critical Control Point (HACCP) system to identify biological, chemical, and other potential food-safety hazards and to control these hazards at each step from cultivation through processing to distribution and sales.[3] Initially developed for NASA to prevent contamination of food sent on space flights, the HACCP is mandatory for producers of certain high-risk foods such as meats, fish, and juices, and encouraged for use by producers of other foods as well as by restaurants and other food retailers.

The Environmental Protection Agency (EPA) also plays a role in food safety by regulating the use of pesticides, water quality, and other environmental concerns. The roles of these agencies are identified in TABLE 12.1.

In 2009, President Barack Obama announced the creation of an interagency Food Safety Working Group to coordinate the food-safety efforts of these and other federal agencies; however, the group met for only two years. In 2015, the president proposed

foodborne illness An illness transmitted by food or water contaminated by a pathogenic microorganism, its toxic secretions, or a toxic chemical.

TABLE 12.1 Government Agencies That Regulate Food Safety

Name of Agency	Year Founded	Role in Food Regulations	Website
U.S. Department of Agriculture (USDA) Food Safety and Inspection Service (FSIS)	1785	Oversees safety of meat, poultry, and processed egg products; also ensures accuracy of meat and poultry labeling	www.fsis.usda.gov
U.S. Food and Drug Administration (FDA)	1862	Regulates food standards of food products (except meat, poultry, and eggs) and bottled water; regulates food labeling and enforces pesticide use as established by EPA	www.fda.gov
Centers for Disease Control and Prevention (CDC)	1946	Works with public health officials to promote and educate the public about health and safety; is able to track information needed in identifying foodborne illness outbreaks	www.cdc.gov
U.S. Environmental Protection Agency (EPA)	1970	Regulates use of pesticides and which crops they can be applied to; establishes standards for water quality	www.epa.gov

consolidating food-safety responsibilities into a new agency, but as of 2016, this consolidation has not yet been achieved.[2]

In January 2011, the U.S. Congress passed into law a new food-safety bill, the Food Safety Modernization Act. This bill provided for increased federal inspections of food-production facilities, new regulations to prevent contamination of foods, and more robust enforcement tools. It may be too soon to judge the effectiveness of these provisions; however, the most recent food-safety progress report from the CDC shows no change or an increase in foodborne illness incidents involving four of six major pathogens, and modest progress (22–32% decline) in incidents involving the remaining two.[4]

The CDC reports that contaminated seafood, chicken, and dairy are responsible for the greatest percentage of foodborne illness outbreaks.[5] However, beef, pork, fresh fruits and vegetables, and even nuts and seeds are also commonly involved. Raw vegetables are a common source of illness: in 2016, 15 people in eight states were hospitalized and 1 died after consuming a packaged fresh salad mix contaminated with a bacterium called *Listeria monocytogenes*. Many mixed foods can be unsafe, especially when they include a combination of ingredients from a variety of fields, feedlots, and processing facilities. These various sources can remain hidden not only to consumers, but even to the food companies using the ingredients. Contamination can occur at any point from farm to table **(FIGURE 12.1)** (page 428), and thus is often difficult to trace.

Among outbreaks associated with a single known setting, restaurants are implicated in about 60% of cases, another 14% involve caterers or banquet facilities, and about 12% occur in homes.[5] Later in this chapter we'll explore ways to reduce your risks.

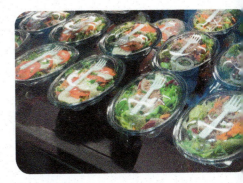

◀ Mixed foods can become contaminated with microbial pathogens at any point from the farm to the packaging center.

recap Foodborne illness arises from the ingestion of food or water contaminated with pathogenic microorganisms, their toxins, or environmental pollutants. It affects 48 million Americans a year, but because the human immune system has evolved effective defenses against it, most cases resolve quickly. Still, each year, about 128,000 Americans require hospitalization for foodborne illness, and about 3,000 die. Contamination can occur at any point from farm to table. Responsibilities for maintaining a safe food supply are currently shared among 15 different federal agencies. The Hazard Analysis Critical Control Point (HACCP) system is required by the FDA and USDA to identify potential food-safety hazards and the critical control points at which these hazards can be prevented. The Food Safety Modernization Act of 2011 increased the inspection and regulation of food production facilities; however, the most recent progress report from the CDC shows either no reduction or an increase in foodborne illness from four of six major pathogens tracked.

▶ **FIGURE 12.1** Food is at risk for contamination at any of the five stages from farm to table, but following food-safety guidelines can reduce the risks.

Farms

Animals raised for meat can harbor harmful microorganisms, and crops can be contaminated with pollutants from irrigation, runoff from streams, microorganisms or toxins in soil, or pesticides. Contamination can also occur during animal slaughter or from harvesting, sorting, washing, packing, and/or storage of crops.

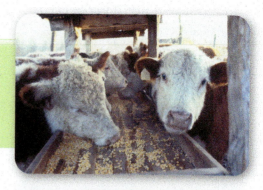

Processing

Some foods, such as produce, may go from the farm directly to the market, but most foods are processed. Processed foods may go through several steps at different facilities. At each site, people, equipment, or environments may contaminate foods. Federal safeguards, such as cleaning protocols, testing, and training, can help prevent contamination.

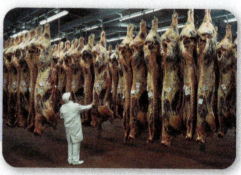

Transportation

Foods must be transported in clean, refrigerated vehicles and containers to prevent multiplication of microorganisms and microbial toxins.

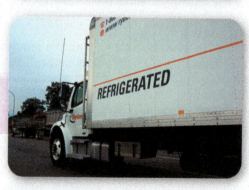

Retail

Employees of food markets and restaurants may contaminate food during storage, preparation, or service. Conditions such as inadequate refrigeration or heating may promote multiplication of microorganisms or microbial toxins. Establishments must follow FDA guidelines for food safety and pass local health inspections.

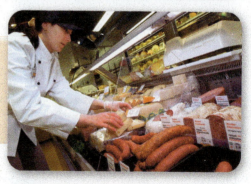

Table

Consumers may contaminate foods with unclean hands, utensils, or surfaces. They can allow the multiplication of microorganisms and microbial toxins by failing to follow the food-safety guidelines for storing, preparing, cooking, and serving foods discussed in this chapter.

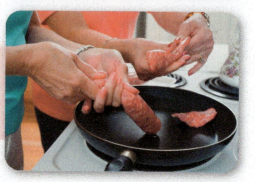

What causes most foodborne illness?

The consumption of food containing pathogenic microorganisms—those capable of causing disease—results in food infections. In contrast, food intoxications result from consuming food in which microorganisms have secreted harmful substances called **toxins**. Naturally occurring plant and marine toxins also contaminate food. Finally, chemical residues in foods, such as heavy metals, pesticides, and packaging residues, can cause illness. Residues are discussed later in this chapter.

Several Types of Microorganisms Contaminate Foods

The microorganisms that most commonly cause food infections are viruses and bacteria.

Viruses Involved in Foodborne Illness

Viruses are extremely tiny noncellular agents that can survive only by infecting living cells. Just one type, norovirus, causes an average of 19 to 21 million infections, well over 50,000 hospitalizations, and up to 800 deaths annually in the United States.[6] In fact, norovirus is behind more than half of all cases of foodborne illness in the United States (**FIGURE 12.2**).[1]

Norovirus is so common and contagious that many people refer to it simply as "the stomach flu"; however, it is not a strain of influenza. Symptoms of infection typically come on suddenly and include stomach cramps as well as both vomiting and diarrhea. Because the vomiting begins abruptly, the person is likely to be in a social setting. Because it is forceful, anyone nearby is likely to become contaminated. Another characteristic that makes norovirus so contagious is that, whereas most viruses perish quickly in a dry environment, norovirus is able to survive on dry surfaces and objects, from countertops to utensils, for days or even weeks. Also, ingestion of even a few "particles" of norovirus can result in full-blown illness.[6]

Healthcare facilities, cruise ships, restaurants, catered events, and college campuses commonly report outbreaks. The best way to prevent the spread of norovirus is to wash your hands, kitchen surfaces, and utensils with warm, soapy water. Alcohol-based hand sanitizers may be used in addition to handwashing, but not as a substitute.[6] If you experience vomiting or diarrhea, immediately clean and disinfect all nearby surfaces and remove and wash laundry thoroughly.

Whereas norovirus infects millions of Americans annually, hepatitis A virus (HAV) infects about 3,500.[7] Like norovirus, HAV can be transmitted person-to-person or via contaminated food and water. The term *hepatitis* means inflammation of the liver. This causes jaundice (a yellowish skin tone), a common sign of HAV infection.[7] Typically, the symptoms of HAV infection include a mild fever, abdominal pain, and nausea and vomiting that lasts a few weeks. Rarely, in elderly patients and those with preexisting liver disease, HAV infection can lead to liver failure and even death.

Bacteria Involved in Foodborne Illness

In contrast to viruses, **bacteria** are cellular microorganisms and are able to reproduce independently, either by dividing in two or by forming reproductive spores. Whereas our resident GI flora contribute to our health and functioning, pathogenic bacteria can cause mild to severe disease.

Foodborne bacterial illness commonly occurs when we ingest pathogenic bacteria living in or on undercooked or raw foods or fluids. These bacteria, which often come from human or animal feces, can damage our cells and tissues either directly or by secreting a destructive toxin. The species of bacteria causing the most illness, hospitalization, and/or death are identified in **TABLE 12.2**. Of these, *Salmonella* is the bacterium responsible for the greatest number of illnesses—nearly 2,600 in 2014. Moreover, of all pathogens, including norovirus, *Salmonella* causes the greatest number of hospitalizations and deaths (**FIGURE 12.3**) (page 430).[1,8]

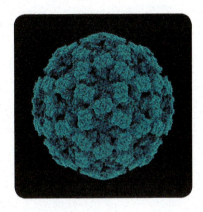

▲ **FIGURE 12.2** Norovirus is responsible for more than half of all cases of foodborne illness in the United States. Infection typically produces a mild illness; however, because it affects so many people, it is the fourth leading cause of foodborne deaths.

To learn more about norovirus infection and how to protect yourself, watch a short video from the CDC at www.cdc.gov/norovirus/.

toxin Any harmful substance; in microbiology, a harmful chemical secretion of a microorganism.

viruses A group of infectious agents that are much smaller than bacteria, lack independent metabolism, and are incapable of growth or reproduction outside of living cells.

bacteria Cellular microorganisms that lack a true nucleus and reproduce by cell division or by spore formation.

TABLE 12.2 Key Bacteria of Concern in Foodborne Illnesses and Deaths

Bacteria	Incubation Period	Duration	Symptoms	Foods Most Commonly Affected	Steps for Prevention
Campylobacter (several species)	1–7 days	2–10 days	Headache Diarrhea Nausea Abdominal cramps	Raw and undercooked meat, poultry, eggs Cake icing Untreated water Unpasteurized milk	Only drink pasteurized milk. Cook foods properly. Avoid cross-contamination.
Clostridium perfringens	8–22 hours	24 hours	Abdominal cramps Diarrhea Dehydration	Beef Poultry Gravies Leftovers	Cook foods thoroughly and serve hot. Refrigerate leftovers promptly. Reheat leftovers thoroughly before serving.
Escherichia coli (some strains produce an enterotoxin)	1–10 days	5–7 days	Abdominal cramps Diarrhea (often bloody) Vomiting	Water; unpasteurized milk, cheese, juice, or cider; undercooked meat; raw produce	Cook foods thoroughly. Avoid cross-contamination. Only drink pasteurized milk and juice. Practice proper handwashing and sanitizing.
Listeria monocytogenes	1–42 days	Days to weeks	Fever Muscle aches Diarrhea Sometimes headache and confusion	Meats, especially hot dogs and deli meats Vegetables Dairy products, especially raw milk and soft cheeses Smoked fish	Cook foods thoroughly and serve hot. Wash produce carefully. If pregnant, do not consume deli meats, smoked fish, or products containing raw milk.
Salmonella (more than 2,300 types)	12–24 hours	4–7 days	Nausea Diarrhea Abdominal pain Chills Fever Headache	Raw or undercooked eggs, poultry, and meat Raw milk and dairy products Seafood Fruits and vegetables	Cook foods thoroughly. Avoid cross-contamination. Only drink pasteurized milk. Practice proper handwashing and sanitizing.
Staphylococcus aureus (which produces an enterotoxin)	1–6 hours	1–2 days	Sudden, severe nausea and vomiting Abdominal cramps Diarrhea may occur	Custard- or cream-filled baked goods Ham Poultry Dressings, sauces, and gravies Eggs Potato salad	Refrigerate foods. Practice proper handwashing and sanitizing.

Sources: Data from Iowa State University Extension, Food Safety. 2015. *What Are the Most Common Foodborne Pathogens?* http://www.extension.iastate.edu/foodsafety/L1.7; U.S. Food and Drug Administration, Foodborne Illnesses: What You Need to Know, 2015, January 29. http://www.fda.gov/Food/FoodborneIllnessContaminants/FoodborneIllnessesNeedToKnow/default.htm; and U.S. Centers for Disease Control and Prevention, Foodborne Outbreak Online Database (FOOD Tool): 1998–2014. 2015, October 8. http://wwwn.cdc.gov/foodborneoutbreaks.

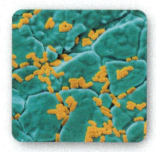

← **FIGURE 12.3** *Salmonella* is the second leading cause of foodborne illness, after norovirus, and the primary cause of foodborne infections requiring hospitalization or resulting in death. Infection can cause fever, diarrhea, and abdominal cramps, and cells of some strains can perforate the intestines and invade the blood.

Listeria monocytogenes, mentioned earlier, causes far fewer illnesses than *Salmonella*—just 55 in 2014. However, *Listeria* infections tend to be more severe. In 2014, over 90% of infections required hospitalization, and nearly 24% resulted in death.[8] Infection is particularly severe in older adults and pregnant women. These populations are advised to avoid soft cheeses or other foods or beverages made with unpasteurized milk, hot dogs and deli meats unless served steaming hot, and refrigerated smoked seafood, because these foods are more likely to harbor *Listeria*. They should also wash their hands, kitchen surfaces, and foods thoroughly as described shortly.

Other Microorganisms Involved in Foodborne Illness

Parasites are microorganisms that simultaneously derive benefit from and harm their host. They are responsible for only about 2% of foodborne illnesses. The most common culprits are helminths and protozoa:

■ **Helminths** are multicellular worms, such as tapeworms **(FIGURE 12.4)**, flukes, and roundworms. They reproduce by releasing their eggs into vegetation or water. When animals consume the contaminated matter, the eggs hatch inside their host. Larvae develop in the host's tissue, where they can survive long after the animal is killed for food. People who eat the food either raw or undercooked consume the larvae, which then mature into adult worms in their small intestine. Some worms cause mild symptoms, such as nausea and diarrhea, whereas others can cause intestinal obstruction or even death. Thoroughly cooking beef, pork, or fish destroys the larvae.

- **Protozoa** are single-celled organisms. One of these, *Toxoplasma gondii*, is one of the top five pathogens responsible for hospitalizations and deaths due to foodborne illness.[1] People typically become infected by eating undercooked, contaminated meat, or by ingesting minute amounts after handling raw meat and then failing to wash their hands.[9] Another protozoan parasite common worldwide is *Giardia*, which lives in the intestines of infected animals and humans and is passed into the environment from their stools. People typically consume *Giardia* by swallowing contaminated water (in lakes, rivers, and so on) or by eating contaminated food. A week or more following ingestion, the person experiences a diarrheal illness, which usually resolves within 2 to 6 weeks.[10]

Fungi are plantlike, spore-forming organisms that can grow as either single cells or multicellular colonies. Three common types are yeasts, which are globular; molds, which are long and thin; and the familiar mushrooms. Very few species of fungi cause serious disease in people with healthy immune systems, and those that do cause disease in humans are not typically foodborne. In addition, unlike bacterial growth, which is invisible and often tasteless, fungal growth typically makes food look and taste so unappealing that we immediately discard it **(FIGURE 12.5)**.

A rare but fatal neurological disease called *variant Creutzfeldt–Jakob disease* (*vCJD*) can occur in people who consume beef or other meat contaminated by **prions**, animal proteins that misfold and become infectious. Over many years, prions destroy normal proteins until the loss of functional nerve tissue progresses to cause neurological disease and eventually death. More than 200 people have died from vCJD, the great majority in Europe before new standards were adopted for animal feeding and surveillance. In the United States, three people have died from vCJD.[11]

Some Foodborne Illness Is Due to Toxins

The microorganisms just discussed cause illness by directly infecting and destroying body cells. In contrast, other bacteria and fungi secrete toxins that bind to body cells and cause a variety of symptoms. Toxins can be categorized according to the type of cell they bind to; neurotoxins damage the nervous system and can cause paralysis, and enterotoxins target the gastrointestinal system and generally cause severe diarrhea and vomiting.

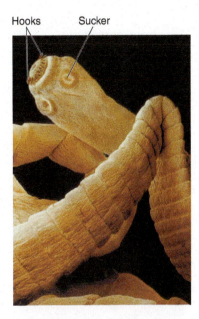

Hooks   Sucker

◆ **FIGURE 12.4** Tapeworms have long bodies with hooks and suckers, which they use to attach to a host's tissue.

parasite A microorganism that simultaneously derives benefit from and harms its host.

helminth A multicellular microscopic worm.

protozoa Single-celled, mobile parasites.

fungi Plantlike, spore-forming organisms that have a true nucleus and can grow as either single cells or multicellular colonies.

prion A protein that misfolds and becomes infectious and destructive; prions are not living cellular organisms or viruses.

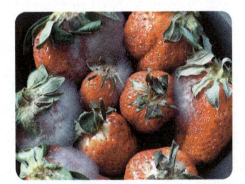

◆ **FIGURE 12.5** Molds rarely cause foodborne illness, in part because they look so unappealing that we throw the food away.

Bacterial Toxins

One of the most common foodborne toxins is produced by the bacterium *Staphylococcus aureus* (see Table 12.2). Although the vomiting it typically provokes is severe, it tends to resolve quickly. In contrast, the neurotoxin produced by the bacterium *Clostridium botulinum* is deadly. This botulism toxin blocks nerve transmission to muscle cells, paralyzing the muscles, including those required for breathing. A common source of contamination is food from a damaged (split, pierced, or bulging) can. If you spot damaged canned goods while shopping, notify the store manager. If you inadvertently purchase food in a damaged can or find that the container spurts liquid when you open it, wash your hands, put on gloves, wrap the can in a sealed plastic bag, and throw it in the trash. Then clean all surfaces with a diluted bleach solution. *Never taste the food, as even a microscopic amount of botulism toxin can be fatal.*[12] Other common sources of *C. botulinum* are foods improperly canned at home, raw honey, oils infused with garlic or herbs, and potatoes baked in foil.

Some strains of *E. coli*, including those involved in the outbreaks mentioned at Chipotle's, produce an enterotoxin toxin called *Shiga toxin*. These types are referred to as *Shiga toxin-producing E. coli,* or STEC. The most common STEC is *E. coli* O157. STECs are likely to require hospitalization because infection can result in bloody diarrhea and kidney failure. In vulnerable populations they can be fatal.[1,8]

Eating spoiled fish—commonly tuna or mackerel—is unwise because the bacteria responsible for the spoilage release toxins into the fish. The result is *scombrotoxic fish poisoning,* which causes headache, vomiting, a rash, sweating, and flushing within a few minutes to 2 hours after consumption. Symptoms usually resolve within a few hours in healthy people.[13]

Fungal Toxins

Some fungi produce poisonous chemicals called *mycotoxins*. (The prefix *myco-* means "fungus.") These toxins are typically found in grains stored in moist environments. In some instances, moist conditions in the field encourage fungi to reproduce and release their toxins on the surface of growing crops. Long-term consumption of mycotoxins can cause organ damage or cancer.

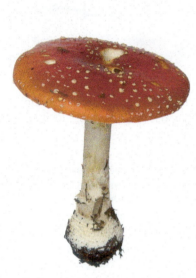

◀ FIGURE 12.6 Some mushrooms, such as this fly agaric, contain fungal toxins that can cause illness or even death.

A highly visible fungus that causes food intoxication is the poisonous mushroom. Most mushrooms are not toxic, but a few, such as the deathcap mushroom (*Amanita phalloides*), can be fatal. Some poisonous mushrooms are quite colorful **(FIGURE 12.6)**, a fact that helps explain why the victims of mushroom poisoning are often children.[14]

Toxic Algae

You may have seen signs warning of a "red tide" along a stretch of coastline. Shellfish beds are closed during a red tide to protect the public from a foodborne illness called *paralytic shellfish poisoning* (PSP).[13] Red tides are caused by the excessive production of certain species of toxic algae, whose bloom turns ocean waters purple, pink, or red. Mussels, clams, and other shellfish consume the toxic algae. When people consume the affected seafood—which typically looks, smells, and tastes normal—PSP results. Symptoms, which typically arise within an hour, range from numbness and tingling to paralysis and respiratory failure.[13]

Ciguatoxins are marine toxins commonly found in large finfish from tropical regions, including grouper, sea bass, and snapper. Symptoms of ciguatoxin poisoning include nausea, vomiting, diarrhea, itching, and blurred vision, but typically resolve within days to several weeks.[13]

Plant Toxins

A variety of plants contain toxins that, if consumed, can cause illness. As humans evolved, we learned to avoid such plants. However, one plant toxin is still commonly found in kitchens. Potatoes that have turned green contain the toxin *solanine,* which forms, along with the harmless green pigment chlorophyll, when the potatoes are exposed to light. Solanine is very toxic even in small amounts, and potatoes that appear green beneath the skin should be thrown away. Toxicity causes vomiting, diarrhea, fever, headache, and other symptoms and can progress to shock. Rarely, the poisoning can be fatal.[15]

You can avoid the greening of potatoes by storing them for only short periods in a dark cupboard or brown paper bag in a cool area. Wash the potato to expose its color, and throw it away if it has turned green.

Certain Conditions Help Microorganisms Multiply in Foods

Given the correct environmental conditions, microorganisms can thrive in many types of food. Four factors affect the survival and reproduction of food microorganisms:

- *Temperature.* Many microorganisms capable of causing human illness thrive at warm temperatures, from about 40°F to 140°F (4°C to 60°C). You can think of this range of temperatures as the **danger zone** (FIGURE 12.7). These microorganisms can be destroyed by thoroughly heating or cooking foods, and their reproduction can be slowed by refrigeration and freezing. Safe cooking and food-storage temperatures are identified later in this chapter.
- *Humidity.* Many microorganisms require a high level of moisture; thus, foods such as boxed dried pasta do not make suitable microbial homes, although cooked pasta left at room temperature would prove hospitable.
- *Acidity.* Most microorganisms have a preferred pH range in which they thrive. Pathogenic bacteria prefer a pH range from slightly acidic to neutral—about 4.6 to 7.0. However, there are exceptions. *Clostridium botulinum*, for example, thrives in alkaline environments, such as fish and most vegetables.
- *Oxygen content.* Many microorganisms require oxygen to function; thus, food-preservation techniques that remove oxygen, such as industrial canning and bottling, keep foods safe for consumption. In contrast, *C. botulinum* thrives in an oxygen-free environment. For this reason, the canning process heats foods to a temperature high enough to destroy this deadly microorganism.

In addition, microorganisms need an entryway into a food. Just as skin protects the body from microbial invasion, the peels, rinds, and shells of many foods seal off access to the nutrients within. Eggshells are a good example of a natural food barrier. Once such a barrier is pierced or removed, however, the food loses its primary defense against contamination. Slicing through an unwashed melon, for example, can contaminate the edible interior.

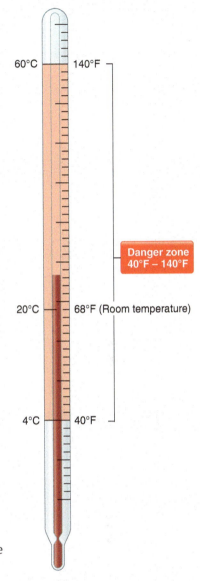

◀ **FIGURE 12.7** The danger zone is a temperature range within which many pathogenic microorganisms thrive. Notice that "room temperature" (about 68°F) is within the danger zone!

Nutri-case | THEO

"I got really sick yesterday after eating lunch in the cafeteria. I had a turkey sandwich, potato salad, and a cola. A few hours later, in the middle of basketball practice, I started to shake and sweat. I felt really nauseated and barely made it to the bathroom before vomiting. Then I went back to my dorm room and crawled into bed. This morning I still feel a little sick to my stomach, and sort of weak. I asked a couple of my friends who ate in the cafeteria yesterday if they got sick, and neither of them did, but I still think it was the food. I'm going off-campus for lunch from now on!"

Do you think that Theo's illness was foodborne? If so, what food(s) do you most suspect? What do you think of his plan to go off-campus for lunch from now on?

danger zone The range of temperature (about 40°F to 140°F, or 4°C to 60°C) at which many microorganisms capable of causing human disease thrive.

recap Food infections result from the consumption of food containing living microorganisms, such as bacteria, whereas food intoxications result from consuming food containing toxins. The top cause of foodborne illness is norovirus. Second in line is the bacterium *Salmonella*, which is also responsible for the greatest number of hospitalizations and deaths. The parasite *Toxoplasma gondii* is one of the top five pathogens responsible for hospitalizations and deaths due to foodborne illness. Prions are self-replicating particles that can contaminate and destroy nerve tissue. *Clostridium botulinum*, "STEC" species of *E. coli*, and other bacteria can produce toxins capable of causing severe illness and even death. Mushrooms, seafood, and potatoes may also contain toxins. In order to reproduce in foods, microorganisms require a precise range of temperature, humidity, acidity, and oxygen content.

LO 3 Discuss strategies for preventing foodborne illness at home and while eating out.

How can you prevent foodborne illness?

The U.S. Department of Health and Human Services' Foodsafety.gov is the nation's gateway to federal food-safety information. Foodsafety.gov identifies four basic rules for food safety (FIGURE 12.8).

Clean: Wash Your Hands and Kitchen Surfaces Often

One of the easiest and most effective ways to prevent foodborne illness is to consistently wash your hands before and after handling food. Most college students believe they know how to wash their hands, but a recent study discovered that they don't! After washing their hands, 58% of students participating in the study still had colonies of microorganisms—some pathogenic—populating their hands![16]

What's the right way to wash? Remove any rings or bracelets before you begin, because jewelry can harbor bacteria. Scrub for at least 20 seconds with a mild soap, being sure to wash underneath your fingernails and between your fingers. Rinse under warm, running water. Although you should wash dishes in hot water, it's too harsh for handwashing: It causes the surface layer of the skin to break down, increasing the risk that microorganisms will be able to penetrate your skin. Dry your hands on a clean towel or fresh paper towel.

Thoroughly wash utensils, containers, and cutting boards with soap and hot water, either in a dishwasher, or by hand, wearing gloves. You can sanitize cutting boards with a solution of 1 tablespoon of chlorine bleach to 1 gallon of water. Flood the surface with the bleach solution and allow it to air dry. Also wash countertops with soap and hot water.

Wash fruits and vegetables thoroughly under running water just before eating, cutting, or cooking them. Prewashed and bagged salad greens clearly marked as ready-to-eat do not need to be washed again. Washing fruits and vegetables with soap or detergent, or using commercial produce washes, is not recommended. Also, do not wash meat, poultry, or fish, as doing so can spread contaminants. Microorganisms in these foods will be destroyed when you thoroughly cook them.[17]

To learn "Clean" tips for preventing foodborne illness, watch a video at www.foodsafety.gov. From the home page, click on the "Clean" logo to find it.

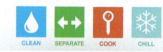

◀ **FIGURE 12.8** This food-safety logo from Foodsafety.gov can help you remember the four steps for reducing your risk of foodborne illness.

Separate: Don't Cross-Contaminate

Cross-contamination is the spread of microorganisms from one food to another. This commonly occurs when raw foods, such as chicken and vegetables, are cut using the same knife or cutting board, or stored or carried to the table on the same plate.[18] Invest in a set of cutting boards of different colors, and reserve one for fresh breads, one for produce, and one for meat, fish, and poultry.

In the refrigerator, keep raw meat, poultry, eggs, and seafood and their juices away from ready-to-eat food. Keep them wrapped in plastic on the lowest shelf of your refrigerator.

When preparing meals with a marinade, reserve some of the fresh marinade in a clean container; then add the raw ingredients to the remainder. In this way, some uncontaminated marinade will be available if needed later in the cooking process. While marinating raw food, keep it in the refrigerator.[18]

Prevent cross-contamination while food shopping. Keep raw meat, poultry, and seafood away from other foods in your cart, and make sure they're wrapped in plastic at the checkout, so their juices won't contaminate other foods. Inspect eggs before putting them in your cart. If a carton has a broken egg, bring it to the store manager. Also, watch out for unsafe practices in the store. For example, the displaying of food products such as cooked shrimp on the same bed of ice as raw seafood is not safe, nor is slicing cold cuts with the same knife used to trim raw meat. Report such practices to your local health authorities.

Chill: Store Foods in the Refrigerator or Freezer

The third rule for keeping food safe from bacteria is to promptly refrigerate or freeze it. Remember the danger zone: microorganisms that cause foodborne illness can reproduce in temperatures above 40°F. To keep them from multiplying in your food, keep it cold. Refrigeration (between 32°F and 40°F) and freezing (at or below 0°F)[19] do not kill all microorganisms, but cold temperatures diminish their ability to reproduce in quantities large enough to cause illness. Also, many naturally occurring enzymes that cause food spoilage are deactivated at cold temperatures.

Shopping for Perishable Foods

When choosing perishable foods, check the "sell by" or "best used by" date on the label. The "sell by" date indicates the last day a product can be sold and still maintain its quality during normal home storage and consumption. The "best used by" date tells you how long a product will maintain best flavor and quality before eating.[20] The "use by" date indicates the last day recommended to consume the food. No matter the type, if the stamped date has passed, don't purchase the item and notify the store manager. These foods should be promptly removed from the shelves.

When shopping for food, purchase refrigerated and frozen foods last. After you check out, get perishable foods home and into the refrigerator or freezer within 1 hour. If your trip home will be longer than an hour, take along a cooler to transport them.

Refrigerating Foods at Home

As soon as you get home from shopping, put meats, eggs, cheeses, milk, and any other perishable foods in the refrigerator. Store meat, poultry, and seafood in the back of the refrigerator away from the door, so that they stay cold, and on the lowest shelf, so that their juices do not drip onto any other foods. If you are not going to use raw poultry, fish, or ground beef within 2 days of purchase, store it in the freezer. A guide for refrigerating foods is provided in **FIGURE 12.9** on page 436.

After a meal, refrigerate leftovers promptly—even if still hot—to discourage microbial growth. The standard rule is to refrigerate leftovers within 2 hours of serving. If the ambient temperature is 90°F or higher, such as at a picnic, foods should be refrigerated within 1 hour.[19] A larger quantity of food takes longer to cool, so divide and conquer: separate leftovers into shallow containers for quicker cooling.[19] Finally, avoid keeping leftovers for more than a few days (see Figure 12.9). If you don't plan to finish a dish within the recommended time frame, freeze it.

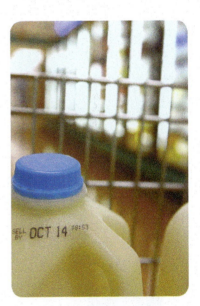

▲ The "sell by" date tells the store how long to display the product for sale.

cross-contamination Contamination of one food by another via the unintended transfer of microorganisms through physical contact.

▶ **FIGURE 12.9** While it's important to keep a well-stocked refrigerator, it's also important to know how long foods will keep.

Source: Data from U.S. Department of Agriculture, Food Safety and Inspection Service. 2015, March. Food safety information. Refrigeration and food safety. www.fsis.usda.gov.

Safe zone 32°F – 40°F

Food	Keeps for...
Uncooked hamburger	1–2 days
Uncooked roasts, steaks, and chops	3–5 days
Uncooked poultry	1–2 days
Uncooked fish	1–2 days
Cooked meats, poultry, and fish	3–4 days
Fresh eggs in shell	3–5 weeks
Hardboiled eggs	1 week
Egg, chicken, tuna, ham, and pasta salads	3–5 days
Soups or stews	3–4 days
Hot dogs and luncheon meats, unopened package	2 weeks
Hot dogs, opened package	1 week
Luncheon meats, opened package	3–5 days

Leftovers are great for lunch the next day, of course, but how do you keep them safe if you pack a lunch at 8 AM and eat it on campus or at work several hours later? Find food-safety strategies for packed lunches in the **Quick Tips** feature on this page.

Freezing and Thawing Foods

The temperature in your freezer should be set at or below 0°F. Use a thermometer and check it periodically. If your electricity goes out, avoid opening the freezer until the power is restored. When the power does come back on, check the temperature. If it is at or below 40°F, or if the food contains ice crystals, the food should still be safe to eat, or refreeze.[21]

As with refrigeration, smaller packages will freeze more quickly. Rather than attempting to freeze an entire casserole, divide the food into multiple, small portions in freezer-safe containers; then freeze.

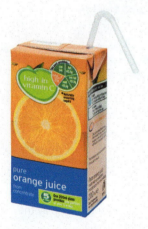

⬆ Freeze a 100% juice box overnight, then tuck it into your packed lunch with your perishable foods. By noontime, you'll have a cold, nutritious drink—and a safer lunch.

QuickTips

Packing a Food-Safe Lunch

✔ **Insulate.** Invest in an insulated lunch box or soft-sided case.

✔ **Keep it cold.** When packing meat or any other perishable, include a freezer pack as well as another ice source. A frozen juice box or small bottle of water works well, and should make a refreshing drink by lunchtime.

✔ **Pack it hot.** For leftovers, soups, and other hot foods, use a thermos: Fill it with boiling water. Let it stand while you heat the food until it's piping hot. When it's ready, drain the water and fill the thermos.

✔ **Wash and wipe.** When it's time for lunch, wash your hands before eating. Pack disposable wipes and, once you've finished eating, discard used food wraps and wipe out the lunch box—as well as your hands. At home, wash reusable containers, thermos, utensils, and the lunch box with hot water and soap.

Source: Data from FoodSafety.gov. Back to School. www.foodsafety.gov/keep/events/backtoschool/

Sufficient thawing will ensure adequate cooking throughout, which is essential to preventing foodborne illness. The safest way to thaw meat, poultry, and seafood is to place the frozen package on the bottom shelf of the refrigerator, on a large plate or in a large bowl to catch its juices. It should be ready to cook within 24 hours. Never thaw frozen meat, poultry, or seafood on a kitchen counter or in a basin of warm water. Room temperatures allow the growth of bacteria on the surface of food. You can also thaw foods in your microwave, following the manufacturer's instructions. Another option is to cook the food without first thawing it. Just allow for a cooking time about 50% longer than usual.[19]

Dealing with Molds in Refrigerated Foods

Some molds like cool temperatures. Mold spores are common in the atmosphere, and they randomly land on food in open containers. If the temperature and acidity of the food are hospitable, they will grow.

If the surface of a small portion of a firm, solid food, such as hard cheese, becomes moldy, it is generally safe to cut off that section down to about an inch and eat the unspoiled portion. However, if soft cheese, sour cream, tomato sauce, a leftover casserole, or another soft or fluid product becomes moldy, discard it entirely, as foods with a high moisture content may be contaminated below the surface.[22]

Cook: Heat Foods Thoroughly

Thoroughly cooking food is a sure way to kill the intestinal worms discussed earlier and many other microorganisms. Color and texture are unreliable indicators of safety. Use a food thermometer to ensure that you have cooked food to a safe minimum internal temperature to destroy any harmful bacteria. The minimum temperatures vary for the type of food:[23]

- Beef, pork, veal, lamb steaks, roasts, and chops: 145°F with a 3-minute rest time before serving
- Fish: 145°F
- Ground beef: 160°F
- Egg dishes: 160°F
- Poultry, whole, pieces, and ground: 165°F

To learn how to use a food thermometer, watch the video at www.foodsafety.gov. From the home page, click on the "Cook" logo to find it.

Place the thermometer in the thickest part of the food, away from bone, fat, or gristle.

It's end of term and you're planning a lakeside barbecue! To keep it food-safe, check out the **Quick Tips** on transporting, cooking, and serving grilled and cold foods on page 438.

Microwave cooking is convenient, but you need to be sure your food is thoroughly and evenly cooked and that there are no cold spots in the food where bacteria can thrive. For best results, cover food, stir often, and rotate for even cooking. Raw and semi-raw (such as marinated or partly cooked) fish delicacies, including sushi and sashimi, may be tempting, but their safety cannot be guaranteed. Always cook fish thoroughly. When done, fish should be opaque and flake easily with a fork. If you're wondering how sushi restaurants can guarantee the safety of their food, the short answer is they can't. All fish to be used for sushi must be frozen using a method that effectively kills any parasites that are in the fish, but it does not necessarily kill bacteria or viruses. Another myth is that hot sauce can kill microbes in raw foods. It can't.

You may have fond memories of licking cake or brownie batter off a spoon when you were a kid, but such practices are no longer considered safe. That's because most cake batter contains raw eggs, one of the most common sources of *Salmonella*. Cook eggs until they are firm.

Protect Yourself from Toxins in Foods

Killing microorganisms with heat is an important step in keeping food safe, but it won't protect you from their toxins. That's because many toxins are unaffected by

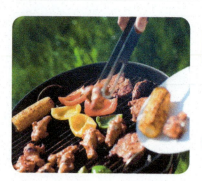

At a barbecue, it's essential to heat foods to the proper temperature.

QuickTips

Staying Food-Safe at a Barbecue

✓ **Keep foods cold—and separate—during transport.** Use small coolers with ice or frozen gel packs to keep food at or below 40°F. Put beverages in one cooler, washed fruits and vegetables and containers of potato salad in another, and wrapped, frozen meat, poultry, and seafood in another. Keep coolers in an air-conditioned part of your car.

✓ **Wash your hands, utensils, and food-preparation surfaces.** Take along a water jug, some soap, and paper towels or a box of moist, disposable towelettes. Keep all utensils and platters clean when preparing foods.

✓ **Grill foods thoroughly.** Use a food thermometer. Burgers should reach 160°F and chicken at least 165°F.

✓ **Avoid contaminating cooked foods.** When taking food from the grill to the table, never use the same platter or utensils that previously held raw meat or seafood.

✓ **Keep grilled food hot.** Move it to the side of the grill, just away from the coals, so that it stays at or above 140°F. If grilled food isn't going to be eaten right away, wrap it well and place it in an insulated container.

✓ **Keep perishable foods on ice.** Drain off water as the ice melts and replace the ice frequently. Don't let any perishable food sit out longer than 2 hours. In temperatures above 90°F, that drops to 1 hour.

Source: Data from U.S. Food and Drug Administration. 2015, November 20. Barbecue basics: Tips to prevent foodborne illness. http://www.fda.gov/forconsumers / ucm094562.htm

heat and are capable of causing severe illness even when the microorganisms that produced them have been destroyed.

For example, let's say you prepare a casserole for a team picnic. Too bad you forget to wash your hands before serving it to your teammates, because you contaminate the casserole with the bacterium *Staphylococcus aureus,* which is commonly found on skin. You and your friends go off and play soccer, leaving the food in the sun, and a few hours later you take the rest of the casserole home. At supper, you heat the leftovers thoroughly, thinking that this will kill any bacteria that multiplied while it was left out. That night you experience nausea, severe vomiting, and abdominal pain. What happened? While your food was left out, *Staphylococcus* multiplied in the casserole and produced a toxin **(FIGURE 12.10)**. When you reheated the food, you killed the microorganisms, but their toxin was unaffected. When you then ate the food, the toxin made you sick.

Be Choosy When Eating Out—Close to Home or Far Away

When choosing a place to eat out, avoid restaurants that don't look clean. Grimy tabletops and dirty restrooms indicate indifference to hygiene. Pay attention to the food service workers, too. If they appear to be ill, or their hands don't look clean, or they're handling both raw and ready-to-eat foods, go elsewhere. Although public health inspectors randomly visit and inspect the food-preparation areas of all businesses that serve food, these inspections don't guarantee safety the day of your visit.

Another way to protect yourself when dining out is by ordering foods to be cooked thoroughly. If you order a hamburger and it arrives pink in the middle, or scrambled eggs and they arrive runny, send the food back. If you order potato,

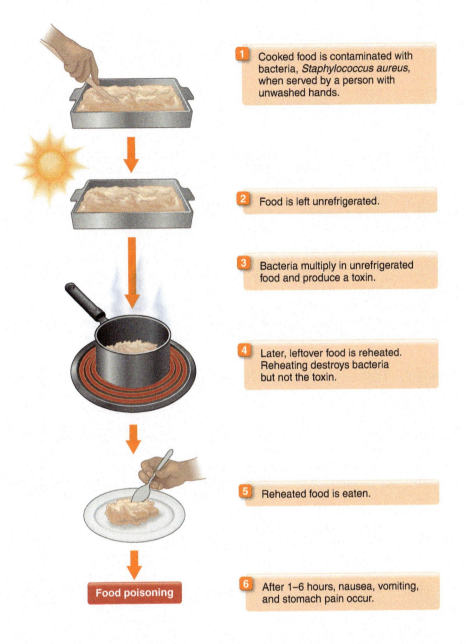

1. Cooked food is contaminated with bacteria, *Staphylococcus aureus*, when served by a person with unwashed hands.

2. Food is left unrefrigerated.

3. Bacteria multiply in unrefrigerated food and produce a toxin.

4. Later, leftover food is reheated. Reheating destroys bacteria but not the toxin.

5. Reheated food is eaten.

Food poisoning

6. After 1–6 hours, nausea, vomiting, and stomach pain occur.

◀ FIGURE 12.10 Food contamination can occur long after the microorganism itself has been destroyed.

egg, tuna, or chicken salad or a dish with a cream sauce, and it arrives looking somewhat congealed or simply less than fresh, it may have been left out too long. Send it back.

When planning a trip, tell your physician your travel plans and ask about vaccinations you need or any medications you should take along in case you get sick. Pack a waterless antibacterial hand cleanser and use it frequently. When dining, choose cooked foods and bottled and canned beverages or tea or coffee made with boiling water (see Chapter 3). All raw food has the potential for contamination.

recap Foodborne illness can be prevented at home by following four tips: (1) Clean: wash your hands and kitchen surfaces often. (2) Separate: isolate foods to prevent cross-contamination. (3) Chill: store foods in the refrigerator or freezer. (4) Cook: heat foods long enough and at the correct temperatures to ensure proper cooking. When eating out, avoid restaurants with areas that don't look clean or workers who appear ill or indifferent to hygiene, and ask that all food be cooked thoroughly.

LO 4 Compare and contrast the various methods manufacturers use to preserve foods.

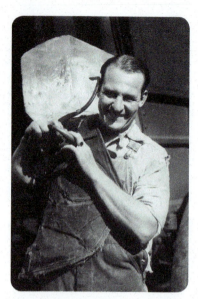

⬥ Before the modern refrigerator, an iceman would deliver ice to homes and businesses.

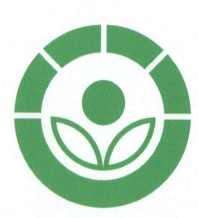

⬥ **FIGURE 12.11** The U.S. Food and Drug Administration requires the Radura—the international symbol of irradiated food—to be displayed on all irradiated food sold in the United States.

pasteurization A form of sterilization using high temperatures for short periods of time.

How is food spoilage prevented?

Any food that has been harvested and that people aren't ready to eat must be preserved in some way or, before long, it will degrade enzymatically and become home to a variety of microorganisms. Even processed foods—foods that are manipulated mechanically or chemically—have the potential to spoil.

The most ancient methods of preserving foods are salting, sugaring, drying, and smoking, all of which draw the water out of plant or animal cells. By dehydrating the food, these methods make it inhospitable to microorganisms and dramatically slow the action of enzymes that would otherwise degrade the food. We still use many of these methods today to preserve and prepare foods and meats, such as salted or smoked fish ham.

Natural methods of cooling have also been used for centuries, including storing foods in underground cellars, caves, running streams, and even "cold pantries"—north-facing rooms of the house that were kept dark and unheated, often stocked with ice. The forerunner of the modern refrigerator—the miniature icehouse, or icebox—was developed in the early 1800s, and in cities and towns a local iceman would make rounds delivering ice to homes.

More recently, technological advances have helped food producers preserve the integrity of their products for months and even years between harvesting and consumption. These include the addition of preservatives such as vitamins C and E, as well as the following:

- *Canning.* Developed in the late 1700s, canning involves washing and blanching food, placing it in cans, siphoning out the air, sealing the cans, and then heating them to a very high temperature. Canned food has an average shelf life of at least 2 years from the date of purchase.
- *Pasteurization.* The technique called **pasteurization** exposes a beverage or other food to heat high enough to destroy microorganisms, but for a short enough period of time that the taste and quality of the food are not affected. For example, in flash pasteurization, milk or other liquids are heated to 162°F (72°C) for 15 seconds.
- *Aseptic packaging.* You probably know aseptic packaging best as "juice boxes." Food and beverages are first heated, then cooled, then placed in sterile containers. The process uses less energy and materials than traditional canning, and the average shelf life is about 6 months.
- *Modified atmosphere packaging.* In this process, the oxygen in a package of food is replaced with an inert gas, such as nitrogen or carbon dioxide. This prevents a number of chemical reactions that spoil food, and it slows the growth of bacteria that require oxygen. The process can be used with a variety of foods, including meats, fish, vegetables, and fruits.
- *High-pressure processing.* In this technique, the food to be preserved is subjected to an extremely high pressure, which inactivates most bacteria while retaining the food's quality and freshness.
- *Irradiation.* This process exposes foods to gamma rays from radioactive metals. Energy from the rays penetrates food and its packaging, killing or disabling microorganisms in the food. The process does not cause foods to become radioactive! A few nutrients, including thiamin and vitamins A, E, and K, are lost, but these losses are also incurred in conventional processing and preparation. Although irradiated food has been shown to be safe, the FDA requires that all irradiated foods be labeled with a Radura symbol and a caution against irradiating the food again **(FIGURE 12.11)**.

recap Salting, sugaring, drying, smoking, and cooling have been used for centuries to preserve food. Preservatives such as vitamin C and E may be added to foods produced today. In addition, canning, pasteurization, irradiation, and several packaging techniques are used to preserve a variety of foods during shipping, as well as on grocer and consumer shelves.

What are food additives, and are they safe?

Have you ever picked up a loaf of bread and started reading its ingredients? You'd expect to see flour, yeast, water, and some sugar, but what are all those other items? They are collectively called *food additives*, and they are in almost every processed food. **Food additives** are not foods in themselves but, rather, natural or synthetic chemicals added to foods to enhance them in some way. More than 3,000 different food additives are currently used in the United States. **TABLE 12.3** identifies only a few of the most common.

Food Additives Include Nutrients and Preservatives

Vitamins and minerals are added to foods as nutrients and as preservatives. As just noted, vitamin E is usually added to fat-based products to keep them from going rancid, and vitamin C is used as an antioxidant in many foods. Iodine is added to table

TABLE 12.3   Examples of Common Food Additives

Food Additive	Foods Found in
Coloring Agents	
Beet extract	Beverages, candies, ice cream
Beta-carotene	Beverages, sauces, soups, baked goods, candies, macaroni and cheese mixes
Caramel	Beverages, sauces, soups, baked goods
Tartrazine	Beverages, cakes and cookies, ice cream
Preservatives	
Alpha-tocopherol (vitamin E)	Vegetable oils
Ascorbic acid (vitamin C)	Breakfast cereals, cured meats, fruit drinks
BHA	Breakfast cereals, chewing gum, oils, potato chips
BHT	Breakfast cereals, chewing gum, oils, potato chips
Calcium proprionate/sodium proprionate	Bread, cakes, pies, rolls
EDTA	Beverages, canned shellfish, margarine, mayonnaise, processed fruits and vegetables, sandwich spreads
Propyl gallate	Mayonnaise, chewing gum, chicken soup base, vegetable oils, meat products, potato products, fruits, ice cream
Sodium benzoate	Carbonated beverages, fruit juice, pickles, preserves
Sodium chloride (salt)	Most processed foods
Sodium nitrate/sodium nitrite	Bacon, corned beef, lunch meats, smoked fish
Sorbic acid/potassium sorbate	Cakes, cheese, dried fruits, jellies, syrups, wine
Sulfites (sodium bisulfite, sulfur dioxide)	Dried fruits, processed potatoes, wine
Texturizers, Emulsifiers, and Stabilizers	
Calcium chloride	Canned fruits and vegetables
Carageenan/pectin	Ice cream, chocolate milk, soy milk, frostings, jams, jellies, cheese, salad dressings, sour cream, puddings, syrups
Cellulose gum/guar gum/gum arabic/locust gum/xanthan gum	Soups and sauces, gravies, sour cream, ricotta cheese, ice cream, syrups
Gelatin	Desserts, canned meats
Lecithin	Mayonnaise, ice cream
Humectants	
Glycerin	Chewing gum, marshmallows, shredded coconut
Propylene glycol	Chewing gum, gummy candies

food additive A substance or mixture of substances intentionally put into food to enhance its appearance, safety, palatability, and quality.

salt to help decrease the incidence of goiter and birth defects related to iodine deficiency. Vitamin D is added to milk, and calcium is added to milk alternatives and some juices to help preserve healthy bone. Folate is added to cereals, breads, and other foods to help prevent birth defects, and many cereals and breads are also fortified with iron.

The following two preservatives have raised health concerns:

- *Sulfites.* A small segment of the population is sensitive to sulfites, preservatives used in many beers and wines and sometimes on grapes and other fresh foods. Consuming sulfites can prompt asthma, headaches, or other symptoms in sensitive people.
- *Nitrites.* Commonly used to preserve processed meats, nitrites can be converted to nitrosamines during the cooking process. Nitrosamines have been found to be carcinogenic in animals, so the FDA has required all foods with nitrites to contain additional antioxidants to decrease the formation of nitrosamines.

Other Food Additives Include Flavorings, Colorings, and Texturizers

Flavoring agents are used to replace the natural flavors lost during food processing. In contrast, *flavor enhancers* have little or no flavor of their own but accentuate the natural flavor of foods. One of the most common flavor enhancers is monosodium glutamate (MSG). In some people, MSG causes symptoms such as headaches, difficulty breathing, and heart palpitations.

Common food *colorings* include beet extract, which imparts a red color; beta-carotene, which gives a yellow color; and caramel, which adds brown color. The coloring tartrazine (FD&C Yellow #5) causes an allergic reaction in some people, and its use must be indicated on the product packaging.

Texturizers are added to foods to improve their texture. *Emulsifiers* help keep fats evenly dispersed within foods. *Stabilizers* give foods "body" and help them maintain a desired texture or color. *Humectants* keep foods such as marshmallows, chewing gum, and shredded coconut moist and stretchy. *Desiccants* prevent the absorption of moisture from the air; for example, they are used to prevent table salt from forming clumps.[24]

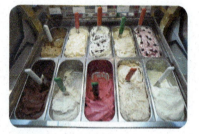

◀ Many foods, such as ice cream, contain colorings.

Are Food Additives Safe?

Federal legislation was passed in 1958 to regulate food additives. Before a new additive can be used in food, the producer of the additive must submit data to the FDA demonstrating its safety. The FDA then determines the additive's safety based on these data. Also in 1958, the U.S. Congress recognized that many substances added to foods do not require stringent testing, as their safety has been established through long-term use or has been recognized by qualified experts through scientific studies. These additives are referred to as **Generally Recognized as Safe (GRAS)**. The GRAS list identifies substances that either have been tested and determined by the FDA to be safe and approved for use in the food industry, or are deemed safe as a result of consensus among experts.

In 1985, the FDA established the Adverse Reaction Monitoring System (ARMS). Under this system, the FDA investigates complaints from consumers, physicians, and food companies about food additives.

The GRAS list is not static; in 2015, for example, the FDA determined that partially hydrogenated oils (PHOs), the main source of *trans* fatty acids in the U.S. diet, are no longer GRAS. Food companies were given until June 2018 to comply, after which time they will no longer be allowed to produce foods containing PHOs.

Generally Recognized as Safe (GRAS) A list of substances approved for use in food production because they have been determined safe for consumption based on a history of long-term use or on the consensus of qualified research experts.

recap Food additives are chemicals intentionally added to foods to enhance their color, flavor, texture, nutrient density, moisture level, or shelf life. Although there is continuing controversy over food additives in the United States, the FDA regulates additives used in our food supply and considers safe those it approves. The GRAS list identifies substances that either have been tested and determined by the FDA to be safe or are deemed safe as a result of consensus among experts.

How is genetic modification used in food production, and is it safe?

LO 6 Describe the processes, uses, benefits, and concerns of genetic modification of foods.

In **genetic modification**, also referred to as *genetic engineering*, the genetic material, or DNA, of an organism is altered to bring about specific changes in its seeds or offspring.

Genetic Modification Includes Selective Breeding and Recombinant DNA Technology

Selective breeding is one example of genetic modification; for example, Brahman cattle, which have poor-quality meat but high resistance to heat and humidity, are bred with English shorthorn cattle, which have good meat but low resistance to heat and humidity. The outcome of this selective breeding process is Santa Gertrudis cattle, which have the desired characteristics of higher-quality meat and resistance to heat and humidity. Although selective breeding is effective, it is a relatively slow process because a great deal of trial and error typically occurs before the desired characteristics are achieved.

Advances in biotechnology have moved genetic modification beyond selective breeding to include the manipulation of the DNA of living cells of one organism to produce the desired characteristics of a different organism. Called **recombinant DNA technology**, the process commonly begins when scientists isolate from an animal, a plant, or a microbial cell a particular segment of DNA—one or more genes—that codes for a protein conferring a desirable trait, such as drought tolerance or increased nutrients **(FIGURE 12.12)**. Scientists then splice the DNA into a "host cell," usually a microorganism. The cell is cultured to produce many copies—a *gene library*—of the beneficial gene. Then, many scientists can readily obtain the gene to modify other organisms that lack the desired trait. The modified DNA causes the plant's cells to build the protein of interest, and the plant expresses the desired trait. The term *genetically modified organism* (GMO) refers to any organism in which the DNA has been altered using recombinant DNA technology.

Cultivation of GMO food crops began in 1996. In the United States, the most common genetic modification in food crops induces tolerance to herbicides, chemicals that kill weeds.[25] Herbicide-tolerant GM crops (HT GMOs) can be sprayed liberally

genetic modification The process of changing an organism by manipulating its genetic material.

recombinant DNA technology A type of genetic modification in which scientists combine DNA from different sources to produce a transgenic organism that expresses a desired trait.

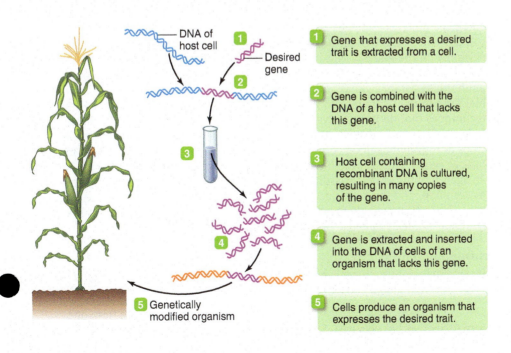

1. Gene that expresses a desired trait is extracted from a cell.

2. Gene is combined with the DNA of a host cell that lacks this gene.

3. Host cell containing recombinant DNA is cultured, resulting in many copies of the gene.

4. Gene is extracted and inserted into the DNA of cells of an organism that lacks this gene.

5. Cells produce an organism that expresses the desired trait.

FIGURE 12.12 Recombinant DNA technology involves producing plants and other organisms that contain modified DNA, which enables them to express desirable traits that are not present in the original organism.

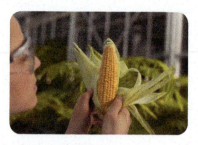

↖ Corn is one of the most widely cultivated genetically modified crops.

with chemicals that previously would have destroyed the crops themselves. The second most common modification induces insect resistance by inserting the gene from the soil bacterium Bt (*Bacillus thuringiensis*).[25] The Bt gene codes for the assembly of a protein that is toxic to specific insects, protecting the plant throughout its life span. The most common GM crops are corn and soybeans. The USDA reports that, in 2015, 89% of all corn crops and 94% of all soybean crops grown in the United States were HT GMOs, and a great majority of these crops were Bt modified as well.[25]

Genetic Modification Has Many Benefits

In 2014, nearly 450 million acres of GM crops were grown in 28 countries worldwide.[26] Many agricultural experts cite numerous benefits resulting from the global adoption of GM technology:[26–28]

- GM crops grow faster and have average yields 22% higher than conventional crops. Crops have been engineered for drought-tolerance, salt-tolerance, and other characteristics that enable them to thrive in challenging climates. As a result, food security for countries struggling to maintain adequate food supplies has increased.
- Cultivation of GM crops has had some environmentally responsible outcomes. These include conservation of water due largely to the development of drought-tolerant species of corn, reduced use of pesticides, reduced energy use, reduced emissions of greenhouse gases, and increased soil conservation due to higher productivity.
- GM crops can be produced with enhanced nutrients, improved digestibility, and lower levels of carcinogens, thereby improving public health.
- Farmer profits have increased by an average of 50% in both developed and developing countries, on both corporate and family farms, the majority owned by resource-poor farmers.

Genetic Modification Poses Certain Risks

As the use of genetic modification increases, however, some public health experts and environmental scientists have become concerned about evidence of its risks. These are discussed here.

Potential Health Risks

The World Health Organization (WHO) has identified several potential health concerns of GM foods:[28–30]

- *Allergenicity.* Theoretically, the transfer of genes from organisms with commonly allergenic proteins—such as fractions of wheat or soy—to nonallergenic organisms could occur. The WHO has not, however, found allergic effects from GM foods currently on the market.
- *Antimicrobial properties.* It is possible that consumption of GM foods containing antibiotic-resistance genes could harm human body cells or the beneficial microbial flora in the GI tract. Although the WHO encourages the use of gene transfer techniques that do not involve antibiotic-resistance genes, the risk remains.
- *Indirect effects on food safety and loss of diversity.* Genes have migrated from GM crops to conventional food crops several miles away (e.g., via wind, birds, or insects).
- *Link to cancer.* In 2015, the International Agency for Research on Cancer (IARC), an agency of the WHO, classified the herbicide glyphosate, commercially known as Roundup, and the herbicide in greatest use in GM crops, as a probable carcinogen. The IARC linked glyphosate specifically to an increased risk for non-Hodgkin lymphoma, a leading cause of cancer death.

Environmental Risks

Environmental scientists have become increasingly concerned about the effects of GM crops on local and global ecologies. We focus on three such concerns here.[28,31–33]

- *Loss of biodiversity.* As already noted, unintentional transfer of genes from one crop to another has occurred. Studies have yielded evidence of transgenes in maize (corn), wheat, and other plants miles away. But even the intentional planting of GM crops promotes the spread of monocultures (genetically identical plants, such as the same variety of wheat or rice), which reduce nutrient and phytochemical variety in our diets, and increase those crops' vulnerability to plant diseases and climate events.

■ *Generation of superweeds.* There is no question that the adoption of HT GMOs—and the liberal application of glyphosate—has led to the generation of *superweeds*; that is, weeds that have evolved a tolerance to herbicides. Superweeds can grow faster, taller, and tougher than typical weeds, requiring farmers to apply more toxic pesticides. These weeds have appeared in 66 countries, including in 22 states in the United States. In 2014, the EPA released new regulations to combat the problem of superweeds, but environmental advocacy groups say they do not go far enough to address the crisis.

■ *Threats to other species.* Ecologists have associated the rise in GM crops to the decline in populations of certain species of birds, insects, and other creatures. One of the most commonly cited examples is the 80% decline in the population of monarch butterflies since 1997. Although climate change and other factors contribute, researchers point out that the butterfly larvae feed on milkweed, which has greatly declined with the increased use of glyphosate in conjunction with increased planting of HT-GMO crops.

Economic Instability

Critics also charge that GMOs have introduced the potential for only a few companies, including Monsanto, the world's largest agricultural biotechnology corporation, to control the majority of world food production. For example, the seed industry has become increasingly dominated by Monsanto, which has bought up smaller seed companies, impeding competition and leading to increased seed prices.

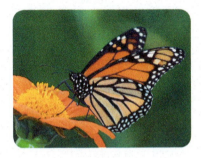

◄ The increased use of glyphosate on HT-GMO corn and soybeans is one factor associated with an 80% decline in the population of monarch butterflies.

Should GM Foods Be Labeled?

Many who oppose genetic engineering—and some who do not—agree that all GM foods should be labeled, so that consumers know what they are purchasing. The European Union (EU) has long required that GM foods be clearly labeled as such. In contrast, as of 2016, the U.S. Food and Drug Administration did not require such labeling. Thus, the only way for consumers to avoid GM foods is to purchase organic foods (discussed shortly).

In contrast, many GM supporters argue that labeling a food as genetically modified would raise consumer concerns about unconfirmed health risks. Globally, most nations, including the United States, perform rigorous assessments of the quality and safety of GM foods.[29] As the WHO notes, similar evaluations are generally not performed for conventional foods. Thus, consumer beliefs that conventional foods are safer than GM foods are not necessarily correct.

Twenty years have now passed since the introduction of GM foods into the marketplace. As more and more of the world's food supply depends on GM crops, the need for rigorous research into their risks, and the development of effective safeguards to reduce those risks, continues to grow as well.

recap In genetic modification, the genetic material, or DNA, of an organism is altered to enhance certain qualities. The process is called recombinant DNA technology. In U.S. agriculture, genetic modification is most often used to induce herbicide tolerance and insect resistance. It may also be used to boost a crop's yield, nutrients, protection from disease, or ability to grow in challenging conditions. GM technology has increased the global food supply and has certain beneficial environmental and economic effects. Concerns include the potential for negative health effects, loss of biodiversity, generation of superweeds, and monopolization of world food production. Many health and consumer groups advocate labeling of all GM foods.

How do residues harm our food supply?

Food residues are chemicals that remain in foods despite cleaning and processing. Residues of global concern include persistent organic pollutants, pesticides, and the hormones and antibiotics used in animals. The health concerns related to residues prompt many consumers to choose organic foods.

Persistent Organic Pollutants Can Cause Illness

Some chemicals released into the atmosphere as a result of industry, agriculture, automobile emissions, and improper waste disposal can persist in soil or water for years or even decades. These chemicals, collectively referred to as **persistent organic pollutants (POPs)**, can travel thousands of miles in gases or as airborne particles, in rain, snow, rivers, and oceans, eventually entering the food supply through the soil or water.[34] If a pollutant gets into the soil, a plant can absorb the chemical into its structure and pass it on as part of the food chain. Animals can also absorb the pollutant into their tissues or consume it when feeding on plants growing in the polluted soil. Fat-soluble pollutants are especially problematic, as they tend to accumulate in the animal's body tissues in ever-greater concentrations as they move up the food chain. This process is called **biomagnification**. The POPs are then absorbed by humans when the animal is used as a food source **(FIGURE 12.13)**.

POP residues have been found in virtually all categories of foods, including baked goods, fruit, vegetables, meat, poultry, fish, and dairy products. Significant levels have been detected all over the Earth, even in pristine regions of the Arctic thousands of miles from any known source.[34]

food residues Chemicals that remain in foods despite cleaning and processing.

persistent organic pollutants (POPs) Chemicals released as a result of human activity into the environment, where they persist for years or decades.

biomagnification The process by which persistent organic pollutants become more concentrated in animal tissues as they move from one creature to another through the food chain.

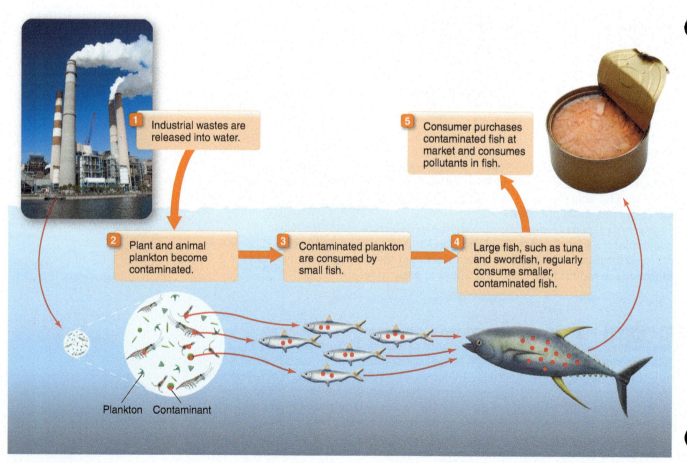

1 Industrial wastes are released into water.

5 Consumer purchases contaminated fish at market and consumes pollutants in fish.

2 Plant and animal plankton become contaminated.

3 Contaminated plankton are consumed by small fish.

4 Large fish, such as tuna and swordfish, regularly consume smaller, contaminated fish.

Plankton   Contaminant

▲ **FIGURE 12.13** Biomagnification of persistent organic pollutants in the food supply.

Health Risks of POPs

POPs are a health concern because of their range of harmful effects on the body. Some are neurotoxins. Many others are carcinogens. Still others act as *endocrine disruptors,* chemicals thought to interfere with the body's endocrine glands and their production of hormones. As you know, hormones play roles in a vast number of body processes, but endocrine disruptors are particularly associated with developmental problems, reproductive system disorders, nerve disorders, and impaired immune function.[34] They disrupt normal body processes by blocking the binding sites for natural hormones on body cells; mimicking natural hormones and thereby augmenting their actions; or altering the synthesis or metabolism of natural hormones.[34]

Some pesticides leave residues that qualify as POPs. Pesticides are discussed shortly.

Heavy Metals

Mercury, a naturally occurring heavy metal element, is found in soil, rocks, and water. It is also released into the air by industry and the burning of garbage and fossil fuels. As mercury falls from the air, it finds its way to rivers, lakes, and the ocean, where it accumulates. Fish absorb mercury as they feed on aquatic organisms, and this mercury is passed on to us when we consume the fish. As mercury accumulates in the body, it has a toxic effect on the nervous system, prompting memory loss and mood swings, as well as impaired vision, hearing, speech, and movement.[35]

Large predatory fish, such as swordfish, shark, king mackerel, and tilefish tend to contain the highest levels of mercury.[35] Because mercury is especially toxic to the developing nervous system of fetuses and growing children, pregnant and breastfeeding women and young children are advised to entirely avoid eating these types of fish. Other fish and shellfish are lower in mercury. The FDA and EPA recommend that pregnant women and young children eat no more than two servings (12 oz) per week of low-mercury fish.[35]

Lead is another heavy metal of concern. You may have heard of the 2015 lead contamination of municipal tap water in Flint, Michigan, and the increased risks to the residents exposed: In children, lead exposure can cause decreased IQ, serious learning and behavioral disorders, and hearing impairment. Adults can experience decreased fertility, nerve disorders, and cardiovascular and kidney disease.[36] Lead is an industrial waste from leaded gasoline, lead-based paints, and lead-soldered cans, now outlawed but decomposing in landfills. Some older homes also have high levels of lead paint dust, or the lead paint may be peeling in chips, which young children may put it their mouths. Some old ceramic mugs and other dishes are fired with lead-based glaze, allowing residues to build up in foods. No amount of lead is safe.

Plasticizers

Chemicals added to paint, varnish, cements, and plastics to increase their workability are collectively known as plasticizers. Two plasticizers found in plastic food containers can leach into foods and act as endocrine disruptors. A chemical called *bisphenol A (BPA)* is routinely used in the linings of canned foods and in some plastic food packaging. BPA is a form of synthetic estrogen, a female reproductive hormone, and research has linked it most conclusively to reproductive and developmental disorders.[37] *Phthalates* are a large group of plasticizers that are found in plastic food packaging, shampoos, carpeting and vinyl flooring, pesticides, and many other products, as well as in animal-based foods and drinking water. Phthalates have also been linked to reproductive and developmental disorders.[37,38]

To limit your exposure to BPA and phthalates:[39]

- Reduce your consumption of canned foods.
- Avoid purchasing food in plastic containers with the recycling codes 3 or 7, as these may contain BPA or phthalates. Do not microwave foods in these containers or use them to hold hot foods or beverages. They are more likely to leach endocrine disruptors when they become heated.
- Whenever possible, choose glass, porcelain, or stainless-steel containers.

Download a free safe-seafood app from the Monterey Bay Aquarium by clicking the link under "What Consumers Can Do" at http://www.seafoodwatch.org.

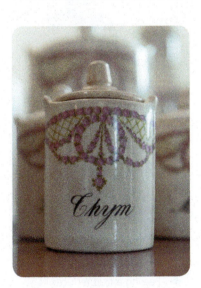

▲ Antique porcelain is often coated with lead-based glaze.

Dioxins

Dioxins are both carcinogens and endocrine disruptors. These industrial pollutants are typically formed as a result of combustion processes, such as waste incineration or the burning of wood, coal, or oil. Dioxins enter the soil and can persist in the environment for many years. There is concern that long-term exposure to dioxins can result in an increased risk for cancer, heart disease, diabetes, reproductive system disorders, and other disorders.[40] Because dioxins easily accumulate in the fatty tissues of animals, most dioxin exposure in humans occurs through dietary intake of animal fats. To reduce your exposure, reduce your consumption of meat, especially fatty meat, and trim the fat from meats before cooking. Choose low-fat milk, yogurt, and cheese, and replace butter with plant oils.

Poly- and Perfluoroalkyl Substances

Concern has also been increasing about persistent residues from poly- and perfluoroalkyl substances (PFASs) that degrade very slowly and have been found all over the globe, including in the tissues of animals and humans. PFASs repel oil and water and are used in food packaging such as pizza boxes, fast food wrappers, and microwave popcorn bags. They also contaminate public tap water. They have been associated with organ damage, cancer, endocrine disorders, and other health problems.[41]

Pesticides Protect Against Crop Losses—But at a Cost

Pesticides are a family of chemicals used in both fields and farm storage areas to decrease the destruction and crop losses caused by weeds, animals, insects, and microorganisms. The three most common types of pesticides used in food production are:

- *Herbicides*, which are used to control weeds and other unwanted plant growth.
- *Insecticides*, which are used to control insects that can infest crops.
- *Fungicides*, which are used to control plant-destroying fungal growth.

Some pesticides used today have a low impact on the environment and are not considered harmful to human health. These include **biopesticides**, which are species-specific and work to suppress a pest's population, not eliminate it. For example, pheromones are a biopesticide that disrupts insect mating by attracting males into traps. Biopesticides do not leave residues on crops—most degrade rapidly and are easily washed away with water.

In contrast, pesticides made from petroleum-based products can persist in the environment, polluting soils, water, plants, and animals. They can also harm agricultural workers and consumers, acting as neurotoxins, carcinogens, and endocrine disruptors. In 2015, the World Health Organization's International Agency for Research on Cancer classified the herbicide glyphosate and the insecticides malathion and diazinon—all commonly used in the United States—as probable carcinogens.[30]

The EPA is responsible for regulating the use of all pesticides in the United States. Although the EPA certifies only pesticides with minimal environmental impact, the agency suggests taking the following steps to reduce your level of exposure to pesticides:[42]

- Wash and scrub all fresh fruits and vegetables thoroughly under running water.
- Peel fruits and vegetables whenever possible, and discard the outer leaves of leafy vegetables, such as cabbage and lettuce. Trim the excess fat from meat and remove the skin from poultry and fish because some pesticide residues collect in the fat.
- Eat a variety of foods from various sources, as this can reduce the risk of exposure to a single pesticide.

You can also reduce your exposure to pesticides by choosing organic foods, as discussed shortly.

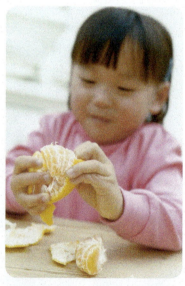

▲ Peeling a fruit reduces its level of pesticide residue; however, you should still scrub fruits before peeling.

pesticides Chemicals used either in the field or in storage to decrease destruction and crop losses by weeds, predators, or disease.

biopesticides Primarily insecticides, these chemicals use natural methods to reduce damage to crops.

Growth Hormones and Antibiotics Are Used in Animals

Introduced in the U.S. food supply in 1994, **recombinant bovine growth hormone (rBGH)** is a genetically engineered growth hormone. It is used in beef herds to induce animals to grow more muscle tissue and less fat. It is also injected into some U.S. dairy cows to increase milk output.

Although the FDA has allowed the use of rBGH in the United States, both Canada and the European Union have banned its use for two reasons:[43]

- The available evidence shows an increased risk for mastitis (inflamed udders), in dairy cows injected with rBGH. Farmers treat mastitis with antibiotics, promoting the development of strains of pathogenic bacteria that are resistant to antibiotics.
- The milk of cows receiving rBGH has higher levels of a hormone called insulin-like growth factor (IGF-1). This hormone can pass into the bloodstream of humans who drink milk from cows that receive rBGH, and some studies have suggested that an elevated level of IGF-1 in humans may increase the risk for certain cancers. However, the evidence from these studies is inconclusive.

The American Cancer Society suggests that more research is needed to help better appraise these health risks. In the meantime, consumer concerns about rBGH have caused a decline in rBGH injection in cows to below 20%.[43]

Antibiotics are also routinely given to animals raised for food. They are added to the feed of swine, for example, to reduce the number of disease outbreaks in overcrowded pork-production facilities. Many researchers are concerned that animals treated with antibiotics have become significant reservoirs for the development of virulent antibiotic-resistant strains of bacteria—so-called superbugs. How does this occur? As conventional antibiotics are repeatedly administered within an animal population, they become less effective because atypical bacterial cells—such as those with advantageous DNA mutations—escape the drugs' effects. These atypical bacteria are enabled to survive and reproduce without competition from the bacterial cells vulnerable to the antibiotics. A particularly dangerous superbug, methicillin-resistant *Staphylococcus aureus* (MRSA), is commonly resident in swine, and about 2% of the U.S. population has been infected.[44] Infection with MRSA can cause symptoms ranging from a fever and skin rash to widespread invasion of tissues, including the bloodstream. MRSA blood infections are sometimes fatal.[44]

In 2013, concerns about the risk of antibiotic use in animals promoting the development of superbugs caused the FDA to restrict the use of antibiotics in food production. Farmers cannot use antibiotics to increase an animal's growth, but only for prevention and treatment of disease.

You can reduce your exposure to growth hormones and antibiotics by choosing organic eggs, milk, yogurt, and cheeses and by eating free-range meat from animals raised without the use of these chemicals. You can also reduce your risk by eating vegetarian and vegan meals more often.

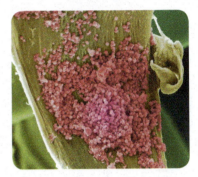

◀ The resistant strain of bacteria responsible for methicillin-resistant *Staphylococcus aureus* (MRSA).

Organic Farming Promotes Ecological Balance

Between 1990 and 2014, sales of organic products in the United States skyrocketed from $1 billion to over $39 billion.[45] About 81% of Americans make at least some organic purchases. But what, exactly, are they buying?

The USDA describes **organic agriculture** as "the application of a set of cultural, biological, and mechanical practices that support the cycling of on-farm resources, promote ecological balance, and conserve biodiversity."[46] Specifically, organic producers cannot use irradiation, sewage sludge, synthetic fertilizers, prohibited pesticides, GMOs, growth hormones, or antibiotics. Animals must be fed certified organic feed and have access to the outdoors.

Any product labeled organic must comply with the following definitions:[46]

- *Organic:* products containing at least 95% organically produced ingredients by weight, excluding water and salt, with the remaining ingredients consisting of those products not commercially available in organic form.
- *Made with organic ingredients:* a product containing at least 70% organic ingredients.

recombinant bovine growth hormone (rBGH) A genetically engineered growth hormone used in beef herds and some dairy cows.

organic agriculture The application of practices that support the cycling of on-farm resources, ecological balance, and biodiversity.

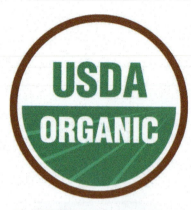

FIGURE 12.14 The USDA organic seal identifies foods that are at least 95% organic.

In products containing less than 70% organically produced ingredients, those ingredients that are organically produced can be specified on the label. Products that are organic may display the USDA organic seal **(FIGURE 12.14)**.

Notice that, in contrast to these strict regulations governing the use of the term *organic*, there is no USDA or FDA standard governing use of the term *natural*. However, the FDA is currently investigating concerns raised by some consumer groups about the potentially misleading use of this unregulated term. Without such regulation, it's wise to assume that a product labeled "All natural" is simply a conventional food.

Farms certified as organic have passed an inspection verifying that they are following all USDA organic standards. Organic farming methods are strict and require farmers to find natural alternatives to many common problems, such as weeds and insects. Contrary to common belief, organic farmers can use pesticides as a "last resort" for pest control when all other methods have failed, but they are restricted to a limited number of approved bio- and synthetic pesticides.[46]

With these safeguards, many people assume that organic foods and beverages are superior to foods produced using conventional methods. Are they right? The **Nutrition Debate** tackles this question.

recap Foodborne persistent organic pollutants (POPs) of greatest concern include the heavy metals mercury and lead, plasticizers, dioxins, and PFASs. Pesticides are used to prevent or reduce food crop losses; however, they too can persist in the environment. POPs and some pesticides can act as neurotoxins, carcinogens, or endocrine disruptors. Research into the health effects of recombinant bovine growth hormone (rBGH) is currently inconclusive. The use of—and residues from—antibiotics in animals raised for food increases the U.S. population's risk for antibiotic-resistant infections. The USDA regulates organic farming standards and inspects and certifies farms that follow all USDA organic standards. Organic producers cannot use irradiation, sewage sludge, synthetic fertilizers, prohibited pesticides, GMOs, growth hormones, or antibiotics. Animals must be fed organic feed, and have access to the outdoors.

Organic Foods: Are They Worth the Cost?

In a recent national survey, 51% of families said that the higher cost of organic foods was a factor limiting their organic purchases. In fact, families who regularly purchase organic foods spend an average of $15 a week more on groceries than families who don't buy organic items.[47] So it's reasonable to ask: Are organic foods worth the cost?

Over the past few decades, hundreds of studies have attempted to compare the nutrient levels of organic foods to those of foods conventionally grown. The results have been inconclusive. For example, two large review studies published in 2011 and 2012 reached opposite conclusions on this issue, one finding consistently higher levels of nutrients in organic produce, and the other finding no nutritional advantage.[48,49] Then, in 2013 and 2015, studies found 62% more omega-3 fatty acids and antioxidants in organic milk as compared to conventional milk,[50,51] and in 2014, a comprehensive review concluded that organically grown produce has a higher level of antioxidant nutrients and phytochemicals.[52]

The lack of conclusive evidence of a nutritional advantage of organic foods may not bother many consumers who choose organic foods to reduce their exposure to pesticide residues. How do organic foods compare on that measure? Two of the studies just mentioned found that organically produced foods were about 30% less likely to be contaminated with detectable pesticide residues or antibiotic-resistant bacteria.[49,52] Another study comparing organically grown soybeans with conventional and HT-GMO soybeans found that the organic beans not only had a much higher nutrient profile but also a much lower pesticide residue; in particular, the HT-GMO soybeans had a high level of glyphosate residue, whereas the organic beans had none.[53] In addition, researchers for the American Academy of Pediatrics recently reviewed all available evidence on organic foods and concluded that "Organic diets have been convincingly demonstrated to expose consumers to fewer pesticides associated with human disease."[54]

Do you think organic foods are worth the extra cost? If you do but you're on a budget, a smart strategy is to spend more for organic when the conventionally grown version is likely to retain a high pesticide residue. TABLE 12.4 identifies the foods that the Environmental Working Group advises should be your priority organic purchases. If your food budget is limited, spend your money on the organically grown versions of these foods. The table also identifies the 15 foods that tend to be lowest in pesticide residues.

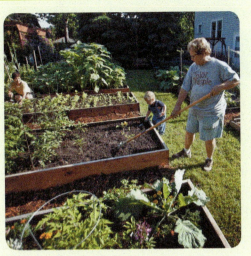

Many urban and suburban residents use techniques such as raised beds to grow their own fruits and vegetables without the use of pesticides.

You can feel confident purchasing conventional versions of these.

What else can you do? Grow some vegetables on your own, even if you have no plot of land, in raised beds in rooftop gardens, on a sunny balcony, or even in a sunny window. Learn more about container gardening at http://www.letsmove.gov/kitchen-garden-checklist.

Be sure to follow the EPA's guidelines for washing produce to reduce your ingestion of pesticide residues. Also try substituting foods on the "Dirty Dozen" list for similar foods among the "Clean Fifteen." For example, skip conventionally grown strawberries, and switch to kiwis. For potatoes, go with sweet potatoes.

CRITICAL THINKING QUESTIONS

1. Do you often purchase organic foods? Why or why not?
2. Given that organic foods are labeled for consumers, should GM foods also be labeled? Support your answer.
3. Search online for the USDA plant hardiness zone in which you live. Identify the length of your region's growing season, and two vegetables you could grow in your region during the summer.

TABLE 12.4 The Environmental Working Group's 2016 Shopper's Guide to Pesticides in Produce

The Dirty Dozen Buy These Organic	The Clean Fifteen Lowest in Pesticides
Strawberries	Avocados
Apples	Corn
Nectarines	Pineapples
Peaches	Cabbage
Celery	Sweet peas
Grapes	Onions
Cherries	Asparagus
Spinach	Mangoes
Tomatoes	Papayas
Bell peppers	Kiwi
Cherry Tomatoes	Eggplant
Cucumbers	Honeydew
	Grapefruit
	Cantaloupe
	Cauliflower

Source: Environmental Working Group. 2016. EWG's Shopper's Guide to Pesticides in Produce. http://www.ewg.org /foodnews/

STUDY PLAN MasteringNutrition™

TEST YOURSELF | ANSWERS

1 F Foodborne illness actually sickens about 48 million Americans each year, and about 3,000 die.

2 F Freezing destroys some microorganisms but only inhibits the ability of other microorganisms to reproduce. When the food is thawed, these cold-tolerant microorganisms resume reproduction.

3 T Although genetic modification can also improve a crop's nutritional profile or yield, the most common use is to increase a crop's ability to tolerate herbicides (weed killers).

review questions

LO 1 **1.** A key reason that foodborne illness has become a serious public health concern in the United States is that

a. an estimated 4.8 million Americans experience foodborne illness each year, and about 300 die.
b. Americans are eating more and more processed foods containing potentially toxic levels of food additives.
c. federal oversight of food safety is fragmented among 15 different agencies.
d. Americans are eating out more frequently, and restaurants are responsible for nearly all cases of foodborne illness.

LO 2 **2.** Among the top microorganisms implicated in foodborne illness,

a. norovirus is responsible for the greatest number of illnesses.
b. *Listeria monocytogenes* is responsible for the greatest number of hospitalizations.
c. Shiga toxin-producing *E. coli* is responsible for the greatest number of deaths.
d. *Toxoplasma gondii* is the only species of helminth.

LO 2 **3.** The majority of foodborne microorganisms reproduce most successfully

a. between 40°F and 140°F.
b. in dry conditions.
c. in alkaline conditions.
d. in an anaerobic environment.

LO 3 **4.** During a 4th of July barbecue on a hot afternoon, a family enjoys grilled fish, potato salad, and coleslaw. Leftovers of these foods should be safe to eat later on as long as they are brought back indoors and refrigerated

a. immediately after serving.
b. within a maximum of 30 minutes after serving.
c. within a maximum of 1 hour after serving.
d. within a maximum of 2 hours after serving.

LO 4 **5.** A food preservation technique in which the oxygen in a food is replaced with an inert gas is

a. aseptic packaging.
b. modified atmosphere packaging.
c. high-pressure processing.
d. irradiation.

LO 5 **6.** Food additives that have raised health concerns include

a. sodium chloride and beta-carotene.
b. sulfites and nitrites.
c. alpha-tocopheral and ascorbic acid.
d. all of the above.

LO 6 **7.** The most common reason that crops in the United States are genetically modified is to

a. confer tolerance to herbicides.
b. protect them from disease.
c. enable them to grow in challenging environmental conditions.
d. boost their concentration of nutrients.

LO 7 8. Residues from heavy metals, plasticizers, dioxins, PFASs, and certain pesticides pose a threat to public health mainly because

a. they promote the development of superbugs.
b. they cause allergies, asthma, and migraine headaches.
c. they can act as neurotoxins, carcinogens, or endocrine disruptors.
d. they can reduce biodiversity.

LO 2 9. **True or false?** A bacterium that commonly contaminates deli meats, smoked fish, and soft cheeses is *Listeria monocytogenes*.

LO 7 10. **True or false?** In the United States, farms certified as organic are allowed to use pesticides under certain conditions.

math review

LO 3 11. Below are the proper cooking temperatures for meat, poultry, and fish from the USDA. Use the following formula to convert each from Fahrenheit to Celsius. Round off.

Formula: $(°\text{Fahrenheit} - 32) \times 5/9 = (°\text{Celsius})$
Example: $(90°\text{F} - 32) \times 5/9 = (°\text{Celsius})$
$90 - 32 = 58$
$58 \times 5/9 = 32°\text{C}$

a. Beef, pork, veal, lamb steaks, roasts, and chops 145° with a 3-minute rest time before serving; fish 145°
b. Ground beef and egg dishes 160°
c. Poultry, whole, pieces, and ground 165°

Answers to Review Questions can be found online in the MasteringNutrition Study Area.

web links

www.foodsafety.gov
Foodsafety.gov
Use this website as a gateway to a range of government food-safety information from tips to outbreak reports.

www.cdc.gov/foodsafety/index.html
CDC Food-Safety Homepage
This section of the larger CDC website focuses on issues specifically related to food safety.

www.fsis.usda.gov/food_safety_education/ index.asp
USDA Food Safety and Inspection Service
Use the Food Safety and Inspection Service area of the larger USDA website to learn more about food safety through a variety of tools and resources.

www.epa.gov/pesticides
U.S. Environmental Protection Agency: Pesticides
This site provides information on agricultural and home-use pesticides, including effects of pesticides on health and the environment.

www.ams.usda.gov
USDA National Organic Program
Click on "National Organic Program" to get to the web page describing the NOP's standards, practices, and labeling.

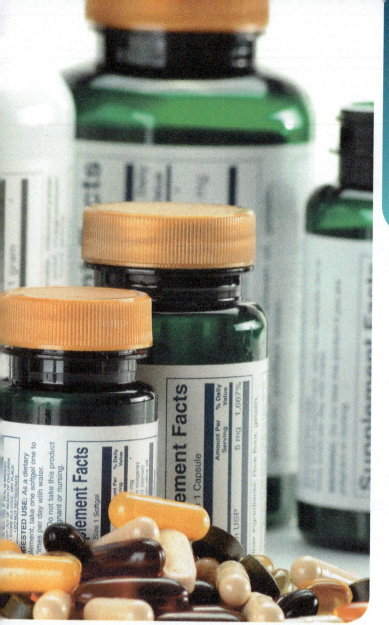

in depth 12.5

The Safety and Effectiveness of Dietary Supplements

learning outcomes

After studying this In Depth, you should be able to:

1 Discuss the limitations in current regulation of dietary supplements sold in the United States, pp. 455–456.

2 Explain what constitutes an herbal supplement and what special precautions are indicated for its use, pp. 456–457.

3 Identify groups of people who might benefit from taking a dietary supplement as well as situations in which dietary supplements are not advised, pp. 457–459.

In April of 2015, 14 U.S. Attorneys General signed a letter to the congressional subcommittee responsible for consumer product safety requesting that Congress launch an investigation into the dietary supplements industry. The action came after DNA testing of several supplements found that they did not contain the ingredients listed on the labels; some were contaminated with high levels of heavy metals including lead and mercury; and some contained allergens such as wheat and grass not identified on the label. Some supplements were labeled as containing natural plant extracts when they actually contained synthetic stimulants. In November 2015, the U.S. Justice Department brought criminal and civil suits against 117 individuals and companies marketing these supplements, some of which had caused illnesses and even deaths.

The Office of Dietary Supplements (ODS) at the National Institutes of Health (NIH) reports that, in 2014, sales of dietary supplements reached nearly $37 billion.[1] A recent survey of students at five U.S. universities found that 66% use a dietary supplement and 12% consume five or more.[2] Is this smart? Dangerous? Who, if anyone, *should* be taking supplements?

How are dietary supplements regulated?

LO 1 Discuss the limitations in current regulation of dietary supplements sold in the United States.

According to the U.S. Food and Drug Administration (FDA), a **dietary supplement** is a product containing ingredients such as vitamins, minerals, herbs, amino acids, or enzymes. They are intended to supplement the diet, not to treat, diagnose, prevent, or cure disease.[3] Supplements come in many forms, including tablets, capsules, softgels, liquids, and powders.

FIGURE 1 shows a label from a multivitamin and mineral (MVM) supplement. There are specific requirements for the information that must be included on the supplement label. Labels bearing a claim must also include the disclaimer "This statement has not been evaluated by the FDA. This product is not intended to diagnose, cure,

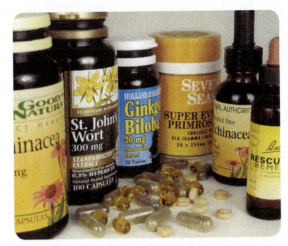

Dietary supplements can be pills, capsules, powders, or liquids and contain micronutrients, amino acids, herbs, or other substances.

or prevent any disease." Any products not meeting these guidelines can be removed from the market.

The Dietary Supplement Health and Education Act (DSHEA) of 1994 classified dietary supplements within the general group of foods, not drugs. This means that the

dietary supplement A product taken by mouth that contains a "dietary ingredient" intended to supplement the diet.

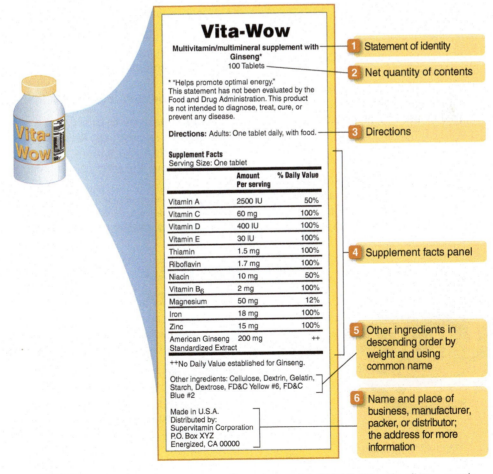

Vita-Wow

Multivitamin/multimineral supplement with Ginseng*

100 Tablets

* "Helps promote optimal energy." This statement has not been evaluated by the Food and Drug Administration. This product is not intended to diagnose, treat, cure, or prevent any disease.

Directions: Adults: One tablet daily, with food.

Supplement Facts
Serving Size: One tablet

	Amount Per serving	% Daily Value
Vitamin A	2500 IU	50%
Vitamin C	60 mg	100%
Vitamin D	400 IU	100%
Vitamin E	30 IU	100%
Thiamin	1.5 mg	100%
Riboflavin	1.7 mg	100%
Niacin	10 mg	50%
Vitamin B$_6$	2 mg	100%
Magnesium	50 mg	12%
Iron	18 mg	100%
Zinc	15 mg	100%
American Ginseng Standardized Extract	200 mg	++

++No Daily Value established for Ginseng.

Other ingredients: Cellulose, Dextrin, Gelatin, Starch, Dextrose, FD&C Yellow #6, FD&C Blue #2

Made in U.S.A.
Distributed by:
Supervitamin Corporation
P.O. Box XYZ
Energized, CA 00000

1. Statement of identity
2. Net quantity of contents
3. Directions
4. Supplement facts panel
5. Other ingredients in descending order by weight and using common name
6. Name and place of business, manufacturer, packer, or distributor; the address for more information

FIGURE 1 A multivitamin and mineral supplement label highlighting the dietary supplement labeling guidelines.

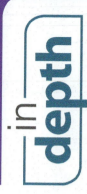

regulation of supplements is much less rigorous than the regulation of drugs. Currently, the FDA is reconsidering how it regulates foods and supplements that are marketed with health claims, but no changes have been finalized at this time. As an informed consumer, you should know that:[3]

- The FDA does not have the authority to review the safety and effectiveness of dietary supplements before they are marketed.
- The company that manufactures a supplement is responsible for determining that the supplement is safe; the FDA does not test any supplement for safety prior to marketing.
- Supplement companies have to notify the FDA if their supplement contains a new dietary ingredient; however, the FDA only reviews such notifications—it does not approve them—and only for safety, not for effectiveness.
- The FDA requires supplements manufacturers to produce products of quality and free of contamination; however, it does not regulate practices to ensure the purity, quality, safety, and composition of dietary supplements.
- Once a supplement is marketed, the FDA can take steps to remove it from the market if it is found to be unsafe or if the claims on the label are false and misleading. Supplements advertisers must be able to substantiate all label claims.

Although many dietary supplements contain the ingredients listed and are safe, the recent investigations mentioned earlier show that many others are dangerous. Because the liver is responsible for clearing toxins from the blood, it is often the organ damaged by use of contaminated supplements. For example, a 2014 study found that, over a 10-year period, eight U.S. medical centers reported more than 100 cases of liver damage caused by dietary supplements. Many of these cases resulted in the need for a liver transplant, and 13% were fatal.[4] How can you avoid purchasing such supplements? The FDA suggests that you keep in mind the nearby **Quick Tips** when evaluating dietary supplements.[5]

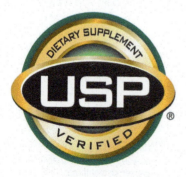

▲ **FIGURE 2** The USP Verified Mark indicates that the manufacturer has followed certain standards for features such as purity, strength, and quality. Registered Trademark of U.S. Pharmacopeial Convention (USP). Used with Permission.

QuickTips

Staying Safe with Supplements

✓ Check with your healthcare provider or an RDN about any nutrients you may need in addition to your regular diet.

✓ Look for the Pharmacopeia (USP) Verified Mark on the label (**FIGURE 2**). Though it doesn't indicate that the supplement is effective in treating any condition, the mark does indicate that the manufacturer followed the standards that the USP has established for features such as purity, quality, and labeling.

✓ Choose recognized brands of supplements. Although not guaranteed, products made by nationally recognized companies more likely have well-established manufacturing standards.

✓ Do not assume that the word *natural* on the label means that the product is safe. Arsenic, lead, and many other natural substances can kill you if consumed in large enough quantities.

✓ Be skeptical of anecdotal information or personal "testimonials."

✓ Ask yourself if the claims for the supplement sound too good to be true; for example, promising that the supplement will enable you to lose a large amount of weight in a short amount of time, or that it is a "miracle cure," or can be used to treat a wide variety of diseases.

✓ Do not hesitate to question a company about how it makes its products. Reputable companies have nothing to hide and are more than happy to inform their customers about the safety and quality of their products.

Source: U.S. Food and Drug Administration (FDA). Center for Food Safety and Applied Nutrition. 2015, September 4. Six tip-offs to rip-offs: Don't fall for health fraud scams. www.fda.gov/forconsumers/consumerupdates/ucm341344.htm

Are there special precautions for herbs?

LO 2 Explain what constitutes an herbal supplement and what special precautions are indicated for its use.

A common saying in India cautions that "A house without ginger is a sick house." Indeed, ginger, echinacea, lavender, and many other **herbs** (also called *botanicals*) have been used for centuries by different cultures throughout the world to promote health and treat discomfort and

herb A plant or plant part used for its scent, flavor, and/or therapeutic properties (also called a *botanical*).

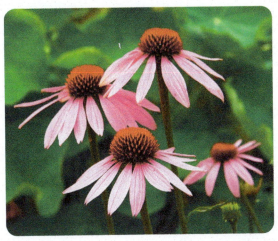

Echinacea, commonly known as purple coneflower, has been used for centuries to prevent colds, flu, and other infections.

disease. Many prescription and over-the-counter drugs are based on botanicals.

The National Center for Complementary and Integrative Health (NCCIH) defines an herb as "a plant or plant part (such as leaves, flowers, or seeds) that is used for its flavor, scent, and/or potential health-related properties."[6] As you would suspect, with a definition this broad there are hundreds of different herbs on the market. Which of these may be effective, and for what disorders, in what forms, and at what dosages? And are some ineffective or even dangerous? To help consumers answer these questions, NCCIH evaluates the most commonly used herbs in "Herbs at a Glance" fact sheets, available at its website (see the **Web Link**s at the end of this chapter).

The use of herbal supplements requires special precautions. In addition to the **QuickTips** for all types of dietary supplements, practice the following strategies offered by the NCCIH specifically for consumers considering the use of herbs:[6]

- Consult a healthcare provider before using any herbal supplement. Herbs can act the same way as drugs; therefore, they can cause medical problems if not prescribed.
- Never take herbal supplements if you have a serious illness, regularly take any prescription or over-the-counter medication, or are pregnant or breastfeeding, unless your physician has approved their use.
- Do not treat children with herbal supplements unless your physician has approved their use.
- Be aware that the active ingredients in many herbal supplements are not known. They may contain dozens, even hundreds, of unknown compounds. Analyses of herbal supplements, like those noted earlier, have routinely found differences between what is listed on the label and what is in the bottle. This means you may be taking less—or more—of the supplement than what the label indicates or

TABLE 1 Potentially Harmful Herbal Supplements

Herb	Potential Risks
Bitter orange	Increased blood pressure and heart rate; heart attack; stroke
Ephedra (also known as *ma huang*, Chinese ephedra, and epitonin)	High blood pressure, irregular heartbeat, nerve damage, insomnia, tremors, headaches, seizures, heart attack, stroke, possible death
Kava (also known as *kava kava*)	Liver damage; death
Licorice root	High blood pressure, fluid retention, hypokalemia
Noni	Liver damage
Thunder god vine	Diarrhea, nausea, skin rash, headache, hair loss, menstrual changes, male infertility; can be fatal if improperly extracted
Willow bark	Reye's syndrome (a potentially fatal reaction that may occur when children take aspirin), allergic reaction in adults
Yohimbe	High blood pressure, increased heart rate, headache, anxiety, dizziness, nausea, vomiting, tremors, insomnia

Source: Data from National Center for Complementary and Integrative Health (NCCIH). 2016. *Herbs at a Glance.* https://nccih.nih.gov/health/herbsataglance.htm

ingesting potentially harmful substances such as grasses, metals, unlabeled prescription drugs, and microorganisms.
- Be aware that the words *standardized, certified,* or *natural* on a label is no guarantee of product quality; in the United States, these terms have no legal definition for supplements.
- Finally, certain herbs are associated with severe—even life-threatening—adverse effects. These should be avoided entirely **(TABLE 1)**.

Should you take a dietary supplement?

LO 3 Identify groups of people who might benefit from taking a dietary supplement as well as situations in which dietary supplements are not advised.

According to a recent survey, 67% of Americans use vitamin or mineral supplements, 35% use "specialty" supplements, 23% use botanicals, and 17% use sports supplements (some of which are ergogenic aids, discussed in more detail in Chapter 11).[7] Many people take more than one. Among supplements users, MVM supplements are the most popular: 71% take an MVM. But contrary to popular belief, a healthful diet can usually provide an adequate level of essential nutrients. Moreover, foods contain a diverse combination of compounds that interact to maintain our health,

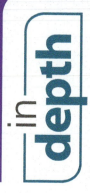

whereas vitamin and mineral supplements contain just the micronutrients identified on the label. Thus, they're not substitutes for a healthful diet.

However, nutritional needs do change throughout the life span, so you may benefit from taking a supplement at certain times for certain reasons. For instance, if you were to adopt a vegan diet, your healthcare provider might prescribe a supplement providing micronutrients absent or less available from plant foods, including riboflavin, vitamin B_{12}, vitamin D, calcium, iron, and zinc. Or if you joined your college soccer team, your team's sport dietitian might review your diet and advise taking a supplement formulated to provide micronutrients that support intense physical activity.

Dietary supplements include hundreds of thousands of products sold for many purposes, so it's impossible to discuss here all of the situations in which their use might be advisable. To simplify this discussion, TABLE 2 identifies groups of people who might benefit from micronutrient supplementation; however, not everyone in these groups needs the supplement indicated. If you fall within one of the groups listed, check with your healthcare provider or a registered dietitian nutritionist (RDN) to find out whether or not you should take the supplement.

The following are instances in which taking supplements is unnecessary or may be harmful:

- Providing fluoride supplements to children who already drink fluoridated water.
- Taking supplements in the belief that they will cure a disease, such as cancer, diabetes, arthritis, or heart disease.
- Taking nonprescribed supplements if you have a serious illness or are taking any prescription medications. For instance, physicians may prescribe micronutrient supplements for their patients with liver or kidney disease to replace nutrients lost during treatment for these diseases. However, these patients should not take any unprescribed supplements because their disease impairs their metabolism, putting them at high risk for toxicity. Similarly, people who take the blood-thinning drug Coumadin should not take any dietary supplements unless their physician has approved them. Vitamin E or K, licorice, St. John's wort, and willow bark are just

TABLE 2 Individuals Who May Benefit from Micronutrient Supplementation

Type of Individual	Specific Supplements That May Help
Newborns	Routinely given a single dose of vitamin K at birth
Infants	Depends on age and nutrition; may need iron, vitamin D, or other nutrients
Children not drinking fluoridated water	Fluoride supplements
Children with poor eating habits or overweight children on an energy-restricted diet	Multivitamin and multimineral supplement that does not exceed the RDA for the nutrients it contains
Pregnant teenagers	Iron and folic acid; other nutrients may be necessary if diet is very poor
Women who may become pregnant	Multivitamin or multivitamin and multimineral supplement that contains 0.4 mg of folic acid
Pregnant or lactating women	Multivitamin and multimineral supplement that contains iron, folic acid, zinc, copper, calcium, vitamin B_6, vitamin C, and vitamin D
People on prolonged or highly calorically restrictive weight-reduction diets	Multivitamin and multimineral supplement
People recovering from serious illness or surgery	Multivitamin and multimineral supplement
People with HIV/AIDS or other wasting diseases; people addicted to drugs or alcohol	Multivitamin and multimineral supplement or single-nutrient supplements
People who do not consume adequate calcium	Calcium should be consumed in whole foods and beverages; however, for some populations, supplements may be prescribed
People with low exposure to sunlight	Vitamin D
People eating a vegan diet	Vitamin B_{12}, riboflavin, calcium, vitamin D, iron, and zinc
People who have had portions of their intestinal tract removed; people who have a malabsorptive disease	Depends on the exact condition; may include various fat-soluble and/or water-soluble vitamins and other nutrients
Elderly people	Multivitamin and multimineral supplement, vitamin B_{12}

a few of many supplements that can dangerously alter the effects of Coumadin. People who take aspirin daily should check with their physician before taking any supplements because aspirin also thins the blood.[8]

- Taking beta-carotene supplements if you are a smoker. There is evidence that beta-carotene supplementation increases the risk for lung and other cancers in smokers.
- Taking supplements to increase your energy level. Although many vitamins and minerals assist in energy metabolism, they do not provide energy because they do not contain fat, carbohydrate, or protein (sources of Calories). Moreover, many stimulant supplements that are taken to increase energy levels have been associated with altered heart rhythms, central nervous system disturbances, and even death.[9]
- Taking single-nutrient supplements, unless prescribed by your physician for a diagnosed medical condition (e.g., prescribing iron supplements for someone with anemia). These supplements contain high amounts of the given nutrient, and taking them can quickly lead to toxicity. Especially harmful in high doses are vitamin A, which can cause liver damage; vitamin B_6, which can injure nerves; niacin, which can cause

vomiting, diarrhea, and damage to muscles, liver, and heart; and the mineral selenium, which can cause tissue damage.

MVM supplements are unlikely to cause harm, so should you take one, just for "insurance"? A recent editorial in the *Annals of Internal Medicine* advised most Americans to stop wasting their money on MVM supplements.[10] It cited other articles published in the same issue of the journal that illustrated no clear evidence of a beneficial effect of dietary supplementation on all-cause mortality, CVD, cancer,[11] or cognitive decline.[12,13] The U.S. Preventive Services Taskforce finds that current evidence is insufficient to support the use of MVMs or single- or paired-nutrient supplements.[11] If you do decide to take an MVM, select one that contains no more than 100% of the recommended levels for the nutrients it contains, but be aware: you might be wasting your money.

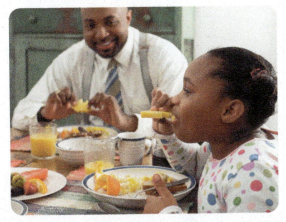

One of the best strategies for maintaining good health is to eat a diet that provides a variety of whole foods. If you do that, you probably won't need supplements.

nutri-case | THEO

"You know, I never thought I needed to take a multivitamin and mineral supplement because I'm healthy and I eat all different kinds of foods. But now I've learned in my nutrition course about what these vitamins and minerals do in the body, and I'm thinking, heck, maybe I should take one just for insurance. I mean, I use up a lot of fuel playing basketball and working out. Maybe if I popped a pill every day, I'd have an easier time keeping my weight up!" Do you think Theo should take a multivitamin and mineral supplement "just for insurance"? Why or why not? Would taking one be likely to have any effect on Theo's weight?

web links

www.dietary-supplements.info.nih.gov
Office of Dietary Supplements

Search this website to find reports evaluating individual supplements you might be considering as well as general information about the health benefits, safety, and regulation of dietary supplements.

www.cfsan.fda.gov
U.S. Food and Drug Administration Center for Food Safety and Applied Nutrition

This site provides information on how to make informed decisions and evaluate information related to dietary supplements.

https.nccih.nih.gov
National Center for Complementary and Integrative Health

From the menu on the left side of the home page, click on "Herbs at a Glance" to find information about an herb you might be considering using.

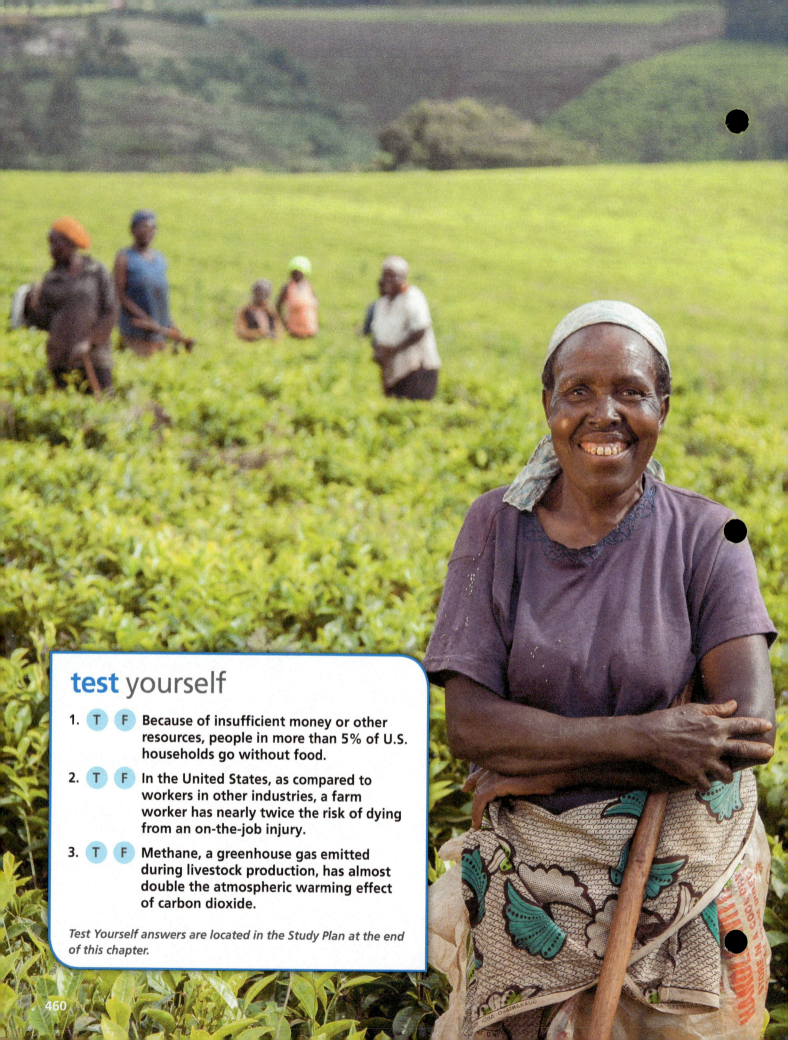

test yourself

1. **T** **F** Because of insufficient money or other resources, people in more than 5% of U.S. households go without food.

2. **T** **F** In the United States, as compared to workers in other industries, a farm worker has nearly twice the risk of dying from an on-the-job injury.

3. **T** **F** Methane, a greenhouse gas emitted during livestock production, has almost double the atmospheric warming effect of carbon dioxide.

Test Yourself answers are located in the Study Plan at the end of this chapter.

13 Food Equity, Sustainability, and Quality

The challenge of "good food"

In an affluent suburb in the United States, shoppers at a farmers market select organic meats, eggs, cheeses, produce, flour, and even freshly baked bread from nearby farms. When asked why they shop there, they say that they want to provide their families "good food." Across the globe in a village in Kenya, a group of neighbors are members of a farming cooperative that grows corn and beans, raises chickens for eggs and cows and goats for milk. Members boast of their ability to feed their families "good food" for breakfast, lunch, and dinner every day.

What is "good food"? Although farmers, chefs, and public health experts would likely propose very different definitions, in this chapter, we define "good food" as nutrient-dense food that is equitably and sustainably produced, distributed, and sold. That might sound like a tall order, but such foods do exist. The challenge is to make them in large enough quantities to feed the world, and make sure that consumers have the ability and the desire to obtain them.[1]

Equity means fairness, and we begin this chapter by looking at inequities in the production, distribution, and sale of the world's food supply. We then discuss the effects of industrial agriculture on our environment and on the quality and diversity of our food. Finally, we identify some ways that nations and organizations are meeting the challenge of "good food," and how you can help.

LO 1 Compare and contrast levels of food insecurity globally and in the United States.

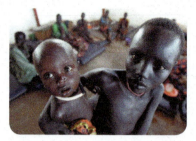

⬆ Hunger and malnutrition are still experienced by many people around the world today.

food insecurity Unreliable access to a sufficient supply of nourishing food.

How prevalent is food insecurity?

In Namibia, a nation in southern Africa, more than 42% of the population is undernourished.[2] Forty-six out of every 1,000 Namibian infants die before reaching their first birthday, and among those who survive to age 5, 13% are underweight. Average life expectancy is 52 years.[3] In the United States, infant mortality is only 6 per 1,000, and instead of being underweight, over 8% of children age 2 to 5 are obese.[3,4] Average life expectancy is now over 78 years; however, the average life expectancy of the poorest Americans is 10 years shorter (for women) and 15 years shorter (for men) than the average for the wealthiest Americans.[5]

Although a variety of factors contribute to disparities in infant mortality, body weight, and life expectancy, one of the most important is a population's level of **food insecurity**—unreliable access to a sufficient supply of nourishing food. Globally, the greatest health disparities are found between populations that are impoverished and those with a dependable supply of nourishing food. As the above comparisons illustrate, however, these disparities exist not only between poor and wealthy nations, but also between poor and wealthy people in developed countries like the United States. Are food distribution and access equitable? Let's have a look.

About 795 Million People Worldwide Are Hungry

The Food and Agricultural Organization of the United Nations (FAO) estimates that about 795 million people (one in nine people) worldwide are chronically undernourished, and 98% of these people live in developing nations.[6] Although this is a disturbing statistic, it represents considerable progress: in 1990, over 1 billion people were undernourished. Then, in September of 2000, the United Nations (UN) and heads of state from around the world committed to a coordinated effort to reduce poverty. Using 1990 as a baseline, they set eight Millennium Development Goals, the first of which was to halve by the year 2015 the proportion of the world's people who suffer from hunger. Significant progress was made toward this goal: The share of undernourished people in the global population fell from 18.6% in 1990–92 to 10.9% in 2014–16, a reduction of nearly 45%.[6]

Still, hunger is endemic to many nations of the world **(FIGURE 13.1)**. About 64% of the world's hungry people live in Asia, and sub-Saharan Africa—the region

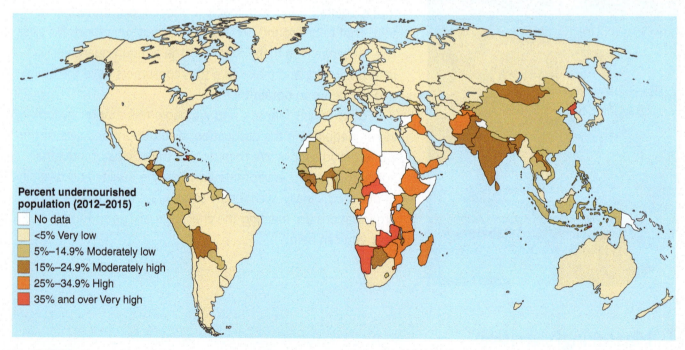

Percent undernourished population (2012–2015)
- No data
- <5% Very low
- 5%–14.9% Moderately low
- 15%–24.9% Moderately high
- 25%–34.9% High
- 35% and over Very high

⬆ **FIGURE 13.1** Although people throughout the world—including in North America—are undernourished, parts of Asia and sub-Saharan Africa have the greatest prevalence of undernourishment overall.

Source: Food and Agricultural Organization of the United Nations (FAO). 2015. FAO Hunger Map 2015. http://www.fao.org/hunger/en/

with the highest prevalence of hungry people—23%—accounts for almost 28%.[6] Closer to home, at least 10% of people in some regions of Central and South America are undernourished, and in Haiti, the prevalence is greater than 50%. The physical and societal consequences of malnutrition are explored **In Depth** following this chapter.

Over 17 Million American Households Are Food Insecure

Although the United States is one of the top 20 richest countries in the world,[3] many of our poorest citizens go hungry. As shown in **FIGURE 13.2**, the Economic Research Service of the U.S. Department of Agriculture (USDA) estimates that 14% of U.S. households (17.4 million households) experienced food insecurity in 2014.[7] This means that, at times during the year, members of these households were uncertain of having, or unable to acquire, enough food to meet their needs, because they had insufficient money or other resources for food.[7]

Of these 17.4 million households, 6.9 million had *very low food security*; that is, in 5.6% of U.S. households, one or more members had to reduce not only the quality, variety, or desirability of their food choices, but also the amount they were able to eat. In other words, people in these homes, at times, were hungry. How do "households" translate into human beings? In 2014, 12.4 million adults and 914,000 children (1.2% of U.S. children), experienced very low food security.[7]

Those at higher risk for food insecurity are households with incomes below 185% of the official U.S. poverty threshold (which was $24,008 for a family of four in 2014), families consisting of single mothers or single fathers and their children, African American households, and Hispanic households. Rural areas have slightly higher prevalence of food insecurity than urban or suburban areas, and prevalence in the South is higher than elsewhere in the U.S.[7]

Sometimes physical, psychological, or social factors contribute to food insecurity among Americans. For instance, people with chronic diseases or disabilities may lose paid work hours due to illness, have to accept lower-wage jobs, or have medical expenses that limit money for food. Depression, addiction to alcohol or other substances, and other psychological disorders can similarly limit productivity and reduce income. Divorce frequently leads to financial stressors, especially for women, who may be unable to collect alimony or child support payments and may have jobs that do not provide an income sufficient to provide fully for the family's needs.

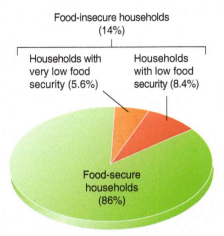

Food-insecure households
(14%)

Households with very low food security (5.6%)

Households with low food security (8.4%)

Food-secure households (86%)

▲ **FIGURE 13.2** Prevalence of food insecurity in U.S. households in 2014.

Source: Coleman-Jensen, A., M. P. Rabbitt, C. Gregory, and A. Singh. 2015, September. *Household Food Security in the United States in 2014.* Economic Research Service. United States Department of Agriculture. http://www.ers.usda.gov/

To read the FAO's 2015 report of The State of Food Insecurity in the World, visit www.fao.org/.

recap Health disparities exist between poor and wealthy nations, and between poor and wealthy regions within the same nation. Food insecurity, which is unreliable access to a sufficient supply of nourishing food, contributes to health disparities. Although significant progress has been made toward the millennium development goal to halve the 1990 prevalence of global hunger by the year 2015, about 795 million people worldwide are still chronically undernourished. In 2014, 14% of U.S. households experienced food insecurity, and over 13 million Americans, including 1.2% of all U.S. children, had very low food security. Low-income families and families headed by a single parent are among those with the highest rates of food insecurity.

Why don't all people have access to nourishing food?

LO 2 Identify several ways in which human behavior contributes to food insecurity.

Weather events and human activity can result in a food supply that is inadequate to support the needs of all of the people in a particular place. Moreover, a recent and ongoing concern is the effect of climate change on the global food supply.

nutri-case | JUDY

"I never seem to be able to make ends meet. I keep hoping next month will be different, but rent and utilities eat up most of my paycheck, so when something unexpected happens, I'm short. Last week, my car broke down and I'm way behind on my credit card payments. Today, a collections guy called and said that, if I didn't pay at least $100 right away, they'd take me to court. When I got off the phone, I started to cry, and Hannah asked me what was wrong. When I told her how bad the money situation is, she thought we might qualify for food stamps. I have a full-time job, so I don't think we'll qualify, but even if we do, I wonder if it'll help much."

In 2015, the federal minimum wage was $7.25 an hour. As a nurse's aide, Judy earns $9 an hour, or $1,560 a month. She is eligible for the Supplemental Nutrition Assistance Program (food stamps). Are you surprised that someone making almost 25% more than the minimum wage, and working full-time, qualifies for food assistance?

Before you're too certain that Judy's eligibility will solve her problems, consider that the average SNAP allotment in 2015 was $127.90 per person per month, or about $30 per week.* If you had just $30 to keep yourself fed for a week, what would you buy?

Take this challenge one step further and follow the example of some U.S. college students to raise local awareness of food insecurity: For 1 week, restrict yourself to just $30 for all your food purchases. Let your campus newspaper and local media outlets know what you're doing, and ask readers to make donations to local food banks.

*Congressional Budget Office. 2015, March. Supplemental Nutrition Assistance Program March 2015 Baseline. http://www.cbo.gov

Acute Food Shortages Are Often Caused by Weather Events and Wars

A **famine** is a severe food shortage affecting a large percentage of the population in a limited geographic area at a particular time. Famines have occurred throughout human history and typically result from a combination of factors, including weather events and human miscalculations. For example, an estimated 20–43 million people died in the so-called great famine in China from 1958 to 1961 when disastrous government land-use policies, combined with both floods and droughts, dramatically limited crop yields. When a population is already living in extreme poverty, even a minor climate event such as high winds or a severe frost can have dire consequences. Other natural disasters that can quickly destroy crops are tsunamis, hurricanes, drought, pest infestations, and plant diseases.

Wars can induce acute food shortages when they interfere with planting or harvest times, when they destroy standing crops, or when populations are forced to flee. Since the civil war in Syria began in 2011, for example, there have been numerous reports of starvation, either because of insufficient funds for food relief to refugees or as a deliberate tactic of oppression.

The Major Cause of Chronic Hunger Is Unequal Distribution of Food

The world produces enough food to meet everyone's needs. Even developing nations currently produce about 2,600 kcal per person per day. Worldwide, the leading cause of longstanding hunger in a region is unequal distribution of this adequate

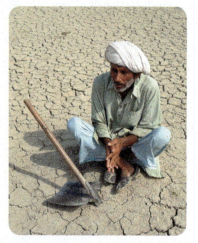

▲ An Indian farmer inspects what is left of his crop during a drought.

famine A severe food shortage affecting a large percentage of the population in a limited geographic area at a particular time.

food supply, largely because of poverty.[8] The most at-risk populations are the rural poor. Lacking sufficient land to grow their own foods, the rural poor must work for others to earn money to buy food, but because they live in rural areas, employment opportunities are limited.

Unequal distribution also occurs because of cultural biases. In many countries, limited food is distributed first to men and boys and only secondarily to women and girls. In such situations, pregnant women and growing girls are the most vulnerable because of their increased needs. Food distribution to the elderly is sometimes also limited, particularly in countries where nutrition services are primarily directed toward pregnant and lactating women, infants, and young children. Access to food can also differ by ethnicity and religion. For example, officials in authority may order that food aid be distributed preferentially to areas where their own ethnic or religious group dominates.

Overpopulation Contributes to Chronic Food Shortages

Experts estimate that, in the year 1000 BCE, the world population was about 50 million people. Nearly 3,000 years would pass before, in the year 1804, world population reached 1 billion. Yet by the year 2011, world population had passed 7 billion; and by 2050, it is projected to reach 9.7 billion.[9] Can the Earth sustain this many inhabitants?

An area is said to experience **overpopulation** when its resources are insufficient to support the number of people living there. In parts of the world with fertile land and adequate rainfall or irrigation systems to support abundant harvests, food shortages rarely happen. However, in more arid climates, especially in areas with high birthrates and low access to imported foods, seasonal and chronic food shortages are common. Of course, resources other than food may become depleted in overpopulated areas. Clean water, clean air, arable land (land suited to growing crops), safe housing, jobs, health care, quality education, and many other resources can be insufficient for the population's needs.

Is the world already overpopulated? Or will it soon become so? No one can answer these questions with absolute certainty, because we cannot predict how advances in technology will affect our depletion of the Earth's natural resources, our generation of pollution and wastes, or our ability to produce more food with fewer resources. However, reducing the demand for food within a region by slowing population growth is one way of improving an area's food supply, and one of the most effective methods of reducing birthrates is to improve education and career opportunities for girls and women.[10] Their increased earning potential, access to contraception, and better health practices lead to smaller, healthier, more economically stable families. Other methods of improving an area's food supply are to increase food production and to import foods into the area.

Local Conditions Can Contribute to Chronic Hunger

Agricultural practices, lack of infrastructure, and the burden of disease can also contribute to hunger in regions around the world.

Agricultural Practices

Some traditional farming practices have the potential to destroy arable land. Deforestation by burning or any other means and overgrazing pastures and croplands destroy the trees and grass roots that preserve soils from wind and water erosion. Growing the same crop year after year on the same plot of ground can deplete the soil of nutrients and reduce crop yield. Use of arable land for **cash crops**, such as cotton, coffee, and tobacco, may replace land use for local food crops, or food crops such as corn and soybeans may be diverted to industrial uses. Also harmful is the practice of growing food for livestock, which compared to food crops feed far fewer people for the resources used. We compare the environmental costs of livestock versus food crops later in this chapter.

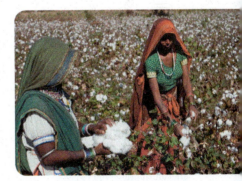

Cotton is a cash crop that farmers often grow instead of local food crops.

overpopulation Condition in which a region's available resources are insufficient to support the number of people living there.

cash crops Crops grown to be sold rather than eaten, such as cotton or tobacco.

Lack of Infrastructure

Exacerbating the scarcity of food production in some areas is a lack of infrastructure. For example, many developing countries lack roads and transportation into rural areas. This limits available food to whatever can be produced locally. In addition, lack of electricity and refrigeration can limit storage of perishable foods before they can be used.

Water management is another aspect of infrastructure that influences nutrition. In dry areas, irrigation can improve food production, but it must be managed carefully to avoid increasing the numbers of mosquitoes, intestinal parasites, and other pests, which can spread infectious diseases. The provision of safe drinking water and sewage systems is another aspect of water management that helps prevent disease.

Impact of Disease

Disease and lack of healthcare resources to fight disease reduce the work capacity of individuals, and this in turn reduces their ability to ward off poverty and malnutrition. This economic phenomenon is demonstrated by the AIDS epidemic. The World Health Organization (WHO) reports that there were nearly 37 million people living with HIV at the end of 2014. That year, about 1.2 million people died from AIDS.[11] HIV is most likely to affect young, sexually active adults who are the primary wage earners in their families. Thus, their illness or death can orphan and impoverish their children, as well as create populations in which children and the elderly predominate.

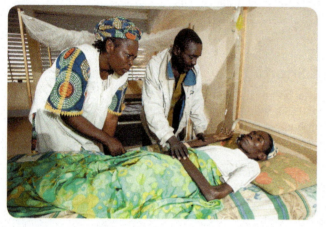

⬆ HIV/AIDS is most severe in under-nourished populations, especially in Africa.

Climate Change Threatens Global Food Security

Global warming is the general term used for the increase of about 1.5°F (0.85°C) in temperature that has occurred near the Earth's surface over the past century.[12] The great majority of climate scientists agree that it has been caused by human activities that have released large amounts of carbon dioxide and other heat-trapping *greenhouse gases* into the atmosphere.[12] Global warming is, in turn, the most significant factor contributing to **climate change**, which the U.S. Environmental Protection Agency (EPA) defines as any significant change in the measures of climate—such as temperature, precipitation, or wind patterns—that occurs over several decades or longer.[13] A 2015 analysis, for example, attributed 75% of heat extremes and 18% of precipitation extremes to global warming.[14]

The United Nations' Intergovernmental Panel on Climate Change (IPCC) reports that global warming and climate change are affecting global food security in a number of ways:[15]

- Reduced crop yields. Higher average temperatures and elevations in greenhouse gases have reduced crop yields in many regions of the world.
- Crop destruction. Heat waves, droughts, tornados, hurricanes, and floods have all destroyed standing crops outright. During the last few decades, for example, California has experienced both its hottest and driest as well as its wettest years on record,[16] causing billions of dollars of crop losses. Crops have also been destroyed by emerging varieties of pests such as fungal species that thrive in higher heat and humidity.
- Impacts on seafood availability. Climate change is reducing the abundance and distribution of seafood in tropical and temperate regions.

In contrast, very northern and southern latitudes of the globe have seen some minimal benefits from warmer temperatures. However, negative impacts of climate trends have been more common.[15] Moreover, a 2015 report found that global food security is becoming increasingly susceptible to the effects of climate change and population growth.[17]

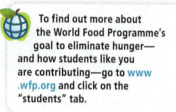

To find out more about the World Food Programme's goal to eliminate hunger—and how students like you are contributing—go to www .wfp.org and click on the "students" tab.

global warming The increase of about 1.5°F (0.85°C) in temperature that has occurred near the Earth's surface over the past century.

climate change Any significant change in the measures of climate—such as temperature, precipitation, or wind patterns—that occurs over several decades or longer.

recap The world produces enough food to meet everyone's needs. Famines are widespread, severe food shortages that can result in starvation and death. They are most commonly caused by natural disasters or wars. Worldwide, the leading cause of longstanding hunger in a region is unequal distribution of an adequate food supply, largely because of poverty. Chronic food shortages can be influenced by regional overpopulation. Increasing educational and career opportunities for women and girls is an effective method of reducing birthrates. Poor agricultural practices, lack of infrastructure, and the burden of disease also contribute to chronic food shortages. Climate change reduces crop yields, destroys crops, and changes availability of seafood.

Is our food equitably produced and sold?

Most people consider the fresh fruits and vegetables, meats, and other nutritious foods available in U.S. supermarkets and restaurants "good food." But if we're defining "good" as equitably produced and sold, then much of the food we eat each day doesn't qualify. Why not? Let's take a look at the working conditions for those who labor in America's agricultural, food retail, and food service industries, which a recent report from the Rockefeller Foundation called "grossly inequitable."[18]

LO 3 Discuss inequities in agricultural and food retail and service labor, and their effects on workers and the consumers they serve.

Farm Labor Is Dangerous and Poorly Paid

Throughout the U.S. labor market, in retail, industry, and even white-collar professions such as college teaching, more and more businesses are hiring "contingent workers." These positions typically offer little job security; no healthcare insurance, accrued sick- or vacation-leave, or retirement benefits; and low wages. This trend is nowhere more clearly seen than in agriculture, where about 20% of the workforce is contingent, up from 14% in the early 1990s.[19] Often referred to as "migrant workers" because they move from one region to another with changing harvest times, agricultural contingent workers also face hazardous conditions in the field. Consider these statistics:[18-21]

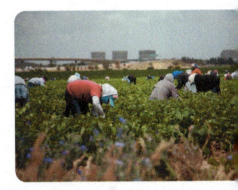

◄ Contingent farm workers are inadequately compensated for their labor, receive few benefits, and have high rates of occupational injury and disease.

- The average annual income for a contingent U.S. farm worker is $10,000–$12,500. Large farms are required to pay minimum wage, but small farms are not, and a majority of contingent farm workers live below the poverty line.
- Under federal law, young people aged 16 years and older are allowed to work on farms during school hours, and children aged 12 years and older may work on farms after school and on weekends with parental permission.
- Farm workers are not entitled to breaks for rest or meals mandated for other U.S. workers by the Fair Labor Standards Act (FLSA).
- Only 17% have any form of healthcare insurance and few have paid sick leave.
- Agriculture ranks as one of the most dangerous industries, with a fatality rate 7 times higher than the average for all workers in private industry. On average, more than 100 youths (under age 20) die each year from farm-labor injuries. Deaths are most commonly due to tractor overturns and other traumatic injuries, and heat stroke.
- Long-term exposure to pesticides, crop dusts, and excessive UV radiation causes lung disease and cancer, and constant bending and stooping causes musculoskeletal injuries.
- Contingent farm worker housing is often overcrowded and substandard, with some units lacking electricity, toilets, and running water.

Food Retail and Service Work Maintains the "Working Poor"

Conditions are only marginally better for the over 7 million cashiers and food and beverage service workers in the United States.[22] The median hourly wage for retail cashiers is $9.14, an amount that puts even a single person with no dependents at increased risk for food insecurity.[7,22] The median hourly wage for restaurant and other food service workers is even lower, just $8.96, and in many states, workers who earn more than $30 a month in tips may lawfully be paid just $2.13 an hour.[22] Thus, it's not surprising that a majority of food retail and service workers live near or even below the poverty line, accounting for many of America's "working poor."

Low wages in the food retail and service industry affect everyone. Among the 52 million Americans who receive government assistance such as Medicaid and Supplemental Nutrition Assistance Program (SNAP) benefits, a majority are unemployed or not in the labor market; however, 6.7% of full-time workers in the U.S. (about 1 out of every 15 full-time workers) receive government assistance.[23] In essence, this means that the average American taxpayer is subsidizing grocery stores, fast-food chains, and other food-service corporations, "making up the difference" in the inadequate wages they pay their employees. This situation has recently led cities and states across the United States to reexamine their minimum wage laws. Although the federal minimum wage has been stuck at $7.25 an hour since 2009, in 2015, Seattle, Washington, increased its minimum wage to $15 an hour, and in 2016, both California and Massachusetts raised the state minimum wage to $10 an hour.[24]

Many workers in food retail and service also have no paid sick leave. These workers are likely to show up for work even when ill with an infectious disease. You've learned (in Chapter 12) that the leading culprit in foodborne illness is norovirus, and the primary way that norovirus spreads is through infected food service workers. Foodborne illness is also a risk when farm workers don't receive paid sick leave. Farm workers infected with norovirus, hepatitis A virus, *Salmonella enteriditis*, and other foodborne microbes can contaminate produce during harvesting, and meat during processing.

Inequities in food security and labor can be discouraging and even distressing. Later in this chapter (pages 474–476) we'll explore some ways you can help promote the equitable production, distribution, and sale of food.

recap Working conditions in America's agricultural and food retail and service industries are inequitable. Contingent farm workers are inadequately paid, receive few benefits considered standard in other industries, and face much greater risks for occupational injury, chronic disease, and workplace fatality. Because farm and food retail and service workers are not paid a living wage, many receive Medicaid, SNAP benefits, and other government assistance funded by all Americans. The majority of these workers also lack paid time off for illness, and therefore are likely to work even when they risk contaminating foods during harvesting, production, preparation, and service.

LO 4 Discuss the effects of industrial agriculture on food security, food diversity, and the environment.

How does industrial agriculture affect the security, sustainability, and diversity of our food supply?

Sustainability is the ability to satisfy humanity's basic needs now and in the future without undermining the natural resource base and environmental quality on which life depends. Whereas some people view sustainability as a lofty but impractical ideal, others point out that it's a necessary condition of human survival. That's because sustainable practices can reduce pollution of our air, soil, and water and preserve resources for future generations. Is our current system of food production sustainable? Let's begin with some history.

sustainability The ability to meet or satisfy basic economic, social, and security needs now and in the future without undermining the natural resource base and environmental quality on which life depends.

Industrial Agriculture Has Increased Food Security but Threatens Our Environment

Like other modern wars, World War II led to innovations in industrial technology, engineering, and chemistry. After the war ended, these innovations were directed toward agriculture, specifically toward increasing worldwide food production to meet the food needs of a dramatically increasing postwar population. Together, the new technologies and practices became known as the **Green Revolution**, a massive program that has led to improved seed quality, fertilizers, pesticides, and farming techniques, which have boosted crop yields throughout the world. As part of the Green Revolution, for example, new **high-yield varieties (HYVs)** of grain were produced by cross-breeding plants and selecting for the most desirable traits. The first HYVs were rice and wheat, but now corn, beans, and many other crops are HYVs.

Industrial techniques were also applied to livestock production. As the total number of livestock and poultry farms with small numbers of animals declined, fewer but much larger operations increased. Between 1964 and 2012, for example, the number of farms raising cattle declined from over 2 million to just 26,500.[25,26] Cattle, pigs, and chickens are now increasingly raised in huge and crowded *confined animal feeding operations* (CAFOs) where their movement is restricted and they are fattened with high-energy feed often containing growth hormones and—until recently banned in the United States by the Food and Drug Administration—growth-promoting antibiotics.

These increases in food crop and animal production have vastly increased the global food supply and improved nutrition for millions of formerly undernourished people. This improvement in global nutrition—and the millions of lives it has saved—is important to bear in mind as we consider the environmental costs it has incurred. These include the following:[27,28]

- Depletion of topsoil due to erosion from heavy tilling leading to desertification of once-arable land
- Pollution of soils and water from salt build-up due to excessive irrigation, pesticide and fertilizer residues, animal waste, and other run-off, leading to loss of clean water and abandonment of once-arable land
- Depletion of ground water supplies from irrigation techniques requiring heavy water consumption
- Development of insecticide-resistant species of insects and herbicide-resistant varieties of weeds resulting from intensified use of agrochemical products
- Increased release of greenhouse gases from increasingly mechanized production and from methane released from animals in CAFOs

Beef production is a particular concern. Research data point to the inefficiency of eating meat from grain-fed cattle instead of eating the grains themselves, including in terms of the resources required and the level of greenhouse gas emissions generated. For corn-fed animals, for example, the efficiency of converting grain Calories to meat and dairy Calories ranges from roughly 3% to 40%, meaning that, on average, a crop capable of sustaining four to five people per acre will sustain only one person.[29] Livestock production also leads to deforestation, as forests are cut down to clear land for grazing or for production of animal feed. The contribution of meat consumption to global warming and resource depletion is discussed further in the **Nutrition Debate** on page 477.

Monopolization of Agriculture Reduces Food Diversity

Industrial agriculture has also reduced **food diversity**—that is, the variety of different species of food crops available. Beginning in the 1960s, revisions of the federal Agricultural Adjustment Act, commonly called the "farm bill," provided financial incentives for America's farmers to grow **monocultures**, single crops cultivated on a massive scale. The number of small farms dwindled, and the remaining industrial operations focused on increasing their production of the few subsidized crops, especially corn, soybeans, wheat, and rice. These few crops then began to monopolize the food supply. Because no subsidies were paid for production of fresh fruits and vegetables, their availability and variety plummeted, and they became more expensive.

As a result of this monopolization, the average American diet lost its variety. As you know, variety is a key component of a healthful diet: different species of fruits, vegetables, and whole grains provide different combinations of nutrients, fiber, and

To learn more about the true costs of livestock production, go to www.sustainabletable .org. In the search bar, type "industrial livestock production" to get started.

Green Revolution The tremendous increase in global productivity between 1944 and 2000 due to selective cross-breeding or hybridization to produce high-yield grains and industrial farming techniques.

high-yield varieties (HYVs) Semi-dwarf varieties of plants that are unlikely to fall over in wind and heavy rains and thus can carry larger amounts of seeds, greatly increasing the yield per acre.

food diversity The variety of different species of food crops available.

monoculture A single crop species cultivated over a large area.

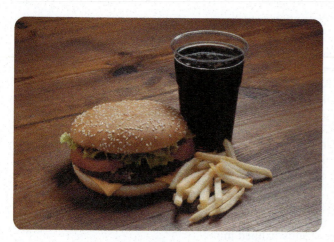

↟ Corn in the American diet doesn't always look like corn. The French fries are deep-fried in corn oil, the cola and bun are sweetened with high-fructose corn syrup, and corn is commonly used to feed beef cattle..

phytochemicals that support our health. Moreover, variety reduces the vulnerability of crops to pests; in contrast, monoculture farming requires heavier application of stronger pesticides. Similarly, because growing the same crop year after year depletes the soil of natural plant nutrients, monocultures require the application of heavy doses of synthetic fertilizers. Finally, different plants respond differently to variations in temperature, rainfall, and other climate conditions. Thus, agricultural variety decreases a region's vulnerability to dramatic food shortages during heat waves, droughts, or other climate events.

The loss of food diversity is not limited to the United States. A 2014 study found that, worldwide, over the past 50 years, national food supplies have become increasingly similar, based on a dwindling number of crop plants, and as a result, global food security is threatened.[30]

The Food Industry Influences America's Diet

When the preliminary report on the *2015–2020 Dietary Guidelines for Americans* was released early in 2015, it proposed to include in the final Guidelines a recommendation that Americans consume less red meat and processed meat. In response, meat industry lobbyists sprang into action, meeting with officials at the USDA and the Department of Health and Human Services (HHS) to request that the Guidelines recommend that Americans eat lean meats. The final Guidelines include seemingly conflicting messages about red and processed meats: one passage assures Americans unambiguously that they are part of a healthful eating pattern, whereas a different passage states that "lower intakes of meats as well as processed meats" are healthful.[31]

This influence of food industry lobbyists on the American diet is not an isolated incident. The Center for Responsive Politics reports the following spending on lobbying efforts by segments of the food industry in 2015:[32]

- Livestock: $2.9 million
- Dairy: $7 million
- Sugar: $10.3 million
- Food manufacturers: $18.3 million
- Beer, wine, and liquor: nearly $25 million

Large corporations, from McDonald's to Nestle, may spend $1 million or more annually. Similarly, individuals and political action committees associated with the food and beverage industries contributed almost $16.9 million to the 2014 campaign cycle.[32]

The food and beverage industries also spend considerable sums to influence voters directly. The soft drink industry, for example, has spent millions of dollars to try to block proposed taxes on sugary drinks in Philadelphia, San Francisco, Berkeley, and New York State. In all but Berkeley, the industry efforts succeeded.

In addition to lobbying, the food and beverage industries influence the American diet through advertising. For example, the Yale Rudd Center for Food Policy and Obesity reports that, in 2012, the fast-food industry spent over $4.6 billion to advertise their products, a figure which is more than 12 times higher than the costs for advertising spent on fruits, vegetables, milk, and bottled water combined.[33]

Marion Nestle, PhD, MPH, and professor of nutrition at New York University, points out that the bottom line is simple: The U.S. food industry produces about twice as many Calories per capita per year than Americans require; thus, to continue to make a profit, the industry must encourage consumers to overeat.[34]

recap Sustainability is the ability to satisfy humanity's basic needs now and in the future without undermining the natural resource base and environmental quality on which life depends. The Green Revolution, a set of innovations in agricultural technologies and practices, has vastly increased the global food supply. Its environmental costs include depletion and pollution of soils and water, the evolution of pesticide-resistant insects and weeds, and increased emissions of greenhouse gases. Industrial agriculture has also reduced food diversity and increased the vulnerability of our food supply to pests and climate events. The food industry spends billions of dollars annually on lobbying efforts, campaign contributions, advertising, and other efforts to influence America's diet.

What initiatives are addressing the challenges of "good" food?

LO 5 Discuss international, governmental, philanthropic, corporate, and local initiatives aimed at increasing the world's supply of and access to "good" food.

By now it should be clear that everyone, from world leaders to food-industry executives to farmers to consumers, plays a role in addressing the complex and interconnected challenges of ensuring everyone's access to "good" food. The UN acknowledges the efforts of "the international community, national governments, civil society, and the private sector" to eradicate global poverty and ensure universal access to ample, nourishing food.[35] Here, we address large-scale efforts to promote food security and sustainability. We'll discuss what you can do as an individual in the section that follows.

Many International Initiatives Increase Access to Nourishing Food

One of the most effective ways to improve the health and nutrition of children worldwide is to encourage breastfeeding. Breast milk not only provides optimal nutrition for healthy growth of the newborn but also contains antibodies that protect against infections. Moreover, infants who are breastfed exclusively are not exposed to the contaminants that may be present in local water and foods. In 1991, WHO and UNICEF initiated the Baby Friendly Hospital Initiative to increase breastfeeding rates worldwide. Under this initiative, new mothers are educated about the benefits of breast milk, and are encouraged to breastfeed exclusively for the first 6 months of the child's life and as part of the child's daily diet until the child is at least 2 years old.

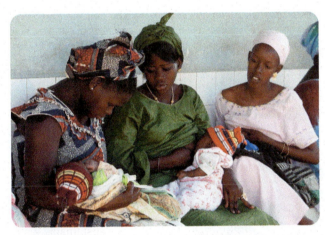

◀ Breastfeeding is highly recommended worldwide.

Breastfeeding is one step among many that can significantly reduce a child's risk for infectious disease. Another important step is supplementation with key micronutrients such as vitamin A, iron, zinc, iodine, and folic acid, all of which are important to the immune system. As part of an international Micronutrient Initiative (MI), the WHO and several other national and international organizations collaborate to provide such supplements to children in developing countries. In addition, programs for deworming and mosquito control combat helminth and malarial infections along with their accompanying iron deficiency.

During famines or other acute food shortages, for example as a result of natural disasters and wars, the United Nations World Food Programme delivers food and other emergency aid. It also helps communities develop new technologies and practices to reduce chronic food shortages and increase resilience in the face of challenging climate conditions. The United States and other nations also donate food and other emergency aid independently.

In addition, many international organizations help improve food security by assisting communities and families to produce their own foods. For example, both USAID and the Peace Corps have agricultural education programs, the World Bank provides loans to fund small business ventures, and many nonprofit and nongovernmental organizations (NGOs) support community and family farms and gardens.

National and Local Programs Help Nourish Americans

In the United States, several USDA programs help low-income citizens acquire food over extended periods of time. Among these are the SNAP benefits mentioned earlier, which provides an allotment to low-income individuals of all ages to purchase food. In addition, the Special Supplemental Nutrition Program for Women, Infants, and Children (WIC) helps pregnant women and children to age 5; the National School Lunch and National School Breakfast Programs provide low-income schoolchildren with free or low-cost meals; and the Summer Food Service Program provides meals to low-income children during the summer months.

The USDA's Commodity Supplemental Food Program distributes surplus foods to charitable agencies for distribution to low-income adults at least 60 years of age. The available items are typically limited to shelf-stable foods: canned fruits, vegetables, meats, and fish; dry beans, pasta, and rice and other grains; ready-to-eat cereals; peanut butter; and instant dry milk. Thus, the program is meant to supplement the fresh foods purchased by the individual.

Both federal health agencies and local governments can provide financial incentives to encourage markets selling fresh produce and other healthful foods to move into low-income areas, or to encourage stores already serving the area to offer more healthful foods. The CDC's Healthful Corner Stores initiative, for example, is helping communities from Philadelphia to Sacramento to invest in corner stores to increase city residents' access to healthy foods such as fresh produce. In addition, a new "urban agriculture" movement is helping to decrease the number of food deserts. Across the United States, city governments are changing zoning codes to encourage the cultivation of vegetable gardens on rooftops, in abandoned parking lots, and even as part of the landscaping on municipal properties.

The United States also has a broad network of local soup kitchens and food pantries that provide meals and food items to needy families. They are supported by volunteers, individual donations, and food contributions from local grocery stores and restaurants.

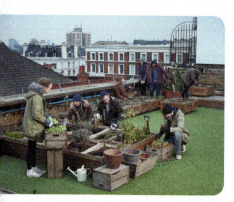

▲ Eagle Street Rooftop Farm is a 6,000-square foot organic vegetable garden located on top of a warehouse in Brooklyn, New York.

Sustainable Agriculture Reduces Environmental Impact and Increases Food Diversity

In response to the environmental problems and loss of food diversity associated with industrial agriculture, a new global movement toward **sustainable agriculture** has evolved. The goal of sustainable agriculture is to develop local, site-specific farming methods that improve soil conservation, crop yields, food security, and food diversity in a sustainable manner. For example, soil erosion can be controlled by **crop rotation**, by terracing sloped land for the cultivation of crops, and by tillage that minimizes disturbance to the topsoil. Organic farming is one method of sustainable agriculture, because to be certified organic, farms must commit to sustainable agricultural practices, including avoiding the use of synthetic fertilizers and toxic and persistent pesticides. Organic meats are produced without the use of antibiotics and hormones for animal growth. Sustainable agriculture also promotes the use of otherwise unusable plants for high-quality animal feed, recycles animal wastes for fertilizers and fuel, and practices humane treatment of animals.

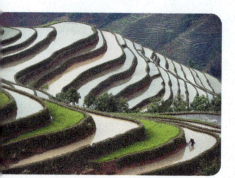

▲ Terracing sloped land to avoid soil erosion is one practice of sustainable agriculture.

The sustainable agriculture movement has led to an increase in family farms and a variety of farming programs, some of which you probably recognize:

- *Family farms.* For three decades, the number of farms in the United States has been decreasing, from 2.48 million in 1982 to 2.11 million in 2012.[26] However, since 2007, the number of small farms (1 to 9 acres) has not declined, and in some states, mainly in New England and the Southwest, they have increased. Some small farmers are taking advantage of programs offering land at reduced prices, community support, and mentoring. Many of these small farms are dedicated to organic farming, crop diversity, and other practices of sustainable agriculture.
- *Community supported agriculture (CSA).* In CSA programs, a farmer sells a certain number of "shares" to the public. Shares typically consist of a box of produce from the farm on a regular basis, such as once weekly throughout the growing season. Farmers get cash early on, as well as guaranteed buyers. Consumers get fresh, locally grown food. Together, farmers and consumers develop ongoing relationships as they share the bounty in a good year, and the losses when weather

sustainable agriculture Term referring to techniques of food production that preserve the environment indefinitely.

crop rotation The practice of alternating crops in a particular field to prevent nutrient depletion and erosion of the soil and to help with control of crop-specific pests.

extremes or blight reduces yield. Although there is no national database on CSA programs, the organization LocalHarvest lists over 4,000.[36]

- *Farmers markets.* There are now more than 8,400 farmers markets in the United States, more than four times the number when the USDA began compiling these data in 1994.[37] With the help of the USDA, many farmers markets are now able to accept SNAP benefits for payment. Thus, farmers markets are helping to increase everyone's access to nourishing food.

- *School gardens.* The School Garden Association of America was founded in 1910, and during World Wars I and II, school gardening became part of the war effort; however, in the postwar decades, school gardens dwindled. Recently, school garden programs have been increasing across the United States. In addition to introducing students to a variety of fruits and vegetables and promoting their acceptance, school garden programs teach valuable lessons in nutrition, agriculture, and even cooking. In many schools, cafeterias incorporate the foods into the school lunch menu.

- *Slow food.* Experts in sustainable agriculture and public health are increasingly challenging our loss of food quality and diversity by advocating "slow food"; that is, nutritious, fresh food produced in ways that preserve biodiversity, sustain the environment, ensure animal welfare, and are affordable by all while respecting the dignity of labor from field to fork.[38] Slow food, to the extent possible, is locally grown, a term that typically refers to food grown within a few hundred miles of the consumer. Although growing a healthful variety of local food from fall through spring is not possible in cold climates, consuming local food when available limits energy use and greenhouse gas emissions from transportation (so-called "food miles"). Also, because these foods move much more quickly from farm to table, they tend to be fresher, retaining more of their micronutrients.

Find a farmers market near you! Go to the USDA's Agricultural Marketing Service home page at http://www.ams.usda.gov. Type "National Farmers Market Directory" in the search bar to get started.

Corporate and Philanthropic Initiatives Are Promoting "Good" Food

Many individuals and venture capital firms are now investing in food technologies dedicated to increasing food security and preserving human health and the environment. Howard Buffett, son of investor Warren Buffett, is supporting no-till farming, crop rotation, and other techniques of sustainable agriculture to help relieve food insecurity in Africa, whereas philanthropist Bill Gates is supporting companies producing vegan versions of chicken, eggs, and other high-protein foods. Other investors are funding indoor agricultural growing systems that do not require soil, food-waste recycling programs, crop monitoring systems that identify specific pests and reduce the random use of pesticides, and services that bring fresh produce from local farms directly to consumers' doors.

Whereas many smaller natural-food companies have long made "good" food part of their company identity, only recently has this goal moved into corporate America. In the past few years, Walmart, Kellogg's, McDonald's, and several other corporations have begun to partner with local growers to promote sustainable agriculture, and in 2016, Walmart modestly increased their workers' minimum wage to $10 per hour.

recap Programs encouraging breastfeeding and providing micronutrient supplementation can significantly improve children's nutrition and reduce their risk for infectious disease. The World Food Programme and other efforts provide emergency food aid and support for investments in long-term food security. In the United States, SNAP, the Commodity Supplemental Food Program, the Healthy Corner Stores initiative, and many other national and local programs help increase access for low-income Americans to nourishing food. The goal of sustainable agriculture is to develop local, site-specific farming methods that improve soil conservation, crop yields, food security, and food diversity in a sustainable manner. Some of its more familiar efforts are organic farming, farmers markets, school gardens, and slow food. Individual investors and corporations are beginning to support or implement initiatives aimed at increasing the equity, sustainability, and quality of America's food.

How can you promote "good" food?

This chapter has reviewed only a handful of the thousands of local to global initiatives comprising the so-called "food movement," in which millions of ordinary consumers are involved. Here, we review some simple steps you can take to join them.

Support Food Security

Have you ever wondered whether efforts you make locally can help feed people thousands of miles away? Let's take a look.

Eating just the Calories you need to maintain a healthful weight leaves more of the global harvest for others and will also likely reduce your use of medical resources. So to raise your consciousness about the physical experience of hunger, try turning off your cell phone and other devices and keeping silent during each meal for a day, so that you can more fully appreciate the food you're eating and reflect on those who are hungry. Also check in with your body before and as you eat: are you really hungry, and if so, how much and what type of food does your body really need right now?

Try to stay aware of how much food you throw away, and ask yourself why. Do you put more food on your plate than you can eat? Do you purchase more food than you can eat and as a result, allow foods stored in your refrigerator to spoil?

Join a community garden or shared farming program, with the goal of donating a portion of your produce each week to a local food pantry. While you're there, consider volunteering to help!

Donate to or raise money for one of the international agencies that work to relieve global hunger. Or join other students fighting food insecurity in the United States by becoming a member of the National Student Campaign Against Hunger and Homelessness. Visit www.studentsagainsthunger.org to learn more. The hungry people you work to help might be closer than you think. A recent study of over 4,000 community college students found that, in the previous 30 days, 22% had gone hungry because of lack of money.[39] One way to help such students is to advocate for an on-campus food bank. Contact the College and University Food Bank Alliance for more information, at www.cufba.org.

Whatever you do, get the word out! If you find an organization whose goals you share, recommend them on your social networking page. Or send a short article about the organization's work to your campus news site, with suggestions about how other students can support their work.

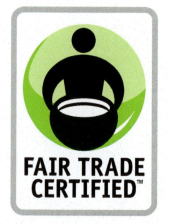

▲ **FIGURE 13.3** The Fair Trade Certified logo guarantees that the product has been produced equitably without exploitation of workers or the environment.

fair trade A trading partnership promoting equity in international trading relationships and contributing to sustainable development by securing the rights of marginalized producers and workers.

Purchase Fair Trade Goods

The **fair trade** movement was born in response to the exploitation of farm laborers around the world. It began decades ago in North America and Europe, and has become a global effort that depends on support from consumers worldwide to purchase fruits, vegetables, coffee, tea, cocoa, wine, and many other products that display the Fair Trade Certified logo[40] **(FIGURE 13.3)**. Fair trade empowers farm laborers to demand living wages and humane treatment. It also reduces child labor and increases children's access to education, because parents earning higher wages are able to allow their children to leave the fields and attend school. Profits from fair trade purchases also support the building of schools and health clinics, provide funds to help farmers adopt sustainable agricultural practices, and provide financial assistance to women so they can set up small businesses.[40]

The choices you make when you shop can contribute to food equity, because your purchases influence local and global markets. To support equitable production worldwide, purchase Fair Trade goods whenever possible, whether at your grocery store or shopping online. The Fair Trade USA website has a handy shopping guide where you can check out what's available, from hundreds of brands of coffee to chocolate, produce, and even fair trade clothing!

Choose Foods That Are Healthful for You and the Environment

Any grocery store manager will tell you that your purchases influence the types of foods that are manufactured and sold. In our global economy, your food choices can even influence the types of foods that are imported. So to the extent that you can:

- Buy organic foods to reduce the use of synthetic pesticides and fertilizers.
- Buy produce from a local farmers market to encourage greater local availability of fresh foods. This reduces the costs and resources devoted to distribution, transportation, and storage of foods.
- Choose whole or less processed versions of packaged foods. This encourages their increased production and saves energy.
- Look to see if your grocery store displays candy and other junk foods at children's eye level—for example, beside the check-out line. If it does, complain to the store manager.
- Avoid empty-Calorie foods and beverages when you're shopping and eating out to discourage their profitability.
- When you eat at a fast-food restaurant, ask for information about the nutritional value of their menu items. Analyze the information. If you see aspects that concern you, take a few minutes to send the company an email sharing your concerns and asking for improved recipes.

In a recent national survey, 33% of college students said that their finances were "traumatic or difficult to handle."[41] If you're one of them, you might be concerned that purchasing organic, local, and whole foods is beyond your budget. If so, you should know that healthful eating doesn't always have to be expensive. Some of the lowest-cost foods currently available in stores are also some of the most nutritious. To find them, check out the **Quick Tips** on this page.

QuickTips

Spending Less to Eat Right

✔ Buy whole grains, such as cereals, brown rice, and pastas in bulk—they store well for longer periods and provide a good base for meals and snacks.

✔ Buy fresh fruits and vegetables in season; otherwise, buy them frozen. They're just as healthful as fresh vegetables, require less preparation, and are typically cheaper.

✔ If lower-sodium options of canned beans and other vegetables are more expensive, buy the less expensive regular option and drain the juice from the vegetables before cooking.

✔ Consume leaner meats in smaller amounts—by eating less, you'll not only save money but reduce the environmental costs of your meal while still obtaining the nutrients that support good health.

✔ Choose frozen fish or canned salmon or tuna packed in water as an alternative to fresh fish.

✔ Avoid frozen or dehydrated prepared meals. They are usually expensive; high in sodium, saturated fats, and energy; and low in fiber and important nutrients.

✔ Buy generic or store brands of foods—be careful to check the labels to ensure that the foods are similar in nutrient value to the higher-priced options.

✔ Cut coupons from local newspapers and magazines, and watch the sale circulars, so that you can stock up on healthful foods you can store.

✔ Consider cooking more meals at home; you'll have more control over what goes into your meals and you'll be able to cook larger amounts and freeze leftovers for future meals.

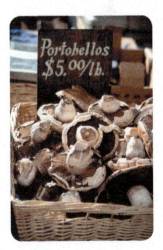

Some specialty foods (such as organic or imported products) can be expensive, but lower-cost alternatives can be just as nutritious.

The amount of meat you eat also affects the environment and the global food supply, because the production of plant-based foods uses fewer natural resources and releases fewer greenhouse gases than the production of animal-based foods. To promote reduced meat consumption on campus, talk with your food services manager about sponsoring "Meatless Mondays." See the **Web Links** for a link to the Meatless Monday website, where you can download a *Meatless Monday Goes to College* toolkit. For more information on the link between meat production and climate change, see the **Nutrition Debate** on the following page.

Pay attention to packaging. As we discussed in Chapter 7, plastics often end up in landfills or as ocean debris. Moreover, their manufacture uses energy and releases greenhouse gases. So resist the urge to purchase a six-pack of bottled water, and purchase a reusable stainless steel or other BPA-free water bottle instead. If you don't like the taste of tap water, install an inexpensive carbon filter on your faucet to improve the taste. In general, purchase foods with the least packaging possible. For instance, skip the bakery products in plastic trays, purchase milk in cartons instead of plastic, and get your take-out from restaurants that use paper containers instead of polystyrene (Styrofoam) or other types of plastic. You won't be able to entirely avoid purchasing foods in plastic packaging, of course, so make it a habit to recycle those you do buy. Finally, carry your food purchases home in your own washable canvas bags.

You know that physical activity is important in maintaining health, but walking, biking, and taking public transportation also limit your consumption of nonrenewable fossil fuels and the emission of greenhouse gases. When it's time to purchase a car, research your options and choose the one with the best fuel economy. With the recent fall in gas prices, the price of many electric vehicles has been falling, too. But electric vehicles aren't your only option, as fuel economy has been improving on traditional vehicles for years. To research the average miles-per-gallon on a new or used car you're considering, visit the U.S. Department of Energy's www.fueleconomy.gov.

As Francis Moore Lappe, author of the groundbreaking *Diet for a Small Planet*, explains, the food movement encourages us to think with an "eco-mind," refusing to accept scarcity, oppression, pollution, and depletion of natural resources in the name of production and profit. By promoting the values of equity, sustainability, and quality, the food movement encourages us to make choices in ways that can positively change our world.[42]

recap Increasing your awareness of your own food cues and food waste can help motivate you to make choices that reduce your use of resources. Consider donating to or volunteering for a food relief organization, or advocating for a food bank on campus. Make fair trade purchases whenever possible, and when you're shopping for food, eating at your campus dining hall, or eating out, choose and request healthful foods. Consider eating vegetarian meals at least one day a week, reduce your purchases of foods in plastic packaging, and walk, bike, or take public transportation as often as possible.

The surge in the world's population has been accompanied by increased meat consumption, particularly in nations transitioning out of poverty. In the United States, we consumed 24.1 billion pounds of beef in 2014.[43] Why is this a concern?

According to the Food and Agricultural Organization of the United Nations, globally, livestock production generates 18% of the greenhouse gases (GHGs) responsible for global warming.[44] These GHGs include not only carbon dioxide (CO_2), but methane (CH_4), which livestock release through belching, flatulence, and their manure. The global-warming potential of CH_4 is 23 times greater than that of CO_2 over a 100-year period.[44]

Other emissions of concern in livestock production are reactive nitrogen compounds (Nr), which have nearly 300 times the global warming potential of CO_2[44] and contribute to smog and acid rain, damaging crops and decreasing biodiversity.

So precisely how different are emissions from beef versus plant foods? One of the most recent studies to tackle this question found that beef production releases 5 to 6 times more GHGs than the average of four other animal-based foods (pork, poultry, eggs, and dairy).[45] However, as compared to the average of three plant-based foods (wheat, potatoes, and rice), the emissions from beef production are far greater (FIGURE 13.4).

The Cattlemen's Beef Board and National Cattlemen's Beef Association website offers a different perspective.[46] They state that GHGs released by U.S. beef production represent 3% of all U.S. GHG emissions, versus 26% for transportation. Still, comparing cows to cars may be more distracting than helpful. We choose what to eat several times a day, and each of these choices can either contribute to or help mitigate climate change.

In addition to being a major source of GHG emissions, livestock production contributes to land degradation, using 30% of the earth's land surface for pasture or feed production.[47] The analysis mentioned earlier found that beef production uses 28 times more land than non-meat animal foods and 160 times more land than plant foods.[45] This loss has global effects, as it reduces the capture of CO_2 performed by plants during photosynthesis. Livestock's presence in vast tracts of land and its demand for feed crops also have contributed significantly to a reduction in biodiversity and a decline in ecosystems.

Another environmental concern is the effect of livestock production on the global water supply. Beef production uses 11 times more water than non-meat animal foods and 8 times more water than plant foods.[45] Moreover, animal waste can run off into neighboring waterways and onto irrigation fields used to produce crops for human consumption.

Although some individuals choose vegetarianism to protect the environment, it is not practical or realistic to expect every human around the world to adopt this lifestyle. Animal products provide important nutrients: the beef industry website points out that a 3-ounce serving of beef supplies 51% of the Daily Value (DV) for protein, 38% of the DV for zinc, and 14% of the DV for iron.[46]

Still, if most Americans were to reduce their consumption of meat even modestly, the change would have a powerful collective impact. A 2014 study of the contribution of a variety of 2,000 kcal diets to climate change concluded that reducing meat consumption could "make a valuable contribution to climate change mitigation."[48] Moreover, as we noted earlier in this chapter, replacing meat with plant proteins would improve food security because, Calorie for Calorie, growing crops for human consumption rather than conversion to meat is much more efficient.

As researchers debate the precise extent of environmental harm attributable to meat consumption, one thing is clear: You can help reduce the damage, starting with your next meal.

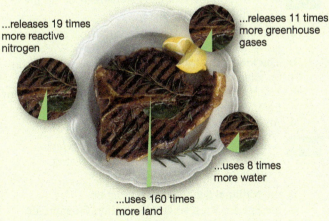

1,000 kcal of beef...

...releases 19 times more reactive nitrogen

...releases 11 times more greenhouse gases

...uses 8 times more water

...uses 160 times more land

● ...than 1,000 kcal of plant foods
(wheat, potatoes, rice)

⬆ **FIGURE 13.4** Comparison of resource use and emissions for beef versus plant foods.

Source: Data from Eshel, G., A. Shepon, T. Makov, and R. Milo. 2014. Land, irrigation water, greenhouse gas, and reactive nitrogen burdens of meat, eggs, and dairy production in the United States. *PNAS* 111(33):11996–12001. doi:10.1073/pnas.1402183111

CRITICAL THINKING QUESTIONS

1. Given the accelerated pace of climate change, as well as land and water degradation, do we have an ethical responsibility to others with whom we share the planet, especially children, to reduce our consumption of meat?

2. What adverse impact might reducing meat consumption have on farmers and ranchers? Would this be greater or worse than the impact of climate change?

3. Would eating less meat be practical for you? Why or why not?

1 T In 2014, the most recent year for which data is available, 5.6% of U.S. households experienced very low food security, meaning that at least some members of those households reduced food intake because of insufficient money or other resources.

2 F The occupational fatality rate for U.S. farm workers is seven times higher than the average for workers in other industries.

3 F Methane emissions are 23 times more potent greenhouse gases than carbon dioxide. In the United States, beef production alone is responsible for 18% of all methane emissions.

review questions

LO 1 **1.** Which of the following statements about food insecurity is true?

a. Between 1990–92 and 2014–16, the share of undernourished people worldwide fell by nearly 45%.
b. About 64% of the world's hungry people live in Africa.
c. About 14% of U.S. children experience hunger.
d. The greatest prevalence of very low food security in the U.S. is in inner cities in the Northeast.

LO 2 **2.** The leading cause of longstanding hunger in a region is

a. famine.
b. war.
c. unequal distribution of food, largely because of poverty.
d. overpopulation.

LO 3 **3.** Which of the following statements about food system labor is true?

a. In many states in the United States, grocery store cashiers may lawfully be paid just $2.13 an hour.
b. A majority of contingent farm workers in the United States live below the poverty line.
c. On average, nearly 100 workers die each year from farm-labor injuries in the United States.
d. About 1 out of every 50 full-time workers in the United States receives government assistance.

LO 4 **4.** Which of the following statements about the Green Revolution is true?

a. It has increased global production of organic foods.
b. It has dramatically increased food security throughout South America, Asia, and Africa.
c. It has ended the loss of topsoil that had been common with traditional farming methods.
d. It has reduced the depletion and pollution of ground water.

LO 4 **5.** Which of the following statements about the food industry is true?

a. The only crop that U.S. farmers receive subsidies to grow is corn.
b. The food industry spends about $4.6 billion a year on advertising.
c. The U.S. food industry produces about twice as many Calories per capita per year than Americans require.
d. All of the above are true.

LO 5 **6.** Of the following federal programs, which provides food assistance to low-income individuals of all ages?

a. the National School Lunch Program
b. the Special Supplemental Nutrition Program for Women, Infants, and Children
c. the Commodity Supplemental Food Program
d. the Supplemental Nutrition Assistance Program (SNAP)

LO 6 7. Which of the following purchases would optimally support food equity, sustainability, and quality?

a. a fair trade certified t-shirt
b. a bottle of cherry soda you buy at a farmers market
c. a certified organic beef burger on a whole-grain bun from an organic foods restaurant
d. a pint of strawberries you pick yourself at an organic farm

LO 1 8. **True or false?** Adults over age 65 years are at greatest risk for food insecurity in the United States.

LO 3 9. **True or false?** The blackberries on your morning cereal could have been harvested by a 12-year-old.

LO 5 10. **True or false?** Crop rotation and terracing are farming methods used in sustainable agriculture.

math review

LO 3 11. In the Rodgers family, Steve works 40 hours a week, all year, at a fast-food restaurant. He earns the federal minimum wage of $7.25. He has one week of paid vacation a year. Steve and his wife, Diane, have struggled to make ends meet since the birth of their son, now 5 months old, so Diane has decided to return to work at the same fast-food restaurant where her husband works. They have decided to stagger their schedules in order to avoid the cost of daycare for their son. The federal poverty threshold in 2016 was $20,160 for a family of three. Answer these questions: Are Steve, Diane, and their son currently living above, at, or below the federal poverty line? If Diane were to return to work 40 hours a week, would the family be characterized as at increased risk for food insecurity? Why or why not?

Answers to Review Questions can be found online in the MasteringNutrition Study Area.

web links

www2.epa.gov/learn-issues/green-living
Environmental Protection Agency's Sustainability Tips
This site offers a wide variety of tips and tools to help you reduce your environmental footprint.

www.freefromhunger.org
Freedom from Hunger
Visit this site to learn about an established international development organization, founded in 1946, that works toward sustainable self-help against chronic hunger and poverty.

www.fooddemocracynow.org
Food Democracy Now
Visit this grassroots community dedicated to building a sustainable, equitable food system.

www.slowfoodusa.org/
Slow Food USA
Slow Food links the pleasure of growing, preparing, and consuming food with commitment to our communities and environment. Visit this site to learn more about the slow food movement and get involved.

www.fairtradeusa.org
Fair Trade USA
Visit this website to find out why "Every Purchase Matters!"

www.meatlessmonday.com/
Meatless Monday
This website offers information on the environmental and health benefits of going meatless one day a week, as well as recipes for vegetarian meals and a toolkit to promote Meatless Mondays on your campus.

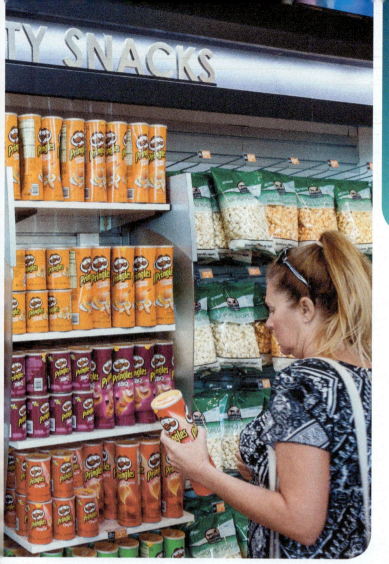

Malnutrition

Hailey knows she should eat more fresh fruits and vegetables, but she doesn't have a car, and the nearest grocery store is several miles away, over busy roads without sidewalks. Besides, she tells herself, even if she took the bus there, she wouldn't be able to afford fresh produce. The few dollars in her purse have to last until the end of the month. And she's running out of her blood pressure medication, and owes her landlord last month's rent. Still, she's hungry. So she walks two blocks to a corner store where she purchases a steamed hot dog and a large bag of corn chips.

Why would someone with very little money purchase foods that are not nutritious? Why are so many of the world's poor—whether they live in developing nations or the United States—obese?

We begin this **In Depth** essay by discussing the broad range of health and societal problems linked to undernourishment, the most dramatic form of malnutrition. We then explore a variety of theories attempting to explain the troubling link between obesity and limited access to nourishing food.

learning outcomes

After studying this In Depth, you should be able to:

1 Describe the health and societal problems associated with undernourishment, pp. 481–483.

2 Explain how obesity can result from limited access to nourishing food, pp. 483–485.

What problems are linked to undernourishment?

LO 1 Describe the health and societal problems associated with undernourishment.

Undernourishment may mean that an individual is unable to consume adequate energy to maintain weight and physiologic functioning; or the individual may consume enough energy, but experience deficiencies of one or more nutrients. In some cases, especially in wealthier nations, limited access to nourishing foods can actually promote simultaneous obesity and deficiency—in an individual who has an excessive intake of high-energy, nutrient-poor foods.

Low Energy Intake Promotes Wasting, Stunting, and Mortality

About 51 million children worldwide don't weigh enough for their height.[1] This is because they suffer from **severe acute malnutrition (SAM)**, a condition in which energy intake is so inadequate that the child experiences **wasting**, a lower than expected body weight. Approximately 161 million of the world's children also experience **stunted growth**; they are shorter than expected for their age.[1] Stunting occurs when energy intake or specific nutrients are inadequate to sustain normal linear growth. In some impoverished communities, the great majority of residents are very short and small; thus, community members may not perceive their stunted growth as unusual or recognize it as a sign of chronic undernourishment.

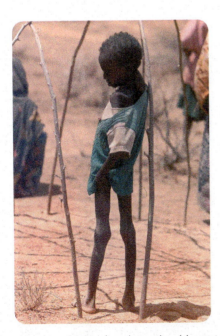

◀ Wasting (extreme thinness) and stunting (short stature for age) are commonly seen in undernourished children.

SAM also dramatically increases a population's rate of **maternal mortality** (deaths of a woman during pregnancy, childbirth, or in the immediate postpartal period) and **infant mortality** (the death of infants between birth and 1 year). For example, the infant mortality rate in industrialized countries of Western Europe ranges from about 2 to 5 per 1,000, whereas in Afghanistan and Mali, two of the world's poorest countries, the infant mortality rate is more than 100 per 1,000.[2]

Worldwide, 43 of every 1,000 children die before reaching age 5. About 45% of these deaths of young children are due to malnutrition.[3] Decreased resistance to infection as a result of undernourishment is a leading factor in these deaths.[3] Protein and many micronutrients are essential to an effective immune response; therefore, in undernourished children, infections occur more frequently and take longer to resolve. These prolonged infections exacerbate malnutrition by decreasing appetite, causing vomiting and diarrhea, producing weight loss, and further weakening the immune system. A vicious cycle of malnutrition, infection, worsening malnutrition, and increased vulnerability to infection develops. **FIGURE 1** (page 482) summarizes the effects of SAM throughout the life cycle.

Micronutrient Deficiencies Lead to Preventable Diseases

In impoverished countries, micronutrient deficiencies are major public health concerns. These are some of the most severe:

- Iron deficiency is the most common micronutrient deficiency in the world.[4] Although it occurs in both males and females of all ages, it is more prevalent in pregnant women and young children because of the demands of fetal and childhood growth. Iron-deficiency anemia contributes to 20% of maternal deaths.
- Prenatal iodine intake is particularly important for fetal brain development, and severe iodine deficiency is the single largest cause of preventable mental

---

severe acute malnutrition (SAM) A state of severe energy deficit defined as a weight for height more than 3 standard deviations below the mean, or the presence of nutrition-related edema.

wasting A physical condition of very low body-weight-for-height or extreme thinness.

stunted growth A condition of shorter stature than expected for chronological age, often defined as 2 or more standard deviations below the mean reference value.

maternal mortality A population's rate of deaths of a woman during pregnancy, childbirth, or in the immediate postpartal period.

infant mortality A population's rate of death of infants between birth and 1 year of age.

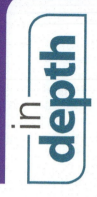

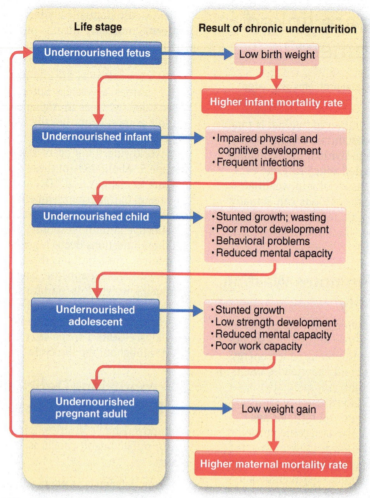

FIGURE 1 Acute and long-term effects of chronic undernourishment throughout the life cycle.

impairment worldwide. Nearly a third of the world's population is iodine deficient.[5] Iodine-deficiency disorders have largely been eliminated in areas of the world with access to iodized salt or oil, and areas where iodine is added to irrigation water.

■ Vitamin A deficiency is the leading cause of blindness in children.[4] An estimated 250 million children worldwide are vitamin A deficient. In addition, because vitamin A supports immune function, these children are highly vulnerable to severe, often fatal infections. The WHO and other global health agencies provide vitamin A supplements, promote breastfeeding, and support family and community vegetable gardens. These efforts have reduced mortality by 23%.[4]

Undernourishment Promotes Socioeconomic Problems

Undernourishment has long been known to diminish work capacity. Iodine, vitamin B_{12}, folate, certain essential fatty acids, and many other nutrients contribute to the development and maintenance of a healthy nervous system; thus,

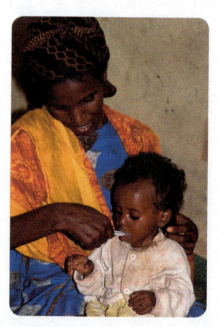

In developing nations, providing vitamin A supplements twice a year to children under age 5 has significantly reduced mortality.

nutri-case | LIZ

"It was really hard spending last summer with my parents, because we kept arguing over food! Even though I'd told them that I'm a vegetarian, they kept serving meals with meat! Then they'd get mad when I'd fix myself a hummus sandwich! When it was my turn to cook, I made lentils with brown rice, whole-wheat pasta primavera, vegetarian curries, and lots of other yummy meals, but my dad kept insisting, 'You have to eat meat or you won't get enough iron!' I told him that plant foods have lots of iron, but he wouldn't listen. Was I ever glad to get back onto campus this fall!"

Recall that Liz is a ballet dancer who trains daily. If she eats a vegetarian diet including meals such as the ones she describes here, will she be at risk for iron deficiency? Why or why not? Are there any other micronutrients that might be low in Liz's diet because she avoids meat? If so, what are they? Overall, will Liz get enough energy to support her high level of physical activity on a vegetarian diet? How would she know if she were low energy?

undernourishment—especially during fetal development, infancy, and early childhood—can permanently reduce cognitive functioning and an individual's ability to contribute to a community's economy. Similarly, the vision loss caused by vitamin A deficiency can severely limit an individual's work capacity.

Inadequate energy intake and micronutrient deficiency can also prompt debilitating weakness, which is especially detrimental when manual labor is the main source of income. The reduced earning capacity of poor, undernourished adults often regenerates a cycle of poverty onto the next generation. Iron-deficiency anemia is particularly debilitating because of iron's role in oxygen transport. Because iron deficiency is a problem among women of childbearing age in both developed and developing countries, it is a global drain on work capacity and productivity.

How could limited access to good food promote obesity?

LO 2 Explain how obesity can result from limited access to nourishing food.

Throughout the world, the prevalence of obesity is increasing at an alarming rate and, along with it, obesity-related chronic diseases. The WHO estimates that the worldwide prevalence of obesity more than doubled between 1980 and 2014. Currently, 1.9 billion people worldwide are overweight, and 600 million of these are obese. Moreover, overweight and obesity are now linked to more deaths worldwide than underweight.[6]

Obesity used to be considered a disease of affluence, but in recent decades, public health researchers have observed an increasing prevalence of obesity in impoverished communities. If food is still scarce in many developing nations, how has the global rate of obesity more than doubled? And if an individual is poor and undernourished, how could he or she also be obese? Let's explore these two paradoxes.

A Nutrition Paradox Is Evident in Transitioning Populations

The **nutrition paradox** is characterized by the coexistence of stunting and overweight/obesity within the same region, the same household, and even the same person. People born in developing nations who were undernourished when young are likely to be short (due to growth stunting) but experience rapid weight gain when their country transitions out of poverty. The nutrition paradox is especially common in China, India, Mexico, and South America. In Colombia, for example, 5% of households have both an overweight or obese mother and a stunted child, and in Ecuador, researchers found that 2.8% of children nationwide exhibited both stunting and overweight or obesity.[7,8]

The WHO identifies two key factors behind the nutrition paradox in transitioning nations:[6]

A trend toward decreased physical activity due to the increasingly sedentary nature of many forms of work, changing modes of transportation, and increasing urbanization.
A global shift toward increased consumption of energy-dense foods high in saturated fats and added sugars but low in micronutrients and fiber.

In effect, all nations have been exposed to a nutritional transition over the past 30 years, as international food companies have made processed, energy-dense foods available at lower cost to more people worldwide.

Another factor contributing to the nutrition paradox may be poor nutrition in previous generations in a population. Maternal undernourishment certainly affects the mother's offspring *in utero*, but researchers are increasingly convinced that the effect continues throughout childhood, into adulthood, and probably into succeeding generations.

---

nutrition paradox The coexistence of aspects of both stunting and overweight/obesity within the same region, household, family, or person.

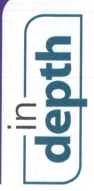

This "fetal origins of adult disease" theory proposes that biological adjustments to poor maternal nutrition made by a malnourished fetus as its organs are developing may be helpful to the child during times of food shortages, but make the child susceptible to obesity and chronic disease when food is plentiful. For example, when a mother is malnourished during the pregnancy, her baby will tend to have a low birth weight but be relatively fat. This occurs because the fetal body preserves fat tissue as a source of energy for growth of the brain; as a result, muscle tissue is reduced. The imbalance promotes abdominal adiposity and metabolic disease later in life; there is now significant evidence supporting this theory. (See the In Depth essay following Chapter 14, pages 524–527, for a detailed discussion of this theory.)

These effects can also be passed on to future generations when affected children of the current generation grow up and start their own families. For this reason, immigrants to richer nations and the poor in developing nations may need four or more generations of improved conditions to overcome all past risks for both short stature and overweight.

Physical and Socioeconomic Factors May Promote Obesity Among the Poor

Could poverty be an independent risk factor for obesity? Even among established (non-immigrant) populations in developed nations, some research has suggested a **poverty–obesity paradox** in which obesity is more prevalent in low-income populations. In the United States, for example, studies following children over time have found that a reduction in family income during early childhood increases the child's risk for becoming overweight or obese, whereas a shift to a higher family income increases the likelihood of weight loss.[9,10] Some researchers have also observed a so-called *hunger–obesity paradox*, in which low-income people are obese while also deficient in one or more nutrients, and in some cases even hungry. For example, the studies in Columbia and Ecuador cited earlier found an increased prevalence of iron-deficiency anemia in impoverished households whose members were also overweight or obese.

What factors could explain these associations? Research is inconclusive, but several hypotheses are being studied. One of the most common hypotheses proposes that low-income people purchase energy-dense foods with longer shelf lives, such as vegetable oils, sugar, refined flour, snack foods, soft drinks, and canned goods, because they are less expensive than perishable foods such as meats, fish, milk, and fresh fruits and vegetables. Choosing such inexpensive, shelf-stable foods may be an important money-saving strategy especially for the rural poor.

A second hypothesis suggests that individuals with limited money to spend are more likely to purchase low-cost, high-volume, energy-dense foods high in carbohydrates and fats, and low in protein. An adequate level of protein intake triggers the body's satiety mechanisms. Thus, in order to reach satiety, individuals who choose cheap foods low in protein end up consuming more total Calories than they would if they were to consume foods higher in protein.[11,12]

Third, the link between obesity and poverty might be explained in part by stress. That is, the stress of having insufficient resources to meet day-to-day expenses results in chronic release of stress hormones—such as cortisol—that slow metabolism and increase appetite, while simultaneously prompting short-sighted decision-making.[13,14] Moreover, some research suggests that self-control itself is a limited resource. People who must continually make difficult economic decisions may "deplete" their ability to make thoughtful, healthful decisions around eating.[15] Thus, the person may be more likely to overeat or eat empty-Calorie "comfort foods." A recent study also suggests that sugar may be particularly appealing to people experiencing chronic stress: Sugar consumption appears to trigger a negative feedback loop that "turns off" the stress response, prompting a measurable decrease in cortisol levels. In other words, for people under stress, sugar may be calming.[16]

Fourth, low-income people's high rates of obesity may reflect their environment. Many obese people live in so-called **food deserts**, defined by the USDA as geographic areas where people lack access to fresh, healthful, and affordable food.[17] Rural food deserts may have no access to any foods, whereas inner-city food deserts may be served only by fast food restaurants and convenience stores that offer few healthful options. A recent study of more than 18,000 U.S. households in 2,100 counties found a significant association between residence in a food desert and prevalence of obesity, even when controlling for other factors such as the food environment within the home.[18] The USDA's Economic Research Service estimates that 23.5 million Americans live in food

Do you live in a food desert? Go to the USDA site, http://ams.usda.gov/ and type in "food desert" in the search box to find out!

---

poverty–obesity paradox The high prevalence of obesity in low-income populations.

food desert A geographic area where people lack access to fresh, healthful, and affordable food.

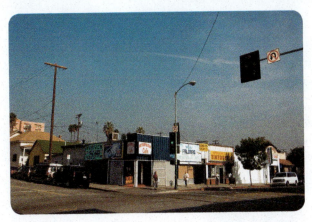

↑ "Food deserts" are geographic areas where people lack access to affordable, nutritious food, typically because of an absence of grocery stores.

deserts.[17] More than half of those people (13.5 million) are low-income. Living in a food desert might limit not only options for nourishing food but also options for physical activity; that is, a neighborhood that is separated from the nearest supermarket by freeways is also likely to have low walkability.[15]

In summary, then, although not all factors contributing to the coincidence of poverty and obesity are entirely clear, there is now substantial evidence of a global burden of overweight and obesity among the poor.

web links

www.care.org
Care

Since 1945, this organization has been working to relieve hunger and improve economic conditions around the world.

www.feedingamerica.org
Feeding America

Visit this site to learn more about hunger and poverty in the United States, and click on Map the Meal Gap to find levels of food insecurity in your state and county.

www.unicef.org/nutrition
United Nations Children's Fund

Visit this site to learn about international concerns affecting the world's children, including nutrient deficiencies and hunger.

www.who.int/nutrition/en
World Health Organization Nutrition

Visit this site to learn about global malnutrition, micronutrient deficiencies, and the nutrition transition.

www.ers.usda.gov
Economic Research Service

The ERS plays a leading role in research into food insecurity in the United States. Visit their page entitled Food Security in the U.S. for annual updates and related reports.

endseniorhunger.aarp.org
AARP Drive to End Hunger Campaign

Visit this site and click on the Recent Research tab to access AARP's report on food insecurity among older Americans.

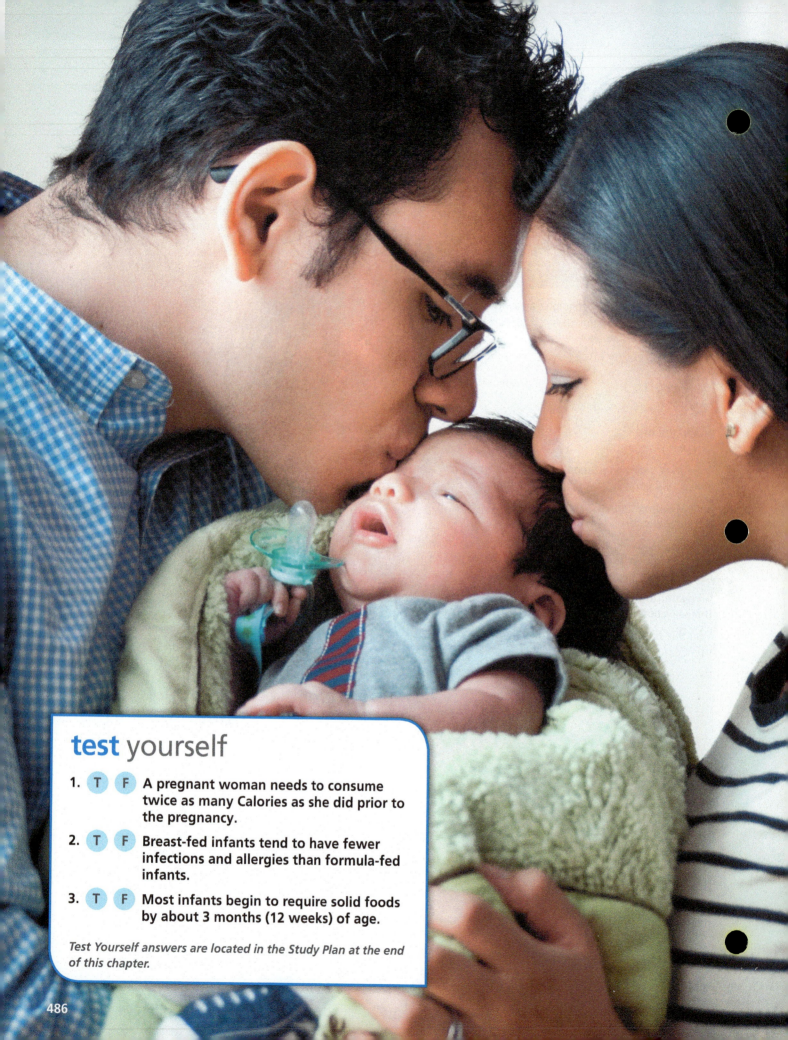

test yourself

1. **T** **F** A pregnant woman needs to consume twice as many Calories as she did prior to the pregnancy.

2. **T** **F** Breast-fed infants tend to have fewer infections and allergies than formula-fed infants.

3. **T** **F** Most infants begin to require solid foods by about 3 months (12 weeks) of age.

Test Yourself answers are located in the Study Plan at the end of this chapter.

486

14 Nutrition Through the Life Cycle

Pregnancy and the first year of life

The birth of baby Tomas brought joy to his parents and extended family. However, little Tomas weighed just over 3 pounds, 5 ounces at birth—about half of what an average full-term newborn weighs. Fortunately, with early nutrition support in the neonatal intensive care unit, Tomas gained weight rapidly and within two weeks was discharged home.

Although the United States has an extensive and expensive healthcare system, the prevalence of low-, very-low-, and extremely low-birth-weight infants, such as Tomas, remains around 8%.[1] In addition, the U.S. infant mortality rate is just over 6 infant deaths for every 1,000 live births,[2] a number that is higher than that of many other developed nations, including most countries of Europe.

What contributes to these troubling statistics? More broadly, what role does prenatal diet play in determining the future health and well-being of the child? In this chapter, we'll discuss how adequate nutrition supports embryonic and fetal development, maintains a pregnant woman's health, and contributes to lactation. We'll then explore the nutrient needs of breastfeeding and formula-feeding infants.

LO 1 Explain how a healthful diet supports conception and normal embryonic and fetal development.

How does a healthful diet support conception and gestation?

From conception through the end of the first year of life, adequate nutrition is essential for tissue formation, neurologic development, and bone growth, modeling, and remodeling. The ability to reach peak physical and intellectual potential in adult life is in part determined by the nutrition received during the earliest stages of development.

A Healthful Diet Is Critical Before Conception

Several factors make adequate nutrition important even before **conception**, the point at which a woman's ovum (egg) is fertilized with a man's sperm. First, some deficiency-related problems develop extremely early in the pregnancy, typically before the mother even realizes she is pregnant. An adequate and varied preconception diet reduces the risk for such early onset problems. For example, inadequate levels of folate during the first few weeks following conception can result in brain and spinal cord defects. This problem is discussed in more detail shortly. To reduce the incidence of such defects, federal guidelines advise all women capable of becoming pregnant to consume 400 µg of folic acid daily, whether or not they plan to become pregnant.

Second, adopting a healthful diet prior to conception includes the avoidance of alcohol, illegal drugs, and other known **teratogens** (substances that cause birth defects). Women should also consult their healthcare provider about their consumption of caffeine, medications, herbs, and supplements, and if they smoke they should attempt to quit.

Third, a healthful diet and an appropriate level of physical activity can help women achieve and maintain an optimal body weight prior to pregnancy. Women with a prepregnancy body mass index (BMI) between 19.8 and 26.0 kg/m^2 have the best chance of a successful pregnancy. Women who are under- or overweight are at greater risk for infertility as well as complications when pregnancy does occur.[3] For example, obesity is associated with a condition called polycystic ovary syndrome (PCOS), which is characterized by abnormal hormone levels, irregular or absent menstrual cycles, and/or impaired ovulation.[4] Women diagnosed with this condition have lower fertility rates. Many, although not all, are overweight or obese and are insulin resistant. If successful in becoming pregnant, women with PCOS have three to four times the risk for pregnancy-related forms of hypertension and diabetes than healthy women, and twice the risk for preterm birth.[5] In women with PCOS who are overweight or obese, weight loss is often the first step of a treatment plan. Achieving and maintaining a healthful weight prior to conception should be the goal of all women seeking a successful pregnancy.

Finally, maintaining a balanced and nourishing diet before conception reduces a woman's risk of experiencing any of several nutrition-related concerns during her pregnancy. These concerns, which are discussed later in the chapter, can affect the health of the pregnant woman as well as her newborn.

The man's nutrition and health prior to pregnancy is important as well. Paternal obesity contributes to abnormalities in sperm, impaired male fertility, alterations in gene expression, increased risk of pregnancy loss, and increased risk for chronic disease in offspring.[6,7] Also, both sperm number and motility (ability to move) are reduced by alcohol consumption as well as by the use of certain prescription and illegal drugs. A man's reproductive health is supported by a diet rich in zinc, calcium, vitamin D, folic acid, and dietary antioxidants such as vitamin C.

During conception, a sperm fertilizes an egg, creating a zygote.

conception The uniting of an ovum (egg) and sperm to create a fertilized egg, or zygote. Also called *fertilization*.

teratogen Any substance that can cause a birth defect.

gestation The period of intrauterine development from conception to birth; typically 38 to 42 weeks.

A Healthful Diet Supports Embryonic and Fetal Development

A balanced, nourishing diet is important throughout **gestation**—the period from conception to birth—to provide the nutrients needed to support fetal development without depriving the mother of the nutrients she needs to maintain her own health. A healthful diet also minimizes the risk of excess energy intake. A full-term pregnancy

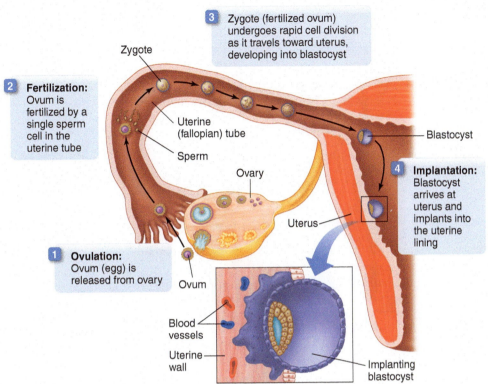

3 Zygote (fertilized ovum) undergoes rapid cell division as it travels toward uterus, developing into blastocyst

Zygote

2 **Fertilization:** Ovum is fertilized by a single sperm cell in the uterine tube

Uterine (fallopian) tube

Sperm

Ovary

Blastocyst

4 **Implantation:** Blastocyst arrives at uterus and implants into the uterine lining

Uterus

1 **Ovulation:** Ovum (egg) is released from ovary

Ovum

Blood vessels

Uterine wall

Implanting blastocyst

FIGURE 14.1 Ovulation, conception, and implantation. The time between fertilization of the ovum and implantation of the blastocyst into the uterine lining is about 10 days.

lasts 38 to 42 weeks and is divided into three **trimesters**, with each trimester lasting about 13 to 14 weeks.

The First Trimester

About once each month, a nonpregnant woman of childbearing age experiences **ovulation**, the release of an ovum from an ovary. The ovum is then drawn into the uterine tube. The first trimester of pregnancy begins when the ovum and sperm unite to form a single, fertilized cell called a **zygote**. As the zygote travels through the uterine tube, it divides into a ball of 12 to 16 cells, which, at about day 4, arrives in the uterus **(FIGURE 14.1)**. By day 10, the inner portion of the zygote, called the *blastocyst*, has implanted into the uterine lining. The outer portion becomes part of the placenta, which is discussed shortly.

Further cell growth, multiplication, and differentiation occur, resulting in the formation of an **embryo**. Over the next 6 weeks, embryonic tissues continue to differentiate and fold into a primitive, tubelike structure, which eventually develops limb buds, organs, and facial features **(FIGURE 14.2)**. The embryo is most vulnerable to

trimester Any one of three stages of pregnancy, each lasting 13 to 14 weeks.

ovulation The release of an ovum (egg) from a woman's ovary.

zygote A fertilized ovum (egg) consisting of a single cell.

embryo The human growth and developmental stage lasting from the third week to the end of the eighth week after fertilization.

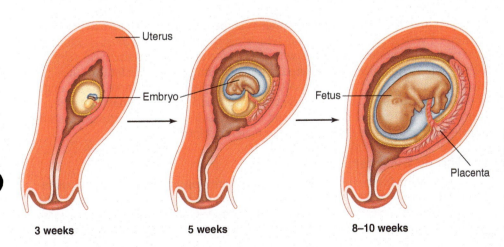

Uterus

Embryo

Fetus

Placenta

3 weeks

5 weeks

8–10 weeks

FIGURE 14.2 Human embryonic development during the first 10 weeks after conception. Organ systems are most vulnerable to teratogens during this time, when cells are dividing and differentiating.

▶ **FIGURE 14.3** Placental development. The placenta is formed from both embryonic and maternal tissues. When the placenta is fully functional, fetal blood vessels and maternal blood vessels are intimately intertwined, allowing the exchange of nutrients and wastes between the two. The mother transfers nutrients and oxygen to the fetus, and the fetus transfers wastes to the mother for disposal.

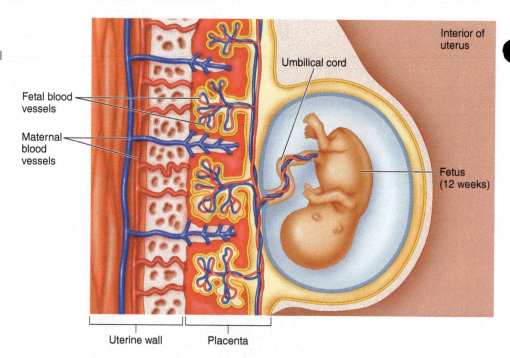

Interior of uterus

Umbilical cord

Fetal blood vessels

Maternal blood vessels

Fetus (12 weeks)

Uterine wall

Placenta

spontaneous abortion The natural termination of a pregnancy and expulsion of pregnancy tissues because of a genetic, developmental, or physiologic abnormality that is so severe that the pregnancy cannot be maintained. Also called *miscarriage*.

placenta A pregnancy-specific organ formed from both maternal and embryonic tissues. It is responsible for oxygen, nutrient, and waste exchange between mother and fetus.

fetus The human growth and developmental stage lasting from the beginning of the ninth week after conception to birth.

umbilical cord The cord containing the arteries and veins that connect the baby (from the navel) to the mother via the placenta.

teratogens during this time. Not only alcohol and illegal drugs, but also some prescription and over-the-counter medications, certain dietary supplements, some viruses and infections, cigarette smoking, and radiation can interfere with embryonic development and cause birth defects. A recent example is the increased risk of microcephaly (abnormally small brain) and other birth defects in the infants of pregnant women infected with the Zika virus. In some cases, the damage from teratogen exposure is so severe that the pregnancy ends in a **spontaneous abortion** (*miscarriage*), most of which occur in the first trimester.

During the first weeks of pregnancy, the embryo obtains its nutrients from cells lining the uterus. But by the fourth week, a primitive **placenta** has formed in the uterus from both embryonic and maternal tissue. Within a few more weeks, the placenta will be a fully functioning organ through which the mother will provide nutrients and remove fetal wastes **(FIGURE 14.3)**.

By the end of the embryonic stage, about 8 weeks postconception, the embryo's tissues and organs have differentiated dramatically. A primitive skeleton has formed and muscles have begun to develop, making movement possible. A primitive heart has begun to beat, and the digestive organs are becoming distinct. The brain has differentiated, and the head has a mouth, eyespots with eyelids, and primitive ears.

The third month of pregnancy marks the transition from embryo to **fetus**. To support its dramatic growth, the fetus requires abundant nutrients from the placenta. It is connected to the fetal circulatory system via the **umbilical cord**, an extension of fetal blood vessels emerging from the fetus's navel (called the *umbilicus*). Blood rich in oxygen and nutrients flows through the placenta and into the umbilical vein (see Figure 14.3). Wastes are excreted in blood returning from the fetus to the placenta via the umbilical arteries. Although many people think there is a mixing of blood from the fetus and the mother, the two blood supplies remain separate. Nutrients move from the maternal blood into the fetal blood and waste products are transferred out of the fetal blood into the maternal blood.

The Second Trimester

During the second trimester (weeks 14 to 27 of pregnancy), the fetus continues to grow and mature **(FIGURE 14.4)**. It develops the ability to suck its thumb, hear, and open and close its eyes in response to light. At the beginning of the second trimester, the fetus is about 3 inches long and weighs about 1.5 pounds. By the end of this

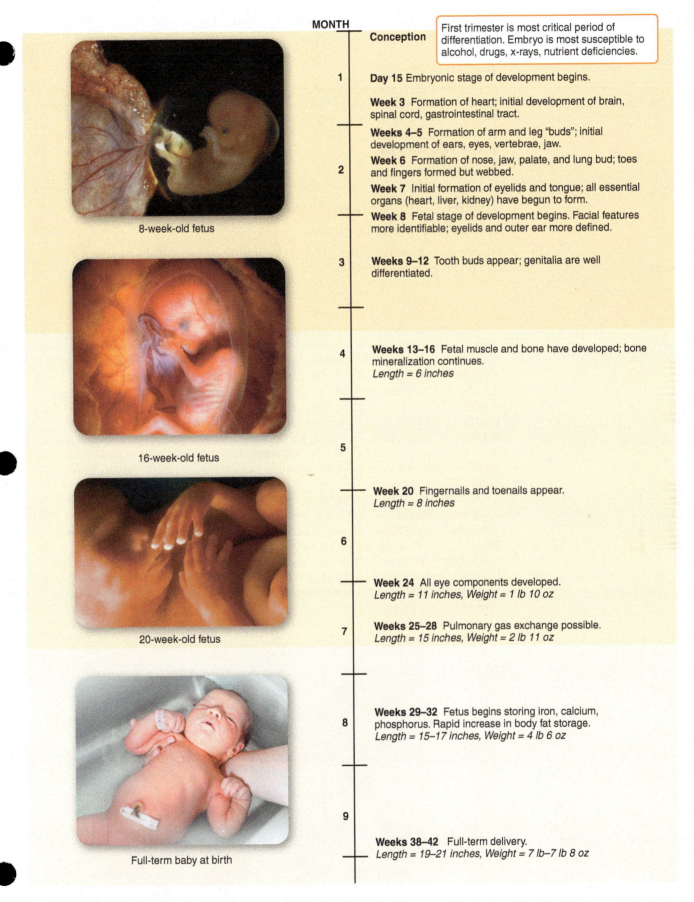

MONTH

Conception

First trimester is most critical period of differentiation. Embryo is most susceptible to alcohol, drugs, x-rays, nutrient deficiencies.

1 **Day 15** Embryonic stage of development begins.

Week 3 Formation of heart; initial development of brain, spinal cord, gastrointestinal tract.

Weeks 4–5 Formation of arm and leg "buds"; initial development of ears, eyes, vertebrae, jaw.

2 **Week 6** Formation of nose, jaw, palate, and lung bud; toes and fingers formed but webbed.

Week 7 Initial formation of eyelids and tongue; all essential organs (heart, liver, kidney) have begun to form.

Week 8 Fetal stage of development begins. Facial features more identifiable; eyelids and outer ear more defined.

3 **Weeks 9–12** Tooth buds appear; genitalia are well differentiated.

8-week-old fetus

4 **Weeks 13–16** Fetal muscle and bone have developed; bone mineralization continues.
Length = 6 inches

5

16-week-old fetus

Week 20 Fingernails and toenails appear.
Length = 8 inches

6

Week 24 All eye components developed.
Length = 11 inches, Weight = 1 lb 10 oz

7 **Weeks 25–28** Pulmonary gas exchange possible.
Length = 15 inches, Weight = 2 lb 11 oz

20-week-old fetus

8 **Weeks 29–32** Fetus begins storing iron, calcium, phosphorus. Rapid increase in body fat storage.
Length = 15–17 inches, Weight = 4 lb 6 oz

9

Weeks 38–42 Full-term delivery.
Length = 19–21 inches, Weight = 7 lb–7 lb 8 oz

Full-term baby at birth

FIGURE 14.4 A timeline of embryonic and fetal development.

trimester, it is generally over a foot long and weighs more than 2 pounds. Some babies born prematurely in the last weeks of the second trimester survive with intensive care.

The Third Trimester

During the third trimester (weeks 28 to birth), the fetus gains nearly half its body length and three-quarters of its body weight! Average birth length is approximately 18 to 22 inches and average birth weight about 7.5 pounds (see Figure 14.4). Brain growth (which continues to be rapid for the first 2 years of life) is also quite remarkable and the lungs become fully mature. The fetus acquires eyebrows, eyelashes, and hair on the head.

Appropriate Maternal Weight Gain Supports a Healthy Birth Weight

An adequate, nourishing diet is one of the most important variables under a woman's control for increasing the chances for birth of a mature newborn (38 to 42 weeks' gestation). Proper nutrition also increases the likelihood that the newborn's weight will be appropriate for his or her gestational age. Generally, a birth weight of at least 5.5 pounds is considered a marker of a successful pregnancy.

An undernourished mother who gains too little weight during her pregnancy is more likely to give birth to a **low-birth-weight** baby than a woman with appropriate nutritional intake. An infant weighing less than 2,500 g (about 5.5 pounds) at birth is considered to be of low birth weight and an infant weighing less than 1,500 g (about 3.3 pounds) is termed very low birth weight. Both groups are at increased risk for infection, learning disabilities, impaired physical development, and death in the first year of life (FIGURE 14.5). Many low- and very-low-birth-weight babies are born **preterm**—that is, before 38 weeks' gestation. Others are born at term but are small for gestational age; in other words, they weigh less than would be expected. Although nutrition is not the only factor contributing to maturity and birth weight, its role cannot be overstated.

Recommendations for weight gain vary according to a woman's weight *before* she became pregnant and whether she is expecting a single or multiple birth (TABLE 14.1). The average recommended weight gain for women of normal prepregnancy weight is 25 to 35 pounds; underweight women should gain a little more than this amount, and overweight and obese women should gain less. Adolescents should follow the same recommendations as those for adult women.[8] Women of normal prepregnancy weight who are pregnant with twins are advised to gain 37 to 54 pounds.[8]

low birth weight Having a weight of less than 5.5 pounds at birth.

preterm The birth of a baby prior to 38 weeks' gestation.

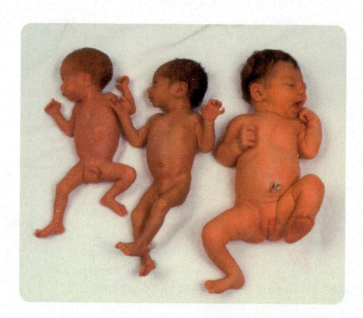

▶ **FIGURE 14.5** A healthy 2-day-old infant (right) compared to two low-birth-weight infants.

TABLE 14.1 Recommended Weight Gain for Women During Pregnancy

Prepregnancy Weight Status	Body Mass Index (kg/m^2)	Recommended Weight Gain (lb)
Normal	18.5–24.9	25–35
Underweight	<18.5	28–40
Overweight	25.0–29.9	15–25

Source: Data adapted from Rasmussen, K. M., and A. L. Yaktine, eds. 2009. *Weight Gain During Pregnancy: Reexamining the Guidelines.* Institute of Medicine; National Research Council. Washington, DC: National Academies Press.

Women who have a low prepregnancy BMI (<18.5 kg/m^2) or gain too little weight during pregnancy increase their risk of having a preterm or low-birth-weight baby; the pregnancy may also dangerously deplete their own nutrient reserves.

Gaining *too* much weight or being overweight (BMI ≥25 kg/m^2) or obese (BMI ≥30 kg/m^2) prior to conception is also risky and much more common. Excessive prepregnancy weight or prenatal weight gain increases the risk that the fetus will be large for gestational age, increasing the likelihood of trauma during vaginal delivery and of cesarean birth. Also, children born to overweight or obese mothers have higher rates of childhood obesity and metabolic abnormalities.[9] In addition, the more weight a woman gains during pregnancy, the more difficult it will be for her to return to prepregnancy weight and the more likely it is that her weight gain will be permanent.

In addition to amount of weight, the *pattern* of weight gain is important. During the first trimester, a woman of normal weight should gain no more than 3 to 5 pounds. During the second and third trimesters, about 1 pound a week is considered healthful. Overweight women should gain only 0.6 pound per week and, for obese women, a gain of 0.5 pound per week is appropriate.[8] If weight gain is excessive in a single week, month, or trimester, the woman should not attempt to lose weight. Instead, the woman should merely attempt to slow the rate of weight gain. In short, weight gain throughout pregnancy should be slow and steady.

In a society obsessed with thinness, it is easy for pregnant women to worry about weight gain. Focusing on the quality of food consumed, rather than the quantity, can help women feel more in control. In addition, following a physician-approved exercise program helps women maintain a positive body image and prevent excessive weight gain. The *2015–2020 Dietary Guidelines for Americans* offers the following guidance: "Before becoming pregnant, women are encouraged to achieve and maintain a healthy weight, and women who are pregnant are encouraged to gain weight within gestational weight gain guidelines" as defined by the Health and Medicine Division of the National Academies of Science (see Table 14.1).[10]

A pregnant woman may also feel less anxious about her weight gain if she understands how that weight is distributed. Of the total weight gained in pregnancy, 10 to 12 pounds are accounted for by the fetus itself, the amniotic fluid, and the placenta (**FIGURE 14.6**) (page 494). In addition, the woman's blood volume increases 40% to 50%, accounting for another 3 to 4 pounds. A woman can expect to be about 10 to 12 pounds lighter immediately after the birth and, within about 2 weeks, another 5 to 8 pounds lighter because of fluid loss. After that, losing the remainder of pregnancy weight depends on more energy being expended than is taken in. Although the production of breast milk requires significant energy, the effect of breastfeeding on postpartum weight loss varies. Moderate weight loss while breastfeeding is safe and will not interfere with the weight gain of the nursing infant.

For an individualized pregnancy weight gain calculator, go to www.choosemyplate.gov. From the home page, search the list under "Online Tools." Click on "Pregnancy Weight Gain Calculator."

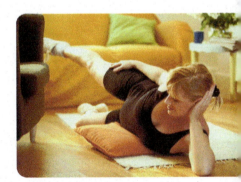

▲ Following a physician-approved exercise program helps pregnant women maintain a positive body image and prevent excess weight gain.

recap Conception is the point at which a woman's ovum is fertilized with a man's sperm. A healthful diet prior to conception is important to reduce the risk for infertility, to prevent nutrient-deficiency disorders that can arise very early in the pregnancy, and to minimize the risk for nutrition-related concerns during pregnancy. A healthful body weight and a nourishing diet is also important for male fertility. A full-term pregnancy lasts from 38 to 42 weeks

▶ **FIGURE 14.6** The weight gained during pregnancy is distributed between the mother's own tissues and the pregnancy-specific tissues.

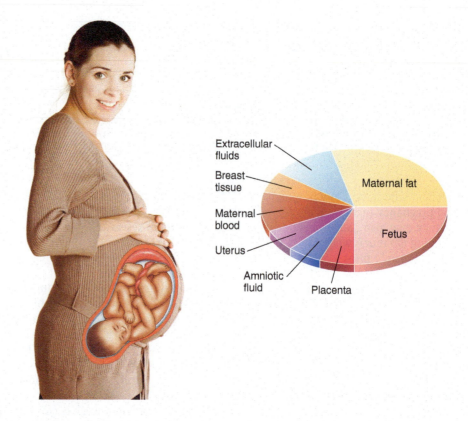

and is traditionally divided into trimesters lasting 13 to 14 weeks. During the first trimester, cells differentiate and divide rapidly to form the various tissues of the human body. Vulnerability to nutrient deficiencies, toxicities, and teratogens is highest during this trimester. The second and third trimesters are characterized by continued growth and maturation of organ systems. Nutrition is important before and throughout pregnancy to maintain the mother's health, support fetal development, and increase the likelihood that the baby will be born after 37 weeks and will weigh at least 5.5 pounds.

LO 2 Identify the nutrient recommendations that change during pregnancy.

What are a pregnant woman's nutrient needs?

The requirement for nearly all nutrients increases during pregnancy to accommodate the growth and development of the fetus without depriving the mother of the nutrients she needs to maintain her own health. With the exception of iron, most of these increased needs can be met by carefully selecting foods high in nutrient density. The ChooseMyPlate.gov website provides useful information that emphasizes the need for dietary adequacy, balance, and variety in food choices; it also suggests food patterns for pregnant women (see the **Web Links** at the end of this chapter).

Macronutrients Provide Energy and Build Tissues

During pregnancy, macronutrients provide necessary energy and building blocks for developing embryonic and fetal tissues as well as other pregnancy-associated tissues.

Recommendations for Energy Intake

Energy requirements increase only modestly during pregnancy.[11] In fact, during the first trimester, a woman should consume approximately the same number of Calories daily as during her nonpregnant days. Instead of eating more, she should attempt to maximize the nutrient density of what she eats. For example, drinking low-fat milk is preferable to drinking soft drinks. Low-fat milk provides valuable protein, vitamins, and minerals to feed the fetus's rapidly dividing cells, whereas soft drinks provide nutritionally empty Calories.

During the last two trimesters of pregnancy, caloric needs increase by about 350 to 450 kcal per day. For a woman consuming 2,000 kcal per day, an extra 400 kcal represents only a 20% increase in Calorie intake. For example, 1 cup of low-fat yogurt and a graham cracker with jam is about 400 kcal. At the same time, some vitamin and mineral needs increase by as much as 50%, so again, the key for getting adequate micronutrients while not consuming too many extra Calories is choosing nutrient-dense foods.

Recommendations for Protein and Carbohydrate Intake

During pregnancy, protein needs increase to 1.1 g per day per kg body weight (an additional 25 g or so of protein per day).[11] Many women already eat this much protein each day. Dairy products, meats, eggs, and soy products are all rich sources of protein, as are legumes, nuts, and seeds.

Carbohydrate intake should be at least 175 g per day.[11] The majority of carbohydrate intake should come from whole grains, fruits, and legumes and other vegetables. These foods are good sources of the B-vitamins and other micronutrients, phytochemicals, and fiber. Fiber-rich foods are satiating, thereby helping to prevent excessive weight gain, and may lower the risk of constipation.

Recommendations for Fat Intake

The guideline for the percentage of daily Calories that comes from fat does not change during pregnancy.[11] Consumption of the right kinds of fats is important. Like anyone else, pregnant women should limit their intakes of saturated and *trans* fats because of their negative impact on cardiovascular health (see Chapter 5). The omega-3 polyunsaturated fatty acid *docosahexaenoic acid* (*DHA*) and the omega-6 arachidonic acid (*ARA*) have been linked in some, but not all, studies to both enhanced brain growth and eye development. Because the fetal brain grows dramatically during the third trimester, DHA is especially important in the maternal diet. Good sources of DHA are oily fish, such as salmon, sardines, anchovies, and mackerel. It is also found in smaller amounts in tuna, chicken, and eggs enhanced by feeding hens a DHA-rich diet. ARA is found in most types of meat, fish, and poultry.

Pregnant women who eat fish should be aware of the potential for mercury contamination because even a limited intake of mercury during pregnancy can impair a fetus's developing nervous system. Although pregnant women should avoid large fish, such as swordfish, shark, tile fish, and king mackerel, they can safely consume up to 12 ounces of most other types of fish per week, as long as it is properly cooked. Albacore tuna, however, should be limited to 6 ounces per week because it is higher in mercury than other types of tuna.[12]

Micronutrients Support Increased Energy Needs and Tissue Growth

During pregnancy, expansion of the mother's blood supply and growth of the uterus, placenta, breasts, body fat stores, and the fetus itself all contribute to an increased need for micronutrients. In addition, the increased need for energy during pregnancy correlates with an increased need for the micronutrients involved in energy metabolism. Discussions of the micronutrients that are most critical during pregnancy follow. See TABLE 14.2 for an overview of the changes in micronutrient needs with pregnancy.

Recommended Folate Intake

Because folate is necessary for cell division, it follows that, during a time when both maternal and fetal cells are dividing rapidly, the requirement for this vitamin increases. Adequate folate is especially critical during the first 28 days after

Watch a video on the history of folic acid fortification of foods at http://www.cdc.gov. From the home page, type "folic acid fortification video" into the search bar, then click on the link.

TABLE 14.2   Changes in Nutrient Recommendations with Pregnancy for Adult Women

Micronutrient	Prepregnancy	Pregnancy	% Increase
Folate	400 µg/day	600 µg/day	50
Vitamin B$_{12}$	2.4 µg/day	2.6 µg/day	8
Vitamin C	75 mg/day	85 mg/day	13
Vitamin A	700 µg/day	770 µg/day	10
Vitamin D	600 IU/day	600 IU/day	0
Calcium	1,000 mg/day	1,000 mg/day	0
Iron	18 mg/day	27 mg/day	50
Zinc	8 mg/day	11 mg/day	38
Sodium	1,500 mg/day	1,500 mg/day	0
Iodine	150 µg/day	220 µg/day	47

neural tube Embryonic tissue that forms a tube, which eventually becomes the brain and spinal cord.

anencephaly A fatal neural tube defect in which there is partial absence of brain tissue, most likely caused by failure of the neural tube to close.

spina bifida The embryotic neural tube defect that occurs when the spinal vertebrae fail to completely enclose the spinal cord, allowing it to protrude.

conception, when it is required for the formation and closure of the **neural tube**, an embryonic structure that eventually becomes the brain and spinal cord. Folate deficiency is associated with neural tube defects, such as **anencephaly**, a fatal defect in which brain tissue is partially or fully absent, and **spina bifida**, in which a portion of the spinal cord protrudes through the spinal vertebrae, causing varying degrees of paralysis **(FIGURE 14.7)**. Adequate folate intake does not guarantee normal neural tube development because the precise cause of neural tube defects is unknown, and there is a genetic component in some cases. Still, it is estimated that 70% of all neural tube defects could be prevented if all women of childbearing age consumed enough folate or folic acid.[13]

To reduce the risk for a neural tube defect, all women capable of becoming pregnant are encouraged to consume 400 µg of folic acid per day. Of course, folate remains very important even after the neural tube has closed. The RDA for folate for pregnant women is therefore 600 µg per day, a full 50% increase over the RDA for a nonpregnant female.[14] A deficiency of folate during pregnancy can result in macrocytic anemia (see Chapter 9) and has been associated with low birth weight, preterm delivery, and failure of the fetus to grow properly. Sources of folate include fortified cereals and grains, spinach, and lentils.

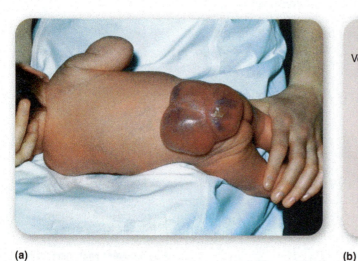

(a)

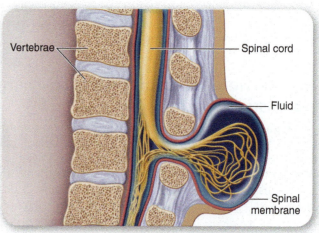

(b)

◆ **FIGURE 14.7**   Spina bifida, a common neural tube defect. **(a)** An external view of an infant with spina bifida. **(b)** An internal view of the protruding spinal membrane and fluid-filled sac.

Recommended Vitamin B$_{12}$ Intake

Vitamin B$_{12}$ (cobalamin) is vital during pregnancy because it regenerates the active form of folate. Not surprisingly, deficiencies of vitamin B$_{12}$ can also result in macrocytic anemia. Yet the RDA for vitamin B$_{12}$ for pregnant women is only 2.6 μg per day, a mere 8% increase over the RDA of 2.4 μg per day for nonpregnant women.[14] How can this be? One reason is that, during pregnancy, absorption of vitamin B$_{12}$ is more efficient. The required amount of vitamin B$_{12}$ can easily be obtained from animal food sources. However, deficiencies have been observed in women who follow a vegan diet. Fortified foods or supplements provide these women with the needed B$_{12}$.

Recommended Vitamin C Intake

Vitamin C is necessary for the synthesis of collagen, a component of connective tissue (including skin, blood vessels, and tendons) and part of the organic matrix of bones. The RDA for vitamin C during pregnancy is increased by a little more than 10% over the RDA for nonpregnant women (from 75 to 85 mg/day).[15] A deficiency of vitamin C during pregnancy increases the risk for preterm birth and other complications. Abundant amounts of vitamin C are found in many food sources, such as citrus fruits and juices and numerous other fruits and vegetables.

Recommended Vitamin A Intake

Vitamin A needs increase during pregnancy by about 10%, to 770 μg per day.[16] However, excess preformed vitamin A can cause fetal abnormalities, particularly heart defects and facial malformations. A well-balanced diet supplies sufficient vitamin A, so supplementation during pregnancy is not recommended. Beta-carotene (which is converted to vitamin A in the body) has not been associated with birth defects.

Recommended Vitamin D Intake

Despite the role of vitamin D in calcium absorption, the RDA for this nutrient does not increase during pregnancy.[17] Pregnant women who receive adequate exposure to sunlight do not need vitamin D supplements. However, pregnant women with darkly pigmented skin and/or limited sun exposure who do not regularly drink vitamin D-fortified milk will benefit from vitamin D supplementation. Most prenatal vitamin supplements contain 10 μg per day of vitamin D, which is considered safe and acceptable. Pregnant women should avoid consuming excessive vitamin D because toxicity can cause developmental disability in the newborn.

Recommended Calcium Intake

Growth of the fetal skeleton requires a significant amount of calcium. However, the RDA for adult pregnant women is the same as that for nonpregnant women, 1,000 mg per day, for two reasons.[17] First, pregnant women absorb calcium from the diet more efficiently than do nonpregnant women. Second, the extra demand for calcium has not been found to cause demineralization of the mother's bones or to increase fracture risk; thus, there is no justification for higher intakes. Sources of calcium include milk, yogurt, and cheese; nondairy foods, such as kale, collard greens, and broccoli; and calcium-fortified soy milk, juices, and cereals.

Recommended Iron Intake

Recall (from Chapter 9) the importance of iron in the formation of red blood cells, which transport oxygen throughout the body. During pregnancy, the demand for red blood cells increases to accommodate the needs of the mother's expanded blood volume, the growing uterus, the placenta, and the fetus itself. Thus, more iron is needed. Fetal demand for iron increases even further during the last trimester, when the fetus stores iron for use during the first few months of life.

Severely inadequate iron intake has the potential to harm the fetus, resulting in an increased risk for low birth weight, preterm birth, and death of the newborn. However, in most cases, the fetus builds adequate stores by "robbing" maternal iron, prompting iron-deficiency anemia in the mother. During pregnancy, maternal iron

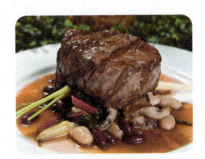

Meats provide protein, vitamin B$_{12}$, heme iron, and zinc.

deficiency causes paleness and exhaustion, but at birth it endangers her life: anemic women are more likely to die during or shortly following childbirth because they are less able to tolerate blood loss and fight infection.

The RDA for iron for pregnant women is 27 mg per day, compared to 18 mg per day for nonpregnant women and 15 mg per day for nonpregnant adolescents.[16] This represents a 50% to 80% increase, despite the fact that iron loss is minimized during pregnancy because menstruation ceases. Typically, women of childbearing age have poor iron stores, and the demands of pregnancy are likely to produce a deficiency. To ensure adequate iron stores during pregnancy, an iron supplement (as part of, or distinct from, a total prenatal supplement) is routinely prescribed during the last two trimesters. Vitamin C enhances iron absorption, as do dietary sources of heme iron; however, substances in coffee, tea, milk, bran, and oxalate-rich foods decrease iron absorption. Therefore, many healthcare providers recommend taking iron supplements with foods high in vitamin C and/or heme iron. Sources of iron include meats, seafood, poultry, fortified cereals, legumes, spinach and other dark green leafy vegetables, and dried fruits.

Recommended Zinc Intake

The RDA for zinc for adult pregnant women increases by about 38% over the RDA for nonpregnant women, from 8 mg per day to 11 mg per day.[16] Zinc is critical in DNA, RNA, and protein synthesis, and inadequate intake can lead to malformations in the fetus, premature labor, and extended labor. The absorption of zinc from supplements may be inhibited by high intakes of non-heme iron, such as high-potency iron supplements, when these two minerals are taken together.[18] However, when food sources of iron and zinc are consumed together in a meal, absorption of zinc is not affected. In addition, the heme form of iron does not appear to inhibit zinc absorption.

Recommended Sodium and Iodine Intake

During pregnancy, the AI for sodium is the same as for a nonpregnant adult woman, or 1,500 mg (1.5 g) per day.[19] Although too much sodium is associated with fluid retention, bloating, and high blood pressure, an increase in body fluids is a normal and necessary part of pregnancy, and as during any life stage, some sodium is necessary to maintain fluid and electrolyte balance.

Iodine needs increase significantly during pregnancy, but the RDA of 220 μg per day is easy to achieve by using a modest amount of iodized salt (sodium chloride) during cooking.

Do Pregnant Women Need Supplements?

Prenatal multivitamin and mineral supplements are not strictly necessary during pregnancy, but most healthcare providers recommend them. Meeting all the nutrient needs would otherwise take careful and somewhat complex dietary planning. Prenatal supplements are especially good insurance for specific populations, such as vegans, adolescents, and others whose diet might normally be low in one or more micronutrients. It is important that pregnant women understand, however, that supplements are to be taken *in addition to*, not as a substitute for, a nutrient-rich diet.

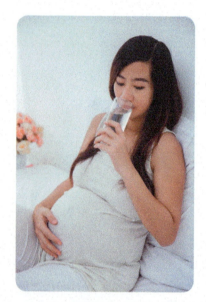

◆ It's important for pregnant women to drink about 10 cups of fluid a day.

amniotic fluid The watery fluid contained within the innermost membrane of the sac containing the fetus. It cushions and protects the growing fetus.

urinary tract infection A bacterial infection of the urethra, the tube leading from the bladder to the body exterior.

Fluid Needs of Pregnant Women Increase

Increased fluid allows for the necessary increase in the mother's blood volume, aids in regulating body temperature, and helps maintain the **amniotic fluid** that surrounds, cushions, and protects the fetus in the uterus. The AI for total fluid intake, which includes drinking water, beverages, and food, is 3 liters per day (or about 12.7 cups). This recommendation includes approximately 2.3 liters (10 cups) of fluid as total beverages, including drinking water.[19]

Drinking adequate fluid also helps combat two common discomforts of pregnancy: fluid retention and, possibly, constipation. Drinking lots of fluids may also lower the risk for **urinary tract infections**, which are common in pregnancy. Fluids also combat dehydration, which can develop if a woman has frequent bouts of vomiting. For these women, fluids such as soups, juices, and sports beverages are usually well tolerated.

recap During the last two trimesters of pregnancy, caloric needs increase by about 350 to 450 kcal per day. The Calories consumed during pregnancy should be nutrient dense. Protein needs increase by about 25 grams a day. Protein, carbohydrates, and healthful unsaturated fats—especially the essential fatty acids DHA and ARA—provide the energy and building blocks for fetal growth. Folate deficiency has been associated with neural tube defects: The RDA increases to 600 μg per day during pregnancy, a full 50% increase over the RDA for nonpregnant women. The requirements for vitamins A, B_{12}, and C increase modestly during pregnancy. Calcium and vitamin D are micronutrients that support bone growth, but intake recommendations do not increase during pregnancy. The requirements for iodine, iron, and zinc all increase to support fetal growth and development while maintaining the mother's health. Most healthcare providers recommend prenatal supplements for pregnant women. Fluid provides for increased maternal blood volume and amniotic fluid.

What are some common nutrition-related concerns of pregnancy?

LO 3 Discuss some common nutrition-related concerns of pregnancy as well as recommendations for engaging in exercise.

Pregnancy-related conditions involving a particular nutrient, such as iron-deficiency anemia, have already been discussed. The following sections describe some of the most common discomforts and disorders of pregnant women that are related to their general nutrition.

Morning Sickness, Cravings, and GI Discomfort Are Common

Although many women look forward to becoming a mother, pregnancy is commonly accompanied by a variety of conditions that, while rarely life-threatening, may be very uncomfortable.

Morning Sickness

Morning sickness, or *nausea and vomiting of pregnancy* (NVP), is a condition characterized by varying degrees of nausea, from occasional mild queasiness to constant nausea with bouts of vomiting. In truth, "morning sickness" is not an appropriate term because the nausea and vomiting can begin at any time of the day and may last all day. NVP usually peaks between weeks 8 and 12, then resolves by weeks 12 to 16, but some women experience it throughout the pregnancy. Usually, the mother and fetus do not suffer lasting harm. However, NVP can become threatening in women who experience such frequent vomiting that they are unable to nourish or hydrate themselves or their fetus adequately.[20] These women may require hospitalization or in-home intravenous (IV) therapy.

There is no cure for morning sickness. However, some women find the following strategies helpful for reducing its severity:

- Eating small, frequent meals and snacks throughout the day. An empty stomach can trigger nausea.
- Consuming the majority of fluids between meals. Frozen ice pops, watermelon, gelatin desserts, and mild broths are some well-tolerated sources of fluid.
- Keeping snacks such as dry cereal or crackers at the bedside to ease nighttime queasiness or nausea before rising.
- Taking prenatal supplements at a time of day when vomiting is least likely.
- Avoiding sights, sounds, smells, and tastes that bring on or worsen queasiness. Cold or room-temperature foods are often easier to tolerate than hot foods.

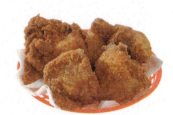

▲ Deep-fried foods are often unappealing to pregnant women.

morning sickness Varying degrees of nausea and vomiting associated with pregnancy, most commonly in the first trimester.

For some women, alternative therapies, such as acupuncture, acupressure wrist bands, biofeedback, meditation, and hypnosis, help. Women should always verify with their healthcare provider that the therapy they are using is safe and does not interact with other treatments, medications, or supplements.

Cravings

It seems like nothing is more stereotypical about pregnancy than the image of a frazzled husband getting up in the middle of the night to run to the convenience store to get his pregnant wife some pickles and ice cream. This image, although humorous, is far from reality for most women. Although some women have specific cravings, most crave a general type of food ("something sweet" or "something salty") rather than a particular food.

Why do pregnant women crave certain tastes? Does a desire for salty foods mean that the woman is experiencing a sodium deficit? Although some people believe that we crave what we need, scientific evidence is lacking. It is more likely that cravings during pregnancy are due to hormonal fluctuations or physiologic changes or have familial or cultural roots. Most cravings are, of course, for edible substances. But a surprising number of pregnant women crave nonfoods, such as laundry starch and clay. This craving, called **pica**, can result in nutritional or health problems for the mother and fetus.[21]

Gastroesophageal Reflux

Gastroesophageal reflux (GER) is common during pregnancy because pregnancy-related hormones relax the smooth muscle of the lower esophagus.[22] During the last two trimesters, the enlarging uterus pushes up on the stomach, worsening the problem. Practical tips for minimizing GER are discussed in detail in Chapter 3. In addition, the woman's healthcare provider may be able to suggest an antacid that is safe for use during pregnancy.

Constipation

Hormone production during pregnancy causes the smooth muscles to relax, including the muscles of the large intestine, slowing colonic movement of food residue.[22] In addition, pressure exerted by the growing uterus on the colon can slow movement even further, making elimination difficult. Practical hints that may help a pregnant woman avoid constipation include consuming 25 to 35 g of fiber each day, concentrating on fresh fruits, legumes and other vegetables, and whole grains. The woman should also make sure to drink the recommended 10 cups of water and other beverages a day, and eat water-rich fruits and vegetables, such as melons, citrus, and lettuce. Regular exercise can also help, as it increases motility of the large intestine. Pregnant women should not use laxatives without the approval of their healthcare provider.

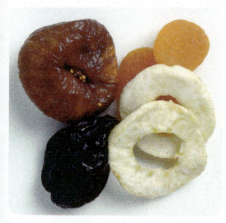

◆ Foods high in fiber, such as dried fruits, reduce the chances of constipation.

Serious Disorders Include Diabetes, Hypertension, and Foodborne Illness

Although most pregnancies are uncomplicated, serious disorders can develop, especially in women who have health challenges before becoming pregnant.

Gestational Diabetes

Gestational diabetes is increasingly common in the United States,[23] diagnosed in as many as 10% of U.S. pregnancies. It is generally a temporary condition in which a pregnant woman is unable to produce sufficient insulin or becomes insulin resistant, resulting in elevated levels of blood glucose. Screening for gestational diabetes is a routine aspect of prenatal care because the symptoms, which include frequent urination, fatigue, and an increase in thirst and appetite, appear to be the same as normal pregnancy symptoms.

Fortunately, gestational diabetes has no ill effects on either the mother or the fetus if blood glucose levels are strictly controlled through diet, exercise, and/or medication.[23] If not controlled, gestational diabetes can result in a baby who is too large as a result of receiving too much glucose across the placenta during fetal life.

pica An abnormal craving to eat nonfood substances such as clay, paint, or chalk.

gestational diabetes A condition of insufficient insulin production or insulin resistance that results in consistently high blood glucose levels, specifically during pregnancy; the condition typically resolves after birth occurs.

nutri-case | JUDY

"Back when I was pregnant with Hannah, the doctor told me I had gestational diabetes but said I shouldn't worry about it. He said I didn't need any medication, and I don't remember changing my diet. In fact, I just kept eating whatever I wanted, and by the time Hannah was born, I had gained almost 60 pounds! I never did lose all that extra weight."

Review what you learned about diabetes in the **In Depth** essay following Chapter 4 (pages 130–137). What information would have been important for Judy to learn while she was pregnant? Is it common for women with gestational diabetes to develop type 2 diabetes later? What are some things Judy could have done to lower her risk for type 2 diabetes?

Inappropriately large infants are at risk for early delivery and trauma during vaginal birth, and they may need to be born by cesarean section. There is also evidence that exposing a fetus to maternal diabetes significantly increases the risk for overweight, obesity, and metabolic disorders such as type 2 diabetes later in life.[23]

Women who are obese, women who are age 35 years or older, and women of Native American, African American, or Hispanic origin have a greater risk of developing gestational diabetes as compared to Caucasian women. Any woman who develops gestational diabetes has a 40% to 60% risk of developing type 2 diabetes within the next 5 to 10 years—particularly if she is obese or overweight. As with any form of diabetes, a healthful diet and regular physical activity reduce the risk for gestational diabetes.

Hypertensive Disorders of Pregnancy

Up to 10% of U.S. pregnancies are complicated by some form of hypertension, yet it accounts for almost 16% of pregnancy-related deaths in developed nations such as the United States.[24] The term *hypertensive disorders of pregnancy* encompasses several different conditions. A woman who develops high blood pressure, with no other symptoms, during her pregnancy is said to have *gestational hypertension*. **Preeclampsia** is characterized by a sudden increase in maternal blood pressure, edema, which leads to excessive and rapid weight gain unrelated to food intake, and protein in the urine. If left untreated, it can progress to *eclampsia*, a very serious condition characterized by seizures, kidney failure, and, potentially, fetal and/or maternal death.

No one knows exactly what causes the various hypertensive disorders of pregnancy, but deficiencies in dietary protein, vitamin C, vitamin E, calcium, and magnesium seem to increase the risk. Other risk factors include first pregnancy, age over 40, African American race, obesity, diabetes, multifetal pregnancy, and a family history of preeclampsia.[24] Management focuses mainly on blood pressure control. Typical treatments include medication and close monitoring, with hospitalization if necessary. Ultimately, only childbirth will cure the condition. Today, with good prenatal care, gestational hypertension is nearly always detected early and can be appropriately managed, and outcomes for both mother and fetus are usually very good. In nearly all women without prior chronic high blood pressure, maternal blood pressure returns to normal within about a day after the birth.

Foodborne Illness

Pregnancy alters a woman's immune system in a way that leaves her more vulnerable to infectious diseases, including foodborne illness. A developing fetus is also at high risk. The bacterium *Listeria monocytogenes,* which causes **listeriosis**, is of particular concern to a pregnant woman and her fetus. Listeriosis is the third leading cause of death from foodborne illness, and 90% of people who contract the disease are in highly vulnerable groups, including pregnant women. In the fetus, listeriosis can result in severe infection that triggers miscarriage or premature birth. The Centers for

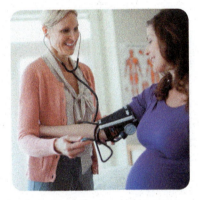

▲ Pregnant women should have their blood pressure measured regularly to test for gestational hypertension.

preeclampsia High blood pressure that is pregnancy specific and accompanied by protein in the urine, edema, and unexpected weight gain.

listeriosis Serious and sometimes fatal illness caused by infection with the bacterium *Listeria monocytogenes,* typically from consumption of contaminated food.

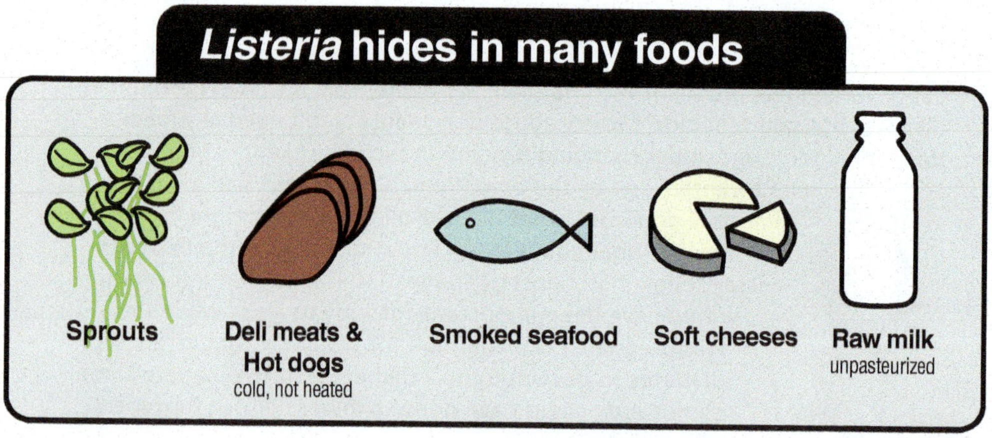

Listeria hides in many foods

Sprouts

Deli meats & Hot dogs
cold, not heated

Smoked seafood

Soft cheeses

Raw milk
unpasteurized

FIGURE 14.8 Certain foods are more likely to be contaminated with *Listeria monocytogenes*, a bacterium that causes listeriosis, a serious illness in pregnant women.

Disease Control and Prevention recommends that pregnant women avoid foods that are more likely to be contaminated with the bacterium (**FIGURE 14.8**).

As discussed earlier, pregnant women are also advised to avoid eating large fish and to limit their intake of canned albacore tuna because of their high mercury content. Pregnant women should consult their state or county health department for information on the safety of locally caught fish.

Safe food-handling practices, discussed in Chapter 12, should be carefully followed by pregnant women and their families.

Maternal Age Can Affect Pregnancy

The adolescent birth rate in the United States has declined by nearly one-third since 1991 and is currently 24 births for every 1,000 adolescents.[25] Although this is the lowest rate in the past 60 years, it is still one of the highest among all industrialized nations.

Throughout the adolescent years, a woman's body continues to change and grow. Peak bone mass has not yet been reached. Full physical stature may not have been attained, and teens are more likely to be underweight than are young adult women. Thus, pregnant adolescents have higher needs for Calories and bone-related nutrients, such as calcium. Teens also commonly begin pregnancy in an iron-deficient state and so have an increased iron need. In addition, many adolescents have not established healthful nutritional patterns. At the same time, higher rates of alcohol use, smoking, and drug use contribute to a greater frequency of nutritional deficiencies.

With regular prenatal care and close attention to proper nutrition and other healthful behaviors, the likelihood of a positive outcome for both the adolescent mother and the infant is similar to that for other mothers and their infants.

Although there is no strict definition of an "older" pregnant woman, many healthcare workers use age 35 as a cut-off point. Older women typically have reduced fertility and an increased risk for miscarriage, stillbirth, gestational diabetes, and hypertension. The risk for chromosomal and other birth defects is also increased. However, on average, older women have higher incomes and more education than younger women, and these can support a healthy pregnancy. Overall, the majority of pregnancies in women over age 35 have the best possible outcome: a healthy baby!

A Careful Vegetarian Diet and Regular Exercise Are Safe During Pregnancy

Pregnant women who are vegetarians often worry about the quality of their diet, and many pregnant women—and their family members—wonder about the safety of vigorous physical activity. These concerns are discussed here.

Vegetarianism

A recent review of maternal and birth outcomes among pregnant vegetarians and vegans reported no increased risk for complications of pregnancy or birth defects among women following a vegetarian or vegan diet.[26] With the possible exception of iron, zinc, and the fatty acids EPA and DHA, vegetarian women who consume dairy products and/or eggs (lacto-ovo-vegetarians) have no nutritional concerns beyond those encountered by every pregnant woman. In contrast, vegan women need to be more vigilant than usual about their intake of nutrients that are derived primarily or wholly from animal products. These include vitamin D (unless fair skinned and regularly exposed to adequate sunlight throughout pregnancy), riboflavin, vitamin B_6, vitamin B_{12}, calcium, iron, and zinc as well as EPA and DHA. Supplements containing these nutrients are usually necessary. A regular prenatal supplement will fully meet the vitamin and iron needs of a vegan woman but does not fulfill calcium needs, so a separate calcium supplement or consumption of calcium-fortified milk alternatives or orange juice, is usually required. Non-animal-based EPA and DHA supplements are also available for vegans.

Exercise

Physical activity during pregnancy is recommended for all women experiencing normal pregnancies.[27] Women who rarely, if ever, exercised before becoming pregnant, and overweight or obese women, can benefit greatly from increased activity but should begin slowly and progress gradually under the guidance of their healthcare provider.

Exercise during pregnancy benefits both mother and fetus in the following ways:

- Reduces risk of gestational diabetes and preeclampsia
- Helps prevent excessive prenatal weight and body fat gain
- Improves mood, energy level, sleep patterns
- Enhances posture and balance
- Improves muscle tone, strength, and endurance
- Reduces lower back pain and shortens the duration of active labor
- Reduces the risk of preterm birth and large-for-gestational age infants

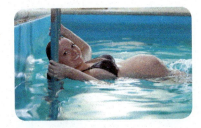

⬆ During pregnancy, women should adjust their physical activity toward comfortable low-impact exercises such as swimming.

Recent guidelines suggest exercises that engage large muscle groups in a continuous manner, including a combination of moderate- and vigorous-intensity aerobic activity, and muscle-strengthening activities.[28,29] (See Chapter 11.) The more vigorous the activity, the less total time is needed to reap its benefits: 6.5 hours per week of brisk walking versus fewer than 3 hours per week of stationary cycling.

Recommendations for muscle-strengthening exercise during pregnancy are straightforward:

- Choose lighter weights and more repetitions.
- Opt for resistance bands over free weights, which might accidently hit or fall on the abdomen.
- Don't lift weights while lying on your back because this might compress a major blood vessel and restrict blood flow to the fetus.
- Avoid sudden movements that might place you off balance, such as lunges or twists.
- Pay attention to your body's signals!

What about yoga and pilates? Both offer classes tailored to pregnant women, adapting certain exercises to accommodate the body's changing center of gravity and increased joint flexibility. Activities that strengthen body core, abdominals, and pelvic floor or Kegel muscles make for an easier pregnancy and birth.

Pregnant women should avoid activities such as horseback riding, scuba diving, water or snow skiing, hockey, gymnastics, and soccer. They should also avoid exercising vigorously in hot and humid weather, dress comfortably, and stay hydrated. If symptoms of stress, such as dizziness, shortness of breath, chest pain, vaginal bleeding or leakage, or uterine contractions occur, all physical activity should stop and a healthcare provider contacted immediately.

> **Want more details on maintaining fitness while pregnant?** Watch this slideshow on exercise during and after pregnancy: **www.webmd.com.** Enter "slideshow pregnancy fitness" into the search bar, then click on the link.

Many Substances Can Harm the Embryo or Fetus

Anything a pregnant woman takes into her body has the potential to reach and affect her fetus; however, the following substances are of particular concern.

Caffeine Consumption

Caffeine, a stimulant found primarily in coffee, tea, soft drinks, and chocolate, crosses the placenta and thus reaches the fetus. Current thinking holds that women who consume less than about 200 to 300 mg per day (the equivalent of one to two cups of coffee) are very likely causing no harm to the fetus.[30,31] However, some studies have linked maternal intakes as low as 100 mg per day to an increased risk for miscarriage, stillbirth, preterm birth, and decreased birth weight.[31] In addition, sweetened coffees, teas, chocolate, and soft drinks provide considerable Calories. A low- or nonfat decaf latte, known to Latinas as *café con leche,* offers a more healthful nutrient profile than coffee alone.

Alcohol Consumption

Frequent drinking (more than seven drinks per week) or occasional binge drinking (more than four to five drinks on one occasion) during pregnancy increases the risk for miscarriage, complications during delivery, preterm birth, and sudden infant death syndrome. In addition, alcohol is a known teratogen, and its consumption during pregnancy increases the risk that the baby will be born with any of a variety of birth defects, including heart, skeletal, kidney, ear, and eye malformations as well as a range of lifelong developmental, behavioral, and mental problems (e.g., hyperactivity and attention deficit disorder). Heavy drinking (more than three to four drinks per day) throughout pregnancy can result in a condition called fetal alcohol syndrome. (See the **In Depth** essay on Alcohol following Chapter 7.) Despite these known dangers, 10% of pregnant women in the United States reported drinking alcohol at some point over the last 30 days while 3% admitted to binge drinking.[32]

Although some women do have the occasional alcoholic drink with no apparent ill effects, there is no amount of alcohol that is known to be safe. The best advice regarding alcohol during pregnancy is to abstain, if not from before conception, then as soon as pregnancy is suspected.

Smoking

Although the dangers of smoking are well known, about 10% of pregnant women smoke during pregnancy.[33] Maternal smoking exposes the fetus to toxins such as lead, cadmium, cyanide, nicotine, and carbon monoxide. Fetal blood flow is reduced, which limits the delivery of oxygen and nutrients, resulting in impaired fetal growth and development. Maternal smoking greatly increases the risk for miscarriage, stillbirth, placental abnormalities, preterm delivery, and low birth weight. Rates of sudden infant death syndrome, respiratory illness, and allergies are higher in the infants and children of smokers compared to those of nonsmokers.

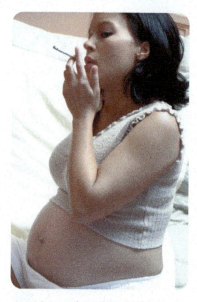

◀ Maternal smoking is extremely harmful to the developing fetus.

Illegal Drug Use

Despite the fact that the use of illegal drugs is unquestionably harmful to the fetus, nearly 5% of pregnant women in the United States report having used illicit drugs and as many as 20% of pregnant women abuse prescription medications.[34,35] Most drugs pass through the placenta into fetal blood, where they accumulate. Prenatal use of illegal drugs also impairs placental blood flow and increases the risk for low birth weight, premature delivery, miscarriage, and placental defects. Newborns suffer signs of withdrawal, including tremors, excessive crying, sleeplessness, and poor feeding. All women are strongly advised to stop taking drugs before becoming pregnant. There is no safe level of use for illegal drugs during pregnancy.

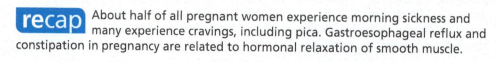

recap About half of all pregnant women experience morning sickness and many experience cravings, including pica. Gastroesophageal reflux and constipation in pregnancy are related to hormonal relaxation of smooth muscle.

Gestational diabetes and hypertensive disorders can seriously affect maternal and fetal well-being. Listeriosis is a foodborne illness that is particularly serious in pregnant women. The nutrient needs of pregnant adolescents are so high that adequate nourishment becomes difficult. A careful vegetarian diet can be healthful during pregnancy, but pregnant women who follow a vegan diet usually need to consume supplements. Exercise (provided the mother has no contraindications) can enhance the health of a pregnant woman. Caffeine intake should be limited and the use of alcohol, cigarettes, and illegal drugs should be completely avoided during pregnancy.

How does nutrition support lactation?

LO 4 Describe the physiology of lactation and the nutrient recommendations for lactating women.

Throughout most of human history, infants have thrived on only one food: breast milk. But during the first half of the 20th century, commercially prepared infant formulas slowly began to replace breast milk as the mother's preferred feeding method. Aggressive marketing campaigns promoted formula-feeding as a status symbol, proof of the family's wealth and modern thinking. In the 1970s, this trend began to reverse as several public health organizations, including the World Health Organization, the American Academy of Pediatrics, and La Leche League, began to promote the nutritional, immunologic, financial, and emotional advantages of breastfeeding and sponsored initiatives to support it.[36] These efforts have paid off: In 2014, almost 80% of new mothers in the United States initiated breastfeeding; nearly 50% of mothers were still breastfeeding their babies at 6 months of age; and 19% of mothers were still exclusively breastfeeding at 6 months.[37]

Lactation Is Maintained by Hormones and Infant Suckling

Lactation, the production of breast milk, is a process that is set in motion during pregnancy in response to estrogen and progesterone, which are produced by the placenta. In addition to performing various functions to maintain the pregnancy, these hormones prepare the breasts physically for lactation. The breasts increase in size, and milk-producing glands (alveoli) and milk ducts are formed **(FIGURE 14.9)**. Toward the end of pregnancy, the hormone *prolactin* increases. Prolactin is released by the anterior pituitary gland and is responsible for milk synthesis.

lactation The production of breast milk.

colostrum The first fluid made and secreted by the breasts from late in pregnancy to about a week after birth. It is rich in immune factors and protein.

Production of Colostrum

By the time a pregnancy has come to full term, the level of prolactin is about 10 times higher than it was at the beginning of pregnancy. At birth, the suppressive effect of estrogen and progesterone ends, and prolactin is free to stimulate milk production. The first substance released is **colostrum**, sometimes called pre-milk or first milk. It is thick, yellowish in color, and rich in protein and micronutrients, and it includes antibodies that help protect the newborn from infection. Colostrum also contains a factor that fosters the growth of a particular species of "friendly" bacteria in the infant gastrointestinal tract. These bacteria in turn prevent the growth of other, potentially harmful bacteria. Finally, colostrum has a laxative effect in infants, helping the infant expel *meconium*, the sticky "first stool."

Within 4 to 6 days, colostrum is fully replaced by mature milk. Mature breast milk contains protein, fat, and carbohydrate (lactose) as well as all the essential vitamins and minerals. Much of the protein and fat is synthesized in the breast, while the rest enters the milk from the mother's bloodstream.

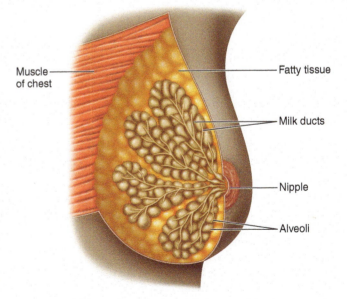

Muscle of chest — Fatty tissue — Milk ducts — Nipple — Alveoli

▲ **FIGURE 14.9** Anatomy of the breast. During pregnancy, estrogen and progesterone secreted by the placenta foster the preparation of breast tissue for lactation. This process includes breast enlargement and development of the milk-producing glands, or alveoli.

Production of Breast Milk

Continued, sustained breast milk production depends entirely on infant suckling (or a similar stimulus, such as a mechanical breast pump). Infant suckling stimulates the continued production of prolactin, which in turn stimulates more milk production. The longer and more vigorous the feeding, the more milk will be produced. Thus, even multiples (twins, triplets) can be successfully breastfed.

Prolactin allows for milk to be produced, but that milk has to move through the milk ducts to the nipple in order to reach the baby's mouth. The hormone responsible for this "let down" of milk is *oxytocin*. Like prolactin, oxytocin is produced by the pituitary gland, and its production is dependent on the suckling stimulus at the beginning of a feeding **(FIGURE 14.10)**. This response usually occurs within 10 to 30 seconds but can be significantly inhibited by stress. Finding a relaxed environment in which to breastfeed is therefore important.

Breastfeeding Woman Have High Nutrient Needs

Breastfeeding requires even more energy than pregnancy, as well as increased intakes of certain micronutrients.

Energy and Macronutrient Recommendations

Milk production requires an estimated 700 to 800 kcal per day. It is generally recommended that lactating women 19 and older consume 330 kcal per day above their pre-pregnancy energy needs during the first 6 months of lactation and 400 additional kcal per day during the second 6 months.[11] This additional energy is sufficient to support adequate milk production. The remaining energy deficit will assist in the gradual loss of excess fat and body weight gained during pregnancy, approximately 1 to 4 pounds per month. It is critical that lactating women avoid severe energy restriction because it can result in decreased milk production. **MEAL FOCUS FIGURE 14.11** compares two sets of meals providing the additional 400 kcal per day required to support the second

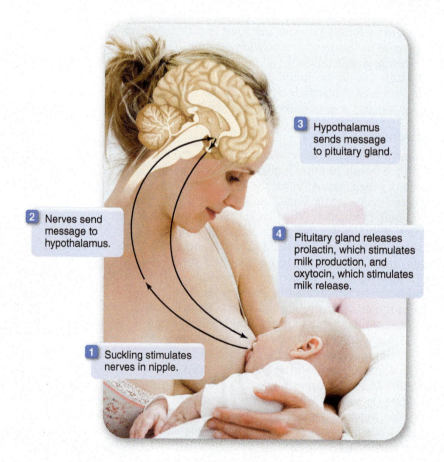

3 Hypothalamus sends message to pituitary gland.

2 Nerves send message to hypothalamus.

4 Pituitary gland releases prolactin, which stimulates milk production, and oxytocin, which stimulates milk release.

1 Suckling stimulates nerves in nipple.

▶ **FIGURE 14.10** Sustained milk production depends on the mother–child interaction during breastfeeding, specifically the suckling of the infant. Suckling stimulates the continued production of prolactin, which is responsible for milk production, and oxytocin, which is responsible for the let-down response.

a day of meals

low NUTRIENT DENSITY

high NUTRIENT DENSITY

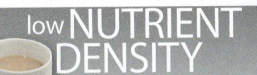

BREAKFAST

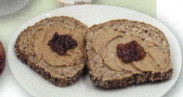

1 cinnamon raisin bagel with
  2 tbsp. cream cheese
8 fl. oz coffee with
  2 tbsp. cream

1 cup Raisin Bran Cereal with
  1/2 cup nonfat milk
2 slices of whole grain bread with
  peanut butter and jam
Medium apple
1 cup orange juice
8 fl. oz decaf nonfat latte

LUNCH

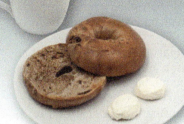

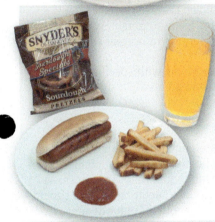

1 cup low-sodium lentil soup
Mixed salad with spinach:
1 hard-boiled egg
1/2 tomato
1/2 green pepper
2 oz cheddar cheese
1 cup raw baby carrots
2 tbsp. low-fat salad dressing

1 beef hot dog
1 white bun
Medium french fries
2 tbsp. catsup
2 oz bag of pretzels
16 fl. oz orange soda

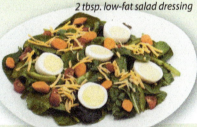

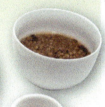

DINNER

2 beef tacos
2 oz tortilla chips with
  1/2 cup guacamole
16 fl. oz unsweetened ice tea
One brownie

2 grilled salmon tacos (3 oz each)
1/2 cup black beans
1/2 cup brown rice
1 cup steamed broccoli
2 oz dark chocolate
1/2 cup fresh strawberries
8 fl. oz decaf nonfat latte

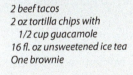

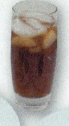

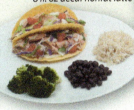

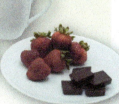

nutrient analysis

2,600 kcal
60 grams of protein
22 grams of dietary fiber
468 micrograms of folate
20 milligrams of vitamin C
540 milligrams of calcium
7 milligrams of zinc
3,570 milligrams of sodium

Provides the DRI for ALL nutrients even before snacks!

nutrient analysis

2,600 kcal
80 grams of protein
48 grams of dietary fiber
983 micrograms of folate
240 milligrams of vitamin C
1,550 milligrams of calcium
12 milligrams of zinc
2,163 milligrams of sodium

6 months of breastfeeding. Notice that the meals on the right meet all of the lactating woman's DRIs even before snacks. One set of meals is low in nutrient density whereas the other meets the nutrient recommendations for breastfeeding mothers.

Of the macronutrients, protein and carbohydrate needs are different from pregnancy requirements. Increases of 15 to 20 g of protein per day and 80 g of carbohydrate per day above prepregnancy requirements are recommended during lactation.[11] Women who breastfeed also need good dietary sources of the essential fatty acids.

Micronutrient Recommendations

The needs for several vitamins and minerals increase over the requirements of pregnancy. These include vitamins A, C, and E, riboflavin, vitamin B_{12}, biotin, and choline, as well as the minerals copper, chromium, manganese, iodine, selenium, and zinc. The requirement for folate during lactation is 500 μg per day, which is decreased from the 600 μg per day required during pregnancy, but it is still higher than prepregnancy needs (400 μg/day).[14]

Requirements for iron decrease significantly during lactation to a mere 9 mg per day.[16] This is because breast milk is relatively low in iron and breastfeeding usually suppresses menstruation for at least a few months, minimizing iron losses.

Calcium is a significant component of breast milk; however, as in pregnancy, calcium absorption is enhanced during lactation, and urinary loss of calcium is decreased. Thus, the recommended intake for calcium for a lactating woman is unchanged from pregnancy and nonpregnant guidelines; that is, 1,000 mg per day for mothers over age 18 and 1,300 mg per day for teen mothers.[17] Typically, if calcium intake is adequate, a woman's bone density returns to normal shortly after lactation ends.

ChooseMyPlate.gov provides a Daily Food Plan for Moms with specific, individualized dietary advice for women who are pregnant, or who are exclusively or partially breastfeeding their infants (see **Web Links** at the end of this chapter).

Do Breastfeeding Women Need Supplements?

If a breastfeeding woman appropriately increases her energy intake, and does so with nutrient-dense foods, her nutrient needs can usually be met without supplements. However, there is nothing wrong with taking a basic multivitamin for insurance, as long as it is not considered a substitute for proper nutrition. Lactating women should consume fish to increase the levels of DHA in their breast milk in order to support the infant's developing nervous system. Vegetarian and vegan women can boost their DHA intake with non-animal-based supplements. Women who don't consume dairy products should monitor their calcium intake carefully.

Fluid Recommendations for Breastfeeding Women

Because extra fluid is expended with every feeding, lactating women need to consume about an extra quart (about 1 liter) of fluid per day.[19] This extra fluid facilitates milk production and reduces risk for dehydration. Breastfeeding women are encouraged to drink a nutritious beverage, such as water, juice, or milk, each time they nurse their baby. However, it is not good practice to drink hot beverages while nursing because accidental spills could burn the infant.

recap Lactation is the result of the coordinated effort of several hormones, including estrogen, progesterone, prolactin, and oxytocin. Breasts are prepared for lactation during pregnancy, and infant suckling provides the stimulus that sustains the production of the prolactin and oxytocin needed to maintain the milk supply. It is recommended that lactating women consume an extra 300 to 400 kcal per day above prepregnancy energy intake, including increased protein, DHA, and fluids. The intake recommendations for vitamins A, C, and E, riboflavin, vitamin B_{12}, biotin, and choline, as well as the minerals copper, chromium, manganese, iodine, selenium, and zinc, increase over the requirements of pregnancy. The intake recommendations for folate and iron decrease from the requirements of pregnancy.

What are some advantages and challenges of breastfeeding?

This section explains why breastfeeding is considered the perfect way to nourish a baby for the first 6 months of life. It also explores factors that may make breastfeeding a difficult choice.

Breast Milk Is Nutritionally Superior to Infant Formula

As adept as formula manufacturers have been at simulating the components of breast milk, an exact replica has never been produced. First, the amount and types of protein in breast milk are ideally suited to the human infant. The main protein in breast milk, lactalbumin, is easily digested in infants' immature gastrointestinal tracts, reducing the risk for gastric distress. Certain proteins in human milk improve the absorption of iron; this is important because breast milk is low in iron. Other proteins in breast milk bind iron and prevent the growth of harmful bacteria that require iron. Antibodies from the mother are proteins that help prevent infection while the infant's immune system is still immature.

The primary carbohydrate in milk is lactose. Lactose provides energy and prevents ketosis in the infant, promotes the growth of beneficial bacteria, and increases the absorption of calcium.

The amounts and types of fats in breast milk are ideally suited to the human infant. DHA and ARA have been shown in many studies to be essential for growth and development of the infant's nervous system and for development of the retina. The concentration of DHA in breast milk reflects the amount of DHA in the mother's diet, and is highest in women who regularly consume fish.

The fat content of breast milk changes according to the age of the infant and during the course of every feeding: The milk that is initially released (*foremilk*) is watery and low in fat, and is thought to satisfy the infant's initial thirst. As the feeding progresses, the milk increases in fat content. Finally, the very last 5% or so of the milk produced during a feeding (*hindmilk*) is very high in fat, similar to cream. This milk is thought to satiate the infant. It is important to let infants suckle for at least 20 minutes at each feeding, so that they get this hindmilk. Breast milk is also relatively high in cholesterol, which supports the rapid growth and development of the brain.

Another important aspect of any type of feeding is the fluid it provides the infant. Because of their small size, infants are at risk for dehydration, which is one reason feedings must be consistent and frequent. This topic is discussed at greater length in the section on infant nutrition.

Breast milk is a good source of readily absorbed calcium and magnesium. It is low in iron, but the iron it does contain is easily absorbed. Because healthy full-term infants store iron in preparation for the first few months of life, most experts agree that their iron needs can be met by breast milk alone for the first 6 months, after which iron-rich foods are needed. Although breast milk provides some vitamin D, the American Academy of Pediatrics and other professional groups recommend that all infants, including those who are breastfed, be provided a vitamin D supplement, particularly those infants with highly pigmented skin.[36] Research suggests that providing a vitamin D supplement to breastfeeding women effectively maintains the vitamin D status of breastfed infants without the need to supplement the infant.[38,39]

Breast milk composition changes as the infant grows and develops. Because of this adaptation, breast milk alone is entirely sufficient to sustain infant growth for the first 6 months of life. In addition, exclusively breast-fed infants maintain total control over their food intake, allowing them to self-regulate energy intake during a critical period of growth and development. Some researchers believe this self-regulation accounts for the finding that breast-fed babies grow in length and weight at a slower rate than formula-fed infants while still maintaining excellent health; they also have a lower risk of obesity throughout their life.

Throughout the next 6 months of infancy, as solid foods are gradually introduced, breast milk remains the baby's primary source of superior-quality nutrition.

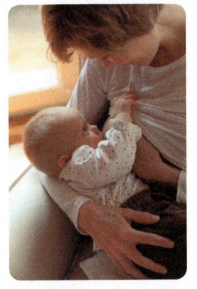

◄ Breastfeeding has benefits for both the mother and her infant.

The American Academy of Pediatrics recommends exclusive breastfeeding for the first 6 months of life, continuing breastfeeding for at least the first year of life, and, if acceptable within the family, into the second year of life.[36]

Breastfeeding Has Many Other Benefits for the Infant and Mother

In addition to its nutritional advantages, breast milk provides a variety of other healthful compounds, and breastfeeding itself has benefits.

Protection from Infections, Allergies, and Residues

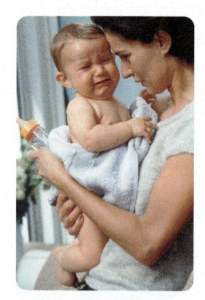

⬆ Breast-fed infants have a lower incidence of respiratory, gastrointestinal, and ear infections than formula-fed infants.

Immune factors from the mother are passed directly to the newborn through breast milk. These factors provide important disease protection for the infant while its immune system is immature. Breast-fed infants have lower rates of respiratory tract, gastrointestinal tract, and ear infections than formula-fed infants. Even a few weeks of breastfeeding is beneficial, but the longer a child is breastfed, the greater the level of passive immunity from the mother. In the United States, exclusive breastfeeding for 6 months has the potential to lower healthcare costs by as much as $13 billion per year, in large part due to a reduction in infant mortality rates related to **sudden infant death syndrome (SIDS)** and necrotizing enterocolitis (a disorder that causes tissue death in the intestine) in breast-fed infants.[40]

In addition, breast milk is nonallergenic, and breastfeeding is associated with a reduced risk for allergies during childhood and adulthood. Breast-fed babies also have a decreased risk of developing diabetes, overweight and obesity, and chronic digestive disorders.[41]

Breast-fed infants are known to have a different profile of gastrointestinal flora compared to formula-fed infants. They have greater numbers of health-promoting *Bifidobacteria* and lower counts of infection-producing bacteria. Moreover, it is thought that the microbiome of breast-fed infants reduces future risk of obesity[42] as well as protecting against infections and diabetes.[43]

Exclusively breast-fed infants are also protected from exposure to known and unknown contaminants and residues that may be present in infant formulas or introduced by caregivers preparing them. For example, a bacterium called *Cronobacter* can contaminate powdered infant formulas. It causes several cases of sepsis (blood infection) and an often fatal meningitis in infants each year.[44] Past concerns centered on bisphenol A (BPA), a toxic chemical that the U.S. Food and Drug Administration banned in 2012 from all baby bottles and toddler's cups. Baby bottles or cups manufactured before 2012 should be discarded unless they are BPA free.

Physiologic Benefits for Mother

Breastfeeding causes uterine contractions, which quicken the return of the uterus to prepregnancy size and reduces bleeding. Many women also find that breastfeeding helps them lose the weight they gained during pregnancy, particularly if it continues for more than 6 months. In addition, breastfeeding appears to be associated with a decreased risk for breast cancer and possibly type 2 diabetes and ovarian cancer.[43]

Breastfeeding also suppresses ovulation, lengthening the time between pregnancies and giving a mother's body the chance to recover before she conceives again.[43] This benefit can be lifesaving for malnourished women living in countries that discourage or outlaw the use of contraceptives. Ovulation may not cease completely, however, so healthcare providers typically recommend the use of contraceptives while breastfeeding to avoid another conception occurring too soon to allow a mother's body to recover from the earlier pregnancy.

Mother–Infant Bonding

Breastfeeding is among the most intimate of human interactions. Ideally, it is a quiet time away from distractions when mother and baby begin to develop an enduring bond of affection known as *attachment*. Breastfeeding enhances attachment by providing the opportunity for frequent, direct skin-to-skin contact, which stimulates the

sudden infant death syndrome (SIDS) The sudden death of a previously healthy infant; the most common cause of death in infants over 1 month of age.

baby's sense of touch and is a primary means of communication. The cuddling and intense watching that occur during breastfeeding begin to teach the mother and baby about the other's behavioral cues. Breastfeeding also reassures the mother that she is providing the best possible nutrition for her baby. Most hospitals now encourage round-the-clock rooming-in of newborns in order to encourage breastfeeding. Attachment can also occur with bottle-feeding, of course, as long as the caregivers provide closeness, cuddling, and skin and eye contact.

Convenience and Cost

Breast milk is always ready, clean, at the right temperature, and available on demand, whenever and wherever it's needed. In the middle of the night, when the baby wakes up hungry, a breastfeeding mother can respond almost instantaneously, and both are soon back to sleep. In contrast, formula-feeding is a time-consuming process: parents have to continually wash and sterilize bottles, and each batch of formula must be mixed and heated to the proper temperature.

In addition, breastfeeding costs nothing other than the price of a modest amount of additional food for the mother. In contrast, formula can be relatively expensive, and there are the additional costs of bottles and other supplies as well as the cost of energy used for washing and sterilization. Finally, breastfeeding is environmentally responsible, using no external energy and producing no external wastes.

Physical and Social Concerns Can Make Breastfeeding Challenging

For some women and infants, breastfeeding is easy from the very first day. Others experience some initial difficulty, but with support from an experienced nurse, lactation consultant, or volunteer from La Leche League, the experience becomes successful and pleasurable. In contrast, some families encounter difficulties that make formula-feeding their best choice. This section discusses some challenges that may impede the success of breastfeeding.

Effects of Drugs and Other Substances on Breast Milk

Many substances, including illegal, prescription, and over-the-counter drugs, as well as herbal and other dietary supplements, pass into breast milk. Breastfeeding mothers should inform their physicians that they are breastfeeding. If a safe and effective form of a necessary medication cannot be found, the mother will have to avoid breastfeeding while she is taking the drug. During this time, she can pump and discard her breast milk, so that her milk supply will be adequate when she resumes breastfeeding.

Caffeine, alcohol, nicotine, and illegal drugs also enter breast milk. Caffeine, nicotine, and other stimulant drugs can make the baby fussy and disturb sleep. Breastfeeding women should reduce their caffeine intake to no more than two or three cups of coffee per day (or the equivalent of other caffeine containing beverages and foods) and avoid caffeine intake within 2 hours prior to nursing their infant. They should also quit smoking and avoid the use of illegal drugs. Alcohol can make the baby sleepy, depress the central nervous system, and slow motor development, in addition to inhibiting the mother's milk supply. Breastfeeding women should abstain from alcohol in the early stages of lactation because it easily passes into the breast milk and infants 0 to 3 months of age metabolize alcohol at a rate half that of adults. It takes about 2 to 3 hours for the alcohol from a single serving of beer or wine to be eliminated from the body, so it is possible but challenging for breastfeeding women to coordinate moderate alcohol intake with their breastfeeding schedule.

Environmental contaminants, including pesticides, industrial solvents, and heavy metals such as lead and mercury, can pass into breast milk when breastfeeding mothers are exposed to these chemicals. Mothers can limit their infants' exposure to these harmful substances by controlling their own environments. Fresh fruits and vegetables should be thoroughly washed and peeled to minimize exposure to pesticides and fertilizer residues. Exposure to paint fumes, gasoline, solvents, and similar products should be greatly limited. Even with some exposure to these environmental contaminants, U.S. and international health agencies agree that the benefits of breast-feeding almost always outweigh potential concerns.

Components that pass into the breast milk from certain foods, such as garlic, onions, peppers, broccoli, and cabbage, may be distasteful enough to the infant to prevent proper feeding. Some babies have allergic reactions to foods the mother has eaten, such as wheat, cow's milk, eggs, or citrus, and suffer gastrointestinal upset, diaper rash, or other reactions. The offending foods must then be identified and avoided.

Maternal HIV Infection

HIV, which causes AIDS, can be transmitted from mother to baby through breast milk. Thus, HIV-positive women in the United States and Canada are encouraged to feed their infants formula. This recommendation does not apply to all women worldwide, however, because the low cost and sanitary nature of breast milk, as compared to the potential for waterborne diseases with formula-feeding, often make breastfeeding the best choice for women in developing countries.

Maternal Obesity

There is strong evidence that maternal obesity significantly reduces the rate of successful breastfeeding.[45] Fewer obese women plan to breastfeed and fewer actually initiate breastfeeding compared to normal weight women. Among those obese women who do breastfeed, they do so for shorter durations and produce a less adequate supply of milk. Obese women report more problems, such as cracked nipples and difficulty initiating breastfeeding, and are more likely to feel uncomfortable breastfeeding in front of others. These findings are particularly troubling because breastfeeding helps a woman lose some of her pregnancy weight, and has been shown to reduce the risk of overweight and obesity in the child, whereas children of obese mothers are, on average, at increased risk for overweight and obesity later in life.

Employment Conflicts

Breast milk is absorbed more readily than formula, making more frequent feedings necessary. Newborns commonly require breastfeedings every 1 to 3 hours versus every 2 to 4 hours for formula-feedings. Mothers who are exclusively breastfeeding and return to work within the first 6 months after the baby's birth must leave several bottles of pumped breast milk for others to feed the baby in their absence. They must then pump their breasts to express the breast milk during the workday and maintain their milk production. Federal legislation now requires "reasonable" break time (typically unpaid) and a private space other than a bathroom for breastfeeding mothers to express their milk.[46]

Work-related travel is also a concern: If the mother needs to be away from home for longer than 24 to 48 hours, she can typically pump and freeze enough breast milk for others to give the baby in her absence. When longer business trips are required, some mothers take the baby with them and arrange for childcare at their destination. Understandably, many women cite returning to work as the reason they switch to formula-feeding.

Some working women successfully combine breastfeeding with commercial formula-feeding. For example, a woman might breastfeed in the morning before she leaves for work, as soon as she returns home, and once again before going to bed. The remainder of the feedings is formula given by the infant's father or a childcare provider. Women who choose supplemental formula-feedings usually find that their body adapts quickly to the change and produces sample milk for the remaining breastfeedings.

Social Concerns

In North America, women have been conditioned to keep their breasts covered in public, even when feeding an infant. Over the past decade, however, both social customs and state laws have become more accommodating and supportive of nursing mothers. Some states have even passed legislation preserving a woman's right to breastfeed in public. With both legal and cultural support, as well as ongoing support

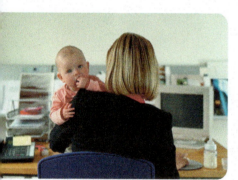

▲ Working moms can be discouraged from—or supported in—breastfeeding in a variety of ways.

from the health care team, women feel free to nurse their infants upon demand, whether they are at home or out in public.[46,47]

What About Bonding for Fathers and Siblings?

With all the attention given to attachment between a breastfeeding mother and her infant, it is easy for fathers and siblings to feel left out. One option that allows other family members to participate in infant feeding is to supplement breastfeedings with bottle-feedings of stored breast milk or formula. If a family decides to share infant feeding in this manner, bottle-feedings can begin as soon as breastfeeding has become well established. That way, the infant will not become confused by the artificial nipple. Fathers and other family members can also bond with the infant when bathing and/or dressing the infant as well as through everyday cuddling and play.

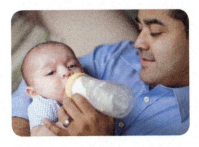

◆ Fathers and siblings can bond with infants through bottle-feeding and other forms of close contact.

recap Breastfeeding provides many benefits to both mother and newborn, including superior nutrition, heightened immunity, mother–infant bonding, convenience, and cost. However, breastfeeding may not be the best option for every family. The mother may need to use a medication that enters the breast milk and makes it unsafe for consumption. HIV-positive women in the United States and Canada are encouraged to feed their infants formula. Obese women report more difficulties with breastfeeding and tend to breastfeed for shorter durations and produce a less adequate supply of milk. A mother's job may interfere with the baby's requirement for frequent feedings. The infant's father and siblings can participate in feedings using a bottle filled with either pumped breast milk or formula.

What are an infant's nutrient needs?

Most first-time parents are amazed at how rapidly their infant grows. Optimal nutrition is extremely important during the first year, as the baby's organs and nervous system continue to develop and the baby grows physically. In fact, physicians use length and weight measurements as the main tools for assessing an infant's nutritional status. These measurements are plotted on growth charts for boys and girls, which track an infant's growth over time **(FIGURE 14.12)** (page 514). Although every infant is unique, in general, physicians look for a correlation between length and weight. In other words, an infant who is in the 60th percentile for length is usually in about the 50th to 70th percentile for weight. An infant who is in the 90th percentile for weight but is in the 20th percentile for length might be overfed. Consistency over time is also a consideration; for example, an infant who suddenly drops well below her established profile for weight might be underfed or ill.

LO 6 Relate the growth and activity patterns of infants to their nutrient needs and the nutrient profile of infant formulas.

Nutrition Fuels Infant Growth and Activity

Babies' basal metabolic rates are high, in part because their body surface area is large compared to their body size. Still, their limited physical activity keeps total energy expenditure relatively low. For the first few months of life, their activities consist mainly of eating and sleeping. As the first year progresses, they begin rolling over, sitting up, crawling, standing, and finally taking the first few wobbly steps. Nevertheless, relatively few Calories are expended in movement, and the primary use of energy is to support growth.

In the first year of life, an infant generally grows about 10 inches in length and triples in weight—a growth rate more rapid than will ever occur again. Not surprisingly, energy needs per unit body weight are also the highest in order to support this phenomenal growth and metabolism.

The infant's growth surge includes the brain. To accommodate such a large increase in brain size, the bones of the skull do not fuse until the second year of life. An infant's head is typically quite large in proportion to the rest of the body. Pediatricians use head circumference as an additional tool for the assessment of growth and nutritional status. After around 18 months of age, the rate of brain growth slows, and gradually the body "catches up" to head size.

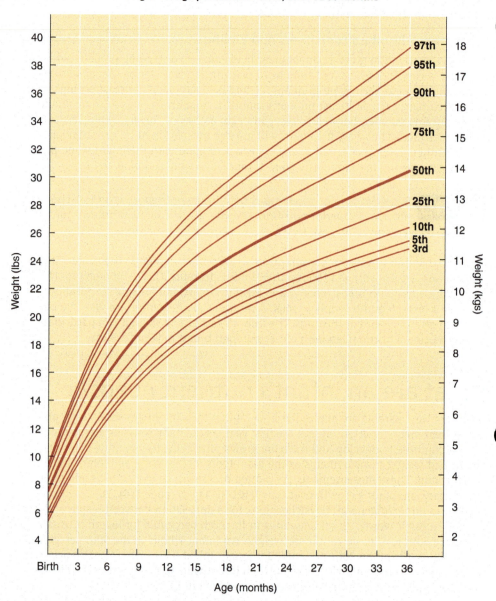

Weight-for-age percentiles: Girls, birth to 36 months

FIGURE 14.12 This weight-for-age growth chart is a much smaller version of charts used by healthcare providers to monitor and assess the growth of an infant/toddler from birth to 36 months. This example shows the growth curves of girls over time, each at different percentiles.

Source: Data adapted from "Clinical Growth Charts: Infants, Birth to 36 Months." Centers for Disease Control and Prevention.

Infants Have Unique Nutrient Needs

Three characteristics of infants combine to make their nutritional needs unique: (1) their high energy needs per unit body weight to support rapid growth, (2) their immature digestive tract and kidneys, and (3) their small size.

Energy and Macronutrient Recommendations

An infant needs to consume about 40 to 50 kcal per pound of body weight per day.[11] This amounts to about 600 to 650 kcal per day at around 6 months of age. Given the immature digestive tract and kidneys of infants, as well as their high fluid needs, providing this much energy may seem difficult. Fortunately, breast milk and commercial formulas are energy dense, contributing about 650 kcal per liter of fluid. When complementary (solid) foods are introduced at 4 to 6 months of age, they provide additional energy.

Infants are not merely small versions of adults. The proportions of macronutrients they require differ from adult proportions, as do the types of food they can tolerate. About 40% to 50% of an infant's energy should come from fat during the first year of life; fat intake below this level can be harmful before the age of 2. Given the high energy needs of infants, it makes sense to take advantage of the energy density of fat (9 kcal/g) to help meet these requirements. Breast milk and commercial formulas are both high in fat (about 50% of total energy). As noted earlier, breast milk is an excellent source of the fatty acids ARA and DHA, although DHA levels vary considerably with the mother's diet. Many formula manufacturers now add ARA and DHA to their products.

Infants 0 to 6 months of age need approximately 9 g of protein per day, whereas infants 7 to 12 months need almost 10 g per day to support their rapid growth.[11] Infants' immature kidneys are not able to process and excrete the excess nitrogen groups from higher-protein diets; thus, no more than 20% of an infant's daily energy requirement should come from protein. Breast milk and commercial formulas both provide adequate total protein and appropriate essential amino acids to support growth and development.

The recommended intake for carbohydrate is set at 60 g per day for infants 0 to 6 months of age and 95 g per day for infants 7 to 12 months old.[11] These levels reflect the lactose content of human milk, which is used as the reference point for most infant nutrient guidelines.

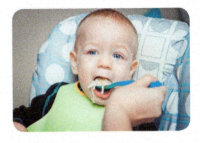

▲ Infants 7 to 12 months old need almost 10 g of protein and 95 g of carbohydrate a day.

Micronutrient Recommendations

Infants need micronutrients to accommodate their rapid growth and development. The micronutrients of particular concern are iron, vitamin D, zinc, fluoride, and iodine. Fortunately, breast milk and commercial formulas provide most of the micronutrients needed for infant growth and development, with some special considerations, discussed shortly.

In addition, all infants are routinely given an injection of vitamin K shortly after birth. This provides vitamin K until the infant's intestine can develop its own healthful bacteria, which then contribute to the infant's supply of vitamin K.

Do Infants Need Supplements?

Breast milk and commercial formulas provide most of the vitamins and minerals infants need. However, several micronutrients may warrant supplementation.

For breast-fed infants, a supplement containing vitamin D is commonly prescribed from birth to around 6 months of age, even in sunny climates, because exposure of a young infant's skin to adequate direct sunlight for vitamin D synthesis is not advised. Vitamin D deficiency is actually quite common among breast-fed infants,[48] especially those with dark skin and limited sunlight exposure. It has been estimated that exclusively breast-fed infants receive less than 20% of the recommended intake of vitamin D, reinforcing the importance of vitamin D supplementation for these infants or their breastfeeding mothers.[48,49]

Iron is extremely important for cognitive development and prevention of iron-deficiency anemia. Breast-fed infants require additional iron beginning no later than 6 months of age because the infant's iron stores become depleted and breast milk is a poor source of iron. At 4 to 6 months of age, breast-fed infants should be started on complementary (solid) foods that are high in iron, such as pureed meats or iron-fortified infant rice cereal.

If the mother is a vegan, her breast milk may be low in vitamin B_{12}, and a supplement of this vitamin should be given to the baby. Fluoride is important for strong tooth development, but fluoride supplementation is not recommended during the first 6 months of life.

For formula-fed infants, supplementation depends on the formula composition and the water supply used to make the formula. Many formulas are already fortified with iron, for example, and some municipal water supplies contain fluoride. If this is the case, and the baby is getting adequate vitamin D through the intake of at least 1 liter of formula per day, then an additional supplement may not be necessary.

Consultation with the infant's pediatrician is essential before giving a supplement. The supplement should be formulated specifically for infants, and the daily dose should not be exceeded. High doses of micronutrients can be dangerous. Too much iron can be fatal, too much fluoride can cause discoloration and pitting of the teeth, and too much vitamin D can lead to calcification of soft tissue, such as the kidneys.

Fluid Recommendations for Infants

Fluid is critical for everyone, but for infants the balance is more delicate for two reasons. First, because infants are so small, they proportionally lose more water through evaporation than adults. Second, their kidneys are immature and unable to concentrate urine. Thus, they are at even greater risk for dehydration. An infant needs about 2 ounces of fluid per pound of body weight, and either breast milk or formula is almost always enough to provide this amount. Experts recently confirmed that "infants exclusively fed human milk do not require supplemental water."[19]

Certain conditions, such as diarrhea, vomiting, fever, or hot weather, can greatly increase fluid loss. In these instances, supplemental fluid, ideally as water, may be necessary. Because too much fluid can be particularly dangerous for an infant, supplemental fluids (whether water or an infant electrolyte formula) should be given only under the advice of a physician. Generally, it is advised that supplemental fluids not exceed 4 ounces per day, and parents should avoid giving sugar water, fruit juices, or any sweetened beverage in a bottle. Parents can be sure that their infant's fluid intake is appropriate if the infant produces six to eight wet diapers per day.

Infant Formula Is a Nutritious Alternative to Breast Milk

If breastfeeding is not feasible, several types of commercial formulas provide nutritious alternatives. By law, U.S. formula manufacturers must meet standards for 29 different nutrients. Although formula companies try to mimic the nutritional value of breast milk, their formulas still cannot duplicate the immune factors, enzymes, and other unique components of human milk.

Most formulas are based on cow's milk that has been modified to make it more appropriate for human infants. The amount of protein is reduced and the balance of the proteins casein and whey are modified to improve digestibility. The sugars lactose (naturally occurring) and sucrose (added), alone or in combination, provide carbohydrates, and vegetable oils and/or synthetic fatty acids replace the naturally occurring butterfat. Recently, some manufacturers have added other nutrients, such as taurine, carnitine, and the fatty acids ARA and DHA, to more closely mimic the nutrient profile of human milk. This chapter's **Nutrition Label Activity** feature identifies some of these ingredients.

Soy-based formulas are a viable alternative for infants who are lactose intolerant (although this is rare in infants) or cannot tolerate the proteins in cow's milk–based formulas. Soy formulas may also satisfy the requirements of families who are strict vegans. However, soy contains isoflavones, phytochemicals that act as estrogens and may alter infant growth and development. Babies can also have allergic reactions to soy-based formulas.

There are also specialized formula preparations for infants with certain medical conditions. Some contain proteins that have been predigested, for example, or have been specially formulated for preterm infants, older infants, and toddlers. The final choice of formula should depend on infant tolerance, stage of infant development, and the advice of the infant's pediatrician.

It is important to note that the use of cow's milk (fresh, dried, evaporated, or condensed) is inappropriate for infants under the age of 1 year. Infants also should not be fed goat's milk, or any plant-based milk alternative such as soymilk, rice milk, or nut milks, as none of these will meet their nutrient needs and can lead to severe nutrient deficiencies.[50]

Reading Infant Food Labels

Imagine that you are a new parent shopping for infant formula. **FIGURE 14.13** shows the label from a typical can of formula. As you can see, the ingredients list is long and has many technical terms. Even well-informed parents would probably be stumped by many of them. Fortunately, with the information you learned in previous chapters, you can probably answer the following questions.

- One of the ingredients listed is a modified form of *whey protein concentrate*. What common food is the source of *whey*?

- The second ingredient listed is *lactose*. Is lactose a form of protein, fat, or carbohydrate? Why is lactose important for infants?

- The front label states the formula has added DHA (docosahexaenoic acid). Is DHA a form of protein, fat, or carbohydrate? Why is this nutrient thought to be important for infants?

- The label also claims that this formula is "Our closest formula to mature breast milk." Can you think of some differences between breast milk and this formula that still exist?

Also, look at the list of nutrients on the label. You'll notice that there is no "% Daily Value" column, which you see on most food labels. Next time you are at the grocery store, look at other baby food items, such as baby cereal or pureed fruits. Do their labels simply list the nutrient content or is the "% Daily Value" column used? Why do you think infant formula has a different label format?

Let's say you are feeding a 6-month-old infant who needs about 500 kcal per day. Using the information from the nutrition section of the label, you can calculate the number of fluid ounces of formula the baby

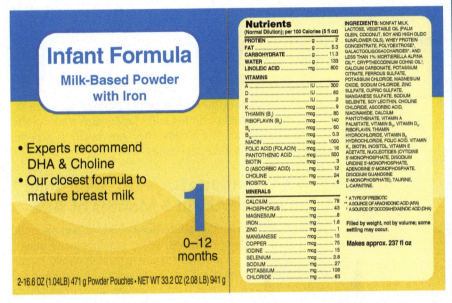

FIGURE 14.13 An infant formula label. Notice that there is a long list of ingredients and no % Daily Value.

needs (this assumes that no cereal or other foods are eaten):

There are 100 kcal (Calories) per 5 fluid ounces.

100 kcal ÷ 5 fl. oz = 20 kcal/fl. oz
500 kcal ÷ 20 kcal/fl. oz = 25 fl. oz of formula per day to meet the baby's energy needs

A 6-month-old infant needs about 210 mg calcium per day. Based on an intake of 25 fluid ounces of formula per day, as just calculated, you can use the label nutrition information to calculate the amount of calcium that is provided:

There are 78 mg calcium per 5 fluid ounce serving of formula.

78 mg ÷ 5 fl. oz = 15.6 mg calcium per fl. oz
15.6 mg calcium per fl. oz × 25 fl. oz = 390 mg of calcium per day

You can see that the infant's need for calcium is easily met by the formula alone.

recap Infancy is characterized by the most rapid growth a human being will ever experience, and appropriate growth is the most reliable long-term indicator of adequate infant nutrition. Three characteristics of infants combine to make their nutritional needs unique: (1) their high energy needs—40 to 50 kcal per pound of body weight—to support rapid growth, (2) their immature digestive tract and kidneys, and (3) their small size. Breast milk is the ideal infant food for the first 6 months of life; infant formula is also a nutritious choice. About 40% to 50%

of an infant's energy intake should come from fat, and no more than 20% from protein. Infants need about 2 ounces of fluid per pound of body weight. Breast milk and commercial formulas provide most of the vitamins and minerals infants need. However, vitamin D, iron, and for infants of vegan mothers, vitamin B_{12} may warrant supplementation.

LO 7 Discuss some common nutrition-related concerns for infants.

What are some common nutrition-related concerns of infancy?

Nutrition is one of the primary concerns of new parents. Many are uncertain when to begin offering solid foods, and what to offer. Moreover, as infants begin to consume a variety of foods, they may begin to experience allergic reactions or other disorders or feeding challenges.

Infants Begin to Need Solid Foods at About 6 Months of Age

Infants begin to need solid, or complementary, foods at around 6 months of age. Before this age, several factors make most infants unable to consume solid food.

One factor is the *extrusion reflex*. In early infancy, the suckling response depends on a particular movement of the tongue that draws liquid out of the breast or bottle. But when solid foods are introduced with a spoon, the extrusion reflex causes the baby to push most of the food back out of the mouth. The extrusion reflex begins to lessen around 4 to 5 months of age.

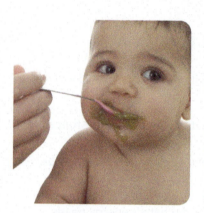

Another factor is the development of appropriate muscle control and oral skills.[51] To minimize the risk for choking, infants must have gained muscular control of the head and neck and be able to sit up (with or without support). In addition, they must be able to signal readiness to eat by opening their mouth, and to move the food from the front of the mouth to the back, where it can be safely swallowed.

Still another part of being ready for solid foods is sufficient maturity of the digestive and kidney systems. Although infants can digest and absorb lactose from birth, they do not develop the ability to digest starch until the age of 3 to 4 months. Feeding cereal, for example, before an infant can digest the starch may cause diarrhea and discomfort. Finally, the kidneys must have matured so that they are better able to process nitrogen wastes from proteins and concentrate urine.

▲ The extrusion reflex will push solid food out of an infant's mouth.

The need for solid foods is also related to nutrient needs. At about 6 months of age, if not fed iron-fortified formula, infant iron stores become depleted; thus, iron-fortified infant cereals are often the first foods introduced. Iron-fortified rice cereal, a source of non-heme iron, rarely provokes an allergic response and is easy to digest. Once a child reaches 6 months of age, pureed meats and poultry can provide well-absorbed heme iron. At this point, overreliance on breast milk or formula can limit the infant's intake of iron-rich foods, resulting in a condition known as *milk anemia*.

Delaying the introduction of infant foods until at least 4 months of age reduces the risk of food allergies. Infant foods should be introduced one at a time, with no other new foods for about 1 week, so that parents can watch for signs of allergies, such as a rash, gastrointestinal problems, a runny nose, or wheezing. The appropriate delaying of solid foods is also associated with a reduced risk of child obesity.[52]

Between 6 months and the time of weaning (from breast or bottle), solid foods should gradually make up an increasing proportion of the infant's diet. A variety of single-grain cereals, strained vegetables, fruits, and protein sources should be introduced by the end of the first year. During this time, food textures can advance from purees to very soft foods and eventually harder or textured foods. Commercial baby foods are convenient, nutritious, typically made without added salt or sugar, and come in a range of age-appropriate textures. However, home-prepared baby foods are usually cheaper and reflect the cultural food patterns of the family. Even throughout the first year, however, solid foods should be a supplement to, not a substitute for, breast milk or iron-fortified formula.

Some Foods and Beverages Are Not Safe for Infants

The following foods should never be offered to an infant:

- **Foods that can cause choking.** Infants cannot adequately chew foods such as grapes, hot dogs, cheese sticks, nuts, popcorn, raw carrots, raisins, and hard candies. These can cause choking.
- **Corn syrup and honey.** These may contain spores of the bacterium *Clostridium botulinum*. These spores can germinate and grow into viable bacteria in the immature digestive tract of infants. The bacteria secrete the potent botulism toxin, which can be fatal. Children older than 1 year can safely consume corn syrup and honey because their digestive tract is mature enough to kill any *C. botulinum* bacteria.
- **Cow's milk, goat's milk, and plant-based milk alternatives.** As noted earlier, these milks do not have a nutrient profile that meets infants' needs. Infants can begin to consume them after the age of 1 year. Infants and toddlers should not be given reduced-fat milks before the age of 2 because they do not contain enough fat. Infants should not be given evaporated milk or sweetened condensed milk.
- **Too much salt and sugar.** Infant foods should not be seasoned with salt or spices. Naturally occurring sugars, such as those found in fruits, are acceptable, but cookies and other processed desserts high in added sugar should be avoided.

> For a list of foods and objects associated with choking, visit the American Academy of Pediatrics' www.healthychidlren.org. Enter "choking prevention" into the search bar, then click on the link.

Several Nutrition-Related Disorders Are Concerns for Infants

Infants cannot speak, and their cries are sometimes indecipherable. Feeding time can therefore be very frustrating for parents if the child is not eating, is not growing appropriately, or has problems such as colic, diarrhea, vomiting, or persistent skin rashes. The following are some nutrition-related concerns for infants.

Allergies

Many foods have the potential to stimulate an allergic reaction. Breastfeeding helps reduce the risk of food allergies, as does delaying the introduction of solid foods until the age of 4 to 6 months. One of the most common allergies in infants is to the proteins in cow's milk–based formulas. Egg white, peanut, and wheat are other common triggers of food allergies. Symptoms vary but may include diarrhea, constipation, bloating, blood in the stool, and vomiting. As stated earlier, every new food should be introduced in isolation, so that any allergic reaction can be identified and the offending food avoided. New techniques to prevent food allergies in infants are the subject of some controversy, as discussed in the **Nutrition Debate** at the end of this chapter.

Dehydration

Whether the cause is diarrhea, vomiting, or inadequate fluid intake, dehydration is extremely dangerous to infants and, if left untreated, can quickly result in death. Treatment includes providing fluids, a task that is difficult if vomiting is occurring. In some cases, the physician may recommend that a pediatric electrolyte solution be administered on a temporary basis. In more severe cases, hospitalization may be necessary. If possible, breastfeeding should continue throughout an illness. A physician should be consulted concerning formula-feeding and solid foods.

Colic

Perhaps nothing is more frustrating to new parents than the relentless crying spells of some infants, typically referred to as **colic**. In this condition, newborns and young infants who appear happy, healthy, and well-nourished suddenly begin to cry or even shriek, continuing for several minutes to 3 hours or more, no matter what their caregiver does to console them. The spells tend to occur at the same time of day, typically late in the afternoon or early in the evening, and often occur daily for a period of several weeks. Overstimulation of the nervous system, feeding too rapidly, swallowing of air, and intestinal gas pain are considered possible culprits, but the precise cause is unknown.

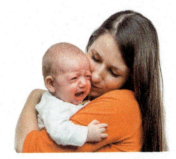

◄ Colicky babies will begin crying for no apparent reason, even if they otherwise appear well nourished and happy.

colic A condition of inconsolable infant crying that lasts for hours at a time.

As with allergies, if a colicky infant is breastfed, breastfeeding should be continued, but the mother should try to determine whether eating certain foods seems to prompt crying and, if so, eliminate the offending food(s) from her diet. Formula-fed infants may benefit from a change in type of formula. In the worst cases of colic, a physician may prescribe medication. Fortunately, most cases disappear spontaneously, possibly because of the maturity of the gastrointestinal tract, around 3 months of age.

Anemia

As stated earlier, full-term infants are born with sufficient iron stores to last for approximately the first 6 months of life. In older infants and toddlers, however, iron is the mineral most likely to be deficient. Iron-deficiency anemia causes pallor, lethargy, and impaired growth. Commercial formulas are fortified with iron. For breastfed infants, some pediatricians prescribe an iron supplement; however, iron for older infants is also supplied by iron-fortified rice cereal.

Nursing Bottle Syndrome

Infants should not be left alone with a bottle, whether lying down or sitting up. As infants manipulate the nipple of the bottle in their mouth, the high-carbohydrate fluid (whether breast milk, formula, or fruit juice) drips out, coming into prolonged contact with the developing teeth. This high-carbohydrate fluid provides an optimal food source for the bacteria that are the underlying cause of **dental caries** (cavities). Severe tooth decay can result **(FIGURE 14.14)**. Encouraging the use of a cup around the age of 8 months helps prevent nursing bottle syndrome, along with weaning the baby from a bottle entirely by the age of 15 to 18 months.

Lead Poisoning

The heavy metal lead is a neurotoxin that is especially harmful to infants and children because their brains and central nervous systems are still developing. Lead poisoning can result in decreased mental capacity, behavioral problems, impaired growth, impaired hearing, and other problems. Unfortunately, leaded pipes and lead paint can still be found in older homes and buildings, and as occurred in the city of Flint, Michigan, in 2015, lead can even leach into the municipal water supply. The following measures can reduce lead exposure:

- Use only cold tap water for drinking, mixing with foods, or cooking. Hot tap water is more likely to leach lead. After a faucet has not been used for a few hours, or overnight, allow the water to run for a minute or so to clear the pipes of any lead-contaminated water before using the water for consumption or cooking. The water should be very cold.
- Replace old plumbing with lead-free fixtures.
- Have lead-based paint professionally removed, or paint over it with latex paint.

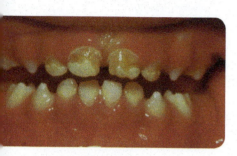

FIGURE 14.14 Leaving a baby alone with a bottle can result in the tooth decay of nursing bottle syndrome.

recap Breast milk or iron-fortified formula provides all necessary nutrients for the first 6 months of life. After that, solid foods can gradually be introduced into an infant's diet. Iron-fortified cereal or strained meats are typical choices, and single-item vegetables and fruits are appropriate. Foods and beverages with added sugars should be avoided. Micronutrient supplements should be given only if prescribed. Parents must avoid giving their infants foods that could trigger choking, such as hot dogs, grapes, and other firm foods. New foods should be introduced slowly, and infants must be monitored for allergies. Colic typically resolves by 3 months of age. Dehydration is a significant risk in infants and must be treated at the earliest signs. To prevent dental caries, infants should not be left alone with a bottle, whether lying down or sitting up. Infants and children are highly vulnerable to lead in paints or contaminated water. Lead poisoning can result in neurological problems.

dental caries Dental erosion and decay caused by acid-secreting bacteria in the mouth and on the teeth. The acid produced is a by-product of bacterial metabolism of carbohydrates deposited on the teeth.

Preventing Food Allergies in Infants: Allergen Avoidance or Introduction?

Recently, the incidence of food allergies (see Chapter 3) among U.S. children has increased by 50 percent, with an annual cost of nearly $25 billion.[53] An estimated 10 percent of infants and toddlers and 8 percent of children in the United States are affected by food allergies,[54] and nearly 40 percent of these children experience a severe reaction.[55] The three most common food triggers of pediatric allergies are peanut, cow's milk, and shellfish; soy, wheat, tree nuts, egg, and fin fish are other common allergens. Whereas many infants grow out of food allergies, children with peanut allergies often remain reactive for decades, if not their entire life.

Historically, the risk for food allergies in infants and toddlers has been linked to early exposure to the food(s). Therefore, national guidelines have recommended—and continue to recommend—delaying the introduction of solid foods until the infant is 4 to 6 months of age.[56] Many concerned parents avoid giving foods with common allergens even to their older infants and toddlers. In one study, nearly half of mothers of 8- to 10-month-old infants withheld nuts, while a small percentage withheld eggs, dairy, and/or fish.[57] Over the past decade, however, there has been growing evidence that this "avoidance" approach has failed to reduce the incidence of food allergies, and may have increased it.[55]

As a result, some allergy and immunology specialists have been encouraging parents to repeatedly feed very small amounts of potentially allergenic foods, such as peanut butter, to their infants.[58] This practice has been shown to reduce the incidence of allergic reactions.[58,59] In one study, parents in the experimental group gave their high-risk infants (4 to 11 months of age) about 1 teaspoon of peanut butter at least three times per week (equal to about 1 tablespoon of peanut butter per week). Parents in the control group completely withheld all peanut-containing foods until the children reached the age of 5. Those who were exposed to peanut early in life had an 80% lower rate of peanut allergy at age 5 years compared to those who had avoided peanuts. A follow-up study showed that the "early exposure" children remained at low risk for peanut allergy even after avoiding peanuts for 1 year.[60] Another study began introducing very small amounts of potentially allergenic foods to breast-fed infants when they were only 3 months old. When reexamined between the ages of 1 and 3 years, the children exposed to the potential allergens were less likely to demonstrate food allergies compared to controls, but only if the parents carefully followed the feeding schedule.[58] Otherwise, there was no protective effect compared to the infants who were exposed at 6 months of age or older. Unfortunately, less than half of the parents were able to adhere to the feeding schedule, so it is unlikely that this approach could be widely adopted.

Based on this evidence, a group of 10 national and international medical groups released new recommendations

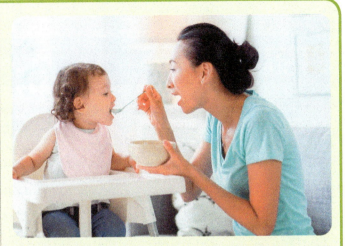

Early introduction of foods containing common allergens—such as peanut butter, wheat biscuits, or plain yogurt—may help reduce the risk for food allergies in childhood.

on how and when to introduce peanut to high-risk infants in order to prevent peanut allergies.[61] While supportive of the "early introduction" approach, the recommendations included "evaluation by an allergist or physician trained in management of allergic diseases in this age group" in order to assess the safety of early introduction of potential allergens.

Thus, parents of infants at low risk (based on family history and other factors) should not withhold common allergens because, as we have seen, prolonged avoidance appears to increase the risk of subsequent food allergies. In contrast, infants considered "at risk" should be evaluated by a specialist who may consider the early introduction approach.

CRITICAL THINKING QUESTIONS

1. Imagine that one of your relatives known to have a peanut allergy recently gave birth to a baby and told you she would *never* feed her child peanuts until 6 years of age. Would you share with her this new research on pediatric allergies? Why or why not?

2. Why do you think it was so difficult for many parents in the pediatric allergy studies to follow for 1 year the schedule for introducing the potentially allergenic foods?

3. Other than a family history of food allergies, what are other factors that increase the risk of food allergies for children? For example, does income, race, geography, or health history of the child make a difference? Go online to review the research and help you identify risk factors.

1 F Pregnant women need only 350 to 450 additional Calories per day, and only during the second and third trimesters of pregnancy. This is an increase of only 20% or less, not a doubling of Calories.

2 T Breast milk contains various immune factors (antibodies and immune system cells) from the mother that protect the infant against infection. The nutrients in breast milk are structured to be easily digested by an infant, resulting in fewer symptoms of gastrointestinal distress and fewer allergies.

3 F Most infants do not have a physiologic need for solid food until about 6 months of age.

review questions

LO 1
1. Folate deficiency in the first weeks after conception has been linked with which of the following problems in the newborn?
a. anemia
b. neural tube defects
c. low birth weight
d. preterm delivery

LO 2
2. During the last two trimesters of pregnancy, about how many extra Calories per day does a woman need over her pre-pregnancy intake?
a. 350 to 450 kcal/day
b. 450 to 550 kcal/day
c. 550 to 650 kcal/day
d. 650 to 750 kcal/day

LO 3
3. Which of the following is a valid recommendation for reducing symptoms of morning sickness?
a. Eat as much as possible at each meal, as a full stomach can reduce nausea.
b. Consume fluids only at mealtimes because fluids on an empty stomach can increase nausea.
c. Keep dry cereal or crackers at the bedside to ease nighttime and morning nausea.
d. Drink colas and other caffeinated, carbonated beverages because these reduce nausea.

LO 4
4. Which of the following hormones is responsible for the letdown response?
a. progesterone
b. estrogen
c. oxytocin
d. prolactin

LO 4
5. Which of the following statements about maternal nutrition is true?
a. Lactating women need more Calories than pregnant women.
b. Lactating women need more iron than pregnant women.
c. Lactating women need more folate than pregnant women.
d. Lactating women must entirely avoid caffeine and alcohol.

LO 5
6. Which of the following statements about breast milk is true?
a. Most carbohydrate in breast milk is in the form of glucose.
b. The fat content of breast milk is lower than that of cow's milk.
c. Breast milk is cholesterol-free.
d. Certain proteins in breast milk help protect the newborn from infection.

LO 6
7. Which of the following micronutrients should be added to the diet of breast-fed infants when they are around 6 months of age?
a. vitamin K
b. calcium
c. iron
d. vitamin A

LO 7
8. After 6 months of age, it is safe and healthful to give infants
a. non-fat milk.
b. a cheese stick or chunks of cheese.
c. honey.
d. none of the above.

LO 1 9. **True or false?** Major developmental errors and birth defects are most likely to occur in the first trimester of pregnancy.

LO 3 10. **True or false?** If gestational diabetes is uncontrolled, the fetus may not receive enough glucose and may be born small for gestational age.

math review

LO 5 11. Mature breast milk averages about 700 kcal per liter, with 35 g of fat and 9 g of protein. Calculate the % of kcal from fat and protein. How do these values compare to those recommended for a healthy young adult? Why are the nutrient proportions of breast milk appropriate for infants?

Answers to Review Questions and Math Review are located at the back of this text and in the MasteringNutrition Study Area.

web links

www.aap.org
American Academy of Pediatrics
Visit this website for information on infants' and children's health. Searches can be performed for topics such as "neural tube defects" and "infant formulas."

www.emedicine.com
eMedicine: Pediatrics
Enter "Pediatrics" into the search bar, then select "toxicology," and then "iron toxicity" to learn about accidental iron poisoning in children and infants.

www.marchofdimes.com
March of Dimes
Click on "During Your Pregnancy" to find links on nutrition during pregnancy, exercise, and things to avoid.

www.diabetes.org
American Diabetes Association
Search for "gestational diabetes" to find information about diabetes that develops during pregnancy.

www.choosemyplate.gov
USDA ChooseMyPlate
Search on the term "Daily Food Plan for Moms" and enter your information to get specific, individualized dietary advice for pregnant, or exclusively or partially breastfeeding, women via the Supertracker feature.

www.lalecheleague.org
La Leche League
Search this site to find multiple articles on the health effects of breastfeeding for mother and infant.

www.nofas.org
National Organization on Fetal Alcohol Syndrome
This site provides news and information relating to fetal alcohol syndrome.

www.helppregnantsmokersquit.org
The National Partnership for Smoke-Free Families
This site was created for healthcare providers and smokers with the purpose of educating about the dangers of smoking while pregnant and providing tools to help pregnant smokers quit.

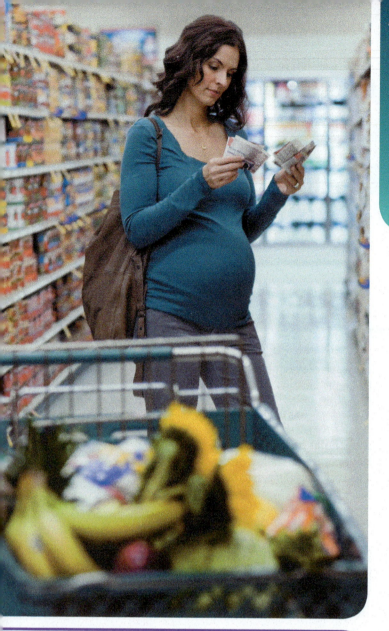

The Fetal Environment

learning outcomes

After studying this In Depth, you should be able to:

1 Identify three health problems seen in adults whose mothers were exposed to famine during their first trimester of pregnancy, pp. 525–526.

2 Describe the effects seen later in life among children born to mothers with specific nutrient deficiencies, obesity, or gestational diabetes, pp. 526–527.

Would you be surprised to learn that your risk of developing obesity, metabolic syndrome, and certain chronic diseases as an adult might have been influenced by what happened before your birth? Over the last several decades, a growing body of evidence has revealed that the fetal environment, including the mother's nutritional status, influences the health of her offspring not only during the first few weeks of life, but also as the infant grows into a child and adult.

In this **In Depth** essay, we explore this relationship, often referred to as the "fetal origins of adult disease" theory. Although it's based on studies of populations that have endured famine, it has broad-ranging implications, including for immigrants from developing nations who move to the United States. We also describe the enduring effects of a variety of other nutritional imbalances in the fetal environment, including specific micronutrient deficiencies and maternal obesity.

How does fetal adaptation to famine affect adult health?

LO 1 Identify three health problems seen in adults whose mothers were exposed to famine during their first trimester of pregnancy.

Some of the earliest research into the fetal origins theory investigated the health of adults born during or shortly after a famine in the Netherlands from 1944 to 1945. During World War II, the Dutch population had been relatively well nourished until October 1944, when the Germans placed an embargo on all food transport into the western Netherlands. At the same time, an unusually early and harsh winter set in. As a result, a severe famine hit the western Netherlands. For the next several months, energy intakes were as low as 500 kcal/day. In May 1945, with the liberation of the country, food supplies were once again plentiful and dietary intake rapidly normalized. Luckily for scientists, the Dutch maintained excellent healthcare records, providing important information not only about pregnancy outcomes but also the health of the offspring over the next 60 years. Not surprisingly, maternal weight gain and infant birth weight were much lower than normal. What was unexpected, however, was the long-term impact of the famine as these "embargo babies" progressed through adulthood.[1,2]

Exposure to famine during the first trimester of pregnancy resulted in a much higher risk among the offspring for obesity, abdominal obesity, hypertension, coronary heart disease, abnormal blood lipids, and metabolic syndrome during adulthood. Exposure during mid-gestation increased the risk of kidney disorders. There is also evidence that prenatal exposure to famine affected the health not only of the individuals deprived *in utero*, but also of their children.[1,2]

Why, you might wonder, would low pregnancy weight gain and low birth weight lead to an increased risk of obesity and other diseases some 50 years later? Most of the proposed mechanisms relate to a process known as **fetal adaptation**. A fetus exposed to a stressful environment, such as maternal starvation or malnutrition, goes into survival mode. Fetal production of hormones shifts in favor of those that promote energy storage, the activity of certain enzymes may change, and the size and functioning of body organs such as the liver, kidney, and pancreas are affected. There may even be changes in the expression of certain genes. Although these adaptations enable the fetus to survive the harmful prenatal environment, these same hormonal, enzymatic, organ, and genetic changes may contribute to the development of chronic diseases over the life span.

The results of other "natural experiments" suggest that the effects of the prenatal environment on adult health depend quite heavily on the precise circumstances in each situation. For example, Leningrad (now St. Petersburg) was under siege by the Germans during World War II for over 2 1/2 years, and as a result the population experienced starvation—over a million people died. And yet, adults who were born during this period did not have the same increased disease risks as found in those exposed, in utero, to the Dutch famine.[3] How could this be, since the Leningrad babies were exposed to conditions far worse than those experienced by the Dutch babies?

Researchers theorize that the impact of fetal exposure to malnutrition is actually worsened if followed by high nutrient intakes shortly after birth.[3] This was a key difference between the Netherlands and Leningrad famines: once the Dutch embargo was lifted, the population returned to a nourishing, adequate diet. This allowed the underweight infants to experience rapid weight gain and catch-up growth during their first year of life **(FIGURE 1)**. In contrast, the Leningrad infants who survived into adulthood may have continued to suffer from malnutrition throughout infancy and even into toddlerhood, remaining underfed and underweight until they were in their childhood years.

How do other nutritional imbalances in utero affect adult health?

LO 2 Describe the effects seen later in life among children born to mothers with specific nutrient deficiencies, obesity, or gestational diabetes.

By definition, a famine is a widespread lack or severe reduction in all food. Thus, research on the long-term health effects of famines cannot identify or describe the impact of in utero deficiencies of specific nutrients. Other studies, however, have been able to look at the impact of specific food patterns or nutrient deficiencies.[4] For example:

- Evidence suggests that poor maternal intake of calcium increases risk of hypertension in adult offspring.
- Poor maternal folate status has been linked not only to neural tube defects in the newborn but also to increased risk of insulin resistance in the child. This, in turn, increases the child's risk for developing diabetes and other metabolic abnormalities.[5]

---

fetal adaptation The process by which fetal metabolism, hormone production, and other physiologic processes shift in response to factors, such as inadequate energy intake, in the maternal environment.

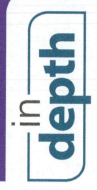

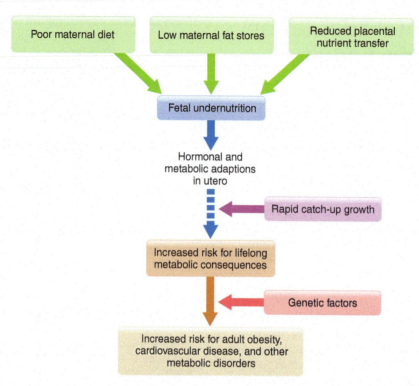

FIGURE 1 Fetal adaptation to undernutrition can lead to a variety of diseases in childhood and throughout adulthood.

■ Given the role of vitamin D in calcium regulation, it may not be surprising that low vitamin D status of pregnant women is associated with reduced bone density in their children.[6]

Research with rats has revealed other links between micronutrient deficiencies and adult health.[6] Thus, fetal stressors that influence adult health include not only starvation and inadequate energy but also specific micronutrient deficiencies.

Strong evidence also links maternal dietary excesses to health problems in adult offspring. Maternal obesity has been linked not only to an increased risk of childhood and adult obesity,[7,8] but also to changes in the "programming" of the fetal brain, resulting in altered feeding behaviors. Maternal obesity is also linked to a higher risk of birth defects, including neural tube defects, many of which have lifelong implications for health.[9] Population studies have also reported an association between high birth weight, common in infants born to obese women, and an increased risk of breast cancer in adulthood.

Maternal diabetes, with its high-glucose environment, has been shown to greatly increase the risk of type 2 diabetes, overweight, abdominal adiposity, high blood triglycerides, hypertension, and metabolic syndrome in adult offspring.[1,10–12] The children of diabetic women are up to eight times more likely to develop type 2 diabetes or pre-diabetes as adults compared to the general population.

Prenatal exposure to excessive levels of individual nutrients also has lifelong implications. A high maternal intake of *trans* and/or saturated fatty acids is associated with increases for heart disease, hypertension, and type 2 diabetes in offspring.[13] Scientists continue to investigate the possible lifelong effects of other nutrient excesses, including the impact of high maternal intake of sodium on risk of hypertension and the effect of high maternal saturated fat intake on risk for congenital heart defects.

nutri-case | HANNAH

"In my nutrition class, I learned that having a mother with diabetes increases the risk that you'll develop diabetes in childhood or adulthood. That helps me understand why my blood sugar test showed I have pre-diabetes, but it doesn't help me understand what to do about it."

Is Hannah destined to develop type 2 diabetes? Why or why not? Identify the factors that increase her risk, as well as the steps she can take to reduce her blood glucose levels and avoid the disease. (Review the **In Depth** on diabetes on pages 130–137.)

In short, research suggests that there are lifelong consequences to any type of nutrient imbalance during pregnancy, whether the imbalance is a total energy deficit, a single nutrient deficiency, or an energy or nutrient excess.

If your mother experienced some type of nutritional imbalance during pregnancy, you certainly are not doomed to suffer from one or more of the health problems mentioned here. That's because most research reports on large groups of people, not individuals. It calculates increases in risk of—or susceptibility to—certain conditions, but it does not and cannot predict health outcomes for individuals. Moreover, fetal adaptation is just one factor in your personal wellness. Much more significant are your lifestyle choices, especially your eating pattern, activity level, alcohol intake, and whether or not you smoke. In short, you have the power to influence your genetics and biology every day.

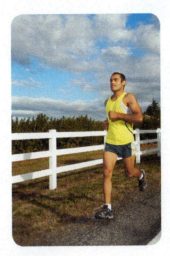

▲ Regular physical activity is one of the most significant factors in maintaining wellness.

web links

www.marchofdimes.com
March of Dimes

This website provides information on the potential risks of maternal dietary imbalances.

www.acog.org/Patients/FAQs/Nutrition-During-Pregnancy
American College of Obstetrics and Gynecology

Visit this web page to find comprehensive information on nutrition during pregnancy, as well as links to related pages.

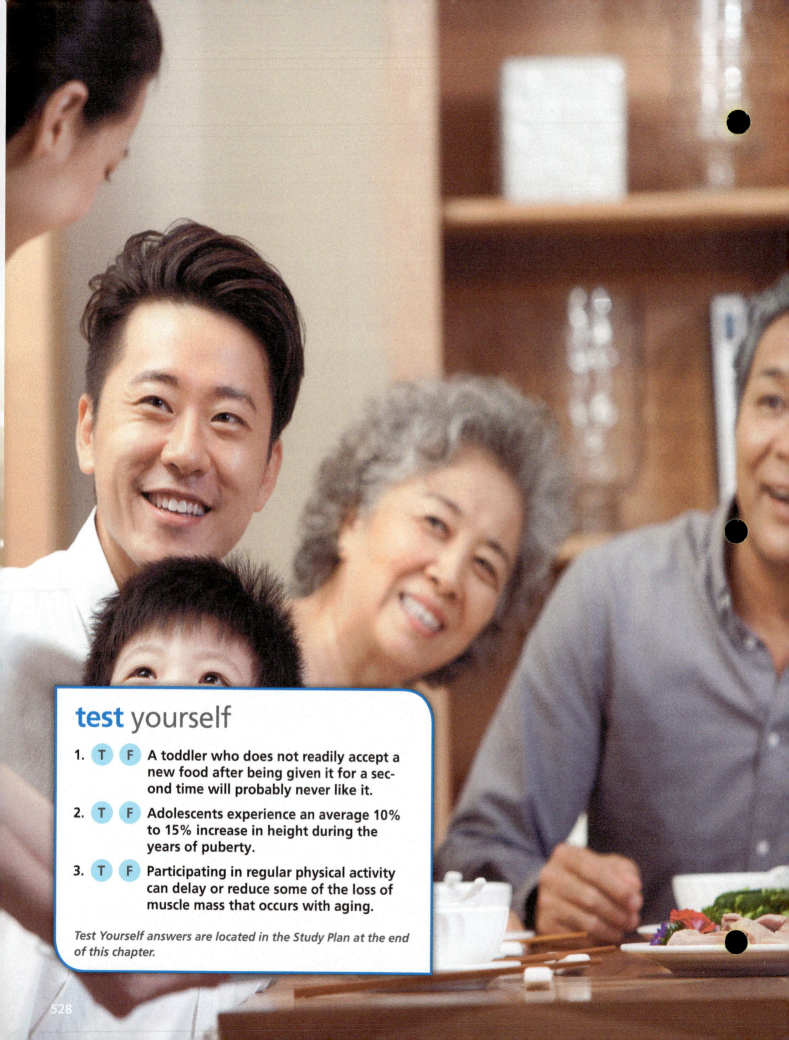

test yourself

1. T F A toddler who does not readily accept a new food after being given it for a second time will probably never like it.

2. T F Adolescents experience an average 10% to 15% increase in height during the years of puberty.

3. T F Participating in regular physical activity can delay or reduce some of the loss of muscle mass that occurs with aging.

Test Yourself answers are located in the Study Plan at the end of this chapter.

15 Nutrition Through the Life Cycle

Childhood to late adulthood

On Sunday afternoons, the Hsiao family gathers for dinner at the Long Beach apartment of their 88-year-old matriarch, Leng. Leng is petite and slender, as are her 70-year-old daughter and 67-year-old son. But when her granddaughters, who are cooking the family meal, send everyone to the table, a change becomes evident. Many of Leng's grandchildren and their spouses are obese, as are some of her great-grandchildren. Leng worries about everyone's weight. One of her grandsons has had a heart attack, and some in her family have been diagnosed with type 2 diabetes. Leng's family isn't alone in their weight problems: in the United States, although the prevalence of obesity has recently stabilized and has actually decreased in preschool children, rates remain unacceptably high.[1] Currently, about 17% of U.S. children and adolescents age 2 to 19 years are classified as obese, leading to both short- and long-term health problems.[1]

Why are the rates of obesity and its associated chronic diseases so high, and what can be done to promote weight management across the life span? How do our nutrient needs change as we grow and age, and what other nutrition-related concerns develop in each life stage? This chapter will help you answer these questions.

LO 1 Describe nutrient recommendations, appropriate food choices, and the risks of a vegan diet for toddlers.

What are the nutritional needs and concerns of toddlerhood?

As babies begin to walk and explore, they transition out of infancy and into the active world of toddlers. From their first to their third birthday, a toddler will grow a total of about 5.5 to 7.5 inches and gain an average of 9 to 11 pounds. Like people of all ages, toddlers need to consume a nutrient-dense diet. But feeding a toddler raises new challenges for parents and caregivers.

Body Size and Activity Increase Toddlers' Nutrient Needs

Nutrient needs increase as a child progresses from infancy to toddlerhood. Although toddlers' rates of growth have slowed, their increased nutrient needs reflect their larger body size and increased activity. Refer to **TABLE 15.1** for a review of specific nutrient recommendations.

Energy and Macronutrient Recommendations for Toddlers

Although the energy requirement per kilogram of body weight for toddlers is slightly less than for infants, *total* energy requirements are higher because toddlers are larger and much more active than infants. The estimated energy requirements (EERs) vary according to the toddler's age, body weight, and level of activity.[2] In general, toddlers should consume a diet that provides enough energy to sustain a healthy and appropriate rate of growth.

Healthy toddlers of appropriate body weight need to consume 30% to 40% of their total daily energy intake as fat.[2] We know that fat provides a concentrated source of energy in a relatively small amount of food, and this is important for toddlers, especially those who are fussy eaters or have little appetite. Moreover, fats, especially the unsaturated fatty acids AA and DHA, support the toddler's still developing nervous system.

Toddlers' protein needs increase modestly because they weigh more than infants and are still growing rapidly. The RDA for protein for toddlers is 1.10 g/kg body weight per day, or approximately 13 g of protein daily.[2] Remember that 2 cups of milk alone provide 16 g of protein; thus, most toddlers have little trouble meeting their protein needs.

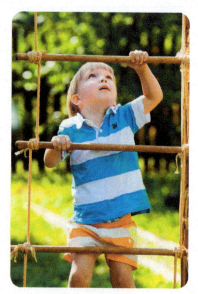

▲ Toddlers expend significant amounts of energy exploring their world.

TABLE 15.1 Nutrient Recommendations for Children and Adolescents

Nutrient	Toddlers (1–3 Years)	Children (4–8 Years)	Children (9–13 Years)	Adolescents (14–18 Years)
Fat	No RDA	No RDA	No RDA	No RDA
Protein	1.10 g/kg body weight per day	0.95 g/kg body weight per day	0.95 g/kg body weight per day	0.85 g/kg body weight per day
Carbohydrate	130 g/day	130 g/day	130 g/day	130 g/day
Vitamin A	300 µg/day	400 µg/day	600 µg/day	Boys: 900 µg/day Girls: 700 µg/day
Vitamin C	15 mg/day	25 mg/day	45 mg/day	Boys: 75 mg/day Girls: 65 mg/day
Vitamin E	6 mg/day	7 mg/day	11 mg/day	15 mg/day
Calcium	700 mg/day	1,000 mg/day	1,300 mg/day	1,300 mg/day
Iron	7 mg/day	10 mg/day	8 mg/day	Boys: 11 mg/day Girls: 15 mg/day
Zinc	3 mg/day	5 mg/day	8 mg/day	Boys: 11 mg/day Girls: 9 mg/day
Fluid	1.3 liters/day	1.7 liters/day	Boys: 2.4 liters/day Girls: 2.1 liters/day	Boys: 3.3 liters/day Girls: 2.3 liters/day

The RDA for carbohydrate for toddlers is 130 g/day, and carbohydrate intake should be about 45% to 65% of total energy intake.[2] As with older children and adults, most of the carbohydrates eaten should be complex, and refined carbohydrates from high-fat/high-sugar items, such as desserts and snack foods, should be kept to a minimum. Fruits and 100% fruit juices are nutritious sources of simple carbohydrates; however, too much fruit juice can displace other foods, including milk and whole fruits, and can cause diarrhea. The American Academy of Pediatrics recommends that the intake of fruit juice be limited to 4 to 6 fl. oz/day for children 1 to 6 years of age.[3]

Adequate fiber is important for toddlers to maintain bowel regularity. The adequate intake (AI) is 14 g of fiber per 1,000 kcal of energy, or, on average, 19 g/day.[2] Whole-grain breads and cereals and fresh fruits and vegetables are healthful choices for toddlers. Too much fiber, however, can inhibit the absorption of iron, zinc, and other essential nutrients; can harm the toddler's small digestive tract; and can cause toddlers to feel full before they have consumed adequate nutrients.

Determining the macronutrient requirements of toddlers can be challenging. See the **You Do the Math** box on page 532 for an analysis of the macronutrient levels in one toddler's daily diet.

Micronutrient Recommendations for Toddlers

As toddlers grow, their micronutrient needs increase (see Table 15.1). Of particular concern with toddlers are adequate intakes of the nutrients associated with fruits and vegetables. In addition, vitamin D, calcium, and iron have been identified as "priority nutrients" for children aged 2 to 4 years. Vitamin D intake, which often decreases in toddlers, is closely linked to milk consumption. The American Academy of Pediatrics recommends vitamin D supplements for all children who consume less than 1 liter of vitamin D–fortified dairy products each day—a group that includes the majority of U.S. children.[3] Vitamin D–fortified soymilk and other milk alternatives, in adequate amounts, are also acceptable.

Adequate calcium is necessary for children to build optimal bone mass, which continues to accumulate until early adulthood. For toddlers, the RDA for calcium is 700 mg/day.[4] Dairy products are excellent sources of calcium. When a child reaches the age of 1 year, whole cow's milk can be given; however, reduced-fat milk (2% or less) should *not* be given until age 2 due to the relatively high need for total energy in young children. If consumption of dairy products is not feasible, calcium-fortified orange juice or soymilk can supply calcium, or children's calcium supplements can be given. Toddlers generally cannot consume enough dark-green vegetables and similar plant foods to depend on them for adequate calcium.

Iron-deficiency anemia is the most common nutrient deficiency in young children in the United States and around the world. Iron-deficiency anemia can affect a child's energy level, attention span, and mood. The RDA for iron for toddlers is 7 mg/day.[5] Good sources of well-absorbed heme iron include lean meats, fish, and poultry; non-heme iron is provided by eggs, legumes, greens, and fortified foods, such as breakfast cereals. When toddlers consume non-heme sources of iron, eating vitamin C at the same meal will enhance the absorption of iron from these sources.

Given toddlers' typically erratic eating habits, pediatricians often recommend an age-appropriate multivitamin and mineral supplement, providing no more than 100% of the Daily Value per dose for any nutrient, as a precaution against deficiencies. Toddlers who are fed a vegan diet, live in a household that cannot afford adequate amounts of nourishing food, or have certain medical issues often benefit from supplements. The toddler's physician or dentist may also prescribe a fluoride supplement if the community water supply is not fluoridated. Toddlers are at particularly high risk of overdosing on iron supplements, so parents must be careful to keep such products out of reach of their children.

Fluid Recommendations for Toddlers

Toddlers lose less fluid from evaporation than infants, and their more mature kidneys are able to concentrate urine, conserving the body's fluid when intake is low. However, as toddlers become active, they start to lose significant fluid through sweat, especially in hot weather. Parents need to make sure an active toddler is drinking

you do the math

Is This Menu Good for a Toddler?

A dedicated mother and father want to provide the best nutrition for their son, Ethan, who is now 1 1/2 years old and has just been completely weaned from breast milk. Ethan weighs about 26 pounds (11.8 kg). In the accompanying table is a typical day's menu for Ethan. Grams of protein, fat, and carbohydrate are given for each food. The day's total energy intake is 1,168 kcal.

Meal	Foods	Protein (g)	Fat (g)	Carbohydrate (g)
Breakfast	Oatmeal (1/2 cup, cooked)	2.5	1.5	13.5
	Brown sugar (1 tsp.)	0	0	4
	Milk (1%, 4 fl. oz)	4	1.25	5.5
	Grape juice (4 fl. oz)	0	0	20
Mid-morning snack	Banana slices (1 small banana)	0	0	16
	Yogurt (nonfat, fruit-flavored 1.3 fl. oz)	5.5	0	15.5
	Orange juice (4 fl. oz)	1	0	13
Lunch	Whole-wheat bread (1 slice)	1.5	0.5	10
	Peanut butter (1 tbsp.)	4	8	3.5
	Strawberry jam (1 tbsp.)	0	0	13
	Carrots (cooked, 1/8 cup)	0	0	2
	Applesauce (sweetened, 1/4 cup)	0	0	12
	Milk (1%, 4 fl. oz)	4	1.25	5.5
Afternoon snack	Bagel (1/2)	3	1	20
	American cheese product (1 slice)	3	5	1
	Water	0	0	0
Dinner	Scrambled egg (1)	11	5	1
	Baby food spinach (3 oz)	2	0.5	5.5
	Whole-wheat toast (1 slice)	1.5	0.5	10
	Mandarin orange slices (1/4 cup)	0.5	0	10
	Milk (1%, 4 fl. oz)	4	1.25	5.5

Calculate the percentage of Ethan's Calories that come from protein, fat, and carbohydrate (the numbers may not add up to exactly 100% because of rounding). In what areas are Ethan's parents doing well, and where can they improve?

Note: This activity focuses on the macronutrients. It does not ask you to consider Ethan's intake of micronutrients or fluids.

Calculations:
There is a total of 47.5 g protein in Ethan's menu.

$$47.5 \text{ g} \times 4 \text{ kcal/g} = 190 \text{ kcal}$$
$$190 \text{ kcal protein}/1{,}168 \text{ total kcal} \times 100 = 16\% \text{ protein}$$

There is a total of 25.75 g fat in Ethan's menu.

$$25.75 \text{ g} \times 9 \text{ kcal/g} = 232 \text{ kcal}$$
$$232 \text{ kcal fat}/1{,}168 \text{ total kcal} \times 100 = 20\% \text{ fat}$$

There is a total of 186.5 g carbohydrate in Ethan's menu.

$$186.5 \text{ g} \times 4 \text{ kcal/g} = 746 \text{ kcal}$$
$$746 \text{ kcal carbohydrate}/1{,}168 \text{ total kcal} \times 100$$
$$= 64\% \text{ carbohydrate}$$

Analysis:
Ethan's parents are doing very well at offering a wide variety of foods from various food groups; they are especially doing well with fruits and vegetables. Also, according to his estimated energy requirement, Ethan requires about 970 kcal/day, and he is consuming 1,168 kcal/day, thus meeting his energy needs.

Ethan's total carbohydrate intake for the day is 186.5 g, which is higher than the RDA of 130 g/day; however, this value falls within the recommended 45% to 65% of total energy intake that should come from carbohydrates. Thus, high carbohydrate intake is adequate to meet his energy needs.

However, Ethan is being offered far more than enough protein. The DRI for protein for toddlers is about 13 g/day, and Ethan is eating more than three times that much!

It is also readily apparent that Ethan is being offered too little fat for his age. Toddlers need at least 30% to 40% of their total energy intake from fat, and Ethan is consuming only about 20% of his Calories from fat. He should be drinking whole milk, not 1% milk. He should occasionally be offered higher-fat foods, such as cheese for his snacks or macaroni and cheese for a meal. Yogurt is fine, but it shouldn't be nonfat at Ethan's age. In conclusion, Ethan's parents should continue to offer a variety of nutritious foods but should shift some of the energy Ethan currently consumes as protein and carbohydrate to fat.

adequately. The recommended fluid intake for toddlers—about 4 cups as beverages, including drinking water—is listed in Table 15.1.[6] Suggested beverages are plain water, milk and calcium-fortified milk alternatives and 100% juices, and foods high in water content, such as vegetables and fruits.

Encourage Nutritious Food Choices with Toddlers

Parents and pediatricians have long known that toddlers tend to be choosy about what they eat. Some avoid entire food groups, such as all meats or vegetables. Others will refuse all but one or two favorite foods (such as peanut butter on crackers) for several days or longer. These behaviors frustrate and worry many parents, but in fact, as long as a variety of healthful food is available, most toddlers have the ability to match their food intake with their needs. A toddler will most likely make up for one day's deficiency later on in the week. Parents who offer only nutritious foods can usually feel confident that their children are being well fed, even if a child's choices seem odd or erratic on any particular day. Food should never be "forced" on a child because doing so sets the stage for eating and control issues later in life.

Toddlers' stomachs are very small, and they cannot consume all of the Calories they need in three meals. They need small meals alternated with nutritious snacks every 2 to 3 hours. A successful technique is to create a snack tray filled with small portions of nutritious food choices, such as one-third of a banana, a few cubes of tofu, and two whole-grain crackers, and leave it within reach of the child's play area. The child can then "graze" on these healthful foods while he or she plays. A snack tray plus a spill-proof cup of milk or water is particularly useful on car trips. Even at mealtime, portion sizes should be small. One tablespoon of a food for each year of age constitutes a serving throughout the toddler and preschool years **(FIGURE 15.1)**. Realistic portion sizes can give toddlers a sense of accomplishment when they "eat it all up" and minimize parents' fears that their child is not eating enough.

Foods prepared for toddlers should be developmentally appropriate. Nuts, carrots, grapes, raisins, cherry tomatoes, and firm cheese are difficult for a toddler to chew and pose a choking hazard. Foods should be soft and sliced into thin strips or wedges that are easy for children to grasp. As the child develops more teeth and becomes more coordinated, the range of food can expand.

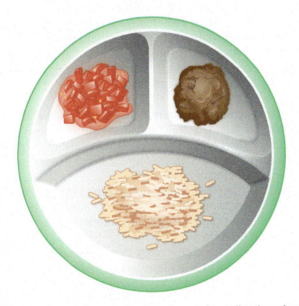

FIGURE 15.1 Portion sizes for preschoolers are much smaller than those for older children. Use the following guideline: 1 tbsp. of the food for each year of age equals 1 serving. For example, 2 tbsp. of rice, 2 tbsp. of black beans, and 2 tbsp. of chopped tomatoes is appropriate for a 2-year-old.

▲ **FIGURE 15.2** Most toddlers are delighted by food prepared in a fun way.

Foods prepared for toddlers can also be fun **(FIGURE 15.2)**. Parents can use cookie cutters to turn a peanut butter sandwich into a pumpkin face, or arrange cooked peas or carrot slices to look like a smiling face on top of mashed potatoes. Juice and yogurt can be frozen into "popsicles" or blended into "milkshakes."

New foods should be introduced gradually. Most toddlers are leery of new foods, spicy foods, hot (temperature) foods, mixed foods such as casseroles, and foods with strange textures. A helpful rule is to encourage the child to eat at least one bite of a new food: if the child does not want the rest, nothing negative should be said and the child should be praised just for the willingness to try. The food should be reintroduced a few weeks later. Toddlers may need as many as 15 exposures to a new food before accepting it. Parents should never bribe with food—for example, promising dessert if the child finishes her squash. Bribing teaches children that food can be used to reward and manipulate. Instead, parents can try to positively reinforce good behaviors—for example, "Wow! You ate every bite of your squash! That's going to help you grow big and strong!"

Role modeling is important because toddlers mimic older children and adults: if they see their parents eating a variety of healthful foods, they are likely to do so as well. Adults have a major impact on the nutritional quality of their children's choices.[7]

Offering two different but healthful snacks will also help toddlers make nutritious food choices. For example, parents might say, "It's snack time! Would you like apples and cottage cheese or bananas and yogurt?"

Finally, toddlers are more likely to eat food they help prepare. Encourage them to assist in the preparation of simple foods, such as helping to pour a bowl of cereal or arrange vegetables on a plate.

Vegan Diets May Not Be Healthful for Toddlers

For toddlers, a lacto-ovo-vegetarian diet, in which dairy foods and eggs are included, can be as wholesome as a diet that includes meats and fish.[8] However, because red meat is an important source of zinc and heme iron, families who do not serve red meat must be careful to include enough zinc and iron from other sources in their child's diet.

In contrast, a vegan diet, in which no foods of animal origin are consumed, poses several potential nutritional risks for toddlers:

- **Protein.** Vegan diets can be too low in total protein or protein quality for toddlers, who need adequate amounts of high-quality protein for growth and increasing activity. Few toddlers can consume enough legumes and whole grains to provide sufficient protein. The high fiber content of legumes and whole grains results in a rapid sense of fullness for toddlers, decreasing their total food intake. Soymilk, tofu, and other soy-based products are excellent sources of complete dietary protein.
- **Calcium.** Children who consume no milk, yogurt, or cheese are at risk for calcium deficiency. As with protein, few children can consume enough calcium from plant sources to meet their daily requirement. Although most brands of soymilk and other milk alternatives, and certain fruit juices and cereals, are now fortified with calcium, supplementation may be necessary.
- **Zinc and Iron.** These minerals, which are abundant in meat, poultry, and seafood, are commonly low in vegan diets. Although both zinc and iron are found in legumes, young children simply cannot eat enough legumes to meet their needs, and supplementation is advised.
- **Vitamins D and B$_{12}$.** Children consuming strict vegan diets are at risk for deficiencies of both of these vitamins. Some cereals and soymilks are fortified with vitamin D; however, many toddlers may still need a vitamin D–containing supplement. Vitamin B$_{12}$ is not available in any amount from plant foods and must be obtained from fortified foods such as soymilk or from supplements.
- **Fiber.** Vegan diets often contain a higher amount of fiber than is recommended for toddlers, resulting in lowered absorption of iron and zinc, as well as the early onset of fullness or satiety.

Although adults who follow a vegan diet have the ability to choose alternative foods and/or supplements to meet the demands for these nutrients, toddlers depend on their parents to make appropriate food choices for them. If parents are determined to maintain a vegan diet for their toddler, choosing to include fortified juices, soymilk, and other soy products, along with an appropriate pediatric supplement and ongoing consultation with a pediatrician or pediatric dietitian, can ensure adequate nutrition in the toddler's diet. With proper planning, vegan children demonstrate appropriate growth, comparable with that of nonvegetarian children.[9]

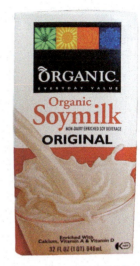

recap Growth during toddlerhood is slower than it is during infancy; however, toddlers are highly active, and total energy, fat, and protein requirements are higher for toddlers than for infants. Although all forms of milk can be used to meet calcium requirements, until age 2, toddlers should drink whole milk. Iron deficiency can be avoided by feeding toddlers lean meats/fish/poultry, eggs, and iron-fortified foods. Toddlers need to drink about 4 cups of water or other beverages per day. Toddlers require small, frequent, nutritious meals and snacks, and food should be soft and cut in small pieces, so that it is easy to handle, mash, and swallow without choking. Role modeling by parents and access to ample healthful foods can help toddlers make nutritious choices. Feeding vegan diets to toddlers poses the potential for deficiencies in protein, calcium, zinc, iron, vitamin D, and vitamin B_{12}.

⬆ Enriched and fortified foods, such as fortified soymilk, should be given to toddlers consuming vegan diets to ensure they get adequate amounts of key nutrients.

What are the nutritional needs and concerns of childhood?

During the preschool and school-age years, children become even more active, but their growth rate slows. Children grow at a slow and steady rate, averaging 2 to 4 inches per year until the rapid growth of adolescence begins.

LO 2 Discuss the nutrient needs of children, the role of school attendance, and nutrition-related concerns of childhood.

Growth and Development Increase Children's Nutrient Needs

Until the age of 8 or 9 years, the nutrient needs of young boys and girls do not differ; because of this, the Dietary Reference Intake (DRI) values for the macronutrients, fiber, and micronutrients are grouped together for children ages 4 to 8 years. The beginning of sexual maturation, however, has a dramatic impact on the nutrient needs of children. Boys' and girls' bodies develop differently in response to gender-specific hormones. These changes in sexual maturation can begin subtly between the ages of 8 and 9 years; thus, the DRI values are separately defined for boys and girls ages 9 to 13 years.[2,4–6,10] Table 15.1 identifies the nutrient needs of children and adolescents.

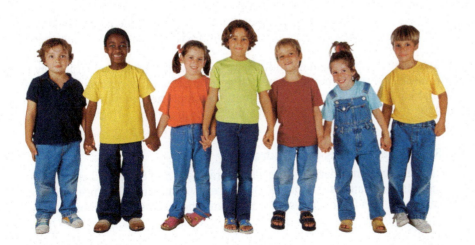

◀ School-age children grow an average of 2 to 4 inches per year.

Energy and Macronutrient Recommendations for Children

Total energy requirements continue to increase throughout childhood because of increasing body size and, for some children, higher levels of physical activity.[2] The EER varies according to the child's age, body weight, and level of activity. Activity levels among children vary dramatically; however, all children can be encouraged to have fun using their muscles in various ways that suit their interests. Parents should provide diets that support normal growth and appropriate physical activity while minimizing the risk for excess weight gain. The U.S. Department of Agriculture (USDA) has produced a Daily Food Plan for preschoolers, helping parents to support their children in maintaining a healthful eating pattern (**FIGURE 15.3**).

Although dietary fat remains a key macronutrient in the preschool years, total fat intake should gradually be reduced to a level closer to that of an adult, 25% to 35% of total energy.[2] One easy way to start reducing saturated fat is to serve lean protein choices, introduce lower-fat dairy products, such as 2% or 1% milk, and minimize the intake of fried foods. A diet providing less than 25% of Calories from fat is not recommended for children because they are still growing, developing, and maturing. In fact, parents should avoid putting too much emphasis on fat at this age. Impressionable and peer-influenced children may be prone to categorize foods as "good" or "bad," leading to skewed views of food and inappropriate eating habits.

The RDA for carbohydrate for children is 130 g/day, which is about 45% to 65% of total daily energy intake.[2] Complex carbohydrates from whole grains, fruits, vegetables, and legumes should be emphasized. Simple sugars should come from fruits and 100% fruit juices, with foods high in refined sugars, such as cakes, cookies, and candies, saved for occasional indulgences. The AI for fiber for children is 14 g/1,000 kcal of energy consumed.[2] As is the case with toddlers, too much fiber can be harmful because it can make a child feel prematurely full and interfere with adequate food intake and nutrient absorption.

As seen in Table 15.1, the protein recommendation for boys and girls is 0.95 g/kg body weight per day.[2] Lean meats, fish, poultry, lower-fat dairy products, soy-based foods, and legumes are nutritious sources of protein that can be provided to children of all ages.

Micronutrient Recommendations for Children

The need for most micronutrients increases slightly for children up to age 8 because of their increasing size. A sharper increase in micronutrient needs occurs during the transition into full adolescence; this increase is due to the beginning of sexual maturation and in preparation for the impending adolescent growth spurt. Children who fail to consume the USDA-recommended 4 cups of fruits and vegetables each day may become deficient in vitamins A, C, and E. Offering fresh fruits and vegetables during meals or as snacks will also improve intakes of fiber and potassium, which are often low in the diets of low-income children. Minerals of concern continue to be calcium, iron, and zinc, which come primarily from animal-based foods.[4,5] Notice that the RDA for iron is based on the assumption that most girls do not begin menstruation until after age 13.[5] Refer again to Table 15.1 for a review of the nutrient needs of children.

If there is any concern that a child's nutrient needs are not being met for any reason (for instance, breakfasts are skipped, lunches are traded, or parents lack money for nourishing food), a pediatric vitamin/mineral supplement that provides no more than 100% of the Daily Value for the micronutrients may help correct any existing deficit.

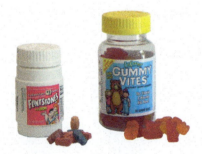

▲ Children's multivitamins often appear in shapes or bright colors.

Fluid Recommendations for Children

The daily fluid recommendations for children are about 5 to 8 cups of beverages, including drinking water (see Table 15.1).[6] The exact amount of fluid needed varies according to a child's level of physical activity and the weather conditions. At this

Healthy Eating for Preschoolers Daily Food Plan

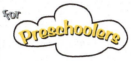

Use this Plan as a general guide.

- These food plans are based on average needs. Do not be concerned if your child does not eat the exact amounts suggested. Your child may need more or less than average. For example, food needs increase during growth spurts.

- Children's appetites vary from day to day. Some days they may eat less than these amounts; other days they may want more. Offer these amounts and let your child decide how much to eat.

Food group	2 year olds	3 year olds	4 and 5 year olds	What counts as:
Fruits	1 cup	1 - 1½ cups	1 - 1½ cups	½ cup of fruit? ½ cup mashed, sliced, or chopped fruit ½ cup 100% fruit juice ½ medium banana 4-5 large strawberries
Vegetables	1 cup	1½ cups	1½ - 2 cups	½ cup of veggies? ½ cup mashed, sliced, or chopped vegetables 1 cup raw leafy greens ½ cup vegetable juice 1 small ear of corn
Grains Make half your grains whole	3 ounces	4 - 5 ounces	4 - 5 ounces	1 ounce of grains? 1 slice bread 1 cup ready-to-eat cereal flakes ½ cup cooked rice or pasta 1 tortilla (6" across)
Protein Foods	2 ounces	3 - 4 ounces	3 - 5 ounces	1 ounce of protein foods? 1 ounce cooked meat, poultry, or seafood 1 egg 1 Tablespoon peanut butter ¼ cup cooked beans or peas (kidney, pinto, lentils)
Dairy Choose low-fat or fat-free	2 cups	2 cups	2½ cups	½ cup of dairy? ½ cup milk 4 ounces yogurt ¾ ounce cheese 1 string cheese

Some foods are easy for your child to choke on while eating. Skip hard, small, whole foods, such as popcorn, nuts, seeds, and hard candy. Cut up foods such as hot dogs, grapes, and raw carrots into pieces smaller than the size of your child's throat—about the size of a nickel.

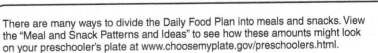

There are many ways to divide the Daily Food Plan into meals and snacks. View the "Meal and Snack Patterns and Ideas" to see how these amounts might look on your preschooler's plate at www.choosemyplate.gov/preschoolers.html.

▲ FIGURE 15.3 The MyPlate Healthy Eating for Preschoolers: Daily Food Plan provides families with an easy-to-use guide to healthful meals.

Source: U.S. Department of Agriculture Food and Nutrition Service.

point in life, children are mostly in control of their own fluid intake. However, as they engage in physical activity at school and in sports and play, young children in particular may need reminders to drink in order to stay properly hydrated, especially if the weather is hot.

Encourage Nutritious Food Choices with Children

Peer pressure can be extremely difficult for both parents and their children to deal with during this life stage. Most children want to feel as if they "belong," and they admire and like to mimic children they believe to be popular. If the popular children at school are eating chips and drinking grape soda, it may be hard for a child to consume a peanut butter on whole-wheat sandwich, an apple, and a low-fat milk without embarrassment. One strategy for combating peer pressure is to introduce kids to appropriate role models, such as star athletes and popular entertainers who follow nutritious diets.

In addition, adults should consistently model healthful eating patterns, and involve children in growing their own food, shopping, and planning and preparing meals. If children have input into what is going into their body, they may be more likely to take an active role in their health. Research suggests that children whose families who prepare and eat meals together on average consume a better quality diet and have a healthier body weight.[11] Moreover, family meals encourage shared conversations that help family members connect. The "Eat Better, Eat Together" nutrition education program promotes family mealtime (FIGURE 15.4).

School Attendance Influences Children's Nutrition

Children's school attendance can affect their nutrition in several ways. First, hectic morning schedules cause many children to minimize or skip breakfast completely. Many nutrition and education experts believe that children who skip breakfast are at increased risk for behavioral and learning problems associated with hunger in the classroom.

Second, with no one monitoring what they eat, children in school do not always consume appropriate types or amounts of food. If they purchase a school lunch, they might not like all the foods being served, or their friends might influence them to skip certain foods with comments such as "This broccoli's nasty!" Even homemade lunches that contain nutritious foods may be left uneaten or traded for less nutritious fare. Some children rush through lunch in order to spend more time on the playground. For this reason, some schools send students to the playground first, giving them time to burn off their excess energy as well as build their hunger and thirst.

Finally, some schools continue to sell foods with low nutrient value at bake sales and other fund-raisers. Also, despite recent legislation and industry-sponsored

Find games, coloring sheets, videos, and songs promoting nutrition and physical activity at the MyPlate Kids' Place. Go to www .choosemyplate.gov/kids.

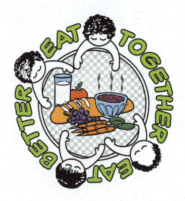

◄ **FIGURE 15.4** *Eat Better, Eat Together* promotes family mealtimes as a way to improve children's diets.

Source: Eat Together, Eat Better image courtesy of Washington State University.

initiatives, some schools still have vending machines offering snacks that are high in empty Calories.

The federally funded School Breakfast Program (SBP) and the National School Lunch Program (NSLP) are administered by the USDA's Food and Nutrition Service. Meals for all students are subsidized; in addition, students from families with incomes at or below 185% of the federal poverty level qualify for reduced-price or free meals. Most research suggests that participation in the School Breakfast Program improves academic achievement,[12,13] particularly among children at risk for food insecurity. A growing number of schools now offer a free "in-class breakfast" to all students, regardless of family income, improving school attendance and program participation as compared to cafeteria-based breakfasts offered only to qualified students.[12] The impact of the SBP and NSLP on children's diets is enormous: over 100,000 schools, including 99% of public schools, participate, serving over 32 million children in 2015.[14]

SBP and NSLP meals must meet the nutritional standards of the 2010 Healthy, Hunger-Free Kids Act:

- Students must be offered both fruits and vegetables every day and must *select* at least one serving for the school to be reimbursed for the meal. In addition, schools must offer dark green and red/orange vegetables and legumes each week. Breakfast meals must offer at least one cup of fruit daily.
- Milk must be fat-free or low fat.
- All grains must be whole-grain-rich.
- Calories, averaged over a week, and portion sizes must be appropriate for the age of the children being served.
- Sodium, saturated fats, and *trans* fats must be reduced to specified levels.

In addition, vending machines and other sources of food on school campuses must meet specific nutrient guidelines.

To comply with these standards, schools nationwide are introducing innovations such as salad bars, baked potato bars, and soup stations to entice students into more healthful choices. Many schools now cultivate a garden on school grounds or even on the school rooftop where children help to grow the vegetables that will be used in their lunches.[15] Many have implemented USDA programs that encourage children to increase their consumption of fruits and vegetables by providing less familiar choices they might not otherwise have the chance to try. Schools that succeed in improving their meals earn additional federal funding.

On the surface, it would appear that, by following these standards, school meals would improve children's diets. However, the nutrients a student *gets* depends on what the student actually *eats*. So, a child might eat the slice of whole-wheat veggie pizza and the low-fat milk but skip the carrot sticks and apple. Also keep in mind that children can still bring high-fat and high-sugar snacks and beverages from home or trade with classmates who bring them.

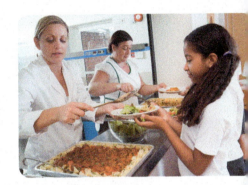

⬆ School-age children may receive a standard school lunch, but many choose less healthful foods when given the opportunity.

Childhood Brings Unique Nutrition-Related Concerns

In addition to the potential nutrient deficiencies that have already been discussed, new concerns arise during childhood. Foremost among these are overweight and obesity, a topic we discuss in detail ahead.

Dental Caries

Dental caries, or cavities, occur when bacteria in the mouth feed on carbohydrates deposited on teeth. As a result of metabolizing the carbohydrates, the bacteria then secrete acid, which begins to erode tooth enamel, leading to tooth decay. The development of dental caries can be minimized by limiting children's intake of sweets, especially those such as jelly beans that stick to teeth, and of sugary drinks. Among one group of third-grade students, one additional serving of a sugar-sweetened beverage per day increased the incidence of caries by over 20%.[16] Finally, frequent brushing helps eliminate the sugars on teeth as well as the bacteria that feed on them.

Fluoride, through a municipal water supply, through fluoridated toothpaste or mouthwash, or through supplements, also helps deter the development of dental caries. Even though the teeth of a young child will be replaced by permanent teeth in several years, it is critical to keep them healthy and strong. This is because they make room for and guide the permanent teeth into position. Children should start having regular dental visits at the age of 3.

Inadequate Calcium Intake

Another nutrition-related concern for children is an inadequate intake of calcium. Adequate calcium is necessary to achieve optimal bone density as well as for numerous other critical body and cell functions. Because peak bone mass is achieved by the late teens or early twenties, inadequate calcium intake during childhood and adolescence can set the stage for poor bone health and potentially osteoporosis in later years.

Dairy products are the most common source of calcium for children in the United States.[4] However, nearly 60% of U.S. children consume fewer than two servings of dairy per day.[17] During the infant, toddler, and preschool years, milk consumption can largely be monitored by parents and other caregivers. Older children often choose soft drinks, sports beverages, fruit punch, and other sugary drinks in place of milk. This "milk displacement" is associated with lower intakes of protein, calcium, phosphorus, magnesium, potassium, and vitamin A, increasing subsequent risk for poor bone health.

Childhood Food Insecurity

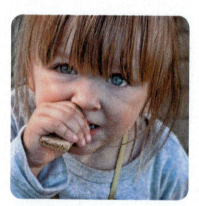

Although most children in the United States grow up with an abundant and healthful supply of food, nearly 4 million households with children, representing 16 million American children, are faced with *food insecurity* and hunger.[18] Food insecurity occurs when a household lacks a consistent, dependable supply of safe and nutritious food. Rates of food insecurity are more than double among African-American and Latino households compared to Caucasian households. These statistics are definitely at odds with America's image as "the land of plenty."

The effects of food insecurity can be very harmful to children, including poorer health, more hospitalizations, greater emotional distress and lower academic achievement.[19,20] Many, but not all, studies find a link between child food insecurity and obesity or overweight.[20] Impaired nutrient status can blunt children's immune responses, making them more susceptible to common childhood illnesses, as well as anemia and poor bone density.

Options for families facing food insecurity include a number of government and privately funded programs, including school breakfast and lunch programs and the Supplemental Nutrition Assistance Program (SNAP; previously known as the Food Stamp program). Community food pantries and kitchens can provide a narrow range of foods for a limited period but cannot be relied on to meet the nutritional needs of children and their families over a prolonged time.

▲ Both children and adults were food insecure in about 9.4% of U.S. households in 2014.

Source: Economic Research Service, September 8, 2015, *Food Security Status of U.S. Households with Children*, www.ers.usda.gov.

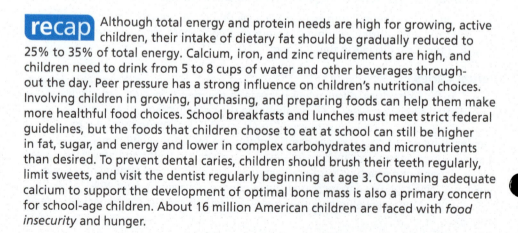

recap Although total energy and protein needs are high for growing, active children, their intake of dietary fat should be gradually reduced to 25% to 35% of total energy. Calcium, iron, and zinc requirements are high, and children need to drink from 5 to 8 cups of water and other beverages throughout the day. Peer pressure has a strong influence on children's nutritional choices. Involving children in growing, purchasing, and preparing foods can help them make more healthful food choices. School breakfasts and lunches must meet strict federal guidelines, but the foods that children choose to eat at school can still be higher in fat, sugar, and energy and lower in complex carbohydrates and micronutrients than desired. To prevent dental caries, children should brush their teeth regularly, limit sweets, and visit the dentist regularly beginning at age 3. Consuming adequate calcium to support the development of optimal bone mass is also a primary concern for school-age children. About 16 million American children are faced with *food insecurity* and hunger.

What are the nutritional needs and concerns of adolescence?

LO 3 Explain how puberty influences the nutrient needs and health concerns of adolescents.

Although there is no consensus on the exact age range corresponding to the term *adolescence,* this life stage begins with the onset of **puberty**, the period in life in which secondary sexual characteristics develop and we become capable of reproducing, and continues through age 18. The nutritional needs of adolescents are influenced by their rapid growth in height, increased weight, changes in body composition, and individual levels of physical activity.

Puberty Triggers Dramatic Growth and Maturation

Growth during adolescence is driven primarily by hormonal changes, including increased levels of testosterone for boys and estrogen for girls. Both boys and girls experience growth spurts, or periods of accelerated increase in height, during later childhood and adolescence. The timing and length of these growth spurts vary by race, gender, nutritional status, and other factors. Growth spurts for girls tend to begin between 10 to 11 years of age, and for boys around 12 to 13 years.

Skeletal growth ceases once closure of the **epiphyseal plates** occurs **(FIGURE 15.5)**. These are plates of cartilage located toward the end of the long bones that provide for their growth in length. Although most girls reach their full adult height by about age 18, some continue to increase in height past age 19, although the rate of growth slows considerably. Most boys continue to grow up to the age of 21, although their rate of growth also slows over time.

In some circumstances, the epiphyseal plates close early and the adolescent fails to reach full stature. The most common causes of this failure are malnutrition, such as may occur with an eating disorder, and the use of anabolic steroids during this critical growth period.

Weight and body composition also change dramatically. The average weight gained by girls and boys during this time is 35 and 45 pounds, respectively; however, weight gain is extremely variable, reflecting the adolescent's energy intake, physical activity level, and genetics. The weight gained by girls and boys is dramatically different in terms of its composition. Girls tend to gain significantly more body fat than boys, with this fat accumulating around the buttocks, hips, breasts, thighs, and upper arms. Although many girls are uncomfortable or embarrassed by these changes, they are a natural result of maturation. Boys gain significantly more muscle mass than girls, and they experience an increase in muscle definition.

The physical activity levels of adolescents are highly variable. Many are physically active in sports or other organized physical activities, whereas others become less interested in sports and more interested in intellectual or artistic pursuits. This variability in activity levels results in highly individual energy needs. Although the rapid growth and maturation that occur during puberty require a significant amount of energy, adolescence is often a time in which overweight begins.

Rapid Growth Increases an Adolescent's Nutrient Needs

The nutrient needs of adolescents are influenced by rapid growth, weight gain, and sexual maturation, in addition to the demands of physical activity (see Table 15.1).

Energy and Macronutrient Recommendations for Adolescents

Adequate energy intake is necessary to maintain adolescents' health, support their dramatic growth and maturation, and fuel their physical activity. Because of these competing demands, the energy needs of adolescents can be quite high. Although it is possible to calculate estimated energy requirements of an adolescent by using a published equation, it is more practical to monitor the growth pattern of the adolescent to ensure that weight remains in proportion to height.[2]

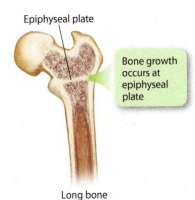

Epiphyseal plate

Bone growth occurs at epiphyseal plate

Long bone

FIGURE 15.5 Skeletal growth ceases once closure of the epiphyseal plates occurs.

puberty The period of life in which secondary sexual characteristics develop and people become biologically capable of reproducing.

epiphyseal plates Plates of cartilage located toward the end of long bones that provide for growth in the length of long bones.

The AMDR for fat is 25% to 35% of total energy. Like adults, adolescents should consume less than 10% of total energy from saturated fats.[2]

The RDA for carbohydrate for adolescents is 130 g/day.[2] As with adults, this amount of carbohydrate covers what is needed to supply adequate glucose to the brain, but it does not cover the amount of carbohydrate needed to support daily activities. Thus, it is recommended that adolescents consume about 45% to 65% of their total energy as carbohydrate, and most should come from fiber-rich carbohydrates. The AI for fiber for adolescents is 26 g/day, which is similar to adult values.

The RDA for protein for adolescents is only slightly higher than that of adults, 0.85 g of protein per kilogram of body weight per day.[2] This amount is assumed to be sufficient to support health and to cover the additional needs of growth and development during the adolescent stage. As with adults, most U.S. adolescents consume protein in amounts that far exceed the RDA.

Micronutrient Recommendations for Adolescents

The micronutrients of particular concern for adolescents are calcium, iron, and vitamins A and D.

Calcium   Adolescence is a critical time to support the achievement of optimal peak bone density. The RDA for calcium for adolescents 14 to 18 years of age therefore increases to 1,300 mg/day.[4] This amount of calcium can be difficult for adolescents to consume if they don't follow a healthful eating pattern. Milk is the leading food source of both calcium and vitamin D, yet average milk intake has decreased significantly over the past decade.[21,22] By age 18, average milk consumption has fallen by more than 25% compared to intake at age 8 years, whereas soda intake has tripled.

Vitamin D   The RDA for vitamin D for adolescents is 600 IU/day.[4] Most foods are naturally low in vitamin D; thus, fortified foods, such as milk and cereals, are important sources of this vitamin. If an adolescent is not consuming adequate vitamin D and does not get enough sunlight year-round, he or she may need to take a supplement.

Iron   The iron requirements of adolescents are relatively high; this is because iron is needed to replace the blood lost during menstruation in girls and to support the increase in blood volume and growth of muscle mass in boys. Between the ages of 14 and 18 years, the RDA for iron for boys is 11 mg/day, whereas the RDA for girls is 15 mg/day.[5] If energy intake is adequate and adolescents consume food sources of heme iron, such as lean meat/fish/poultry, each day, they should be able to meet the RDA for iron. However, many young people adopt a vegetarian lifestyle during this life stage, or they consume foods that have limited amounts of iron. Both of these situations can prevent adolescents from meeting the RDA for iron and, particularly in females, can increase their risk for iron-deficiency anemia.

Vitamin A   Vitamin A is critical to support the rapid growth and development that occur during adolescence. The RDA for vitamin A is 900 µg/day for boys and 700 µg/day for girls ages 14 to 18 years.[5] The RDA can be met by consuming at least 5 servings of dark-green, yellow, and orange fruits and vegetables each day. As with iron and calcium, meeting the RDA for vitamin A can be a challenging goal if the adolescent fails to make healthful food choices. In such cases, a multivitamin and mineral supplement that provides no more than 100% of the Daily Value for the micronutrients can be beneficial as a safety net. As with younger children and adults, a supplement should never be considered to be a substitute for a balanced, healthful diet.

Fluid Recommendations for Adolescents

The fluid needs of adolescents are higher than those of children because of their higher physical activity levels and the extensive growth and development that occur during this phase of life. The AI for total fluid for adolescent girls and boys is listed in Table 15.1; it includes about 9 and 11 cups, respectively, as beverages, including drinking water.[6] Boys require a higher fluid intake because they are often more active than girls and have more lean tissue. Highly active adolescents of either gender who are exercising in the heat may have higher fluid needs than the AI, and these individuals should be encouraged to drink water and other unsweetened beverages often to quench their thirst and avoid dehydration.

Encourage Nutritious Food Choices with Adolescents

At this point in their lives, adolescents are making most of their own food choices, and many are buying and preparing a significant amount of the foods they consume. Although parents can still be effective role models, adolescents are generally strongly influenced by their peers, their personal food preferences, and their own developing sense of which foods constitute a healthful and adequate diet. Adolescents are anxious to develop their own identity and establish a more self-reliant lifestyle. The decision to adopt a vegetarian diet, for example, may represent an adolescent's effort to establish some distance from the family unit.

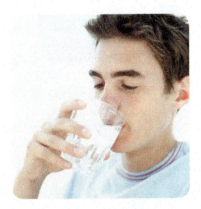

◀ Adolescents have higher fluid needs than younger children.

One area of concern in most adolescents' diets is a lack of vegetables, fruits, and whole grains. Many teens eat on the run, skip meals, and select fast foods and convenience foods because they are inexpensive, are accessible, and taste good. High school students are often allowed to leave campus for lunch, increasing their opportunities to eat high-fat, low-nutrient fast foods. Parents and school food service personnel can capitalize on adolescents' preferences for pizza, burgers, spaghetti, and sandwiches by providing more healthful meat and cheese alternatives, whole-grain breads, and plenty of appealing vegetable-based sides or additions to these foods. In addition, keeping healthful snacks accessible, such as fruits and vegetables that are cleaned and prepared in easy-to-eat pieces, may encourage adolescents to choose more of these foods as between-meal snacks. Teens should also be encouraged to consume adequate milk and other calcium-enriched beverages, while minimizing sodas, sports drinks, and other sugary drinks.

As adolescents leave the family home for college or their own apartments, it is important that they set the foundation for healthful eating. One question teens often have is how to stock their first kitchen. What basic foods—or staples—should they always have on hand, so that they can quickly and easily assemble healthful meals and snacks? The **Quick Tips** list (page 544) includes the foods that many Americans consider to be staples. It can be modified to include items that are staples in non-Western cultures and to address vegetarian, vegan, low-fat, low-sodium, or other diets.

Appearance and Substance Use Are Key Concerns of Adolescence

Nutrition-related concerns for adolescents include body image and acne, as well as cigarette smoking and the use of alcohol and illegal drugs.

Body Image and Eating Disorders

Preoccupation with body weight, height, muscle mass, complexion, hair, and other aspects of physical appearance is common and normal among adolescent boys and girls. But in some teens, an initially healthful concern about body image and weight can turn into a dangerous obsession during this emotionally challenging life stage. Body image and eating disorders frequently begin during adolescence and can occur in boys as well as in girls. Parents, teachers, and friends should be aware of the warning signs, which include restricted eating patterns; excessive exercise; rapid and extreme weight loss; regular trips to the bathroom after meals; and signs of frequent vomiting or laxative use. (For more information, see the **In Depth** essay following Chapter 11.)

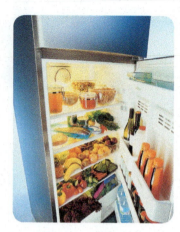

▲ Keeping a well-stocked refrigerator allows you to quickly and easily assemble healthful meals.

QuickTips

Stocking Your First Kitchen

Keep your refrigerator stocked with:

✓ Low-fat or skim milk or soymilk

✓ Calcium-enriched orange juice

✓ Hard cheeses

✓ Eggs

✓ Lean deli meats or soy meat alternatives

✓ Hummus, peanut butter, and other healthful, perishable spreads

✓ A 2- to 3-day supply of dark-green lettuce and other salad fixings, or ready-to-eat salads

✓ A 2- to 3-day supply of other fresh veggies

✓ A 2- to 3-day supply of fresh fruits

✓ Low-fat salad dressings, mustards, and salsas

✓ Whole-grain breads, rolls, bagels, pizza crusts, and tortillas

Stock your freezer with:

✓ Individual servings of chicken breast, extra-lean ground beef, pork loin chops, fish fillets, or soy meat alternatives

✓ Lower-fat frozen entrées ("boost" with salad, whole-grain roll, and extra veggies)

✓ Frozen veggies (no sauce)

✓ Frozen cheese or veggie pizza ("boost" with added mushrooms, green peppers, and other veggie toppings)

✓ Low-fat ice cream, sherbet, or sorbet

Stock your pantry with:

✓ Staples such as potatoes, sweet potatoes, onions, and garlic

✓ Canned or vacuum-packed tuna, salmon, and crab (in water, not oil)

✓ Canned legumes, such as black beans, refried beans, pinto/kidney beans, and garbanzo beans

✓ Low-sodium, low-fat, high-fiber canned soups (read the label!)

✓ Dried beans and/or lentils

✓ Whole-grain pasta and rice

✓ Tomato-based pasta sauces

✓ Canned fruit in juice with no added sugar

✓ Dried fruits, such as golden raisins, cranberries, and apricots

✓ Nuts, such as peanuts, almonds, and walnuts

✓ Whole-grain ready-to-eat cereals or oatmeal

✓ Whole-grain, low-fat crackers

✓ Low-salt pretzels, low-fat tortilla/corn chips, and low-fat or nonfat microwave popcorn

✓ Salt, pepper, balsamic vinegar, low-sodium soy sauce, and similar condiments and spices

✓ Olive and canola oils

Adolescent Acne

Another concern related to appearance is the acne flare-ups that plague many adolescents. The hormonal changes that occur during puberty are largely responsible, although stress, genetic factors, and personal hygiene may be secondary contributors. But what about foods?

For years, chocolate, fried foods, and fatty foods were linked to acne. In the 1960s, however, these theories were discounted and researchers came to agree that diet had virtually no role in its development. However, there is now strong evidence that dietary choices may indeed influence the risk or severity of acne.[23,24] Whereas some studies have found an association between a high glycemic-load diet and increased acne (see Chapter 4),[23] others have found a reduced risk for acne among people following a Mediterranean dietary pattern (see the **In Depth** essay following Chapter 2).[24] These studies are not conclusive; however, the Mediterranean diet is rich in fruits, vegetables, whole grains, olive oil, and fish—foods that provide vitamin A, vitamin C, zinc, and other nutrients that help to maintain skin health and immune function.

Prescription medications, including the vitamin A derivative 13-*cis*-retinoic acid (Accutane), effectively control severe forms of acne. Over-the-counter and prescription topical medications, applied directly to the skin, may also be used. Neither Accutane nor any other prescription vitamin A derivative should be used by women who are pregnant, are planning a pregnancy, or may become pregnant. Accutane is a known teratogen, causing severe fetal malformations. Adolescent females who treat their acne with vitamin A–derivative prescription drugs must protect themselves against pregnancy and immediately contact their physician if they discover or believe they are pregnant. Incidentally, vitamin A taken in supplement form is not effective in acne treatment and, due to its own risk for toxicity, should not be used in amounts that exceed 100% of the Daily Value.

Use of Tobacco, Alcohol, and Illegal Drugs

Adolescents are naturally curious and many are open to experimenting with tobacco, alcohol, and illegal drugs. Smoking, including tobacco and e-cigarettes, diminishes appetite and is often used by adolescent girls to achieve or maintain a lower body weight.[25] Cigarettes can also interfere with nutrient metabolism. Other effects of smoking on young people include the following:

- Addiction to nicotine
- Reduced rate of lung growth
- Impaired athletic performance and endurance
- Shortness of breath
- Early signs of heart disease and stroke
- Increased risk for lung cancer and other smoking-related cancers

Among adolescents, smoking is also associated with an increased incidence of participation in other risky behaviors, such as abusing alcohol and other drugs, fighting, and engaging in unprotected sex. There is also a link between adolescent smoking and early onset of depression and anxiety disorders.[26]

Alcohol and illegal drug use can start at early ages, even in school-age children. Motor vehicle accidents are the leading cause of death among adolescents; the risk of being involved in an accident is greatly increased by using alcohol and illegal drugs. Alcohol can also interfere with proper nutrient absorption and metabolism, and it can take the place of foods in an adolescent's diet; these adverse effects of alcohol put adolescents at risk for various nutrient deficiencies. Alcohol consumption and the use of certain illegal drugs are also associated with "the munchies," a feeling of food craving that usually results in the intake of large quantities of high-fat, high-sugar, nutrient-poor foods. This behavior can result in overweight or obesity, and it increases the risk for nutrient imbalance. Teens who use illegal drugs and alcohol are often in poor physical condition, are either underweight or overweight, have poor appetites, and perform poorly in school.

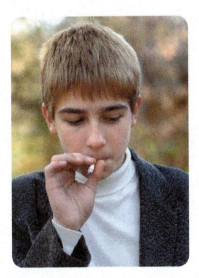

Cigarette smoking can interfere with nutrient metabolism, in addition to having other harmful effects.

nutri-case | LIZ

"High school was really hard for me. Because dance took up such a big part of my life, I just didn't make a lot of friends. When I looked at the popular girls, I always noticed how slender they all were. So I started skipping lunch and eating less at dinner. This went on until I went to an audition for a production of *The Nutcracker*. I wanted so badly to dance in it, but I was feeling so spaced out—I guess from hunger—that before I knew what had happened, I was on the floor! I sprained my ankle and didn't get to dance at all that year! So that's why, while I've been preparing for my audition with the City Ballet, I made sure I'm getting at least 1,000 Calories a day. The audition's tomorrow, and I'm not going to end up on the floor this time!"

Do you—or does someone you know—equate body weight with popularity and desirability? Why are adolescents or young adults particularly prone to this type of thinking? If Liz succeeds in getting into the City Ballet—given what you've learned throughout this text—what health risks do you think she is likely to face in the future? How could she reduce these risks?

recap Puberty is the period in life in which secondary sexual characteristics develop and the ability to reproduce begins. Adolescents experience rapid increases in height, weight, and lean body mass and fat mass. Energy needs can be very high. Fat intake should be 25% to 35% of total energy, and carbohydrate intake should be 45% to 65%. The RDA for protein is 0.85 g per kg body weight. Calcium is needed to optimize bone growth and to achieve peak bone density, and iron needs are increased due to increased muscle mass in boys and to menstruation in girls. Adolescents need to drink about 8 cups (girls) and 11 cups (boys) of water or other beverages daily. Adolescents are at risk of skipping meals and selecting fast foods and snack foods in place of whole grains, fruits, and vegetables. Milk is commonly replaced with sugary drinks. Body image and eating disorders, acne, cigarette smoking, and use of alcohol and illegal drugs are also concerns for this age group.

LO 4 Discuss the problem of pediatric obesity, including medical issues and preventive measures.

Why is pediatric obesity harmful, and what can be done?

Although the prevalence of obesity has stabilized for U.S. children and adolescents since 2007, rates remain unacceptably high.[1] The problem can begin as early as the toddler years: Over 20% of children 2 to 5 years old are classified as overweight, while 8% are categorized as obese.[1] As mentioned at the beginning of this chapter, overall, about 17% of U.S. children and adolescents ages 2 to 19 years—nearly 13 million children—are currently classified as obese.

Obesity Impairs Children's Health

We may feel shocked at the sight of an obese child, but children's health experts point out that we should be more concerned by underlying medical issues.[27] Even in early childhood, obesity can worsen asthma, increase risk of dental caries, cause sleep apnea, impair the child's mobility, reduce academic performance, and lead to intense teasing, low self-esteem, depression, and social isolation. Fatty liver is diagnosed in one-half of obese adolescents, and increasing numbers of obese children are experiencing abnormal blood lipids, high blood pressure, high blood glucose, metabolic syndrome, skeletal disorders, and other medical problems.[27] Also, it has been estimated that about 70% of children who are obese maintain their higher weight as adults, thus prevention or treatment of pediatric obesity will positively impact rates of adult obesity.

Parents should not be offended if the child's pediatrician or other healthcare provider expresses concern over the child's weight status; early intervention is often the most effective measure against lifelong obesity. Pediatricians use growth charts published by the Centers for Disease Control and Prevention (CDC) to track a child's growth over time and identify children at risk for overweight or obesity. The charts aid clinicians in assessing a child's stature-for-age, weight-for-age, and BMI-for-age (see Appendix E). The charts are also available for families at the CDC website listed in the **Web Links**. The CDC classifies as obese children over the age of 2 who are at or above the 95th percentile for their gender-specific BMI-for-age; that is, their BMI is higher than that of 95% of U.S. children of the same age and gender. Children at or above the 85th percentile but below the 95th percentile on BMI-for-age charts are defined as overweight. Recently, the CDC added two new categories to describe severe obesity among children and adolescents:

- Class 2 obesity is a BMI greater than or equal to 120% of the 95th percentile or a BMI greater than or equal to 35; approximately 6% of U.S. children meet the criteria for class 2 obesity.
- Class 3 obesity is a BMI greater than or equal to 140% of the 95th percentile or a BMI greater than or equal to 40; approximately 2% of U.S. children meet the criteria for class 3 obesity.

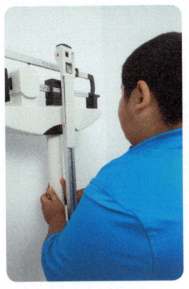

The rates of obesity among U.S. children remain unacceptably high.

Unfortunately, rates of class 2 and 3 obesity have increased over the past several years, particularly among girls.[28]

Using growth charts, pediatricians and parents can easily observe the pattern that develops from year to year. Children who begin to track toward higher and higher BMI-for-age percentiles should be encouraged and supported in healthful, balanced eating and increased physical activity.

Encourage Healthful Eating Patterns

The introduction and retention of healthful eating patterns within the family unit are among the most effective strategies in the fight against pediatric obesity.[29] Rather than singling out overweight children and placing them on restrictive diets, experts encourage family-wide improvements in food choices and mealtime habits. Parents should strive to consistently provide nutritious food choices, limit access to sugary drinks, and sit down to a shared family meal as often as possible. Using the MyPlate model, parents and children can work together to "diagram" meals that include brightly colored vegetables, deep-brown whole grains, lean plant and animal protein sources, and dairy or dairy substitutes. A meal that includes prewashed bagged salad, frozen vegetables, instant brown rice, and deli-prepared broiled chicken is a quick and healthful option. Television and other electronic distractions should be off limits throughout mealtimes to encourage attentive eating and true enjoyment of the food.

Parents should retain control over the purchase and preparation of foods until older children and teens are responsible and knowledgeable enough to make healthful decisions. As the "gatekeepers" for household food supplies, parents' choices to buy or not to buy chips, sweets, fried foods, and sugary drinks influence their family members' health. Parents can keep a supply of nonperishable snacks—such as granola bars, dried fruits and nuts, and kid-friendly fruits, including apples, bananas, and oranges—to grab as everyone dashes out the door. Whenever possible, parents should minimize the number of meals eaten in restaurants, especially fast-food franchises. When families do eat out, large portion sizes can be shared; moreover, the family can order grilled, broiled, or baked foods instead of fried foods. Sugary drinks should be replaced with low-fat milk or water.

Finally, parents remain important role models, even through the often turbulent adolescent years. Parents themselves should follow a healthful eating pattern, engage in regular physical activity, and avoid substance abuse.

As discussed earlier, schools play a role in shaping eating behaviors. Parents can work with local school boards to eliminate or restrict the sale of soda, candy,

Download a free, 112-page cookbook chock-full of healthy, kid-friendly recipes from the National Heart, Lung, and Blood Institute. Go to www.nhlbi.nih .gov, enter "keep the beat heart healthy recipes" into the search box, then click on the link.

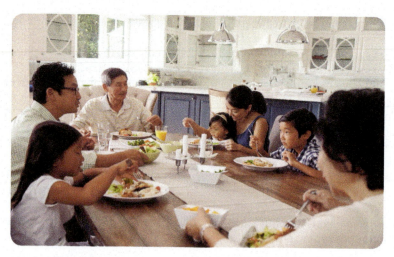

▲ Families should try to have shared meals whenever possible.

chips, and pastries. Schools can set aside land or construct raised beds for vegetable gardens, and food service providers can use the produce in breakfasts and lunches. Consistent and repeated school-based messages on good nutrition can reinforce the efforts of parents and healthcare providers.

Tips on family fitness can be found at www.verywell.com. From the home page, enter "family fitness" into the search box and choose a link.

Encourage Physical Activity

Television, computer use, and electronic games often tempt children into a sedentary lifestyle, but increased energy expenditure through increased physical activity is essential for successful weight management. The Physical Activity Guidelines for Americans recommend bone- and muscle-strengthening activities for children at least 3 days each week,[30] in addition to at least 1 hour of moderate to vigorous physical activity each day. For younger children, daily activity can be divided into two or three shorter sessions, allowing them to regroup, recoup, and refocus between activity sessions. Overweight children are more likely to engage in physical activities that are noncompetitive, fun, and structured in a way that allows them to proceed at their own pace. All children can be encouraged to have fun using their muscles in various ways that suit their interests (TABLE 15.2). Activity-based interactive DVD games are ideal for children who must remain indoors for extended periods.

As with healthful eating patterns, parents play an important role in establishing and maintaining an active lifestyle for the family. Shared family activities such as bicycle riding, volleyball or basketball games, hikes, and water sports encourage physical activity throughout the year. Parents can establish daily limits on the use of electronic games, television, recreational use of computers, and other sedentary activities in order to minimize sitting time. These approaches can help reduce children's and adolescents' obesity risk.

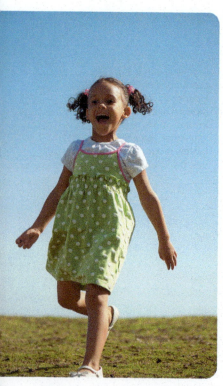

▲ Active, healthy-weight children are less likely to become over-weight adults.

recap Obesity is an important concern for children of all ages, their families, and their communities. About 17% of U.S. children and adolescents ages 2 to 19 years—nearly 13 million children—are currently classified as obese. Complications of obesity include more severe asthma, sleep apnea, impaired mobility, metabolic syndrome, reduced academic performance, low self-esteem, depression, and many other problems. Parents should model healthful eating and activity behaviors. Schools play an important role in providing nutritious breakfasts and lunches and varied opportunities for daily physical activity. Children should engage in bone- and muscle-strengthening activities for at least 3 days each week, in addition to at least 1 hour of moderate to vigorous physical activity each day.

TABLE 15.2 Examples of Physical Activities for Children and Adolescents*

Type of Physical Activity	Age Group: Children	Age Group: Adolescents
Moderate-intensity aerobic	■ Active recreation, such as hiking, skateboarding, rollerblading ■ Bicycle riding ■ Brisk walking	■ Active recreation, such as canoeing, hiking, skateboarding, rollerblading ■ Brisk walking ■ Bicycle riding (stationary or road bike) ■ Housework and yard work, such as sweeping or pushing a lawn mower ■ Games that require catching and throwing, such as baseball and softball
Vigorous-intensity aerobic	■ Active games involving running and chasing, such as tag ■ Bicycle riding ■ Jumping rope ■ Martial arts, such as karate ■ Running ■ Sports such as soccer, ice or field hockey, basketball, swimming, tennis ■ Cross-country skiing	■ Active games involving running and chasing, such as flag football ■ Bicycle riding ■ Jumping rope ■ Martial arts, such as karate ■ Running ■ Sports such as soccer, ice or field hockey, basketball, swimming, tennis ■ Vigorous dancing ■ Cross-country skiing
Muscle-strengthening	■ Games such as tug-of-war ■ Modified push-ups (with knees on the floor) ■ Resistance exercises using body weight or resistance bands ■ Rope or tree climbing ■ Sit-ups (curl-ups or crunches) ■ Swinging on playground equipment/bars	■ Games such as tug-of-war ■ Push-ups and pull-ups ■ Resistance exercises with exercise bands, weight machines, hand-held weights ■ Climbing wall ■ Sit-ups (curl-ups or crunches)
Bone-strengthening	■ Games such as hopscotch ■ Hopping, skipping, jumping ■ Jumping rope ■ Running ■ Sports such as gymnastics, basketball, volleyball, tennis	■ Hopping, skipping, jumping ■ Jumping rope ■ Running ■ Sports such as gymnastics, basketball, volleyball, tennis

Note: Some activities, such as bicycling, can be moderate or vigorous intensity, depending on level of effort.

Source: Data from *2008 Physical Activity Guidelines for Americans,* U.S. Department of Health and Human Services.

What characterizes aging?

Throughout this book, our exploration of nutrition and physical activity has focused mainly on young and middle-age adults. In the following section, we discuss aging, including the ways in which diet and lifestyle affect the aging process.

Americans Are Getting Older

The U.S. population is getting older each year. Consider the following statistics:

- In 2014, average life expectancy at birth was projected at 78.8 years.[31]
- The elderly (those 65 years and above) number over 45 million and account for about 14% of the American population.[32]
- People 85 years of age and older currently represent the fastest-growing U.S. population subgroup, projected to increase from 6 million in 2015 to nearly 20 million by the year 2050.[32] These so-called very elderly or oldest old account for the majority of healthcare expenditures and nursing home admissions in the United States.

LO 5 Describe the growth of the older adult population in the United States and the physiologic changes that accompany normal aging.

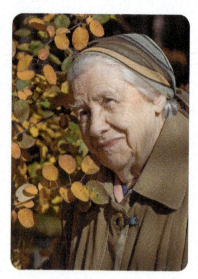

Centenarians represent the future of U.S. elderly.

■ The number of *centenarians,* persons over the age of 100 years, and *super centenarians,* over 110 years, continues to grow as well. Between 2000 and 2014, the number of centenarians grew by over 40%, and there are now more than 72,000 centenarians in the United States.

These statistics have important nutrition-related implications for you, even if you're a young adult. That's because a nutritious diet and regular physical activity throughout life can delay the onset of chronic diseases, and help you to maintain a better quality of life as you age.

Characteristic Physiologic Changes Accompany Aging

Older adulthood is a time in which body systems begin to slow and degenerate. If the following discussion of this degeneration seems disturbing or depressing, remember that the changes described are at least partly within an individual's control. For instance, some of the decrease in muscle mass, bone mass, and muscle strength is due to low physical activity levels. In addition, there are intriguing lines of research actively searching for a modern-day "fountain of youth," some of which are discussed in the **In Depth** essay following this chapter.

Age-Related Changes in Sensory Perception

For most individuals, eating is a social and pleasurable process; the sights, sounds, odors, and textures associated with food stimulate and enhance one's appetite. However, odor, taste, touch, and vision all decline with age and negatively affect the food intake and nutritional status of older adults.

It has been estimated that over half of older adults experience a significant impairment in their sense of smell. The nerve receptors for taste and smell are complementary; thus, enjoyment of food relies heavily on the sense of smell. Older adults who cannot adequately appreciate the appealing aromas of food may be unable to fully enjoy the foods offered in a meal. Although often a simple consequence of aging, loss of odor perception can also be caused by a zinc deficiency or a medication. If this is the case, a zinc supplement or change of medication may be a simple solution.

Because the sense of smell contributes significantly to the sense of taste, *dysgeusia,* or an impaired sense of taste, is also common. Most often diminished are the abilities to detect salt and bitter tastes. The perception of sweetness and sourness also declines, but to a lesser extent.

Loss of visual acuity has unexpected consequences for the nutritional health of older adults. Many have difficulty reading food labels, including nutrient information and "pull dates" for perishable foods. Driving skills decline, limiting the ability of some older Americans to get to a market offering healthful, affordable foods. Older adults with vision loss may not be able to see the temperature knobs on stoves or the controls on microwave ovens and may therefore choose cold meals, such as sandwiches, rather than meals that require heating. Also, the visual appeal of a colorful, attractively arranged plate of food is lost to visually impaired elderly people, further reducing their desire to eat healthful meals.

Age-Related Changes in Gastrointestinal Function

Significant changes in the mouth, stomach, intestinal tract, and related organs occur with aging. Some of these changes can increase the risk for nutrient deficiency and excessive weight loss.

With increasing age, salivary production declines. A dry mouth reduces taste perception, increases tooth decay, and makes chewing and swallowing more difficult. Thus, a diet rich in moist foods, including fruits and vegetables; sauces or gravies on meats; and high-fluid desserts, such as puddings, is advised. Difficulty swallowing, clinically known as *dysphagia,* can also result from a stroke or a condition such as Parkinsonism. Smooth, thick foods, such as cream soups, applesauce, milkshakes, fruit nectars, yogurt, and puddings, are usually well tolerated.

Older adults are also at risk for a reduced secretion of gastric hydrochloric acid, which limits the absorption of minerals such as calcium, iron, and zinc and food sources of folic acid and vitamin B_{12}. A decline in intrinsic factor also reduces the absorption of vitamin B_{12} (see Chapter 8). Thus, vitamin B_{12} supplements and/or B_{12} injections are advised.

Age-Related Changes in Body Composition

With aging, body fat increases and muscle mass declines, leading to impaired physical functioning in the elderly. It has been estimated that women and men lose 20% to 25% of their lean body mass, respectively, as they age from 35 to 70 years. The decreased production of certain hormones, including testosterone and growth hormone, and chronic diseases contribute to this loss of muscle, as do poor diet and an increasingly sedentary lifestyle. Adequate protein intake and regular physical activity, including strength or resistance training, can help older adults maintain their muscle mass and strength.[33,34]

Body fat increases from young adulthood through middle age, peaking at approximately 55 to 65 years of age, then declining in persons over the age of 70. With aging, body fat shifts from subcutaneous stores, just below the skin, to internal, or visceral, fat stores. Older men and women tend to deposit more fat in their abdominal region compared to younger adults. Among women, this shift in body fat stores is most dramatic after the onset of menopause and coincides with an increased risk for heart disease, diabetes, and metabolic syndrome.

Bone mineral density declines with age and may eventually drop to the critical fracture zone. Among older women, the onset of menopause leads to a sudden and dramatic loss of bone due to the lack of estrogen. Although it is less dramatic, elderly men also experience this loss of bone, due in part to decreasing levels of testosterone. In addition to the well-known benefits of calcium and vitamin D, intakes of vitamins A, C, and K, phosphorus, magnesium, fluoride, and protein are recognized as influencing bone density. As noted in the **Nutrition Debate** on physical activity in the elderly (page 559), bone health can be promoted through regular weight-bearing activity in adults well into their 90s and beyond.

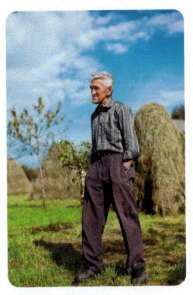

▲ Age-related changes in sensory as well as gastrointestinal function can lead to inappropriate weight loss in older adults.

recap The U.S. population is getting older. Adults age 65 and older account for about 14% of the U.S. population. The physiologic changes that can occur with aging include sensory declines; an impaired ability to chew, swallow, and absorb and metabolize various nutrients; a loss of muscle mass and lean tissue; increased fat mass; and decreased bone density. These age-related changes influence the nutritional needs of older adults and their ability to consume a healthful diet.

What are the nutritional needs and concerns of older adults?

LO 6 Explain how aging influences the nutrient needs and health concerns of older adults.

The energy and nutrient needs of older adults reflect their reduced physical activity and the physiologic changes of aging. At the same time, several nutrition-related health concerns arise.

Some Nutrient Recommendations Increase or Decrease with Aging

The requirements for many nutrients are the same for older adults as for young and middle-aged adults. A few nutrient requirements increase, and a few are actually lower. TABLE 15.3 identifies the nutrient recommendations that change as well as the physiologic reasons behind these changes.

TABLE 15.3 Nutrient Recommendations That Change with Increased Age

Changes in Nutrient Recommendations	Rationale for Changes
Vitamin D Increased need for vitamin D from 600 IU/day for adults age 18–70 years to 800 IU/day for adults over age 70 years	Decreased bone density Decreased ability to synthesize vitamin D in the skin
Calcium Increased need for calcium from 1,000 mg/day for adults 19–50 years to 1,200 mg/day for women 51 years of age and older, and men 71 years and older	Decreased bone density Decreased absorption of dietary calcium
Fiber Decreased need for fiber from 38 g/day for young men to 30 g/day for men 51 years and older; decreases for women from 25 g/day for young women to 21 g/day for women 51 years and older	Decreased energy intake
B-Vitamins Increased need for vitamin B_6 and need for vitamin B_{12} as a supplement or from fortified foods	Lower levels of gastric juice Decreased absorption of food B_{12} from gastrointestinal tract Increased need to reduce homocysteine levels and to optimize immune function

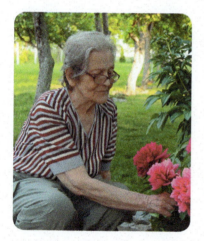

⬆ Older adults have lower total energy requirements as a result of several factors, including a less physically active lifestyle.

Energy and Macronutrient Recommendations for Older Adults

The energy needs of older adults are lower than those of younger adults. This decrease is due to a loss of muscle mass and lean tissue, a reduction in thyroid hormones, and an increasingly sedentary lifestyle. It is estimated that total daily energy expenditure decreases approximately 10 kcal each year for men and 7 kcal each year for women ages 19 and older.[2] This adds up over time; for example, a woman who needs 2,000 kcal at age 20 needs just 1,650 at age 70. Some of this decrease in energy expenditure is an inevitable response to aging, but some of the decrease can be delayed or minimized by staying physically active.

To avoid weight gain, older adults need to consume a diet high in nutrient-dense foods. The USDA MyPlate model can be adapted to reflect the needs of older adults and help guide their food choices **(FIGURE 15.6)**. See the **In Depth** essay following this chapter to learn more about the theories of Caloric restriction and intermittent fasting, which propose that low-energy diets may significantly prolong life.

To reduce their risk for cardiovascular and other chronic diseases, it is recommended that older adults maintain a total fat intake within 20% to 35% of total daily energy intake, with less than 10% of total energy intake coming from saturated fat.

The RDA for carbohydrate is the same for adults of all ages: 130 g/day.[2] Fiber-rich carbohydrates should be emphasized over refined carbohydrates: it is recommended that older individuals consume a diet that contains no more than 25% of total energy intake as sugars.[2] The fiber recommendations are slightly lower for older adults than for younger adults because older adults eat less energy. After age 50, 30 g of fiber per day for men and 21 g for women is assumed sufficient to reduce the risks for constipation and diverticular disease, maintain healthful blood levels of glucose and lipids, and provide good sources of nutrient-dense, low-energy foods.

The DRI for protein is the same for adults of all ages: 0.80 g protein/kg body weight per day.[2] Some researchers have argued for a protein allowance of 1.0 to 1.2 g per kg body weight for older adults in order to optimize their protein status; however, the issue remains unresolved.[35,36] Protein is important to help minimize the loss of muscle and lean tissue, optimize healing after injury or disease, maintain immunity, and help prevent excessive bone loss. Many protein-rich foods are also important sources of the vitamins and minerals that are typically low in the diets of older adults; thus, protein is an important nutrient for this age group.

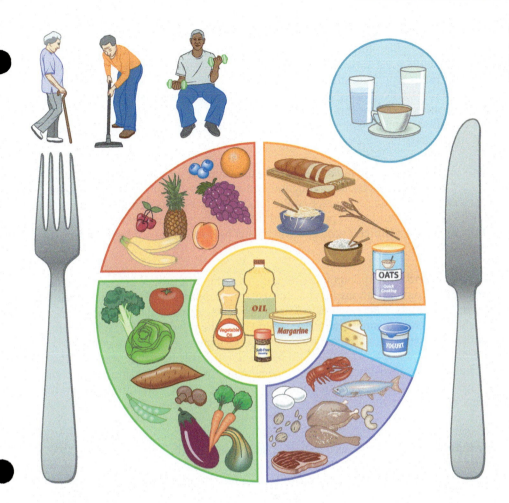

Micronutrient Recommendations for Older Adults

The vitamins and minerals of particular concern for older adults are identified in Table 15.3.

Calcium Preventing or minimizing the consequences of osteoporosis is a top priority for older adults. The RDA for calcium is higher for all adults over the age of 70 years and for women aged 51 to 70 years compared to younger adults.[4] The calcium requirement increases at an earlier age for women compared to men due to the earlier onset of bone loss, typically at the onset of menopause.

Vitamin D Older adults living in long-term care facilities are at increased risk for vitamin D deficiency because they may not be exposed to amounts of sunlight adequate for vitamin D synthesis in the skin. Even among older adults leading active lives, the use of sunscreen may block the sunlight needed for vitamin D synthesis. It is critical, therefore, that older adults consume foods that are high in calcium and vitamin D and, when needed, use supplements in appropriate amounts and under the guidance of a healthcare provider. Adequate vitamin D not only enhances bone health but optimizes immunity and supports normal muscle and pancreatic function. A deficiency of vitamin D may increase the older adult's risk of falls, cognitive impairment, and overall mortality.[37]

Iron Iron needs decrease with aging. This decrease is primarily due to reduced muscle and lean tissue in both men and women and the cessation of menstruation in women. The decreased need for iron in older men is not significant enough to change the recommendations for iron intake in this group; thus, the RDA for iron is the same for older and younger men, 8 mg/day. However, the RDA for iron for older women is 8 mg/day, which is 10 mg/day lower than the RDA for younger women.[5] Heme iron from meat, fish, and poultry represents the most available source of dietary iron; however, some older adults reduce their intake of these foods because of cost or difficulties in chewing and swallowing. Fortified grains and cereals, as well as legumes, greens, and dried fruits, can provide additional iron in the diet.

Zinc   Although zinc recommendations are the same for all adults, it is a critical nutrient for optimizing immune function and wound healing in older adults. Zinc intake can be inadequate in older adults for the same reasons that heme iron intake may be deficient: red meats, poultry, and fish are relatively expensive, and older adults may have a difficult time chewing meats because of loss of teeth and/or the use of dentures.

Vitamins C and E   Although it is thought that older adults have increased oxidative stress, the recommendations for the antioxidant vitamins C and E are the same as for younger adults.[38] Researchers continue, however, to investigate the potential benefits of dietary or supplemental vitamin C and the roles it may play in lowering the risk of hypertension, impaired physical performance, and other age-related disorders. Vitamin E also continues to be evaluated for its potential to reduce the risk of cataracts and age-related macular degeneration, two types of vision impairment discussed shortly, as well as other forms of oxidative stress.[39] Overall, however, the ability of dietary or supplemental vitamin C or E to lower risk of age-related disorders remains uncertain.

B-vitamins   Older adults need to pay close attention to their intake of the B-vitamins—specifically, vitamin B_{12}, vitamin B_6, and folate.[10] Inadequate intakes of these nutrients increase the levels of the amino acid homocysteine in the blood. This state has been linked to an increased risk for cardiovascular disease, age-related dementia (including Alzheimer's disease), and loss of cognitive function in the elderly.[10]

The RDA for both folate and vitamin B_{12} is the same for younger and older adults, but up to 30% of older adults cannot absorb enough vitamin B_{12} from foods because of reduced production of gastric juice. It is recommended that older adults consume supplements or foods that are fortified with vitamin B_{12} because the vitamin B_{12} in these products is absorbed more readily. Vitamin B_{12} is also available via injection. Vitamin B_6 recommendations are slightly higher for adults age 51 and older because these higher levels appear necessary to reduce homocysteine levels, decrease risk of depression, and optimize cognitive function in this population.

Vitamin A   Vitamin A requirements are the same for adults of all ages; however, older adults should be careful not to consume more than the RDA because the absorption of vitamin A is actually greater in older adults. Thus, this group is at greater risk for vitamin A toxicity, which can cause liver damage and neurologic problems. In addition, high intakes of vitamin A by older adults have been linked to increased risk for hip fractures.[5] Although older adults should avoid high dietary vitamin A and high-potency vitamin A supplements, consuming fruits and vegetables high in beta-carotene or other carotenoids is safe and does not lead to vitamin A toxicity.

Supplementation   A variety of factors may limit an older adult's ability to eat healthfully. These include limited financial resources, reduced appetite, social isolation, an inability to prepare foods, and illnesses and physiologic changes that limit the absorption and metabolism of many nutrients. Thus, some older adults may benefit from taking a multivitamin and mineral supplement that contains no more than the RDA for all the nutrients contained in the supplement. Additional supplementation may be necessary for nutrients such as calcium, vitamin D, and vitamin B_{12}. However, supplementation with individual nutrients should be done only under the supervision of the individual's primary healthcare provider because the risk of nutrient toxicity is high in this population.

Fluid Recommendations for Older Adults

The AI for fluid is the same for older and younger adults.[6] Men should consume 3.7 liters of total water per day, which includes 3.0 liters (about 13 cups) as beverages, including drinking water. Women should consume 2.7 liters of total water per day, which includes 2.2 liters (about 9 cups) as beverages. Kidney function changes with age, and the thirst mechanism of older people can be impaired. These changes can result in chronic dehydration and hypernatremia (elevated blood sodium levels) in this population. Some older adults intentionally limit their beverage intake because they have urinary incontinence or don't want to be awakened for nighttime urination. This practice can endanger their health, so it is important for them to seek treatment for the incontinence and continue to drink plenty of fluids.

Older Adults Have Many Unique Nutrition-Related Concerns

In addition to overweight and underweight, older adults commonly face dental problems, eye disorders, and potential interactions between nutrients and medications. Also, some older adults face financial difficulties that affect their nutritional choices. Each of these concerns is discussed briefly in the following sections.

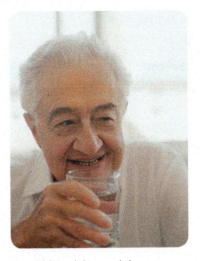

Older adults need the same amount of fluids as other adults.

Obesity and Underweight

In the United States, nearly 41% of adults between the ages of 65 and 74 years are obese; however, the incidence drops to just below 28% for those 75 years and older.[40] The elderly population as a whole has a high risk for cardiovascular disease, type 2 diabetes, and cancer, all of which are more prevalent in older adults who are obese. Obesity also increases the severity and consequences of osteoarthritis, limits mobility, and is associated with functional declines in daily activities.

Underweight is also risky for older adults; mortality rates are actually higher in the underweight elderly (BMI below 18.5) than in the overweight elderly (BMI 25.0 to 29.9). Significantly underweight older adults have fewer protein reserves to call upon during periods of catabolic stress, such as post-surgery or trauma, and are more susceptible to infection. Inappropriate weight loss suggests inadequate energy intake, which also implies inadequate nutrient intake. Chronic deficiencies of protein, vitamins, and minerals leave older adults at risk for poor wound healing and a depressed immune response.

Gerontologists have identified "nine Ds" that account for most cases of geriatric weight loss **(FIGURE 15.7)** (page 556). Several of these factors promote weight loss by reducing energy intake, others by increasing energy expenditure or loss of nutrients. A condition known as *geriatric failure-to-thrive*—also called "the dwindles"—illustrates the complexity of inappropriate age-related weight loss and related health issues.

Dental Health Issues

Diet plays an important role in the maintenance of dental health in the elderly. Deficiencies of the B-vitamins can lead to irritation, inflammation, and cracking of the lips and tongue, whereas vitamin C deficiency increases the risk for periodontal (gum) disease. A lack of adequate calcium, vitamin D, and protein contributes to bone loss in the oral cavity, which increases risk for tooth loss. Saliva helps neutralize the decay-promoting acids produced by oral bacteria; however, with aging, saliva production decreases.

Despite great advances in dental health, older adults remain at high risk of losing some or all of their teeth, suffering from gum disease, or having poorly fitting dentures, which cause considerable mouth pain and make chewing difficult. Adults with poorly fitted dentures or chewing problems tend to avoid meats and firm fruits and vegetables, leading to nutrient deficiencies. Older adults can compensate for a loss of chewing ability by selecting soft, protein-rich foods, such as eggs, peanut

▶ **FIGURE 15.7** The nine Ds of geriatric weight loss. These are among the most significant factors contributing to inappropriate weight loss in the elderly.

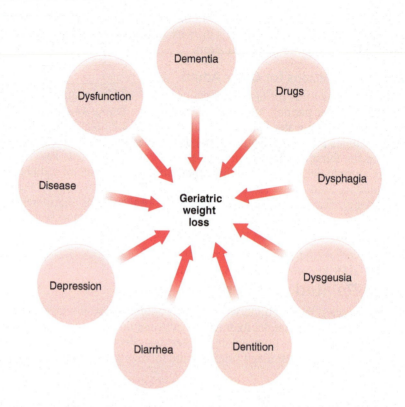

butter, cheese, yogurt, ground meat, fish, and well-cooked legumes. Red meats and poultry can be stewed or cooked in liquid for a long period. Oatmeal and other whole-grain cooked cereals can provide needed fiber, as do mashed berries and bananas, ripened melons, and canned vegetables. Shredded and minced raw vegetables can be added to dishes. With planning, older adults with oral health problems can maintain a varied, healthful diet.

Age-Related Eye Diseases

Two age-related eye disorders are responsible for vision impairment and blindness in older adults. **Macular degeneration** is damage to the macula, the portion of the retina of the eye that enables us to see the center of the visual field and to see details **(FIGURE 15.8a)**. Affecting more than 1.75 million U.S. adults, it is the leading cause of blindness in the elderly. A **cataract** is a cloudiness in the lens of the eye (Figure 15.8b). This condition affects 20% of adults in their 60s and almost 70% of those in their 80s. Although these are different conditions, sunlight exposure and smoking are lifestyle practices that increase the risk for both.

Recent research suggests, but does not prove, that dietary choices may slow the progress of these two degenerative eye diseases, saving millions of dollars and preventing or delaying the functional losses associated with impaired vision. Several studies have shown the beneficial effects of antioxidants, including vitamins C and E, on cataract formation, whereas others have reported no significant benefit.[41] Two phytochemicals, lutein and zeaxanthin, have also been identified as protective by some, but not all, studies.[42] These four antioxidants, as well as zinc and omega-3 fatty acids, may also provide protection against macular degeneration.[41] Although the research is not yet conclusive, older adults can benefit by consuming foods rich in these nutrients, primarily colorful fruits and vegetables, nuts, and whole grains. Vision-enhancing nutrient supplements, the formulations of which are based on the results of two large research studies (AREDS 1 and 2), may help delay the progression of macular degeneration and cataracts.[43]

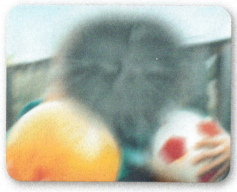

(a)

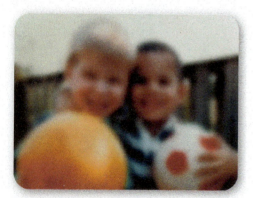

(b)

◆ **FIGURE 15.8** These photos simulate two forms of vision loss common in older adults. **(a)** Macular degeneration results in a loss of central vision. **(b)** Cataracts impair vision across the visual field.

Interactions Between Medications and Nutrition

Although persons 65 years of age and older account for only 13% of the U.S. population, they are prescribed about 35% of all medications, and they experience almost 40% of all adverse drug effects.[44] Between 2006 and 2011, the incidence of major drug-drug interactions among older adults doubled from 8% to 15%.[45] At least in part, these statistics reflect the risks of **polypharmacy**, or the use of five or more prescription drugs at any given time. Nearly 40% of Americans age 65 and older take five or more prescription medications, meeting the definition of polypharmacy.[45] A small but significant number of older adults use 10 or more medications, a practice known as *excessive polypharmacy*. The more medications older adults take, the greater their risk for cognitive decline, falls, drug-drug interactions, medication errors, and rehospitalization.[46] Medications can interact not only with each other, but also with herbs and other dietary supplements.

Medications can also reduce or increase appetite, thereby promoting weight loss or weight gain. Moreover, they can affect nutrient digestion, absorption, activation, or excretion. A number of medications reduce the absorption of certain vitamins and minerals, including calcium, iron, and fat-soluble vitamins. Other medications reduce the activation of vitamin D, vitamin B_6, folate, and other vitamins. Certain anticoagulants interfere with vitamin K metabolism, which means that healthcare providers must carefully balance drug dosage in order to minimize risk of vitamin K deficiency. Finally, some medications, such as diuretics, increase urinary excretion of potassium or other nutrients.

From the opposite perspective, food and supplement choices can negatively impact medication activity and effectiveness. Individual foods such as grapefruit juice, spinach, and aged cheese are known to react negatively with a number of drugs. A compound in grapefruit juice, for example, inhibits the breakdown of as many as 85 different drugs, leading to as much as a tenfold increase in blood drug levels and potential overdose. High calcium foods and calcium supplements decrease the absorption of many antibiotics, greatly reducing their therapeutic value. Foods high in vitamin K, such as dark green leafy vegetables, greatly reduce the effectiveness of certain anticoagulants, leading to the potential for abnormal clot formation. **TABLE 15.4** summarizes some of the more common drug–nutrient interactions.

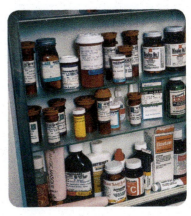

◆ Medications taken by older adults can interact in a harmful way with one another and with nutrients and foods.

TABLE 15.4 Examples of Common Drug–Nutrient Interactions

Category of Drug	Interactions
Antacids	May decrease the absorption of iron, calcium, folate, vitamin B_{12}
Antibiotics	May reduce the absorption of calcium, fat-soluble vitamins; reduces the production of vitamin K by gut bacteria
Anticonvulsants	Interfere with activation of vitamin D
Anticoagulants ("blood thinners")	Reduce the activity of vitamin K
Antidepressants	May cause weight gain as a result of increased appetite
Antiretroviral agents (used in treatment of HIV/AIDS)	Reduce absorption of most nutrients
Aspirin	Lowers blood folate levels; increases iron loss due to gastrointestinal bleeding
Diuretics	May increase urinary excretion of potassium, sodium, calcium, magnesium; may cause retention of potassium, other electrolytes
Laxatives	Increase fecal excretion of dietary fat, fat-soluble vitamins, calcium, and other minerals

macular degeneration A vision disorder characterized by deterioration of the macula, the central portion of the retina, and marked by loss or distortion of the center of the visual field.

cataract A damaged portion of the eye's lens, which causes cloudiness that impairs vision.

polypharmacy The use of five or more prescription drugs at any one time.

Financial Problems

Over 8% of elderly men and women in the United States, or 4 million adults over the age of 60 years, experience some form of food insecurity. At greatest risk are African American, Hispanic, and other minorities; those living in the South; and those living alone. In response to this problem, the federal government has developed a network of food and nutrition services for older Americans. These services are typically coordinated with state and local governments as well as nonprofit or community organizations. They include the following:

- **Supplemental Nutrition Assistance Program (SNAP):** Previously known as the Food Stamp program, this USDA program provides food assistance for low-income households. It is designed to meet the basic nutritional needs of eligible people of all ages. Participants are provided with a monthly allotment, typically in the form of a prepaid debit card or food coupons. Unfortunately, only 67% of older Americans who are eligible for SNAP participate, a rate below that of younger groups.[47]

- **Congregate Nutrition Services Program:** This program is administered by the Administration on Aging, a unit within the Department of Health and Human Services (HHS).[48] Each year, it provides more than 200 million meals to disabled, low-income, minority, and rural elderly, as well as those with limited English language skills, and those at risk for institutionalization.[49] Nearly 60% of the participants report that one meal represents half or more of their total daily food intake.[50]

- **Nutrition Services Incentive Program:** This USDA-administered program provides a limited number of "commodity foods" to nearly 600,000 low-income adults 60 years and older. Foods are distributed to state-level agencies, then to community organizations. They include cereals, peanut butter, dry beans, rice or pasta, and canned juice, fruits, vegetables, meat, poultry, and tuna. The foods distributed are rich in nutrients typically lacking in the diets of low-income elderly.

- **Senior Farmers' Market Nutrition Program:** This program, sponsored by the USDA, provides funds to states and Indian tribal governments to distribute coupons to 865,000 low-income seniors, so that they can buy eligible foods such as fruits and vegetables at farmers' markets and roadside stands. Seniors enjoy the nutritional benefits of fresh local produce and the opportunity to increase the variety of their meals.[51]

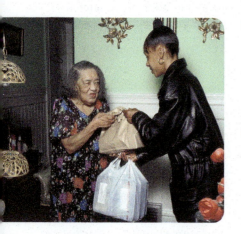

◀ For many homebound, disabled, and low-income older adults, community programs are lifelines that provide nourishing meals as well as vital social contact.

recap Because of their loss of lean tissue and lower physical activity levels, older adults need less total energy than younger adults. Their macronutrient intake levels are the same as for younger adults, but some researchers believe that older adults need more protein. The micronutrients of concern are calcium, vitamin D, iron, zinc, vitamin B_6, vitamin B_{12}, and folate. Supplementation may be necessary. Older adults are at risk for chronic dehydration. Men need to drink about 13 cups of water and other beverages per day, and women need about 9 cups. Both obesity and underweight increase the risk for disease and disability in older adults. Dental and vision problems can limit the intake of meats, fruits, and vegetables, leading to nutrient deficiencies. Medications can interact with each other in harmful ways, and certain medications and foods or nutrients can have adverse interactions. More than 8% of older adults in the United States experience food insecurity. Several government and community programs are available for older adults in need of food assistance.

Physical Activity in Older Adulthood: What Amounts, Types, and Intensities Are Appropriate?

A minority of older adults exercise. Fewer than 44% of the "young elderly" (65–74 years) and only 27% of the "older elderly" (75 years and above) report participating in any regular leisure-time physical activity.[52] Even fewer—about 14% of young elderly and 8% of older elderly—meet federal (CDC) guidelines for aerobic and muscle-strengthening activities.[53] These statistics are unfortunate, because we know that physically active elders live longer and have a reduced risk for cardiovascular disease, type 2 diabetes, obesity, depression, and cognitive decline. The complications of arthritis and osteoporosis can also be reduced with appropriate exercise, as can the risk for falls and bone fractures.[54] The need for healthcare visits is also reduced with regular exercise.

How much physical activity do older adults need in order to achieve these health benefits—and does moderate activity count, or should seniors "go for the gold"? Here are the most recent CDC guidelines:[55]

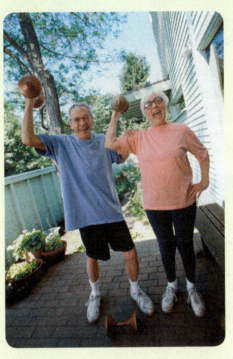

Engaging in regular physical activity is one of the best strategies for maintaining quality of life before and throughout the senior years.

- *Aerobic activity:* Seniors should engage in a minimum of 150 minutes of moderate-intensity aerobic activity (brisk walking, bicycling, swimming) or 75 minutes of vigorous aerobic activity (running or jogging) every week.

- *Muscle strengthening:* Seniors should engage in resistance or strength training on 2 or more days a week. The activities should work all the major muscle groups. Free weights, weight machines, resistance bands, push-ups, and heavy physical work are all strengthening.

- *Flexibility and balance:* Seniors should do a few minutes of flexibility exercises, such as stretches, tai chi, Pilates, or yoga, most days of the week. Daily balance exercises are also important to reduce the risk for falls. In addition to tai chi, toe raises, side leg raises, and rear leg swings are examples of effective balance activities.

Older adults who cannot meet these standards should engage in whatever level of physical activity is tolerable, as any increase in activity among sedentary elderly can improve their health and mobility.[54]

Are older adults more susceptible to injury or harm from vigorous exercise? At greatest risk are people who perform activities at an intensity or a duration they are not used to. Think of the "weekend warrior": a person who is very sedentary most days of the week but goes "all out" on a Saturday afternoon. This person is at high risk for a heart attack or sudden cardiac death during or shortly after vigorous activity. A second vulnerable group includes older adults with diagnosed or undiagnosed heart disease and those with diabetic foot ulcers. Seniors may also be more vulnerable to dehydration, heat stress, fractures, falls, knee pain, and muscle soreness or stiffness with intense exercise.[54]

To minimize the risk for exercise-related cardiac events and other complications of vigorous exercise, older adults should follow these guidelines:

- Work with a qualified healthcare provider to determine the types, intensities, and duration of physical activities appropriate for them.

- Become familiar with the signs of cardiac impairment: shortness of breath, chest pain, neck pain, dizziness or palpitations, and unusual fatigue.

- Recognize the need to modify activity patterns under conditions of stress, such as very cold temperatures, high heat or humidity, or during recovery from an illness.

- Exercise in rooms with appropriate temperature, ventilation, and lighting; wear appropriate clothing and comfortable shoes; and have water readily available.

- Engage in supervised warm-up and cool-down activities.

For most older adults, the risks of vigorous exercise are outweighed by the benefits—better health, more independence, less disability, and a longer, happier life!

CRITICAL THINKING QUESTIONS

1. What might encourage an older adult to start a regular program of physical activity after a lifetime of mostly sedentary behavior?
2. If you were the manager of a fitness center popular with young adults, what modifications to the facility might you propose to make it more attractive to older adults? Do you think one fitness center can effectively serve both young and older adults? Why or why not?
3. How might communities increase exercise opportunities for the elderly?

review questions

LO 1 1. Which of the following breakfasts would be most appropriate to serve a 20-month-old child?

a. 1/2 cup of iron-fortified cooked oat cereal, 2 tbsp. of mashed pineapple, and 1 cup of whole milk
b. 2 tbsp. of nonfat yogurt, 2 tbsp. of applesauce, one slice of melba toast spread with strawberry preserves, and 1 cup of calcium-fortified orange juice
c. 1/2 cup of iron-fortified cooked oat cereal, 1/4 cup of cubed pineapple, and 1 cup of low-fat milk
d. two small link sausages cut in 1-inch pieces, 2 tbsp. of scrambled egg, one slice of whole-wheat toast, four cherry tomatoes, 2 tbsp. of applesauce, and 1 cup of whole milk

LO 1 2. Which of the following is most likely to be deficient in the diet of a vegetarian toddler?

a. carbohydrate and fat
b. vitamin C
c. iron and zinc
d. fiber

LO 2 3. Which of the following statements about the nutrient needs of preschool and school-age children is true?

a. Children's estimated energy requirement (EER) is 1,200 kcal per day.
b. Children require a diet providing between 25% to 35% of total energy as fat.
c. Children's RDA for protein is 0.8 g per kg body weight.
d. It is recommended that all children take a pediatric multivitamin/multimineral supplement.

LO 3 4. An adolescent continues to grow in height until

a. production of testosterone and estrogen ceases.
b. the epiphyseal plates close.
c. peak bone density is reached.
d. approximately age 13 in girls and age 16 in boys.

LO 3 5. The RDA for calcium is 1,300 mg for which of the following groups?

a. both boys and girls, ages 4 to 18
b. girls only, ages 9 to 18
c. both boys and girls, ages 9 to 18
d. girls only, ages 14 to 18

LO 4 6. Which of the following statements about pediatric obesity is true?

a. Fewer than 10% of U.S. children and adolescents are obese.
b. To control energy intake, parents should encourage obese children to skip breakfast.
c. Among adolescents, cigarette smoking increases the risk for obesity.
d. None of the above is true.

LO 5 7. Which of the following events occurs with normal aging?

a. Absorption of vitamin B_{12} from foods in the gastrointestinal tract is reduced.
b. A reduced sense of smell contributes to dysgeusia, which together make food less appealing.
c. Muscle mass decreases.
d. All of the above occur with normal aging.

LO 6 8. Among older adults

a. cataracts are the most common cause of blindness.
b. those living alone have a lower rate of food insecurity than those living with others.
c. the need for vitamin A is two times greater than for younger adults.
d. the prevalence of obesity declines after age 75.

LO 2 9. **True or false?** The food choice patterns of children are heavily influenced by the food choices of their parents.

LO 6 10. **True or false?** Mortality rates are higher in the underweight elderly than in the overweight elderly.

math review

LO 5 **11.** While helping her 72-year-old grandmother put away groceries, Kristina notices three new supplement bottles. One is a single-nutrient vitamin A supplement, which provides 3,333 µg/dose. The second is a "Healthy Skin Formula" providing 1,500 µg vitamin A/dose. The third is a multivitamin-mineral supplement that provides 2,200 µg vitamin A/dose. When Kristina asks her grandmother about these new products, her grandmother explains that she read online that vitamin A makes your skin look younger, so she was taking the three supplements every day to make her wrinkles go away faster. If Kristina's grandmother takes one dose of each of the three supplements per day, what percentage of the RDA does she consume? Of the UL? Do you see any potential problems with this level of vitamin A intake?

Answers to Review Questions and Math Review are located at the back of this text and in the MasteringNutrition Study Area.

web links

www.cdc.gov
The Centers for Disease Control and Prevention
In the Search bar, type "parent information children." From the index page, select any topic of interest, from growth charts to school health.

www.nutrition.gov/life-stages
Nutrition.gov
This USDA site lets you select from Toddlers, Children, and Teen sections; each provides age-specific information, age-appropriate activities, nutrition web links, and consumer and nutrition news.

www.vrg.org
The Vegetarian Resource Group
Learn more about vegetarianism for all ages. Included on the site are sections for teens and kids as well as recipes and eating guides.

www.nutrition.wsu.edu
Eat Better, Eat Together
This website offers educational materials for strengthening family meal time. Suggestions for community events, media interviews, and educational materials are available. Enter "eat better" into the search bar to get underway.

www.aoa.gov
Administration on Aging
Find statistics on aging, as well as information and resources on healthy aging.

www.fns.usda.gov
USDA Food & Nutrition Service
Read about government programs to provide food to people of all ages, including school meal programs, SNAP, and the Nutrition Services Incentive Program.

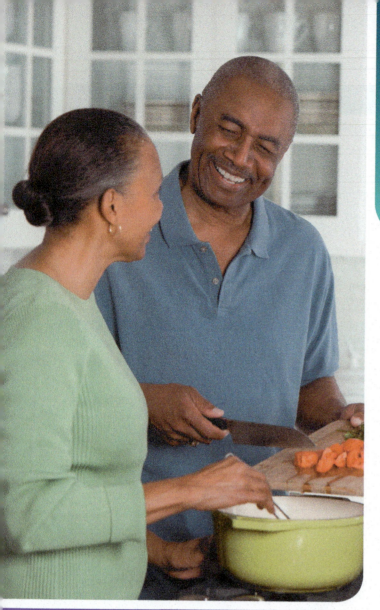

in depth 15.5

Searching for the Fountain of Youth

learning outcomes

After studying this In Depth, you should be able to:

1 Discuss the proposed mechanisms by which Calorie restriction may increase life span, as well as challenges and alternatives, pp. 563–564.

2 Refute the claim that single-nutrient, herbal, and other dietary supplements increase longevity, p. 565.

3 Evaluate the potential of your current health-related behaviors to increase or reduce the likelihood of your living a long and healthy life, p. 566.

Throughout human history, legends have told of a "fountain of youth" that reverses decades of aging in anyone who drinks its waters. One 16th century myth claimed that the Spanish explorer Ponce de León sought for these restorative waters throughout Florida, and a 15-acre archaeological park in Saint Augustine, Florida, still commemorates this mythical journey. Of course, no one believes such tales any longer, but modern equivalents persist: anti-aging diets, supplements, cosmetics, and spa treatments. If you were to read that you could live to celebrate your 100th birthday in good health by eating about a quarter less than the average energy intake for your gender and height, would you do it? Would you try anti-aging micronutrients, phytochemicals, herbs, or hormones? Or would you assume that the claims for these therapies were just fairy tales, too?

In this **In Depth** essay, we'll discuss the science behind anti-aging diets and supplements. We'll also identify lifestyle changes you can make right now to live longer in good health. What other actions can you take right now to live longer in good health? Let's find out.

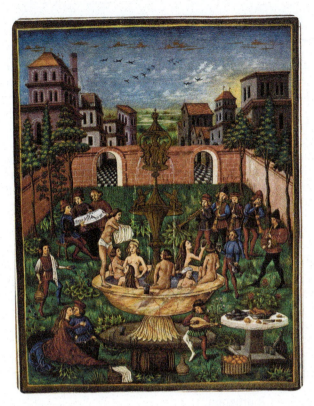

We may no longer believe in an actual "fountain of youth," but our search for health and longevity continues today.

Does calorie restriction increase life span?

LO 1 Discuss the proposed mechanisms by which Calorie restriction may increase life span, as well as challenges and alternatives.

A practice known as *Calorie restriction* (CR) has been getting a great deal of press lately. CR involves consuming 20% to 30% fewer Calories than would be typical for your weight, body composition, and level of activity, while still getting enough nutrients to keep your body functioning in good health.

Research has shown that CR can significantly extend the life span of rats, mice, fish, flies, and yeast cells as well as non-human primates such as monkeys.[1] But only in the past few years have researchers begun to design and conduct studies of CR in humans. The results of these preliminary studies suggest that CR can also improve metabolic measures of health in humans and thus may be able to extend the human life span.[2-7]

Calorie Restriction May Reduce Production of Free Radicals

How might CR prolong life span? Although not fully understood, the reduction in metabolic rate that occurs with restricted caloric intake results in a much lower production of free radicals, which in turn reduces oxidative damage throughout the body, possibly lowering chronic disease risk and prolonging life. Several, but not all, human studies show that CR also improves insulin sensitivity and decreases blood glucose, LDL cholesterol, and blood pressure, reducing the risk for cardiovascular disease, stroke, and diabetes. There is also evidence that CR can alter gene expression in ways that reduce the effects of aging and lower the risk of cancer and other diseases. Other metabolic effects of CR reported in several, but not all, human studies include:[1-5,7]

- Decreased fat mass and lean body mass
- Increased serum high-density lipoprotein (HDL) cholesterol
- Decreased core body temperature
- Decreased energy expenditure beyond that expected for the weight loss that occurred, which suggests a generalized slowing of metabolic rate
- Reduced levels of DNA damage
- Lower levels of chronic inflammation
- Protective changes in various hormone levels

It is important to emphasize that, in laboratory studies, species found to live longer with CR are fed highly nutritious diets. Situations such as starvation, anorexia nervosa, and extreme fad dieting, in which both energy and nutrient intakes are severely restricted, do not result in prolonged life but are associated with an increased risk for premature death. It's also essential to understand that the benefits of CR are thought to correlate to the age at which the program begins. The later in life the CR protocol is started, the lower the expected benefit.

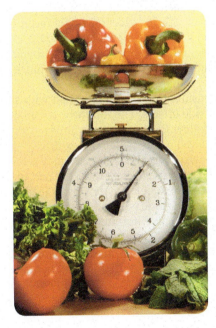

On a Calorie-restricted diet, all food must be highly nutritious, and both nutrients and energy must be calculated precisely.

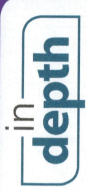

Calorie Restriction Presents Significant Challenges

Although the benefits listed previously appear promising, the research data supporting these benefits in humans are only preliminary. Research that can precisely study CR in humans over decades might never be conducted because of logistical and ethical concerns, including an increased risk for malnutrition. Currently, the most extensive study examined the impact of CR over only a two-year period, and participants achieved only a 12% reduction in usual Caloric intake, not the target 20% to 30% reduction typically associated with CR.[7]

In the absence of prolonged high-quality human studies, several CR groups, including the "CRONies" (Caloric Restriction with Optimal Nutrition), have provided researchers with some data. Most of the CRONies are males in their late 30s to mid 50s. One report indicated that most CRONies had followed the CR diet for about 10 years and reduced their caloric intake by about 30%. Overall, members report improved blood lipids and the other health benefits listed earlier. Still, researchers lack specific data on how well free-living adults actually follow the rigid and extensive demands of CR protocols. In addition, researchers now question if the caloric restriction alone led to the metabolic improvements or if the largely vegetarian, Mediterranean-like diet of the CRONies, along with their active lifestyle, contributed to the metabolic improvements.[3,5]

It has been estimated that humans would need to restrict their typical energy intake by at least 20% for 40 years or more in order to gain a potential 4 to 5 additional years of healthy living.[8] If you normally eat about 2,000 kcal/day, a 20% reduction would result in an energy intake of about 1,600 kcal per day. Although at first this might not seem difficult, bear in mind that you would need to maintain this lower Calorie/high nutrient-density pattern every day for 40 years.

Also consider that CR is associated with several unpleasant side effects. The top three complaints of those who follow CR are constant hunger, frequently feeling cold, and a loss of libido (sex drive).[1] In addition, CR impairs wound healing and may reduce immune response. There is concern that, if initiated in early adulthood, CR might reduce bone density or lead to inappropriate loss of muscle mass. And because the production of female reproductive hormones is linked to a certain level of body fat, CR could result in amenorrhea and/or impair a woman's fertility. Interestingly, as noted earlier, most of the members of the CRONies are males. Finally, it is well known that being significantly underweight is associated with increased mortality, especially among older adults.

Alternatives to Calorie Restriction Show Similar Benefits

As researchers continue to question the effectiveness and practicality of CR, alternative approaches have been developed and studied. *Intermittent fasting* (*IF*), also known as *every-other-day-feeding* (*EODF*), *alternate-day fasting* (*ADF*), or *time-restricted feeding*, does *not* reduce average energy intake but simply alters the pattern of food intake.[9-12] These approaches been shown, in animals, to prolong life span and improve a range of metabolic measures of health. Although not as well studied as CR, ADF, for example, has produced beneficial changes in metabolic profile including blood lipid levels.[11]

Additionally, some researchers have proposed that the lower and largely plant protein intake of CR drives some of the metabolic improvements. Even without caloric restriction, vegan diets are known to lower blood pressure, LDL cholesterol, triglycerides, and fasting glucose levels. Most people would find it much easier to simply reduce their total protein intake and/or convert to a largely vegan diet than to maintain a lifelong 20% to 30% reduction in their energy intake. Finally, the combination of a healthful diet with adequate physical activity can decrease inflammation and oxidative stress without the need for the more extreme CR program.

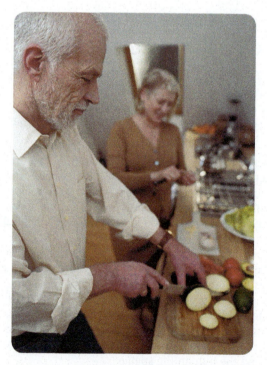

Maintaining either a Calorie-restricted or vegan diet requires significant meal planning, but both appear to have similar health benefits.

Can supplements slow aging?

LO 2 Refute the claim that single-nutrient, herbal, and other dietary supplements increase longevity.

Recently, some researchers have speculated that consuming the optimum level of nutrients could extend a person's healthy life span. Could micronutrient supplements take the place of whole foods in providing this "optimum level of nutrients"? And could other ingredients, besides vitamins and minerals, also slow aging?

The global anti-aging market accounts for nearly $125 billion in sales, with some individuals spending as much as $20,000 a year on various products and services.[13] Among the most popular are "anti-aging" supplements, many of which provide specific combinations of vitamins and minerals marketed with claims that the product has powerful antioxidant effects, or will boost memory, reduce fine lines and wrinkles, or maintain joint health. Are these micronutrient supplements worth the investment? Unfortunately, not even one trial of such supplements has shown them to be effective.[14] In fact, some studies actually have reported a *higher* risk of death with high doses of vitamin A, vitamin E, or beta-carotene supplements.[15] Nevertheless, a quick Internet search will open up a world of promises of better health and longer life if you use the advertised supplements!

In addition to micronutrients, supplements that claim to enhance longevity often contain:

- Food extracts, such as resveratrol from red wines and other foods
- Herbs, including Siberian ginseng, ginkgo biloba, and various combinations of botanicals from Asia
- Animal extracts, such as royal jelly and dried glandulars
- Hormone-based preparations, such as DHEA (dehydroepiandrosterone), HGH (human growth hormone), and melatonin
- Metabolites, such as alpha-lipoic acid

Manufacturers promote these products with claims such as "revered in the Far East for centuries" and "nature's own therapeutic powers." However, as with micronutrient supplements, no well-designed research studies support the claims of life-extending effectiveness for any of these products in humans. More disturbingly, like antioxidant supplements, many of these non-nutrient supplements have serious side effects. For example, ginkgo biloba can cause gastrointestinal upset, nausea, diarrhea, headache, dizziness, abnormal bleeding, or an allergic reaction and is known to interact with several medications.[16] HGH can contribute to high cholesterol levels, increase the risk of diabetes and hypertension, and cause joint pain, muscle weakness, and other symptoms.[17] Despite concerns such as these, sales of anti-aging supplements continue to grow.

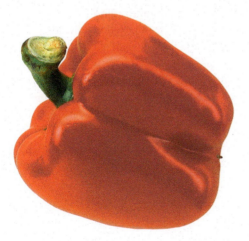

Anyone can benefit from the antioxidant nutrients in fresh fruits and vegetables.

nutri-case | GUSTAVO

"I don't believe in taking pills. If you eat good food, you get everything you need and it's the way nature intended it. My daughter kept nagging my wife and me to start taking B vitamins and some kind of Chinese herb with a name I can't pronounce. She said we need this stuff because when people get to be our age they have problems with their nerves and circulation. I didn't fall for it, but my wife did, and then her doctor told her she needs calcium pills and vitamin D, too. The kitchen counter is starting to look like a medicine cabinet! Our ancestors never took pills their whole lives! So how come we need them? I think the whole thing is a hoax to get you to empty your wallet."

Would you support Gustavo's decision to avoid taking supplements? Given what you have learned in previous Nutri-Cases about Gustavo's wife, would you support or oppose her taking ginkgo biloba, B-vitamins, calcium, or vitamin D? Explain your choices.

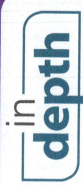

Are your actions today promoting a longer, healthier life?

LO 3 Evaluate the potential of your current health-related behaviors to increase or reduce the likelihood of your living a long and healthy life.

If none of these options interest you, is there anything else you can do to increase your chances of living a long and healthful life? The Centers for Disease Control and Prevention (CDC) reminds us that chronic disease is responsible for seven out of every ten deaths of Americans.[18] Moreover, just five behaviors within your control are key to the prevention of chronic disease:

- Getting adequate amounts of physical activity on a regular basis
- Maintaining a healthful body weight and composition
- Never smoking
- Consuming no or only moderate amounts of alcohol
- Obtaining sufficient sleep on a daily basis

So, if you want to live a longer, healthier life, the CDC advises that you adopt the health habits identified in the nearby **Quick Tips** box.

QuickTips
Promoting Your Longevity

✔ Engage in at least 30 minutes of moderate or vigorous physical activity most days of the week.

✔ Consume a diet based on the *2015–2020 Dietary Guidelines for Americans,* the Mediterranean diet, or a vegan/vegetarian diet.

✔ Use only the nutrient supplements that have been recommended to you by your healthcare provider and within the recommended amounts.

✔ Achieve and maintain a healthful weight and body composition.

✔ If you smoke or use any other form of tobacco, stop. If you don't smoke, don't start.

✔ If you drink alcohol, do so only in moderation, meaning no more than two drinks per day for men and one drink per day for women.

✔ Maintain a healthy sleep schedule, aiming for at least 7 hours of uninterrupted sleep every 24 hours.

web links

www.nia.nih.gov
The National Institute on Aging

The National Institute on Aging provides information about how older adults can benefit from physical activity and a healthful diet.

www.nihseniorhealth.gov
National Institutes of Health, Senior Health

This website, written in large print, offers up-to-date information on popular health topics for older Americans.

www.aarp.org
The American Association of Retired Persons

Visit this gateway site for a wide range of articles on nutrition, physical activity, and other health-related topics for older adults.

https://nccih.nihgov/health/aging
National Institutes of Health, National Center for Complementary and Integrative Health

This website provides information on supplements for older adults, health scams targeting older adults, and complementary health interventions for chronic diseases common among older adults.

Appendices

Appendix A

2015–2020 Dietary Guidelines, Dietary Reference Intakes, and Dietary Guidelines Recommendations

Daily Nutritional Goals for Age-Sex Groups Based on Dietary Reference Intakes & *Dietary Guidelines* Recommendations

	Source of Goal[a]	Child 1–3	Female 4–8	Male 4–8	Female 9–13	Male 9–13	Female 14–18	Male 14–18	Female 19–30	Male 19–30	Female 31–50	Male 31–50	Female 51+	Male 51+
Calorie Level(s) Assessed		1,000	1,200	1,400, 1,600	1,600	1,800	1,800	2,200, 2,800, 3,200	2,000	2,400, 2,600, 3,000	1,800	2,200	1,600	2,000
Macronutrients														
Protein, g	RDA	13	19	19	34	34	46	52	46	56	46	56	46	56
Protein, % kcal	AMDR	5–20	10–30	10–30	10–30	10–30	10–30	10–30	10–35	10–35	10–35	10–35	10–35	10–35
Carbohydrate, g	RDA	130	130	130	130	130	130	130	130	130	130	130	130	130
Carbohydrate, % kcal	AMDR	45–65	45–65	45–65	45–65	45–65	45–65	45–65	45–65	45–65	45–65	45–65	45–65	45–65
Dietary Fiber, g	14 g/1,000 kcal	14	16.8	19.6	22.4	25.2	25.2	30.8	28	33.6	25.2	30.8	22.4	28
Added Sugars, % kcal	DGA	<10%	<10%	<10%	<10%	<10%	<10%	<10%	<10%	<10%	<10%	<10%	<10%	<10%
Total Fat, % kcal	AMDR	30–40	25–35	25–35	25–35	25–35	25–35	25–35	20–35	20–35	20–35	20–35	20–35	20–35
Saturated Fat, % kcal	DGA	<10%	<10%	<10%	<10%	<10%	<10%	<10%	<10%	<10%	<10%	<10%	<10%	<10%
Linoleic Acid, g	AI	7	10	10	10	12	11	16	12	17	12	17	11	14
Linolenic Acid, g	AI	0.7	0.9	0.9	1	1.2	1.1	1.6	1.1	1.6	1.1	1.6	1.1	1.6
Minerals														
Calcium, mg	RDA	700	1,000	1,000	1,300	1,300	1,300	1,300	1,000	1,000	1,000	1,000	1,200	1,000[b]
Iron, mg	RDA	7	10	10	8	8	15	11	18	8	18	8	8	8
Magnesium, mg	RDA	80	130	130	240	240	360	410	310	400	320	420	320	420
Phosphorus, mg	RDA	460	500	500	1,250	1,250	1,250	1,250	700	700	700	700	700	700
Potassium, mg	AI	3,000	3,800	3,800	4,500	4,500	4,700	4,700	4,700	4,700	4,700	4,700	4,700	4,700
Sodium, mg	UL	1,500	1,900	1,900	2,200	2,200	2,300	2,300	2,300	2,300	2,300	2,300	2,300	2,300
Zinc, mg	RDA	3	5	5	8	8	9	11	8	11	8	11	8	11
Copper, mcg	RDA	340	440	440	700	700	890	890	900	900	900	900	900	900
Manganese, mg	AI	1.2	1.5	1.5	1.6	1.9	1.6	2.2	1.8	2.3	1.8	2.3	1.8	2.3
Selenium, mcg	RDA	20	30	30	40	40	55	55	55	55	55	55	55	55
Vitamins														
Vitamin A, mg RAE	RDA	300	400	400	600	600	700	900	700	900	700	900	700	900
Vitamin E, mg AT	RDA	6	7	7	11	11	15	15	15	15	15	15	15	15
Vitamin D, IU	RDA	600	600	600	600	600	600	600	600	600	600	600	600[c]	600[c]
Vitamin C, mg	RDA	15	25	25	45	45	65	75	75	90	75	90	75	90
Thiamin, mg	RDA	0.5	0.6	0.6	0.9	0.9	1	1.2	1.1	1.2	1.1	1.2	1.1	1.2
Riboflavin, mg	RDA	0.5	0.6	0.6	0.9	0.9	1	1.3	1.1	1.3	1.1	1.3	1.1	1.3
Niacin, mg	RDA	6	8	8	12	12	14	16	14	16	14	16	14	16
Vitamin B_6, mg	RDA	0.5	0.6	0.6	1	1	1.2	1.3	1.3	1.3	1.3	1.3	1.5	1.7
Vitamin B_{12}, mcg	RDA	0.9	1.2	1.2	1.8	1.8	2.4	2.4	2.4	2.4	2.4	2.4	2.4	2.4
Choline, mg	AI	200	250	250	375	375	400	550	425	550	425	550	425	550
Vitamin K, mcg	AI	30	55	55	60	60	75	75	90	120	90	120	90	120
Folate, mcg DFE	RDA	150	200	200	300	300	400	400	400	400	400	400	400	400

[a] RDA = Recommended Dietary Allowance, AI = Adequate Intake, UL = Tolerable Upper Intake Level, AMDR = Acceptable Macronutrient Distribution Range, DGA = *2015–2020 Dietary Guidelines* recommended limit; 14 g fiber per 1,000 kcal = basis for AI for fiber.
[b] Calcium RDA for males ages 71+ years is 1,200 mg.
[c] Vitamin D RDA for males and females ages 71+ years is 800 IU.
Sources: Institute of Medicine. Dietary Reference Intakes: The essential guide to nutrient requirements. Washington (DC): The National Academies Press; 2006.
Institute of Medicine. Dietary Reference Intakes for Calcium and Vitamin D. Washington (DC): The National Academies Press; 2010.

Appendix B

Calculations and Conversions

Calculation and Conversion Aids

Commonly Used Metric Units

millimeter (mm): one-thousandth of a meter (0.001)
centimeter (cm): one-hundredth of a meter (0.01)
kilometer (km): one-thousand times a meter (1000)
kilogram (kg): one-thousand times a gram (1000)
milligram (mg): one-thousandth of a gram (0.001)
microgram (μg): one-millionth of a gram (0.000001)
milliliter (ml): one-thousandth of a liter (0.001)

International Units

Some vitamin supplements may report vitamin content as International Units (IU).

To convert IU to:

- Micrograms of vitamin D (cholecalciferol), divide the IU value by 40 or multiply by 0.025.
- Milligrams of vitamin E (alpha-tocopherol), divide the IU value by 1.5 if vitamin E is from natural sources. Divide the IU value by 2.22 if vitamin E is from synthetic sources.
- Vitamin A: 1 IU = 0.3 μg retinol or 3.6 μg beta-carotene.

Retinol Activity Equivalents

Retinol Activity Equivalents (RAE) are a standardized unit of measure for vitamin A. RAE account for the various differences in bioavailability from sources of vitamin A. Many supplements will report vitamin A content in IU, as just shown, or Retinol Equivalents (RE).

1 RAE = 1 μg retinol
        12 μg beta-carotene
        24 μg other vitamin A carotenoids

To calculate RAE from the RE value of vitamin carotenoids in foods, divide RE by 2.

For vitamin A supplements and foods fortified with vitamin A, 1 RE = 1 RAE.

Folate

Folate is measured as Dietary Folate Equivalents (DFE). DFE account for the different factors affecting bioavailability of folate sources.

1 DFE = 1   μg food folate
        0.6 μg folate from fortified foods
        0.5 μg folate supplement taken on an empty stomach
        0.6 μg folate as a supplement consumed with a meal

To convert micrograms of synthetic folate, such as that found in supplements or fortified foods, to DFE:

$$\mu g \text{ synthetic} \times \text{folate } 1.7 = \mu g \text{ DFE}$$

For naturally occurring food folate, such as spinach, each microgram of folate equals 1 microgram DFE:

$$\mu g \text{ folate} = \mu g \text{ DFE}$$

Conversion Factors

Use the following table to convert U.S. measurements to metric equivalents:

Original Unit	Multiply by	To Get
ounces avdp	28.3495	grams
ounces	0.0625	pounds
pounds	0.4536	kilograms
pounds	16	ounces
grams	0.0353	ounces
grams	0.002205	pounds
kilograms	2.2046	pounds
liters	1.8162	pints (dry)
liters	2.1134	pints (liquid)
liters	0.9081	quarts (dry)
liters	1.0567	quarts (liquid)
liters	0.2642	gallons (U.S.)
pints (dry)	0.5506	liters
pints (liquid)	0.4732	liters
quarts (dry)	1.1012	liters
quarts (liquid)	0.9463	liters
gallons (U.S.)	3.7853	liters
millimeters	0.0394	inches
centimeters	0.3937	inches
centimeters	0.03281	feet
inches	25.4000	millimeters
inches	2.5400	centimeters
inches	0.0254	meters
feet	0.3048	meters
meters	3.2808	feet
meters	1.0936	yards
cubic feet	0.0283	cubic meters
cubic meters	35.3145	cubic feet
cubic meters	1.3079	cubic yards
cubic yards	0.7646	cubic meters

Length: U.S. and Metric Equivalents

1/4 inch	=	0.6 centimeter
1 inch	=	2.5 centimeters
1 foot	=	0.3048 meter
		30.48 centimeters
1 yard	=	0.91144 meter
1 millimeter	=	0.03937 inch
1 centimeter	=	0.3937 inch
1 decimeter	=	3.937 inches
1 meter	=	39.37 inches
		1.094 yards
1 micrometer	=	0.00003937 inch

Weights and Measures

Food Measurement Equivalencies from U.S. to Metric

Capacity

1/5 teaspoon	=	1 milliliter
1/4 teaspoon	=	1.25 milliliters
1/2 teaspoon	=	2.5 milliliters
1 teaspoon	=	5 milliliters
1 tablespoon	=	15 milliliters
1 fluid ounce	=	28.4 milliliters
1/4 cup	=	60 milliliters
1/3 cup	=	80 milliliters
1/2 cup	=	120 milliliters
1 cup	=	225 milliliters
1 pint (2 cups)	=	473 milliliters
1 quart (4 cups)	=	0.95 liter
1 liter (1.06 quarts)	=	1,000 milliliters
1 gallon (4 quarts)	=	3.84 liters

Weight

0.035 ounce	=	1 gram
1 ounce	=	28 grams
1/4 pound (4 ounces)	=	114 grams
1 pound (16 ounces)	=	454 grams
2.2 pounds (35 ounces)	=	1 kilogram

U.S. Food Measurement Equivalents

3 teaspoons	=	1 tablespoon
1/2 tablespoon	=	1-1/2 teaspoons
2 tablespoons	=	1/8 cup
4 tablespoons	=	1/4 cup
5 tablespoons + 1 teaspoon	=	1/3 cup
8 tablespoons	=	1/2 cup
10 tablespoons + 2 teaspoons	=	2/3 cup
12 tablespoons	=	3/4 cup
16 tablespoons	=	1 cup
2 cups	=	1 pint
4 cups	=	1 quart
2 pints	=	1 quart
4 quarts	=	1 gallon

Volumes and Capacities

1 cup	=	8 fluid ounces
		1/2 liquid pint
1 milliliter	=	0.061 cubic inch
1 liter	=	1.057 liquid quarts
		0.908 dry quart
		61.024 cubic inches
1 U.S. gallon	=	231 cubic inches
		3.785 liters
		0.833 British gallon
		128 U.S. fluid ounces

1 British Imperial gallon	=	277.42 cubic inches
		1.201 U.S. gallons
		4.546 liters
		160 British fluid ounces
1 U.S. ounce, liquid or fluid	=	1.805 cubic inches
		29.574 milliliters
		1.041 British fluid ounces
1 pint, dry	=	33.600 cubic inches
		0.551 liter
1 pint, liquid	=	28.875 cubic inches
		0.473 liter
1 U.S. quart, dry	=	67.201 cubic inches
		1.101 liters
1 U.S. quart, liquid	=	57.75 cubic inches
		0.946 liter
1 British quart	=	69.354 cubic inches
		1.032 U.S. quarts, dry
		1.201 U.S. quarts, liquid

Energy Units

1 kilocalorie (kcal)	=	4.2 kilojoules
1 millijoule (MJ)	=	240 kilocalories
1 kilojoule (kJ)	=	0.24 kcal
1 gram carbohydrate	=	4 kcal
1 gram fat	=	9 kcal
1 gram protein	=	4 kcal

Temperature Standards

	°Fahrenheit	°Celsius
Body temperature	98.6°	37°
Comfortable room temperature	65–75°	18–24°
Boiling point of water	212°	100°
Freezing point of water	32°	0°

Temperature Scales

To Convert Fahrenheit to Celsius:
$[(°F − 32)\ 5]/9$

1. Subtract 32 from °F.
2. Multiply (°F − 32) by 5, then divide by 9.

To Convert Celsius to Fahrenheit:
$[(°C × 9)/5] + 32$

1. Multiply °C by 9, then divide by 5.
2. Add 32 to (°C × 9/5).

Appendix C

Foods Containing Caffeine | Data from: USDA Nutrient Database for Standard Reference, Release 23.

Beverages

Food Name	Serving	Caffeine/Serving (mg)
Beverage mix, chocolate flavor, dry mix, prepared w/milk	1 cup (8 fl. oz)	7.98
Beverage mix, chocolate malt powder, fortified, prepared w/milk	1 cup (8 fl. oz)	5.3
Beverage mix, chocolate malted milk powder, no added nutrients, prepared w/milk	1 cup (8 fl. oz)	7.95
Beverage, chocolate syrup w/o added nutrients, prepared w/milk	1 cup (8 fl. oz)	5.64
Beverage, chocolate syrup, fortified, mixed w/milk	1 cup milk and 1 tbsp syrup	2.63
Cocoa mix w/aspartame and calcium and phosphorus, no sodium or vitamin A, low kcal, dry, prepared	6 fl. oz water and 0.53-oz packet	5
Cocoa mix w/aspartame, dry, low kcal, prepared w/water	1 packet dry mix with 6 fl. oz water	1.92
Cocoa mix, dry mix	1 serving (3 heaping tsp. or 1 envelope)	5.04
Cocoa mix, dry, w/o added nutrients, prepared w/water	1-oz packet with 6 fl. oz water	4.12
Cocoa mix, fortified, dry, prepared w/water	6 fl. oz H_2O and 1 packet	6.27
Cocoa, dry powder, high-fat or breakfast, plain	1 piece	6.895
Cocoa, hot, homemade w/whole milk	1 cup	5
Coffee liqueur, 53 proof	1 fl. oz	9.048
Coffee liqueur, 63 proof	1 fl. oz	9.05
Coffee w/cream liqueur, 34 proof	1 fl. oz	2.488
Coffee mix w/sugar (cappuccino), dry, prepared w/water	6 fl. oz H_2O and 2 rounded tsp. mix	74.88
Coffee mix w/sugar (French), dry, prepared w/water	6 fl. oz H_2O and 2 rounded tsp. mix	51.03
Coffee mix w/sugar (mocha), dry, prepared w/water	6 fl. oz and 2 round tsp. mix	33.84
Coffee, brewed	1 cup (8 fl. oz)	94.8
Coffee, brewed, prepared with tap water, decaffeinated	1 cup (8 fl. oz)	2.37
Coffee, instant, prepared	1 cup (8 fl. oz)	61.98
Coffee, instant, regular, powder, half the caffeine	1 cup (8 fl. oz)	30.99
Coffee, instant, decaffeinated	1 cup (8 fl. oz)	1.79
Coffee and cocoa (mocha) powder, with whitener and low-Calorie sweetener	1 cup	405.48
Coffee, brewed, espresso, restaurant-prepared	1 cup (8 fl. oz)	502.44
Coffee, brewed, espresso, restaurant-prepared, decaffeinated	1 cup (8 fl. oz)	2.37
Energy drink, with caffeine, niacin, pantothenic acid, vitamin B_6	1 fl. oz	9.517
Milk beverage mix, dairy drink w/aspartame, low kcal, dry, prep	6 fl. oz	4.08
Milk, low-fat, 1% fat, chocolate	1 cup	5
Milk, whole, chocolate	1 cup	5
Soft drink, cola w/caffeine	1 fl. oz	2
Soft drink, cola, w/higher caffeine	1 fl. oz	8.33
Soft drink, cola or pepper type, low kcal w/saccharin and caffeine	1 fl. oz	3.256
Soft drink, cola, low kcal w/saccharin and aspartame, w/caffeine	1 fl. oz	4.144
Soft drink, lemon-lime soda, w/caffeine	1 fl. oz	4.605
Soft drink, low kcal, not cola or pepper, with aspartame and caffeine	1 fl. oz	4.44
Soft drink, pepper type, w/caffeine	1 fl. oz	3.07
Tea mix, instant w/lemon flavor, w/saccharin, dry, prepared	1 cup (8 fl. oz)	16.59
Tea mix, instant w/lemon, unsweetened, dry, prepared	1 cup (8 fl. oz)	26.18
Tea mix, instant w/sugar and lemon, dry, no added vitamin C, prepared	1 cup (8 fl. oz)	28.49
Tea mix, instant, unsweetened, dry, prepared	1 cup (8 fl. oz)	30.81
Tea, brewed	1 cup (8 fl. oz)	47.36
Tea, brewed, prepared with tap water, decaffeinated	1 cup (8 fl. oz)	2.37
Tea, instant, unsweetened, powder, decaffeinated	1 tsp.	1.183
Tea, instant, w/o sugar, lemon-flavored, w/added vitamin C, dry prepared	1 cup (8 fl. oz)	26.05
Tea, instant, with sugar, lemon-flavored, decaffeinated, no added vitamin	1 cup	9.1

Cake, Cookies, and Desserts

Food Name	Serving	Caffeine/serving (mg)
Brownie, square, large (2–3/4″ × 7/8″)	1 piece	1.12
Cake, chocolate pudding, dry mix	1 oz	1.701
Cake, chocolate, dry mix, regular	1 oz	3.118
Cake, German chocolate pudding, dry mix	1 oz	1.985
Cake, marble pudding, dry mix	1 oz	1.985
Candies, chocolate-covered, caramel with nuts	1 cup	35.34
Candies, chocolate-covered, dietetic or low-Calorie	1 cup	16.74
Candy, milk chocolate w/almonds	1 bar (1.45 oz)	9.02
Candy, milk chocolate w/rice cereal	1 bar (1.4 oz)	9.2
Candy, raisins, milk-chocolate-coated	1 cup	45
Chocolate chips, semisweet, mini	1 cup chips (6-oz package)	107.12
Chocolate, baking, unsweetened, square	1 piece	22.72
Chocolate, baking, Mexican, square	1 piece	2.8
Chocolate, sweet	1 oz	18.711
Cookie Cake, Snackwell Fat Free Devil's Food, Nabisco	1 serving	1.28
Cookie, Snackwell Caramel Delights, Nabisco	1 serving	1.44
Cookie, chocolate chip, enriched, commercially prepared	1 oz	3.118
Cookie, chocolate chip, homemade w/margarine	1 oz	4.536
Cookie, chocolate chip, lower-fat, commercially prepared	3 pieces	2.1
Cookie, chocolate chip, refrigerated dough	1 portion, dough spooned from roll	2.61
Cookie, chocolate chip, soft, commercially prepared	1 oz	1.985
Cookie, chocolate wafers	1 cup, crumbs	7.84
Cookie, graham crackers, chocolate-coated	1 oz	13.041
Cookie, sandwich, chocolate, cream-filled	3 pieces	3.9
Cookie, sandwich, chocolate, cream-filled, special dietary	1 oz	0.85
Cupcake, chocolate w/frosting, low-fat	1 oz	0.86
Donut, cake, chocolate w/sugar or glaze	1 oz	0.284
Donut, cake, plain w/chocolate icing, large (3–1/2″)	1 each	1.14
Fast food, ice cream sundae, hot fudge	1 sundae	1.58
Fast food, milk beverage, chocolate shake	1 cup (8 fl. oz)	1.66
Frosting, chocolate, creamy, ready-to-eat	2 tbsp creamy	0.82
Frozen yogurt, chocolate	1 cup	5.58
Fudge, chocolate w/nuts, homemade	1 oz	1.984
Granola bar, soft, milk-chocolate-coated, peanut butter	1 oz	0.85
Granola bar, with coconut, chocolate-coated	1 cup	5.58
Ice cream, chocolate	1 individual (3.5 fl. oz)	1.74
Ice cream, chocolate, light	1 oz	0.85
Ice cream, chocolate, rich	1 cup	5.92
M&M's Peanut Chocolate	1 cup	18.7
M&M's Plain Chocolate	1 cup	22.88
Milk chocolate	1 cup chips	33.6
Milk-chocolate-coated coffee beans	1 NLEA serving	48
Milk dessert, frozen, fat-free milk, chocolate	1 oz	0.85
Milk shake, thick, chocolate	1 fl. oz	0.568
Pastry, eclair/cream puff, homemade, custard-filled w/chocolate	1 oz	0.567
Pie crust, chocolate-wafer-cookie-type, chilled	1 crust, single 9″	11.15
Pie, chocolate mousse, no bake mix	1 oz	0.284
Pudding, chocolate, instant dry mix prepared w/reduced-fat (2%) milk	1 oz	0.283
Pudding, chocolate, regular dry mix prepared w/reduced-fat (2%) milk	1 oz	0.567
Pudding, chocolate, ready-to-eat, fat-free	4 oz can	2.27
Syrups, chocolate, genuine chocolate flavor, light, Hershey	2 tbsp.	1.05
Topping, chocolate-flavored hazelnut spread	1 oz	1.984
Yogurt, chocolate, nonfat milk	1 oz	0.567
Yogurt, frozen, chocolate, soft serve	0.5 cup (4 fl. oz)	2.16

Starch List

1 starch choice = 15 g carbohydrate, 0–3 g protein, 0–1 g fat, and 80 cal

Icon Key

☺ = More than 3 g of dietary fiber per serving.

! = Extra fat, or prepared with added fat. (Count as 1 starch + 1 fat.)

▮ = 480 mg or more of sodium per serving.

Food	Serving Size
Bread	
Bagel, 4 oz	¼ (1 oz)
! Biscuit, 2½"across	1
Bread	
☺ reduced-calorie	2 slices (1½ oz)
white, whole-grain, pumpernickel, rye, unfrosted raisin	1 slice (1 oz)
Chapatti, small, 6" across	1
! Cornbread, 1¾" cube	1 (1½ oz)
English muffin	½
Hot dog bun or hamburger bun	½ (1 oz)
Naan, 8" by 2"	¼
Pancake, 4" across, ¼" thick	1
Pita, 6" across	½
Roll, plain small	1 (1 oz)
! Stuffing, bread	⅓ cup
! Taco shell, 5" across	2
Tortilla	
Corn, 6" across	1
Flour, 6" across	1
Flour, 10" across	⅓ tortilla
! Waffle, 4"-square or 4" across	1
Cereals and Grains	
Barley, cooked	⅓ cup
Bran, dry	
☺ oat	¼c
☺ wheat	½ c

Food	Serving Size
☺ Bulgur (cooked)	½ c
Cereals	½ c
☺ bran	½ c
cooked (oats, oatmeal)	½ c
puffed	1½ c
shredded wheat, plain	½ c
sugar-coated	½ c
unsweetened, ready-to-eat	¾ c
Couscous	⅓ c
Granola	
low-fat	¼ c
! regular	¼ c
Grits, cooked	½ c
Kasha	½ c
Millet, cooked	⅓ c
Muesli	¼ c
Pasta, cooked	⅓ c
Polenta, cooked	⅓ c
Quinoa, cooked	⅓ c
Rice, white or brown, cooked	⅓ c
Tabbouleh (tabouli), prepared	½ c
Wheat germ, dry	3 tbs
Wild rice, cooked	½ c
Starchy Vegetables	
Cassava	⅓ c
Corn	½ c
on cob, large	½ cob (5 oz)

Food	Serving Size	Food	Serving Size
☺ Hominy, canned . . . . ¾ c		! whole-wheat regular . . . . 2–5 (¾ oz)	
☺ Mixed vegetables with corn, peas, or pasta . 1 c		! whole-wheat lower fat or crispbreads 2–5 (¾ oz)	
☺ Parsnips. . . . . ½ c		Graham crackers, 2½" square 3	
☺ Peas, green . . . . ½ c		Matzoh. . . . . ¾ oz	
Plantain, ripe . . . . ⅓ c		Melba toast, about 2" by 4" piece 4 pieces	
Potato		Oyster crackers. 20	
baked with skin. . . . . ¼ large (3 oz)		Popcorn . . . . 3 c	
boiled, all kinds . . . . ½ c or ½ medium (3 oz)		! ☺ with butter. . . . . 3 c	
! mashed, with milk and fat . . . . ½ c		☺ no fat added . . . . 3 c	
French fried (oven-baked) . . . . 1 cup (2 oz)		☺ lower fat . . . . 3 c	
☺ Pumpkin, canned, no sugar added . . . . . 1 c		Pretzels. . . . . ¾ oz	
Spaghetti/pasta sauce . . . . ½ c		Rice cakes, 4" across 2	
☺ Squash, winter (acorn, butternut). . . . . . 1 c		Snack chips	
☺ Succotash. . . . . ½ c		fat-free or baked (tortilla, potato),	
Yam, sweet potato, plain . . . . ½ c		baked pita chips . . . . 15–20 (¾ oz)	
		! regular (tortilla, potato). . . . . 9–13 (¾ oz)	

Crackers and Snacks

Animal crackers. 8
Crackers
!   round-butter type. 6
    saltine-type 6
!   sandwich-style, cheese or peanut
    butter filling 3

Beans, Peas, and Lentils
(Count as 1 starch + 1 lean meat)
☺ Baked beans . . . . ⅓ c
☺ Beans, cooked (black, garbanzo,
    kidney, lima, navy, pinto, white). . . . . . . ½ c
☺ Lentils, cooked (brown, green, yellow). . . ½ c
☺ Peas, cooked (black-eyed, split). . . . . ½ c
❙ ☺   Refried beans, canned . . . . ½ c

Fruit List

1 fruit choice = 15 g carbohydrate, 0 g protein, 0 g fat, and 60 cal
Weight includes skin, core, seeds, and rind.

Icon Key
☺ = More than 3 g of dietary fiber per serving.
! = Extra fat, or prepared with added fat.
❙ = 480 mg or moreof sodium per serving.

Food	Serving Size	Food	Serving Size
Apples		Dried fruits (blueberries,	
unpeeled, small . . . . 1 (4 oz)		cherries, cranberries, mixed	
dried. . . . . 4 rings		fruit, raisins). . . . . 2 tbs	
Applesauce, unsweetened. . ½ c		Figs	
Apricots		dried. 1½	
canned . . . . ½ c		☺ fresh. . . . . 1½ large or 2 medium (3½ oz)	
dried . . . . 8 halves		Fruit cocktail . . . . ½ c	
❙ fresh. . . . . 4 whole (5½ oz)		Grapefruit	
Banana, extra small. . . . . . . 1 (4 oz)		large. . . . . ½ (11 oz)	
Blackberries . . . . ¾ c		sections, canned . . . . . . ¾ c	
❙ Blueberries . . . . ¾ c		Grapes, small . . . . 17 (3 oz)	
Cantaloupe, small . . . . ⅓ melon or 1 c cubed (11 oz)		Honeydew melon . . . . 1 slice or 1 c cubed (10 oz)	
Cherries		☺ Kiwi . . . . 1 (3½ oz)	
sweet, canned . . . . ½ c		Mandarin oranges, canned. . ¾ c	
sweet, fresh . . . . 12 (3 oz)		Mango, small. . . . . ½ fruit (5½ oz) or ½ c	
Dates 3		Nectarine, small. . . . . 1 (5 oz)	

Food	Serving Size	Food	Serving Size
☺ Orange, small	1 (6½ oz)	☺ Raspberries	1 c
Papaya	½ fruit or 1 c cubed (8 oz)	☺ Strawberries	1 ¼ c whole berries
Peaches		☺ Tangerines, small	2 (8 oz)
canned	½ c	Watermelon.	1 slice or 1¼ c
fresh, medium	1 (6 oz)		cubes (13½ oz)
Pears			
canned	½ c	**Fruit Juice**	
fresh, large.	½ (4 oz)	Apple juice/cider	½ c
Pineapple		Fruit juice blends, 100%	
canned	½ c	juice	⅓ c
fresh	¾ c	Grape juice.	⅓ c
Plums		Grapefruit juice	½ c
canned	½ c	Orange juice	½ c
dried (prunes)	3	Pineapple juice	½ c
small.	2 (5 oz)	Prune juice.	⅓ c

Milk and Yogurts

1 milk choice = 12 g carbohydrate and 8 g protein

Food	Serving Size	Count As
Fat-Free or Low-Fat (1%)		
(0–3 g fat per serving, 100 calories per serving)		
Milk, buttermilk, acidophilus milk, Lactaid	1c	1 fat-free milk
Evaporated milk	½ c.	1 fat-free milk
Yogurt, plain or flavored with an artificial sweetener	⅔ c (6 oz)	1 fat-free milk
Reduced-Fat (2%)		
(5 g fat per serving, 120 calories per serving)		
Milk, acidophilus milk, kefir, Lactaid	1 c	1 reduced-fat milk
Yogurt, plain	⅔ c (6 oz)	1 reduced-fat milk
Whole		
(8 g fat per serving, 160 calories per serving)		
Milk, buttermilk, goat's milk	1 c	1 whole milk
Evaporated milk	½ c.	1 whole milk
Yogurt, plain	8 oz	1 whole milk
Dairy-Like Foods		
Chocolate milk		
fat-free.	1 c	1 fat-free milk + 1 carbohydrate
whole	1 c	1 whole milk + 1 carbohydrate
Eggnog, whole milk	½ c.	1 carbohydrate + 2 fats
Rice drink		
flavored, low-fat	1 c	2 carbohydrates
plain, fat-free.	1 c	1 carbohydrate
Smoothies, flavored, regular	10 oz	1 fat-free milk + 2½ carbohydrates
Soy milk		
light	1c	1 carbohydrate + ½ fat
regular, plain	1c	1 carbohydrate + 1 fat
Yogurt		
and juice blends.	1 c	1 fat-free milk + 1 carbohydrate
low carbohydrate (less than 6 g carbohydrate per choice)	⅔ c (6 oz)	½ fat-free milk
with fruit, low-fat	⅔ c (6 oz)	1 fat-free milk + 1 carbohydrate

Sweets, Desserts, and Other Carbohydrates List

1 other carbohydrate choice = 15 g carbohydrate and variable protein, fat, and calories.

Icon Key

▮ = 480 mg or more of sodium per serving.

Food	Serving Size	Count As
Beverages, Soda, and Energy/Sports Drinks		
Cranberry juice cocktail	½ c	1 carbohydrate
Energy drink	1 can (8.3 oz)	2 carbohydrates
Fruit drink or lemonade	1 c (8 oz)	2 carbohydrates
Hot chocolate		
regular	1 envelope added to 8 oz water	1 carbohydrate + 1 fat
sugar-free or light	1 envelope added to 8 oz water	1 carbohydrate
Soft drink (soda), regular	1 can (12 oz)	2½ carbohydrates
Sports drink	1 cup (8 oz)	1 carbohydrate
Brownies, Cake, Cookies, Gelatin, Pie, and Pudding		
Brownie, small, unfrosted	1¼" square, ⅞", high (about 1 oz)	1 carbohydrate + 1 fat
Cake		
angel food, unfrosted	1½ of cake (about 2 oz)	2 carbohydrates
frosted	2" square (about 2 oz)	2 carbohydrates + 1 fat
unfrosted	2" square (about 2 oz)	1 carbohydrate + 1 fat
Cookies		
chocolate chip	2 cookies (2¼" across)	1 carbohydrate + 2 fats
gingersnap	3 cookies	1 carbohydrate
sandwich, with creme filling	2 small (about ⅔ oz)	1 carbohydrate + 1 fat
sugar-free	3 small or 1 large (¾ oz–1 oz)	1 carbohydrate + 1–2 fats
vanilla wafer	5 cookies	1 carbohydrate + 1 fat
Cupcake, frosted	1 small (about 1¾ oz)	2 carbohydrates + 1–1½ fats
Fruit cobbler	½ c (3½ oz)	3 carbohydrates + 1 fat
Gelatin, regular	½ c	1 carbohydrate
Pie		
commercially prepared fruit, 2 crusts	⅙ of 8" pie	3 carbohydrates + 2 fats
pumpkin or custard	⅛ of 8" pie	1½ carbohydrates + 1½ fats
Pudding		
regular (made with reduced-fat milk)	½ c	2 carbohydrates
sugar-free, or sugar-free and fat-free (made with fat-free milk)	½ c	1 carbohydrate
Candy, Spreads, Sweets, Sweeteners, Syrups, and Toppings		
Candy bar, chocolate/peanut	2 "fun size" bars (1 oz)	1½ carbohydrates + 1½ fats
Candy, hard	3 pieces	1 carbohydrate
Chocolate "kisses"	5 pieces	1 carbohydrate + 1 fat
Coffee creamer		
dry, flavored	4 tsp	½ carbohydrate + ½ fat
liquid, flavored	2 tbs	1 carbohydrate
Fruit snacks, chewy (pureed fruit concentrate)	1 roll (¾ oz)	1 carbohydrate
Fruit spreads, 100% fruit	1½ tbs	1 carbohydrate
Honey	1 tbs	1 carbohydrate

Food	Serving Size	Count As
Jam or jelly, regular	1 tbs	1 carbohydrate
Sugar	1 tbs	1 carbohydrate
Syrup		
chocolate	2 tbs	2 carbohydrates
light (pancake type)	2 tbs	1 carbohydrate
regular (pancake type)	1 tbs	1 carbohydrate

Condiments and Sauces

Food	Serving Size	Count As
Barbeque sauce	3 tbs	1 carbohydrate
Cranberry sauce, jellied	¼ c	1½ carbohydrates
Gravy, canned or bottled	½ c	½ carbohydrate + ½ fat
Salad dressing, fat-free, low-fat, cream-based	3 tbs	1 carbohydrate
Sweet and sour sauce	3 tbs	1 carbohydrate

Doughnuts, Muffins, Pastries, and Sweet Breads

Food	Serving Size	Count As
Banana nut bread	1″ slice (1 oz)	2 carbohydrates + 1 fat
Doughnut		
cake, plain	1 medium, (1½ oz)	1½ carbohydrates + 2 fats
yeast type, glazed	3¾″ across (2 oz)	2 carbohydrates + 2 fats
Muffin (4 oz)	¼ muffin (1 oz)	1 carbohydrate + ½ fat
Sweet roll or Danish	1 (2½ oz)	2½ carbohydrates + 2 fats

Frozen Bars, Frozen Dessert, Frozen Yogurt, and Ice Cream

Food	Serving Size	Count As
Frozen pops	1	½ carbohydrate
Fruit juice bars, frozen, 100% juice	1 bar (3 oz)	1 carbohydrate
Ice cream		
fat-free	½ c	1½ carbohydrates
light	½ c	1 carbohydrate + 1 fat
no sugar added	½ c	1 carbohydrate + 1 fat
regular	½ c	1 carbohydrate + 2 fats
Sherbet, sorbet	½ c	2 carbohydrates
Yogurt, frozen		
fat-free	⅓ c	1 carbohydrate
regular	½ c	1 carbohydrate + 0–1 fat

Granola Bars, Meal Replacement Bars/Shakes, and Trail Mix

Food	Serving Size	Count As
Granola or snack bar, regular or low-fat	1 bar (1 oz)	1½ carbohydrates
Meal replacement bar	1 bar (1⅓ oz)	1½ carbohydrates + 0–1 fat
Meal replacement bar	1 bar (2 oz)	2 carbohydrates + 1 fat
Meal replacement shake, reduced-calorie	1 can (10–11 oz)	1½ carbohydrates + 0–1 fat
Trail mix		
candy/nut-based	1 oz	1 carbohydrates + 2 fats
dried-fruit-based	1 oz	1 carbohydrate + 1 fat

Nonstarchy Vegetable List

1 vegetable choice = 5 g carbohydrate, 2 g protein, 0 g fat, 25 cal

Icon Key

☺ = More than 3 g of dietary fiber per serving.

▮ = 480 mg or more of sodium per serving.

Amaranth or Chinese spinach	Kohlrabi
Artichoke	Leeks
Artichoke hearts	Mixed vegetables (without corn, peas, or pasta)
Asparagus	Mung bean sprouts
Baby corn	Mushrooms, all kinds, fresh
Bamboo shoots	Okra
Beans (green, wax, Italian)	Onions
Bean sprouts	Oriental radish or daikon
Beets	Pea pods
▮ Borscht	☺ Peppers (all varieties)
Broccoli	Radishes
☺ Brussels sprouts	Rutabaga
Cabbage (green, bok choy, Chinese)	▮ Sauerkraut
Carrots	Soybean sprouts
Cauliflower	Spinach
Celery	Squash (summer, crookneck, zucchini)
☺ Chayote	Sugar pea snaps
Coleslaw, packaged, no dressing	▮ Swiss chard
Cucumber	Tomato
Eggplant	Tomatoes, canned
Gourds (bitter, bottle, luffa, bitter melon)	▮ Tomato sauce
Green onions or scallions	▮ Tomato/vegetable juice
Greens (collard, kale, mustard, turnip)	Turnips
Hearts of palm	Water chestnuts
Jicama	Yard-long beans

Meat and Meat Substitutes List

Icon Key

! = Extra fat, or prepared with added fat. (Add an additional fat choice to this food.)

▮ = 480 mg or more of sodium per serving (based on the sodium content of a typical 3 oz serving of meat, unless 1 or 2 is the normal serving size).

Food	Amount	Food	Amount
Lean Meats and Meat Substitutes		*Fish, fresh or frozen, plain:* catfish, cod,	
(1 lean meat choice = 7g protein, 0–3 g		flounder, haddock, halibut, orange	
fat, 45 calories)		roughy, salmon, tilapia, trout, tuna..	1 oz
Beef: Select or Choice grades trimmed		▮ *Fish, smoked:* herring or salmon	
of fat: ground round, roast (chuck,		(lox)	1 oz
rib, rump), round, sirloin, steak		*Game:* buffalo, ostrich, rabbit,	
(cubed, flank, porterhouse, T-bone),		venison.	1 oz
tenderloin . . . . 1 oz		▮ Hot dog with 3 g of fat or less per oz (8	
▮ Beef jerky . . . . 1 oz		dogs per 14 oz package) *(Note: May*	
Cheeses with 3 g of fat or less per oz. . . . . . 1 oz		*be high in carbohydrate.)*	1
Cottage cheese . . . . ¼ cup		*Lamb:* chop, leg, or roast	1 oz
Egg substitutes, plain . . . . ¼ cup		*Organ meats:* heart, kidney, liver *(Note:*	
Egg whites. 2		*May be high in cholesterol)*	1 oz

Food	Amount	Food	Amount

Oysters, fresh or frozen. . . . . 6 medium

Pork, lean
- ▮ Canadian bacon . . . . 1 oz
  rib or loin chop/roast, ham,
    tenderloin . . . . 1 oz

Poultry without skin: Cornish hen,
  chicken, domestic duck or goose
  (well drained of fat), turkey . . . . 1 oz

*Processed sandwich meats with 3 g of
  fat or less per oz:* chipped beef,
  deli thin-sliced meats, turkey ham,
  turkey kielbasa, turkey pastrami . . . 1 oz

Salmon, canned. . . . . 1 oz

Sardines, canned . . . . 2 medium

▮ Sausage with 3 g or less fat per oz . . . . . 1 oz

Shellfish: clams, crab, imitation shellfish,
  lobster, scallops, shrimp . . . . 1 oz

Tuna, canned in water or oil, drained . . 1 oz

Veal: Lean chop, roast. . . . . 1 oz

Medium-Fat Meat and Meat Substitutes

*(1 medium-fat meat choice = 7g
protein, 4–7g fat, and 75 calories)*

Beef: corned beef, ground beef,
  meatloaf, Prime grades trimmed of
  fat (prime rib), short ribs, tongue . . . 1 oz

Cheeses with 4–7 g of fat per oz: feta,
  mozzarella, pasteurized processed
  cheese spread, reduced-fat cheeses,
  string . . . . 1 oz

Egg *(Note: High in cholesterol, limit to
  3 per week.)* 1

Fish, any fried product . . . . 1 oz

Lamb: ground, rib roast . . . . 1 oz

Pork: cutlet, shoulder roast. . . . . 1 oz

Poultry: chicken with skin; dove,
  pheasant, wild duck, or goose; fried
  chicken; ground turkey. . . . . 1 oz

Ricotta cheese . . . . 2 oz or ¼ c

▮ Sausage with 4–7 g fat per oz . . . . 1 oz

Veal: Cutlet (no breading) . . . . 1 oz

High-Fat Meat and Meat Substitutes[a]

*(1 high-fat meat choice = 7g protein,
8 + g fat, 100 calories)*

Bacon
- ▮ pork. . . . . 2 slices (16 slices per lb or 1 oz each, before cooking)
- ▮ turkey . . . . 3 slices (½ oz each before cooking)

Cheese, regular: American, bleu, brie,
  cheddar, hard goat, Monterey Jack,
  queso, Swiss. 1 oz

▮! *Hot dog:* beef, pork, or combination
  (10 per lb-sized package) 1

▮ *Hot dog:* turkey or chicken (10 per
  lb-sized package) 1

Pork: ground, sausage, spareribs . . . . . . 1 oz

*Processed sandwich meats with 8 g
  of fat or more per oz:* bologna,
  pastrami, hard salami . . . . 1 oz

▮ *Sausage with 8 g of fat or more per
  oz:* bratwurst, chorizo, Italian,
  knockwurst, Polish, smoked,
  summer . . . . 1 oz

[a]These foods are high in saturated fat, cholesterol, and calories and may raise blood cholesterol levels if eaten on a regular basis. Try to eat 3 or fewer servings from this group per week.

Plant-Based Proteins

Because carbohydrate and fat content varies among plant-based proteins, you should read the food label.

Icon Key

☺ = More than 3 g of dietary fiber per serving; 7 g protein; calories vary.

▮ = 480 mg or more of sodium per serving (based on the sodium content of a typical 3-oz serving of meat, unless 1 or 2 oz is the normal serving size).

Food	Amount	Count As
"Bacon" strips, soy-based	3 strips	1 medium-fat meat
☺ Baked beans.	⅓ c	1 starch + 1 lean meat
☺ Beans, cooked: black, garbanzo, kidney, lima, navy, pinto, white	½ c	1 starch + 1 lean meat
☺ "Beef" or "sausage" crumbles, soy-based.	2 oz.	½ carbohydrate + 1 lean meat
"Chicken" nuggets, soy-based	2 nuggets (1½ oz).	½ carbohydrate + 1 medium-fat meat

Food		Amount	Count As
☺	Edamame	½ c	½ carbohydrate + 1 lean meat
	Falafel (spiced chickpea and wheat patties)	3 patties (about 2 inches across)	1 carbohydrate + 1 high-fat meat
	Hot dog, soy-based	1 (1½ oz)	½ carbohydrate + 1 lean meat
☺	Hummus	⅓ c	1 carbohydrate + 1 high-fat meat
☺	Lentils, brown, green, or yellow	½ c	1 carbohydrate + 1 lean meat
☺	Meatless burger, soy-based	3 oz	½ carbohydrate + 2 lean meats
☺	Meatless burger, vegetable- and starch-based	1 patty (about 2½ oz)	1 carbohydrate + 2 lean meats
	Nut spreads: almond butter, cashew butter, peanut butter, soy nut butter	1 tbs	1 high-fat meat
☺	*Peas, cooked:* black-eyed and split peas	½ c	1 starch + 1 lean meat
▮☺	Refried beans, canned	½ c	1 starch + 1 lean meat
	"Sausage" patties, soy-based	1 (1½ oz)	1 medium-fat meat
	Soy nuts, unsalted	¾ oz	½ carbohydrate + 1 medium-fat meat
	Tempeh	¼ cup	1 medium-fat meat
	Tofu	4 oz (½ cup)	1 medium-fat meat
	Tofu, light	4 oz (½ cup)	1 lean meat

Fat List

1 fat choice = 5 g fat, 45 cal

Icon Key

▮ = 480 mg or more of sodium per serving.

Food	Serving Size
Unsaturated Fats—Monounsaturated Fats	
Avocado, medium	2 tbs (1 oz)
Nut butters (trans fat-free): almond butter, cashew butter, peanut butter (smooth or crunchy)	1½ tsp
Nuts	
almonds	6 nuts
Brazil	2 nuts
cashews	6 nuts
filberts (hazelnuts)	5 nuts
macadamia	3 nuts
mixed (50% peanuts)	6 nuts
peanuts	10 nuts
pecans	4 halves
pistachios	16 nuts
Oil: canola, olive, peanut	1 tsp
Olives	
black (ripe)	8 large
green, stuffed	10 large
Polyunsaturated Fats	
Margarine: lower-fat spread (30% to 50% vegetable oil, *trans* fat-free)	1 tbs
Margarine: stick, tub (*trans* fat-free), or squeeze (*trans* fat-free)	1 tsp

Food	Serving Size
Mayonnaise	
reduced-fat	1 tbs
regular	1 tsp
Mayonnaise-style salad dressing	
reduced-fat	1 tbs
regular	2 tsp
Nuts	
Pignolia (pine nuts)	1 tbs
walnuts, English	4 halves
Oil: corn, cottonseed, flaxseed, grape seed, safflower, soybean, sunflower	1 tsp
Oil: made from soybean and canola oil—Enova	1 tsp
Plant stanol esters	
light	1 tbs
regular	2 tsp
Salad dressing	
▮ reduced-fat (*Note: May be high in carbohydrate.*)	2 tbs
▮ regular	1 tbs
Seeds	1 tbs
flaxseed, whole	1 tbs
pumpkin, sunflower	1 tbs
sesame seeds	1 tbs
Tahini or sesame paste	2 tsp

Food	Serving Size	Food	Serving Size

Saturated Fats

Bacon, cooked, regular or turkey....	1 slice
Butter	
reduced-fat	1 tbs
stick	1 tsp
whipped....................	2 tsp
Butter blends made with oil	
reduced-fat or light............	1 tbs
regular	1½ tsp
Chitterlings, boiled	2 tbs (½ oz)
Coconut, sweetened, shredded	2 tbs
Coconut milk	
light	¼ c
regular	1½ tbs
Cream	
half and half	2 tbs
heavy	1 tbs

light	1½ tbs
whipped.....................	2 tbs
whipped, pressurized	¼ c
Cream cheese	
reduced-fat	1½ tbs (¾ oz)
regular	1 tbs (½ oz)
Lard	1 tsp
Oil: coconut, palm, palm kernel.....	1 tsp
Salt pork......................	¼ oz
Shortening, solid	1 tsp
Sour cream	
reduced-fat or light............	3 tbs
regular	2 tbs

Free Foods List

A *free food* is any food or drink that has less than 20 calories and 5 g or less of carbohydrate per serving. Foods with a serving size listed should be limited to three servings per day. Foods listed without a serving size can be eaten as often as you like.

Icon Key

▪ = 480 mg or more of sodium per serving.

Food	Serving Size	Food	Serving Size

Low Carbohydrate Foods

Cabbage, raw.....................	½ c
Candy, hard (regular or sugar-free)...	1 piece
Carrots, cauliflower, or green beans, cooked..........................	¼ c
Cranberries, sweetened with sugar substitute	½ c
Cucumber, sliced	½ c
Gelatin	
dessert, sugar-free	
unflavored	
Gum	
Jam or jelly, light or no sugar added..	2 tsp
Rhubarb, sweetened with sugar substitute........................	½ c
Salad greens	
Sugar substitutes (artificial sweeteners)	
Syrup, sugar-free..................	2 tbs

Modified Fat Foods with Carbohydrate

Cream cheese, fat-free	1 tbs (½ oz)
Creamers	
nondairy, liquid................	1 tbs
nondairy, powdered	2 tsp

Margarine spread	
fat-free.......................	1 tbs
reduced-fat	1 tsp
Mayonnaise	
fat-free.......................	1 tbs
reduced-fat	1 tsp
Mayonnaise-style salad dressing	
fat-free.......................	1 tbs
reduced-fat	1 tsp
Salad dressing	
fat-free or low-fat..............	1 tbs
fat-free, Italian	2 tbs
Sour cream, fat-free, reduced-fat.....	1 tbs
Whipped topping	
light or fat-free	2 tbs
regular	1 tbs

Condiments

Barbecue sauce	2 tsp
Catsup (ketchup).................	1 tbs
Honey mustard	1 tbs
Horseradish	
Lemon juice	
Miso	1½ tsp
Mustard	

Food	Serving Size	Food	Serving Size
Parmesan cheese, freshly grated	1 tbs	▮ Soy sauce, regular or light	1 tbs
Pickle relish	1 tbs	Sweet and sour sauce	2 tsp
Pickles		Sweet chili sauce	2 tsp
▮ dill	1½ medium	Taco sauce	1 tbs
sweet, bread and butter	2 slices	Vinegar	
sweet, gherkin	¾ oz	Yogurt, any type	2 tbs
Salsa	¼ c		

Drinks/Mixes

Any food on this list—without serving size listed—can be consumed in any moderate amount.

Icon Key

▮ = 480 mg or more of sodium per serving.

▮ Bouillon, broth, consommé	Diet soft drinks, sugar-free
Bouillon or broth, low sodium	Drink mixes, sugar-free
Carbonated or mineral water	Tea, unsweetened or with sugar substitute
Club soda	Tonic water, diet
Cocoa powder, unsweetened (1 tbs)	Water
Coffee, unsweetened or with sugar substitute	Water, flavored, carbohydrate free

Seasonings

Any food on this list can be consumed in any moderate amount.

Flavoring extracts (for example, vanilla, almond, peppermint)	Spices
Garlic	Hot pepper sauce
Herbs, fresh or dried	Wine, used in cooking
Nonstick cooking spray	Worcestershire sauce
Pimento	

Combination Foods List

Icon Key

☺ = More than 3 g of dietary fiber per serving.

▮ = 600 mg or more of sodium per serving (for combination food main dishes/meals).

Food	Serving Size	Count As
Entrées		
▮ Casserole type (tuna noodle, lasagna, spaghetti with meatballs, chili with beans, macaroni and cheese)	1 c (8 oz)	2 carbohydrates + 2 medium-fat meats
▮ Stews (beef/other meats and vegetables)	1 c (8 oz)	1 carbohydrate + 1 medium-fat meat + 0–3 fats
Tuna salad or chicken salad	½ c (3½ oz)	½ carbohydrate + 2 lean meats + 1 fat

Food	Serving Size	Count As
Frozen Meals/Entrées		
☺ Burrito (beef and bean)	1 (5 oz)	3 carbohydrates + 1 lean meat + 2 fats
Dinner-type meal	generally 14–17 oz	3 carbohydrates + 3 medium-fat meats + 3 fats
Entrée or meal with less than 340 calories	about 8–11 oz	2–3 carbohydrates + 1–2 lean meats
Pizza		
cheese/vegetarian thin crust	¼ of 12″ (4½ to 5 oz)	2 carbohydrates + 2 medium-fat meats
meat topping, thin crust	¼ of 12″ (5 oz)	2 carbohydrates + 2 medium-fat meats, + 1½ fats
Pocket sandwich	1 (4½ oz)	3 carbohydrates + 1 lean meat + 1–2 fats
Pot pie	1 (7 oz)	2½ carbohydrates + 1 medium-fat meat + 3 fats
Salads (Deli-Style)		
Coleslaw	½ c	1 carbohydrate + 1½ fats
Macaroni/pasta salad	½ c	2 carbohydrates + 3 fats
Potato salad	½ c	$1^1/_2$ carbohydrates + 1–2 fats
Soups		
Bean, lentil, or split pea	1 cup	1 carbohydrate + 1 lean meat
Chowder (made with milk)	1 c (8 oz)	1 carbohydrate + 1 lean meat + 1½ fats
Cream (made with water)	1 c (8 oz)	1 carbohydrate + 1 fat
Instant	6 oz prepared	1 carbohydrate
with beans or lentils	8 oz prepared	2½ carbohydrates + 1 lean meat
Miso soup	1 c	½ carbohydrate + 1 fat
Oriental noodle	1 c	2 carbohydrates + 2 fats
Rice (congee)	1 c	1 carbohydrate
Tomato (made with water)	1 c (8 oz)	1 carbohydrate
Vegetable beef, chicken noodle, or other broth-type	1 c (8 oz)	1 carbohydrate

Fast Foods List[a]

Icon Key
☺ = More than 3 g of dietary fiber per serving.
ꜜ = Extra fat, or prepared with added fat.
ꞁ = 600 mg or more sodium per serving (for fast food main dishes/meals).

Food	Serving Size	Exchanges per Serving
Breakfast Sandwiches		
Egg, cheese, meat, English muffin	1 sandwich	2 carbohydrates + 2 medium-fat meats
Sausage biscuit sandwich	1 sandwich	2 carbohydrates + 2 high-fat meats + 3½ fats
Main Dishes/Entrées		
☺ Burrito (beef and beans)	1 (about 8 oz)	3 carbohydrates + 3 medium-fat meats + 3 fats

[a]The choices in the Fast Foods list are not specific fast food meals or items, but are estimates based on popular foods. You can get specific nutrition information for almost every fast food or restaurant chain. Ask the restaurant or check its website for nutrition information about your favorite fast foods.

Food	Serving Size	Exchanges per Serving
▮ Chicken breast, breaded and fried	1 (about 5 oz)	1 carbohydrate + 4 medium-fat meats
Chicken drumstick, breaded and fried	1 (about 2 oz)	2 medium-fat meats
▮ Chicken nuggets	6 (about 3½ oz)	1 carbohydrate + 2 medium-fat meats + 1 fat
▮ Chicken thigh, breaded and fried	1 (about 4 oz)	½ carbohydrate + 3 medium-fat meats + 1½ fats
▮ Chicken wings, hot	6 (5 oz)	5 medium-fat meats + 1½ fats

Oriental

Food	Serving Size	Exchanges per Serving
▮ Beef/chicken/shrimp with vegetables in sauce	1 c (about 5 oz)	1 carbohydrate + 1 lean meat + 1 fat
▮ Egg roll, meat	1 (about 3 oz)	1 carbohydrate + 1 lean meat + 1 fat
Fried rice, meatless	½ c	1½ carbohydrates + 1½ fats
▮ Meat and sweet sauce (orange chicken)	1 c	3 carbohydrates + 3 medium-fat meats + 2 fats
▮☺ Noodles and vegetables in sauce (chow mein, lo mein)	1 c	2 carbohydrates + 1 fat

Pizza

Food	Serving Size	Exchanges per Serving
▮ Cheese, pepperoni, regular crust	⅛ of 14″ (about 4 oz)	2½ carbohydrates + 1 medium-fat meat + 1½ fats
▮ Cheese/vegetarian, thin crust	¼ of 12″ (about 6 oz)	2½ carbohydrates + 2 medium-fat meats + 1½ fats

Sandwiches

Food	Serving Size	Exchanges per Serving
▮ Chicken sandwich, grilled	1	3 carbohydrates + 4 lean meats
▮ Chicken sandwich, crispy	1	3½ carbohydrates + 3 medium-fat meats + 1 fat
Fish sandwich with tartar sauce	1	2½ carbohydrates + 2 medium-fat meats + 2 fats
Hamburger		
▮ large with cheese	1	2½ carbohydrates + 4 medium-fat meats + 1 fat
regular	1	2 carbohydrates + 1 medium-fat meat + 1 fat
▮ Hot dog with bun	1	1 carbohydrate + 1 high-fat meat + 1 fat
Submarine sandwich		
▮ less than 6 grams fat	6″ sub	3 carbohydrates + 2 lean meats
▮ regular	6″ sub	3½ carbohydrates + 2 medium-fat meats + 1 fat
Taco, hard or soft shell (meat and cheese)	1 small	1 carbohydrate + 1 medium-fat meat + 1½ fats

Salads

Food	Serving Size	Exchanges per Serving
▮☺ Salad, main dish (grilled chicken type, no dressing or croutons)	Salad	1 carbohydrate + 4 lean meats
Salad, side, no dressing or cheese	Small (about 5 oz)	1 vegetable

Food	Serving Size	Exchanges per Serving
Sides/Appetizers		
❙ French fries, restaurant style	Small	3 carbohydrates + 3 fats
Medium		4 carbohydrates + 4 fats
Large		5 carbohydrates + 6 fats
❙ Nachos with cheese	Small (about 4½ oz)	2½ carbohydrates + 4 fats
❙ Onion rings	1 serving (about 3 oz)	2½ carbohydrates + 3 fats
Desserts		
Milkshake, any flavor	12 oz	6 carbohydrates + 2 fats
Soft-serve ice cream cone	1 small	2½ carbohydrates + 1 fat

Alcohol List

In general, 1 alcohol choice (½ oz absolute alcohol) has about 100 calories.

Alcoholic Beverage	Serving Size	Count As
Beer		
light (4.2%)	12 fl. oz	1 alcohol equivalent + ½ carbohydrate
regular (4.9%)	12 fl. oz	1 alcohol equivalent + 1 carbohydrate
Distilled spirits: vodka, rum, gin, whiskey, 80 or 86 proof	1½ fl. oz	1 alcohol equivalent
Liqueur, coffee (53 proof)	1 fl. oz	1 alcohol equivalent + 1 carbohydrate
Sake	1 fl. oz	½ alcohol equivalent
Wine		
dessert (sherry)	3½ fl. oz	1 alcohol equivalent + 1 carbohydrate
dry, red or white (10%)	5 fl. oz	1 alcohol equivalent

Stature-for-Age Charts

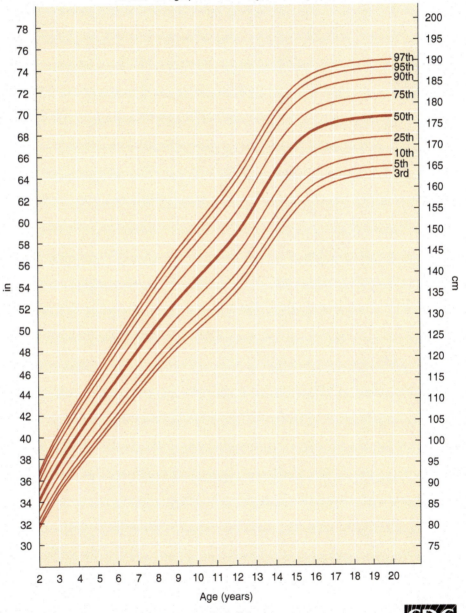

CDC Growth Charts: United States
Stature-for-age percentiles: Boys, 2 to 20 years

Source: "CDC Growth Charts, United States" Developed by the National Center for Health Statistics in collaboration with the National Center for Chronic Disease Prevention and Health Promotion, from the Centers For Disease Control and Prevention website, 2000.

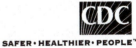

SAFER · HEALTHIER · PEOPLE™

CDC Growth Charts: United States
Stature-for-age percentiles: Girls, 2 to 20 years

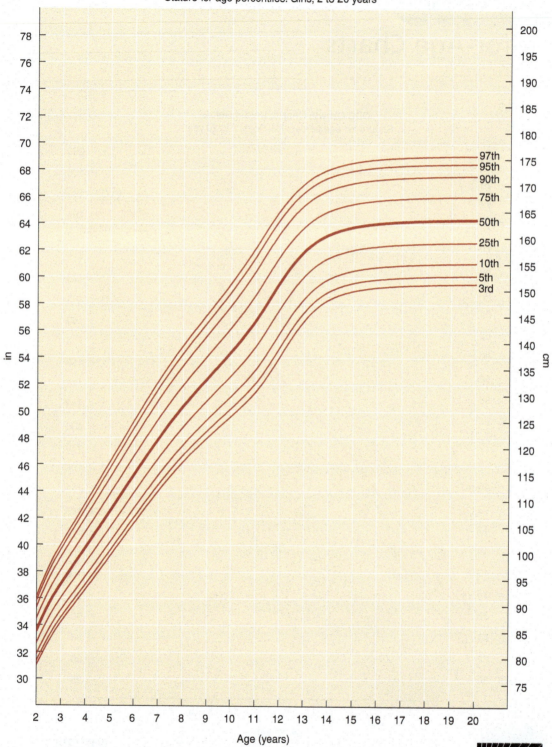

Age (years)

Source: "CDC Growth Charts, United States" Developed by the National Center for Health Statistics in collaboration with the National Center for Chronic Disease Prevention and Health Promotion,from the Centers For Disease Control and Prevention website, 2000.

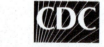

SAFER • HEALTHIER • PEOPLE™

The USDA Food Guide Evolution

Early History of Food Guides

Did you know that in the United States food guides in one form or another have been around for over 125 years?

That's right. Back in 1885 a college chemistry professor named Wilber Olin Atwater helped bring the fledgling science of nutrition to a broader audience by introducing dietary standards that became the basis for the first U.S. food guide. Those early standards focused on defining the daily needs of an "average man" for proteins and Calories. They soon expanded into food composition tables with three sweeping categories: protein, fat, and carbohydrate; mineral matter; and "fuel values." As early as 1902, Atwater advocated for three foundational nutritional principles that we still support today: variety, proportionality, and moderation in food choices and eating.

These ideas were adapted a few years later by a nutritionist named Caroline Hunt, who developed a food "buying" guide divided into five categories: meats and proteins; cereals and starches; vegetables and fruits; fatty foods; and sugar.

From the 1930s to the early 1970s, these guidelines kept changing—from twelve food groups to seven to four, and from there to a "Hassle-Free" guide that briefly increased the number of groups back up to five. Although critics identified many drawbacks of these approaches, they were necessary attempts to provide Americans with reliable guidelines based on the best scientific data and practices available at the time.

Contemporary Food Guides: From Pyramid to Plate

By the early 1980s, public health experts began to recognize that, to be effective, a national food guide had to reflect key philosophical values. These core values included the following:

- it must encompass a broad focus on *overall health;*
- it should emphasize the use of *current research;*
- it should be an approach that includes the *total diet,* rather than parts or pieces;
- it should be *useful;*
- it should be *realistic;*
- it should be *flexible;*
- it should be *practical;*
- and it must be *evolutionary,* able to adapt as new information comes to light.

These values guided the development of the USDA Food Guide Pyramid, released in 1992, which also was the first guide to include a graphic representation of the Dietary Guidelines

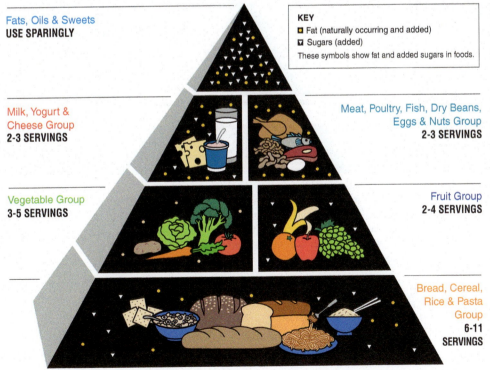

Fats, Oils & Sweets
USE SPARINGLY

KEY
◻ Fat (naturally occurring and added)
▽ Sugars (added)
These symbols show fat and added sugars in foods.

Milk, Yogurt & Cheese Group
2-3 SERVINGS

Meat, Poultry, Fish, Dry Beans, Eggs & Nuts Group
2-3 SERVINGS

Vegetable Group
3-5 SERVINGS

Fruit Group
2-4 SERVINGS

Bread, Cereal, Rice & Pasta Group
6-11 SERVINGS

Source: U.S. Department of Agriculture/U.S. Department of Health and Human Services

The 1992 Food Guide Pyramid. This representation of the USDA guidelines took several years to develop and attempted to convey in a single image all the key aspects of a nutritional guide.

Data from: The 1992 Food Guide Pyramid.

for Americans—in the shape of a pyramid. The 1992 Guide included the following components:

- Nutritional Goals
- Food Groups
- Serving Sizes
- Nutrient Profiles
- Numbers of Servings

The 1992 Guide did not have an enthusiastic reception. Instead, critics quickly began pointing out flaws in the design, recommendations, and ease of use. Many nutritionists trying to use the Guide to teach different population groups basic nutrition messages found that it was out of touch with people's day-to-day lives. Back to the drawing board!

The USDA addressed these complaints by revising—and then radically reinventing—the 1992 Guide. Let's take a look at this evolution of the USDA Food Guide over the past two decades by examining the following graphics.

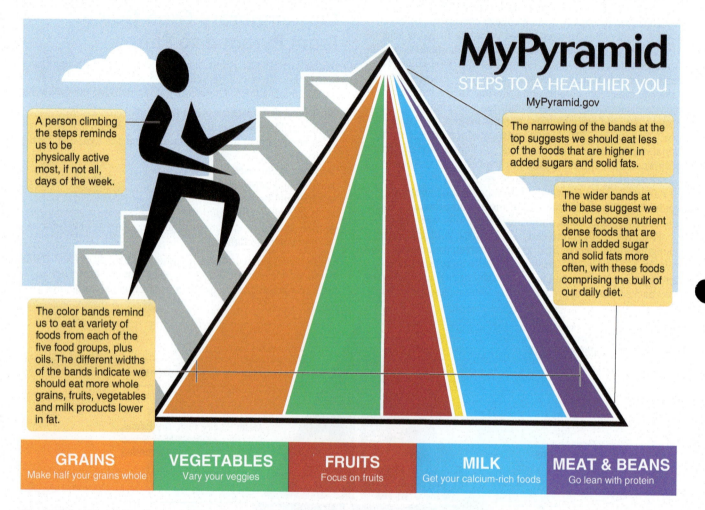

The USDA revised the Guide in 2005 to address concerns regarding the recommendations and ease of use for a general audience. The result was the MyPyramid Food Guidance System, which retained the "pyramid" graphic, but in a simpler presentation that included an emphasis on daily physical activity, and introduced an interactive MyPyramid website where consumers could enter personal data and print out a personalized guide.

Data from: USDA ChooseMyPlate. www.choosemyplate.org

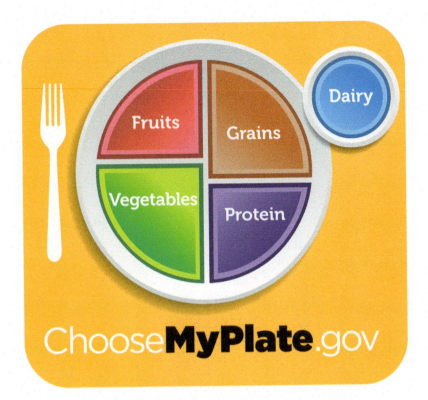

In May 2011 the USDA again changed the food guide—this time dramatically. Dropping the pyramid concept, as well as the previous attempts to teach detailed lessons about foods and physical activity, the new MyPlate guide uses simple icons to directly convey a few key pointers for maintaining a healthy diet. The accompanying website, www.choosemyplate.gov, includes more detailed information as well as interactive tools and multimedia for professionals and consumers.

Data from: www.nal.usda.gov and www.choosemyplate.gov.

references

Chapter 1

1. Office of Disease Prevention and Health Promotion. 2015. HealthyPeople.gov. Healthy People 2020. www.HealthyPeople.gov.
2. Institute of Medicine, Food and Nutrition Board. 2003. *Dietary Reference Intakes: Applications in Dietary Planning*. Washington, DC: National Academies Press.
3. Institute of Medicine, Food and Nutrition Board. 2002. *Dietary Reference Intakes for Energy, Carbohydrates, Fiber, Fat, Protein and Amino Acids (Macronutrients)*. Washington, DC: National Academies Press.
4. Cochrane Bias Methods Group. Addressing reporting bias. https://bmg.cochrane.org/addressing-reporting-biases.
5. Fogel, J., and S. B. S. Shlivko. 2010. Weight problems and spam e-mail for weight loss products. *South. Med. J.* 103(1):31–36.
6. Winterfeldt, E. A., M. L. Bogle, and L. L. Ebro. 2013. Dietetics. Practice and Future Trends. 4th edn. Sudbury, MA: Jones and Bartlett.
7. O'Connor, A. 2015. Coca-Cola funds scientists who shift blame for obesity away from bad diets. *The New York Times*, August 9, 2015. http://well.blogs.nytimes.com/2015/08/09/coca-cola-funds-scientists-who-shift-blame-for-obesity-away-from-bad-diets/?_r=0
8. Global Energy Balance Network. 2015. http://gebn.org/
9. Bes-Rastrollo, M., M. B. Schulze, M. Ruiz-Canela, and M. A. Martinez-Gonzalez. 2013. Financial conflicts of interest and reporting bias regarding the association between sugar-sweetened beverages and weight gain: A systematic review of systematic reviews. *PLOS Med.* 10(12):e1001578.
10. Belluz J., and S. Oh. 2015. Look at who Coca-Cola funded over the past 5 years. *VOX Science & Health*, September 25, 2015. http://www.vox.com/2015/9/25/9396921/coke-research-funding#vox-coca-cola-funding__graphic

In Depth: New Frontiers in Nutrition and Health

1. Waterland, R. A., and R. L. Jirtle. 2003. Transposable elements: Targets for early nutritional effects on epigenetic gene regulation. *Mol. Cell. Biol.* 23(15):5293–5300.
2. Soubry, A, J. M. Schildkraut, A. Murtha, et al. 2013, February 6. Paternal obesity is associated with IGF2 hypomethylation in newborns: Results from a Newborn Epigenetics Study (NEST) cohort. *BMC Medicine* 11:29. doi: 10.1186/1741-7015-11-29
3. Keijer, J., F. P. Hoevenaars, A. Nieuwenhuizen, and E. M. van Schothorst, 2014, October 21. Nutri-genomics of body weight regulation: A rationale for careful dissection of individual contributors. *Nutrients* 6(10):4531-51. doi: 10.3390/nu6104531
4. Khalil, C. A. 2014, July. The emerging role of epigenetics in cardiovascular disease. *Ther Adv Chronic Dis.* 5(4):178–187.
5. Ohlhorst, S. D., R. Russell, D. Bier, et al. 2013. September. Nutrition research to affect food and a healthy lifespan. *Adv Nutr.* 4(5):579–584.
6. Neeha, V. S. and P. Kinth, 2013, June. Nutrigenomics research: A review. *J Food Sci Technol.* 50(3): 415–428.
7. National Human Genome Research Institute. 2014. National DNA Day. Updated March 2014. https://www.genome.gov/26525485
8. Sender, R., S. Fuchs, and R. Milo. 2016, January. Are we really vastly outnumbered? Revisiting the ratio of bacterial to host cells in humans. *Cell* 164(3):337-340. doi: http://dx.doi.org/10.1016/j.cell.2016.01.013
9. Hemarajata, P. and J. Versalovic, 2013. Effects of probiotics on gut microbiota: Mechanisms of intestinal immunomodulation and neuromodulation. *Therap Adv Gastroenterol.* 6(1):39–51. http://www.ncbi.nlm.nih.gov/pmc/articles/PMC3539293/
10. Krajmalnik-Brown, R., Z. E. Ilhan, D. W. Kang, and J. K DiBaise. 2012. Effects of gut microbes on nutrient absorption and energy regulation. *Nutr. Clin. Pract.* 27(2):201–214.
11. Yoon, M. Y., K. Lee, and S. S. Yoon. 2014. Protective role of gut commensal microbes against intestinal infections. *J. Microbiol.* 52(12):983–989. doi: 10.1007/s12275-014-4655-2.
12. Munyaka, P., A. E. Khafipou, and J. E. Ghia. 2014. External influence of early childhood establishment of gut microbiota and subsequent health implications. *Front. Pediatr.* 2:109.
13. Mueller, N. T., R. Whyaat, L. Hoepner, et al. 2015, April. Prenatal exposure to antibiotics, cesarean section and risk of childhood obesity. *Intl. J. Obes.* 39(4):665-670. doi: 10.1038/ijo.2014.180
14. Arrieta, M. C., L. T. Stiemsma, P. A. Dimitriu, et al. 2015, September 30. Early infancy microbial and metabolic alterations affect risk of childhood asthma. *Science Translational Medicine.* 7(307):307ra152. doi: 10.1126/scitranslmed.aab2271
15. Magro, D. O. 2014. Effect of yogurt containing polydextrose, Lactobacillus acidophilus NCFM and Bifidobacterium lactis HN019: A randomized, double-blind, controlled study in chronic constipation. *Nutri. J.* 13:75. doi: 10.1186/1475-2891-13-75
16. Chen, M., Q. Sun, E. Giovannucci, et al. 2014. Dairy consumption and risk of type 2 diabetes: 3 cohorts of U.S. adults and an updated meta-analysis. *BMC Med.* 12:215. doi:10.1186/s12916-014-0215-1
17. Langkamp-Henken, B., C. C. Rowe, A. L. Ford, et al. 2015. Bifidobacterium bifidum R0071 results in a greater proportion of healthy days and a lower percentage of academically stressed students reporting a day of cold/flu: A randomised, double-blind, placebo-controlled study. *Br. J. Nutr.* 113(3):426–434.
18. Produce for Better Health Foundation. 2013, November 10. What are phytochemicals? Fruits and veggies: More matters. http://www.fruitsandveggiesmorematters.org/what-are-phytochemicals
19. Rodriguez-Casado, A. 2014, September 16. The health potential of fruits and vegetables phytochemicals: Notable examples. *Crit Rev Food Sci Nutr.* 0. [Epub ahead of print] doi: 10.1080/10408398.2012.755149
20. Bellik, Y., S. M. Hammoudi, F. Abdellah et al. 2012. Phytochemicals to prevent inflammation and allergy. *Recent Pat. Inflamm. Allergy Drug Discov.* 6(2):147–158.
21. Vasanthi, H. R., N. Shrishrimal, and D. K. Das. 2012. Phytochemicals from plants to combat cardiovascular disease. *Curr. Med. Chem.* 19(14):2242–2251.
22. Rossi, T., C. Gallo, B. Bassani, et al. 2014. Drink your prevention: Beverages with cancer preventive phytochemicals. *Pol Arch Med Wewn.* 124(12):713–722. http://pamw.pl/sites/default/files/PAMW%202014_12_Albini_0.pdf
23. Luo, W. P., Y. J. Fang, M. S. Lu, et al. 2015, March 16. High consumption of vegetable and fruit colour groups is inversely associated with the risk of colorectal cancer: A case-control study. *Br J Nutr:* 0:1–10. [Epub ahead of print].
24. Gostner, J. M., K. Becker, F. Ueberall, and D. Fuchs. 2015, February 16. The good and bad of antioxidant foods: An immunological perspective. *Food Chem Toxicol.* pii: S0278-6915(15)00058-7. [Epub ahead of print]. doi: 10.1016/j.fct.2015.02.012
25. The Alpha-Tocopherol, Beta-Carotene Cancer Prevention Study Group. 1994. The effect of vitamin E and beta carotene on the incidence of lung cancer and other cancers in male smokers. *N. Engl. J. Med.* 330(15):1029–1035.
26. Omenn, G. S., G. E. Goodman, M. D. Thornquist, et al. 1996. Risk factors for lung cancer and for intervention effects in CARET, the Beta-Carotene and Retinol Efficacy Trial. *J. Natl. Cancer Inst.* 88(21):1550–1559.

Chapter 2

1. U.S. Department of Health and Human Services and U.S. Department of Agriculture. 2015, December. *2015–2020 Dietary Guidelines for Americans*, 8th ed. http://health.gov/dietaryguidelines/2015/guidelines/

2. U.S. Department of Agriculture, Economic Research Service. 2014. Data products. food expenditures. http://www.ers.usda.gov/data-products/food-expenditures.aspx#26636

3. Mandala Research. 2011. LivingSocial dining out survey. Key findings. http://mandalaresearch.com/index.php/purchase-reports/download_form/24-livingsocial-dining-out-survey-key-findings

4. Ogden, C. L., M. D. Carroll, B. K. Kit, and K. M. Flegal. 2014. Prevalence of childhood and adult obesity in the United States, 2011–2012. *JAMA*, 311(8):806–814.

5. Swartz, J. J., D. Braxton, and A. J. Viera. 2011. Calorie menu labeling on quick-service restaurant menus: An updated systematic review of the literature. *Int. J. Behav. Nutr. Phys. Act.* 8:135.

6. Sinclair, S. E., M. Cooper, and E. D. Mansfield. 2014. The influence of menu labeling on calories selected or consumed: A systematic review and meta-analysis. *J. Acad. Nutr. Diet.* 114:1375–1388, e15.

7. Bleich, S. N., C. L. Barry, T. L. Gary-Webb, and B. J. Herring. 2014. Reducing sugar-sweetened beverage consumption by providing caloric information: How black adolescents alter their purchases and whether the effects persist. *Am. J. Public Health.* 104(12): 2417–2424.

8. Phares, E. H. 2016. New Dietary Guidelines remove restriction on total fat and set limit for added sugars but censor conclusions of the scientific advisory committee. 2016, January 7. *The Nutrition Source.* http://www.hsph.harvard.edu/nutritionsource/2016/01/07/new-dietary-guidelines-remove-restriction-on-total-fat-and-set-limit-for-added-sugars-but-censor-conclusions/

9. Wright, J. D., and C. Y. Wang. 2011. Awareness of federal dietary guidance in persons aged 16 years and older: Results from the National Health and Nutrition Examination Survey 2005–2006. *J. Am. Diet. Assoc.* 111:295–300.

10. Epstein, S. B., K. Jean-Pierre, S. Lynn, and A. K. Kant. 2013. Media coverage and awareness of the 2010 Dietary Guidelines for Americans and MyPlate. *Am. J. Health Prom.* 28(1):e30–e39.

11. U.S. Department of Health and Human Services and U.S. Department of Agriculture. 2015, December. *2015–2020 Dietary Guidelines for Americans*, 8th ed. http://health.gov/dietaryguidelines/2015/guidelines/

12. Scientific Report of the 2015 Dietary Guidelines Advisory Committee. 2015. Advisory report to the Secretary of Health and Human Services and the Secretary of Agriculture. http://health.gov/dietaryguidelines/2015-scientific-report/

In Depth: Healthful Eating Patterns

1. U.S. Department of Health and Human Services and U.S. Department of Agriculture. 2015, December. *2015–2020 Dietary Guidelines for Americans*, 8th ed. http://health.gov/dietaryguidelines/2015/guidelines/

2. Scientific Report of the 2015 Dietary Guidelines Advisory Committee. 2015. Advisory report to the Secretary of Health and Human Services and the Secretary of Agriculture. http://health.gov/dietaryguidelines/2015-scientific-report/

3. Trichpoulou, A., M. A. Martínez-González, T. Y. N. Tong, et al. 2014. Definitions and potential health benefits of the Mediterranean diet: Views from experts around the world. *BMC Medicine* 12:112. doi: 10.1186/1741-7015-12-112.

4. Estruch, R., E. Ros, J. Salas-Salvadó, et al. 2013. Primary prevention of cardiovascular disease with a Mediterranean diet. *N. Engl. J. Med.* 368:1279–1290.

5. Féart, C., C. Samieri, B. Allès, and P. Barberger-Gateau. 2013. Potential benefits of adherence to the Mediterranean diet on cognitive health. *Proc. Nutr. Soc.* 72(1):140–152.

6. Physician's Committee for Responsible Medicine. n.d. Power Plate *All in One* Guide. http://www.pcrm.org/health/diets/pplate/power-plate

Chapter 3

1. Haleem, D. J. 2015, December 9. Drug targets for obesity and depression: From serotonin to leptin. *Curr. Drug Targets* 17:1–10. doi: 10.2174/1389450117666151209123049

2. Gosby, A. K., A. D. Conigrave, D. Aubenheimer, and S. J. Simpson. 2014, March. Protein leverage and energy intake. *Obes. Rev.* 15(3):183–191. doi: 10.1111/obr.12131

3. LeBlanc, J. G., C. Milani, G. S. de Giori, et al. 2013, April. Bacteria as vitamin suppliers to their host: A gut microbiota perspective. *Curr. Opin. Biotech.* 24(2):160–168. doi: 10.1016/j.copbio.2012.08.005

4. Linares, D. M., P. Ross, and C. Stanton. 2015, December. Beneficial microbes: The pharmacy in the gut. *Bioengineered* 28:1–28. doi: 10.1080/21655979.2015.1126015

5. Zaura, E., B. W. Brandt, M. J. Teixeira de Mattos, et al. 2015. Same exposure but two radically different responses to antibiotics: Resilience of the salivary microbiome versus long-term microbial shifts in feces. *mBio* 6(6):e01693-15. doi:10.1128/mBio.01693-15

6. National Digestive Diseases Information Clearinghouse (NDDIC). 2014, November 13. Symptoms and causes of GER and GERD. www.niddk.nih.gov

7. National Digestive Diseases Information Clearinghouse (NDDIC). 2014, August. Peptic ulcer disease and NSAIDs. www.niddk.nih.gov

8. National Digestive Diseases Information Clearinghouse (NDDIC). 2013, November. Diarrhea. www.niddk.nih.gov

9. National Digestive Diseases Information Clearinghouse (NDDIC). 2015, February 23. Irritable bowel syndrome. www.niddk.nih.gov

10. American Cancer Society. 2016. *Cancer Facts and Figures 2016.* www.cancer.org

11. Hussain, S. A. and S. Hamid. 2014. *Helicobacter pylori* in humans: Where are we now? *Adv. Biomed. Res.* 3:63. doi: 10.4103/2277-9175.125844

12. Vaz, L. E., K. P. Kleinman, M. A. Raebel, et al. 2014, March. Recent trends in outpatient antibiotic use in children. *Pediatrics* 133(3):375–385. doi:10.1542/peds.2013-2903

13. Pacifico, L., J. F. Osborn, V. Tromba, et al. 2014, February 14. Helicobacter pylori infection and extragastric disorders in children: A critical update. *World J. Gastroenterol.* 20(6):1379–1401.

14. Trasande, L., J. Blustein, M. Liu, et al. 2013. Infant antibiotic exposures and early-life body mass. *Int. J. Obesity* 37(1):16–23.

In Depth: Disorders Related to Specific Foods

1. National Institute of Diabetes and Digestive and Kidney Diseases. 2014, June. Lactose intolerance. www.niddk.nih.gov

2. U.S. Food and Drug Administration. 2015, September 2. Food allergies: What you need to know. www.fda.gov

3. National Institute of Diabetes and Digestive and Kidney Diseases. 2015, June. Celiac disease. www.niddk.nih.gov

4. Tian, N., G. Wei, D. Schuppan, and E. J. Helmerhorst. 2014. Effect of *Rothia mucilaginosa* enzymes on gliadin (gluten) structure, deamidation, and immunogenic epitopes relevant to celiac disease. *Am. J. Physiol: Gastrointest. Liver Physiol.* 15;307(8):G769–76. doi: 10.1152/ajpgi.00144.2014

5. Fasano, A., A. Sapone, V. Zevallos, and D. Schuppan. 2015. Non-celiac gluten sensitivity. *Gastroenterology.* pii: S0016-5085(15)00029-3. doi: 10.1053/j.gastro.2014.12.049

6. Ludvigsson, J. F., D. A. Leffler, J. C. Bai, et al. 2013. The Oslo definitions for coeliac disease and related terms. *Gut* 62:43–52. doi:10.1136/gutjnl-2011-301346

7. Mansueto, P., A. Seidita, A. D'Alcamo, and A. Carrocio. 2014. Non-celiac gluten sensitivity: A literature review. *J. Am. Coll. Nutr.* 33(1):39–54. doi: 10.1080/07315724.2014.869996

Chapter 4

1. Humphreys, K. J., M. A. Conlon, G. P. Young, et al. 2014. Dietary manipulation of oncogenic microRNA expression in human rectal mucosa: A randomized trial. *Cancer Prev. Res.* 7(8):786–795.

2. Institute of Medicine, Food and Nutrition Board. 2002. *Dietary Reference Intakes for Energy, Carbohydrates, Fiber, Fat, Protein and*

Amino Acids (Macronutrients). Washington, DC: The National Academy of Sciences.

3. U.S. Department of Health and Human Services and U.S. Department of Agriculture. 2015, December. *2015–2020 Dietary Guidelines for Americans*, 8th edn. http://health.gov/dietaryguidelines/2015/guidelines/

4. Ben, Q., Y. Sun, R. Chai, et al. 2015. Dietary fiber intake reduces risk for colorectal adenoma: A meta-analysis. *Gastroenterol.* 146(3):689–699.

5. Harvard T. H. Chan School of Public Health. 2016. The nutrition source. *Fiber and Colon Cancer: Following the Scientific Trail.* http://www.hsph.harvard.edu/nutritionsource/fiber-and-colon-cancer/

6. Hackett, R. A., M. Kivimaki, M. Kumari, and A. Steptoe. 2015. Diurnal cortisol patterns, future diabetes and impaired glucose metabolism in the Whitehall II cohort study. *J. Clin. Endocrinol. Metab.* doi: http://dx.doi.org/10.1210/jc.2015-2853 [Epub ahead of print]

7. Peters, A., and B. S. McEwan. 2015. Stress habituation, body shape and cardiovascular mortality. *Neurosci. Biobehav. Rev.* 56:139–150.

8. Goff, L. M., D. E. Cowland, L. Hooper, and G. S. Frost. 2013. Low glycaemic index diets and blood lipids: A systematic review and meta-analysis of randomized controlled trials. *Nut. Metab. Cardiovasc. Dis.* 23(1):1–10.

9. De Koning, L., V. S. Malik, M. D. Kellogg, et al. 2012. Sweetened beverage consumption, incident coronary heart disease, and biomarkers of risk in men. *Circulation.* 125:1735–1741.

10. Yang, Q., Z. Zhang, E. W. Gregg, et al. 2014. Added sugar intake and cardiovascular diseases mortality among U.S. adults. *JAMA Intern. Med.* 174(4):516–524.

11. Basu, S., P. Yoffee, N. Hills, and R. H. Lustig. 2013. The relationship of sugar to population-level diabetes prevalence: An econometric analysis of repeated cross-sectional data. *PLoS ONE.* 8(2):e57873. doi:10.1371/journal.pone.0057873

12. Te Moranga, L., S. Mallard, and J. Mann. 2013. Dietary sugars and body weight: Systematic review and meta-analyses of randomized controlled trials and cohort studies. *BMJ.* 346:e7492.

13. Hoy, M. K., and J. D. Goldman. 2014, September. Fiber intake of the U.S. population: What we eat in America, NHANES 2009–2010. *Food Surveys Research Group Dietary Data Brief No. 12.* http://www.ars.usda.gov/SP2UserFiles/Place/80400530/pdf/DBrief/12_fiber_intake_0910.pdf

14. Moore, L. V., and F. E. Thompson. 2015. Adults meeting fruit and vegetable intake recommendations—United States, 2013. *Morbid. Mortal. Weekly Rep.* 64(26):709–713.

15. American College Health Association. 2015. *National College Health Assessment II: Reference Group Executive Summary Spring 2015.* Hanover, MD: American College Health Association.

16. International Food Information Council Foundation. 2014. Facts About Low-Calorie Sweeteners. http://www.foodinsight.org/articles/facts-about-low-calorie-sweeteners

17. International Food Information Council Foundation. 2014. Everything You Need to Know About Aspartame. http://www.foodinsight.org/Everything_You_Need_to_Know_About_Aspartame

18. Miller, P. E., and V. Perez. 2014. Low-calorie sweeteners and body weight and composition: A meta-analysis of randomized controlled trials and prospective cohort studies. *Am. J. Clin. Nutr.* 100(3):765–777.

19. Peters, J., H. Wyatt, G. Foster, et al. 2014. The effects of water and non-nutritive sweetened beverages on weight loss during a 12-week weight loss treatment program. *Obesity.* 22(6):1415–1421.

20. Malik, V. S., and F. B. Hu. 2015. Fructose and cardiometabolic health: What the evidence from sugar-sweetened beverages tells us. *J. Am. Coll. Cardiol.* 66(14):1615–1624.

21. U.S. Department of Health and Human Services and U.S. Department of Agriculture. 2015, December. *2015–2020 Dietary Guidelines for Americans*, 8th edn. http://health.gov/dietaryguidelines/2015/guidelines/

22. Te Moranga, L., S. Mallard, and J. Mann. 2013. Dietary sugars and body weight: Systematic review and meta-analyses of randomized controlled trials and cohort studies. *BMJ.* 346:e7492.

23. Bray G. A., S. J. Nielsen, and B. M. Popkin. 2004. Consumption of high-fructose corn syrup in beverages may play a role in the epidemic of obesity. *Am. J. Clin. Nutr.* 79:537–543.

24. White, J. S. 2013. Challenging the fructose hypothesis: New perspectives on fructose consumption and metabolism. *Adv. Nutr.* 4:246–256.

25. Vos, M. B., and J. E. Lavine. 2013. Dietary fructose in nonalcoholic fatty liver disease. *Heptology.* 57(6):2525–2531.

26. Stanhope, K. L., J.-M. Schwarz, and P. J. Havel. 2013. Adverse metabolic effects of dietary fructose: results from recent epidemiological, clinical, and mechanistic studies. *Curr. Opin. Lipidol.* 24(3):198–206.

In Depth: Diabetes

1. Centers for Disease Control and Prevention. National Center for Chronic Disease Prevention and Health Promotion. Division of Diabetes Translation. 2014. *National Diabetes Statistics Report.* http://www.cdc.gov/diabetes/pubs/statsreport14/national-diabetes-report-web.pdf

2. Blackwell, D. L., J. W. Lucas, and T. C. Clarke. 2014. Summary health statistics for U.S. adults: National health interview survey, 2012. National Center for Health Statistics. *Vital and Health Stat.* 10(260).

3. Murphy, S. L., M. A. Kochanek, J. Xu, and M. Heron. 2015, August 31. *National Vital Statistics Reports 63*(9). Centers for Disease Control and Prevention. http://www.cdc.gov

4. American Diabetes Association. 2014. Genetics of diabetes. http://www.diabetes.org/diabetes-basics/genetics-of-diabetes.html

5. American College Health Association. 2015, Spring. National College Health Assessment II: Undergraduate Student Reference Group Executive Summary Hanover, MD: American College Health Association.

6. Basu, S., P. Yoffe, N. Hills, and R. H. Lustig. 2013. The relationship of sugar to population-level diabetes prevalence: An economic analysis of repeated cross-sectional data. *PLoS ONE.* 8(2):e57873. doi:10.1371/journal.pone.0057873

7. Cho, S. S., L. Qi, G. C. Fahey, Jr., and D. M. Klurfeld. 2013. Consumption of cereal fiber, mixtures of whole grains and bran, and whole grains and risk reduction in type 2 diabetes, obesity, and cardiovascular disease. *Am. J. Clin. Nutr.* 98(2):594–619.

8. Aune, D., T. Norat, P. Romundstad, and L. J. Vatten. 2013. Whole grain and refined grain consumption and the risk of type 2 diabetes: A systematic review and dose-response meta-analysis of cohort studies. *Eur. J. Epidemiol.* 28:845–858.

9. The InterAct Consortium. 2013. Association between dietary meat consumption and incident type 2 diabetes: The EPIC-InterAct study. *Diabetologia.* 56:47–59.

10. Pan, A., Q. Sun, A. M. Bernstein, et al. 2013. Changes in red meat consumption and subsequent risk of type 2 diabetes mellitus. Three cohorts of U.S. men and women. *JAMA Int. Med.* 173(14):1328–1335.

11. Crump, C., J. Sundquist, M. A. Winkleby, W. Sieh, and K. Sundquist. 2016, March 8. Physical fitness among Swedish military conscripts and long-term risk for type 2 diabetes mellitus: A cohort study. *Ann. Intern. Med.* doi: 10.7326/M15-2002

12. American College of Sports Medicine and the American Diabetes Association. 2010. Exercise and type 2 diabetes: American College of Sports Medicine and American Diabetes Association joint position statement. *Med. Sci. Sports Exerc.* 42(12):2282–2303.

13. Centers for Disease Control and Prevention. 2015. Tips from former smokers. Smoking and diabetes. http://www.cdc.gov/tobacco/campaign/tips/diseases/diabetes.html

14. Academy of Nutrition and Dietetics. 2014. Diabetes and diet. http://www.eatright.org/resource/health/diseases-and-conditions/diabetes/diabetes-and-diet

Chapter 5

1. U.S. Food and Drug Administration (FDA). 2015. Food facts. Talking about trans fats: What you need to know. http://www.fda.gov/downloads/Food/IngredientsPackagingLabeling/UCM239579.pdf

2. Pan, A., M. Chen, R. Chowdhury, et al. 2012. a-Linolenic acid and risk of cardiovascular disease: A systematic review and meta-analysis. *The American Journal of Clinical Nutrition* 96(6): 1262–1273.

3. Mozaffarian, D., and J. H. Wu. 2011. Omega-3 fatty acids and cardiovascular disease: Effects on risk factors, molecular pathways, and clinical events. *Journal of the American College of Cardiology* 58(20):2047–2067.

4. Jump, D. B., C. M. Depner, and S. Tripathy. 2012. Omega-3 fatty acid supplementation and cardiovascular disease. Thematic Review Series: New lipid and lipoprotein targets for the treatment of cardiometabolic diseases. *Journal of Lipid Research* 53(12): 2525–2545.

5. Baum, S. J., P. M. Kris-Etherton, W. C. Willett, et al. 2012. Fatty acids in cardiovascular health and disease: A comprehensive update. *Journal of Clinical Lipidology.* 6(3):216–234.

6. Johnson, R. K., L. J. Appel, M. Brands, et al. 2009. Dietary sugars intake and cardiovascular health: A scientific statement from the American Heart Association. *Circulation* 120(11):1011–1020.

7. DiNicolantonio, J. J., S. C. Lucan, and J. H. O'Keefe. 2015. The evidence for saturated fat and for sugar related to coronary heart disease. *Progress in Cardiovascular Diseases.* doi: 10.1016/j.pcad.2015.11.006

8. Singh, G. M., R. Micha, S. Khatibzadeh, et al. 2015. Estimated global, regional, and national disease burdens related to sugar-sweetened beverage consumption in 2010. *Circulation* 132(8): 639–666.

9. Institute of Medicine (IOM) Food and Nutrition Board, ed. 2005. *Dietary Reference Intakes for Energy, Carbohydrate, Fiber, Fat, Fatty Acids, Cholesterol, Protein, and Amino Acids.* Washington, DC: The National Academies Press.

10. Rodriguez, N. R., N. M. DiMarco, and S. Langley. 2009. Nutrition and athletic performance. *Medicine and Science in Sports and Exercise* 41(3):709–731.

11. National Heart Lung and Blood Institute (NHLBI), National Institutes of Health (NIH). 2005. In brief: Your guide to lowering your blood pressure with DASH. http://www.nhlbi.nih.gov/health/resources/heart/hbp-dash-in-brief-html

12. U.S. Department of Health Human Services and U.S. Department of Agriculture. 2015, December. *2015–2020 Dietary Guidelines for Americans,* 8th ed. http://health.gov/dietaryguidelines/2015/guidelines/

13. U.S. Department of Health and Human Services (DHHS). 2015, February. Scientific Report of the 2015 Dietary Guidelines Advisory Committee. http://health.gov/dietaryguidelines/2015-scientific-report/

14. Mozaffarian, D., M. B. Katan, A. Ascherio, et al. 2006. *Trans* fatty acids and cardiovascular disease. *The New England Journal of Medicine* 354(15):1601–1613.

15. Willett, W. C. 2012. Dietary fats and coronary heart disease. *Journal of Internal Medicine* 272(1):13–24.

16. Clapp, J., C. J. Curtis, A. E. Middleton, and G. P. Goldstein. 2014. Prevalence of partially hydrogenated oils in U.S. packaged foods, 2012. *Preventing Chronic Disease* 11:E145.

17. Othman, R. A., M. H. Moghadasian, and P. J. Jones. 2011. Cholesterol-lowering effects of oat b-glucan. *Nutrition Reviews* 69(6):299–309.

18. Lichtenstein, A. H., and P. J. Jones. Lipids: Absorption and transport. In: Erdman, J. W., I. A. MacDonald, and S. H. Zeisel, eds. 2012. *Present Knowledge of Nutrition,* 10th ed. Oxford, UK: Wiley-Blackwell.

19. Flock, M. R., M. H. Green, and P. M. Kris-Etherton. 2011. Effects of adiposity on plasma lipid response to reductions in dietary saturated fatty acids and cholesterol. *Advances in Nutrition* 2(3):261–274.

20. Fernandez, M. L., and M. Calle. 2010. Revisiting dietary cholesterol recommendations: Does the evidence support a limit of 300 mg/d? *Current Atherosclerosis Reports* 12(6):377–383.

21. Mozaffarian, D., T. Hao, E. B. Rimm, et al. 2011. Changes in diet and lifestyle and long-term weight gain in women and men. *New England Journal of Medicine* 364(25):2392–2404.

22. Mattes, R. D., P. M. Kris-Etherton, and G. D. Foster. 2008. Impact of peanuts and tree nuts on body weight and healthy weight loss in adults. *The Journal of Nutrition* 138(9):1741S–1745S.

23. Baer, D. J., S. K. Gebauer, and J. A. Novotny. 2015. Walnuts consumed by healthy adults provide less available energy than predicted by the Atwater factors. *The Journal of Nutrition* 146(1): 9–13. doi: 10.3945/ jn.115.217372

24. Mhurchu, C. N., C. Dunshea-Mooij, D. Bennett, and A. Rodgers. 2005. Effect of chitosan on weight loss in overweight and obese individuals: a systematic review of randomized controlled trials. *Obes Rev.* 6(1):35–42.

25. Mhurchu, C. N., C. A. Dunshea-Mooij, D. Bennett, and A. Rodgers. 2005. Chitosan for overweight or obesity. Cochrane database of systematic reviews (Online) (Cochrane Database Syst Rev). 2005(3):CD003892.

26. Jull, A. B., C. Ni Mhurchu, D. A. Bennett, C. A. Dunshea-Mooij, and A. Rodgers. 2008. Chitosan for overweight or obesity. Cochrane database of systematic reviews (Online) (Cochrane Database Syst Rev). 2008(3):CD003892 3.

27. Dombrowski, S. U., K. Knittle, A. Avenell, V. Araujo-Soares, and F. F. Sniehotta. 2014. Long term maintenance of weight loss with non-surgical interventions in obese adults: systematic review and meta-analyses of randomised controlled trials. BMJ 348.

28. Chowdhury, R., S. Warnakula, S. Kunutsor, et al. 2014. Association of dietary, circulating, and supplement fatty acids with coronary risk: A systematic review and meta-analysis. *Annals of Internal Medicine* 160:6.

29. Mozaffarian, D., R. Micha, and S. Wallace. 2010. Effects on coronary heart disease of increasing polyunsaturated fat in place of saturated fat: A systematic review and meta-analysis of randomized controlled trials. *PLoS Medicine* 7(3):e1000252.

30. Dawczynski, C., M. E. Kleber, W. März, G. Jahreis, and S. Lorkowski. 2014. Association of dietary, circulating, and supplement fatty acids with coronary risk. *Annals of Internal Medicine* 161(6):453–454.

31. Liebman, B. F., M. B. Katan, and M. F. Jacobson. 2014. Association of dietary, circulating, and supplement fatty acids with coronary risk. *Annals of Internal Medicine* 161(6):454–455.

32. Willett, W. C., M. J. Stampfer, and F. M. Sacks. 2014. Association of dietary, circulating, and supplement fatty acids with coronary risk. *Annals of Internal Medicine* 161(6):453.

33. Astrup, A. 2014. A changing view on saturated fatty acids and dairy: From enemy to friend. *The American Journal of Clinical Nutrition* 100(6):1407–1408.

34. Astrup, A. 2014. Yogurt and dairy product consumption to prevent cardiometabolic diseases: Epidemiologic and experimental studies. *The American Journal of Clinical Nutrition* 99(5):1235S–1242S.

35. Chandra, A., and A. Rohatgi. 2014. The role of advanced lipid testing in the prediction of cardiovascular disease. *Current Atherosclerosis Reports* 16(3):394.

36. Dutheil, F., G. Walther, R. Chapier, et al. 2014. Atherogenic subfractions of lipoproteins in the treatment of metabolic syndrome by physical activity and diet—the RESOLVE trial. *Lipids in Health and Disease* 13(1):112.

37. Dutheil, F., G. Lac, B. Lesourd, et al. 2013. Different modalities of exercise to reduce visceral fat mass and cardiovascular risk in metabolic syndrome: The RESOLVE* randomized trial. *International Journal of Cardiology* 168(4):3634–3642.

In Depth: Cardiovascular Disease

1. Murphy, S. L., K. D. Kochanek, J. Xu, and M. Heron. 2015. National vital statistics reports. *National Vital Statistics Reports* 63(9). www.cdc.gov

2. Mizuno, Y., R. F. Jacob, and R. P. Mason. 2011. Inflammation and the development of atherosclerosis. *Journal of Atherosclerosis and Thrombosis* 18(5):351–358.

3. Center for Disease Control and Prevention (CDC). 2015. Stroke facts. http://www.cdc.gov/stroke/facts.htm

4. Mozaffarian, D., E. J. Benjamin, A. S. Go, et al. 2016. Heart disease and stroke statistics—2016 update: A report from the American Heart Association. *Circulation*. CIR. 0000000000000350.

5. Marwick, T. H., M. D. Hordern, T. Miller, et al. 2009. Exercise training for type 2 diabetes mellitus: Impact on cardiovascular risk: A scientific statement from the American Heart Association. *Circulation* 119(25):3244–3262.

6. Department of Health and Human Services (DHHS). 2008. *2008 Physical Activity Guidelines for Americans*. Department of Health and Human Services. 2008(ODPHP Publication No U0036. http://health.gov/paguidelines/guidelines/

7. Hohensinner, P. J., A. Niessner, K. Huber, C. M. Weyand, and J. Wojta. 2011. Inflammation and cardiac outcome. *Current Opinion in Infectious Diseases* 24(3):259–264.

8. Dallmeier, D., and W. Koenig. 2014. Strategies for vascular disease prevention: The role of lipids and related markers including apolipoproteins, low-density lipoproteins (LDL)-particle size, high sensitivity C-reactive protein (hs-CRP), lipoprotein-associated phospholipase A 2 (Lp-PLA 2) and lipoprotein (a)(Lp (a)). *Best Practice & Research Clinical Endocrinology & Metabolism* 28(3): 281–294.

9. Flock, M. R., W. S. Harris, and P. M. Kris-Etherton. 2013. Long-chain omega-3 fatty acids: Time to establish a dietary reference intake. *Nutrition Reviews* 71(10):692–707.

10. Kromhout, D., and J. de Goede. 2014. Update on cardiometabolic health effects of omega-3 fatty acids. *Current Opinion in Lipidology* 25(1):85–90.

11. Eckel, R. H., J. M. Jakicic, J. D. Ard, et al. 2014. 2013 AHA/ACC guideline on lifestyle management to reduce cardiovascular risk: A report of the American College of Cardiology/American Heart Association Task Force on Practice Guidelines. *Journal of the American College of Cardiology* 63(25):2960–2984.

12. Singh, G. M., R. Micha, S. Khatibzadeh, et al. 2015. Estimated global, regional, and national disease burdens related to sugar-sweetened beverage consumption in 2010. *Circulation* 132(8): 639–666.

13. Jump, D. B., C. M. Depner, and S. Tripathy. 2012. Omega-3 fatty acid supplementation and cardiovascular disease Thematic Review Series: New lipid and lipoprotein targets for the treatment of cardiometabolic diseases. *Journal of Lipid Research* 53(12): 2525–2545.

14. Mann, S., C. Beedie, and A. Jimenez. 2013. Differential effects of aerobic exercise, resistance training and combined exercise modalities on cholesterol and the lipid profile: review, synthesis and recommendations. *Sports Medicine* 44(2):211–221.

15. U.S. Department of Health Human Services and U.S. Department of Agriculture. 2015, December. *2015–2020 Dietary Guidelines for Americans*, 8th ed. http://health.gov/dietaryguidelines/2015/guidelines/.

16. Centers for Disease Control and Prevention (CDC). 2015. Peventing heart disease: healthy living habits. http://www.cdc.gov/heartdisease/healthy_living.htm

17. Institute of Medicine (IOM) Food and Nutrition Board, ed. 2005. *Dietary reference intakes for energy, carbohydrate, fiber, fat, fatty acids, cholesterol, protein, and amino acids*. Washington, DC: The National Academies Press.

18. Othman, R. A., M. H. Moghadasian, and P. J. Jones. 2011. Cholesterol-lowering effects of oat b-glucan. *Nutrition Reviews* 69(6):299–309.

19. Lumeng, C. N., and A. R. Saltiel. 2011. Inflammatory links between obesity and metabolic disease. *The Journal of Clinical Investigation* 121(6):2111–2117.

20. Dutheil, F., G. Lac, B. Lesourd, et al. 2013. Different modalities of exercise to reduce visceral fat mass and cardiovascular risk in metabolic syndrome: The RESOLVE* randomized trial. *International Journal of Cardiology* 168(4):3634–3642.

21. Appel, L. J., M. W. Brands, S. R. Daniels, et al. 2006. Dietary approaches to prevent and treat hypertension: A scientific statement from the American Heart Association. *Hypertension* 47(2):296–308.

22. Blumenthal, J. A., M. A. Babyak, A. Sherwood, et al. 2010. Effects of the dietary approaches to stop hypertension diet alone and in combination with exercise and caloric restriction on insulin sensitivity and lipids. *Hypertension* 55(5):1199–1205.

Chapter 6

1. Rafii, M., M. Chapman, J. Owens, et al. 2015. Dietary protein requirement of female adults >65 years determined by the indicator amino acid oxidation technique is higher than current recommendations. *Journal of Nutrition* 145(1):18–24.

2. American College of Sports Medicine, Academy of Nutrition and Dietetics, and Dietitians of Canada. 2016. Joint Position Statement. Nutrition and athletic performance. *Medicine and Science in Sports and Exercise* 48(3):543–568.

3. National Center for Health Statistics. 2015. *Health, United States, 2014: With Special Feature on Adults Aged 55–64*. Hyattsville, MD.

4. Ford, E. S., and W. H. Dietz. 2013. Trends in energy intake among adults in the United States: Findings from NHANES. *The American Journal of Clinical Nutrition* 97:848–853.

5. U.S. Department of Health and Human Services and U.S. Department of Agriculture. December 2015. *2015–2020 Dietary Guidelines for Americans*, 8th ed. http://health.gov/dietaryguidelines/2015/guidelines/

6. Bao, Y., J. Han, F. B. Hu, et al. 2013. Association of nut consumption with total and cause-specific mortality. *The New England Journal of Medicine* 369:2001–2011.

7. Lu, H. N., W. J. Blot, Y-B. Xiang, et al. 2015. Prospective evaluation of the association of nut/peanut consumption with total and cause-specific mortality. *JAMA Internal Medicine*. Epub ahead of print, doi:10.1001/jamainternmed.2014.8347

8. Pan, A., Q. Sun, J. E. Manson, W. C. Willett, and F. B. Hu. 2013. Walnut consumption is associated with lower risk of type 2 diabetes in women. *The Journal of Nutrition* 143:512–518.

9. Calvez, J., N. Poupin, C. Chesneau, C. Lassale, and D. Tomé. 2012. Protein intake, calcium balance and health consequences. *European Journal of Clinical Nutrition* 66:281–295.

10. Evert, A. B., J. L. Boucher, M. Cypress, et al. 2013. Nutrition therapy recommendations for the management of adults with diabetes. *Diabetes Care* 36:3821–3842.

11. Phillips, S. M. 2014. A brief review of higher protein diets in weight loss: A focus on athletes. *Sports Medicine* 44(Suppl. 2):S149–S153.

12. Chowdhury, R., S. Warnakula, S. Kunutsor, et al. 2014. Association of dietary, circulating, and supplement fatty acids with coronary risk: A systematic review and meta-analysis. *Annals of Internal Medicine* 160(6):398–406.

13. van Bussel, B. C. T., R. M. A. Henry, I. Ferreira, et al. 2015. A healthy diet is associated with less endothelial dysfunction and less low-grade inflammation over a 7-year period in adults at risk of cardiovascular disease. *Journal of Nutrition* 145(3):532–540.

14. Smith, M. I., T. Yatsunenko, M. J. Manary, et al. 2013. Gut microbiomes of Malawian twin pairs discordant for kwashiorkor. *Science* 339:548–554.

15. The Vegetarian Resource Group. 2015, May 29. How often do Americans eat vegetarian meals? And how many adults in the U.S. are vegetarian? www.vrg.org

16. The Vegetarian Resource Group. 2014, May 30. How many teens and other youth are vegetarian and vegan? The Vegetarian Resource Group asks in a 2014 national poll. www.vrg.org

17. The Vegetarian Resource Group. 2016. Veganism in a nutshell. https://www.vrg.org/nutshell/vegan.htm

18. National Institutes of Health, National Cancer Institute. 2015. About cancer. *Chemicals in Meat Cooked at High Temperatures and Cancer Risk*. http://www.cancer.gov/about-cancer/causes-prevention/risk/diet/cooked-meats-fact-sheet

19. Le, L. T., and J. Sabaté. 2014. Beyond meatless, the health effects of vegan diets: Findings from the Adventist cohorts. *Nutrients* 6(6):2131–2147.

20. Bardone-Cone, A. M., E. E. Fitzsimmons-Craft, M. B. Harney, et al. 2012. The inter-relationships between vegetarianism and

eating disorders among females. *Journal of the American Dietetic Association* 112(8):1247–1252.

21. Institute of Medicine, Food and Nutrition Board. 2005. *Dietary Reference Intakes for Energy, Carbohydrate, Fiber, Fat, Fatty Acids, Cholesterol, Protein, and Amino Acids (Macronutrients)*. Washington, DC: National Academies Press.

22. Marini, J. C. 2015. Protein recommendations: Are we ready for new recommendations? *Journal of Nutrition* 145(1):5–6.

23. Rafii, M., M. Chapman, J. Owens, et al. 2015. Dietary protein requirement of female adults <65 years determined by the indicator amino acid oxidation technique is higher than current recommendations. *Journal of Nutrition* 145(1):18–24.

24. Tang, M., G. P. McCabe, R. Elango, et al. 2014. Assessment of protein requirements in octogenarian women with use of the indicator amino acid oxidation technique. *American Journal of Clinical Nutrition* 99:891–898.

25. Deutz, N. E. P., J. M. Bauer, R. Barazzoni, et al. 2014. Protein intake and exercise for optimal muscle function with aging: Recommendations from the ESPEN Expert Group. *Clinical Nutrition* 33:929–936.

26. Elango, R., M. A. Humayun, R. O. Ball, and P. B. Pencharz. 2011. Protein requirement of healthy school-aged children determined by the indicator amino acid oxidation method. *American Journal of Clinical Nutrition* 94:1545–1552.

In Depth: Vitamins and Minerals: Micronutrients with Macro Powers

1. Institute of Medicine, Food and Nutrition Board. 2001. *Dietary Reference Intakes for Vitamin A, Vitamin K, Arsenic, Boron, Chromium, Copper, Iodine, Iron, Manganese, Molybdenum, Nickel, Silicon, Vanadium, and Zinc*. Washington, DC: National Academies Press.

2. Bjelakovic, G., N. D. Nikolova, and C. Gluud. 2014. Antioxidant supplements and mortality. *Current Opinion in Clinical Nutrition & Metabolic Care* 17:40–44.

3. Burckhardt, P. 2015. Vitamin A and bone health. In: M. F. Holick and J. W. Nieves, eds. *Nutrition and Bone Health*. New York, NY: Springer.

4. Sinck, J. W. R., M. de Groh, and A. J. MacFarlane. 2015. Genetic modifiers of folate, vitamin B-12, and homocysteine status in a cross-sectional study of the Canadian population. *American Journal of Clinical Nutrition* 101:1295–1304.

Chapter 7

1. Sanchis-Gomar, F., H. Parej-Galeano, G. Cervellin, G. Kippi, and C. P. Earnest. 2015. Energy drink overconsumption in adolescents: Implications for arrhythmnias and other cardiovascular events. *Canadian Journal of Cardiology* 31:572–575.

2. Center for Science in the Public Interest. 2014. Documents link more deaths to energy drinks. http://www.cspinet.org/new/201406251.html

3. Tucker, M. A., M. S. Ganio, J. D. Adams, et al. 2015. Hydration status over 24-H is not affected by ingested beverage composition. *Journal of the American College of Nutrition* 34:318–327.

4. Maughan, R. J., P. Watson, P. A. A. Cordery, et al. 2016. A randomized trial to assess the potential of different beverages to affect hydration status: Development of a beverage hydration index. *American Journal of Clinical Nutrition*. doi:10.3945/ajcn.115.114769. Available at http://ajcn.nutrition.org/content/early/2015/12/23/ajcn.115.114769.short.

5. Institute of Medicine, Food and Nutrition Board. 2004. *Dietary Reference Intakes for Water, Potassium, Sodium, Chloride, and Sulfate*. Washington, DC: National Academy Press.

6. Casa, D. J., J. K. DeMartini, M. F. Bergeron, et al. 2015. National Athletic Trainers' Association position statement: Exertional heat illnesses. *Journal of Athletic Training* 50:986–1000.

7. International Bottled Water Association. 2016. Bottled water market. http://www.bottledwater.org/economics/bottled-water-market

8. Seppa, N. 2015. Coffee reveals itself as an unlikely elixir. *Science News* 188:16–20.

9. 2015 Dietary Guidelines Advisory Committee. 2015. *Scientific Report of the 2015 Dietary Guidelines Advisory Committee*. http://health.gov/dietaryguidelines/2015-scientific-report/

10. Pang, J., Z. Zhang, T. Zheng, et al. 2016. Green tea consumption and risk of cardiovascular and ischemic related diseases: A meta-analysis. *International Journal of Cardiology* 202:967–974.

11. Sarin, S., C. Marya, R. Nagpal, S. S. Oberoi, and A. Rekhi. 2015. Preliminary clinical evidence of the antiplaque, antigingivitis efficacy of a mouthwash containing 2% green tea—a randomized clinical trial. *Oral Health & Preventive Dentistry* 13:197–203.

12. Sansone, R., A. Rodriguez-Mateos, J. Heuel, et al. for the Flaviola Consortium, European Union 7th Framework Program. 2015. Cocoa flavanol intake improves endothelial function and Framingham Risk Score in healthy men and women: A randomized, controlled, double-masked trial: The Flaviola Health Study. *British Journal of Nutrition* 114:1246–1255.

13. Mastroiacovo, D., C. Kwik-Uribe, D. Grassi, S. Necozione, et al. 2015. Cocoa flavanol consumption improves cognitive function, blood pressure control and metabolic profile in elderly subjects: The Cocoa, Cognition, and Aging (CoCoA) Study—a randomized controlled trial. *American Journal of Clinical Nutrition* 101:538–548.

14. Ali, F., H. Rehman, Z. Babayan, D., Stapleton, and D. D. Joshi. 2015. Energy drinks and their adverse health effects: A systematic review of the current literature. *Postgraduate Medicine*. doi: 10.1080/00325481.2015.1001712

15. DiNicolantonio, J. J., S. C. Lucan, and J. H. O'Keefe. 2015. The evidence for saturated fat and for sugar related to coronary heart disease. *Prog Cardiovascular Disease* [Epub ahead of print]. doi: 10.1016/j.pcad.2015.11.006

16. Singh, G. M., R. Micha, S. Khatibzadeh, et al. 2015. Estimated global, regional, and national disease burdens related to sugar-sweetened beverage consumption in 2010. *Circulation* 132:639–666.

17. Zytnick, D., S. Park, and S. J. Onufrak. 2016. Child and caregiver attitudes about sports drinks and weekly sports drink intake among U.S. youth. *American Journal of Health Promotion* 30:e110–e119.

18. U.S. Department of Health and Human Services and U.S. Department of Agriculture. 2015, December. *2015–2020 Dietary Guidelines for Americans*, 8th ed. http://health.gov/dietaryguidelines/2015/guidelines/

19. Center for Nutrition and Health Policy. 2000. *Dietary Guidelines for Americans, 1980–2000*. http://www.health.gov/dietaryguidelines/1980_2000_chart.pdf

20. Gardner, T. J. 2009. Letter to C. Davis, U.S. Department of Agriculture and K. McMurry, Department of Health and Human Services. http://www.heart.org/idc/groups/heart-public/@wcm/@adv/documents/downloadable/ucm_312853.pdf

21. World Health Organization. 2012. *Guideline: Sodium intake for adults and children*. Geneva: World Health Organization [WHO]. http://www.who.int/nutrition/publications/guidelines/sodium_intake_printversion.pdf

22. Graudal, N., G. Jurgens, B. Baslund, and M. H. Alderman. 2014. Compared with usual sodium intake, low- and excessive-sodium diets are associated with increased mortality: A meta-analysis. *Am J Hypertens*. 27(9):1129–1137. doi: 10.1093/ajh/hpu028

In Depth: Alcohol

1. Centers for Disease Control and Prevention. 2015. Alcohol Poisoning Deaths. http://www.cdc.gov/vitalsigns/alcohol-poisoning-deaths/index.html. 6.

2. U.S. Department of Health and Human Services and U.S. Department of Agriculture. 2015, December. *2015–2020 Dietary Guidelines for Americans*, 8th ed. http://health.gov/dietaryguidelines/2015/guidelines/

3. Schrieks, I. C., A. Stafleu, S. Griffioen-Roose, et al. 2015. Moderate alcohol consumption stimulates food intake and food reward of savoury foods. *Appetite* 89:77–83.

4. Handing, E. P., R. Andel, P. Kadlecova, M. Gatz, and N. L. Pedersen. 2015. Midlife alcohol consumption and risk of dementia over 43 years of follow-up: a population-based study from the Swedish Twin Registry. *J Gerontol A Biol Sci Med Sci.* 70: 1248–1254.

5. Poli, A., and F. Visioli. 2015. Moderate alcohol use and health: An update a consensus document. BIO Web of Conferences. 5:04001. doi: 10.1051/bioconf/20150504001

6. Singh, C. K., X. Liu, and N. Ahmad. 2015. Resveratrol, in its natural combination in whole grape, for health promotion and disease management. *Ann. N.Y. Acad. Sci.* 1348:150–160.

7. Park, S-Y., L. N. Kolonel, U. Lim, K. K. et al. 2014. Alcohol consumption and breast cancer risk among women of five ethnic groups with light to moderate intakes: The Multiethnic Cohort Study. *Interntl. J. Cancer.* 134:1504–1510.

8. Jones, S. B., L. Loehr, C. L. et al. 2015. Midlife alcohol consumption and the risk of stroke in the atherosclerosis risk in communities study. *Stroke.* 46:3124–3130.

9. Chakraborty, S. 2014. Analysis of NHANES 1999–2002 data reveals noteworthy association of alcohol consumption with obesity. *Ann. Gastroenterol.* 27:250–257.

10. National Institute on Alcohol Abuse and Alcoholism. 2014. Harmful interactions: Mixing alcohol with medicines. NIH Publication No. 13-5329. Revised. http://pubs.niaaa.nih.gov/publications/Medicine/medicine.htm

11. National Institute on Alcohol Abuse and Alcoholism. 2015. Alcohol Facts and Statistics. http://www.niaaa.nih.gov/alcohol-health/overview-alcohol-consumption/alcohol-facts-and-statistics

12. Centers for Disease Control and Prevention. 2015. Fact Sheets—Binge Drinking. http://www.cdc.gov/alcohol/fact-sheets/binge-drinking.htm

13. White, A., and R. Hingson. 2014. The burden of alcohol use: Excessive alcohol consumption and related consequences among college students. *Alcohol Res.* 35:201–218. http://pubs.niaaa.nih.gov/publications/arcr352/201-218.htm

14. Feldstein Ewing, S. W., A. Sakhardande, and S-J. Blakemore. 2014. The effect of alcohol consumption on the adolescent brain: A systematic review of MRI and fMRI studies of alcohol-using youth. *NeuroImage: Clinical.* 5:420–437.

15. Risher, M. L., R. L. Fleming, W. C. Risher, et al. 2015. Adolescent intermittent alcohol exposure: Persistence of structural and functional hippocampal abnormalities into adulthood. *Alcohol Clin. Exp. Res.* 39:989–997.

16. Molina, P. E., J. D. Gardner, F. M. Souza-Smith, and A. M. Whitaker. 2014. Alcohol abuse: Critical pathophysiological processes and contributions to disease burden. *Physiology.* 29:203–215.

17. Bagnardi, V., M. Rota, E. Botteri, I. et al. 2014. Alcohol consumption and site-specific cancer risk: A comprehensive dose-response. *Brit. J. Cancer.* 12:580–593. doi: 10.1038/bjc.2014.579

18. Stahre, M., J. Roeber, D. Kanny, R. D. Brewer, and X. Zhang. 2014. Contribution of excessive alcohol consumption to deaths and years of potential life lost in the U.S. *Prev. Chronic. Dis.* doi: 10.5888/pcd11.130293

19. National Institute on Alcohol Abuse and Alcoholism. 2013. A snapshot of annual high-risk college drinking consequences. www.collegedrinkingprevention.gov/statssummaries/snapshot.aspx

20. National Institute on Alcohol Abuse and Alcoholism. n.d. Rethinking drinking: How to reduce your risks. http://rethinkingdrinking.niaaa.nih.gov/Thinking-about-a-change/Strategies-for-cutting-down/Tips-To-Try.aspx

Chapter 8

1. Bettendorff, L. 2012. Thiamin. In: Erdman, J. W., I. A. Macdonald, S. H. Zeisel, eds. *Present Knowledge in Nutrition*, 10th ed., pp. 261–279. Washington, DC: ILSI Press.

2. McCollum, E. V. 1957. *A History of Nutrition.* Boston: Houghton Mifflin Co.

3. Institute of Medicine (IOM), Food and Nutrition Board. 1998. *Dietary Reference Intakes for Thiamin, Riboflavin, Niacin, Vitamin B6, Folate, Vitamin B12, Pantothenic Acid, Biotin, and Choline.* Washington, DC: National Academies Press.

4. McCormick, D. B. 2012. Riboflavin. In: Erdman, J. W., I. A. Macdonald, S. H. Zeisel, eds. *Present Knowledge in Nutrition*, 10th ed., pp. 280–292. Washington, DC: ILSI Press.

5. Penberthy, W. T., and J. B. Kirkland. 2012. Niacin. In: Erdman, J. W., I. A. Macdonald, and S. H. Zeisel, eds. *Present Knowledge in Nutrition*, 10th ed., pp. 293–306. Washington, DC: ILSI Press.

6. Da Silva, V. R., K. A. Russel, and J. F. Gregory. 2012. Vitamin B6. In: Erdman, J. W., I. A. Macdonald, and S. H. Zeisel, eds. *Present Knowledge in Nutrition*, 10th ed., pp. 307–320. Washington, DC: ILSI Press.

7. Stover, P. J. 2014. Folic Acid. In: Ross, A. C., B. Caballer, R. Cousins, K. L. Tucker, and T. R. Ziegler, eds. *Modern Nutrition in Health and Disease*, 11th ed., pp. 358–368. Philadelphia: Lippincott Williams & Wilkins.

8. Gropper, S. S., and J. L. Smith. 2012. Folate. In *Advanced Nutrition and Human Health*, 6th ed., pp. 344–354. Belmont, CA: Wadsworth.

9. Stabler, S. P. 2012. Vitamin B12. In: Erdman, J. W., I. A. Macdonald, and S. H. Zeisel, eds. *Present Knowledge in Nutrition*, 10th ed., pp. 343–358. Washington, DC: ILSI Press.

10. Holligan S. D., C. E. Berryman, L. Wang, et al. 2012. Atherosclerotic Cardiovascular Disease. In: Erdman, J. W., I. A. Macdonald, and S. H. Zeisel, eds. *Present Knowledge in Nutrition*, 10th ed., pp. 745–805. Washington, DC: ILSI Press.

11. Huang, T., Y. Chen, B. Yang, et al. 2012. Meta-analysis of B vitamin supplementation on plasma homocysteine, cardiovascular and all-cause mortality. *Clinical Nutrition.* 31(4):448–454.

12. Nicoll, R., J. M. Howard, and M. Y. Henein. 2015. A review of the effect of diet on cardiovascular calcification. *International Journal of Molecular Sciences*, 16(4):8861–8883. doi: http://dx.doi.org/10.3390/ijms16048861

13. Carmel, R. 2014. Cobalamin (Vitamin B_{12}). In: Ross, A. C., B. Caballer, R. Cousins, K. L. Tucker, and T. R. Ziegler, eds. *Modern Nutrition in Health and Disease*, 11th ed., pp. 369–389. Philadelphia: Lippincott Williams & Wilkins.

14. Miller, J. W., and R. B. Rucker. Pantothenic Acid. 2013. In: Erdman, J. W., I. A. Macdonald, and S. H. Zeisel, eds. *Present Knowledge in Nutrition*, 10th ed., pp. 375–390. Washington, DC: ILSI Press.

15. World Health Organization (WHO). 2014. WHO I Guideline: Fortification of Food-grade Salt with Iodine for the Prevention and Control of Iodine Deficiency Disorders. Geneva: WHO. http://apps.who.int/iris/bitstream/10665/136908/1/9789241507929_eng.pdf?ua=1

16. National Institutes of Health (NIH) Office of Dietary Supplements. 2016. Chromium Dietary Supplement Fact Sheet. http://ods.od.nih.gov/factsheets/Chromium-HealthProfessional/

17. Institute of Medicine (IOM). Food and Nutrition Board. 2000. *Dietary Reference Intakes for Vitamin C, Vitamin E, Selenium and Carotenoids.* Washington, DC: National Academy Press.

18. Kristal, A. R., A. K. Darke, J. S. Morris, et al. 2014. Baseline selenium status and effects of selenium and vitamin E supplementation on prostate cancer risk. *The Journal of the National Cancer Institute* 106(3):djt456.

19. Bjelakovic, G., D. Nikolova, and C. Gluud. 2013. Meta-regression analyses, meta-analyses, and trial sequential analyses of the effects of supplementation with beta-carotene, vitamin A, and vitamin E singly or in different combinations on all-cause mortality: Do we have evidence for lack of harm? *PLoS ONE* 8(9):e74558. doi: 10.1371/journal.pone.0074558

20. Fashner, J., K. Ericson, and S. Werner. 2012. Treatment of the common cold in children and adults. *American Family Physician* 86(2):153–159.

21. National Institutes of Health (NIH). U.S. National Library of Medicine. 2015. MedlinePlus. Beta-carotene. https://www.nlm.nih.gov/medlineplus/druginfo/natural/999.html.

22. World Health Organization (WHO). 2016. Micronutrient Deficiencies. Vitamin A Deficiency. http://www.who.int/nutrition/topics/vad/en/

23. U.S. Food and Drug Administration. 2016, July 8. FDA approves Differin Gel 0.1% for over-the-counter use to treat acne. www.fda.gov

24. Albanes, D., O. P. Heinonen, J. K. Huttunen, et al. 1995. Effects of alpha-tocopherol and beta-carotene supplements on cancer incidence in the Alpha-Tocopherol Beta-Carotene Cancer Prevention Study. *The American Journal of Clinical Nutrition* 62(suppl.):1427S–1430S.

25. Omenn, G. S., G. E. Goodman, M. D. Thornquist, et al. 1996. Effects of a combination of beta carotene and vitamin A on lung cancer and cardiovascular disease. *New England Journal of Medicine* 334:1150–1155.

26. Druesne-Pecollo, N., P. Latino-Martel, T. Norat, et al. 2010. Beta-carotene supplementation and cancer risk: a systematic review and meta-analysis of randomized controlled trials. *International Journal of Cancer* 127(1):172–184.

27. Joshipura, K. J., F. B. Hu, J. E. Manson, et al. 2001. The effect of fruit and vegetable intake on risk for coronary heart disease. *Annals of Internal Medicine* 134:1106–1114.

28. Liu, S., I.-M. Lee, U. Ajani, et al. 2001. Intake of vegetables rich in carotenoids and risk of coronary heart disease in men: The Physicians' Health Study. *International Journal of Epidemiology* 30:130–135.

29. The Alpha-Tocopherol, Beta-Carotene Cancer Prevention Study Group (The ATBC Study Group). 1994. The effect of vitamin E and beta carotene on the incidence of lung cancer and other cancers in male smokers. *New England Journal of Medicine* 330:1029–1035.

30. Sesso, H. D., J. E. Buring, W. G. Christen, et al. 2008. Vitamins E and C in the prevention of cardiovascular disease in men: The Physicians' Health Study II randomized controlled trial. *JAMA* 300(18):2123–2133.

31. Lee, I. M., N. R. Cook, J. M. Gaziano, et al. 2005. Vitamin E in the primary prevention of cardiovascular disease and cancer: The Women's Health Study: A randomized controlled trial. *JAMA* 294(1):56–65.

32. Kokubo, Y., H. Iso, I. Saito, et al. 2013. The impact of green tea and coffee consumption on the reduced risk of stroke incidence in Japanese population. *Stroke* 44:1369–1374.

33. Gardener, H., T. Rundek, C. B. Wright, M. S. V. Elkind, and R. L. Sacco. 2013. Coffee and tea consumption are inversely associated with mortality in a multiethnic urban population. *Journal of Nutrition* 143(8):1299–1308.

In Depth: Cancer

1. American Cancer Society. 2016. *Cancer Facts and Figures, 2016.* Atlanta: American Cancer Society. http://www.cancer.org/research/cancerfactsstatistics/cancerfactsfigures2016/.

2. American Cancer Society. 2015. Infections That Can Lead to Cancer. http://www.cancer.org/cancer/cancercauses/othercarcinogens/infectiousagents/infectiousagentsandcancer/index

3. Colantonio, S., M. B. Bracken, and J. Beecker. 2014. The association of indoor tanning and melanoma in adults: Systematic review and meta-analysis. *Journal of the American Academy of Dermatology* 70(5):847–857.

4. Wehner, M. R., M. M. Chren, D. Nameth, et al. 2014. International prevalence of indoor tanning: A systematic review and meta-analysis. *JAMA Dermatology* 150(4):390–400.

5. American Cancer Society. 2014. Signs and Symptoms of Cancer. http://www.cancer.org/cancer/cancerbasics/signs-and-symptoms-of-cancer

6. American Cancer Society. 2016. Eat Healthy. http://www.cancer.org/healthy/eathealthygetactive/eathealthy/index

7. Tong, X., and J. Pelling. 2013. Targeting the PI3K/Akt/mTOR axis by apigenin for cancer prevention. *Anticancer Agents in Medicinal Chemistry* 13(7):971–978.

8. Arango, D., K. Morohashi, A. Yilmaz, et al. 2013. Molecular basis for the action of a dietary flavonoid revealed by the comprehensive identification of apigenin human targets. *PNAS* 110(24):E2153–E2162.

9. Abdull Razis, A. F., and N. M. Noor. 2013. Cruciferous vegetables: Dietary phytochemicals for cancer prevention. *Asian Pacific Journal of Cancer Prevention* 14(3):1565–1570.

10. Bjelakovic, G., D. Nikolova, L. L. Gluud, R. G. Simonetti, and C. Gluud. 2012. Antioxidant supplements for prevention of mortality in healthy participants and patients with various diseases. *Cochrane Database of Systematic Reviews* 3: CD007176. doi: 10.1002/14651858.CD007176.pub2

Chapter 9

1. World Health Organization (WHO) Nutrition. 2015. Micronutrient deficiencies: Iron deficiency anemia. http://www.who.int/nutrition/topics/ida/en/#

2. Aggett, P. J. 2012. Iron. In: Erdman, J. W., I. A. Macdonald, S. H. Zeisel, eds. *Present Knowledge in Nutrition*, 10th ed., pp. 506–520. Washington, DC: ILSI Press.

3. Gropper, S. S., and J. L. Smith. 2013. *Advanced Nutrition and Human Health*, 6th ed. Belmont, CA: Wadsworth.

4. Institute of Medicine (IOM), Food and Nutrition Board. 2002. *Dietary Reference Intakes for Vitamin A, Vitamin K, Arsenic, Boron, Chromium, Copper, Iodine, Iron, Manganese, Molybdenum, Nickel, Silicon, Vanadium, and Zinc.* Washington, DC: National Academies Press.

5. Sharp, P. A. 2010. Intestinal iron absorption: Regulation by dietary and systemic factors. *International Journal for Vitamin and Nutrition Research* 80(4–5)231–242.

6. Spanierman, C. S. 2014. Iron toxicity in emergency medicine. *Medscape Reference. Drugs, Disease and Procedures.* http://emedicine.medscape.com/article/815213-followup

7. Duchini, A. 2016. Hemochromatosis. *Medscape Reference. Drugs, Disease and Procedures.* http://emedicine.medscape.com/article/177216-overview

8. Milman, N. 2012. Postpartum anemia II: Prevention and treatment. *Annals of Hematology* 91(2):143–154. PubMed PMID: PMID: 22160256.

9. Science, M., J. Johnstone, D. E. Roth, G. Guyatt, and M. Loeb. 2012. Zinc for the treatment of the common cold: a systematic review and meta-analysis of randomized controlled trials. *CMAJ: Canadian Medical Association Journal* 184(10):E551–561.

10. Singh, M., and R. R. Das. 2012. Zinc for the common cold. *Cochrane Database of Systemic Reviews* 2. Art. No. Cd001364. doi:10.1002/14651858

11. Institute of Medicine (IOM), Food and Nutrition Board. 1998. *Dietary Reference Intakes for Thiamin, Riboflavin, Niacin, Vitamin B6, Folate, Vitamin B12, Pantothenic Acid, Biotin, and Choline.* Washington, DC: National Academies Press.

12. Ferland, G. 2012. Vitamin K. In: Erdman, J. W., I. A. Macdonald, S. H. Zeisel, eds. *Present Knowledge in Nutrition*, 10th ed., pp. 230–247. Washington, DC: ILSI Press.

13. Hemilä, H., and E. Chalker. 2013. Vitamin C for preventing and treating the common cold. *Cochrane Database of Systemic Reviews* 1. Art. No. CD000980. doi:10.1002/14651858.CD000980.pub4.

14. NIH Osteoporosis and Related Bone Diseases National Resource Center. 2015. Osteoporosis: Peak bone mass in women. http://www.niams.nih.gov/Health_Info/Bone/Osteoporosis/bone_mass.asp

15. Institute of Medicine, Food and Nutrition Board. 1997. *Dietary Reference Intakes for Calcium, Phosphorus, Magnesium, Vitamin D, and Fluoride.* Washington, DC: National Academies Press.

16. Hoy, M. K., and J. D. Goldman. 2014. Calcium intake of the U.S. population. *What We Eat in America*, NHANES 2009–2010. Food Surveys Research Group, Dietary Data Brief No. 13.

17. U.S. Department of Health and Human Services, National Kidney and Urologic Diseases Information Clearinghouse. 2013. Diet for kidney stone prevention. NIH Publication No. 13-6425. http://www.niddk.nih.gov

18. Chang, A. R., M. Lazo, L. J. Appel, O. M. Gutiérrez, and M. E. Grams. 2014. High dietary phosphorus intake is associated with all-cause mortality: results from NHANES III. *American Journal of Clinical Nutrition* 99:320–327.

19. Qu, X., F. Jin, Y. Hao, Z. Zhu, H. Li, T. Tang, and K. Dai. 2013. Nonlinear association between magnesium intake and the risk of colorectal cancer. *Journal of Gastroenterology and Hepatology* 25(3):309–318.

20. Institute of Medicine, Food and Nutrition Board. 2010. *Dietary Reference Intakes for Calcium and Vitamin D.* Washington, DC: National Academies Press.

21. Vimaleswaran, V. S., D. J. Berry, C. Lu, E., et al. 2013. Causal relationship between obesity and vitamin D status: Bi-directional Mendelian randomization analysis of multiple cohorts. *PLoS Medicine* 10(2):e1001383.

22. Thacher, T. D., P. R. Fischer, P. J. Tebben, et al. 2013. Increasing incidence of nutritional rickets: A population-based study in Olmsted County, Minnesota. *Mayo Clinic Proceedings* 88(2): 176–183.

23. Fang, Y., C. Hu, X. Tao, Y. Wan, and F. Tao. 2012. Effect of vitamin K on bone mineral density: A meta-analysis of randomized controlled trials. *Journal of Bone and Mineral Metabolism* 30(1):60–68.

24. Forrest, K. Y., and W. L. Stuhldreher. 2011. Prevalence and correlates of vitamin D deficiency in US adults. *Nutrition Research* 31(1): 48–54.

25. Song, Y., L. Wang, A. G. Pittas, et al. 2013. Blood 25-hydroxy vitamin D levels and incident type 2 diabetes. *Diabetes Care* 36(5):1422–1428.

26. Zittermann, A., S. Iodice, S. Pilz, et al. 2012. Vitamin D deficiency and mortality risk in the general population: A meta-analysis of prospective cohort studies. *American Journal of Clinical Nutrition* 95:91–100.

27. Holick, M. F., N. C. Binkley, H. A. Bischoff-Ferrari, C. M. Gordon, D. A. Hanley, et al. 2012. Guidelines for preventing and treating vitamin D deficiency and insufficiency revisited. *Journal of Clinical Endocrinology & Metabolism* 97(4):1153–1158.

28. Holick, M. F., N. C. Binkley, H. A. Bischoff-Ferrari, et al. 2011. Evaluation, treatment, and prevention of vitamin D deficiency: An Endocrine Society Clinical Practice Guideline. *Journal of Clinical Endocrinology & Metabolism* 96:1911–1930.

29. International Osteoporosis Foundation. 2014, December 16. Are skin cancer prevention campaigns scaring people away from healthy sun exposure? *News Stories.* http://www.iofbonehealth.org/news/are-skin-cancer-prevention-campaigns-scaring-people-away-healthy-sun-exposure

In Depth: Osteoporosis

1. National Osteoporosis Foundation. 2016. What is osteoporosis and what causes it? https://www.nof.org/patients/what-is-osteoporosis/

2. International Osteoporosis Foundation. 2015. Facts and statistics. http://www.iofbonehealth.org/facts-statistics

3. Urano, T., and S. Inoue. 2015, April 11. Recent genetic discoveries in osteoporosis, sarcopenia and obesity. *Endocrine Journal.* epub ahead of print. doi:10/1507/endocrj.EJ15-0154.

4. Yoon, V., N. M. Maalouf, and K. Sakhaee. 2012. The effects of smoking on bone metabolism. *Osteoporosis International* 23:2081–2092.

5. Maurel, D. B., N. Boisseau, C. L. Benhamou, and C. Jaffre. 2012. Alcohol and bone: Review of dose effects and mechanisms. *Osteoporosis International* 23(1):1–16.

6. Hallström, H., L. Byberg, A. Glynn, et al. 2013. Long-term coffee consumption in relation to fracture risk and bone mineral density in women. *American Journal of Epidemiology* 178(6):898–909.

7. Xie, H. L., B. H. Wu, W. Q. Xue, et al. 2013. Greater intake of fruit and vegetables is associated with a lower risk of osteoporotic hip fractures in elderly Chinese: A 1:1 matched case-control study. *Osteoporosis International* 24(11):2827–2836.

8. Boeing, H., A. Bechthold, A. Bub, et al. 2012. Critical review: Vegetables and fruit in the prevention of chronic diseases. *European Journal of Nutrition* 51(6):637–663.

9. Dawson-Hughes, B., and S. S. Harris. 2002. Calcium intake influences the association of protein intake with rates of bone loss in elderly men and women. *American Journal of Clinical Nutrition* 75:773–779.

10. Calvez, J., N. Poupin, C. Chesneau, C. Lassale, and D. Tomé. 2012. Protein intake, calcium balance and health consequences. *European Journal of Clinical Nutrition* 66:281–295.

11. Moyer, V.A., on behalf of the U.S. Preventive Services Task Force. 2013. Vitamin D and calcium supplementation to prevent fractures in adults: U.S. Preventive Services Task Force Recommendation statement. *Annals of Internal Medicine* 158(9):691–696.

12. Park, S. M., J. Jee, J. Y. Joung, et al. 2014. High dietary sodium intake assessed by 24-hour urine specimen increase urinary calcium excretion and bone resorption marker. *Journal of Bone Metabolism* 21(3):189–194.

13. Institute of Medicine, Food and Nutrition Board. 1997. *Dietary Reference Intakes for Calcium, Phosphorus, Magnesium, Vitamin D, and Fluoride.* Washington, DC: National Academies Press.

14. Evans, R. K., C. H. Negus, A. J. Centi, et al. 2012. Peripheral QCT sector analysis reveals early exercise-induced increases in tibial bone mineral density. *Journal of Musculoskeletal and Neuronal Interactions* 12(3):155–164.

15. Marques, E. A., J. Mota, and J. Carvalho. 2012. Exercise effects on bone mineral density in older adults: A meta-analysis of randomized controlled trials. *AGE* 34(6):1493–1515.

16. National Osteoporosis Foundation (NOF). 2016, April 11. NOF responds to *The New York Times* article, "Exercise is Not the Path to Strong Bones." https://www.nof.org/news/nof-responds-to-the-new-york-times-article-exercise-is-not-the-path-to-strong-bones/

17. National Institute of Arthritis and Musculoskeletal and Skin Diseases. 2014. Bone health for life: Easy-to-read information for patients and families. http://www.niams.nih.gov/Health_Info/Bone_Health/default.asp#6

18. Bolam, K. A., J. G. Z. van Uffelen, and D. R. Taaffe. 2013. The effect of physical exercise on bone density in middle-aged and older men: A systematic review. *Osteoporosis International* 24(11):2749–2762.

19. Wilhelm, M., G. Roskovensky, K. Emery, et al. Effect of resistance exercises on function in older adults with osteoporosis or osteopenia: A systematic review. *Physiotherapy Canada* 64(4): 386–394.

20. Real J., G. Galindo, L. Galván, et al. 2015. Use of oral bis-phosphonates in primary prevention of fractures in postmenopausal women: A population-based cohort study. *PLoS ONE* 10(4):e0118178.

21. Lee, S., R. V. Yin, H. Hirpara, et al. 2015. Increased risk for atypical fractures associated with bisphosphonate use. *Family Practice* 32(3):276–281.

22. Writing Group for the Women's Health Initiative Investigators. 2002. Risks and benefits of estrogen plus progestin in healthy postmenopausal women. Principal results from the Women's Health Initiative randomized control trial. *JAMA* 288:321–332.

23. U.S. Preventive Services Task Force. 2013. Understanding task force recommendations. Menopausal hormone therapy for the primary prevention of chronic conditions: U.S. Preventive Services Task Force recommendation statement. *Annals of Internal Medicine* 158(1):47–54.

24. Bolland, M. J., A. Grey, A. Avenell, G. D. Gamble, and I. R. Reid. 2011. Calcium supplements with or without vitamin D and risk of cardiovascular events: Reanalysis of the Women's Health Initiative limited dataset and meta-analysis. *BMJ* 342:d2040, doi:10.1136/bmj.d2040.

25. Prentice, R. L., M. B. Pettinger, R. D. Jackson, et al. 2013. Health risks and benefits from calcium and vitamin D supplementation: Women's Health Initiative clinical trial and cohort study. *Osteoporosis International* 24(12):567–580.

26. Paziana, K., and S. Pazaianas. 2015. Calcium supplements controversy in osteoporosis: A physiological mechanism supporting cardiovascular adverse effects. *Endocrine* 48(3):776–778.

27. National Institutes of Health. Office of Dietary Supplements. 2016. Vitamin D. Fact Sheet for Health Professionals. https://ods.od.nih.gov/factsheets/VitaminD-HealthProfessional/

Chapter 10

1. Flegal, K. M., B. K. Kit, H. Orpana, and B. I. Graubard. 2013. Association of all-cause mortality with overweight and obesity using standard body mass index categories. A systematic review and meta-analysis. *JAMA* 309(1):71–82.

2. Willett, W. C., F. B. Hu, and M. Thun. 2013. Letters. Overweight, obesity and all-cause mortality. *JAMA* 309(16):1681–1682.

3. Hughes, V. 2013. The big fat truth. *Nature* 497(23 May 2013):428–430. www.nature.com/news/the-big-fat-truth-1.13039#/b9

4. Pettitt, D. J., J. Talton, D. Dabelea, et al. 2014. Prevalence of diabetes in U.S. youth in 2009: The SEARCH for Diabetes in Youth Study. *Diabetes Care* 37(2):402–408.

5. Chen, L., D. J. Magliano, and P. Z. Zimmet. 2012. The worldwide epidemiology of type 2 diabetes mellitus—present and future perspectives. *Nature Reviews Endocrinology* 8:228–236.

6. Hall, K. D., S. B. Heymsfield, J. W. Kemnitz, et al. 2012. Energy balance and its components: implications for body weight regulation. *American Journal of Clinical Nutrition* 95(4):989–994.

7. von Loeffelholz, C. The role of non-exercise activity thermogenesis in human obesity. 2014. Endotext www.ncbi.nlm.nih.gov/books/NBK279077/

8. Keane, E., R. Layte, J. Harrington, P. M. Kearney, and I. J. Perry. 2012. Measured parental weight status and familial socio-economic status correlates with childhood overweight and obesity at age 9. *PLoS One.* http://dx.doi.org/10.1371/journal.pone.0043503

9. Manco, M., and B. Dallapiccola. 2012. Genetics of pediatric obesity. *Pediatrics* 130:123–133.

10. Locke, A. E., B. Kahali, S. I. Berndt, et al. 2015. Genetic studies of body mass index yield new insights for obesity biology. *Nature* 518:197–206.

11. Harbron, J., L. van der Merwe, M. G. Zaahl, M. J. Kotze, and M. Senekal. 2014. Fat mass and obesity-associated (FTO) gene polymorphisms are associated with physical activity, food intake, eating behaviors, psychological health, and modeled change in body mass index in overweight/obese Caucasian adults. *Nutrients* 6(8):3130–3152.

12. Fothergill, E., J. Guo, L. Howard, et al. 2016. Persistent metabolic adaptation 6 years after "The Biggest Loser" competition. *Obesity.* doi:10.1002/oby.21538.

13. Speakman, J. R. 2014. If body fatness is under physiological regulation, then how come we have an obesity epidemic? *Physiology* 29(2):88–98.

14. Gosby, A. K., A. D. Conigrave, D. Raubenheimer, and S. J. Simpson. 2014. Protein leverage and energy intake. *Obesity Reviews* 15:183–191.

15. Booth, S. 2015. Are your meds making you gain weight? 2015. WebMD. www.webmd.com/diet/obesity/medication-weight-gain.

16. Briggs, D. I., S. H. Lockie, Q. Wu, et al. 2013. Calorie-restricted weight loss reverses high-fat diet-induced ghrelin resistance, which contributes to rebound weight gain in a ghrelin-dependent manner. *Endocrinology* 154:700–717.

17. Perry, B., and Y. Wang. 2012. Appetite regulation and weight control: The role of gut hormones. *Nutrition and Diabetes* 2:e26. doi:10.1038/nutd.2011.21.

18. Babakus, W. S., and J. L. Thompson. 2012. Physical activity among South Asian women: a systematic, mixed-methods review. *International Journal of Behavioral Nutrition and Physical Activity* 9:150. doi: 10.1186/1479-5868-9-150.

19. Komar-Samardzija, M., L. T. Braun, J. K. Keithley, and L. T. Quinn. 2012. Factors associated with physical activity levels in African-American women with type 2 diabetes. *Journal of the American Academy of Nurse Practitioners* 24:209–217.

20. Pan, L., B. Sherry, R. Njai, and H. M. Blanck. 2012. Food insecurity is associated with obesity among US adults in 12 states. *Journal of the Academy of Nutrition and Dietetics* 112(9):1403–1409.

21. Jerrett, M., R. McConnell, J. Wolch, et al. 2014. Traffic-related air pollution and obesity formation in children: A longitudinal, multilevel analysis. *Environmental Health* 13:49. www.ehjournal.net/content/13/1/49

22. Ding, D., T. Sugiyama, and N. Owen. 2012. Habitual active transport, TV viewing and weight gain: A four-year follow-up study. *Preventive Medicine* 54:201–204.

23. Brixval, C. S., S. L. B. Rayce, M. Rasmussen, B. E. Holstein, and P. Due. 2012. Overweight, body image and bullying—An epidemiological study of 11- to 15-years-olds. *European Journal of Public Health* 22(1):126–130.

24. Academy of Nutrition and Dietetics. 2016. Staying Away from Fad Diets. www.eatright.org/resource/health/weight-loss/fad-diets/staying-away-from-fad-diets

25. Prentice, R. L., B. Caan, R. T. Chlebowski, et al. 2006. Low-fat dietary pattern and risk of invasive breast cancer: The Women's Health Initiative randomized controlled dietary modification trial. *JAMA* 295:629–642.

26. Beresford, S. A., K. C. Johnson, C. Ritenbaugh, et al. 2006. Low-fat dietary pattern and risk of colorectal cancer: The Women's Health Initiative randomized controlled dietary modification trial. *JAMA* 295:643–654.

27. Howard, B. V., L. Van Horn, J. Hsia, et al. 2006. Low-fat dietary pattern and risk of cardiovascular disease: The Women's Health Initiative randomized controlled dietary modification trial. *JAMA* 295:655–666.

28. Howard, B. V., J. E. Manson, M. L. Stefanick, et al. 2006. Low-fat dietary pattern and weight change over 7 years: The Women's Health Initiative dietary modification trial. *JAMA* 295:39–49.

29. Hu, T., K. T. Mills, L. Yao, et al. 2012. Effects of low-carbohydrate diets versus low-fat diets on metabolic factors: A meta-analysis of randomized controlled clinical trials. *American Journal of Epidemiology* 176(Suppl 7):S44–S54.

30. Piernas, C., and B. M. Popkin. 2011. Food portion patterns and trends among U.S. children and the relationship to total eating occasion size, 1977–2006. *Journal of Nutrition* 141(6):1159–1164.

31. Freedman, M. R., and C. Brochado. 2012. Reducing portion size reduces food intake and plate waste. *Obesity* 18(9):1864–1866.

32. Pérez-Escamilla, R., J. E. Obbagy, J. M. Altman, et al. 2012. Dietary energy density and body weight in adults and children: A systematic review. *Journal of the Academy of Nutrition and Dietetics.* 112(5):671–684.

33. The National Weight Control Registry. NWCR Facts. www.nwcr.ws/Research/default.htm Accessed August 29, 2016.

34. Timmerman, G. M., and A. Brown. 2012. The effect of a *Mindful Restaurant Eating* intervention on weight management in women. *Journal of Nutrition Education and Behavior* 44:22–28.

35. Miller, C. K., J. L. Kristeller, A. Headings, H. Nagaraja, and W. F. Miser. 2012. Comparative effectiveness of a mindful eating intervention to a diabetes self-management intervention among adults with type 2 diabetes: A pilot study. *Journal of the Academy of Nutrition and Dietetics.* 112:1835–1842.

36. Howard, B. V., L. Van Horn, J. Hsia, et al. 2006. Low-fat dietary pattern and risk of cardiovascular disease: The Women's Health Initiative randomized controlled dietary modification trial. *JAMA* 295(6):655–666.

37. Prentice, R. L., B. Caan, R. T. Chlebowski, et al. 2006. Low-fat dietary pattern and risk of invasive breast cancer: The Women's Health Initiative randomized controlled dietary modification trial. *JAMA* 295(6):629–642.

38. Beresford, S. A. A., K. C. Johnson, C. Ritenbaugh, et al. 2006. Low-fat dietary pattern and risk of colorectal cancer: The Women's Health Initiative randomized controlled dietary modification trial. *JAMA* 295(6):643–654.

39. Howard, B. V., J. E. Manson, M. L. Stefanick, et al. 2006. Low-fat dietary pattern and weight change over 7 years: The Women's Health Initiative dietary modification trial. *JAMA* 295(6):39–49.

40. Krebs, J. D., C. R. Elley, A. Parry-Strong, H. Lunt, P. L. Drury, et al. 2012. The Diabetes Excess Weight Loss (DEWL) Trial: A randomized controlled trial of high-protein versus high-carbohydrate diets over 2 years in type 2 diabetes. *Diabetologia* 55:905–914.

41. de Souza, R. J., G. A. Bray, V. J. Carey, et al. 2012. Effects of four weight-loss diets differing in fat, protein, and carbohydrate on fat mass, lean mass, visceral adipose tissue, and hepatic fat: Results from the POUNDS LOST trial. *American Journal of Clinical Nutrition* 95:614–625.

42. Harvard School of Public Health. 2016. Low-fat diet not a cure-all. *The Nutrition Source.* www.hsph.harvard.edu/nutritionsource/low-fat/

43. Manheimer, E. W., E. J. van Zuuren, Z. Fedorowicz, and H. Pijl. 2015. Paleolithic nutrition for metabolic syndrome: Systematic

review and meta-analysis. *American Journal of Clinical Nutrition.* Epub ahead of print, doi:10.3945/ajcn.115.113613.

44. Academy of Nutrition and Dietetics. 2015. Should we eat like our caveman ancestors? www.eatright.org/resource/health/weight-loss/fad-diets/should-we-eat-like-our-caveman-ancestors

In Depth: Obesity

1. Ogden, C. L., M. D. Carroll, B. K. Kit, and K. M. Flegal. 2014. Prevalence of childhood and adult obesity in the United States, 2011–2012. *JAMA* 311(8):806–814.
2. Beltrán-Sánchez, H., M. O. Harhay, M. M. Harhay, and S. McElligott. 2013. Prevalence and trends of metabolic syndrome in the adult U.S. population, 1999–2010. *Journal of the American College of Cardiology* 62(8):697–703.
3. MyHealthyWaist.org. 2016. The concept of CMR. www.myhealthywaist.org/the-concept-of-cmr/
4. Michaud, M., L. Balardy, G. Moulis, et al. 2013. Proinflammatory cytokines, aging, and age-related diseases. *Journal of Post-Acute Long-Term Care Medicine* 14(12):877–882.
5. Foresight. Government Office for Science. 2007. Tackling obesities: Future choices—project report. 2nd ed. https://www.gov.uk/government/uploads/system/uploads/attachment_data/file/287937/07-1184x-tackling-obesities-future-choices-report.pdf
6. Nicklas, J. M., K. W. Huskey, R. B. Davis, and C. C. Wee. 2012. Successful weight loss among obese U.S. adults. *American Journal of Preventive Medicine* 42(5):481–485.
7. Thomas, J. G., D. S. Bond, S. Phelan, J. O. Hill, and R. R. Wing. 2014. Weight-loss maintenance for 10 years in the National Weight Control Registry. *American Journal of Preventive Medicine* 46(1):17–23.
8. Institute of Medicine, Food and Nutrition Board. 2002. *Dietary Reference Intakes for Energy, Carbohydrate, Fiber, Fat, Fatty Acids, Cholesterol, Protein, and Amino Acids (Macronutrients).* Washington, DC: National Academies Press.
9. Mayo Clinic. 2015. Healthy Lifestyle. Weight loss. Prescription weight loss drugs. www.mayoclinic.org/healthy-lifestyle/weight-loss/in-depth/weight-loss-drugs/art-20044832
10. National Institutes of Health. Office of Dietary Supplements. 2015. Dietary supplements for weight loss. Fact sheet for health professionals. http://ods.od.nih.gov/factsheets/WeightLoss-HealthProfessional/#en8
11. Chang, S.-H., C. R. T. Stoll, J. Song, et al. 2014. The effectiveness and risks of bariatric surgery. An updated systematic review and meta-analysis, 2003–2012. *JAMA Surgery* 149(3):275–287.

Chapter 11

1. Caspersen, C. J., K. E. Powell, and G. M. Christensen. 1985. Physical activity, exercise, and physical fitness: Definitions and distinctions for health-related research. *Public Health Reports* 100:126–131.
2. American College of Sports Medicine. 2014. *ACSM's Health-Related Physical Fitness Assessment Manual*, 4th ed. Philadelphia: Lippincott Williams & Wilkins.
3. Heyward, V. H., and A. Gibson. 2014. *Advanced Fitness Assessment and Exercise Prescription*, 7th ed. Champaign, IL: Human Kinetics.
4. Nutrition, Physical Activity and Obesity Data, Trends and Maps website. 2015. U.S. Department of Health and Human Services, Centers for Disease Control and Prevention (CDC), National Center for Chronic Disease Prevention and Health Promotion, Division of Nutrition, Physical Activity and Obesity, Atlanta, GA, 2015. Available at www.cdc.gov/nccdphp/DNPAO/index.html
5. U.S. Department of Health and Human Services. 2009. 2008 Physical Activity Guidelines for Americans. http://health.gov/paguidelines/guidelines/default.aspx#toc
6. Institute of Medicine, Food and Nutrition Board. 2002. *Dietary Reference Intakes for Energy, Carbohydrates, Fiber, Fat, Protein and Amino Acids (Macronutrients)*. Washington, DC: National Academy of Sciences.

7. Gunnell, K. E., P. R. E. Crocker, D. E. Mack, P. M. Wilson, and B. D. Zumbo. 2014. Goal contents, motivation, psychological need satisfaction, well-being and physical activity: A test of self-determination theory over 6 months. *Psychology of Sport and Exercise* 15(1):19–29.
8. Teixeira, P. J., M. N. Silva, J. Mata, A. L. Palmeira, and D. Markland. 2012. Motivation, self-determination, and long-term weight control. *The International Journal of Behavioral Nutrition and Physical Activity* 9:22. www.ijbnpa.org/content/9/1/22
9. Centers for Disease Control and Prevention. 2015. Target Heart Rate and Estimated Maximum Heart Rate. www.cdc.gov/physicalactivity/basics/measuring/heartrate.htm
10. Bogdanis, G. C. 2012. Effects of physical activity and inactivity on muscle fatigue. *Frontiers in Physiology* 3:142. www.ncbi.nlm.nih.gov/pmc/articles/PMC3355468/
11. Glenn, T. C., N. A. Martin, D. L. McArthur, et al. 2015. Endogenous nutritive support after traumatic brain injury: Peripheral lactate production for glucose supply via gluconeogenesis. *Journal of Neurotrauma* 32(11):811–819.
12. Gibala, M. J., J. P. Little, M. J. MacDonald, and J. A. Hawley. 2012. Physiological adaptations to low-volume, high-intensity interval training in health and disease. *The Journal of Physiology* 590:1077–1084.
13. Pritchett, K., and R. Pritchett. 2013. Chocolate milk: A post-exercise recovery beverage for endurance sports. *Medicine and Sport Science* 59:127–134.
14. American College of Sports Medicine, Academy of Nutrition and Dietetics, and Dietitians of Canada. 2016. Nutrition and Athletic Performance. Joint Position Statement. *Medicine and Science in Sports and Exercise* 48(3):543–568.
15. Broeder, C. E., J. Quindry, K. Brittingham, et al. 2000. The Andro Project: Physiological and hormonal influences of androstenedione supplementation in men 35 to 65 years old participating in a high-intensity resistance training program. *Archives of Internal Medicine* 160:3093–3104.
16. Burrows, T., K. Pursey, M. Neve, and P. Stanwell. 2013. What are the health implications associated with the consumption of energy drinks? A systematic review. *Nutrition Reviews* 71(3):135–148.
17. Blancquaert, L., I. Everaert, and W. Derave. 2015. Beta-alanine supplementation, muscle carnosine and exercise performance. *Current Opinion in Clinical Nutrition and Metabolic Care* 18(1):63–70.
18. U.S. Department of Health and Human Services. 1996. *Physical Activity and Health: A Report of the Surgeon General.* Atlanta: U.S. Department of Health and Human Services, Centers for Disease Control and Prevention, National Centers for Chronic Disease Prevention and Health Promotion.
19. Arem, H., S. C. Moore, A. Patel, et al. 2015. Leisure time physical activity and mortality: A detailed pooled analysis of the dose-response relationship. *JAMA Internal Medicine.* 175(6):959–967.
20. Gebel, K., D. Ding, T. Chey, et al. 2015. Effect of moderate to vigorous physical activity on all-cause mortality in middle-aged and older Australians. *JAMA Internal Medicine* 175(6):970–977.

In Depth: Disorders Related to Body Image, Eating, and Exercise

1. Advertising Standards Authority of Britain. 2016. Rulings. www.asa.org.uk
2. American College Health Association. 2015. *National College Health Assessment II: Reference Group Executive Summary Spring, 2015.* Hanover, MD: American College Health Association.
3. van Vliet, J. S., P. Q. Gustafsson, and N. Nelson. 2016. Feeling "too fat" rather than being "too fat" increases unhealthy eating habits among adolescents—even in boys. *Food & Nutrition Research* 60. doi:10.3402/fnr.v60.29530.
4. Cook, B., T. A. Karr, and C. Zunker, 2015. The influence of exercise identity and social physique anxiety on exercise dependence. *Journal of Behavioral Addictions* 4(3):195–199.

5. Scribner, C., and K. A. Beals. 2016. Disordered eating in athletes. In: Karpinski, C., and C. A. Rosenbloom, eds. *Sports Nutrition. A Practice Manual for Professionals*, 6th ed. Chicago, IL: Academy of Nutrition and Dietetics.

6. Landolfi, E. 2013. Exercise addiction. *Sports Medicine* 43(2):111–119. doi:10.1007/s40279-012-0013-x

7. Weinstein, A., G. Maayan, and Y. Weinstein. 2015. A study on the relationship between compulsive exercise, depression and anxiety. *Journal of Behavioral Addictions* 4(4):315–318.

8. Mufaddel, A., O. T. Osman, F. Almugaddam, and M. Jafferany. 2013. A review of body dysmorphic disorder and its presentation in different clinical settings. *Primary Care Companion for CNS Disorders* 15(4):PCC.12r01464.

9. Phillipou, A., and D. Castle. 2105. Body dysmorphic disorder in men. *Australian Family Physician* 44(11):798–801.

10. Suffolk, M. T., T. M. Dovey, H. Goodwin, and C. Meyer. 2013. Muscle dysmorphia: methodological issues, implications for research. *Eating Disorders* 21(5):437–457. doi:http://dx.doi.org/10.1080/10640266.2013.828520

11. Weltzin, T. E. 2012. A silent problem: Males with eating disorders in the workplace. National Association of Anorexia Nervosa and Associated Disorders. www.anad.org.

12. Browne, H. A., S. L. Gair, J. M. Scharf, and D. E. Grice. 2014. Genetics of obsessive-compulsive disorder and related disorders. *Psychiatric Clinics of North America* 37(3):319–335.

13. Grave, R. D. 2011. Eating disorders: Progress and challenges. *European Journal of Internal Medicine* 22:153–160.

14. Crowther, J., K. E. Smith, and G. A. Williams. 2015. Familial risk factors and eating disorders. *The Wiley Handbook of Eating Disorders*. Hoboken, NJ: Wiley, pp. 338–351.

15. Treasure, J., A. M. Claudino, and N. Zucker. 2010. Eating disorders. *Lancet* 375:583–593.

16. Strasburger, V. C., A. B. Jordan, and E. Donnerstein. 2010. Health effects of media on children and adolescents. *Pediatrics* 125(4): 756–767.

17. Strasburger, V. C., E. Donnerstein, and B. J. Bushman. 2014. Why is it so hard to believe that media influence children and adolescents? *Pediatrics* 133(4):571–573.

18. Tiggemann, M., and A. Slater. 2013. NetGirls: The Internet, Facebook, and body image concern in adolescent girls. *International Journal of Eating Disorders* 46(6):630–633. doi:http://dx.doi.org/10.1002/eat.22141

19. Giordano, S. 2015. Eating disorders and the media. *Current Opinion in Psychiatry* 28(6):478–482.

20. Culbert, K. M., S. E. Racine, and K. L. Klump. 2015. Research review: What we have learned about the causes of eating disorders—a synthesis of sociocultural, psychological, and biological research. *Journal of Child Psychology and Psychiatry, and Allied Disciplines* 56(11):1141–1164. doi:http://dx.doi.org/10.1111/jcpp.12441

21. Fitzsimmons-Craft, E. E. 2011. Social psychological theories of disordered eating in college women: Review and integration. *Clinical Psychology Review* 31(7):1224–1237.

22. Costa-Font, J., and M. Jofre-Bonet. 2011. Anorexia, body image, and peer effects: Evidence from a sample of European women. *Centre for Economic Performance*: CEP discussion paper No. 1098. http://cep.lse.ac.uk/pubs/download/dp1098.pdf

23. Young, S., P. Rhodes, S. Touyz, and P. Hay. 2013. The relationship between obsessive-compulsive personality disorder traits, obsessive-compulsive disorder and excessive exercise in patients with anorexia nervosa: A systematic review. *Journal of Eating Disorders* 1:16.

24. American Psychiatric Association (APA). 2015. Eating disorders. www.psychiatry.org/eating-disorders

25. Koven, N. S., and A. W. Abry. 2015. The clinical basis of orthorexia nervosa: Emerging perspectives. *Neuropsychiatric Disease and Treatment* 11:385–394.

26. Keel, P. K., T. A. Brown, L. A. Holland, and L. D. Bodell. 2012. Empirical classification of eating disorders. *Annual Review of Clinical Psychology* 8:381–404.

27. Murnen, S. K., and L. Smolak. 2015. Gender and eating disorders. *The Wiley Handbook of Eating Disorders*. Hoboken, NJ: Wiley, pp. 352–366.

28. MacLean, A., H. Sweeting, L. Walker, et al. 2015. "It's not healthy and it's decidedly not masculine": A media analysis of UK newspaper representations of eating disorders in males. *BMJ Open* 5(5). doi:http://dx.doi.org/10.1136/bmjopen-2014-007468

29. National Eating Disorders Association. 2016. Get the facts on eating disorders, 2016. www.nationaleatingdisorders.org/get-facts-eating-disorders

30. National Association of Anorexia Nervosa and Associated Disorders. 2016. Eating disorder statistics. www.anad.org/get-information/about-eating-disorders/eating-disorders-statistics/

31. American Psychiatric Association (APA). 2013. *Diagnostic and Statistical Manual of Mental Disorders (DSM-V)*, 5th ed. Washington, DC: Author.

32. National Institutes of Mental Health, National Institutes of Health. 2012. Spotlight on eating disorders. www.nimh.nih.gov/about/director/2012/spotlight-on-eating-disorders.shtml

33. National Institutes of Mental Health, National Institutes of Health. 2014. Eating disorders: About more than food. NIH Publication No. TR 14-4901. www.nimh.nih.gov/health/publications/eating-disorders-new-trifold/eating-disorders-pdf_148810.pdf

34. National Institutes of Mental Health, National Institutes of Health. 2016. Eating disorders. https://www.nimh.nih.gov/health/topics/eating-disorders/index.shtml

35. Vander Wal, J. S. 2012. Night eating syndrome: A critical review of the literature. *Clinical Psychology Review* 32:49–59.

36. Gallant, A. R., J. Lundgren, and V. Drapeau. 2012. The night-eating syndrome and obesity. *Obesity Reviews* 13(6):528–536. doi:http://dx.doi.org/10.1111/j.1467-789X.2011.00975.x

37. Mountjoy, M., J. Sundgot-Borgen, L. Burke, et al. 2014. International Olympic Committee Consensus Statement: Beyond the female athlete triad-relative energy deficiency in sport (Red-S). *British Journal of Sports Medicine* 48(7):491–497. doi:http://dx.doi.org/10.1136/bjsports-2014-093502

38. Nattiv, A., A. B. Loucks, M. M. Manore, et al. 2007. The female athlete triad. *Medicine & Science in Sports & Exercise* 39(10):1867–1882.

39. Reiter, S. C., and L. Graves. 2010. Nutrition therapy for eating disorders. *Nutrition in Clinical Practice* 25:122–136.

Chapter 12

1. U.S. Centers for Disease Control and Prevention [CDC]. 2014, January 8. Estimates of foodborne illness in the United States. www.cdc.gov/foodborneburden/index.html

2. U.S. Government Accountability Office [GAO]. 2015. Improving federal oversight of food safety. www.gao.gov/highrisk/revamping_food_safety/why_did_study#t = 0

3. U.S. Food and Drug Administration [FDA]. 2015, September 3. Hazard Analysis Critical Control Point [HACCP]. www.fda.gov/Food/GuidanceRegulation/HACCP/default.htm

4. U.S. Centers for Disease Control and Prevention [CDC]. 2015. Food Safety Progress Report for 2014. www.cdc.gov/foodnet/pdfs/progress-report-2014-508c.pdf

5. U.S. Centers for Disease Control and Prevention [CDC]. 2015, May 27. New CDC data on foodborne illness outbreaks. www.cdc.gov/features/foodborne-diseases-data/

6. U.S. Centers for Disease Control and Prevention [CDC]. 2015, December 10. Norovirus. www.cdc.gov/norovirus/index.html

7. U.S. Centers for Disease Control and Prevention [CDC]. 2015, May 31. Viral hepatitis. www.cdc.gov/hepatitis/

8. U.S. Centers for Disease Control and Prevention [CDC]. 2015, October 8. Foodborne Outbreak Online Database (FOOD Tool): 1998–2014. www.cdc.gov/foodborneoutbreaks/

9. U.S. Centers for Disease Control and Prevention [CDC]. 2015, March 26. Parasites—toxoplasmosis: *Epidemiology and risk factors*. www.cdc.gov/parasites/toxoplasmosis/epi.html

10. U.S. Centers for Disease Control and Prevention [CDC]. 2015, July 21. Parasites—*Giardia: epidemiology and risk factors*. www.cdc.gov/parasites/giardia/epi.html

11. U.S. Centers for Disease Control and Prevention [CDC]. 2014, October 7. vCJD (Variant Creutzfeldt-Jakob Disease). www.cdc.gov/ncidod/dvrd/vcjd/qa.htm

12. U.S. Centers for Disease Control and Prevention [CDC]. 2014, April 25. Botulism. www.cdc.gov/nczved/divisions/dfbmd/diseases/botulism/

13. Ansdell, V. E. 2015, July 10. Food poisoning from marine toxins. U.S. Centers for Disease Control and Prevention [CDC]. wwwnc.cdc.gov/travel/yellowbook/2016/the-pre-travel-consultation/food-poisoning-from-marine-toxins

14. Horowitz, B. Z. 2013, April 3. Mushroom toxicity. *Medscape Reference*. http://emedicine.medscape.com/article/167398-overview 10

15. National Institutes of Health [NIH]. 2013, October 21. Potato plant poisoning: Green tubers and sprouts. MedlinePlus. www.nlm.nih.gov/medlineplus/ency/article/002875.htm

16. Prater, K. J., C. A. Fortuna, J. L. McGill, et al. 2016. Poor hand hygiene by college students linked to more occurrences of infectious diseases, medical visits, and absence from classes. *American Journal of Infection Control* 44(1): 66–70.

17. U.S. Department of Health & Human Services. n.d. Clean: Wash hands and surfaces often. www.foodsafety.gov/keep/basics/clean/index.html

18. U.S. Department of Health & Human Services. n.d. Separate: Don't cross-contaminate. www.foodsafety.gov/keep/basics/separate/index.html

19. U.S. Department of Health & Human Services. n.d. Chill: Refrigerate promptly. www.foodsafety.gov/keep/basics/chill/index.html

20. U.S. Department of Agriculture Food Safety and Inspection Service. 2015, March 24. Food product dating. www.fsis.usda.gov/wps/portal/fsis/topics/food-safety-education/get-answers/food-safety-fact-sheets/food-labeling/food-product-dating/food-product-dating

21. U.S. Department of Health and Human Services. n.d. Frozen food and power outages: When to save and when to throw out. www.foodsafety.gov/keep/charts/frozen_food.html

22. U.S. Department of Agriculture Food Safety and Inspection Service. 2013, August 22. Molds on food: Are they dangerous? www.fsis.usda.gov/wps/portal/fsis/topics/food-safety-education/get-answers/food-safety-fact-sheets/safe-food-handling/molds-on-food-are-they-dangerous-_/

23. U.S. Department of Agriculture Food Safety and Inspection Service. 2013, May. Is it done yet? www.fsis.usda.gov/wps/wcm/connect/c825bac8-c024-4793-be76-159dfb56a88f/IsItDoneYet_Brochure.pdf?MOD = AJPERES

24. Center for Science in the Public Interest [CSPI]. 2014. Chemical cuisine. Learn about food additives. www.cspinet.org/reports/chemcuisine.htm

25. U.S. Department of Agriculture Economic Research Service. 2015, July 9. Adoption of genetically engineered crops in the U.S.: Recent trends in GE adoption. www.ers.usda.gov/data-products/adoption-of-genetically-engineered-crops-in-the-us/recent-trends-in-ge-adoption.aspx

26. International Service for the Acquisition of Agri-Biotech Applications [ISAAA]. 2014. *Global Status of Commercialized Biotech/GM Crops: 2014.* ISAAA Brief No. 49-2014: Executive summary. Ithaca, NY: ISAAA. www.isaaa.org/resources/publications/briefs/49/executivesummary/default.asp

27. Klumper, W., and M. Qaim. 2014. A meta-analysis of the impacts of genetically modified crops. *PLOS One* e111629. doi:10.1371/journal.pone.0111629

28. Gilbert, N. 2013. Case studies: A hard look at GM crops. *Nature* 497:7447. www.nature.com/news/case-studies-a-hard-look-at-gm-crops-1.12907

29. World Health Organization [WHO]. 2014, May. *Frequently asked questions on genetically modified foods.* www.who.int/foodsafety/areas_work/food-technology/Frequently_asked_questions_on_gm_foods.pdf?ua = 1

30. International Agency for Research on Cancer [IARC]. 2015, March 20. IARC Monographs Volume 112: Evaluation of five organophosphate insecticides and herbicides. www.iarc.fr/en/media-centre/iarcnews/pdf/MonographVolume112.pdf

31. Bjerga, A. 2013, May 29. Monsanto modified wheat not approved by USDA found in field. *Bloomberg News.* www.bloomberg.com/news/articles/2013-05-29/monsanto-modified-wheat-unapproved-by-usda-found-in-oregon-field

32. Heap, I. 2015. The international survey of herbicide resistant weeds. www.weedscience.org

33. Xerces Society. 2015. Monarchs in peril. www.xerces.org/wp-content/uploads/2014/01/WesternMonarchsInPeril_XercesSociety.pdf

34. U.S. Environmental Protection Agency [EPA]. 2014, June 12. Persistent organic pollutants: A global issue, a global response. www2.epa.gov/international-cooperation/persistent-organic-pollutants-global-issue-global-response

35. National Institute of Environmental Health Sciences. 2015, October 20. Mercury. www.niehs.nih.gov/health/topics/agents/mercury/index.cfm

36. National Institute of Environmental Health Sciences. 2016, February 4. Lead. www.niehs.nih.gov/health/topics/agents/lead/index.cfm

37. National Institute of Environmental Health Sciences. 2016, January 8. Endocrine disruptors. www.niehs.nih.gov/health/topics/agents/endocrine/index.cfm

38. U.S. Environmental Protection Agency [EPA]. 2015, October 24. Phthalates. www.epa.gov/assessing-and-managing-chemicals-under-tsca/phthalates

39. National Institute of Environmental Health Sciences. 2015, January 21. Bisphenol A (BPA). www.niehs.nih.gov/health/topics/agents/sya-bpa/index.cfm

40. National Institute of Environmental Health Sciences. 2016, February 11. Dioxins. www.niehs.nih.gov/health/topics/agents/dioxins/index.cfm

41. Blum, A., S. A. Balan, M. Scheringer, et al. 2015. The Madrid statement on poly- and perfluoroalkyl substances (PFASs). *Environmental Health Perspectives* 123:A107–A111. http://dx.doi.org/10.1289/ehp.1509934

42. U.S. Environmental Protection Agency [EPA]. 2015, March 19. Pesticides and food: Healthy, sensible food practices. www.epa.gov/pesticides/food/tips.htm

43. American Cancer Society. 2014, September 10. Recombinant bovine growth hormone. www.cancer.org/cancer/cancercauses/othercarcinogens/athome/recombinant-bovine-growth-hormone

44. U.S. Centers for Disease Control and Prevention [CDC]. 2015, January 8. Methicillin-resistant *Staphylococcus aureus* (MRSA) infections. www.cdc.gov/mrsa/

45. Organic Trade Association. 2016. Market analysis. https://ota.com/resources/market-analysis

46. U.S. Department of Agriculture Agricultural Marketing Service. 2015, September. National organic program. Introduction to organic practices. https://www.ams.usda.gov/sites/default/files/media/Organic%20Practices%20Factsheet.pdf

47. Organic Trade Association. 2015. Media: Quick stats. https://ota.com/media/quick-stats

48. Brandt, K., C. Leifert, R. Sanderson, and C. J. Seal. 2011. Agro-ecosystem management and nutritional quality of plant foods: The case of organic fruits and vegetables. *Critical Reviews in Plant Sciences* 30(1–2):177–197.

49. Smith-Spangler C., M. L. Brandeau, G. E. Hunter, et al. 2012. Are organic foods safer or healthier than conventional alternatives? A systematic review. *Annals of Internal Medicine* 157(5):348–366. doi:10.7326/0003-4819-157-5-201209040-00007

50. Benbrook, C. M., G. Butler, M. A. Latif, C. Leifert, and D. R. Davis. 2013. Organic production enhances milk nutritional quality by shifting fatty acid composition: A United States-wide, 18-month study. *PLoS One* 8(12):e82429. doi:10.1371/journal.pone.0082429

51. Kusche, D., K. Kuhnt, K. Ruebesam, et al. 2015. Fatty acid profiles and antioxidants of organic and conventional milk from low- and high-input systems during outdoor period. *Journal of the Science of Food and Agriculture* 95(3):529–539.

52. Baranski, M., D. Srednicka-Tober, N. Volakakis, et al. 2014. Higher antioxidant and lower cadmium concentrations and lower incidence of pesticide residues in organically grown crops: A

systemic literature review and meta-analyses. *British Journal of Nutrition* 26:1–18.

53. Bohn, T., M. Cuhra, T. Traavik, et al. 2014. Compositional differences in soybeans on the market: Glyphosate accumulates in Roundup Ready GM soybeans. *Food Chemistry* 153:207–215.

54. Forman, J., and J. Silverstein. 2012. Organic foods: Health and environmental advantages and disadvantages. *Pediatrics* 130(5):e1406–e1415. doi: 10.1542/peds.2012-2579

In Depth: The Safety and Effectiveness of Dietary Supplements

1. Office of Dietary Supplements. 2016, February 11. Fact sheet for health professionals: Multivitamin/mineral supplements. http://ods .od.nih.gov

2. Lieberman, H. R., B. P. Marriott, C. Williams, et al. 2015. Patterns of dietary supplement use among college students. *Clinical Nutrition* 34(5):976–985. doi:10.1016/j.clnu.2014.10.010.

3. U.S. Food and Drug Administration [FDA]. Center for Food Safety and Applied Nutrition. 2008. FDA 101: dietary supplements.

4. Navarro, V. J., H. Barnhart, H. L. Bonkovsky, et al. 2014. Liver injury from herbals and dietary supplements in the U.S. Drug-Induced Liver Injury Network. *Hepatology* 60(4):1399–1408.

5. U.S. Food and Drug Administration [FDA]. Center for Food Safety and Applied Nutrition. 2015, September 4. Six tip-offs to rip-offs: Don't fall for health fraud scams. www.fda.gov/forconsumers/ consumerupdates/ucm341344.htm

6. National Center for Complementary and Integrative Health [NCCIH]. 2016, February 24. Using dietary supplements wisely. https://nccih.nih.gov/health/supplements/wiseuse.htm

7. Dickinson, A., J. Blatman, N. El-Dash, and J. C. Franco. 2014. Consumer usage and reasons for using dietary supplements: Report of a series of surveys. *Journal of the American College of Nutrition* 33(2):176–182.

8. National Institutes of Health [NIH]. 2012. Important information to know when you are taking Warfarin (Coumadin) and Vitamin K. www.cc.nih.gov/ccc/patient_education/drug_nutrient/coumadin1.pdf

9. Jabbar, S. B., and M. G. Hanly. 2013. Fatal caffeine overdose: A case report and review of the literature. *American Journal of Forensic Medicine and Pathology* 34(4):321–324.

10. Guallar, E., S. Stranges, C. Mulrow, L. J. Appel, and E. R. Miller III. 2013. Enough is enough: Stop wasting money on vitamin and mineral supplements. *Annals of Internal Medicine* 159(12):850–851.

11. Fortmann, S. P., B. U. Burda, C. A. Senger, J. S. Lin, and E. P. Whitlock. 2013. Vitamin and mineral supplements in the primary prevention of cardiovascular disease and cancer: An updated systematic evidence review for the U.S. Preventive Services Task Force. *Annals of Internal Medicine* 159:824–834.

12. Grodstein, F., J. O'Brien, J. H. Kang, et al. 2013. Long-term multivitamin supplementation and cognitive function in men: A randomized trial. *Annals of Internal Medicine* 159:806–814.

13. Lin, J. S., E. O'Connor, R. C. Rossom, L. A. Perdue, and E. Eckstrom. 2013. Screening for cognitive impairment in older adults: A systematic review for the U.S. Preventive Services Task Force. *Annals of Internal Medicine* 159:601–612.

Chapter 13

1. James, S. W., and S. Friel. 2015. An integrated approach to identifying and characterising resilient urban food systems to promote population health in a changing climate. *Public Health Nutr.* 2015 Sep; 18(13):2498–2508. doi: 10.1017/S1368980015000610

2. Food and Agricultural Organization of the United Nations (FAO). 2015. *FAO Hunger Map 2015.* Available at http://www.fao.org/ hunger/en.

3. Central Intelligence Agency. 2016, February 25. *The World Factbook.* Available at https://www.cia.gov/library/publications/the-world-factbook/

4. U.S. Centers for Disease Control and Prevention (CDC). 2015, June 19. Childhood Obesity Facts. Available at http://www.cdc.gov/ obesity/data/childhood.html.

5. Chetty, R., M. Stepner, S. Abraham, et al. 2016. The association between income and life expectancy in the United States, 2001–2014. *Journal of the American Medical Association.* April 10, 2016; doi:10.1001/jama.2016.4226.

6. Food and Agricultural Organization of the United Nations (FAO). 2015. *The State of Food Insecurity in the World.* Available at http:// www.fao.org/3/a-i4646e.pdf.

7. Coleman-Jensen, A., M. P. Rabbitt, C. Gregory, and A. Singh. 2015, September. *Household Food Security in the United States in 2014.* Economic Research Report No. 194. Economic Research Service. United States Department of Agriculture. Available at http://www .ers.usda.gov/.

8. World Hunger Education Service. 2015. *2015 World Hunger and Poverty Facts and Statistics.* Available at http://www.worldhunger .org/.

9. United Nations, Department of Economic and Social Affairs, Population Division. 2015. *World Population Prospects: The 2015 Revision,* Figure 2, page 2. Working Paper No. ESA/P/WP.241. Available at esa.un.org/.

10. Population Reference Bureau. 2015. *2015 World Population Data Sheet—with a special focus on women's empowerment.* Available at http://www.prb.org.

11. World Health Organization. 2015, November. *HIV/AIDS: Fact Sheet No. 360.* Available at http://www.who.int/.

12. U.S. Environmental Protection Agency. 2016, February 23. Climate Change: Basic Information. Available at http://www.epa.gov/.

13. U.S. Environmental Protection Agency. 2016, February 23. Glossary of Climate Change Terms. Available at http://www.epa.gov/.

14. Fischer, E. M., and R. Knutti. 2015. Anthropogenic contribution to global occurrence of heavy-precipitation and high-temperature extremes. *Nature.* 27 April 2015. doi:10.1038/NCLIMATE2617

15. Porter, J. R., L. Xie, A. J. Challinor, et al. 2014. Food security and food production systems. In: Field, C. B., V. R. Barros, D. J. Dokken, et al., eds. *Climate Change 2014: Impacts, Adaptation, and Vulnerability. Part A: Global and Sectoral Aspects. Contribution of Working Group II to the Fifth Assessment Report of the Intergovernmental Panel on Climate Change* Cambridge, United Kingdom and New York, NY, USA: Cambridge University Press, pp. 485–533.

16. Swain, D. L., D. E. Horton, D. Singh, and N. S. Diffenbaugh. 2016. Trends in atmospheric patterns conducive to seasonal precipitation and temperature extremes in California. *Science Advances.* March 2016. doi:10.1126/sciadv.1501344

17. Suweis, S., J. A. Carr, A. Maritan, A. Rinaldo, and P. D'Odorico. 2015. Resilience and reactivity of global food security. *Proceedings of the National Academy of Sciences,* 2015; 201507366. doi: 10.1073/ pnas.1507366112

18. Rockefeller Foundation. 2012, August. Social and Economic Equity in U.S. Food and Agriculture Systems. Available at http://www .fsg.org/Portals/0/Uploads/Documents/PDF/Equity_in_US_Food_ Agriculture_Systems.pdf?cpgn = WP%20DL%20-%20Social%20 and%20Economic%20Equity%20in%20U.S.%20Food%20and%20 Agriculture%20Systems.

19. McCluskey, M., T. McGarity, S. Shapiro, and M. Shudtz. 2013, January. *At the Company's Mercy: Protecting Contingent Workers from Unsafe Working Conditions.* Center for Progressive Reform. White Paper #1301. Available at http://www.progressivereform.org/ articles/contingent_workers_1301.pdf.

20. U.S. Centers for Disease Control and Prevention. 2014, December 15. Agricultural Safety. http://www.cdc.gov/niosh/topics/ aginjury/.

21. United States Department of Labor. 2016, January 1. State Child Labor Laws Applicable to Agriculture. Available at http://www.dol .gov/whd/state/agriemp2.htm.

22. Bureau of Labor Statistics. 2015, December. Food Preparation and Serving; and Cashiers. Available at www.bls.gov/.

23. Irving, S. K., and T. A Loveless. 2015, May. Dynamics of Economic Well-Being: Participation in Government Programs, 2009–2012: Who Gets Assistance? United States Census Bureau. P70-141. Available at www.census.gov/.

24. Economic Policy Institute. April 8, 2016. Minimum Wage Tracker. Available at www.epi.org.

25. U.S. Department of Agriculture. n.d. Census of Agriculture: Historical Archive. Available at http://agcensus.mannlib.cornell.edu/AgCensus/homepage.do.

26. U.S. Department of Agriculture. 2014, May 2. Census of Agriculture: 2012. Available at http://www.agcensus.usda.gov/Publications/2012/.

27. Union of Concerned Scientists. n.d. Hidden Costs of Industrial Agriculture. Available at www.ucsusa.org.

28. World Wildlife Fund. 2016. Environmental Impacts of Farming. Available at wwf.panda.org.

29. Foley, J. 2013, March 5. It's Time to Rethink America's Corn System. *Scientific American*. Available at http://www.scientificamerican.com/article/time-to-rethink-corn/.

30. Khoury, C. K., A. D. Bjorkman, H. Dempewolf, et al. 2014. Increasing homogeneity in global food supplies and the implications for food security. *Proc. Natl. Acad. Sci. U.S.A.* 111(11):4001–4006. doi:10.1073/pnas.1313490111

31. U.S. Department of Health and Human Services and U.S. Department of Agriculture. 2015, December. *2015–2020 Dietary Guidelines for Americans*, 8th edition. Available at http://health.gov/dietaryguidelines/2015/guidelines/.

32. Center for Responsive Politics. 2016, January 22. Influence and Lobbying. Available at http://www.opensecrets.org/.

33. Yale Rudd Center for Food Policy & Obesity. 2013, November. *Fast Food F.a.c.t.s. 2013: Measuring Progress in Nutrition and Marketing to Children and Teens*. Available at http://fastfoodmarketing.org/.

34. Nestle, M. 2013. *Food Politics: How the Food Industry Influences Nutrition and Health: Revised and Expanded 10th Anniversary Edition*. Berkeley: University of California Press, p. 13.

35. United Nations. 2014. The Millennium Development Goals Report 2014. 14-27027. Available at http://www.un.org/.

36. LocalHarvest. 2016. Community Supported Agriculture. www.localharvest.org/csa/.

37. U.S. Department of Agriculture (USDA). 2016, April. Farmers Markets and Direct-to-Consumer Marketing. Available at www.ams.usda.gov/.

38. Slow Food USA. 2016. About Us. Accessed April 15, 2016 at www.slowfoodusa.org/.

39. Goldrick-Rab, S., K. Broton, and D. Eisenberg. 2015, December. Hungry to Learn: Addressing Food & Housing Insecurity Among Undergraduates. *Wisconsin HOPE Lab*. http://wihopelab.com/publications/Wisconsin_hope_lab_hungry_to_learn.pdf.

40. Fair Trade USA. 2016. What Is Fair Trade? Accessed April 15, 2016 at www.fairtradeusa.org/.

41. American College Health Association. 2015. *ACHA-NCHA II: Reference group executive summary, spring 2015*. Available at www.acha-ncha.org.

42. Moore Lappé, F. 2011, September 14. The Food Movement: Its Power and Possibilities. *The Nation*. www.thenation.com/article/163403/food-movement-its-power-and-possibilities.

43. U.S. Department of Agriculture (USDA). 2016, January 26. Cattle & Beef: Statistics & Information. Available at http://www.ers.usda.gov/topics/animal-products/cattle-beef/statistics-information.aspx

44. Food and Agricultural Organization of the United Nations. 2016. The Role of Livestock in Climate Change. Accessed April 18, 2016. Available at http://www.fao.org/agriculture/lead/themes0/climate/en/.

45. Eshel, G., A. Shepon, T. Makov, and R. Milo. 2014. Land, irrigation water, greenhouse gas, and reactive nitrogen burdens of meat, eggs, and dairy production in the United States. *PNAS*. 111(33):11996–12001. doi:10.1073/pnas.1402183111

46. Cattlemen's Beef Board and National Cattlemen's Beef Association. 2015. Explore Beef. http://www.explorebeef.org/environment.aspx

47. Havlik, P, H. Valin, M. Herroro, et al. 2014. Climate change mitigation through livestock system transitions. *PNAS*. 111(10):3709–3714. doi:10.1073/pnas.1308044111 Available at http://www.pnas.org/content/111/10/3709.long

48. Scarborough, P., P. N. Appleby, A. Mizdrak, et al. 2014. Dietary greenhouse gas emissions of meat-eaters, fish-eaters, vegetarians and vegans in the UK. *Clim Change*. 125(2):179–192. Available at http://www.ncbi.nlm.nih.gov/pmc/articles/PMC4372775/

In Depth: Malnutrition

1. International Food Policy Research Institute. 2015. *Global Nutrition Report 2015: Actions and Accountability to Advance Nutrition and Sustainable Development*. Washington, DC. Available at http://ebrary.ifpri.org/utils/getfile/collection/p15738coll2/id/129443/filename/129654.pdf.

2. Central Intelligence Agency. 2016, February 25. *The World Factbook*. Available at https://www.cia.gov/librar/publications/the-world-factbook/

3. World Health Organization. 2016, January. Children: Reducing mortality. www.who.int/mediacentre/factsheets/fs178/en/.

4. World Health Organization. 2015. Micronutrient deficiencies. Available at http://www.who.int/nutrition/topics/

5. Iodine Global Network. 2015. About the Iodine Global Network. Available at http://www.ign.org/p142000253.html

6. World Health Organization. 2015, January. Obesity and Overweight. Fact Sheet No 311. Available at http://www.who.int/mediacentre/factsheets/fs311/en/

7. Sarmiento, O. L., D. C. Parra, S. A. Gonzalez, I. González-Casanova, A. Y. Forero, and J. Garcia. 2014. The dual burden of malnutrition in Colombia. *Am J. Clin. Nutr.* 100(6):1628S–35S. doi:10.3945/ajcn.114.083816. Epub 2014, October 29.

8. Freire, W. B., K. M. Silva-Jaramillo, M. J. Ramirez-Luzuriaga, P. Belmont, and W. F. Waters. 2014. The double burden of undernutrition and excess body weight in Ecuador. *Am. J. Clin. Nutr.* 100(6):1636S–43S. doi:10.3945/ajcn.114.083766. Epub 2014, October 29.

9. Demment, M. M., J. D. Haas, and C. M. Olson. 2014. Changes in family income status and the development of overweight and obesity from 2 to 15 years: a longitudinal study. *BMC Public Health.* 14:417. doi:10.1186/1471-2458-14-417.

10. Oddo, V. M., and J. C. Jones-Smith. 2015. Gains in income during early childhood are associated with decreases in BMI z scores among children in the United States. *Am. J. Clin. Nutr.* 101(6):1225–31. pii: ajcn096693. [Epub ahead of print]

11. Raubenheimer, D., G. E. Machovsky-Capuska, A. K. Gosby, and S. Simpson. 2015. Nutritional ecology of obesity: from humans to companion animals. *British Journal of Nutrition.* 113 Suppl:S26–39. doi:10.1017/S0007114514002323.

12. Gosby, A. K., A. D. Conigrave, D. Raubenheimer, and S. J. Simpson. 2014. Protein leverage and energy intake. *Obesity Reviews.* 15(3):183–91. doi:10.1111/obr.12131.

13. Hemmingsson, E. 2014. A new model of the role of psychological and emotional distress in promoting obesity: conceptual review with implications for treatment and prevention. *Obesity Reviews.* 15(9):769–79. doi:10.1111/obr.12197.

14. Haushofer, J., and E. Fehr. 2014. On the psychology of poverty. *Science* 344(6186):862–867. doi:10.1126/science.1232491.

15. Hruschka, D. J. 2012. Do economic constraints on food choice make people fat? A critical review of two hypotheses for the poverty-obesity paradox. *Am. J. Hum. Bio.* 24:277–285.

16. Tryon, M. S., K. L. Stanhope, E. S. Epel, et al. 2015. Excessive sugar consumption may be a difficult habit to break: a view from the brain and body. *J. Clin. Endocrinol. Metab.* 100(6):2239–47. Available at http://press.endocrine.org/doi/abs/10.1210/jc.2014-4353.

17. U.S. Department of Agriculture Agricultural Marketing Service. n.d. Food Deserts. Available at http://apps.ams.usda.gov/fooddeserts/fooddeserts.aspx.

18. Chen, D., E. C. Jaenicke, and R. J. Volpe. 2016. Food environments and obesity: Household diet expenditure versus food deserts. *American Journal of Public Health.* 106(5):881–888. doi:10.2105/AJPH.2016.303048.

Chapter 14

1. Centers for Disease Control and Prevention [CDC]. 2015. National Vital Statistics System: Birth Data. http://www.cdc.gov/nchs/births.htm

2. Mathews, T. J., M. F. MacDorman, M. E. Thoma. 2015. Infant mortality statistics from the 2013 period linked birth/infant death data set. *National vital statistics reports* 64(9). Hyattsville, MD: National Center for Health Statistics.

3. Dickey, R. P. 2015. Evaluation of women with unexplained infertility. In: Schattman, G. L., S. C. Esteves, and A. Agarwal, eds. *Unexplained Infertility*. New York: Springer.

4. Carmina, E. 2015. Reproductive system outcome among patients with polycystic ovarian syndrome. *Endocrinology and Metabolism Clinics of North America* 44:787–797.

5. Palomba, S., M. A. de Wilde, A. Falbo et al. 2015. Pregnancy complications in women with polycystic ovary syndrome. *Human Reproduction Update.* doi: 10.1093/humupd/dmv029

6. Louis, G. M. B., K. J. Sapra, E. F. Schisterman et al. 2016. Lifestyle and pregnancy loss in a contemporary cohort of women recruited before conception: The LIFE study. *Fertility and Sterility.* http://dx.doi.org/10.1016/j.fertnstert.2016.03.009

7. Soubry, A., J. M. Schildkraut, A. Murtha et al. 2013. Parental obesity is associated with *IGF2* hypomethylation in newborns: Results from a Newborn Epigenetics Study (NEWT) cohort. *BMC Medicine* 11:29–38.

8. Rasmussen, K. M., and A. L. Yaktine, eds. 2009. *Weight Gain During Pregnancy: Reexamining the Guidelines*. Washington, DC: National Academies Press.

9. Gaillard, R., E. A. P. Steegers, L. Duijts, et al. 2014. Childhood cardiometabolic outcomes of maternal obesity during pregnancy—The generation R study. *Hypertension* 63:683–691.

10. U.S. Department of Health and Human Services and U.S. Department of Agriculture. 2015, December. *2015–2020 Dietary Guidelines for Americans*, 8th ed. http://health.gov/dietaryguidelines/2015/guidelines/

11. Institute of Medicine, Food and Nutrition Board. 2002. *Dietary Reference Intakes for Energy, Carbohydrate, Fiber, Fat, Fatty Acids, Cholesterol, Protein, and Amino Acids*. Washington, DC: National Academies Press.

12. Food and Drug Administration. 2014. Food safety for moms-to-be: While you're pregnant—methylmercury. http://www.fda.gov/Food/ResourcesForYou/HealthEducators/ucm083324.htm

13. Spina Bifida Association. 2015. Lower the risk. http://spinabifidaassociation.org/lower-the-risk/

14. Institute of Medicine, Food and Nutrition Board. 1998. *Dietary Reference Intakes for Thiamin, Riboflavin, Niacin, Vitamin B6, Folate, Vitamin B12, Pantothenic Acid, Biotin, and Choline*. Washington, DC: National Academies Press.

15. Institute of Medicine, Food and Nutrition Board. 2000. *Dietary Reference Intakes for Vitamin C, Vitamin E, Selenium, and Carotenoids*. Washington, DC: National Academies Press.

16. Institute of Medicine, Food and Nutrition Board. 2001. *Dietary Reference Intakes for Vitamin A, Vitamin K, Arsenic, Boron, Chromium, Copper, Iodine, Iron, Manganese, Molybdenum, Nickel, Silicon, Vanadium, and Zinc*. Washington, DC: National Academies Press.

17. Institute of Medicine, Food and Nutrition Board. 2011. *Dietary Reference Intakes for Calcium and Vitamin D*. Washington, DC: National Academies Press.

18. Mayo-Wilson, E., A. Imdad, J. Junior, S. Dean, and Z. A. Bhutta. 2014. Preventive zinc supplementation for children, and the effect of additional iron: A systematic review and meta-analysis. *BMJ Open* 4:e004647. doi:10.1136/bmjopen-2013-004647

19. Institute of Medicine, Food and Nutrition Board. 2004. *Dietary Reference Intakes for Water, Potassium, Sodium, Chloride, and Sulfate*. Washington, DC: National Academies Press.

20. Matthews, A., D. M. Haas, D. P. O'Mathuna, T. Dowswell, and M. Doyle. 2014. Interventions for nausea and vomiting in early pregnancy. The Cochrane Library. doi: 10.1002/14651858.CD007575.pub3

21. Miao, D., S. L. Young, and C. D. Golden. 2015. A meta-analysis of pica and micronutrient status. *American Journal of Human Biology* 27:84–93.

22. Zielinski, R., K. Searing, and M. Deibel. 2015. Gastrointestinal distress in pregnancy: Prevalence, assessment, and treatment of 5 common minor discomforts. *Journal of Perinatal & Neonatal Nursing* 29:23–31.

23. American Diabetes Association. 2016. Management of diabetes in pregnancy. *Diabetes Care* 39(Suppl. 1):S94–S98.

24. The American College of Obstetricians and Gynecologists: Committee on Obstetric Practice. 2015. Committee Opinion: First-trimester risk assessment for early-onset preeclampsia. http://www.acog.org/Resources-And-Publications/Committee-Opinions/Committee-on-Obstetric-Practice/First-Trimester-Risk-Assessment-for-Early-Onset-Preeclampsia

25. U.S. Department of Health & Human Services. 2016. Trends in teen pregnancy and childbearing. http://www.hhs.gov/ash/oah/adolescent-health-topics/reproductive-health/teen-pregnancy/trends.html#

26. Piccoli, G. B., R. Clari, F. N. Vigotti et al. 2015. Vegan-vegetarian diets in pregnancy: danger or panacea? A systematic narrative review. *British Journal Obstetrics and Gynaecology* 122:623–633.

27. The American College of Obstetricians and Gynecologists: Committee on Obstetric Practice. 2015. Committee Opinion: Physical activity and exercise during pregnancy and the postpartum period. http://www.acog.org/Resources-And-Publications/Committee-Opinions/Committee-on-Obstetric-Practice/Physical-Activity-and-Exercise-During-Pregnancy-and-the-Postpartum-Period

28. American College of Sports Medicine. n.d. Exercise during pregnancy. https://www.acsm.org/docs/current-comments/exerciseduringpregnancy.pdf

29. Academy of Nutrition and Dietetics. 2014. Position of the Academy of Nutrition and Dietetics: Nutrition and lifestyle for a healthy pregnancy outcome. 114:1099–1103.

30. March of Dimes. 2015. Caffeine in pregnancy. http://www.marchofdimes.org/pregnancy/caffeine-in-pregnancy.aspx

31. Greenwood, D. C., N. J. Thatcher, J. Ye et al. 2014. Caffeine intake during pregnancy and adverse birth outcomes: A systematic review and dose-response meta-analysis. *European Journal of Epidemiology* 29:725–734.

32. Centers for Disease Control and Prevention. 2015. Alcohol use and binge drinking among women of childbearing age—United States, 2011–2013. *Morbidity and Mortality Weekly Report* 64:1042–1046.

33. Centers for Disease Control and Prevention. 2015. How does smoking during pregnancy harm my health and my baby? http://www.cdc.gov/reproductivehealth/maternalinfanthealth/tobaccousepregnancy/

34. Varner, M. W., R. M. Silver, C. J. Rowland Hogue et al. The Eunice Kennedy Shriver National Institute of Child Health and Human Development Stillbirth Collaborative Research Network. 2014. Association between stillbirth and illicit drug use and smoking during pregnancy. *Obstetrics and Gynecology* 123:113–125.

35. Worley, J. 2014. Identification and management of prescription drug abuse in pregnancy. *Journal of Perinatal & Neonatal Nursing* 28:196–203.

36. American Academy of Pediatrics, Section on Breastfeeding. 2012. Breastfeeding and the use of human milk policy statement. *Pediatrics* 129:e827–841.

37. Centers for Disease Control and Prevention. 2014. Breastfeeding ReportCard: United States/2014. www.cdec.gov/breastefeeding/pdf/2014breastfeedingreportcard.pdf

38. March, K. M., N. N. Chen, C. D. Karakochuk et al. 2015. Maternal vitamin D3 supplementation at 50 μg/d protects against low serum 25-hydroxyvitamin D in infants at 8 wk of age: A randomized controlled trial of 3 doses of vitamin D beginning in gestation and continued in lactation. *American Journal Clinical Nutrition* 102:402–410.

39. Hollis, B. W., C. L. Wagner, C. R. Howard et al. 2015. Maternal versus infant vitamin D supplementation during lactation: A randomized controlled trial. *Pediatrics* 136:625–634.

40. Colen, C. G., and D. M. Ramey. 2014. Is breast truly best? Estimating the effects of breastfeeding on long-term child health and wellbeing

in the United States using sibling comparisons. *Social Science & Medicine* 109:55–65.

41. McGuire, S. 2013. Centers for Disease Control and Prevention. *Strategies to prevent obesity and other chronic diseases: The CDC guide to strategies to support breastfeeding mothers and babies.* Atlanta, GA: U.S. Department of Health and Human Services, *Advances in Nutrition* 5:291–292.

42. Koleva, P. T., S. L. Bridgman, and A. L. Kozyrskyj. 2015. The infant gut microbiome: Evidence for obesity risk and dietary intervention. *Nutrients* 7:2237–2260.

43. Victora, C. G., R. Bahl, A. J. D. Barros et al. for the Lancet Breast-feeding Series Group. 2016. Breastfeeding in the 21st century: Epi-demiology, mechanisms, and lifelong effect. *Lancet.* 387:475–490.

44. Centers for Disease Control and Prevention. 2015. Cronobacter. http://www.cdc.gov/cronobacter/technical.html

45. Nommsen-Rivers, L. A. 2016. Does insulin explain the relation between maternal obesity and poor lactation outcomes? An overview of the literature. *Advances in Nutrition* 7:407–414.

46. Yang, Y. T., J. B. Saunders, and K. B. Kozhimannil. 2016. Health policy brief: Workplace and public accommodations for nursing mothers. *Health Affairs.* http://healthaffairs.org/healthpolicybriefs/brief_pdfs/healthpolicybrief_154.pdf

47. The American College of Obstetricians and Gynecologists: Committee on Obstetric Practice. 2016. Committee opinion: Optimizing support for breastfeeding as part of obstetric practice. http://www.acog.org/Resources-And-Publications/Committee-Opinions/Committee-on-Obstetric-Practice/Optimizing-Support-for-Breastfeeding-as-Part-of-Obstetric-Practice

48. Darmawikarta, D., Y. Chen, G. Lebovic et al. 2016. Total duration of breastfeeding, vitamin D supplementation, and serum levels of 25-hydroxyvitamin D. *American Journal of Public Health.* doi: 10.2015/AJPH.2015.303021

49. við Streym, S., C. S. Højskov, U. K. Møller et al. 2016. Vitamin D content in human milk: A 9-mo follow-up study. *American Journal Clinical Nutrition* 103:107–114.

50. Vitoria, I., B. López, J. Gómez et al. 2016. Improper use of a plant-based vitamin C-deficient beverage causes scurvy in an infant. *Pediatrics* 137(2):1–5. doi:10.1542/peds.2015-2781

51. Cichero, J. A. Y. 2016. Introducing solid foods using a baby-led weaning vs. spoon-feeding: A focus on oral development, nutrient intake and quality of research to bring balance to the debate. *Nutrition Bulletin* 41:72–77.

52. Wang, J., Y. Wu, G. Xiong et al. 2016. Introduction of comple-mentary feeding before 4 months of age increases the risk of childhood overweight or obesity: A meta-analysis of prospective cohort studies. *Nutrition Research.* http://dx.doi.org/10.1016/j.nutres.2016.03.003.doi/10.1016/j.nutres.2016.03.003

53. Jackson, K. D., L. D. Howie, and L. J. Akinbami. 2013. Trends in allergic conditions among children: United States, 1997–2011. *NCHS Data Brief* 10:1–8.

54. Stanton, B. F. 2015. Foreword: Management of pediatric food allergy. *Pediatric Clinics of North America* 62:xv–xvi.

55. Wright, B. L., M. Walker, B. P. Vickery, and R. S. Gupta. 2015. Clinical management of food allergy. *Pediatric Clinics of North America* 62:1409–1424.

56. American Academy of Pediatrics. 2016. Infant food and feeding. https://www.aap.org/en-us/advocacy-and-policy/aap-health-initiatives/HALF-Implementation-Guide/Age-Specific-Content/Pages/Infant-Food-and-Feeding.aspx

57. McAndrew, F., J. Thompson, L. Fellows et al. 2012. Infant feeding survey 2010. Leeds, United Kingdom: Health and Social Care Information Centre. http://www.hscic.gov.uk/article/3895/Infant-Feeding-Survey-2010

58. Du Toit, G., G. Roberts, P. H. Sayre et al. 2015. Randomized trial of peanut consumption in infants at risk for peanut allergy. *New England Journal of Medicine* 372:803–813.

59. Perkin, M. R., K. Logan, A. Tseng et al. 2016. Randomized trial of introduction of allergenic foods in breast-fed infants. *New England Journal of Medicine.* doi:10.1056/NEJMoa1514210

60. Du Toit, G., P. H. Sayre, G. Roberts et al. 2016. Effect of avoidance on peanut allergy after early peanut consumption. *New England Journal of Medicine.* doi:10.1056/NEJMoa1514209

61. Fleischer, D. M., S. Sicherer, M. Greenhawt et al. 2015. Consensus communication on early peanut introduction and the prevention of peanut allergy in high-risk infants. *Journal Allergy Clinical Immunology* 136:258–261.

In Depth: The Fetal Environment

1. Langley-Evans, S. C. 2015. Nutrition in early life and the programming of adult disease: A review. *Journal of Human Nutrition and Dietetics* 28(s1):1–14.

2. Lumey, L. H., and F. W. A. van Poppel. 2013. The Dutch Famine of 1944–1945 as a human laboratory: Changes in the early life environment and adult health. In: Humney, L. H., and A. Vaiserman, eds. *Early Life Nutrition and Adult Health and Development.* Hauppauge, NY: Nova Publishers.

3. Stanner, S. A., and J. S. Yudkin. 2001. Fetal programming and the Leningrad siege study. *Twin Research* 4:287–292.

4. Vanhees, K., I. G. C. Vonhögen, F. J. van Schooten, and R. W. L. Godschalk. 2014. You are what you eat, and so are your children: The impact of micronutrients on the epigenetic programming of offspring. *Cellular and Molecular Life Sciences* 71:271–285.

5. McKay, J. A., and J. C. Mathers. 2016. Conference on "Diet, gene regulation and metabolic disease." Symposium 3: Nutrition, epigenetics and the fetal origins of metabolic disease. Maternal folate deficiency and metabolic dysfunction in offspring. *Proceedings of the Nutrition Society* 75:90–95.

6. Javaid, M. K., S. R. Crozier, N. C. Harvey, et al. 2006. Maternal vitamin D status during pregnancy and childhood bone mass at age 9 years: A longitudinal study. *Lancet* 367(9504):36–43.

7. Keane, E., R. Layte, J. Harrington, P. M. Kearney, and U. Perry. 2012. Measured parental weight status and familial socio-economic status correlates with childhood overweight and obesity at age 9. *PLoS One* 7:e43503.

8. Schellong, K., S. Schuylz, T. Harder, and A. Plagemann. 2012. Birth weight and long-term overweight risk: Systematic review and meta-analysis including 643,902 persons from 66 studies and 26 countries globally. *PLoS One* 7:e47776.

9. Weedn, A. E., B. S. Mosley, M. A. Cleves et al. 2014. Maternal reporting of prenatal ultrasounds among women in the National Birth Defects Prevention Study. *Birth Defects Research (Part A)* 100:4–12.

10. Van Kijk, S. J., P. L. Malloy, H. Varinlin, et al. 2015. Epigenetics and human obesity. *International Journal of Obesity* 39: 85–97.

11. Garcia-Vargas, L., S. S. Addison, R. Nistala, D. Kurukulasuriya, and J. R. Sowers. 2012. Gestational diabetes and the offspring: Implications in the development of the cardiorenal metabolic syndrome in offspring. *Cardiorenal Medicine* 2:134–142.

12. Nielsen, G. L., C. Dethlefsen, S. Lundbye-Christensen, et al. 2012. Adiposity in 277 young adult male offspring of women with diabetes compared with controls: A Danish population-based cohort study. *Acta Obstetricia et Gynecologica Scandinavica* 91:838–843.

13. Mennitti, L. V., J. L. Oliveira, C. A. Morais et al. 2015. Type of fatty acids in maternal diets during pregnancy and/or lactation and metabolic consequences of the offspring. *The Journal of Nutritional Biochemistry* 26:99–111.

Chapter 15

1. Centers for Disease Control and Prevention [CDC]. 2015. Overweight and obesity. Childhood obesity facts. www.cdc.gov/obesity/data/childhood.html

2. Institute of Medicine, Food and Nutrition Board. 2002. *Dietary Reference Intakes for Energy, Carbohydrates, Fiber, Fat, Protein and Amino Acids (Macronutrients).* Washington, DC: The National Academy of Sciences.

3. American Academy of Pediatrics. 2011. *Healthy children, fit children: Answers to common questions from parents about nutrition and fitness.* Elk Grove Village, IL: American Academy of Pediatrics.

4. Ross, A. C., C. L. Taylor, A. L. Yaktine, and H. B. Del Valle, eds. 2011. *Dietary Reference Intakes for Calcium and Vitamin D.* Washington, DC: National Academy Press.

5. Institute of Medicine, Food and Nutrition Board. 2001. *Dietary Reference Intakes for Vitamin A, Vitamin K, Arsenic, Boron, Chromium, Copper, Iodine, Iron, Manganese, Molybdenum, Nickel, Silicon, Vanadium, and Zinc.* Washington, DC: National Academy Press.

6. Institute of Medicine, Food and Nutrition Board. 2004. *Dietary Reference Intakes for Water, Potassium, Sodium, Chloride, and Sulfate.* Washington, DC: National Academy Press.

7. Palfreyman, Z., E. Haycraft, and C. Meyer. 2014. Development of the parental modeling behaviours scale (PARM): Links with food intake among children and their mothers. *Maternal & Child Nutrition* 10:617–629.

8. McEvoy, C. T., and J. V. Woodside. 2015. Vegetarian diets. In: Koletzko, B., J. Bhatia, Z. A. Bhutta et al., eds. *Pediatric Nutrition in Practice.* Basel, Switzerland: Karger, pp. 134–138.

9. Academy of Nutrition and Dietetics. 2015. Position of the Academy of Nutrition and Dietetics: Vegetarian diets. *Journal of the Academy of Nutrition and Dietetics* 115:801–810.

10. Institute of Medicine, Food, and Nutrition Board. 1998. *Dietary Reference Intakes for Thiamin, Riboflavin, Niacin, Vitamin B6, Folate, Vitamin B12, Pantothenic Acid, Biotin, and Choline.* Washington, DC: National Academy Press.

11. Flattum, C., M. Draxten, M. Horning et al. 2015. HOME Plus: Program design and implementation of a family-focused, community-based intervention to promote the frequency and healthfulness of family meals, reduce children's sedentary behavior, and prevent obesity. *International Journal of Behavioral Nutrition and Physical Activity* 12(1):53. doi:10.1186/s12966-015-0211-7

12. Anzman-Frasca, S., H. C. Djang, M. M. Halmo, P. R. Dolan, and C. D. Economos. 2015. Estimating impacts of a breakfast in the classroom program on school outcomes. *JAMA Pediatrics* 169:71–77.

13. Adolphus, K., C. L. Lawton, and L. Dye. 2013. The effects of breakfast on behavior and academic performance in children and adolescents. *Frontiers in Human Neuroscience.* doi:10.3389/fnhum.2013.00425

14. U.S. Department of Agriculture. 2016. School lunch participation and meals served. www.fns.usda.gov/sites/default/files/pd/slsummar.pdf

15. Frerichs, L., J. Brittin, D. Sorensen et al. 2015. Influence of school architecture and design on healthy eating: A review of the evidence. *American Journal of Public Health.* 105:e46–e57. doi:10.2105/AJPH.2014.302453

16. Wilder, J. R., L. M. Kaste, A. Handler, T. Chapple-McGruder, and K. M. Rankin. 2016. The association between sugar-sweetened beverages and dental caries among third-grade students in Georgia. *Journal of Public Health Dentistry* 76:76–84.

17. Keast, D. R., K. M. Hill Gallant, A. M. Albertson, C. K. Gugger, and N. M. Holschuh. 2015. Associations between yogurt, dairy, calcium, and vitamin D intake and obesity among U.S. children aged 8–18 years: NHANES 2005–2008. *Nutrients* 7:1577–1593.

18. Coleman-Jensen, A., M. P. Rabbitt, C. Gregory, and A. Singh. 2015. *Household Food Security in the United States in 2014,* ERR-194, U.S. Department of Agriculture, Economic Research Service.

19. American Academy of Pediatrics Council on Community Pediatrics, Committee on Nutrition. 2015. Promoting food security for all children: Policy statement. *Pediatrics* 136:e1431–e1438.

20. Fram, M. S., L. D. Ritchie, N. Rosen, and E. A. Frongillo. 2015. Child experience of food insecurity is associated with child diet and physical activity. *Journal of Nutrition* 145:499–504.

21. Mesirow, M. S. C., and J. A. Welsh. 2015. Changing beverage consumption patterns have resulted in fewer liquid calories in the diets of U.S. children: National Health and Nutrition Examination Survey 2001–2010. *Journal of the Academy of Nutrition and Dietetics* 115:559–566.

22. Quann, E. E., V. L. Fulgoni III, and N. Auestad. 2015. Consuming the daily recommended amounts of dairy products would reduce the prevalence of inadequate micronutrient intakes in the United States: diet modeling student based on NHANES 2007–2010. *Nutrition Journal* 14:90. doi:10.1186/s12937-015-0057-5

23. Çerman, A. A., E. Aktaş, I. K. Altunay et al. 2016. Dietary glycemic factors, insulin resistance, and adiponectin levels in acne vulgaris. *Journal of the American Academy of Dermatology.* http://dx.doi.org/10.1010/j.jaad.2016.02.1220. doi.org/10.1016/j.jaad.2016.02.1220

24. Grossi, E., S. Cazzaniga, S. Crotti et al. 2016. The constellation of dietary factors in adolescent acne: A semantic connectivity map approach. *Journal European Academy of Dermatology and Venereology* 30:96–100.

25. Lange, K., S. Thamotharan, M. Racine, C. Hirko, and S. Fields. 2014. The relationship between weight and smoking in a national sample of adolescents: Role of gender. *Journal of Health Psychology.* http://hpq.sagepub.com/content/early/2014/01/09/1359105313517275.long. doi:10.1177/1359105313517275

26. Arnold, E. M., E. Greco, K. Desmond, and M. J. Rotheram-Borus. 2014. When life is a drag: Depressive symptoms associated with early adolescent smoking. *Vulnerable Children* and *Youth Studies: An International Interdisciplinary Journal* 9:1–9.

27. Armstrong, S., S. Lazorick, S. Hampl et al. 2016. Physical examination findings among children and adolescents with obesity: An evidence-based review. *Pediatrics* 137:1–15.

28. Skinner, A. C., and J. A. Skelton. 2014. Prevalence and trends in obesity and severe obesity among children in the United States, 1999–2012. *JAMA Pediatrics* 168:561–566.

29. Hampl, S., C. Odar Stough, K. Poppert Cordts et al. 2016. Effectiveness of a hospital-based multidisciplinary pediatric weight management program: Two-year outcomes of PHIT Kids. *Childhood Obesity.* doi:10.1089/chi.2014.0119

30. Centers for Disease Control and Prevention [CDC]. 2015. Physical activity: How much physical activity do children need? www.cdc.gov/physicalactivity/everyone/guidelines/children.html

31. Arias, E. 2016. Changes in life expectancy by race and Hispanic origin in the United States, 2013–2014. NCHS data brief, no. 244. Hyattsville, MD: National Center for Health Statistics.

32. Administration on Aging. Projected future growth of the older population: by age: 1900–2050. http://www.aoa.acl.gov/aging_statistics/future_growth/future_growth.aspx#age

33. Loenneke, J. P., P. D. Loprinzi, C. H. Murphy, and S. M. Phillips. 2016. Per meal dose and frequency of protein consumption is associated with lean mass and muscle performance. *Clinical Nutrition.* http://dx.doi.org/10.1016/j.clnu.2016.04.002. doi.org/10.1016/j.clnu.2016.04.002

34. Porter Starr, K. N., C. F. Pieper, M. C. Orenduff et al. 2016. Improved function with enhanced protein intake per meal: a pilot study of weight reduction in frail, obese older adults. *Journal of Gerontology: Medical Sciences.* doi:10.1093/Gerona/glv210

35. Paddon-Jones, D., W. W. Campbell, P. F. Jacques et al. 2015. Protein and healthy aging. *The American Journal of Clinical Nutrition* 101(Suppl):1339S–1345S.

36. Marinia, J. C. 2015. Protein requirements: Are we ready for new recommendations? *Journal of Nutrition* 145:5–6.

37. Hoffmann, M. R., P. A. Senior, and D. R. Mager. 2015. Vitamin D supplementation and health-related quality of life: A systematic review of the literature. *Journal of the Academy of Nutrition and Dietetics* 115:406–418.

38. Institute of Medicine, Food and Nutrition Board. 2000. *Dietary Reference Intakes for Vitamin C, Vitamin E, Selenium, and Carotenoids.* Washington, DC: National Academy Press.

39. Christen, W. G., R. J. Glynn, J. M. Gaziano et al. 2015. Age-related cataract in men in the selenium and vitamin E cancer prevention trial eye endpoints study. *JAMA Ophthalmology* 133:17–24.

40. Fakhouri, T. H. I., C. L. Ogden, M. D. Carroll, B. K. Kit, and K. M. Flegal. 2012. Prevalence of obesity among older adults in the United States, 2007–2010. NCHS data brief, no. 106. Hyattsville, MD: National Center for Health Statistics.

41. McCusker, M. M., K. Durrani, M. J. Payette, and J. Suchecki. 2016. An eye on nutrition: The role of vitamins, essential fatty acids, and antioxidants in age-related macular degeneration, dry eye syndrome and cataract. *Clinics in Dermatology* 34:276–285.

42. Wu, J., E. Cho, W. C. Willett, S. M. Sastry, and D. A. Schaumberg. 2015. Intakes of lutein, zeaxanthin, and other carotenoids and age-related macular degeneration during 2 decades of prospective follow-up. *JAMA Ophthalmology* 133:1415–1424.

43. Schmidl, D., G. Garhöfer, and L. Schmetterer. 2015. Nutritional supplements in age-related macular degeneration. *Acta Ophthalmologica* 93:105–121.

44. Charlesworth, C. J., E. Smit, D. S. H. Lee, F. Alramadhan, and M. C. Odden. 2015. Polypharmacy among adults aged 65 years and older in the United States: 1988–2010. *Journal of Gerontology: Medical Sciences.* doi:10.1093/Gerona/glv013

45. Qato, D. M., J. Wilder, L. P. Schumm, V. Gillet, and G. C. Alexander. 2016. Changes in prescription and over-the-counter medication and dietary supplement use among older adults in the United States, 2005 vs 2011. *JAMA Internal Medicine.* doi:10.1001/jamainternmed.2015.8581

46. Sganga, F., F. Landi, C. Ruggiero et al. 2015. Polypharmacy and health outcomes among older adults discharged from hospital: Results from the CRIME study. *Geriatrics & Gerontology International* 15:141–146.

47. Squires, B. 2014. Why are we encouraging struggling seniors to enroll in SNAP? AARP Foundation. www.aarp.org/aarp-foundation/our-work/hunger/info-2012/snap-food-benefits-help-seniors-enroll.html

48. Lloyd, J. L., and N. S. Wellman. 2015. Older American Act nutrition programs: A community-based nutrition program helping older adults remain at home. *Journal of Nutrition in Gerontology and Geriatrics* 34:90–109.

49. Ziegler, J., N. Redel, L. Rosenberg, and B. Carlson. 2015. Older Americans Act nutrition programs evaluation: Meal cost analysis. Cambridge, MA: Mathematica Policy Research.

50. U.S. Department of Health and Human Services. Administration on Aging. Nutrition Services. www.aoa.acl.gov/AoA_Programs/HPW/Nutrition_Services/index.aspx

51. U.S. Department of Agriculture. Senior Farmers' Market Nutrition Program. 2015. www.fns.usda.gov/sfmnp/senior-farmers-market-nutrition-program-sfmnp

52. Administration on Aging, *Profile of older Americans 2015*, www.aoa.acl.gov/aging_statistics/Profile/2015/14.aspx

53. Centers for Disease Control and Prevention [CDC]. 2015. Early release of selected estimates based on data from the National Health Interview Survey, 2014. www.cdc.gov/nchs/fastats/exercise.htm

54. Sparling, P. B., B. J. Howard, D. W. Dunstan, and N. Owen. 2015. Recommendations for physical activity in older adults. *British Medical Journal.* doi:10.1136/bmj.h100

55. Centers for Disease Control and Prevention [CDC]. 2015. How much physical activity do adults need? www.cdc.gov/physicalactivity/basics/adults/index.htm

In Depth: Searching for the Fountain of Youth

1. de Cabo, R., D. Carmona-Gutierrez, M. Bernier, M. N. Hall, and F. Madeo. 2014. The search for antiaging interventions: From elixirs to fasting regimens. *Cell* 157:1515–1526.

2. Rizza, W., N. Veronese, and L. Fontana. 2014. What are the roles of calorie restriction and diet quality in promoting healthy longevity? *Ageing Research Reviews* 13:38–45.

3. Gilmore, L. A., E. Ravussin, and L. M. Redman. 2015. Anti-aging effects of nutritional modification: The state of the science on caloric restriction. In: Bales, C. W. et al., eds. *Handbook of Clinical Nutrition and Aging.* New York: Springer Science and Business Media.

4. López-Lluch, G., and P. Navas. 2016. Calorie restriction as an intervention in ageing. *Journal of Physiology* 594.8:2043–2060.

5. Sohal, R. S., and M. J. Forster. 2014. Caloric restriction and the aging process: A critique. *Free Radical Biology & Medicine* 73:366–382.

6. Fontana, L., and L. Partridge. 2015. Promoting health and longevity through diet: From model organisms to humans. *Cell* 161:106–118.

7. Ravussin, E., L. M. Redman, J. Rochon et al. 2015. A 2-year randomized controlled trial of human caloric restriction: Feasibility and effects on predictors of health span and longevity. *Journals of Gerontology Series A: Biological Sciences and Medical Sciences* 70:1097–1104.

8. Speakman, J. 2010. Can calorie restriction increase the human lifespan? Oral presentation at *Federation of American Societies of Experimental Biology.* Anaheim, CA. April 2010.

9. Patterson, R. E., A. Z. LaCroix, S. J. Hartman et al. 2015. Intermittent fasting and human metabolic health. *Journal Academy of Nutrition and Dietetics* 115:1203–1212.

10. Hoddy, K. K, C. Gibbons, C. M. Kroeger et al. 2016. Changes in hunger and fullness in relation to gut peptides before and after 8 weeks of alternate day fasting. *Clinical Nutrition.* www.clinicalnutritionjournal.com/article/S0261-5614(16)00102-3/abstract

11. Klemple, M. C., C. M. Kroeger, and K. A. Varady. 2013. Alternate day fasting (ADF) with a high-fat diet produces similar weight loss and cardio-protection as ADF with a low-fat diet. *Metabolism: Clinical and Experimental* 62:137–143.

12. Mattson, M. P., D. B. Allison, L. Fontana et al. 2014. Meal frequency and timing in health and disease. *Proceedings of the National Academy of Sciences.* 111:16647–16653.

13. Transparency Market Research. 2015. Anti-aging market is estimated to be worth USD 191.7 billion globally by 2019: Transparency Market Research.

14. *Consumer Reports.* 2013. Can anti-aging supplements help you look younger? The claims vs. the reality. www.consumerreports.org/cro/2013/08/anti-aging-supplements-claims-vs-reality/index.htm

15. Bjelakovic, G., D. Nikolova, L. L. Gluud, R. G. Simonetti, and C. Gluud. 2013. Antioxidant supplements for prevention of mortality in healthy participants and patients with various diseases. www.consumerreports.org/cro/2013/08/anti-aging-supplements-claims-vs-reality/index.htm

16. Mayo Clinic. 2015. Ginkgo (Ginkgo biloba). www.mayoclinic.org/drugs-supplements/ginkgo/safety/hrb-20059541

17. Mayo Clinic. 2015. Performance-enhancing drugs: Know the risks. www.mayoclinic.org/healthy-living/fitness/in-depth/performance-enhancing-drugs/art-20046134

18. Liu, Y., J. B. Croft, A. G. Wheaton et al. 2016. Clustering of five health-related behaviors for chronic disease prevention among adults, United States, 2013. *Prevention Chronic Disease* 13:160054. www.cdc.gov/pcd/issues/2016/16_0054.htm

answers

Answers to Review Questions

Chapter 1

Review Questions

1. **c.** identifying and preventing diseases caused by dietary deficiencies.
2. **a.** Pellagra is caused by a nutrient deficiency.
3. **d.** micronutrients.
4. **b.** the RDA for vitamin C.
5. **d.** "A high-protein diet increases the risk for porous bones" is an example of a hypothesis.
6. **b.** an observational study.
7. **c.** conflict of interest.
8. **b.** National Institutes of Health.
9. true
10. false

Math Review

11. 24.5% of Kayla's diet comes from fat; this percentage is within the AMDR for fat.

Chapter 2

Review Questions

1. **c.** is based on foods that provide a high level of nutrients and fiber for a relatively low number of Calories.
2. **b.** A conditioned taste aversion to pork sausages could develop in a person who learns how they are made.
3. **d.** the % Daily Value of select nutrients in one serving of the food.
4. **a.** limiting intake of added sugars, saturated fats, and sodium.
5. **d.** fruits and vegetables
6. **b.** a serving that is 1 ounce or equivalent to an ounce for either grains or protein foods.
7. **d.** None of the above is true.
8. true
9. false
10. false

Math Review

11. The total Calorie content of Hannah's lunch is 699 Calories. The sodium content is 1,656 mg, which is 72% of the recommended total daily sodium limit. A simple change Hannah could make to reduce the total Calories and sodium in her lunch would be to replace the packet of Ranch dressing on her salad with a drizzle of olive oil and vinegar.

Chapter 3

Review Questions

1. **c.** atoms, molecules, cells, tissues, organs, systems
2. **b.** two flexible layers of phospholipid molecules.
3. **c.** hypothalamus.
4. **c.** the middle segment of the small intestine.
5. **c.** small intestine.
6. **a.** collectively known as the enteric nervous system.
7. **a.** gastric juice in the esophagus.
8. true
9. false
10. true

Math Review

11. The difference between pH 9 and pH 2 is 7. The alkalinity of baking soda as compared to gastric juice can be expressed as $7 = \log10 (10,000,000)$. In other words, baking soda is 10 million times more alkaline than gastric juice.

Chapter 4

Review Questions

1. **a.** monosaccharides.
2. **d.** Consuming a diet high in fiber-rich carbohydrates may reduce the level of cholesterol in the blood.
3. **b.** is converted to glycogen and stored in the liver and muscles.
4. **b.** the potential of foods to raise blood glucose and insulin levels.
5. **c.** up to 65% of our daily energy intake as carbohydrate.
6. **d.** sweetened soft drinks.
7. **c.** whole-oat cereal
8. **a.** phenylketonuria.
9. false
10. true

Math Review

11. The AMDR for carbohydrate for adults is 45–65% of total daily energy. If Simon wants to make sure he is meeting the minimum (45%), the answers are:
a) 3,500 kcal per day × 0.45 = 1,575 kcal per day of carbohydrate, preferably from fiber-rich sources; and
b) 1,575 kcal per day ÷ 4 kcal per gram of carbohydrate = 393.75 grams. Thus, Simon should consume at least 394 grams of carbohydrate per day.

Chapter 5

Review Questions

1. **d.** produced by the body.
2. **b.** monounsaturated.
3. **c.** both saturated and unsaturated fats.
4. **d.** found in leafy green vegetables, flaxseeds, soy milk, walnuts, and almonds.
5. **b.** are a major source of fuel for the body at rest.
6. **a.** lipoprotein lipase
7. **c.** less than 10% of total energy.
8. **c.** vegetables, fish, and nuts.
9. true
10. false

Math Review

11. Answers will vary.
12. Maria should consume between 400 and 700 kcal/day as total fat. She should consume no more than 200 kcal/day as saturated fat. This would leave about 200 to 500 kcal/day for healthful unsaturated fats. She should keep her intake of *trans* fatty acids to an absolute minimum—ideally, none at all.

Chapter 6

Review Questions

1. **c.** hydrogen, carbon, oxygen, and nitrogen.
2. **d.** None of the above is true.

3. **d.** mutual supplementation.
4. **a.** exert pressure that draws fluid out of tissue spaces, preventing edema.
5. **c.** protease.
6. **c.** The RDA for protein is higher for children and adolescents than for adults.
7. **b.** Protein levels in the blood must be adequate to transport fat.
8. **a.** Rice, pinto beans, acorn squash, soy butter, and almond milk
9. false
10. false

Math Review

11. **(a)** The AMDR for protein is 10% to 35% of total daily energy intake. Thus, the lower level of AMDR for Barry is equal to 3,000 kcal × 0.10 = 300 kcal protein. This is equivalent to 75 g of protein (300 kcal ÷ 4 kcal/g protein). The upper level of AMDR for Barry is equivalent to 262.5 g of protein (1,050 kcal ÷ 4 kcal/g protein). Barry is meeting the AMDR for protein. (b) Assuming Barry is not an athlete, his RDA for protein is 0.8 g of protein per kg body weight per day × 75 kg = 60 g per day. Barry is exceeding the RDA for protein.

Chapter 7
Review Questions

1. **a.** extracellular fluid.
2. **c.** It provides protection for the brain and spinal cord.
3. **b.** It is freely permeable to water but not to electrolytes.
4. **d.** all of the above.
5. **a.** tap water
6. **c.** The kidney's excretion and reabsorption of sodium contribute to blood pressure regulation.
7. **b.** It can be found in fresh fruits and vegetables.
8. **b.** sweating and breathing heavily while active in a hot environment
9. true
10. false

Math Review

11. He should consume 9 cups of fluid.

Chapter 8
Review Questions

1. **c.** a molecule that combines with and activates an enzyme.
2. **d.** vitamin B_6.
3. **d.** vitamin B_{12}.
4. **a.** iodine.
5. **b.** an atom loses an electron.
6. **b.** Both vitamins donate electrons to free radicals.
7. **a.** Beta-carotene is a provitamin precursor of vitamin A.
8. **d.** is regenerated by a form of vitamin A.
9. false
10. true

Math Review

11. **(a)** Each tablet contains 400 IU of the synthetic form of vitamin E. In supplements containing the synthetic form of vitamin E, 1 IU is equal to 0.45 mg α-TE. To convert IU to mg α-TE = 400 IU × 0.45 = 180 mg α-TE, which is equal to 180 mg of active vitamin E.
(b) The RDA for vitamin A is 15 mg alpha-tocopherol per day. To calculate the percentage of the RDA for vitamin E coming from the supplements = (180 mg α-TE ÷ 15 mg α-TE) × 100 = 1200%

(c) The tolerable upper intake level is 1,000 mg alpha-tocopherol per day, and thus the amount coming from the supplement is relatively small at 180 mg. Although in the past up to 18 times the RDA has been shown to be safe (18 × 15 mg = 270 mg of alpha-tocopherol per day), recent evidence suggests that even 400 IU per day could increase the risk for premature mortality. Thus it would be safest for Joey's mother to obtain adequate vitamin E from her diet. If she is taking aspirin each day as prescribed, it is imperative that she stop taking vitamin E supplements, as aspirin is an anticoagulant and taking vitamin E supplements could enhance its action and result in uncontrollable bleeding and hemorrhaging.

Chapter 9
Review Questions

1. **b.** About two-thirds of the body's iron is found in hemoglobin, the oxygen-carrying compound in red blood cells.
2. **a.** iron-deficiency anemia.
3. **b.** vitamin K.
4. **d.** is essential for the synthesis of collagen.
5. **c.** It has a faster turnover rate than cortical bone.
6. **d.** structure of bone, nerve impulse transmission, muscle contraction, and blood clotting.
7. **a.** They regulate the absorption of calcium and phosphorus from the small intestine.
8. **c.** a fair-skinned retired teacher living in a nursing home in Ohio.
9. true
10. false

Math Review

11. This statement is false. Although 20 mg/day × 100 days = 2,000 mg, or 2 g, zinc absorption rates range from just 10% to 35% of dietary intake.

Chapter 10
Review Questions

1. **d.** None of the above.
2. **a.** body mass index.
3. **b.** take in more energy than they expend.
4. **a.** energy expended via basal metabolism, the thermic effect of food, and physical activity equals energy intake.
5. **b.** ghrelin
6. **c.** a low-income single parent who provides child care to other families in their urban apartment block
7. **a.** a realistic, achievable goal.
8. **c.** a peanut-butter sandwich on whole-grain bread with an apple
9. false
10. true

Math Review

11. To calculate Misty's BMI: Convert Misty's height to meters and her weight to kg. Her height is 5 feet 8 inches or 68 inches, which is equal to 1.727 meters (68 inches × .0254 cm/inch). Her weight is 148 pounds, which is equal to 67.27 kilograms (148 lbs × 0.4545 kg/lb). Thus, her BMI is equal to 22.6 kg/m² (67.27 kg/2.982529 meters). Misty's BMI falls into the normal weight category.

There are many questions and bits of advice you could share with Misty. You could inquire as to why she feels she is overweight and suggest she explore the various definitions of a healthful body weight listed in this chapter. You could point out that as she exercises regularly, she is promoting overall health, and she might get her body composition measured to reassure her that her weight is in the healthful range. You could also suggest that she schedule an appointment with a registered dietitian to discuss her dietary intake and views on her personal body image.

To estimate Misty's kcal needs, first calculate her BMR = 0.9 kcal per kg body weight per hour = 0.9 kcal/body weight/hour × 67.27 kg × 24 hours/day = 1,453 kcal/day. Next, estimate the energy cost of Misty's activity. Being moderately active, Misty expends kcal ranging from 50% to 70% of her BMR, or 726 kcal (0.50 × 1,453 kcal) and 1,017 kcal (0.70 × 1,453 kcal). Finally, add together Misty's BMR and energy needed to perform daily activities: 1,453 kcal/day + 726 kcal/day = 2,179 kcal/day to 1,453 kcal/day + 1,017 kcal/day = 2,470 kcal/day.

Chapter 11
Review Questions
1. **c.** Reduces anxiety and mental stress
2. **c.** 50% to 70% of your estimated maximal heart rate.
3. **a.** 1 to 3 seconds.
4. **b.** Fat
5. **b.** Carbohydrate loading results in increased storage of glycogen in muscles and the liver.
6. **b.** somewhat higher than for sedentary adults, about 1.0 to 1.2 g protein per kg body weight.
7. **d.** drink a beverage containing carbohydrate and electrolytes both before and during the event in amounts that balance hydration with energy, carbohydrate, and electrolyte needs.
8. **d.** caffeine
9. true
10. false

Math Review
11. **(a)** Liz's suggested intake for protein is identified as 1.5 grams per kg body weight. Her body weight is equal to 105 lbs ÷ 2.2 = 47.7 kg. Her protein intake (in grams) is equal to 1.5 grams protein/kg body weight × 47.7 kg = 71.6 grams.

    (b) Liz's preferred fat intake is 20% of her total daily energy intake, thus 1,800 kcal × 0.20 = 360 kcal. Because the energy value of fat is 9 kcal per gram, her total intake of fat in grams = 360 kcal ÷ 9 kcal/gram = 40 grams of fat.

    (c) To calculate Liz's carbohydrate intake, you must first determine the amount of kcal of her total energy intake that remains once her protein and fat intake are accounted for.

    - Liz's protein intake is 71.6 grams; as the energy value of protein is 4 kcal per gram, her kcal intake from protein = 71.6 grams × 4 kcal/gram = 286.4 kcal.
    - Liz's fat intake has already been calculated as 360 kcal.
    - As Liz's total energy intake is 1,800 kcal per day, the amount of kcal she'll consume from carbohydrate = 1,800 kcal − 286.4 kcal − 360 kcal = 1,153.6 kcal of carbohydrate.
    - The energy value of carbohydrates is 4 kcal per gram, and thus Liz's intake of carbohydrate in grams is equal to 1,153.6 kcal ÷ 4 kcal/gram = 288.4 grams.

    (d) To determine if Liz's carbohydrate intake falls within the AMDR = (1,153.6 kcal of carbohydrate ÷ 1,800 kcal) × 100 = 64%. Thus her carbohydrate intake does fall within the AMDR.

Chapter 12
Review Questions
1. **c.** federal oversight of food safety is fragmented among 15 different agencies.
2. **a.** norovirus is responsible for the greatest number of illnesses.
3. **a.** between 40°F and 140°F.
4. **c.** within a maximum of 1 hour after serving.
5. **b.** modified atmosphere packaging.
6. **b.** sulfites and nitrites.
7. **a.** confer tolerance to herbicides.
8. **c.** they can act as neurotoxins, carcinogens, or endocrine disruptors.
9. true
10. true

Math Review
11. **a.** 145°F = 63°C
    b. 160°F = 71°C
    c. 165°F = 74°C

Chapter 13
Review Questions
1. **a.** Between 1990-92 and 2014-16, the share of undernourished people worldwide fell by nearly 45%.
2. **c.** unequal distribution of food, largely because of poverty.
3. **b.** A majority of contingent farm workers in the United States live below the poverty line.
4. **b.** It has dramatically increased food security throughout South America, Asia, and Africa.
5. **c.** The U.S. food industry produces about twice as many Calories per capita per year than Americans require.
6. **d.** the Supplemental Nutrition Assistance Program (SNAP)
7. **d.** a pint of strawberries you pick yourself at an organic farm
8. false
9. true
10. true

Math Review
11. Steve earns $15,080 annually ($7.25/hour × 40 hours a week × 52 weeks a year). He and his family are currently living far below the federal poverty threshold, which in 2016 was $20,160 for a family of three. If Diane were to return to work for 40 hours a week, their annual income would double to $30,160 ($15,080 × 2 = $30,160). As you learned in this chapter, families earning at or below 185% of the federal poverty level are at increased risk for food insecurity: 185% of the poverty threshold of $20,160 = $37,296 ($20,160 × 1.85 = $37,296). Even if Steve and Diane both worked full time (80 hours a week combined), they would still be at high risk for food insecurity ($30,160 is significantly less than $37,296).

Chapter 14
Review Questions
1. **b.** neural tube defects
2. **a.** 350 to 450 kcal/day
3. **c.** Keep dry cereal or crackers at the bedside to ease nighttime and morning nausea.
4. **c.** oxytocin
5. **a.** Lactating women need more Calories than pregnant women.

6. **d.** Certain proteins in breast milk help protect the newborn from infection.
7. **c.** iron
8. **d.** none of the above.
9. true
10. false

Math Review

11. **(a)** To calculate the % of kcal in breast milk that comes from fat, first convert grams of fat to fat kcal: 35 g fat/liter × 9 kcal/g = 315 fat kcal/liter. Then calculate the % of total breast milk kcal from fat: [315 fat kcal ÷ 700 total kcal] × 100 (to convert to percentage) = 45% of kcal in breast milk are from fat. **(b)** To calculate the % of kcal in breast milk that come from protein, first convert grams of protein to protein kcal: 9 g protein × 4 kcal/g = 36 protein kcal. Then calculate the % of total breast milk kcal from protein: [36 kcal ÷ 700 total kcal] × 100 (to convert to percentage) = 5% of kcal from protein. **(c)** 45% of kcal from fat is much higher than the range that is recommended for healthy young adults (20–35% of total kcal from fat), but a high fat diet is needed to meet the energy needs of rapidly growing infants. 5% of kcal from protein is much lower than what is recommended for most young adults (10–35% of kcal from protein), but the kidneys of young infants are immature and not able to excrete large amounts of nitrogen. The small gastric capacity of infants and their relatively immature kidneys explain why the proportions of Calories from fat and protein in breast milk are ideally suited for young infants.

Chapter 15

Review Questions

1. **a.** $\frac{1}{2}$ cup of iron-fortified cooked oat cereal, 2 tbsp. of mashed pineapple, and 1 cup of whole milk

2. **c.** iron and zinc
3. **b.** Children require a diet providing between 25% to 35% of total energy as fat.
4. **b.** the epiphyseal plates close.
5. **c.** both boys and girls, age 9 to 18
6. **d.** None of the above is true.
7. **d.** All of the above occur with normal aging.
8. **d.** the prevalence of obesity declines after age 75.
9. true
10. true

Math Review

11. To calculate the total vitamin A intake of Kristina's grandmother, add up the amount of vitamin A in one dose of each of the three supplements: 3,333 + 1,500 + 2,200 = 7,033 μg of vitamin A per day.

   To calculate the % of the RDA consumed by Kristina's grandmother, take her daily total intake, divide by the RDA, and multiply by 100 to convert to a percent: [7,033 μg ÷ 700 μg] × 100 = 1,005% of the UL, or ten times more than the recommended amount.

   To calculate the % of the vitamin A UL consumed by Kristina's grandmother each day, take her total daily intake, divide by the UL, and multiply by 100 to convert to a percent: [7,033 μg ÷ 3,000 μg] × 100 = 234% of the UL, or more than twice the recommended upper limit. This amount of vitamin A, taken on a regular basis, could certainly lead to vitamin A toxicity over time. The UL for adults, including the elderly, is 3,000 μg per day.

NOTE: These calculations reflect the % of the RDA, not % above the RDA.

glossary

A

absorption The physiologic process by which molecules of food cross from the gastrointestinal tract into the circulation.

Acceptable Daily Intake (ADI) An FDA estimate of the amount of a nonnutritive sweetener that someone can consume each day over a lifetime without adverse effects.

accessory organs of digestion The salivary glands, liver, gallbladder, and pancreas, which contribute to GI function but are not anatomically part of the GI tract.

acetylcholine A neurotransmitter that is involved in many functions, including muscle movement and memory storage.

acidosis A disorder in which the blood becomes acidic; that is, the level of hydrogen in the blood is excessive. It can be caused by respiratory or metabolic problems.

added sugars Sugars and syrups that are added to food during processing or preparation.

adenosine triphosphate (ATP) The common currency of energy for virtually all cells of the body.

adipokines Cell signaling proteins secreted by adipose tissue; some promote inflammation.

aerobic exercise Exercise that involves the repetitive movement of large muscle groups, increasing the body's use of oxygen and promoting cardiovascular health.

alcohol abuse A pattern of alcohol consumption, whether chronic or occasional, that results in harm to one's health, functioning, or interpersonal relationships.

alcohol Chemically, a compound characterized by the presence of a hydroxyl group; in common usage, a beverage made from fermented fruits, vegetables, or grains and containing ethanol.

alcohol dependence A disease state characterized by alcohol craving, loss of control, physical dependence, and tolerance.

alcohol hangover A cluster of signs and symptoms, including headache, nausea, and vomiting, that occurs as a consequence of drinking too much alcohol.

alcoholic hepatitis A serious condition of inflammation of the liver caused by alcohol abuse.

alcohol poisoning A potentially fatal condition in which an overdose of alcohol results in cardiac and/or respiratory failure.

alcohol use disorder (AUD) Medical diagnosis for problem drinking that has become severe and is characterized by either abuse or dependence.

alkalosis A disorder in which the blood becomes basic; that is, the level of hydrogen in the blood is deficient. It can be caused by respiratory or metabolic problems.

alpha-linolenic acid (ALA) An essential fatty acid found in leafy green vegetables, flaxseed oil, soy oil, and other plant foods; an omega-3 fatty acid.

amenorrhea The absence of menstruation. In females who had previously been menstruating, it is defined as the absence of menstrual periods for 3 or more continuous months.

amino acids Nitrogen-containing molecules that combine to form proteins.

amniotic fluid The watery fluid contained within the innermost membrane of the sac containing the fetus. It cushions and protects the growing fetus.

anabolic The characteristic of a substance that builds muscle and increases strength.

anaerobic Means "without oxygen"; the term used to refer to metabolic reactions that occur in the absence of oxygen.

anencephaly A fatal neural tube defect in which there is partial absence of brain tissue, most likely caused by failure of the neural tube to close.

anorexia An absence of appetite.

anorexia nervosa A serious, potentially life-threatening eating disorder that is characterized by self-starvation, which eventually leads to a deficiency in the energy and essential nutrients required by the body to function normally.

antibodies Defensive proteins of the immune system. Their production is prompted by the presence of bacteria, viruses, toxins, allergens, and other antigens.

antioxidant A compound that has the ability to prevent or repair the damage caused by oxidation.

appetite A psychological desire to consume specific foods.

ariboflavinosis A condition caused by riboflavin deficiency.

atherosclerosis A condition characterized by accumulation of cholesterol-rich plaque on artery walls; these deposits build up to such a degree that they impair blood flow.

atrophic gastritis A condition in which chronic inflammation of the stomach lining erodes gastric glands, reducing stomach acid secretion and thus absorption of vitamin from foods.

atrophy A decrease in the size and strength of muscles that occurs when they are not worked adequately.

B

bacteria Cellular microorganisms that lack a true nucleus and reproduce by cell division or by spore formation.

bariatric surgery Surgical alteration of the gastrointestinal tract performed to promote weight loss.

basal metabolic rate (BMR) The energy the body expends to maintain its fundamental physiologic functions.

beriberi A disease of muscle wasting and nerve damage caused by thiamin deficiency.

bile Fluid produced by the liver and stored in the gallbladder; it emulsifies fats in the small intestine.

binge drinking The consumption of five or more alcoholic drinks on one occasion for a man, or four or more drinks for a woman.

binge eating Consumption of a large amount of food in a short period of time, usually accompanied by a feeling of loss of self-control.

binge-eating disorder A disorder characterized by binge eating an average of twice a week or more, typically without compensatory purging.

bioavailability The degree to which the body can absorb and utilize any given nutrient.

biomagnification The process by which persistent organic pollutants become more concentrated in animal tissues as they move from one creature to another through the food chain.

biopesticides Primarily insecticides, these chemicals use natural methods to reduce damage to crops.

blood volume The amount of fluid in blood.

body composition The ratio of a person's body fat to lean body mass.

body dysmorphic disorder (BDD) A clinically diagnosed psychiatric disorder characterized by a disabling preoccupation with perceived defects in appearance.

body fat mass The amount of body fat, or adipose tissue, a person has.

body image A person's perception, feelings about, and critique of his or her body's appearance and functioning.

body mass index (BMI) A measurement representing the ratio of a person's body weight to his or her height (kg/m^2).

bolus A mass of food that has been chewed and moistened in the mouth.

bone density The degree of compactness of bone tissue, reflecting the strength of the bones. Peak bone density is the point at which a bone is strongest.

brush border The microvilli projecting from the membrane of enterocytes of the small intestine's villi. These microvilli tremendously increase the small intestine's absorptive capacity.

buffers Proteins that help maintain proper acid–base balance by attaching to, or releasing, hydrogen ions as conditions change in the body.

bulimia nervosa A serious eating disorder characterized by recurrent episodes of binge eating and recurrent inappropriate compensatory behaviors in order to prevent weight gain, such as self-induced vomiting, fasting, excessive exercise, or misuse of laxatives, diuretics, enemas, or other medications.

C

calcitriol The primary active form of vitamin D in the body.

cancer A group of diseases characterized by cells that reproduce spontaneously and independently and may invade other tissues and organs.

carbohydrate loading Also known as glycogen loading. A process that involves altering training and carbohydrate intake, so that muscle glycogen storage is maximized.

carbohydrate One of the three macronutrients, a compound made up of carbon, hydrogen, and oxygen, that is derived from plants and provides energy.

carbohydrates The primary fuel source for our bodies, particularly for our brain and for physical exercise.

carcinogen Any substance capable of causing the cellular mutations that lead to cancer.

cardiovascular disease (CVD) A general term for abnormal conditions involving dysfunction of the heart and blood vessels, which can result in heart attack or stroke.

carotenoid A fat-soluble plant pigment that the body stores in the liver and adipose tissues. The body is able to convert certain carotenoids to vitamin A.

case control studies Observational studies that compare groups with and without a condition, allowing researchers to gain a better understanding of factors that may influence disease.

cash crops Crops grown to be sold rather than eaten, such as cotton or tobacco.

cataract A damaged portion of the eye's lens, which causes cloudiness that impairs vision.

celiac disease An inherited disorder characterized by inflammation of the lining of the small intestine upon consumption of gluten.

cell differentiation The process by which immature, undifferentiated stem cells develop into highly specialized functional cells of discrete organs and tissues.

cell membrane The boundary of an animal cell that separates its internal cytoplasm and organelles from the external environment.

cell The smallest unit of matter that exhibits the properties of living things, such as growth and metabolism.

Centers for Disease Control and Prevention (CDC) The leading federal agency in the United States that protects the health and safety of people.

cephalic phase The earliest phase of digestion, in which the brain thinks about and prepares the digestive organs for the consumption of food.

cholecalciferol Vitamin D_3, a form of vitamin D found in animal foods and the form we synthesize from the sun.

chronic diseases Diseases that come on slowly and can persist for years, often despite treatment.

chylomicron A lipoprotein produced in the enterocyte; transports dietary fat out of the intestinal tract.

chyme A semifluid mass consisting of partially digested food, water, and gastric juices.

cirrhosis of the liver End-stage liver disease characterized by significant abnormalities in liver structure and function; may lead to complete liver failure.

climate change Any significant change in the measures of climate—such as temperature, precipitation, or wind patterns—that occurs over several decades or longer.

clinical trials Tightly controlled experiments in which an intervention is given to determine its effect on a certain disease or health condition.

coenzyme A molecule that combines with an enzyme to activate it and help it do its job.

cofactor A mineral or non-protein compound that is needed to allow enzymes to function properly.

colic A condition of inconsolable infant crying that lasts for hours at a time.

collagen A protein that forms strong fibers in the matrix of bone, blood vessels, and other connective tissues.

colostrum The first fluid made and secreted by the breasts from late in pregnancy to about a week after birth. It is rich in immune factors and protein.

complementary proteins Two or more foods that together contain all nine essential amino acids necessary for a complete protein. It is not necessary to eat complementary proteins at the same meal.

complete protein Food that contains sufficient amounts of all nine essential amino acids to support growth and health.

complex carbohydrate A nutrient compound consisting of long chains of glucose molecules, such as starch, glycogen, and fiber.

conception The uniting of an ovum (egg) and sperm to create a fertilized egg, or zygote. Also called fertilization.

conditionally essential amino acids Amino acids that are normally considered nonessential but become essential under certain circumstances when the body's need for them exceeds the ability to produce them.

conditioned taste aversion Avoidance of a food as a result of a negative experience, such as illness, even if the illness has no relationship with the food consumed.

conflict of interest A situation in which a person is in a position to derive personal benefit and unfair advantage from actions or decisions made in their official capacity.

constipation A condition characterized by the absence of bowel movements for a period of time that is significantly longer than normal for the individual, and stools that are small, hard, and difficult to pass.

cool-down Activities done after an exercise session is completed; should be gradual and allow your body to slowly recover from exercise.

cortical bone (compact bone)   A dense bone tissue that makes up the outer surface of all bones as well as the entirety of most small bones of the body.

creatine phosphate (CP)   A high-energy compound that can be broken down for energy and used to regenerate ATP.

cretinism   A form of mental impairment that occurs in children whose mothers experienced iodine deficiency during pregnancy.

crop rotation   The practice of alternating crops in a particular field to prevent nutrient depletion and erosion of the soil and to help with control of crop-specific pests.

cross-contamination   Contamination of one food by another via the unintended transfer of microorganisms through physical contact.

cytoplasm   The interior of an animal cell, not including its nucleus.

D

danger zone   The range of temperature (about 40°F to 140°F, or 4°C to 60°C) at which many microorganisms capable of causing human disease thrive.

DASH diet   The diet developed in response to research into hypertension funded by the National Institutes of Health: DASH stands for "Dietary Approaches to Stop Hypertension."

deamination   The process by which an amine group is removed from an amino acid. The nitrogen is then transported to the kidneys for excretion in the urine, while the carbon and other components are metabolized for energy or used to make other compounds.

dehydration   The depletion of body fluid. It results when fluid excretion exceeds fluid intake.

denaturation   The process by which proteins uncoil and lose their shape and function when they are exposed to heat, acids, bases, heavy metals, alcohol, and other damaging substances.

denature   The action of the unfolding of proteins in the stomach. Proteins must be denatured before they can be digested.

dental caries   Dental erosion and decay caused by acid-secreting bacteria in the mouth and on the teeth. The acid produced is a by-product of bacterial metabolism of carbohydrates deposited on the teeth.

diabetes   A chronic disease in which the body can no longer regulate glucose normally.

diarrhea   A condition characterized by the frequent passage of loose, watery stools.

dietary fiber   The nondigestible carbohydrate parts of plants that form the support structures of leaves, stems, and seeds.

Dietary Guidelines for Americans   A set of principles developed by the U.S. Department of Agriculture and the U.S. Department of Health and Human Services to assist Americans in designing a healthful diet and lifestyle.

Dietary Reference Intakes (DRIs)   A set of nutritional reference values for the United States and Canada that applies to healthy people.

dietary supplement   A product taken by mouth that contains a "dietary ingredient" intended to supplement the diet.

digestion   The process by which foods are broken down into their component molecules, either mechanically or chemically.

disaccharide   A carbohydrate compound consisting of two sugar molecules joined together.

disordered eating   A general term used to describe a variety of abnormal or atypical eating behaviors that are used to keep or maintain a lower body weight.

diuretic   A substance that increases fluid loss via the urine.

docosahexaenoic acid (DHA)   An omega-3 fatty acid available from marine foods and as a metabolic derivative of alpha-linolenic acid.

drifty gene hypothesis   A hypothesis suggesting that random mutation and drift in the genes that control the upper limit of body fatness can help explain why some people become obese and others do not.

drink   The amount of an alcoholic beverage that provides approximately 0.5 fl. oz of pure ethanol.

dual-energy x-ray absorptiometry (DXA or DEXA)   Currently, the most accurate tool for measuring bone density.

E

eating disorder   A clinically diagnosed psychiatric disorder characterized by severe disturbances in body image and eating behaviors.

edema   A disorder in which fluids build up in the tissue spaces of the body, causing fluid imbalances and a swollen appearance.

eicosapentaenoic acid (EPA)   An omega-3 fatty acid available from marine foods and as a metabolic derivative of alpha-linolenic acid.

electrolyte   A substance that disassociates in solution into positively and negatively charged ions and is thus capable of carrying an electrical current; the ions in such a solution.

electron   A negatively charged particle orbiting the nucleus of an atom.

elimination   The process by which undigested portions of food and waste products are removed from the body.

embryo   The human growth and developmental stage lasting from the third week to the end of the eighth week after fertilization.

empty Calories   Calories from solid fats or added sugars that provide few or no nutrients.

energy cost of physical activity   The energy that is expended on body movement and muscular work above basal levels.

energy expenditure   The energy the body expends to maintain its basic functions and to perform all levels of movement and activity.

energy intake   The amount of energy a person consumes; in other words, the number of kcal consumed from food and beverages.

enriched foods   Foods in which nutrients that were lost during processing have been added back, so that the food meets a specified standard.

enteric nervous system (ENS)   The autonomic nerves in the walls of the GI tract.

enterocytes   The cells lining the wall of the intestine.

enzymes   Small chemicals, usually proteins, that act on other chemicals to speed up body processes but are not apparently changed during those processes.

epidemiological studies   Studies that examine patterns of health and disease in defined populations.

epiphyseal plates   Plates of cartilage located toward the end of long bones that provide for growth in the length of long bones.

ergogenic aids   Substances used to improve exercise and athletic performance.

erythrocytes The red blood cells, which are the cells that transport oxygen in our blood.

esophagus A muscular tube of the GI tract connecting the pharynx to the stomach.

essential amino acids Amino acids not produced by the body that must be obtained from food.

essential fatty acids (EFAs) Fatty acids that must be consumed in the diet because they cannot be made by our body.

exchange system A diet planning tool in which exchanges, or portions, are organized according to the amount of carbohydrate, protein, fat, and Calories in each food.

exercise A subcategory of leisure-time physical activity; any activity that is purposeful, planned, and structured.

extracellular fluid The fluid outside the body's cells, either in the body's tissues or as the liquid portion of blood or lymph.

F

fair trade A trading partnership promoting equity in international trading relationships and contributing to sustainable development by securing the rights of marginalized producers and workers.

famine A severe food shortage affecting a large percentage of the population in a limited geographic area at a particular time.

fats An important energy source for our bodies at rest and during low-intensity exercise.

fat-soluble vitamins Vitamins that are not soluble in water but are soluble in fat. These are vitamins A, D, E, and K.

fatty acids Long chains of carbon atoms bound to each other as well as to hydrogen atoms.

fatty liver An abnormal accumulation of fat in the liver that develops in people who abuse alcohol.

female athlete triad A syndrome that consists of three clinical conditions in some physically active females: low energy availability (with or without eating disorders), menstrual dysfunction, and low bone density.

fermentation A process in which an agent causes an organic substance to break down into simpler substances resulting in the production of ATP.

fetal adaptation The process by which fetal metabolism, hormone production, and other physiologic processes shift in response to factors, such as inadequate energy intake, in the maternal environment.

fetal alcohol syndrome (FAS) The most severe consequence of maternal alcohol consumption; characterized by physical malformations and emotional, behavioral, and learning problems.

fetus The human growth and developmental stage lasting from the beginning of the ninth week after conception to birth.

FITT principle The principle used to achieve an appropriate overload for physical training; FITT stands for frequency, intensity, time, and type of activity.

fluid A substance composed of molecules that move past one another freely. Fluids are characterized by their ability to conform to the shape of whatever container holds them.

fluorosis A condition, marked by staining and pitting of the teeth, caused by an abnormally high intake of fluoride.

food additive A substance or mixture of substances intentionally put into food to enhance its appearance, safety, palatability, and quality.

food allergy An inflammatory reaction to food caused by an immune system hypersensitivity.

foodborne illness An illness transmitted by food or water contaminated by a pathogenic microorganism, its toxic secretions, or a toxic chemical.

food desert A geographic area where people lack access to fresh, healthy, and affordable food.

food diversity The variety of different species of food crops available.

food insecurity Unreliable access to a sufficient supply of nourishing food.

food intolerance Gastrointestinal discomfort caused by certain foods that is not a result of an immune system reaction.

food residues Chemicals that remain in foods despite cleaning and processing.

food The plants and animals we consume.

fortified foods Foods in which nutrients are added that did not originally exist in the food, or which existed in insignificant amounts.

free radical A highly unstable atom with an unpaired electron in its outermost shell.

frequency Refers to the number of activity sessions per week you perform.

fructose The sweetest natural sugar; a monosaccharide that occurs in fruits and vegetables; also called levulose, or fruit sugar.

functional fiber The nondigestible forms of carbohydrates that are extracted from plants or manufactured in a laboratory and have known health benefits.

functional foods Foods that may have biologically active ingredients that provide health benefits beyond basic nutrition.

fungi Plantlike, spore-forming organisms that have a true nucleus and can grow as either single cells or multicellular colonies.

G

galactose A monosaccharide that joins with glucose to create lactose, one of the three most common disaccharides.

gallbladder A saclike accessory organ of digestion, which lies beneath the liver; it stores bile and secretes it into the small intestine.

gastric juice Acidic liquid secreted within the stomach; it contains hydrochloric acid and other compounds.

gastroesophageal reflux disease (GERD) A chronic disease in which episodes of gastroesophageal reflux cause heartburn or other symptoms more than twice per week.

gastrointestinal (GI) tract A long, muscular tube consisting of several organs: the mouth, pharynx, esophagus, stomach, small intestine, and large intestine and rectum.

gene expression The process of using a gene to make a protein.

Generally Recognized as Safe (GRAS) A list of substances approved for use in food production because they have been determined safe for consumption based on a history of long-term use or on the consensus of qualified research experts.

genetic modification The process of changing an organism by manipulating its genetic material.

gestational diabetes A condition of insufficient insulin production or insulin resistance that results in consistently high blood glucose levels, specifically during pregnancy; the condition typically resolves after birth occurs.

gestation The period of intrauterine development from conception to birth; typically 38 to 42 weeks.

ghrelin A protein synthesized in the stomach that acts as a hormone and plays an important role in appetite regulation by stimulating appetite.

global warming The increase of about 1.5°F (0.85°C) in temperature that has occurred near the Earth's surface over the past century.

glucagon The hormone secreted by the alpha cells of the pancreas in response to decreased blood levels of glucose; it causes the breakdown of liver stores of glycogen into glucose.

gluconeogenesis The generation of glucose from the breakdown of proteins into amino acids.

glucose The most abundant sugar molecule, a monosaccharide generally found in combination with other sugars; it is the preferred source of energy for the brain and an important source of energy for all cells.

glycemic index The system that assigns ratings (or values) for the potential of foods to raise blood glucose and insulin levels.

glycemic load The amount of carbohydrate in a food multiplied by the food's glycemic index, divided by 100.

glycerol An alcohol composed of three carbon atoms; it is the backbone of a triglyceride molecule.

glycogen A polysaccharide; the storage form of glucose in animals.

glycolysis The breakdown of glucose; yields two ATP molecules and two pyruvic acid molecules for each molecule of glucose.

goiter Enlargement of the thyroid gland; can be caused by iodine toxicity or deficiency.

grazing Consistently eating small meals throughout the day; done by many athletes to meet their high energy demands.

Green Revolution The tremendous increase in global productivity between 1944 and 2000 due to selective cross-breeding or hybridization to produce high-yield grains and industrial farming techniques.

H

healthful diet A diet that provides the proper combination of energy and nutrients and is adequate, moderate, nutrient-dense, balanced, and varied.

heartburn A painful sensation that occurs over the sternum when gastric juice pools in the lower esophagus.

heat cramps Involuntary, spasmodic, and painful muscle contractions that are caused by electrolyte imbalances occurring as a result of strenuous physical activity in high environmental heat.

heat exhaustion A serious condition, characterized by heavy sweating and moderately elevated body temperature, that develops from dehydration in high heat.

heat stroke A potentially fatal response to high temperature characterized by failure of the body's heat-regulating mechanisms; also commonly called sunstroke.

helminth A multicellular microscopic worm.

heme iron Iron that is a part of hemoglobin and myoglobin; found only in animal-based foods, such as meat, fish, and poultry.

heme The iron-containing molecule found in hemoglobin.

hemoglobin The oxygen-carrying protein found in our red blood cells; almost two-thirds of all the iron in our body is found in hemoglobin.

herb A plant or plant part used for its scent, flavor, and/or therapeutic properties (also called a botanical).

hidden fats Fats that are not apparent, or "hidden" in foods, such as the fats found in baked goods, regular-fat dairy products, marbling in meat, and fried foods.

high-fructose corn syrup A highly sweet syrup that is manufactured from corn and is used to sweeten soft drinks, desserts, candies, and jellies.

high-yield varieties (HYVs) Semi-dwarf varieties of plants that are unlikely to fall over in wind and heavy rains and thus can carry larger amounts of seeds, greatly increasing the yield per acre.

homocysteine An amino acid that requires adequate levels of folate, vitamin B_6, and vitamin B_{12} for its metabolism. High levels of homocysteine in the blood are associated with an increased risk for vascular diseases, such as cardiovascular disease.

hormone A chemical messenger secreted into the bloodstream by a gland. Hormones regulate physiologic processes at sites distant from the glands that secrete them.

human microbiome The complete population of microorganisms, including their genes, that inhabit the human body.

hunger A physiologic drive for food.

hydrogenation The process of adding hydrogen to unsaturated fatty acids, making them more saturated and thereby more solid at room temperature.

hypercalcemia A condition marked by an abnormally high concentration of calcium in the blood.

hyperglycemia A condition in which blood glucose levels are higher than normal.

hyperkalemia A condition in which blood potassium levels are dangerously high.

hypermagnesemia A condition marked by an abnormally high concentration of magnesium in the blood.

hypernatremia A condition in which blood sodium levels are dangerously high.

hypertension A chronic condition characterized by above-average blood pressure levels—specifically, systolic blood pressure over 140 mmHg, or diastolic blood pressure over 90 mmHg.

hypertrophy The increase in strength and size that results from repeated work to a specific muscle or muscle group.

hypocalcemia A condition characterized by an abnormally low concentration of calcium in the blood.

hypoglycemia A condition marked by blood glucose levels that are below normal fasting levels.

hypokalemia A condition in which blood potassium levels are dangerously low.

hypomagnesemia A condition characterized by an abnormally low concentration of magnesium in the blood.

hyponatremia A condition in which blood sodium levels are dangerously low.

hypothalamus A region of the forebrain above the pituitary gland, where visceral sensations, such as hunger and thirst, are regulated.

hypothesis An educated guess as to why a phenomenon occurs.

I

impaired fasting glucose Fasting blood glucose levels that are higher than normal but not high enough to lead to a diagnosis of type 2 diabetes.

incidence The rate of new (or newly diagnosed) cases of a disease within a period of time.

incomplete protein Food that does not contain all of the essential amino acids in sufficient amounts to support growth and health.

infant mortality A population's rate of death of infants between birth and 1 year of age.

inorganic A substance or nutrient that does not contain carbon and hydrogen.

insensible water loss The loss of water not noticeable by a person, such as through evaporation from the skin and exhalation from the lungs during breathing.

insoluble fibers Fibers that do not dissolve in water.

insulin insensitivity (*insulin resistance*) A condition in which the body becomes less sensitive (or more resistant) to a given amount of insulin, resulting in insulin having a biological effect that is less than expected.

insulin The hormone secreted by the beta cells of the pancreas in response to increased blood levels of glucose; it facilitates the uptake of glucose by body cells.

intensity The amount of effort expended during an activity, or how difficult the activity is to perform.

intracellular fluid The fluid held at any given time within the walls of the body's cells.

ion Any electrically charged particle, either positively or negatively charged.

iron-deficiency anemia A form of anemia that results from severe iron deficiency.

irritable bowel syndrome (IBS) A group of symptoms caused by changes in the normal functions of the GI tract.

K

Keshan disease A heart disorder caused by selenium deficiency. It was first identified in children in the Keshan province of China.

ketoacidosis A condition in which excessive ketones, which are acidic, lower the pH of blood, altering basic body functions and damaging tissues.

ketones Substances produced during the breakdown of fat when carbohydrate intake is insufficient to meet energy needs. Ketones provide an alternative energy source for the brain when glucose levels are low.

ketosis The process by which the breakdown of fat during fasting states results in the production of ketones.

kwashiorkor A form of protein-energy malnutrition that is typically seen in malnourished infants and toddlers and is characterized by wasting, edema, and other signs of protein deficiency.

L

lactase A digestive enzyme that breaks lactose into glucose and galactose.

lactation The production of breast milk.

lacteal A small lymph vessel located inside the villi of the small intestine.

lactic acid A compound that results when pyruvic acid is metabolized in the presence of insufficient oxygen.

lactose A disaccharide consisting of one glucose molecule and one galactose molecule. It is found in milk, including human breast milk; also called milk sugar.

lactose intolerance A disorder in which the small intestine does not produce enough lactase enzyme to break down the sugar lactose, which is found in milk and milk products.

large intestine The terminal region of the GI tract, in which most water is absorbed and feces are formed.

lean body mass The amount of fat-free tissue, or bone, muscle, and internal organs, a person has.

leisure-time physical activity Any activity not related to a person's occupation; includes competitive sports, recreational activities, and planned exercise training.

leptin A hormone, produced by body fat, that acts to reduce food intake and to decrease body weight and body fat.

leukocytes The white blood cells, which protect us from infection and illness.

limiting amino acid The essential amino acid that is missing or in the smallest supply in the amino acid pool and is thus responsible for slowing or halting protein synthesis.

linoleic acid An essential fatty acid found in vegetable and nut oils; one of the omega-6 fatty acids.

lipids A diverse group of organic substances that are insoluble in water; lipids include triglycerides, phospholipids, and sterols.

lipoprotein A spherical compound in which fat clusters in the center and phospholipids and proteins form the outside of the sphere.

lipoprotein lipase (LPL) An enzyme that sits on the outside of cells and breaks apart triglycerides in chylomicrons, so that their fatty acids can be removed and taken up by the cell.

listeriosis Serious and sometimes fatal illness caused by infection with the bacterium Listeria monocytogenes, typically from consumption of contaminated food.

liver The largest accessory organ of digestion and one of the most important organs of the body. Its functions include the production of bile and the processing of nutrient-rich blood from the small intestine.

low birth weight Having a weight of less than 5.5 pounds at birth.

M

macrocytic anemia A form of anemia manifested as the production of larger than normal red blood cells containing insufficient hemoglobin; also called megaloblastic anemia.

macronutrients Nutrients that our bodies need in relatively large amounts to support normal function and health. Carbohydrates, fats, and proteins are energy-yielding macronutrients.

macular degeneration A vision disorder characterized by deterioration of the macula, the central portion of the retina, and marked by loss or distortion of the center of the visual field.

major minerals Minerals we need to consume in amounts of at least 100 mg per day and of which the total amount in our bodies is at least 5 g.

maltase A digestive enzyme that breaks maltose into glucose.

maltose A disaccharide consisting of two molecules of glucose. It does not generally occur independently in foods but results as a by-product of digestion; also called malt sugar.

marasmus A form of protein-energy malnutrition that results from grossly inadequate intake of energy and protein and other nutrients and is characterized by extreme tissue wasting and stunted growth and development.

maternal mortality A population's rate of deaths of a woman during pregnancy, childbirth, or in the immediate postpartal period.

maximal heart rate The rate at which your heart beats during maximal-intensity exercise.

meat factor A special factor found in meat, fish, and poultry that enhances the absorption of non-heme iron.

megadose A nutrient dose that is 10 or more times greater than the recommended amount.

megadosing Taking a dose of a nutrient that is 10 or more times greater than the recommended amount.

metabolic syndrome A cluster of five potentially modifiable factors, such as abdominal obesity, that increases the risk for cardiovascular disease and type 2 diabetes.

metabolic water The water formed as a by-product of our body's metabolic reactions.

metabolism The chemical reactions by which large compounds, such as carbohydrates, fats, and proteins, are broken down into smaller units the body can use. Also refers to the assembly of smaller units into larger compounds.

micronutrients Nutrients needed in relatively small amounts to support normal health and body functions. Vitamins and minerals are micronutrients.

mindful eating The nonjudgmental awareness of the emotional and physical sensations one experiences while eating or in a food-related environment.

minerals Inorganic elements that assist in the regulation of many body processes and the maintenance of many body tissues.

moderate drinking Alcohol consumption of up to one drink per day for women and up to two drinks per day for men.

monoculture A single crop species cultivated over a large area.

monosaccharide The simplest of carbohydrates, consisting of one sugar molecule, the most common form of which is glucose.

monounsaturated fatty acid (MUFA) A fatty acid that has two carbons in the chain bound to each other with one double bond; MUFAs are generally liquid at room temperature.

morbid obesity A condition in which a person's body weight exceeds 100% of normal, putting him or her at very high risk for serious health consequences; a BMI = 40 kg/m^2.

morning sickness Varying degrees of nausea and vomiting associated with pregnancy, most commonly in the first trimester.

mouthfeel The tactile sensation of food in the mouth; derived from the interaction of physical and chemical characteristics of the food.

multifactorial disease A disease that may be attributable to one or more of a variety of causes.

mutual supplementation The process of combining two or more incomplete protein sources to make a complete protein.

myoglobin An iron-containing protein similar to hemoglobin except that it is found in muscle cells.

MyPlate The visual representation of the USDA Food Patterns and the website supporting their implementation.

N

National Institutes of Health (NIH) The world's leading medical research center and the focal point for medical research in the United States.

neural tube Embryonic tissue that forms a tube, which eventually becomes the brain and spinal cord.

neurotransmitters Chemical compounds that transmit messages from one nerve cell to another.

night blindness A vitamin A deficiency disorder that results in loss of the ability to see in dim light.

night-eating syndrome Disorder characterized by intake of the majority of the day's energy between 8:00 pm and 6:00 am. Individuals with this disorder also experience mood and sleep disorders.

nonessential amino acids Amino acids that can be manufactured by the body in sufficient quantities and therefore do not need to be consumed regularly in our diet.

non-exercise activity thermogenesis (NEAT) The energy that is expended to do all activities above BMR and TMF, but excluding volitional sporting activities.

non-heme iron The form of iron that is not a part of hemoglobin or myoglobin; found in animal- and plant-based foods.

nonnutritive sweeteners Manufactured sweeteners that provide little or no energy; also called alternative sweeteners.

normal weight Having an adequate but not excessive level of body fat for health.

nucleus The positively charged, central core of an atom. It is made up of two types of particles—protons and neutrons—bound tightly together. The nucleus of an atom contains essentially all of its atomic mass.

nutrient density The relative amount of nutrients and fiber per amount of energy (or number of Calories).

nutrients Chemicals found in foods that are critical to human growth and function.

nutrigenomics A scientific discipline studying the interactions between genes, the environment, and nutrition.

Nutrition Facts panel The label on a food package that contains the nutrition information required by the FDA.

nutrition paradox The coexistence of aspects of both stunting and overweight/obesity within the same region, household, family, or person.

nutrition The science that studies food and how food nourishes our bodies and influences our health.

nutritive sweeteners Sweeteners, such as sucrose, fructose, honey, and brown sugar, that contribute Calories (energy).

O

obesity Having an excess of body fat that adversely affects health, resulting in a person having a weight that is substantially greater than some accepted standard for a given height; a BMI of 30 to 39.9 kg/m^2.

observational studies Studies that indicate relationships between nutrition habits, disease trends, and other health phenomena of large populations of humans.

olfaction Our sense of smell, which plays a key role in the stimulation of appetite.

organ A body structure composed of two or more tissues and performing a specific function; for example, the esophagus.

organelle A tiny "organ" within a cell that performs a discrete function necessary to the cell.

organic agriculture The application of practices that support the cycling of on-farm resources, ecological balance, and biodiversity.

organic A substance or nutrient that contains the elements carbon and hydrogen.

osmosis The movement of water (or any solvent) through a semipermeable membrane from an area where solutes are less concentrated to areas where solutes are highly concentrated.

osteoblasts Cells that prompt the formation of new bone matrix by laying down the collagen-containing component of bone, which is then mineralized.

osteoclasts Cells that erode the surface of bones by secreting enzymes and acids that dig grooves into the bone matrix.

osteomalacia A vitamin D–deficiency disease in adults, in which bones become weak and prone to fractures.

osteoporosis A disease characterized by low bone mass and deterioration of bone tissue, leading to increased bone fragility and fracture risk.

ounce-equivalent (oz-equivalent) A serving size that is 1 ounce, or equivalent to an ounce, for the grains and the protein foods sections of MyPlate.

overhydration The dilution of body fluid. It results when water retention or intake is excessive.

overload principle Placing an extra physical demand on your body in order to improve your fitness level.

overpopulation Condition in which a region's available resources are insufficient to support the number of people living there.

overweight Having a moderate amount of excess body fat, resulting in a person having a weight that is greater than some accepted standard for a given height but is not considered obese; a BMI of 25 to 29.9 kg/m^2.

ovulation The release of an ovum (egg) from a woman's ovary.

oxidation A chemical reaction in which molecules of a substance are broken down into their component atoms. During oxidation, the atoms involved lose electrons.

P

pancreas An accessory organ of digestion located behind the stomach; it secretes digestive enzymes and bicarbonate as well as hormones that help regulate blood glucose.

pancreatic amylase An enzyme secreted by the pancreas into the small intestine that digests any remaining starch into maltose.

parasite A microorganism that simultaneously derives benefit from and harms its host.

parathyroid hormone (PTH) A hormone secreted by the parathyroid gland when blood calcium levels fall. It increases blood calcium levels by stimulating the activation of vitamin D, increasing reabsorption of calcium from the kidneys, and stimulating osteoclasts to break down bone.

pasteurization A form of sterilization using high temperatures for short periods of time.

pellagra A disease that results from severe niacin deficiency.

pepsin An enzyme in the stomach that begins the breakdown of proteins into shorter polypeptide chains and single amino acids.

peptic ulcer An area of the GI tract that has been eroded away by the acidic gastric juice of the stomach.

peptide bond Unique type of chemical bond in which the amine group of one amino acid binds to the acid group of another in order to manufacture dipeptides and all larger peptide molecules.

peptide YY (PYY) A protein produced in the gastrointestinal tract that is released after a meal in amounts proportional to the energy content of the meal; it decreases appetite and inhibits food intake.

peristalsis Waves of squeezing and pushing contractions that move food in one direction through the length of the GI tract.

pernicious anemia A vitamin B$_{12}$ deficiency disease that occurs when immune destruction of parietal cells in the stomach reduces production of intrinsic factor, thereby limiting vitamin B$_{12}$ absorption.

persistent organic pollutants (POPs) Chemicals released as a result of human activity into the environment, where they persist for years or decades.

pesticides Chemicals used either in the field or in storage to decrease destruction and crop losses by weeds, predators, or disease.

pharynx Segment of the GI tract connecting the back of the nose and mouth to the top of the esophagus.

phospholipid A type of lipid in which a fatty acid is combined with another compound that contains phosphate; unlike other lipids, phospholipids are soluble in water.

photosynthesis The process by which plants use sunlight to fuel a chemical reaction that combines carbon and water into glucose, which is then stored in their cells.

physical activity Any movement produced by muscles that increases energy expenditure; includes occupational, household, leisure-time, and transportation activities.

physical fitness The ability to carry out daily tasks with vigor and alertness, without undue fatigue, and with ample energy to enjoy leisure-time pursuits and meet unforeseen emergencies.

phytochemicals Naturally occurring plant compounds believed to have health-promoting effects in humans.

pica An abnormal craving to eat nonfood substances such as clay, paint, or chalk.

placebo An imitation treatment having no active ingredient that is sometimes used in a clinical trial.

placenta A pregnancy-specific organ formed from both maternal and embryonic tissues. It is responsible for oxygen, nutrient, and waste exchange between mother and fetus.

plant-based diet A diet consisting mostly of plant sources of foods, especially whole foods, with only limited amounts, if any, of animal-based and processed foods.

plasma The fluid portion of the blood; needed to maintain adequate blood volume so that the blood can flow easily throughout our body.

platelets Cell fragments that assist in the formation of blood clots and help stop bleeding.

polypharmacy The use of five or more prescription drugs at any one time.

polysaccharide A complex carbohydrate consisting of long chains of glucose.

polyunsaturated fatty acid (PUFA) A fatty acid that has more than one double bond in the chain; PUFAs are generally liquid at room temperature.

poverty–obesity paradox The high prevalence of obesity in low-income populations.

prebiotics Nondigestible food compounds that support the growth and/or activity of one or a limited number of bacteria in the large intestine.

prediabetes A term used synonymously with *impaired fasting glucose*; it is a condition considered to be a major risk factor for both type 2 diabetes and heart disease.

preeclampsia High blood pressure that is pregnancy specific and accompanied by protein in the urine, edema, and unexpected weight gain.

preterm The birth of a baby prior to 38 weeks' gestation.

prevalence The percentage of the population that is affected with a particular disease at a given time.

prion A protein that misfolds and becomes infectious and destructive; prions are not living cellular organisms or viruses.

proteins The only macronutrient that contains nitrogen; the basic building blocks of proteins are amino acids.

probiotics Foods, beverages, or supplements containing living microorganisms that beneficially affect consumers by improving the intestinal microbial balance.

processed foods Foods that have been manipulated in some way to transform raw ingredients into products for consumption.

proof A measure of the alcohol content of a liquid; 100-proof liquor is 50% alcohol by volume, 80-proof liquor is 40% alcohol by volume, and so on.

prooxidant A substance that promotes oxidation and oxidative cell and tissue damage.

proteases Enzymes that continue the breakdown of polypeptides in the small intestine.

protein-energy malnutrition A disorder caused by inadequate consumption of protein. It is characterized by severe wasting.

protein leverage hypothesis A hypothesis suggesting that the body has a fixed daily dietary protein target, and because our current diets are proportionally higher in carbohydrates and fats and lower in protein, we overeat to meet this target.

proteins Large, complex molecules made up of amino acids and found as essential components of all living cells.

protozoa Single-celled, mobile parasites.

provitamin An inactive form of a vitamin that the body can convert to an active form. An example is beta-carotene.

puberty The period of life in which secondary sexual characteristics develop and people become biologically capable of reproducing.

purging An attempt to rid the body of unwanted food by vomiting or other compensatory means, such as excessive exercise, fasting, or laxative abuse.

pyruvic acid The primary end product of glycolysis.

Q

quackery The promotion of an unproven remedy, such as a supplement or other product or service, usually by someone unlicensed and untrained.

R

recombinant bovine growth hormone (rBGH) A genetically engineered growth hormone used in beef herds and some dairy cows.

recombinant DNA technology A type of genetic modification in which scientists combine DNA from different sources to produce a transgenic organism that expresses a desired trait.

registered dietitian (RD) A professional designation that requires a minimum of a bachelor's degree in nutrition, completion of a supervised clinical experience, a passing grade on a national examination, and maintenance of registration with the Academy of Nutrition and Dietetics (in Canada, the Dietitians of Canada). RDs are qualified to work in a variety of settings.

remodeling The two-step process by which bone tissue is recycled; includes the breakdown of existing bone and the formation of new bone.

resistance training Exercise in which our muscles act against resistance.

resorption The process by which the surface of bone is broken down by cells called osteoclasts.

retinal An active, aldehyde form of vitamin A that plays an important role in healthy vision and immune function.

retina The delicate, light-sensitive membrane lining the inner eyeball and connected to the optic nerve. It contains retinal.

retinoic acid An active, acid form of vitamin A that plays an important role in cell growth and immune function.

retinol An active, alcohol form of vitamin A that plays an important role in healthy vision and immune function.

rhodopsin A light-sensitive pigment found in the rod cells that is formed by retinal and opsin.

rickets A vitamin D–deficiency disease in children. Signs include deformities of the skeleton, such as bowed legs and knocked knees. Severe rickets can be fatal.

S

saliva A mixture of water, mucus, enzymes, and other chemicals that moistens the mouth and food, binds food particles together, and begins the digestion of carbohydrates.

salivary amylase An enzyme in saliva that breaks starch into smaller particles and eventually into the disaccharide maltose.

salivary glands A group of glands found under and behind the tongue and beneath the jaw that release saliva continually as well as in response to the thought, sight, smell, or presence of food.

satiety A physiologic sensation of fullness (from the Latin *satis* meaning enough, as in *satisfied*).

saturated fatty acid (SFA) A fatty acid that has no carbons joined together with a double bond; SFAs are generally solid at room temperature.

scientific method The standardized, multistep process scientists use to examine evidence and test hypotheses.

screening test Clinical exam performed on a large population to detect early evidence of disease.

scurvy Vitamin C deficiency disease caused by failure of collagen synthesis.

sensible water loss Water loss that is noticed by a person, such as through urine output and visible sweating.

set-point hypothesis A hypothesis suggesting that the body raises or lowers energy expenditure in response to increased and decreased food intake and physical activity. This action maintains an individual's body weight within a narrow range.

severe acute malnutrition (SAM) A state of severe energy deficit defined as a weight for height more than 3 standard deviations below the mean, or the presence of nutrition-related edema.

simple carbohydrate Commonly called sugar; can be either a monosaccharide (such as glucose) or a disaccharide.

small intestine The longest portion of the GI tract, where most digestion and absorption take place.

soluble fibers Fibers that dissolve in water.

solvent A substance that is capable of mixing with and breaking apart a variety of compounds. Water is an excellent solvent.

sphincter A tight ring of muscle separating some of the organs of the GI tract and opening in response to nerve signals indicating that food is ready to pass into the next section.

spina bifida The embryotic neural tube defect that occurs when the spinal vertebrae fail to completely enclose the spinal cord, allowing it to protrude.

spontaneous abortion The natural termination of a pregnancy and expulsion of pregnancy tissues because of a genetic, developmental, or physiologic abnormality that is so severe that the pregnancy cannot be maintained. Also called miscarriage.

starch A polysaccharide stored in plants; the storage form of glucose in plants.

sterol A type of lipid found in foods and the body that has a ring structure; cholesterol is the most common sterol in our diets.

stomach A J-shaped organ where food is partially digested, churned, and stored until it is released into the small intestine.

stretching Exercise in which muscles are gently lengthened using slow, controlled movements.

stunted growth A condition of shorter stature than expected for chronological age, often defined as 2 or more standard deviations below the mean reference value.

sucrase A digestive enzyme that breaks sucrose into glucose and fructose.

sucrose A disaccharide composed of one glucose molecule and one fructose molecule; sucrose is sweeter than lactose or maltose.

sudden infant death syndrome (SIDS) The sudden death of a previously healthy infant; the most common cause of death in infants over 1 month of age.

sustainability The ability to meet or satisfy basic economic, social, and security needs now and in the future without undermining the natural resource base and environmental quality on which life depends.

sustainable agriculture Term referring to techniques of food production that preserve the environment indefinitely.

system A group of organs that work together to perform a unique function; for example, the gastrointestinal system.

T

teratogen Any substance known to have the potential to harm a developing embryo or fetus.

teratogen Any substance that can cause a birth defect.

theory A conclusion, or scientific consensus, drawn from repeated experiments.

thermic effect of food (TEF) The energy expended as a result of processing food consumed.

thirst mechanism A cluster of nerve cells in the hypothalamus that stimulate the desire to drink fluids in response to an increase in the concentration of blood solutes or a decrease in blood pressure and blood volume.

thrifty gene hypothesis A hypothesis suggesting that some people possess a gene (or genes) that causes them to be energetically thrifty, resulting in their expending less energy at rest and during physical activity.

time of activity How long each exercise session lasts.

tissue A grouping of like cells that performs a function; for example, muscle tissue.

total fiber The sum of dietary fiber and functional fiber.

toxin Any harmful substance; in microbiology, a harmful chemical secretion of a microorganism.

trabecular bone (spongy bone) A porous bone tissue that makes up only 20% of our skeletons and is found within the ends of the long bones, inside the spinal vertebrae, inside the flat bones (sternum, ribs, and most bones of the skull), and inside the bones of the pelvis.

trace minerals Minerals we need to consume in amounts less than 100 mg per day and of which the total amount in our bodies is less than 5 g.

transamination The process of transferring the amine group from one amino acid to another in order to manufacture a new amino acid.

transcription The process through which messenger RNA copies genetic information from DNA in the nucleus.

translation The process that occurs when the genetic information carried by messenger RNA is translated into a chain of amino acids at the ribosome.

transport proteins Protein molecules that help transport substances throughout the body and across cell membranes.

triglyceride A molecule consisting of three fatty acids attached to a three-carbon glycerol backbone.

trimester Any one of three stages of pregnancy, each lasting 13 to 14 weeks.

T-score A comparison of an individual's bone density to the average peak bone density of a 30-year-old healthy adult.

tumor Any newly formed mass of undifferentiated cells.

type 1 diabetes A disorder in which the body cannot produce enough insulin.

type 2 diabetes A progressive disorder in which body cells become less responsive to insulin.

type of activity The range of physical activities a person can engage in to promote health and physical fitness.

U

umbilical cord The cord containing the arteries and veins that connect the baby (from the navel) to the mother via the placenta.

underweight Having too little body fat to maintain health, causing a person to have a weight that is below an acceptable defined standard for a given height; a BMI less than 18.5 kg/m².

urinary tract infection A bacterial infection of the urethra, the tube leading from the bladder to the body exterior.

USDA Food Patterns A set of recommendations for types and amounts of foods to consume from the five major food groups and subgroups to help people meet the Dietary Guidelines for Americans.

V

vegetarianism The practice of restricting the diet to foods and food substances of plant origin, including vegetables, fruits, grains, nuts, and seeds.

viruses A group of infectious agents that are much smaller than bacteria, lack independent metabolism, and are incapable of growth or reproduction outside of living cells.

viscous Having a gel-like consistency; viscous fibers form a gel when dissolved in water.

visible fats Fats that are clearly present and visible in our food, or visibly added to food, such as butter, margarine, cream, shortening, salad dressings, chicken skin, and untrimmed fat on meat.

vitamins Organic compounds that assist in the regulation of many body processes and the maintenance of many body tissues.

vomiting The involuntary expulsion of the contents of the stomach and duodenum from the mouth.

W

warm-up Also called preliminary exercise; includes activities that prepare you for an exercise bout, including stretching, calisthenics, and movements specific to the exercise bout.

wasting A physical condition of very low body-weight-for-height or extreme thinness.

water-soluble vitamins Vitamins that are soluble in water. These include vitamin C and the B vitamins.

wellness A multidimensional, active process by which people make choices that enhance their lives.

whole foods Foods that have been modified as little as possible, remaining in or near their natural state.

Z

zygote A fertilized ovum (egg) consisting of a single cell.

index

Note: Page numbers followed by *f* and *t* indicate figures and tables, respectively.

credits

Chapter 1

Chapter Opener: Cultura Exclusive/Getty Images; p. 4: Anna Hoychuk/Shutterstock; Fig. 1.1: Yeko Photo Studio/Shutterstock; Fig. 1.2 (top): Lester V. Bergman/Getty Images; Fig. 1.2 (bottom): Michael Klein/Getty Images; p. 8: michaeljung/Shutterstock; p. 11: pinonepantone/Fotolia; p. 12: lidante/Shutterstock; Fig. 1.4: Samuel Borges Photography/Shutterstock; p. 14: Comstock Images/Getty Images; p. 15: OJO Images Ltd/Alamy Stock Photo; Fig. 1.5 (top): Alexander Raths/Shutterstock; Fig. 1.5 (middle left): Shutterstock; Fig. 1.5 (middle right): Simone Van Den Berg/Shutterstock; Fig. 1.5 (bottom): Shutterstock; Fig. 1.6 (top): mrks_v/Fotolia; Fig. 1.6 (middle): Sandra Baker/Alamy Stock Photo; Fig. 1.6 (bottom): Miriam Doerr Martin Frommherz/Shutterstock; p. 22: Pearson Education; p. 23: Pearson Education; p. 24: Liquidlibrary/Thinkstock/Getty Images; p. 25: James Gathany/CDC; p. 26: RosaBetancourt 0 people images/Alamy.

Chapter 1.5

Chapter Opener: JGI/Tom Grill/Getty Images; Fig. 1: Randy L. Jirtle; p. 32 (left): Science Photo Library/Alamy Stock Photo; p. 32 (right): OJO Images Ltd/Alamy Stock Photo; p. 33: Pearson Education; p. 35: Rob Bartee/Alamy Stock Photo; Fig. 3 (top): Southern Illinois University/Photo Researchers, Inc.; Fig. 3 (second): DJM-photo/Shutterstock; Fig. 3 (bottom): Image Source/Getty Images; Fig. 3 (top): Pixtal/Age Fotostock; Fig. 3 (top): Joy Brown/Shutterstock.

Chapter 2

Chapter Opener: Bambu Productions/Getty Images; p. 38: Skim New Media Limited/Alamy Stock Photo; Fig. 2.1: Pearson Education; Fig. 2.2: Jon Riley/Stone/Getty Images; p. 41: Brand X Pictures/Photodisc/Getty Images; Fig. 2.3: Pearson Education; Fig. 2.4: Pearson Education; p. 46: Sky Bonillo/PhotoEdit; p. 47: Pearson Education; p. 48: StockFood GmbH/Alamy Stock Photo; Fig. 2.5: ALEAIMAGE/Getty Images; Fig. 2.6: Kelly Cline/Getty Images; Fig. 2.7: iStockphoto/Thinkstock; Fig. 2.8: Hurst Photo/Shutterstock; Fig. 2.9: Natalia Mylova/Fotolia; Fig. 2.7: Pearson Education; Fig. 2.8 (top left): Image Source/Alamy; Fig. 2.8 (top right): bigacis/Fotolia; Fig. 2.8 (bottom left): F. Schussler/PhotoLink/Getty Images; Fig. 2.8 (bottom right): Ragnar Schmuck/Getty Images; p. 54: Ed Ou/Associated Press; p. 55: Koichi Kamoshida/Stringer/Getty Images; p. 56: Alexander Walter/Getty Images.

Chapter 2.5

Chapter Opener: Betsie Van Der Meer/Getty Images; p. 60 (top): Tetra Images/Getty Images; p. 60 (bottom left): Jeff Greenberg/PhotoEdit; p. 60 (bottom right): Pearson Education.

Chapter 3

Chapter Opener: Shutterstock; p. 72: Michael Flippo/Fotolia; p. 78: SPL/Science Source/Photo Researchers, Inc.; p. 80: Bon Appetit/Kröger/Alamy; Fig. 3.18: Dr. E. Walker/Science Source; p. 88 (top): Susan Van Etten/PhotoEdit. All rights reserved.; p. 88 (bottom): Pearson Education; p. 89: Nataliya Peregudova/Fotolia; Fig. 3.13 (top): David Musher/Science Source; Fig. 3.13 (middle): Steve G. Schmeissner/Science Source; Fig. 3.13 (bottom): Don W. Fawcett/Science Source; p. 90: MedicalRF.com/Alamy Stock Photo.

Chapter 3.5

Chapter Opener: Brett Stevens/Getty Images; p. 94: Dorling Kindersley Limited; p. 95: David Murray/Jules Selmes/Dorling Kindersley Ltd.; p. 96 (left): Pearson Education; p. 96 (right): Cordelia Molloy/Science Source.

Chapter 4

Chapter Opener: Jasmina/Getty Images; p. 102: Shutterstock; p. 103: Pearson Education; Stockbyte/Getty Images; Fig. 4.5 (top): Bernd Leitner/Fotolia; Fig. 4.5 (middle): Doug Menuez/Forrester Images/Getty Images; Fig. 4.5 (bottom): E+/Getty Images; Fig. 4.10 (top): Shutterstock; Fig. 4.10 (bottom): Flashon Studio/Shutterstock; p. 112 (left): Steve Shott/Dorling Kindersley; p. 112 (right): Ryan McVay/Getty Images; p. 114: Maridav/Fotolia; p. 115: Foodcollection/Getty Images; p. 119: Dorling Kindersley Limited; p. 120 (left): Giuseppe_R/Shutterstock; p. 120 (right): Diana Taliun/Shutterstock; p. 4.15: Alex459/Shutterstock; Fig. 4.16: Pearson Education; p. 123: Ian O'Leary/Dorling Kindersley, Ltd.; p. 124: Pearson Education; p. 125: joloei/Fotolia; p. 126: Pearson Education; p. 127: Shutterstock.

Chapter 4.5

Chapter Opener: Fertnig/Getty Images; Fig. 2: Scott Camazine/Alamy Stock Photo; Fig. 4: Dmitry Lobanov/Shutterstock; p. 135: sandy young/Alamy Stock Photo; p. 136: Pearson Education.

Chapter 5

Chapter Opener: Brett Stevens/Getty Images; p. 140: Dorling Kindersley Limited; p. 146: Mara Zemgaliete/Fotolia; p. 148: Getty Images Sport; p. 149: Danny E Hooks/Shutterstock; p. 150: Kip Peticolas/Fundamental Photographs; p. 154: Wilmy van Ulft/Shutterstock; p. 156: Pearson Education; p. 157: capacitorphoto/Fotolia; Fig. 5.15: Pearson Education; p. 163: Kip Peticolas/Fundamental Photographs; p. 164: Frances Roberts/Alamy Stock Photo.

Chapter 5.5

Chapter Opener: milanzeremski/Shutterstock; p. 169 (top): Biophoto Associates/Science Source; p. 169 (bottom): Biophoto Associates/Science Source; p. 170: Arthur Tilley/Getty Images; p. 171: 14ktgold/Fotolia; p. 175: altafulla/Shutterstock; p. 176: Pearson Education; p. 177: Pearson Education.

Chapter 6

Chapter Opener: stockcreations/Shutterstock; p. 180: Andresr/Shutterstock; Fig. 6.7: Andrew Syred/Science Source; p. 186: Alena Kogotkova/Shutterstock; Fig. 6.8: Pearson Education; Fig. 6.9 (top): Falater Photo/Fotolia; Fig. 6.9 (bottom): Alamy Stock Photo; p. 193: Dorling Kindersley Limited; Fig. 6.12 (top): Stockbyte/Getty Images; Fig. 6.12 (middle): Mike Goldwater/Alamy Stock Photo; Fig. 6.12 (bottom): Alan K. Bailey/Rubberball/Getty Images; p. 196: Pearson Education; Fig. 6.13: Pearson Education; Fig. 6.13 (top right): Renn Valo, CDV/Pearson Education; Fig. 6.14 (left): REUTERS/Alamy Stock Photo; Fig. 6.14 (right): Christine Osborne Pictures/Alamy Stock Photo; Fig. 6.15: Renn Valo, CDV/Pearson Education; p. 204: BananaStock/Alamy Images; p. 205 (a): Glowimages/Getty Images; p. 205 (b): Danita Delimont/Alamy Stock Photo; p. 206: Dorling Kindersley Limited; p. 207: Pearson Education; p. 208: Colin Underhill/Alamy.

Chapter 6.5

Chapter Opener: Valentyn Volkov/Shutterstock; p. 212: Simon Smith/Dorling